TEXTBOOK OF
GENERAL SURGERY

TEXTBOOK OF
GENERAL SURGERY

BY

WARREN H. COLE, M.D., F.A.C.S.

PROFESSOR AND HEAD OF THE DEPARTMENT OF SURGERY, UNIVERSITY
OF ILLINOIS COLLEGE OF MEDICINE; DIRECTOR OF SURGICAL
SERVICE, ILLINOIS RESEARCH AND EDUCATIONAL
HOSPITALS, CHICAGO

AND

ROBERT ELMAN, M.D.

ASSOCIATE PROFESSOR OF CLINICAL SURGERY, WASHINGTON
UNIVERSITY SCHOOL OF MEDICINE; ASSISTANT SURGEON,
BARNES HOSPITAL; ASSOCIATE SURGEON, ST. LOUIS
CHILDREN'S HOSPITAL; DIRECTOR OF SURGICAL
SERVICE, H. G. PHILLIPS HOSPITAL, ST. LOUIS.

FOURTH EDITION

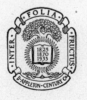

D. APPLETON-CENTURY COMPANY
INCORPORATED

NEW YORK   LONDON

TO

DR. EVARTS AMBROSE GRAHAM

TEACHER, CHIEF AND FRIEND, WHO
HAS EXERTED A GUIDING INFLUENCE FOR
MANY YEARS ON OUR PROFESSIONAL
CAREERS, AND WHO HAS UNSELFISHLY
DEVOTED MUCH TIME AND THOUGHT IN
A CONSULTING CAPACITY DURING THE
PREPARATION OF THIS TEXT

PREFACE

The increasing tempo of world events as it influences surgery is reflected in the present or Fourth Edition. Because of the entrance of this country into the world conflict, an additional chapter has been written entitled War and Catastrophe Surgery. Therein are contained new knowledge as well as supplementary discussions on topics already considered in the original text. Throughout the text many other changes and additions have been made to include the significant surgical advances developing since printing of the last edition. Because of limitations in time and facilities, the same paging is retained except that new pages have been added, in order to include more data on fluid and electrolyte balance, amino-acid therapy, hypoproteinemia, transfusions, chemotherapy and appendicitis. On many other subjects lesser additions were made possible by condensing and eliminating obsolescent material without increasing the text. By revision and rewriting we have also increased emphasis on wounds, burns, surgical shock and other similar subjects related to war casualties. This has been aided by improving many of the illustrations or by replacing them with new ones.

To have enjoyed the invaluable assistance of the same consultant authors in the present edition as in the last was again a pleasure and a privilege. To them has been added Dr. Charles Lund to whom we are indebted for going over the chapter on Thermal Injuries. Several of the consultant authors are now in the armed services and have seen military medical action; we were particularly glad to have the benefit of their additional experiences. Sincere thanks are due other colleagues who have helped in revising smaller parts of the text; among them are Drs. Arthur F. Abt, Edwin F. Gildea, Peter Heinbecker, Carl V. Moore, Eric Oldberg, Nathan Womack and W. Barry Wood.

WARREN H. COLE
ROBERT ELMAN

PREFACE TO THIRD EDITION

Since this book was first published in 1936, a great many advances in surgery have been made. Attempting to keep up with the progress in surgery, important changes were made in the second edition, but the changes made in the present (or third) edition represent a revision of the first as well as second edition, and are so extensive that it has been necessary to completely reset the book.

In accordance with the original plan, detailed consideration of such specialities as ophthalmology, otology and rhinology were eliminated, although many features are included with which the general surgeon must be acquainted. On the other hand, separate chapters are assigned to such allied specialties as genito-urinary surgery and gynecology. Certain features of neurosurgery are included, particularly in regard to head injuries. Because of this scope of the book the term general surgery was used.

The subject matter is presented as far as possible from a physiological point of view, so that the principles underlying both the clinical features and particularly treatment will be better understood. Pathogenesis has been emphasized in order to bring the rationale of treatment into bolder relief. Because of the importance of surgical pathology in the teaching of surgery itself, numerous photomicrographs and illustrations of gross specimens along with the case histories of representative neoplastic and other lesions will be found throughout the text. The details of non-operative therapy have been fully covered. Operations, although discussed in principle, have not been described in detail except a few of the more common ones. Most operations involve such meticulous and extensive detail that there is insufficient space in a single volume to include them in an adequate manner. To present incomplete descriptions of operative technic is often misleading and may actually be dangerous; it would appear unwise therefore to even attempt to include them. Appropriate sources for details of operative therapy are the various systems of surgery.

Because of the influence of war on surgical thought during the past year or two, and of its probable effect for many years to come, we have devoted particular attention to open wounds and burns. Numerous changes or additions have been made in the treatment of fractures, particularly compound fractures. Much more emphasis has been placed on the use of silk in the repair of wounds, and the importance of the adoption of "silk philosophy" in the care of wounds has been stressed. The material on amputations and on anesthesia have each been enlarged into separate chapters. A new chapter on diabetes has been added because the use of insulin has so prolonged the life of diabetics as to make these patients with surgical lesions much more numerous.

The effectiveness of the sulfonamide compounds, especially in accidental wounds and abdominal operations, has required extensive and innumerable additions. Water and electrolyte balance as well as transfusions and the use of plasma, have been discussed at much greater length. More space has been devoted to the differential diagnosis of jaundice. The numerous current contributions to the knowledge of the endocrines have necessitated innumerable changes in this chapter. Numerous illustrations, fifty in number, were changed or replaced by new ones. Several which seemed unimportant were deleted. These many additions have been made without increasing significantly the total text by condensing a few of the earlier chapters on infection and by minor deletion of obsolete or relatively unimportant material elsewhere. Our greatest difficulty was the selection of material for inclusion.

The choice of what is important and what is not important is not easy, particularly in view of the tremendous recent and current advances in surgery. To assist us in these decisions we have had in this edition the help of a number of friends and colleagues, all teachers of surgery, most of them in other schools, thus bringing to the problem different points of views. They have gone over our revised material and have made suggestions and alterations, which we were happy to incorporate in the present edition. The list of these consultants is printed separately; it was a great pleasure to us to have had their advice and counsel.

We are also indebted to many more of our colleagues at Washington University, the University of Illinois and elsewhere. Dr. Barney Brooks made valuable suggestions regarding contents and arrangement of chapters. The chapter on the surgical diseases of the chest which was so unselfishly written by Dr. Evarts Graham, has been completely revised and brought up to date by him with the able assistance of his associate, Dr. Brian B. Blades. As in previous editions Dr. J. B. Brown has made several suggestions as to the various aspects of oral and plastic surgery. To Dr. Leon Bromberg we are again indebted for reading much of the proof especially in the first part of the book, and for other reasons. Dr. W. R. Rainey helped prepare part of the portion devoted to rectal diseases. Dr. Ralph Waters has kindly reviewed our chapter on Anesthesia and offered many valuable suggestions. Other colleagues have aided in numerous ways. We are happy to thank Dr. Malcolm M. Cook for several of the new photographs. Mr. Tom Jones has kindly reviewed our illustrations and offered many suggestions. We are indebted to Miss Sophia Schweich and Mr. Carl Linden for many new drawings. Miss Annabel Wheeler has untiringly contributed secretarial assistance in preparation of the revised manuscript. The publishers have at all times manifested the utmost cooperation and have spared no time or energy on their part in preparation of the revised edition.

WARREN H. COLE
ROBERT ELMAN

FOREWORD

The object of this book has been to present a systematic survey of the field of surgery. Obviously in the space of one volume an attempt could be made only to deal with those aspects of surgery which would seem to be the most important. It is not easy to make a satisfactory selection of those topics which actually are the most important. Different surgeons would doubtless have various opinions concerning what subjects actually are the most important and, therefore, deserve the most emphasis. Especially would this be true in regard to many of the conditions which have now, by more or less common consent, fallen into the realm of some one of the specialized subdivisions of surgery. This book reflects the effort which has consistently been made to give rather more information about those matters with which every general practitioner should be familiar than to attempt to cover the entire field of surgery.

With the enormous development of surgery during the present century it has become increasingly more difficult to prepare a work which could properly be called a *Textbook of General Surgery*. For such a book should be small enough to be encompassed in one volume and at the same time be sufficiently comprehensive to give the student a reasonable amount of information concerning those surgical conditions with which every medical student should be more or less familiar. To prepare such a work has been a challenge which many authors have accepted. Many of the results have been excellent but there is a rather widespread feeling among surgical teachers that the ideal text has not yet been written. Perhaps it never will be. Certainly no book could hold a first rank place for a long period of time without frequent revisions because of the necessity to incorporate within it the rapid changes in points of view, in methods of diagnosis, in the treatment and even in the conceptions of what diseases may properly be regarded as having surgical aspects. As one reviews the changed conceptions concerning what conditions have surgical aspects he is forced to the realization that nowadays there are scarcely any diseases in which the advice of the surgeon may not be sought. Within the years of the present century almost incredible changes have occurred. Pulmonary tuberculosis, certain aspects of nephritis, heart diseases, malignant hypertension, cancer of the lung, hyperinsulinism, hyperparathyroidism, to mention a few, have already been transformed from conditions which presumably had no surgical implications to ones which now demand space and attention in any comprehensive work on surgery. Endocrinology, one of the newest medical sciences, is now, from a therapeutic aspect, largely a surgical problem. When one contrasts the present scope of surgery, therefore, with its scope when it was largely the practice of external medicine, he of necessity realizes that the writing of a satisfactory textbook becomes increasingly difficult as time goes on.

Dr. Cole and Dr. Elman have appreciated that, because of the necessities involved, a textbook of surgery should have certain qualities. In order to encompass the material in a single volume conciseness is a prime requisite and, of necessity, many things have to be omitted which it would be desirable to have in the book. It seems to me that they have carried out their object in a remarkable manner. The various surgical conditions are excellently described as are also the accepted methods of treatment. On the other hand, they have very rightly in such a book paid but scant attention to the conceptions and the treatment of the diseases in question which are too new to have been given a sufficient trial. Moreover, by eliminating many relatively unimportant details, the authors have felt justified in expecting the student to become familiar with all of the material included in the text. Obviously, of course, no limits should ever be placed on the amount of reading of current and other literature; indeed, further outside reading is demanded of the student. To aid him, an extensive bibliography has been included. Elaborate descriptions of operations are not given because such material is presented in the various systems of surgery and it hardly deserves a place in a book of this kind. The principles involved in the various operative procedures, however, are stated. It is futile to attempt to make an undergraduate student a finished surgeon. To accomplish that purpose years of postgraduate study and experience are required. Nothing, therefore, would be gained by including within this book extensive and detailed descriptions of operations.

The book should be found to be very helpful, not only to undergraduate students but also to general practitioners, who desire to obtain in a concise manner information about many of the advances which have been made in surgery. Even the experienced surgeon will find the book helpful for the same reason.

EVARTS A. GRAHAM

CONSULTING AUTHORS

After preparing our revision for the third edition we submitted portions of it to certain of our medical friends who appeared particularly well qualified in the subjects or chapters as indicated below. They have kindly acted as consultants by reading the revised material and making many splendid suggestions and additions. The chapter on Surgical Diseases of the Chest is an exception, since it was originally written entirely by Dr. Evarts A. Graham and revised by him and Dr. Brian B. Blades. For the fourth edition we have had the valuable help of Dr. Charles C. Lund in the chapter on Thermal Injuries. We take this opportunity to express our sincere appreciation for the efforts of the following consultants and collaborators.

WILLARD M. ALLEN, M.D.
PROFESSOR OF OBSTETRICS AND GYNECOLOGY, WASHINGTON UNIVERSITY SCHOOL OF MEDICINE; OBSTETRICIAN AND GYNECOLOGIST, BARNES AND ST. LOUIS MATERNITY HOSPITALS

Gynecology

MAJOR BRIAN B. BLADES*
MEDICAL CORPS, ARMY OF THE UNITED STATES

Surgical Diseases of the Chest

ALFRED BLALOCK, M.D.
PROFESSOR OF SURGERY, JOHNS HOPKINS UNIVERSITY SCHOOL OF MEDICINE; SURGEON-IN-CHIEF, JOHNS HOPKINS HOSPITAL, BALTIMORE, MARYLAND

Shock and Hemorrhage

ALEXANDER BRUNSCHWIG, M.D., F.A.C.S.
PROFESSOR OF SURGERY, UNIVERSITY OF CHICAGO

Neoplasms and Cysts

---

* M.D., In Absentia Assistant Professor of Clinical Surgery, Washington University School of Medicine; Assistant Surgeon, Barnes, St. Louis Children's and St. Louis Maternity Hospitals.

WILLIAM H. CASSELS, M.D.

ASSOCIATE PROFESSOR OF ANESTHESIA, UNIVERSITY OF ILLINOIS COLLEGE OF MEDICINE; CHIEF ANESTHETIST TO ILLINOIS RESEARCH HOSPITAL

Anesthesia

FREDERICK A. COLLER, M.D., F.A.C.S., F.R.C.S.

PROFESSOR OF SURGERY, UNIVERSITY OF MICHIGAN SCHOOL OF MEDICINE; CHAIRMAN, DEPARTMENT OF SURGERY, UNIVERSITY HOSPITAL

The Peritoneal Cavity

EVARTS A. GRAHAM, M.D., F.A.C.S.

BIXBY PROFESSOR OF SURGERY, WASHINGTON UNIVERSITY SCHOOL OF MEDICINE; SURGEON-IN-CHIEF, BARNES AND ST. LOUIS CHILDREN'S HOSPITALS

Surgical Diseases of the Chest

LIEUTENANT COLONEL R. ARNOLD GRISWOLD*

MEDICAL CORPS, ARMY OF THE UNITED STATES

Fractures, Dislocations and Sprains: General Considerations

LIEUTENANT COMMANDER CHARLES G. JOHNSTON**

MEDICAL CORPS, UNITED STATES NAVY

Intestinal Obstruction

J. ALBERT KEY, B.S., M.D.

CLINICAL PROFESSOR OF ORTHOPEDIC SURGERY, WASHINGTON UNIVERSITY SCHOOL OF MEDICINE; ASSOCIATE SURGEON TO BARNES, CHILDREN'S AND JEWISH HOSPITALS, ST. LOUIS

The Organs of Movement

CHARLES C. LUND, M.D.

ASSISTANT PROFESSOR OF SURGERY, HARVARD MEDICAL SCHOOL; VISITING SURGEON, BOSTON CITY HOSPITAL

Thermal, Chemical and Electrical Trauma

---

* M.D., F.A.C.S., In Absentia Professor and Head of Department of Surgery, University of Louisville School of Medicine; Director of Surgery, Louisville City Hospital.
** M.D., In Absentia Professor of Surgery, Wayne University College of Medicine; Director of Surgery, Detroit Receiving Hospital.

CYRIL M. MacBRYDE, M.D.

ASSISTANT PROFESSOR OF CLINICAL MEDICINE, WASHINGTON UNIVERSITY
SCHOOL OF MEDICINE; ASSISTANT PHYSICIAN, BARNES
HOSPITAL, ST. LOUIS

The Endocrine Glands

LIEUTENANT COLONEL JOHN H. MULHOLLAND*

MEDICAL CORPS, ARMY OF THE UNITED STATES

Blood Vessels

HOWARD C. NAFFZIGER, M.D., F.A.C.S.

PROFESSOR OF SURGERY, UNIVERSITY OF CALIFORNIA MEDICAL SCHOOL;
CHAIRMAN, DEPARTMENT OF SURGERY AND SURGEON-IN-CHIEF,
UNIVERSITY OF CALIFORNIA HOSPITAL

The Nervous System

THOMAS G. ORR, M.D., F.A.C.S.

PROFESSOR OF SURGERY, UNIVERSITY OF KANSAS SCHOOL OF MEDICINE;
SURGEON-IN-CHIEF, UNIVERSITY OF KANSAS HOSPITALS

Amputations

DALTON K. ROSE, M.D., F.A.C.S.

PROFESSOR OF CLINICAL GENITOURINARY SURGERY, WASHINGTON UNIVERSITY
SCHOOL OF MEDICINE; ASSOCIATE SURGEON, BARNES AND
ST. LOUIS CHILDREN'S HOSPITALS

The Genito-Urinary System

HARVEY B. STONE, A.B., M.D., F.A.C.S.

ASSOCIATE PROFESSOR OF SURGERY, JOHNS HOPKINS UNIVERSITY SCHOOL OF
MEDICINE; VISITING SURGEON, JOHNS HOPKINS HOSPITAL, UNION
MEMORIAL HOSPITAL, CHURCH HOME AND INFIRMARY AND
HOSPITAL FOR THE WOMEN OF MARYLAND

Stomach, Duodenum, Small Intestine, Appendix, Colon, Rectum

---

* M.D., F.A.C.S., In Absentia Professor of Clinical Surgery and Assistant Dean,
New York University College of Medicine; Associate Visiting Surgeon, Third Surgical
Division, Bellevue Hospital, New York.

ALLEN O. WHIPPLE, M.D., F.A.C.S.
VALENTINE MOTT PROFESSOR OF SURGERY, COLLEGE OF PHYSICIANS AND
SURGEONS, COLUMBIA UNIVERSITY; DIRECTOR OF THE SURGICAL
SERVICE, PRESBYTERIAN HOSPITAL, NEW YORK CITY

Liver, Gallbladder, Pancreas and Spleen

CONTENTS

Chapter I

SURGICAL HISTORY AND EXAMINATIONS

Chapter II

INFLAMMATION AND REPAIR

Chapter III

BACTERIAL INFLAMMATION

Chapter IV

ACUTE SURGICAL INFECTIONS

Chapter V

ACUTE HAND INFECTIONS

CHAPTER VI

MISCELLANEOUS INFECTIONS

CHAPTER VII

ULCER, GANGRENE, SINUS, FISTULA

CHAPTER VIII

SURGICAL METHODS

CHAPTER IX

ANESTHESIA

CHAPTER X

WOUNDS

Chapter XI

AMPUTATIONS

Chapter XII

SURGERY IN DIABETES

Chapter XIII

SHOCK AND HEMORRHAGE

Chapter XIV

THERMAL, CHEMICAL AND ELECTRICAL TRAUMA

Chapter XV

THE EMERGENCY PROSTRATE PATIENT: COMA UNCONSCIOUSNESS, DELIRIUM AND CONVULSIONS

CHAPTER XVIII

FRACTURES, DISLOCATIONS AND SPRAINS: SPECIFIC TYPES

Chapter XIX

THE ORGANS OF MOVEMENT: BONE, JOINT, BURSA, TENDON AND MUSCLE

Chapter XX

BLOOD VESSELS

CHAPTER XXI

THE LYMPHATIC SYSTEM

CHAPTER XXII

THE NERVOUS SYSTEM

CHAPTER XXIII

LIVER, GALLBLADDER, PANCREAS AND SPLEEN

CONTENTS

Chapter XXIV

THE ALIMENTARY TRACT

CONTENTS

CHAPTER XXV

THE PERITONEAL CAVITY

CHAPTER XXVI

INTESTINAL OBSTRUCTION

Chapter XXVII

HERNIA

Chapter XXVIII

THE BREAST

CHAPTER XXIX

SURGICAL DISEASES OF THE CHEST

CHAPTER XXX

THE ENDOCRINE GLANDS

Chapter XXXI

GYNECOLOGY

CHAPTER XXXII

THE GENITO-URINARY SYSTEM

CHAPTER XXXIII

WAR AND CATASTROPHE SURGERY

CONTENTS

TEXTBOOK OF
GENERAL SURGERY

CHAPTER I

THE SURGICAL HISTORY AND EXAMINATION

THE SURGICAL HISTORY

The history of a patient with a surgical disease differs in several respects from that of the usual medical conditions although the main features are similar. With the modern trend toward objective and laboratory methods of diagnosis, laudable as it is, there is apt to be decreasing attention given to the patient's story of his trouble. Yet it is surprising how often a careful and expert history will be all that is necessary to lead to a correct diagnosis. Moreover, a significant history often yields information which aids the surgeon in deciding upon the appropriate type of therapy. It should not be forgotten, finally, that it is often while taking the history that the surgeon establishes his first contact with the patient and that he may foster or destroy thereby that attitude of confidence and coöperation which is so important in the art of medicine; this art together with science raises to the highest plane the practitioner's therapeutic endeavors. Moreover, the surgeon who is able to gain the patient's confidence by his initial verbal contact will find the problem of physical examination greatly simplified because of the added coöperation engendered. This is particularly true of children.

The Chief Complaint.—It is obviously important to know the main clinical manifestation presented by the patient, yet such a statement may not be expressed by the patient's first words. Most individuals complain not of their symptoms but what they interpret the symptoms to mean; many mention but one symptom but really have many others; a few have no real complaint but fear that they are suffering from some dreaded malady; this excessive apprehension may not be detectable until a detailed history is obtained. Thus, the patient may simply complain of "kidney trouble" when actually a back pain is the main manifestation; "appendicitis" may be the patient's answer to the question yet the real symptom is a profuse leukorrhea with mild right lower quadrant pain; many women come to the doctor because they have a "lump in the breast" (which may or may not be present) whereas in reality the main trouble is the fear of cancer, and the normal irregularity of breast tissue is interpreted as a dangerous tumor. In general, therefore, it is important by conversation and judicious questions to elicit from the patient the *real complaint* and if there are more than one, to evaluate which seems more serious to the patient. The surgeon must not forget, however, that every patient, regardless of the presenting complaint, should be questioned in reference to other manifestations of disease. For this purpose a review of the various systems is invaluable.

Of the complaints presented by surgical patients the most prominent are probably pain, and swelling or tumefaction; disability of one type or another and detailed complaints such as superficial ulcers, vomiting, diarrhea, constipation, loss of weight, etc., though less prominent are also important.

Before recording the history it is well to get a general idea of the entire story so that the details may be presented in proper sequence.

The History of the Present Illness.—This must be obtained with an economy of words but with an abundance of significant detail, particularly of positive events. Occasionally negative incidents are mentioned, *e.g.,* the absence of nausea or vomiting after severe abdominal pain is sufficiently significant to be recorded. The onset should be carefully described, whether sudden and definite or gradual and indefinite. In many instances the onset will coincide with some accidental event, *i.e.,* a lump is felt after a slight trauma to the breast whereas it may have been there for a long period previously. When *pain* is a manifestation the surgeon must determine if possible its severity. This is often difficult but such questions as "Does it keep you awake at night?", "Did you have to stop what you were doing and lie down?", "Did you call a doctor?", "Did he give you a hypodermic?" will often aid in estimating the degree of pain. Often the pain is really only a discomfort or ache. Its duration is important, especially if it occurs in attacks varying from a few minutes to hours or days. The location of the pain, particularly when it radiates or moves from one site to another, may be extremely significant. The kind of pain may often be described, whether cramping, dull, sore, throbbing, etc. It is particularly important to inquire if the abdominal pain is of a cramping and intermittent type because the pain associated with intestinal obstruction is apt to be of this kind. In every case the influence, if any, of other activities and of remedies should be detected. Abdominal pain may be worse or better with the ingestion of food, with defecation, with rest or activity, with the stage of the menstrual cycle, etc. When pain is located in an extremity, about the anus or in the chest the obvious influence of the activities associated with the part is determined. Disability of one kind or another is subjected to a similar scrutiny. Of particular importance in the history of neoplasms is the duration of the growth and the rate and constancy of growth, because malignant neoplasms are apt to be of relatively short duration and exhibit a progressive growth. Other complaints should also be scrutinized. The answers to certain questions should not be accepted without qualifications. Thus the statement that pus or blood has never been noticed in the feces means nothing if the patient never looks at the stool after defecation. On the other hand such positive signs as blood in the urine, constipation, diarrhea may be used by patients without conveying an accurate meaning, thereby requiring more detailed questioning on the part of the doctor. Thus the dark urine of dehydration is sometimes described as bloody; in women the presence of blood may be misinterpreted when it is of vaginal rather than of urinary origin. Constipation has a variable significance to many patients; the surgeon should inquire as to the frequency of defecation, the amount of the stool and if possible its character. Similar questions should be asked when diarrhea is a complaint. Bleeding in general, is often exaggerated by many patients in that a mild loss of blood will be described as a "hemorrhage." However, persistent bleeding, though small in amount, will be severe enough to cause anemia.

The progress of the patient's symptoms must be obtained in proper chronologic order and with detailed descriptions of the variations in severity, a list of the various remedies employed and the statements of any attending physician, particularly in regard to his physical findings. The course of the disease can often be mapped from such a careful study, and is frequently of great aid in prescribing further therapy, especially if the diagnosis remains doubtful and further study is required.

A history of trauma is frequent in surgical diseases but cannot be taken at its face value unless the relation between the injury and the complaint is definitely established by detailed questions. Most individuals, particularly in describing the illness of children under their care, will connect an injury with the beginning of symptoms, because it makes the cause easy for them to understand. The average person cannot believe that disease may start in some spontaneous or occult manner and hence searches his memory for some trauma (or dietary indiscretion) as the event immediately preceding his illness. In children slight trauma is so frequent that such a history is often unreliable; on the other hand serious trauma may be sustained by young children and a negative history be obtained because no one observed the injury.

With a history of definite trauma it is important to reconstruct the scene of the accident if possible in order to determine the degree of force sustained by the body, the type of impact and the point of the body involved. For example, detailed questioning may reveal the fact that the trauma was so insignificant that fracture of a bone is unlikely. In the case of deep wounds, especially of compound fractures, it may influence the type of therapy greatly if the surgeon can determine, from the history, the kind and degree of contamination, *i.e.,* whether the wound was sustained outdoors, in a fertilized field or a clean highway and especially whether the clothes of the patient protected the wound. If there were no tears in the clothes over a compound fracture, for example, the contamination is likely to consist only of organisms present on the patient's own skin (*e.g.,* Staphylococcus albus) and hence is of less serious importance.

Important in eliciting a history of trauma is the existence of mental symptoms such as momentary loss of consciousness, etc. It also is necessary to know of preëxisting disease such as epilepsy, etc., which may have played a role in initiating the accident. It is obvious, however, that the emergency treatment of the patient's wounds and general condition are of paramount and primary concern. The history is clearly secondary to such care, but it must not be overlooked, and as soon as possible the significant details should be obtained and recorded.

Family History.—Many irrelevant features are often obtained in the family history, which, however, must be investigated because it may contain information sufficiently important to suggest the correct diagnosis. The cause of death of immediate relatives should be ascertained, if possible, because of the tendency for certain diseases to be prevalent in certain families. Cancer, many diseases of the heart and kidney (*e.g.,* nephritis, polycystic kidney), insanity and numerous other diseases may at times exhibit these hereditary tendencies. Tuberculosis is particularly prone to be disseminated through a family because of contact infection. Stillbirths and miscarriages (occurring without obvious cause) are usually associated with syphilis as the etiologic factor.

Past History.—Information regarding the patient's past health should always be obtained, particularly when the lesion explaining the symptoms is not discernible. Such data will often aid materially in the diagnosis. For example, numerous similar attacks of right lower quadrant pain may suggest a diagnosis of recurrent appendicitis. Again a history of a serious intra-abdominal operation might mean the presence of adhesive bands, producing intestinal obstruction as a cause for cramping abdominal pains.

Lest important data be overlooked, the following routine is useful:

1. Childhood diseases, especially those with complications.
2. Various systems: head and neck, heart and lungs, gastro-intestinal tract, genitourinary organs, nervous system and special senses.
3. Marital history including menstrual and reproductive.
4. Details concerning operations, accidents and serious illnesses.
5. Nutritional history and the personality of the patient (see below).

Nutritional History.—That a healthy person will naturally select a well balanced diet was a commonly held but now thoroughly exploded theory. Ample studies have shown a disturbing incidence of nutritional deficiencies among those who consider themselves well. Among the sick, the percentage, of course, rises sharply. The reasons are many: ignorance, prejudice, poverty. While it is true that most of these deficiencies are sub-clinical and cannot be diagnosed by clinical manifestations, the physician can detect their existence from the dietary history and actually measure their degree by various chemical methods. Detailed questions are necessary in obtaining a history. For example, does the patient eat a fair amount of good proteins such as meat, eggs or milk? Are the vitamin-containing foods such as fruits and vegetables, milk, butter and meat included in their diets regularly? Underweight, it should be emphasized, is not necessarily associated with malnutrition. Many individuals of normal or even excessive weight may actually be suffering from vitamin or protein deficiencies; in these cases the high body weight is merely a manifestation of hidden edema or of large fat deposits.

Surgical diseases are particularly prone to be associated with nutritional deficiencies (see page 150) which must be corrected before adequate therapy is carried out. The normal healing of wounds and the elimination of postoperative complications both depend on the presence in the body of adequate amounts of at least four of the six nutritional elements, water, minerals, vitamins and proteins. The first step in the evaluation of these deficiencies is a good nutritional history.

Personality.—A good clinical history cannot be complete unless it contains information about the patient's personality. Such information may be merely limited to a word, such as phlegmatic, choleric, sanguine or melancholic, the four types of personalities described by Hippocrates. Or it may involve a paragraph or two involving some of the intimate details of the patient's life. These facts often form an excellent background for the interpretation of the significance of the patient's symptoms. For example, pain, sometimes expressed as excruciating in certain asthenic individuals, may be a symptom of emotional maladjustment and not of specific organic disease. By contrast, robust individuals may have only moderate complaints in the presence of a serious lesion. Important clues to the prognosis and ability to survive serious operations can often be derived from knowledge of the patient's personality. The old-fashioned family doctor knew these facts and was able to achieve excellent therapeutic results in many instances without the benefit of modern technics. How much better can the modern surgeon achieve a larger percentage of cures if he but utilize the information gained by knowledge of his patient's personality!

THE SURGICAL EXAMINATION

The surgical examination includes first the physical examination, then the laboratory and special examinations. To this may be added when possible the follow-up examination. By the physical examination one usually includes only such observations as can be made by the surgeon with the aid only of the five senses and perhaps such simple apparatus as a stethoscope, flash light, rubber glove, etc. It comprises what is often called a bedside examination in contrast to the results of special laboratory, x-ray and other tests. There has been some controversy in recent years as to the relative importance of bedside and laboratory studies. Obviously both types of examination should be at the disposal of the well-equipped practitioner. It should be emphasized, however, that the general rule of proceeding from the simple to the complex should be observed. Clearly, if a diagnosis can be made on the basis of the history and simple physical examination alone further tests may be unjustified. To one trained in bedside examination, indeed, no further studies are necessary in a great majority of cases. And even when the complete gamut of laboratory and other data is required, the value of the bedside examination should never be overlooked. Modern surgery does not run the danger of returning to the "horse-and-buggy" days just because it insists upon utilizing the five senses which were all the old practitioner had at his disposal.

The Physical Examination.—During the simple bedside examination a certain routine is often useful. First in importance is the *facies* of the patient which immediately gives an indication of the existence of pain, shock, fever (hectic flush), etc. The study of the patient's facies, of course, requires no time and the information is conveyed while the surgeon is obtaining the history or instituting emergency treatment. The importance of the three basic measurements, *i.e.,* temperature, pulse and respirations (often abbreviated T.P.R.) is obvious and they are usually obtained at the very outset of the examination. To this should be added the measurement of the blood pressure which is obviously important in patients with impaired circulation (surgical shock).

Local examination of the lesion is ordinarily carried out in the following order, inspection, voluntary movements and palpation. The importance of adequate illumination is obvious during all steps in the examination. The surgeon should also, as far as possible, arrange his position and that of the patient so that both are as comfortable as possible; attention to this detail often permits much more accurate observations.

1. *Inspection,* since it inflicts no pain, is carried out first. This is aided by asking the patient to point to the exact site of the pain, swelling, ulcer, etc. Comparison with the opposite side often aids in detecting swelling or deformity. The

color of the part is noted and the results of transillumination are obtained in certain cases. Inspection of the patient must not be confined to the part alone if examination of neighboring structures is indicated. Thus a lymphangitis may not be detected unless the patient with an infected finger is asked to roll up his sleeve.

2. *Voluntary movements* are elicited in order to detect the degree and type of disability present. This also requires the infliction of no pain and thus aids the surgeon in gaining the confidence of his patient. Movements are compared with those on the normal side. Limitation due to pain should be distinguished from that due to other causes (ankylosis, muscle spasm, fear, paralysis, severed tendon, etc.). Special attention is paid to those movements which tend to produce pain.

3. *Palpation* can yield a great deal of information if skilfully carried out. It can, however, if improperly done so completely alienate the patient that further procedures become impossible. Avoidance of pain is obviously the key to a successful palpation, yet the elicitation of tenderness is one of the important findings. Thus gentleness is of extreme importance; this combined with confidence on the part of the patient will permit the coöperation which is so essential. The patient should be apprised of the likelihood of pain but be assured that any manipulations will cease at the first indication of it. For this the facies of the patient should be watched, constantly if possible. If it is possible to divert the attention of the patient during the examination more accurate information can often be obtained; this is especially true of children. Important is the necessity of starting the palpation at a part which is not tender and approaching the lesion gradually, rather than palpating immediately the tender spot. The importance of localizing point tenderness cannot be emphasized too much; when it can be elicited its diagnostic value is considerable.

After the examination of the local lesion, it is, of course, essential that the entire body be examined, except when the lesion is trivial and has no possible relationship to the various systems. If the examiner is relatively inexperienced, he will find it convenient to adopt a definite routine in the sequence of these examinations, such as starting at the head, proceeding downward to the neck, chest, abdomen and lower extremities, lest he omit some important part of the examination.

During abdominal palpation gentleness yet thoroughness is especially important, for here not only is the palpator searching for tenderness but also for voluntary muscle guard, involuntary muscle spasm and muscle rigidity, all various degrees of tenseness on the part of the abdominal muscles which have an important bearing in the diagnosis of peritoneal irritation and infection. The decision as to the necessity of operation frequently depends on the findings obtained during abdominal palpation. The detection of a tumor or mass may be extremely important especially if associated with the signs of infection.

The other findings obtained on palpation include such data as local temperature (compare with the corresponding area on the opposite side), pitting edema, crepitus and fluctuation. Each of these signs requires special and careful palpation. Percussion is often of value over herniations and abdominal enlargement; auscultation is sometimes useful in detecting various bruits in arteriovenous fistulas, toxic thyroids, etc. Under palpation also are included tests for sensation and reflexes which may indicate nerve injury or disease of various types.

The surgeon also counts as part of his examination the inspection and palpation of the various orifices of the body, notably rectal and vaginal examinations which are described in detail later. The mouth and throat also yield information of importance in various injuries and other surgical diseases. The eyes and ears also should not be overlooked in the search for significant findings. Instruments for adequate illumination are of great value.

Of extreme importance to the surgeon in many cases is simple inspection of the urine, stool and vomitus. Much significant data as to the patient's disease may be obtained in this manner. Statements by others as to the presence of blood, the type of stool, the amount or character of the vomitus, the color of the urine, etc., are often inaccurate or unavailable but if specimens are saved the surgeon may often get decisive data by direct inspection alone. When the patient expectorates, the sputum likewise should be inspected for its character and amount, the presence of blood, etc. The importance of discharges of various types, particularly of pus, is obvious; aspiration is often indicated in order to note what type of fluid is present in certain inflammatory and other swellings. While these observations are simple and seem obvious and easy, it is surprising how often they are overlooked, and much important information lost. The alert surgeon utilizes all data available, even the simplest, before or while he asks for the more complicated data which are included under the heading of laboratory and special examinations.

Laboratory Examinations.—A great many laboratory examinations are available and they offer a wide latitude of choice; the possible data obtained thereby are extensive, yet ordinarily only a few should be made, *i.e.,* only those really of importance in arriving at a diagnosis or in avoiding serious errors. The irreducible minimum is, of course, the examination of the urine and blood cells, which should be part of the routine, and because it requires simple apparatus should really be included in the results of the bedside examination. This routine is particularly important in preoperative cases for reasons discussed in more detail elsewhere. In a few patients, however, more complicated laboratory examinations will be indicated, most of them included under the generic term of blood chemistry.

Blood chemical determinations require a well equipped laboratory and careful, well controlled technics. Of those determinations which are apt to be of importance to the surgeon are estimations of blood urea, blood sugar, of serum albumin and globulin, of prothrombin, of serum amylase, icteric index, and concentrations of sulfanilamide and of vitamin C. This type of data is discussed in detail in later chapters. It is probable that biochemical observations will become more and more important as the various unsolved problems in surgery gradually unfold themselves. To keep abreast of these newer developments the well-equipped surgeon will find it necessary to learn more of biochemistry than ever before. Besides blood chemistry, other procedures may be indicated, *e.g.,* urinary excretion of phenolsulfonphthalein, stool examinations, and spinal fluid study.

Special Examinations.—Most of the special examinations in surgical patients are made by means of the x-ray and require the services of an expert radiologist in order to prove of the greatest value to the surgeon. This is not only true of the interpretation of the films but also of the technic of taking them. It should be emphasized that the possession of even the latest and most complete x-ray equipment will not enable the novice to elicit the greatest help this method of examination is capable of affording. This applies not only to such special studies as those of the gastro-intestinal tract but even to ordinary roentgenograms. On the other hand, the surgeon himself should view and study the films in each case, correlating what he sees and what the radiologist sees with the rest of the clinical picture. Consultation with the radiologist is also often of great value. Recent advances in the field of the x-ray in special examinations are the kymograph for the accurate measurement of visceral movements, and the laminograph (planograph) for detailed study of deeply situated shadows. Included also as special examinations are the use of the cystoscope, proctoscope, esophagoscope, bronchoscope and gastroscope; these are described in later chapters. Measurements of vital capacity, the basal metabolic rate, the injection of lipoidol into sinus tracts, spinal canal and the bronchi, electrocardiograms, etc., are frequently indicated in individual cases.

The examination of tissues removed at operation is often assigned to a special field called *surgical pathology*. The most important facts of tissue diagnosis, both gross and microscopic, must be in the possession of every surgeon. This is particularly true of the gross examination of lesions encountered at the operating table. An important decision often depends upon the ability of the surgeon to identify lesions, particularly to distinguish between benign and malignant ones. For example, by external examination it will frequently be impossible to determine accurately, whether or not a breast tumor is malignant or benign; however, the surgeon should be sufficiently well trained in surgical pathology to make that decision by cut section of the tumor in the operating room after its local removal. The proper procedure, *i.e.,* radical or simple mastectomy may then be performed without waiting for a microscopical report; the patient will, therefore, be spared a second operation. For this reason, detailed training in surgical pathology is part of the modern surgeon's education. This responsibility, moreover, should not be shifted to another individual, particularly one who is not himself especially trained in pathology. It should be emphasized, moreover, that this education must be a continuous one. The surgeon should study the microscopic features of each specimen he has removed in order to correlate them with the gross appearance and with the rest of the clinical picture. Only in this way can the surgeon bring to his work all the knowledge necessary to bring his professional proficiency to its highest plane. It is largely because of these considerations that many of the surgical diseases discussed herein will be illustrated by gross and microscopic photographs showing the important features of their surgical pathology.

Follow-up Examinations.—The high percentage of excellent results following most surgical therapy at the present time owes much to systematic follow-up studies in many clinics where patients are examined for months and years at regular intervals after they leave the hospital. In this way only can the end results of surgical procedures be evaluated, *e.g.,* the recurrence rate following herniotomy with various technics is accurately determined only in this manner. Such examinations are not only appreciated by the patients themselves but also serve a useful purpose in the education of students and younger surgeons. Follow-up examinations are especially important in malignant disease in order to determine as early as possible the existence or non-existence of recurrent growths or metastases.

CHAPTER II

INFLAMMATION AND REPAIR

Kinds of Injury   *Factors Influencing Repair*
The Pathology of Inflammation   *Kinds of Repair*
The Process of Healing

The human body is constantly beset by injurious agents of various kinds. Inflammation has been described as the body's response to such injury. In simple cases it consists of vascular, humoral and cellular reactions which aim to fight off and conquer the irritant. But when tissue is killed or even merely removed or divided, the response of the body goes much farther for there is now the problem of removing dead cells, replacing the lost tissue and uniting the separated structures. These last reactions have been described as healing or repair. Together, inflammation and repair represent, therefore, the sum of nature's response to injury. The final result is sometimes satisfactory, but too often the spontaneous efforts of nature are defective, particularly in regard to the healing process. Study of the mechanisms underlying inflammation and repair thus should have a practical value to the surgeon for it will enable him to recognize and improve upon the useful factors as well as to realize the defective ones and take measures against them.

KINDS OF INJURY

The response of the body to injury depends to a large extent on its kind and severity. In general the simplest injuries are those which damage cells without impairing their viability, such as a stroke on the skin with a dull blunt object, or a mild scald or sunburn. The more severe injuries cause actual death of cells, called necrosis, or, when the tissue involved is extensive, gangrene. On the other hand, tissue may be divided or separated with very little or no necrosis. Classified according to type, the various injurious agents may be described as follows:

1. *Mechanical (or traumatic) agents* are perhaps the most common and vary greatly in degree. The lesions produced are called wounds, and are discussed in considerable detail in Chapter X.

2. *Chemical irritants* are often inadvertently used in salves and solutions; especially dangerous are those containing phenol which produces definite cell injury and in some cases actual death of tissue. Ordinarily, the serious chemical injuries are due to accidental contacts with strong acids, alkalis, liquid bromine, etc., which destroy the tissue with which they come in contact. Insect and snake bites are often serious because of the introduction of toxic chemical substances which injure cells directly.

9

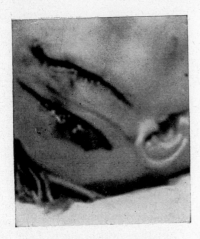

FIG. 1.—TRAUMATIC INJURY.

Two deep lacerations of the scalp sustained by the patient. Severed temporal muscle can be seen in the lower part of the posterior wound.

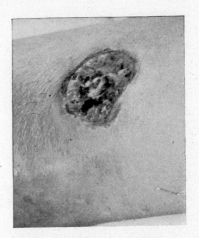

FIG. 2.—CHEMICAL INJURY.

A spreading ulcer of the leg developed in this patient after a simple laceration was treated by repeated application of a salve containing phenol. Rapid healing followed cessation of the chemical irritation.

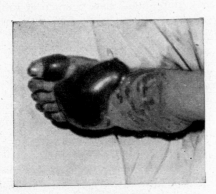

FIG. 3.—THERMAL ENERGY AS AN INJURIOUS AGENT.

This blister has the same appearance as if caused by excessive heat. Actually it was produced by excessive exposure to severe cold; it represents an injury due to frostbite.

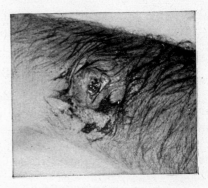

FIG. 4.—BACTERIAL INJURY.

Local necrosis caused by a spontaneous furuncle which has already opened and discharged its content of pus.

3. *Radiant energy* such as heat, and also x-ray and radium have the power to incite an inflammatory reaction and if severe, actually to kill tissue. Electricity of high amperage not only can burn tissue, but also may coagulate cytoplasm and thus kill cells immediately. By chilling, cold can injure tissue, and by freezing, can actually kill it. The effects of these agents will be described in Chapter XIV.

4. *Pathogenic bacteria* and their products of growth or disintegration are far and away the most important and most frequent agents capable of inciting the inflammatory reaction, acting not only as the primary agent, but more commonly entering the field after other agents have started the injury. Bacteria, of course, not only damage cells, but are capable of provoking extensive necrosis, and frequently challenge life itself. The acute bacterial inflammations are discussed in Chapter III; miscellaneous infections are described in Chapter VI.

THE PATHOLOGY OF INFLAMMATION

The essential reactions following injury can best be studied by observing a superficial area of inflammation such as that following a slight burn or stroke on the skin. In recent years the microscopic study of such an area has been especially aided by the use of the motion picture camera. It is Virchow, however, the founder of modern cellular pathology, to whom we owe a great deal of our knowledge of the inflammatory process. Histologists such as Maximow elucidated many of the details and the use of vital dyes has contributed much additional information. Prominent in the more physiological approach is the important monograph by Menkin.[1] A recent study of the physical factors is that of Bellis.[8]

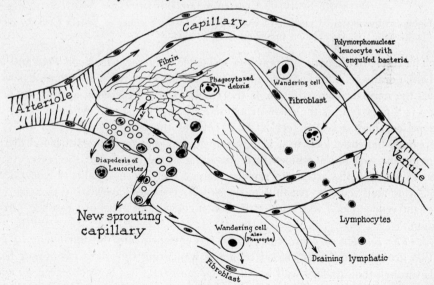

Fig. 5.—Diagram Illustrating the Main Histologic Features of Inflammation and Repair.

To the clinical observer the inflamed area shows the so-called four cardinal signs, first mentioned by Galen:[2] *i.e.*, redness, swelling, heat and pain. These gross effects, however, can best be explained by describing the bodily mechanisms which give rise to them. These consist arbitrarily of four elements, (1) the vascular, (2) the cellular, (3) the humoral and (4) the nerve reactions.

1. *The vascular reaction* is one of dilatation which involves arterioles, capillaries, venules and lymphatics. Primary undoubtedly is the arteriolar dilatation which forces closed capillaries open, widens those already open, and enlarges passively or secondarily the collecting venules and lymphatics. There is some evidence, however, that the capillaries are also capable of independent changes in the caliber of their lumen. Vascular changes are under nervous control, both local and central, and may in part be due to the release, according to Thomas Lewis,[3] of a histamine-like substance into the tissues as a result of the injurious agent.

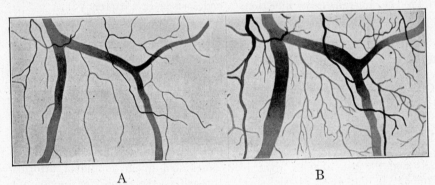

A   B

FIG. 6.—DIAGRAM ILLUSTRATING THE INCREASED CALIBER OF BLOOD VESSELS OCCURRING AFTER THE STIMULUS EXERTED BY AN INFLAMMATORY AGENT.

Note also the increased number of channels, due to the opening of vessels formerly closed. *A,* resting state; *B,* vasodilation following inflammation.

The result of this vasodilation is a tremendous *increase in blood flow* and also in lymph drainage. This has been measured and found to reach a magnitude several times the normal. The red color is the result of this hyperemia and in the acute stage is a fiery red, or the color of arterial blood. The blood flow is so rapid that the patient may actually feel it as a definite throbbing synchronous with the heart beat. Increased local heat is a phenomenon due to rapid flow of blood thereby bringing the part to the temperature prevailing in the interior of the body. As the process subsides the arterioles rapidly resume their normal caliber, whereas the capillaries and venules, reacting more slowly, become somewhat congested with stagnant venous blood which gives the bluish color to all areas of subsiding inflammation.

2. *The cellular response* consists of the entrance into the inflammatory area of two groups of cells, *i.e.,* blood cells and wandering cells; the passage of blood cells through the capillary wall is called *diapedesis* and has been observed by every student in biology who has watched the blood flow in the skin of a frog's web after an irritant such as mustard oil is applied to the part. The mechanism by which cells make their way through the capillary wall probably has something to do with local changes in the permeability of the endothelium, but more potent is the chemotactic power of substances released in the inflamed area.

Attracted also in large numbers are the wandering or tissue cells normally present in tissue everywhere and called by various authors macrophages, histiocytes and endothelial leukocytes. The wandering cell is larger than the lymphocyte and is mononuclear. Both it and the white blood cell are phagocytic, engulfing bacteria and thus playing an important part in the defense in bacterial inflammation. The macrophage, however, is also able to engulf dead tissue and other debris and can form fibroblasts which, as will be pointed out below, are important in repair.

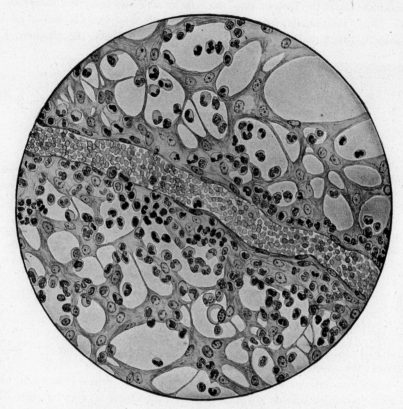

FIG. 7.—THE CELLULAR RESPONSE TO ACUTE INFLAMMATION.

Inflamed omentum showing outwandered leukocytes about a small vessel. (From MacCallum, *Textbook of Pathology,* 1932, W. B. Saunders Co., p. 143.)

3. *The humoral response* consists of the escape of serum through the dilated capillaries along with the cells. This outpouring of fluid is called *exudation.* It is at once taken up by the lymphatics so that there is an increased flow of lymph as well as blood. However, the lymph drainage is rarely rapid enough, and soon the serum fills the tissue spaces giving rise to swelling which sometimes takes the form of a localized lymphedema. If the more superficial layers are involved as in a sunburn the fluid may give rise to a blister. The chemical composition of the fluid which leaves the capillaries approaches that of plasma, *i.e.,* it contains a large amount of plasma protein. When the loss is great as in an extensive injury or burn symptoms of shock may follow (see p. 256). Exudation is of importance in defense

for it serves to dilute toxins, to furnish specific antibodies, to neutralize the bacterial products, and to supply nourishment to the cells which have been mobilized on the field of battle. Later the exudate coagulates and forms a fibrin network along which repair takes place.

4. *The nerve reaction* incites the vascular dilation already mentioned. It also arouses the sense of immediate pain which serves to warn the patient and prevents continuance of the injury in many cases. When swelling occurs the pain fibers are again stimulated and the patient puts the part at rest and becomes concerned with its care. Thus, individuals with anesthetic skin due to various kinds of nerve lesions may, without realizing it, suffer serious injury due to the absence of pain

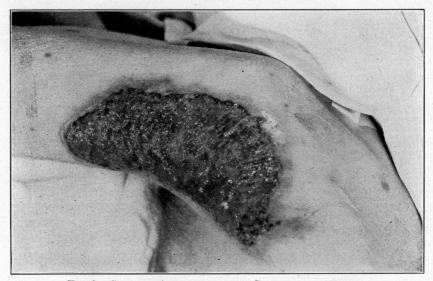

FIG. 8.—CLINICAL APPEARANCE OF A GRANULATING WOUND.

The original injury was a severe burn of the axilla involving the full thickness of the skin (3rd degree); the necrotic tissue has already sloughed away.

fibers. Moreover, nerves are apparently necessary in repair for such patients often exhibit lesions which do not heal and are called trophic; they are discussed in detail later on (see p. 123).

Variations in the degree of pain produced in inflammation depend on variations in the degree and location of the swelling. Thus, soft tissue inflammation is less painful than that developing in some rigid structure such as bone. A rapidly increasing exudation is apt to be more painful than one less acute. Areas well supplied by nerves are obviously more painful when inflamed, as, for example, an injury in the fingers. Sometimes when spontaneous pain is slight in deep seated inflammation it can be elicited by digital pressure over the most accessible part of the lesion. Pain produced in this manner is spoken of as *tenderness*. Even when spontaneous pain is present, palpation will increase its severity and also detect the point of maximum tenderness.

THE PROCESS OF HEALING

The picture of dilatation, diapedesis, and exudation as just described is seen only in relatively simple inflammation. Most injuries seen by the surgeon are much more serious in that they have produced death of cells, and loss or division of tissue. In either case they lead to a defect in the continuity of tissue. To correct such defects is part of the process of repair. In the simple reaction which follows a slight scald in which no cells are killed, a blister may form and perhaps a little pigmentation may finally be seen. The end result in general, however, is undetectable

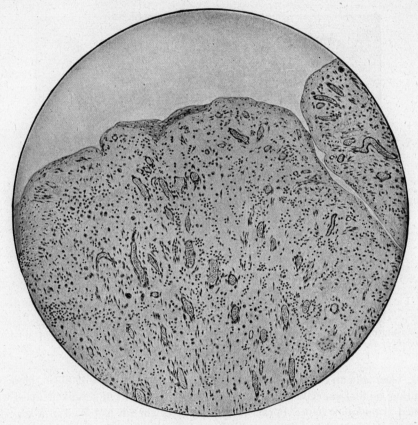

FIG. 9.—MICROSCOPIC APPEARANCE OF CROSS SECTION OF GRANULATION TISSUE FORMED IN THE HEALING OF AN ULCER.

(From MacCallum, *Textbook of Pathology*, 1932, W. B. Saunders Co., p. 213.)

except when permanent functional changes have been produced. But even with the tiniest scratch where tissue is divided, killed or removed, the final stage is detectable as a microscopic scar which represents the end result of repair.

Though healing obviously follows the death or loss of tissue, actually the processes of inflammation and repair are often synchronous. W. G. MacCallum [4] has very aptly emphasized this synchronism by comparing inflammation and repair to a burning house in which firemen are actively fighting the flames in the roof while at the same time workmen are clearing away debris, and masons and carpenters are already mending the damaged parts below.

The spontaneous course of nature in healing is rather direct. Removal of dead tissue occurs by phagocytosis or actual sloughing or both, thus producing a defect. Defects are also produced by actual loss of tissue as when a portion of skin is avulsed. Unless immediately sutured, defects also follow mere division of tissue which retracts because of its elasticity. Into the defect, usually along the fibrin network laid down by coagulated serum, grow cells called fibroblasts which originate from the wandering cell mentioned above, and also from the endothelium of capil-

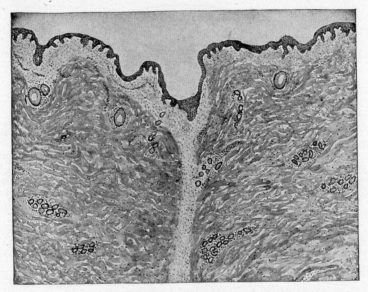

FIG. 10.—MICROSCOPIC SECTION THROUGH A HEALED SURGICAL INCISION OF THE ABDOMINAL WALL.

Note the thin scar binding the two parts of the divided normal tissue. (From MacCallum, *Textbook of Pathology,* 1932, W. B. Saunders Co., p. 207.)

laries. They take an elongated shape as they grow. The mixture of fibrin, blood clot, sprouting capillaries, cells and fibroblasts forms a moist red succulent mass which is called *granulation tissue.* It can be seen as such when it has filled in a superficial defect. Eventually the entire area becomes less vascular, the long fibroblasts lose their nucleus and cytoplasm, and assume the histological appearance of dense fibrous tissue. Grossly a firm cicatrix or scar forms covered by a single layer of epithelium which has grown in from the adjacent normal skin. (See repair of skin and connective tissue on pp. 18 and 19).

This end result in the spontaneous healing of a defect is often far from satisfactory. The scar is large and dense, lacks suppleness and elasticity and tends to contract more and more and when located over a joint often bends it into an abnormal fixed position. Scar, when it develops in the intestinal wall or urethra, is apt to lead to stricture with its resulting obstruction to the lumen. The epithelium covering the scar is also imperfect for it is thin and delicate and withstands normal usage poorly. It, moreover, contains no sweat or sebaceous glands because these structures do not regenerate.

Spontaneous healing is apt to be satisfactory only when there are no defects. Thus excellent healing results when the divided tissue has been perfectly approximated by the surgeon, for the area of granulation tissue is then almost microscopic, just sufficient to glue the wound edges together and finally bind them by a thin fibrous scar. Still more ideal, of course, would be the ability of tissue to reproduce itself and thus to repair by regeneration, just as the lobster which grows a new limb in place of the one that is lost. Regeneration does occur with certain human tissue and under certain circumstances. The liver, for example, regenerates perfectly even when almost all of it has been removed, and so do some other parenchymatous organs, but to a lesser extent. With the other structures more commonly involved in surgical lesions, such as skin, bone, tendon, nerve, etc., various degrees of regeneration are possible under various circumstances. Such knowledge is important to the surgeon for it enables him to improve upon the unsatisfactory results which nature alone achieves. The application of such knowledge to the practical problem of treatment is obvious. The details of treatment are discussed in succeeding chapters. Here the underlying principles are emphasized.

FACTORS INFLUENCING REPAIR

The important factors influencing repair (spontaneous as well as therapeutic), aside from the influence of the degree and kind of injury, are (1) the kind of tissue involved, particularly its vascularity, (2) the surgical technic used in treatment, (3) the presence of pathogenic bacteria in the wound, and (4) certain constitutional factors, not always understood, but quite important in some cases.

1. *The kind of tissue* injured determines first of all the degree of damage sustained because some cells are more sturdy than others. Secondly, the question as to whether regeneration is possible or whether defects must be replaced only by scar depends upon the kind of tissue. Thirdly, the fact that some tissues may be successfully transplanted has a bearing on the surgical treatment because defects may often be best remedied by this procedure. (a) *Nerve cells* are not very resistant to injurious agents, yet are well protected by anatomical and vascular barriers. Circulatory impairment of even a few minutes may suffice to cause their functional death. When actually necrotic they cannot be regenerated, but become replaced by scar tissue which arises from adjacent neuroglial cells. Mammalian nerve cells have not been successfully transplanted. (b) *Nerve fibers,* at least peripheral ones, are also well protected against adjacent inflammation, but are subject, of course, to crushing injuries or actual division. If such an injury involves the death of the axis cylinder which is primarily concerned with the transmission of the nerve impulse, all the fibers distal to the lesion degenerate. This process is spoken of as the reaction of degeneration which takes several days for completion. Repair then occurs by outgrowth from the central end and under favorable circumstances may lead to a complete regeneration of the nerve after many months. Transplantation has never been achieved with functional continuity. Muscle, like nerve fibers, can regenerate by a process of budding from the adjacent normal cells, but ordinarily does not do this, defects being

replaced by scar tissue. (*c*) *Cartilage* behaves differently in different locations. Articular cartilage, when injured, cannot regenerate and is replaced by scar; costal cartilage, on the other hand, is easily transplanted and regenerates provided the perichondrium is intact. The difference is due to the presence in the perichondrium of stem or parent cells capable of forming adult chondrocytes which in themselves are incapable of regeneration. These stem cells are absent in the articular cartilage which does not possess a perichondrium and hence presents a grave problem when severe injury occurs. (*d*) *Skin,* though resistant to injury, is most often subject to

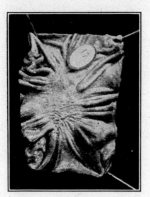

FIG. 11.—REGENERATION OF GASTRIC MUCOSA (EXPERIMENT PERFORMED ON DOGS).

The center of the specimen represents a completely healed defect which had been excised surgically several weeks previously. Microscopic study revealed complete reproduction even of gastric glands. (From Ferguson, *Am. J. Anat.,* 1928, 42:441.)

it, being exposed to the outside world. Skin is composed of two layers, the epidermis or epithelial layer and the dermis or connective tissue layer. When a defect involves both layers completely the regeneration which occurs is far from perfect for the new skin does not possess the tough elastic dermal layer beneath, nor the hornified protective layer outside. Transplantation or skin grafting can be done successfully and is frequently performed. The transplanted skin becomes revascularized rapidly and lives as such. It is necessary, however, that the skin to be transplanted successfully should come from the patient himself. (See also skin grafting, p. 275.) This is a general rule for the transplantation of tissues. (*e*) *Mucous membrane* of the squamous type behaves the same as skin. But the gastro-intestinal tract has tremendous powers of regeneration at least in replacing defects caused by a single injury. Large areas of the gastric mucosa have been removed experimentally and found to regenerate even to the reproduction of the digestive glands. Gastric and duodenal ulcers frequently heal perfectly at least as far as the mucosa is concerned. It is true that strictures do form, but these are due to injury of underlying muscle and connective tissue. The development of strictures is even more likely in the healing of mucosal defects in the biliary tract, ureter and urethra. (*f*) *Bone* is frequently injured and is prone to bacterial inflammation. It has great powers of regeneration which is particularly rapid in children even under unfavorable conditions. Into the hematoma which forms about fractured bone ends grow cells which originate from the periosteum and endosteum of the bone, and form adult chondrocytes similar to the cartilage cells in embryonic and infant life. These are invaded by osteoclasts which soon become replaced by osteoblasts which have the power of taking up calcium phosphate which bestows rigidity to the bone. (See also bone healing, p. 352.) Ordinarily, so complete is bone repair that the site of injury may be impossible to detect after several months. Bone is readily transplantable. Although it probably loses its viability after such transfer, it finally becomes part and parcel of the adjacent bone tissue. Nevertheless, for some reason dead bone is not as successfully transplanted as live bone in most instances. (*g*) *Fat or fatty tissue* is sensitive to injury and is prone to infection. It cannot regenerate, and when necrotic, becomes replaced with scar tissue.

With special care fat has been transplanted. Fibroblasts have been seen to form fat cells. (*h*) The *serous surfaces* are composed of mesothelium, as the peritoneum, for example. It is not often injured, though a frequent site of infection. The serosal cells are able to regenerate; free transplants of omentum take very well and are useful in intra-abdominal surgery. (*i*) *Connective or fibrous tissue* is most important in repair since it is the universal replacement tissue, filling in gaps and uniting divided structures. It is formed from fibroblasts by metaplasia from capillary endothelium and wandering cells which are present in every inflammatory, and hence healing, area. This newly formed fibrous or connective tissue, however, contains collagenous but scarcely any elastic fibers. This accounts for its dense consistency and its distressing tendency to contracture.

Connective tissue in the body occurs in a variety of forms, is very resistant to injury, and is easily and successfully transplanted. It is represented by such tissue as fascia, tendons, blood vessel walls, derma of the skin, subcutaneous tissue, etc. These differ greatly from inflammatory connective tissue since all contain varying amounts of elastic fibers which, though formed by the fibrous cell itself, are a non-viable part of the structure. It is of importance to note that regenerated fibrous tissue cells, *i.e.*, scar, is not the same as the parent cells in that they do not have the power to form elastic fibers. Thus, if a defect is made in fascia the hiatus becomes filled with simple strands of fibrous tissue which does not have the toughness or elasticity of the adjacent fascia. The same is true of regenerated tendon, derma, and ligaments. It is obvious, therefore, if the qualities of strength and elasticity are needed the defect must be filled by a transplant.

Transplantation of fascia, therefore, is frequently performed. Like a bone transplant it probably loses its viability temporarily. The outer edge becomes immediately revascularized, but the center of the graft probably dies. Yet it eventually becomes replaced with living cells and is indistinguishable from normal fascia and retains all the properties of fascia. Narrow strips of living fascia from the patient himself are often used as sutures with which to sew together the edges of large defects in the fascia of the abdominal wall (McArthur, Gallie). There is evidence that such narrow strips remain alive without the death of any part of them.

2. The type of *surgical technic* used in treatment plays a great role in determining the kind of healing (W. S. Halsted[5]). It will be mentioned in some detail in other places. Briefly, we may say here that the rapidity of healing and its completeness, that is, in the sense of returning as closely and rapidly to its normal structure and function as possible, depends in large measure on the kind of surgical technic used in the treatment of the injury. This applies particularly to the injury produced by the surgeon intentionally during the course of an operation but also to his efforts in suturing a wound produced accidentally. Gentle handling of tissue obviously minimizes the extent of the inflammatory reaction by avoiding unnecessary tissue damage. This factor is of extreme importance. Dead spaces which become filled with serum, then granulation tissue and finally with dense scar are likewise responsible for poor healing. Careful hemostasis prevents the need for added phagocytosis in removing blood clots. Undue tension in suturing jeopardizes the blood supply of the tissue, leads to necrosis, and hence increases the intensity of the inflammatory process. To avoid such tension is, therefore, one object of careful surgery. All of

these precautions have an added importance for they minimize the incidence of infection as will be discussed later. The kind of suture and its size also influence healing; catgut, though finally absorbed, provokes a true inflammatory reaction with scarring, even in absence of infection, unlike fine silk. The latter, on the other hand, in the presence of infection may act as a foreign body and may slough out. (See also p. 32.)

3. *The presence of bacteria* in a wound in sufficient numbers and virulence to provoke an infection is by far the most important of all the factors influencing repair. Regeneration of tissue may be prevented by infection, and transplantation fail. Moreover, bacteria may increase the amount of tissue destroyed, prolong in-

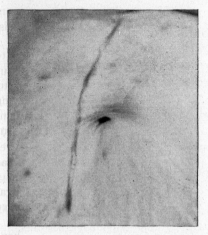

FIG. 12.—HEALING BY FIRST INTENTION.

The abdominal incision was made two months previously for the removal of a diseased gallbladder in a 78 year old woman.

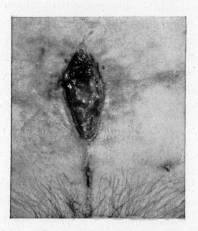

FIG. 13.—HEALING BY SECONDARY INTENTION.

The upper portion of a low midline incision for the performance of a gynecological operation became infected and is healing by granulation tissue.

flammatory and reparative changes and lead to excessive scarring. Their further effects will be considered in some detail in separate chapters.

4. *Constitutional factors* often play an important role in healing. Children have a greater power of cellular repair than adults. On the other hand, very young infants are less resistant to certain infections, though their reparative processes in clean wounds are very rapid. Healing in the aged is notoriously slow. However, there are wide individual variations, the nature of which is not understood. It may be related to the power of growth in general. The fundamental relationship between the healing and growth processes has been especially emphasized by Harvey.[6]

The general condition of the patient is of extreme importance in the process of wound healing. Such factors as vitamin C deficiency, hypoproteinemia, etc., are recognized as extremely significant. Clean wound healing should be the aim of surgeons, regardless of the obstacles placed in its way. An excellent discussion of the factors involved in clean wound healing with a critical analysis of the fundamental principles involved is that of Whipple.[7]

KINDS OF REPAIR

Repair is customarily classified into certain types. *Healing by first intention or per primam* is that which is the closest approach to perfection in that practically no infection has interfered (aseptic healing), and that the structures have been approximated so accurately that practically no defect is apparent. The amount of granulation tissue is just enough to glue and join the opposed surfaces with a thin, almost microscopic scar. In some cases by an actual bridging over through regeneration of the tissue itself, perfect healing results, as for example, in a successfully sutured nerve.

Healing by secondary intention is the term applied to the process which occurs when necrosis is extensive, infection severe, or tissue loss so great that a mass of granulation tissue finally fills in the defect. The resulting scar or cicatrix is usually prominent and sometimes by its contraction leads to permanent disability. Even if the end result is satisfactory, healing by secondary intention is always of longer duration and requires much more care on the part of the patient and surgeon.

BIBLIOGRAPHY

1. MENKIN, VALY. *Dynamics of Inflammation,* Macmillan, 1940.
2. GALEN (131-202 A.D.) quoted by GARRISON, F. H. *Introduction to the History of Medicine,* W. B. Saunders Company, Philadelphia, 1921, Ed. 3, p. 104.
3. LEWIS, THOMAS. *The Blood Vessels of the Human Skin and Their Responses,* Shaw and Sons, London, 1927.
4. MACCALLUM, W. C. *A Textbook of Pathology,* W. B. Saunders Company, Philadelphia, 1916, p. 130.
5. HALSTEAD, W. S. The Treatment of Wounds, etc., *Johns Hopkins Hospital Reports,* 2:255, 1891; Ligature and Suture Material, etc., *J. Am. M. Ass.,* 60; 1119, 1913.
6. HARVEY, S. C. The Velocity of the Growth of Fibroblasts in the Healing Wound, *Arch. Surg.,* 18:1227, 1929.
7. WHIPPLE, A. O. The Essential Principles of Clean Wound Healing, *Surg., Gynec., & Obst.,* 70:257, 1940.
8. BELLIS, C. J. A Study of the Physical Factors Concerned in Inflammation, *Surg.,* 12:251, 1942.

CHAPTER III

BACTERIAL INFLAMMATION

PROPHYLAXIS: ASEPSIS AND ANTISEPSIS

Bacterial inflammation is usually spoken of as infection; because it is one of the greatest enemies we have to fight in surgery our constant aim should be to prevent or minimize it. The prevention of surgical infection in a modern operating room is taken for granted; just as much so perhaps as its presence was taken for granted in the hospitals of the past. It is difficult for present day surgeons to realize the revolting conditions before the Listerian era. The offensive smell emanating from a hospital betrayed the presence of surgical patients. Nearly all operations were followed by suppuration, septicemia, or gangrene. The mortality was often appalling; if a patient with a simple laceration were dressed in such a hospital he would be almost sure to develop a serious infection. It is not surprising that Joseph Lister, as a young surgeon at Glasgow, on seeing these foul-smelling surgical wounds should have thought of the contemporary experiments of Louis Pasteur[1] on fermentation and putrefaction. Indeed the surgical wounds of that day did putrefy. It was undoubtedly the work of Pasteur which influenced Lister, even though it was Schwann[2] in 1837 who first showed that putrefaction could be prevented by heat and was therefore due to living organisms. Lister, by analogy, argued that the putrefying wounds were also due to living organisms, but obviously he could not use heat on patients' tissues. To kill bacteria, therefore, he selected the antiseptic phenol, probably because it was then used to deodorize the putrefying sewers of the nearby city of Carlisle.

Lister, because he emphasized the use of chemicals to combat infection, is credited with being the discoverer of antiseptic surgery. Indeed, his paper in 1867 was entitled, "On the Antiseptic Principle in the Practice of Surgery."[3] Although Lister's teachings now seem so obvious and fundamental, he spent a large part of his life defending his thesis and often found himself in bitter polemics with his English colleagues. In America Lister's technic was also slow to become generally adopted. In Germany, however, his work was hailed with much enthusiasm and acclaim. His visit there in 1875 grew into a triumphal procession.[4] It is to the Germans, moreover, that we owe our present ideas of aseptic surgery which is an extension of Listerism. Von Bergman, by introducing steam sterilization in 1886 and the elaborate aseptic ritual in 1891, is generally credited with originating the conception of aseptic surgery which really, however, is more of an outgrowth of the observations of Oliver Wendel Holmes and the Viennese obstetrician Semmelweiss, than of the teachings of Pasteur and Lister. Pasteur and Lister were concerned with living organisms and their eradication. Dr. Holmes knew nothing of bacteria, but did know that contact between one infected patient and another would result in a transfer of the infection, because something was carried from the first to the second patient and usually by the attending physician's hands; as early as 1842 he wrote advising doctors to cleanse their hands thoroughly before and after attending each parturient woman in order to reduce the incidence of puerperal fever. Semmelweiss in Austria made the same observation independently, although his first paper was not published until 1857. At that time child bed fever often played as much havoc in the lying-in hospitals as surgical infections did in the surgical wards. Like Lister in England, Semmelweiss entered into long controversies with his colleagues who generally refused to listen to his accurate and important teachings, and because of this he is said to have become utterly broken in spirit by the time he died.

The importance of contact contamination still forms one of the backbones of modern aseptic surgery. The principle was well expressed by Theodore Kocher, who was discussing many years ago the then widely debated question as to the necessity of wearing rubber gloves during an operation. His surprising aphorism was to the effect that it was much more important to wear gloves between rather than during operations. This indeed would tend to prevent contact implantation. The use of rubber gloves in surgical operations was introduced by the American surgeon Halsted in 1890. Today the careful surgeon wears rubber gloves not only during an operation, but also whenever he touches infectious material, as, for example, when dressing or examining suppurating wounds. There must be no opportunity of any virulent organism harboring itself on his hands. This should be true even outside of the hospital.

Modern aseptic surgery goes even farther. Theoretically it aims at complete eradication of bacteria (sterility) so that not a single bacterium can reach the wound at any time during and after the operation. In this way healing takes place without infection, *i.e.*, aseptically, or by first intention. The set-up for maintaining such a technic is an elaborate one and requires attention to detail and painstaking daily and hourly watching to see that no loopholes admit any offending organism. Such aseptic surgery is like a chain which is only as strong as the weakest link and it is the problem of the surgeon and operating room personnel to see that no virulent bacteria get into the operative field, and through a break in technic thus create a weak link which destroys the entire scheme.

Such perfection in actual practice is almost impossible to attain, largely because of two sources of contamination. The first is due to the fact that the surgeon's hands and the patient's skin with the ordinary routine cannot be rid of all of their bacterial inhabitants. Although the surface of the skin can be sterilized, the deeper epidermal layers as well as the recesses of the hair follicles, sweat and sebaceous glands harbor organisms which are practically impossible to eradicate.

The second source of contamination is the existence of bacteria in the dust of the air. Lister was much concerned with air contamination and used a carbolic spray which may perhaps have removed the organisms from the air; it proved to be too irritating and poisonous for general adoption. Air contamination may be greatly minimized by limiting the number of individuals walking in the operating room, by ordinary cleanliness and by other means. These have been well discussed by Deryl Hart [5] who also advocates and uses ultraviolet radiation as an additional

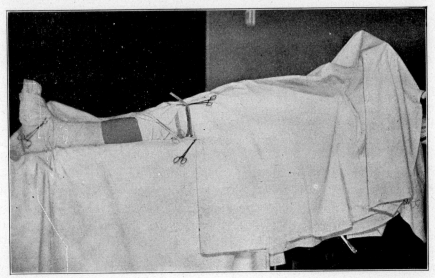

FIG. 14.—PROPER METHOD OF DRAPING FOR AN ASEPTIC OPERATION ON THE LEFT LOWER LEG.

means of minimizing air-borne bacterial contamination. In general, however, it has been found that these two sources of contaminations, *i.e.*, skin and air, do not interfere with perfect healing, provided certain prophylactic measures are carried out. These conditions, as well as other factors which have to do with the prophylaxis of infection in general, will be briefly discussed.

Methods of Surgical Sterilization.—Surgical sterilization, as already mentioned, depends on both asepsis and antisepsis. Asepsis refers to the exclusion of bacteria from the operative field; antisepsis is concerned with the destruction of bacteria already present.

Asepsis is ordinarily sought in clean wounds intentionally inflicted by the surgeon in the operating room. Bacteria are prevented from entering the field by three general means. 1. *Mechanical means* imply ordinary cleanliness by the use of soap, water and scrubbing brush on the walls, floors and ceiling of the operating room. The area of the patient's skin about the proposed incision is also mechanically cleansed by careful shaving and washing. The hands of all members of the surgical team are subject to especially vigorous cleansing, particularly of the crevices under the nails and cuticles. Warm water is important for it promotes sweating, thereby bringing to the surface bacteria embedded in the depths of the sweat and sebaceous glands. It should be emphasized that scrubbing the hands for ten minutes is a much more effective method of sterilization than the use of antiseptics (see Fig. 16). The stirring of dust from the floor is minimized by limiting the number of those walking about and by the use of clean white shoes which have never been used outside. 2. *Heat* is widely used in many ways to destroy bacteria, particularly in the sterilization of dressings, instruments and other apparatus used during the operation. It is important to realize that destruction of bacteria by heat, particularly of spores, is due to coagulation of the bacterial protoplasm. This procedure requires the presence of moisture unless very high temperatures approaching that of an actual flame are used. For this reason wet heat is much more efficient than dry heat; boiling water is much more effective than heated air. Most efficient of all is moist saturated steam vapor which is made to attain a temperature much above that of boiling water by containing the steam in a closed chamber (autoclave) under sufficient pressure. The chief value of the increased pressure is its effect on raising the temperature. Thus, pure steam under a pressure of ten to fifteen pounds will attain a temperature of 115 to 120 C. (240 to 248 F.). Under such conditions the most resistant pathogenic spores will be destroyed in a very short time. Another great advantage of moist steam under pressure is its great penetrating power which enables one to sterilize large amounts of dressings, sheets, etc., if not too tightly packed. The condensation of the steam as it penetrates the cooler layers of fabric also aids greatly, for a thin film of moisture is thereby deposited and the local temperature increased tremendously due to the liberation of heat during condensation. 3. *Chemicals* are of minor importance, but are useful mostly for purposes of surface sterilization, especially on the skin of the scrubbed hands of the operating team and also on the skin of the area to be incised. Tincture of iodine (see Table 1), 70 per cent alcohol, potassium permanganate and bichloride of mercury are used, as well as picric acid and acriflavine. Tincture of iodine is probably used more frequently than any other chemical on the patient's skin preparatory to operation. The iodine is allowed to dry but is so irritating that it must be removed with alcohol to prevent blistering. Ethyl alcohol alone is also an extensively used surface antiseptic. Although most surgeons pay but slight attention to the strength of alcohol used, according to a thorough study by Price,[9] the optimum bacteriacidal concentration is limited to 70 per cent *by weight* and that slight variations in strength seriously diminished its efficiency. If these observations are true it is apparent that precautions are necessary to avoid changes in concentration by either dilution or evaporation. Phenol, the backbone of Lister's antiseptic technic, is rarely used now except to cauterize infected tissue and to sterilize sharp instruments which might be dulled by boiling. Gaseous formaldehyde is often used to sterilize cystoscopic and bronchoscopic instruments.

Antisepsis in contrast to asepsis, finds its modern application in the accident room where wounds are seen which were sustained outside the hospital, and often under conditions of maximum contamination, so that the open tissue is covered with millions of bacteria. To accomplish perfect healing is, nevertheless, the aim even in such cases. Here indeed is practiced true antiseptic surgery after the manner of Lister. If antisepsis is achieved and the wound is rid of the contaminating organisms the necessary surgery can then be done and the wound closed with all the precautions of aseptic surgery and perfect healing will follow.

In open wounds, however, antiseptics may do much damage by injuring tissue cells as well as bacteria so that they have to be diluted in order to prove noninjurious to the patient to a degree which makes them innocuous to the germs as well. A comparative study of various antiseptics is summarized herewith because the investigators (Salle and Lazarus [6]) measured the effect of the chemical on tissue cells as well as on bacteria. The number expressing the relationship between the dilution inhibitory to cell and to bacterial growth was called the toxicity index. These workers found that iodine in aqueous solution (dilute Lugol's solution) was the only antiseptic more toxic to bacteria than to cells, thus confirming the older observations of Lambert.[7] To this should perhaps be added proflavine and 2:7-diamino acridine, two acridine drugs investigated in England,[8] and found to be the only ones among many tested, which, at a 1:1000 concentration, produced a minimal injury to brain tissue *in vivo* and the least effect on the metabolism of brain tissue *in vitro*. While the action of the sulfonamides is quite different from the chemicals here mentioned, they are used locally in open wounds (see page 36).

TABLE 1

COMPARISON OF ACTION AND EFFICIENCY OF VARIOUS ANTISEPTICS
(*After Salle and Lazarus* [6])

Antiseptic	Highest Dilution Showing No Tissue Growth = A	Highest Dilution Showing No Growth of S. aureus = B	Toxicity Index = A/B.	Phenol Coefficient
Iodine (Lugol's Solution)	1-1,800	1-20,000	0.09	308
Hexylresorcinol	1-21,000	1-7,000	3.0	108
Metaphen	1-76,000	1-6,000	12.7	92
Phenol	1-840	1-70	12.0	...
Merthiolate	1-176,400	1-5,000	35.3	70
Mercurochrome	1-10,500	1-40	262.0	0.6

Breaks in Aseptic Surgical Technic.—The development of a post operative wound infection in what should have been a perfectly healed incision means, of course, that bacteria have slipped in through some loophole in spite of the elaborate precautions; the chain has developed a weak link. It is important, therefore, to make careful observations of all such infections even though trivial, and to culture the pus in order to identify the contaminating organism. Each step in the preparation of dressings, solutions, and instruments must be carefully investigated, sterilizers checked, autoclaves examined, and chemical solutions analyzed bacteriologically. Air-borne contamination from dust is also investigated and eliminated as far as possible, along lines already discussed. In most cases, however, the fault lies with the surgeon, operating team or personnel.

These possible breaks in technic permit contamination from six sources:

1. The *mouths and throats* of the operating room personnel emit countless bacteria into the air with each expiration. These cause no trouble ordinarily when

efficient masks are worn. To be effective, masks must efficiently strain the exhaled air of all droplets. Because of this fact masks of cellophane have been devised but have one serious defect in so far as they merely deflect the exhaled air. Much more practical and scientific is the use of substances such as cellucotton (Arnold [10]) or flannel (de Takats [11]) which have more of a tendency to filter the exhaled air. Masks must cover both mouth and nostrils, and of course must be comfortable to the wearer. They must be worn by all entering the operating room. When droplets are ejected while talking, or especially by coughing, sneezing, laughing or clearing the throat, the danger of air contamination becomes real, even though masks are

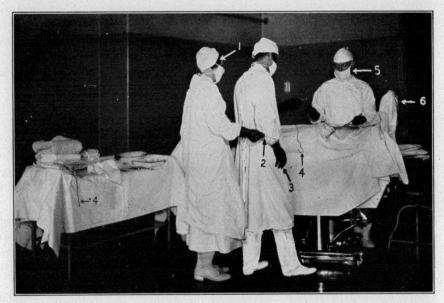

FIG. 15.—COMMON ERRORS AND BREAKS IN TECHNIC, TO BE GUARDED AGAINST IN THE OPERATING ROOM.

1, nurse's hair incompletely covered by cap; 2, passing instruments should never be done behind another person; 3, the gloved hand should not fall to the side but must be kept above the level of the operating table; 4, sutures must not be allowed to drag below the field of operation; 5, the nose as well as the mouth must be covered by the mask; 6, draping over the anesthetic screen must be complete.

worn. Such actions are therefore interdicted in the operating room, especially over an open wound. Regardless of masks, moreover, the presence of any person with a respiratory infection in an operating room courts serious danger, not only because such individuals are likely to cough uncontrollably, but of more importance, the bacteria they exhale are so virulent that the deposition of relatively few on the wound may result in a serious infection. An outbreak of streptococcus wound infections was studied by Meleney and Stevens [12] in which careful bacteriological study revealed the source of the contamination in the pharynx of one of the operating room nurses.

2. The *skin of the surgeon's hands* as well as those of the other members of the team form the second source of contamination. The danger of contact infection has already been emphasized. The presence of infected lesions on the hands, even

if slight, should exclude the individual from scrubbing up for the operation, because rubber gloves are not absolute in their protection. Not only are they porous, but they may become torn or punctured, sometimes without being noticed, and virulent organisms spilled into the wound.

3. The *patient's skin* is a third link which may weaken the chain. Unless the operation is urgent, the presence of even minor infections in the field of the proposed incision contraindicates operation until the furuncle, dermatitis or ulcer is healed. The presence of a large abscess anywhere, even though not in the field of operation, may also be a possible source of contamination. If the patient has a respiratory infection the same danger is present. Such infections may give rise to a bacteriemia which will lead to a wound infection by the deposition of blood-borne organisms in the field traumatized by the surgeon. In such cases when the operation is one of election it is safer to wait until the offending lesion is healed.

4. A fourth loophole is *faulty sterilization* with autoclaves. As mentioned above, only moist heat under pressure effectively destroys spores. The presence of air in the autoclave, improper packing of supplies, etc., may seriously interfere with effective sterilization.

5. *Catgut* is a fifth possible source of contamination since it is prepared from an infected tissue, *i.e.,* the lower small intestine of sheep. Constant and alert precautions on the part of the makers of catgut usually yield sterile sutures, but the danger is nevertheless present and numerous instances of infected catgut have been reported (Meleney and Chatfield [13]).

6. A final loophole in the aseptic scheme may occur by a *gross break in technic, i.e.,* touching a sterile with a nonsterile object. Every surgeon and nurse must have an almost automatic alertness about such sources of contamination, a sort of second nature which makes it literally impossible for any nonsterile object to touch the field of operation or anything which comes in contact with it.

Other Factors in Asepsis.—Although the methods just outlined, if rigidly carried out, will prevent outside bacteria from entering the operative field, they cannot eliminate bacteria already present in the deep layers of the patient's skin or the few which may be circulating in his blood. Most surgeons realize, however, that these few bacteria do not interfere with perfect healing because, with good surgical technic, the wound can easily cope with them without infection. Emphasis must be placed, therefore, on the fact that these bacteria become important only when their multiplication is aided and abetted by faults of operative technic, factors which are never overlooked by careful surgeons. Most of these factors of operative technic are described in detail in later chapters. They comprise such features as the *gentle handling of tissue, careful hemostasis, and avoidance of tension* in placing sutures; emphasis on these and other similar details formed an important part of the teaching of W. S. Halsted and others before the beginning of this century. Halsted also made numerous technical contributions such as rubber gloves, silver foil, gutta percha drains, etc., which are interestingly described in a paper by him already mentioned.[14] Halsted was also an early advocate of the use of silk rather than catgut as sutures because, among other reasons, he felt that silk insured more careful technic. There is at present a great tendency to use silk more and more; an excellent and brief discussion of its value may be found in a paper by

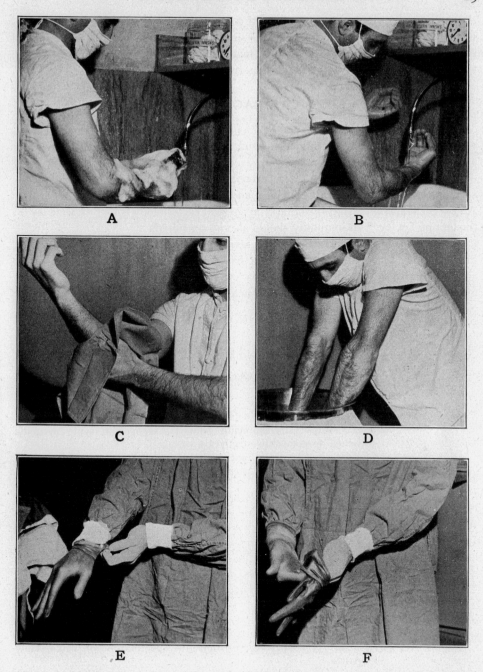

FIG. 16.—VARIOUS STEPS IN THE PROCESS OF "SCRUBBING UP," OR ASEPTIC PREPARATION.

A, scrubbing the hands and arms up to and above the elbows for ten minutes with a brush, soap and running water; *B,* allowing water to drain off the elbows; *C,* drying hands with a sterile towel; *D,* the hands and arms are then bathed in alcohol or acetone solution; *E* and *F,* proper method of putting on gloves unassisted. Note that the outside of the glove is not touched by the skin.

A. O. Whipple [15] and in a more detailed contribution by F. L. Meleney.[16] Experimental studies of the strength of wounds sutured with catgut and silk will be found in a report by Howes.[17] The paper by Harvey [18] on the suture should also be read. A more detailed discussion of suture material will be found on page 202.

SURGICAL BACTERIOLOGY

Surgical bacteriology may be defined as the application of bacteriological knowledge to the diagnosis and treatment of surgical infections. Most surgical infections are associated with wounds; many, however, develop spontaneously or after slight or indetectable injuries. The latter become surgical because they produce lesions such as abscesses which require incision and drainage or other surgical procedures. An excellent and extensive monograph on surgical bacteriology is that of Meleney [19]; the text of Topley [20] on immunity should also be consulted.

Classification of Bacteria.—Only a few of the many bacteria will be discussed in detail; the following classification is based on the shape, staining properties and on anaerobic or aerobic properties of growth. Other features of bacteria may be learned by consulting standard bacteriology texts.

CLASSIFICATION OF BACTERIA

Those of most importance to the surgeon are in italics.
(Modified from Meleney [19])

CLINICAL OCCURRENCE

I. Aerobic Bacteria
  A. Cocci
    (1) Gram-positive
      Streptococcus—erysipelas, acute cellulitis, septicemia, acute pyogenic arthritis, osteomyelitis, empyema
      Staphylococcus—furuncles, carbuncles, osteomyelitis, septicemia
      Pneumococcus—empyema, peritonitis, acute arthritis
    (2) Gram-negative
      Gonococcus—pelvic disease, urethritis, prostatitis, acute joint infection
      Meningococcus—meningitis
  B. Bacilli
    (1) Gram-positive
      B. tuberculosis—infection of bones, joints, meninges, lungs, lymph nodes, peritoneum
      B. anthracis—anthrax
      B. diphtheriae—throat infections, wound infections (very rare)
      B. botulinus—botulism
    (2) Gram-negative
      B. coli—peritonitis, appendiceal abscess, cystitis
      B. typhosus—typhoid fever, osteomyelitis, perforation of ileum, cholecystitis
      B. mucosus capsulatus—pneumonia, empyema
      B. proteus
      B. tularense—tularemia
      B. pyocyaneus—secondary invader of superficial wounds
      B. mallei—glanders
      B. influenzae—acute arthritis, empyema
      B. ducrey—chancroid

II. Anaerobic Bacteria
    A. Cocci
        Streptococcus—peritonitis, mouth infections, pelvic infections.
    B. Bacilli
        B. *welchii* (perfringens) ⎫
        B. novyi   ⎪
        B. sporogenes   ⎬ gas gangrene
        B. histolyticum   ⎪
        B. tetani—tetanus ⎭
    C. *Spirochetes*
        T. pallidum—syphilis of bones, joints, meninges, skin, etc.
III. Higher Bacteria
    A. Mycetes—*Actinomycetes*—actinomycosis

The bacteria of greatest importance in acute surgical infections are the *pyogenic bacteria*. The term pyogenic (pus-forming) is usually applied to all of the following organisms though only the staphylococcus is a typical pus-producer. Moreover, the tubercle bacillus, though not a pyogenic bacterium, may in cold abscesses produce typical thick creamy pus. Nevertheless, the term is generally used to apply to the staphylococcccus, streptococcus, pneumococcus, colon bacillus and pyocyaneus bacillus.

Staphylococcus exists in at least three forms, the aureus, albus and citrus; the modifying terms are based on the color the colonies produce on culture. The aureus is commonly pathogenic in furuncle and superficial wound infections. It causes rapid suppuration, forming thick creamy pus with a sweetish odor which has a tendency to remain localized as an abscess and break through to the outside, eventually healing without difficulty. The favorable outcome which thus followed staphylococcus infections led the ancients to call its pus laudable. Many, in fact believed that healing could not occur without the formation of this pus. On the other hand, it is now known that the staphylococcus may incite serious infections such as septicemia and pyemia, and has been cultivated from the blood stream in such cases. The albus form is a normal resident of the skin where it lives as a saprophyte. Certain strains are known to produce toxins.

Streptococcus occurs in several well known types or strains; *i.e.,* hemolytic, non-hemolytic, viridans, and anaerobic. Other classifications have divided this organism in other groups depending on sugar fermentation and other properties. It is a normal inhabitant of the oral cavity, vaginal tract, and is present in the intestinal contents. When virulent it is a much more serious invader than the staphylococcus, for it tends to spread and involve wide areas of tissue, causing necrosis without localizing tendencies. Moreover, there is much less tendency to form pus; when pus forms it is usually watery in character though later it becomes thick. Streptococcus is the etiological agent in erysipelas, in scarlet fever, acute tonsillitis and a host of other infections. The anaerobic streptococcus is also a serious invader and is encountered in various pelvic infections, peritonitis, symbiotic infections, etc. Sulfanilamide is effective in the treatment of streptococcal infections. (See p. 36.)

B. coli is a normal inhabitant of the lower bowel and as might be expected is the main invader after appendiceal infections. It also escapes through the bowel wall in cases of secondary peritonitis from any other causes such as various types of perforation. Pus produced by this organism has an offensive fecal odor and though in the early stage is thin, brownish and watery, it later becomes thicker. Gas may be associated with it. Infections of the gall bladder, liver and genitourinary tracts, are also often due to the B. coli.

Pneumococcus, though chiefly confined to lung infections, is met with in surgery when such infections are followed by empyema. The pus in such a case, though at first thin, rapidly becomes thick, creamy, mucoid and contains much clotted fibrin. The pneumococcus may also cause primary peritonitis in children and is not infrequently the offending organism in acute pyogenic arthritis and sometimes in meningitis. The meningococcus, however, is the invader in epidemic meningitis.

B. pyocyaneus has little pathogenic importance, but is met with not infrequently over large superficial granulating wounds as a secondary invader. It betrays its presence by the development of a greenish or bluish color to the discharge and by its peculiar musty odor. It can be banished from the wound by the application of weak acid solution (1 per cent acetic acid).

Other bacteria are also important to the surgeon. Mention should be made of anaerobic and microaerophilic organisms, especially, the streptococci which are present in certain puzzling chronic ulcers (see p. 122). Spores are also important because they resist ordinary means of antisepsis and may reside in contaminated wounds for years without activity after healing has occurred. The development of the spores into their active vegetative form may occur subsequently after sufficient trauma. Spores occur commonly in tetanus and gas gangrene which are discussed later. Ordinary pyogenic bacteria may also become dormant under certain special conditions, particularly when they are present in infected compound fractures. Healing may occur, but the organisms remain viable and may set up a severe infection years later if the involved bone is traumatized again for any reason.

The Virulence of Bacteria.—The disease producing powers of bacteria vary tremendously. Only a few of the factors will be discussed; they are really to be considered along with the factors influencing the resistance of the body which are described in the next section. The *strain or kind* of bacterium is obviously important. Many of these differences have already been described. The *number of bacteria* undoubtedly plays a role in virulence. An open wound can ordinarily take care of a certain number of micro-organisms without any perceptible increase in the degree of the inflammatory reaction. Wounds which have healed *per primam* have repeatedly been shown to contain a certain number of bacteria. If the number is too great, phagocytosis may be ineffective and by force of numbers alone the bacteria may set the stage for a real infection. For example Hunt [21] cultured 28 clean abdominal wounds just before closure; colonies numbering from 40 to 1680 were obtained from all but 3 cases, even though 19 of them healed without any evidence of infection and the remainder were associated with only a slight exudate. It is significant, however, that the one with 1680 colonies on the plate developed a mild postoperative thrombophlebitis.

Foreign bodies and necrotic tissue in a wound contribute to the severity of any infection. This was not generally realized until World War I, during which surgeons of many nations were confronted with millions of wound infections. A clean bullet wound through the thigh, for example, was apt to heal perfectly. Shrapnel wounds which nearly always contained much foreign material and jagged necrotic tissue were the most seriously infected. On the other hand, if foreign bodies and devitalized tissue were removed (débridement) within a few hours after the wound was received, the incidence of infection was slight or absent. The medical manuals of all nations finally came to prescribe débridement of such wounds as the primary form of treatment. In acute peritonitis this influence of necrotic material in increasing virulence has been shown experimentally. Dogs will withstand the injection of large numbers of certain bacteria into the peritoneum without infection; only when bits of sterile agar, muscle, or other foreign bodies are implanted at the same time does a fatal peritonitis follow (W. S. Halsted [22]). In chronic draining sinuses the role of foreign bodies in maintaining infection is also well known.

Bacterial symbiosis or synergism has also been shown to increase bacterial virulence in certain sugical infections. Many of these observations have been made by Meleney.[23] Clinically, such symbiosis undoubtedly explains certain extensive spreading ulcers of the abdominal wall and other parts of the body. The serious nature of human bites which inoculate a mixed group of mouth organisms into the wound may perhaps be explained on this basis. Peritonitis, so often due to a mixed infection, may also owe its high mortality to bacteria acting synergistically particularly when there is a perforation of the appendix or other viscus.

The Resistance of the Body.—The possession of resistance by the patient is often spoken of as his immunity, which may be local or general or both. *Local immunity* depends somewhat on the type of tissue, especially its vascularity. The term is mostly used to describe the local resistance which an area develops after fighting off an infection so that the same organism can no longer invade at this point at least, though it may still get a foothold in some other part of the body. After a consideration of the available evidence Topley [24] concludes that "it is possible to induce an immunity which is confined to the neighborhood of the treated area, and is not shared by the body as a whole."

The resistance of the body ordinarily is largely due to a *general immunity*. The possession of such immunity is specific and resides in the body as a whole, although the protein, particularly the globulin, fraction of the plasma and the cells of the so-called reticulo-endothelial system (plus other leukocytic and phagocytic cells), are supposed to be primarily involved in the mechanisms of immunity. A third and important factor in resistance is the protective action of the lymph nodes. The development of leukocytosis during infections is also a manifestation of resistance. *Natural* (innate) *immunity* refers to resistance inherent or at least obtained in some unknown spontaneous way or congenitally. *Acquired immunity,* on the other hand, is the result of defenses built up in fighting a previous infection. *Artificial immunity* is a similar defense obtained, however, by one of two methods of treatment, *i.e.,* passive or active immunization. Of the two, the latter is especially important in the prevention of tetanus (see page 80).

Bacterial Diagnosis.—Identification of the causative bacterium is most important in all surgical infections, not only in diagnosis and prognosis, but especially in therapy. If specific therapy is indicated or if chemotherapy is to be used such identification is not only essential but should be made as early as possible. In order to detect bacterial synergism isolation of more than one organism is obviously necessary.

Examination of pus is the most direct method of bacterial diagnosis but must be carried out immediately after the abscess is opened. Delay often leads to a failure because the lesion becomes rapidly invaded by secondary organisms. The first and easiest step in the study of pus is to make an appropriately stained smear on a glass slide. The smear may show the nature of the leukocytes, whether poly- or mononuclear, as well as bacteria. If the smear shows no bacteria, cultures must be made, preferably under both aerobic and anaerobic conditions. Injection of the pus into guinea pigs or other animals may be important in establishing or ruling out a diagnosis of tuberculosis. For adequate bacteriological examinations it is best to obtain several cubic centimeters of the pus itself. If the amount of pus is small it is preferable to collect it on a cotton swab which should first be moistened with sterile saline inasmuch as a tiny amount of pus will otherwise be soaked up by the cotton and be lost. Cultures should be made promptly or the material kept in an ice box; if left at room temperature the organisms may die by drying.

Blood culture when positive is often the only way of identifying the causative organisms in cases where no pus is obtainable. Unfortunately a blood culture is not always positive even when organisms are present; the power of the blood to rid itself of bacteria is tremendous, at least partially by virtue of the astonishing phagocytic activity of the reticulo-endothelial cells which line the blood channels, especially of the lungs, liver and spleen. Millions of bacteria or tiny foreign particles have been injected into the blood stream of experimental animals only to disappear within a few hours. In general, the greater the number of bacteria found on blood culture the more serious the infection. Aside from the number of organisms a positive blood culture has considerable prognostic value, as shown on analysis of a large series of streptococcus infections by Keefer, Ingelfinger and Spink.[25]

Other methods of bacterial diagnosis are often of considerable importance. Microscopic study of biopsied material may be useful in certain cases, especially in the chronic granulomatous infections, *e.g.,* tuberculosis, actinomycosis and syphilis. Agglutination tests applied to the blood are very useful in typhoid and tularemia. Doubtless with further study many more infections will become thus more easily detected.

Specific Immune Therapy.—Specific therapy with bacteriological material such as antitoxins have in general been of more value in medical than in surgical infections. The use of serums and vaccines must in any case be carefully evaluated before adopting them because of the tendency for therapeutic applications of bacteriological research to far outstrip justifiable indications. *Vaccines* are suspensions of bacteria which have been killed by heat or chemicals and are then injected subcutaneously, intramuscularly or intravenously. As a prophylactic measure against specific infections to which the patient might be exposed in the near future, vaccines have undoubtedly been responsible for saving many lives (*e.g.,* typhoid prophylaxis). Vaccines are also used prophylactically in recurrent staphylococcus infections (furunculosis) in which each focus is assumed to be too mild to instigate sufficient antibody formation. Once an infection has gained a real foothold the value of vaccine is open to question. The wholesale use of vaccines, once heralded as a cure for practically every infection, has rightfully fallen into desuetude. *Bacteriophage* is responsible for the rather rapid dissolution of certain bacteria in culture on addition of Berkfeld filtrates from other cultures. This remarkable breaking up of bacteria has thus far failed to find a proved place in the treatment of infections, although therapeutic claims have been made and much stimulating research is still going on. *Serums* are used as vehicles for administering specific antibodies, such as antitoxins; usually the serum is that of the horse in which antibodies have been produced by previous treatment with specific antigen. Such specific therapy is spoken of as passive immunization. The great disadvantage and even danger in the use of serums to confer passive immunity is due to the possibility of foreign protein reactions.[26] Examples of specific antibodies of value in surgery are largely confined to prophylaxis as in tetanus. The development of an anti-staphylococcus serum promises much in the treatment of severe septicemia due to this bacterium (Julianelle [27]). An excellent review of advances in the specific therapy of staphylococcus sepsis is that of Spink.[28] Much better than passive immunization with antitoxin is the use of active immunization which has achieved widespread success in the prevention of tetanus (see p. 80).

Many surgeons have assumed that specific antibodies may be supplied to a patient suffering from severe septicemia, notably those due to the streptococcus, by giving repeated blood *transfusions* from healthy individuals. Careful study of the evidence by many observers has revealed that this is not true, at least under the usual circumstances; indeed, some observers state that transfusion in sepsis may even be harmful (Doan [29]). Certain donors, it is true, may possess specific antibodies against the particular organism present in a particular patient. This correlation, however, must be determined by serological study, *i.e.,* a selection must be made from a group of donors whose blood definitely agglutinates, or has opsonins against the bacterium isolated from the patient. Indeed, Lyons and Ward [30] studied the blood of normal individuals and found that many of them contained specific opsonins against hemolytic streptococci isolated from humans with septicemia. Selection of a donor in such a manner would probably have great therapeutic value; only by such a procedure can the surgeon expect a beneficial immunological effect from transfusions. The beneficial clinical effects of transfusions as ordinarily carried out in certain patients with septicemia are probably due to the fact that needed serum protein and erythrocytes are supplied, *i.e.,* to correct hypoproteinemia and anemia.

CHEMOTHERAPY

Although chemotherapy includes the use of quinine in malaria, salvarsan in syphilis, etc., the term is now most generally applied to the use of chemicals in combating the invasion of the body by pyogenic bacteria. Entirely unknown until a few years ago, chemotherapy has revolutionized the treatment of many pyogenic infections, including those encountered in surgical diseases. The chemicals used are nearly all members of the sulfonamide group and are often called collectively sulfonamides. More recently metabolic products of mould and soil bacterial growth (penicillin and gramicidin) have been found to have antibacterial activity and they will be discussed under a separate heading.

Chemotherapy with the Sulfonamides.—Gerhard Domagk, a 45-year-old German pathologist and chemist, first observed in 1932 that a red dye, prontosil, the earliest of the sulfonamide drugs, exerted a curative effect on streptococcus infections in mice. His observations were not published until 1935 but led to the extensive use of this series of drugs in human infections. So momentous was this discovery that Domagk was offered but refused the Nobel Prize in 1939.

Several sulfonamide drugs are in more or less common use at the present time. The original sulfonamide, prontosil, is now scarcely used in this country. The first to be introduced and extensively used was sulfanilamide. Next were sulfapyridine and sulfathiazole. The most recent member is sulfadiazine.[31] Sulfaguanidine and sulfasuxidine are of still more recent development, but have a specialized use, *i.e.*, because they are so poorly absorbed when given by mouth, they reduce the bacterial content of the gastro-intestinal tract. A recent review is that of Spink.[32]

The mode of action of the sulfonamides, while not entirely clear, is, of course, not that of a bactericide or antiseptic. The drugs seem to influence bacterial metabolism, depriving the organism of elements necessary for growth, thus enabling the body to combat their invasion more effectively. However, each of the sulfonamides has deleterious effects (which are described below) as well as therapeutic value, and it is essential that knowledge of their action be complete and detailed before extensive use is undertaken. The sulfonamides are all extremely diffusible once they are absorbed and appear rapidly in all body fluids and secretions, in pus, suppurative exudates and even in the cerebrospinal fluid. Because they are more or less promptly excreted in the urine, they require repeated administration for continued effect which may be accurately followed by measuring the blood level of the drug. All the sulfonamides form relatively insoluble acetyl derivatives which may be precipitated in and damage the kidneys, a danger which is greatest with sulfapyridine, which is therefore not used in severe nephritis. Although this danger is minimized by the excretion of a dilute urine, it is important to limit fluid intake in urinary infections to secure a high concentration of the drug in the urine.

The prophylactic use of the sulfonamides is of extreme importance surgically. For such a purpose the drug may be employed locally or systemically (by mouth or parenterally) or by both routes. For example, the drug, when dusted in the peritoneal cavity after colonic surgery, into other wounds after operation, after traumatic contaminations, burns or incisions through infected tissue, etc., will reduce the incidence of post operative infections. In World War II evidence has already been presented in favor of the prophylactic use of sulfanilamide in contaminated war wounds; in one series in which the drug had been used infection was remarkably absent, in contrast to a 70 per cent incidence of streptococcus infection previous to its use.[33] In the American army every soldier has tablets of sulfadiazine which he may take by mouth as well as first aid packets of sulfanilamide to dust into wounds.

The local effect of the sulfonamides must not be confused with the surface action of the antiseptic drugs. The important effect of the sulfonamides is in the tissues; thus they must be absorbed in order to influence invading bacteria. Because it is difficult to predict or control this absorption there is a growing tendency to rely on the systemic administration of the drug which rapidly appears in the exudate of wounds. It should be emphasized, moreover, that the local use of the sulfonamides can never displace the fundamental principles for the treatment of wounds. These drugs should be looked upon as an adjunct to well-established surgical principles and not as a means for displacing or stretching these principles. The local effect of the various sulfonamides varies considerably. Sulfanilamide, for example, has a relatively narrow specificity as compared with the other drugs and is, of course, more soluble and therefore rapidly absorbed. These properties are actually disadvantages as far as the effect of local use of the drug is concerned. On the other hand, sulfathiazole and sulfadiazine, because of their lower solubilities, remain locally for 24 to 48 hours, thus exerting a more prolonged effect than in the case of sulfanilamide, which disappears 4 to 6 hours after application. Moreover, both sulfathiazole and sulfadiazine are less likely to produce toxic manifestations due to rapid absorption. It should be mentioned, however, that slowly absorbed drugs have one possible disadvantage in that, if used in too large quantities, they act as foreign bodies, preventing a contact of the tissues and thus prolonging healing. This objection can be met obviously by limiting the amount of the drug which is used locally, just as one should limit the dose of any drug to its proper level. The present authors are convinced that massive doses of any sulfonamide in a wound may prove harmful. The use of a moderate amount of the drug locally is preferable, particularly when this is supplemented by the systemic administration of the drug in order to maintain a good blood level.

Even when used after the onset of surgical infections there is a growing feeling that the sulfonamides are most effective when the organism has produced cellulitis and before suppuration has occurred. Clinical observation suggests that not only has the drug little curative effect on localized suppuration but that it tends to mask local signs and even seems to inhibit the normal pointing process. This is probably associated with the presence in pus of para-amino benzoic acid or closely related substances, which inhibit the action of the sulfonamides. Thus chemotherapy should not be used as the sole therapeutic agent in the treatment of an abscess; incision and drainage are still necessary.

Significant differences exist in the action of the sulfonamides. *Sulfanilamide* exerts a favorable influence in infections produced primarily by streptococcus, meningococcus and gonococcus. It probably has a beneficial effect in many other infections such as lymphogranuloma venereum, chancroid, etc., which are discussed in detail later. *Sulfapyridine,*[34] in addition to affecting the above mentioned organisms, is superior to sulfanilamide in the treatment of pneumococcal infections. Thus it has more medical than surgical interest, although it has almost been displaced by *sulfathiazole,*[35] which seems to be just as effective but less toxic. Sulfathiazole is gradually displacing the other sulfonamides in the treatment of gonococcal infections. *Sulfadiazine* [31] is probably less toxic and just as effective and is enjoying an increasing use. It is notable that thus far none of the sulfonamides has proved unequivocally effective against the staphylococcus. The parenteral use of the sulfonamides depends on their solubilities, which vary. Sulfanilamide is the most soluble (1 per cent), can thus be readily injected as such even subcutaneously, and has also been given per rectum. Sulfathiazole and sulfadiazine are too insoluble to be given as such parenterally; however, they both form extremely soluble (5 per cent) sodium salts. These salts, because they are extremely alkaline, are commonly used only by intravenous injection. In 5 per cent solution they may produce necrosis if given subcutaneously, but if diluted with Ringer's solution to 0.5 or 1 per cent can be safely given in this way. *Sulfaguanidine* and *sulfasuxidine*,[36] particularly the latter, are useful in reducing the bacterial flora of the gastro-intestinal tract and have thus been indicated in bacterial dysentery and ulcerative colitis, but particularly in preparation for colonic surgery by prophylactically minimizing the degree of bacterial contamination and thus the likelihood of postoperative peritonitis.

The dose of the various sulfonamides when used systemically averages about 0.1 gram per kilo (¾ grain per pound) per day. When the patient is under hospital care, it is a common practice to give a larger initial dose during the first 24 hours, *i.e.*, 1 grain per pound of body weight. Enough of the drug should be given to maintain a blood level varying between 8 and 12 mg. per cent depending somewhat upon the drug used; chemical methods for this determination have been described by Marshall.[37] Untoward reactions are watched for and the drug discontinued if they are sufficiently severe. The deleterious changes are largely in the blood, the most serious being agranulocytosis and anemia. Acidosis, which may follow the use of sulfanilamide, can be prevented by giving alkalis such as NaH_2CO_3. The dusky color which sometimes follows the use of sulfanilamide, especially in children, is due largely to changes in the hemoglobin; methemoglobinemia, when it occurs, can be combated by the intravenous injections of methylene blue,[38] but against sulfhemoglobinemia there is no remedy except discontinuance of the drug. Actually, however, very little injury is produced by these changes in hemoglobin. Hepatic damage has also been described and is manifested by jaundice. The effects on the kidneys have been mentioned above. In individuals sensitive to the sulfonamides a febrile reaction or skin rash occasionally occurs. This may be the precursor of bone marrow depression and calls for immediate discontinuance of the offending drug. On the other hand, once a patient shows signs of sensitivity he is likely to suffer the same reaction immediately after he is given the drug a second time. Under such circumstances the reaction may be avoided by shifting to another sulfonamide, a common and entirely justified practice. Subjective manifestations are numerous and are referable largely to the central nervous system; they include headache, dizziness, visual disturbances, etc.

The authors of this text favor the use of sulfonamides in surgical infections for a limited period of time early in the course of treatment and with rather large initial doses in order to achieve a high blood level for a short period of time in order to combat intensively and promptly the invasive tendencies of the attacking organism. After this effect has been achieved, we feel the dose of the drug should be reduced or discontinued. If the drug has no effect we see no advantage in continuing its use indefinitely. This practice fits in with the principle expressed above, *i.e.*, that the sulfonamides in surgical infections are of great value before actual invasion occurs or early in the course of the invasion.

Penicillin.—This substance, which has still not been isolated as an individual chemical substance, is a metabolic product of the growth of a certain mould and has a remarkable antistaphylococcus activity in addition to being effective against other organisms.[39] Inasmuch as the sulfonamides have little influence on the staphylococcus, penicillin fills a long needed hiatus in the chemotherapy of pyogenic bacteria. Although the use of penicillin is quite recent, sufficient evidence has been obtained to justify its early promise. It is completely nontoxic and can be given in tremendous amounts without any untoward effect. Unfortunately, however, the drug is excreted in the urine extremely rapidly; so much so, in fact, that it must be administered either as a continuous venoclysis or by intramuscular injections every 2 or 4 hours day and night in order to maintain a sufficient high concentration in the tissues to achieve a therapeutic effect. Another difficulty with this substance is its extreme instability as compared with the sulfonamides, requiring special care in its preparation. It exists as sodium and calcium salts, the latter of which is more stable. Penicillin is ineffective when given by mouth.

Gramicidin.—This material, and also tyrothricin, are metabolic products of the growth of certain soil bacteria. Both have also been shown to have definite antibacterial activity. The former has been isolated in pure form and is a polypeptide. Both of these substances are too toxic when injected to be used parenterally and their use is therefore limited entirely to local applications. Considerable promise has emerged from their preliminary use, but sufficient evidence is still forthcoming before they can be recommended for general adoption.

BIBLIOGRAPHY

1. VALLERY-RADOT, R. *The Life of Louis Pasteur,* trans. by Mrs. R. L. Devonshire, Constable & Co., London, 1920.
2. SCHWANN, T. Cited by Garrison, F. H. *History of Medicine,* Saunders, Phila., 1929, 4th ed., p. 456.
3. LISTER, J. On the Antiseptic Principle in the Practice of Surgery, *Lancet,* 2:353, 1867.
4. GODLEE, R. J. *Lord Lister,* London, Macmillan, 1917, 2nd ed.
5. HART, D. Pathogenic Bacteria in the Air of the Operating Room, *Arch. Surg.,* 37:521, 1938.
6. SALLE, A. J. and LAZARUS, A. S. A Comparison of the Resistance of Bacteria and Embyronic Tissue to Germicidal Substances, *Proc. Soc. Exper. Biol. & Med.,* 1934-35; 32:665, 937, 1057, 1119, 1481.
7. LAMBERT, R. A. The Comparative Resistance of Bacteria and Human Tissues to Certain Germicidal Substances, *J. Am. M. Ass.,* 67:1300, 1916.
8. FLEMING, A., RUSSELL, D. S., FALCONER, M. A., MANIFOLD, M. C., and others. Discussion on the Effect of Antiseptics on Wounds, *Proc. Roy. Soc. Med.,* 33:487, 1940.
9. PRICE, P. B. Ethyl Alcohol as a Germicide, *Arch. Surg.,* 38:528, 1939.
10. ARNOLD, L. A New Surgical Mask, *Arch. Surg.,* 37:1008, 1938.
11. de TAKATS, G. and JESSER, J. H. Postoperative Infection. *Surg., Gynec. & Obst.,* 72:1028, 1941.
12. MELENEY, F. L. and STEVENS, F. A. Postoperative Haemolytic Streptococcus Wound Infections and Their Relation to Haemolytic Streptococcus Carriers Among the Operating Personnel, *Surg., Gynec. & Obst.,* 43:338, 1926.
13. MELENEY, F. L. and CHATFIELD, M. The Sterility of Catgut in Relation to Hospital Infections, *Surg. Gynec. & Obst.,* 52:430, 1931.
14. HALSTED, W. S. Ligature and Suture Material. The Employment of Fine Silk in

Preference to Catgut and the Advantages of Transfixion of Tissues and Vessels in Control of Hemorrhage; Also an Account of the Introduction of Gloves, Gutta Percha Tissues and Silver Foil, *J. Am. M. Ass.*, 60:1119, 1913.

15. WHIPPLE, A. O. The Use of Silk in the Repair of Clean Wounds, *Ann. Surg.*, 98:662, 1933.

16. MELENTY, F. L. Infection in Clean Operative Wounds, *Surg., Gynec. & Obst.*, 60:264, 1935.

17. HOWES, E. L. The Strength of Wounds Sutured with Catgut and Silk, *Surg., Gynec. & Obst.*, 57:300, 1933.

18. HARVEY, S. C. Concerning the Suture, *Surg., Gynec & Obst.*, 58:791, 1934.

19. MELENEY, F. L. *Nelson's Loose Leaf Living Surgery*, Vol. I, Chap. III, p. 88, New York, 1927.

20. TOPLEY, W. W. C. *Outline of Immunity*, Baltimore, 1933 (Wm. Wood & Co.).

21. HUNT, E. L. Some Further Observations upon Contamination of Operative Wounds by Air-Borne Bacteria, *N. E. Jour. Med.*, 209:931, 1933.

22. HALSTED, W. S. The Treatment of Wounds, etc., *Johns Hopkins Hosp. Rep.*, 2:255, 1891.

23. MELENEY, F. L. Bacterial Synergism in Disease Processes, *Ann. Surg.*, 94:961, 1931.

24. TOPLEY, W. W. C. *Loc. cit.*, p. 236.

25. KEEFER, C. S., INGELFINGER, F. J. and SPINK, W. W. Significance of Hemolytic Streptococcus Bacteriemia (246 patients), *Arch. Int. Med.*, 60:1084, 1937.

26. MACKENZIE, G. M. and HANGER, F. M. Serum Disease and Serum Accidents, *J. Am. M. Ass.*, 94:260, 1930.

27. JULIANELLE, L. Observations on the Specific Therapy (Type A anti-serum) of Staphylococcus Septicemia, *Ann. Int. Med.*, 13:388, 1939.

28. SPINK, W. W. Specific Therapy in Staphylococcus Sepsis, *Surg.*, 8:483, 1940.

29. DOAN, C. A. The Transfusion Problem, *Physiol. Rev.*, 7:1, 1927.

30. LYONS, C. and WARD, H. K. Studies on the Hemolytic Streptococcus of Human Origin, *J. Exper. Med.*, 61:531, 1935.

31. SADUSK, J. F. and TREDWAY, J. B. Observations on the Absorption, Excretion and Acetylation of Sulfadiazine in Man. *Yale J. Biol. & Med.*, 13:539, 1941.

32. SPINK, W. W. *Sulfanilamide and Related Compounds in General Practice*. The Year Book Publishers. Chicago, 2nd Ed. 1942.

33. FOREIGN LETTERS, London. Chemotherapy of War Wounds, *J. Am. M. Ass.*, 114:1683, 1940.

34. BROWN, W. H., THORNTON, W. B. and WILSON, J. S. Evaluation of the Clinical Toxicity of Sulfanilamide and Sulfapyridine, *J. Am. M. Ass.*, 114:1605, 1940.

35. SADUSK, J. P., BLAKE, F. G. and SEYMOUR, A. Observations on the Absorption, Excretion, Diffusion, and Acetylation of Sulfathiazole in Man, *Yale J. Biol. & Med.*, 12:681, 1940.

36. Editorial: Sulfaguanidine and Succinyl-sulfathiazole for Bacillary Dysentery, *J. Am. Ass.*, 121:1353, 1943.

37. MARSHALL, E. K., JR. Determination of Sulfanilamide in Blood and Urine, *Proc. Soc. Exp. Biol. and Med.*, 36:422, 1937.

38. HARTMANN, A. F., PERLEY, A. M. and BARNETT, H. L. A Study of Some of the Physiological Effects of Sulfanilamid II, Methemaglobin and Its Control, *Jour. Clin. Invest.*, 17:699, 1938.

39. KEEFER, CHESTER S., ET AL. Penicillin in the Treatment of Infections, *J. Am. M. Ass.*, 122:1217, 1943.

CHAPTER IV

ACUTE SURGICAL INFECTIONS

Of the various acute surgical infections, due usually to either the streptococcus or staphylococcus, only those are considered in this chapter which invade the surface of the body through a portal of entry which is associated with either no actual trauma or at most through a slight or trivial wound. Infections of actual wounds are taken up in detail in the chapter on wounds.

The initial stage in acute surgical infections is often spoken of as the stage of invasion. During this stage the process may remain a local one at the portal of entry, although even then it produces systemic effects often so slight as to be unnoticed. More often, systemic manifestations are clearly evident and may even become so pronounced as to occupy the center of the stage, whereas the portal of entry may be insignificant and, indeed, in many instances indetectable. Very important are these systemic or general effects, when present, because they signify invasion of the entire body by the infecting organism or its products, thus jeopardizing life; mortality in the acute surgical infections is due to this process called septicemia, or what the lay person speaks of as blood poisoning. For purposes of clarity the local and systemic effects of acute surgical infections will be described separately.

THE LOCAL LESIONS: CELLULITIS AND SUPPURATION

Whenever there is local evidence of bacterial invasion at the portal of entry the initial stage consists of an area of inflammation which is called cellulitis. This is to be distinguished from suppuration, or the formation of pus, which often but not always follows the initial stage. The distinction between cellulitis and suppuration is important therapeutically because any incision into an area of cellulitis is rarely of value when no pus is present and may actually lead to dangerous spread of the infection. Conversely, when pus is present incision and drainage should, with few exceptions, be promptly carried out. The exceptions to these general rules will be mentioned later.

Cellulitis.—The local manifestations of cellulitis are in general those which have already been described for inflammation except that the signs and symptoms are much more severe and pronounced; so much so, in fact, that ordinarily there

39

is no difficulty in differentiating it from nonbacterial inflammation. Subjectively, the patient will usually complain of pain, redness and swelling, and disability. The *pain* is usually more severe in sensitive tissue such as the tips of the fingers and at sites where swelling results in rapid increase of tension, such as the thick skin at the back of the neck. In lax tissues such as those of the face, pain is apt to be less severe but swelling more evident. Accompanying pain is often a throbbing which, with the pain, is aggravated by a dependent position of the inflamed part. On inspection one sees first the swelling and redness and may feel the heat radiating from the area, all of which are due to the hyperemia and increased blood flow and exudation. The *redness* is of a fiery color, is most intense at the portal of entry and fades

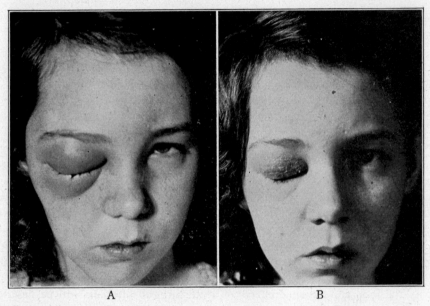

A   B

FIG. 17.—ACUTE CELLULITIS OF THE RIGHT ORBIT WHICH SUBSIDED SPONTANEOUSLY, WITH CONSERVATIVE CARE.

A, at the onset of the swelling; *B*, nine days later. The primary cause of the cellulitis was a right antral infection, which was drained intranasally.

off gradually into normal surrounding skin. The *swelling* often coincides with the redness. Frequently it extends well beyond the area of cellulitis; such swelling is not red or tender and is called lymphedema and is observed especially in infections of the hand and face. On rare occasions the swelling may be so intense as to occlude the arterial supply to the part which is blanched and eventually becomes necrotic. On palpation of the area one can demonstrate *tenderness, i.e.,* induced pain or pain elicited on pressure. Such palpation may be justified in order to detect *point tenderness* which is often valuable, first, in revealing the probable location of a deep infection which has produced no changes on the surface of the skin, and second, in determining the probable portal of entry or site of suppuration in diffuse cellulitis or where spontaneous pain is slight.

Suppuration.—Although acute cellulitis as just described may subside uneventfully, more often the local area suppurates, *i.e.,* it exhibits evidence of liquefaction and softening at the center of the lesion, a process which is accompanied by the formation of pus, which is composed not only of dead bacteria and leukocytes, but also digested and necrotic tissue and exudate. Many other terms are used to describe suppuration such as localization, abscess formation, developing a pyogenic membrane, walling off, coming to a head, pointing.

The local manifestations of suppuration are those of cellulitis as just described plus the added evidence of pus formation, which because of the softening and liquefaction of the tissues becomes clinically demonstrable by fluctuation. *Fluctuation* is the sensation given to the palpating fingers by any localized collection of fluid, provided it is present under not too great tension. One finger compresses the fluid and transmits the impulse to the other stationary examining finger. Lipomas, cysts or other tumefactions may be so soft as to impart a sense of fluctuation, but cause no difficulty in differentiation in the absence of signs of inflammation. Suppuration may, of course, be evident on mere inspection when the pus has reached the surface and shows through the skin. *Point tenderness* is an important sign of suppuration when fluctuation is difficult to elicit, as, for example, in many infections of the hand and in very small areas of inflammation where it is mechanically impossible to test for fluctuation. In such cases the gradual narrowing of the zone of tenderness on successive examinations may be of decisive importance as an indication that pus has formed. Point tenderness is also valuable in deep infections such as those of the ischiorectal space or the deep tissue of the thigh or back. *Aspiration* may be advisable in

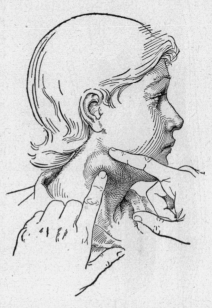

FIG. 18.—THE USE OF TWO FINGERS IN ELICITING FLUCTUATION IN A SWELLING CONTAINING FLUID.

(From Homans, *Textbook of Surgery,* 1931, C. S. Thomas, p. 63.)

detecting pus, especially when the depth or location of the lesion makes fluctuation or point tenderness difficult to elicit. Aspiration may also be used in other situations where questionable fluctuation exists or cannot be detected, *e.g.,* empyema thoracis, pyogenic arthritis. If the pus is thick, aspiration may fail unless a large bore needle is used. Obviously aspiration is contraindicated when it may result in injury to vital or important adjacent structures.

Suppuration as well as cellulitis may be associated with evidences of local extension of the infection. These manifestations, midway between the local and systemic effects of infection, will now be described.

PATHS OF EXTENSION

The local manifestations of acute surgical infections as just described are not infrequently accompanied or followed by evidence of extension. Such extension of the infection may occur by one or more of three ways: lymphatic, venous and by direct extension. In doing so a variety of lesions may be produced.

Lymphangitis and Lymphadenitis.—The invasion of the lymphatic channels leading from the local portal of entry probably begins within a few minutes after the onset of infection (McMaster and Hudack [1]). If the channels themselves become inflamed they are evident clinically as red streaks extending toward the regional lymph nodes (see Fig. 331, page 525). Such red streaks are spoken of as *tubular lymphangitis*. Whether or not the lymphatics show such visible inflammation they practically always act as a pathway for extension because there is nearly always an involvement of the regional lymph nodes, which become the site of an acute lymphadenitis. Both lymphangitis and lymphadenitis are described in more detail in Chapter XXI.

Phlebitis.—The veins carrying blood from the local area of infection undoubtedly act as a passive path of extension in many cases. When a chill occurs it is often due to the entrance of bacteria themselves into the blood stream by way of the venous channels. The spread of the local infection to distant parts of the body even in absence of a chill must largely occur by way of the blood stream. Actual inflammation of the veins may occur and is manifested by a swelling, redness and tenderness along the course of the vessel. Such a lesion is called phlebitis; often the blood in such an inflamed vein becomes thrombosed producing thrombophlebitis. The resulting thrombophlebitis is serious because it sets the stage for embolism, *i.e.*, the breaking off of bits of such thrombi which then enter the blood stream and are carried to the lungs and if arising in the lungs, to the heart and brain. Examples are thrombosis of the angular vein secondary to infections of the lip and saphenous thrombosis secondary to cellulitis of the leg.

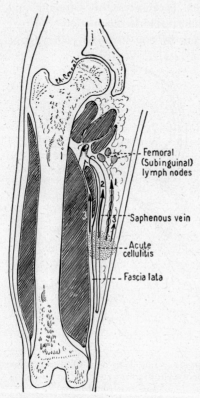

Femoral (Subinguinal) lymph nodes

Saphenous vein

Acute cellulitis

Fascia lata

FIG. 19.—THREE PATHS OF EXTENSION OF A CELLULITIS, LOCATED FOR EXAMPLE, ON THE INNER SIDE OF THE THIGH.

1, by lymphatic spread; 2, by venous channels; and 3, by direct extension into the deeper fascial planes or subcutaneously.

Direct Extension.—Acute surgical infections may spread in all directions by simply invading adjacent tissue until the process is arrested by the local defense mechanisms. Direct extension is perhaps the most common method of spread especially in the subcutaneous tissues but is serious when it takes place by way of fascial planes and tendon sheaths, particularly in the hand. Body cavities such as the peritoneum also permit serious spread of infection by direct extension.

SYSTEMIC EFFECTS: SEPTICEMIA

The general or systemic effects of an acute surgical infection are those produced by an extension of the local process to the rest of the body which is evident by clinical manifestations commonly called septicemia. This term implies the presence of bacteria in the blood stream, although the blood culture is not always positive. Whether or not a positive blood culture can be obtained the clinical manifestations of septicemia are often so clear as to enable one to make a diagnosis at the bedside. An excellent review of septicemia is that of Whitby.[2]

The *clinical manifestations* are now listed somewhat in chronological order.

1. A *chill* not infrequently announces the entrance of the infection into the general blood stream and may be due to the fact that a shower of bacteria suddenly breaks into a blood vessel and is dispersed throughout the body. A chill in its most characteristic form causes the patient to shake violently and the spasmodic contractions of the masseter muscle make his teeth chatter. The sensation of cold is pronounced, being really an aggravated form of ordinary shivering. Because of peripheral vasoconstriction the extremities are cold, whereas the temperature of the deeper tissues may be very high (105° F. or above).

2. *Fever* is almost an invariable accompaniment of systemic infection even when the chill is absent. It is not usually sustained, however, as in pneumonia or typhoid fever but may be of the irregular intermittent type, *i.e.,* elevated in the afternoon, normal in the morning. When this diurnal variation becomes very pronounced the fever is spoken of as *septic* or *spiked,* for the sudden swings of temperature on the chart are represented by almost vertical lines. The peak may reach 40° to 42° C. (104° to 107° F.). The variations, however, are frequently not diurnal, but quite irregular. Fever probably serves a useful purpose, being in some way connected with the development of defenses by the body. It is absent, for example, in some of the very severe fulminating infections, usually in older patients who die within a short time after the organisms have invaded. It is a part of the accelerated metabolism which the body automatically sets up to fight the infection, and it has been shown by Rolly and Meltzer, W. H. Welch and others that the formation of certain antibodies in animals could be accelerated by putting them in a heated environment (MacCallum[3]). There is evidence, however, that this beneficial effect is true only up to 40° C. (104° F.). Above this level deleterious or even fatal effects may occur. Because moderate fever is a reaction which serves a useful purpose antipyretics are no longer used. The temperature sponge as given by the nurse is not so much to reduce the fever *per se* (unless dangerously high), but merely to give symptomatic relief to the patient.

3. *Prostration* is nearly always present in general septicemia, but may vary from a feeling of general malaise to a complete asthenia, sometimes so alarming as to suggest shock. All gradations between these two extremes occur dependent not only on the virulence of the infection, but also to some extent on the personality or vigor of the patient.

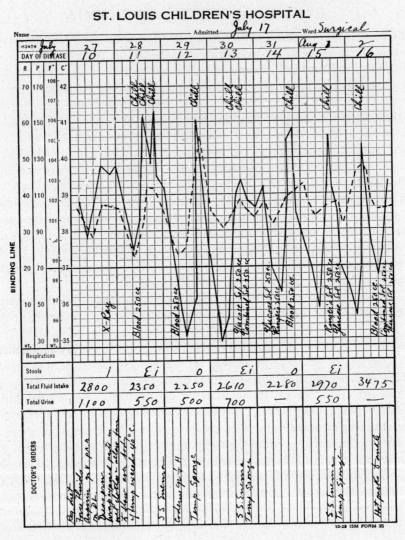

CHART I.—SEPTICEMIA DUE TO HEMOLYTIC STREPTOCOCCUS.

Note the septic (spiked) temperature curve. The disease started as an apparently innocent infection of the thumb. The patient, a ten-year-old boy, then developed a deep axillary abscess, later an osteomyelitis of the tibia and died one month later. At autopsy abscesses and infected infarcts were found in the liver, kidneys, lungs, etc. At the present time the fatal outcome in this case would undoubtedly not have occurred due to the introduction of sulfanilamide, especially if it were used early in the course of the infection.

4. *Leukocytosis* is a common sign and may reach 20,000 or more leukocytes per cubic millimeter. The differential count is also characteristic and may be of prognostic value (the Schilling count shows an increased "stab" count or shift to the left). In agranulocytosis or in a fulminating infection when the patient has no resistance, leukocytosis is absent. Leukocytosis, moreover, may be one of the first manifestations of infection, before the development of fever and other signs of general invasion of the body.

5. *Blood culture* should show a positive growth in all cases of general invasion. This is not always true, however, although the likelihood is increased by repeating the test (see p. 34).

6. The *sensorium* is usually depressed, the patient being listless, apathetic and uninterested in his surroundings. On the other hand, he may be alert, apprehensive, restless and even delirious. Sometimes both extremes may be present in the same patient (at different times), often depending on the extent of the fever. More or less general hyperesthesia of the skin everywhere is often observed. Loss of morale is a prominent symptom in long drawn-out cases.

7. *Digestive symptoms* are frequent in children. Anorexia is the rule, and nausea and vomiting are not unusual in young patients with any sort of general infection. These symptoms are not so apt to occur in adults.

8. Evidence of *metastatic foci* are often noted in septicemia, such as abscesses, empyema, osteomyelitis, acute suppurative arthritis, etc. This is important therapeutically because incision and drainage are usually indicated in such lesions. Unfortunately many of these metastatic foci remain occult and inaccessible, *e.g.*, infected infarcts of lungs, kidneys, multiple abscesses of the lung, retroperitoneal fat, endocarditis, etc.

VARIETIES OF TERMINATION (PROGNOSIS)

The course of acute surgical infections depends both on the treatment and on certain unpredictable factors concerned with the mysteries of immunity and resistance. The differences in the clinical course may be classified as follows:

1. *Abortion or spontaneous resolution* of the local lesion may occur, *i.e.*, the acute cellulitis gradually fades away leaving no trace of the often intense inflammatory battle which had taken place in the tissues. This is the normal manner in which erysipelas (see p. 83) terminates. Furuncles also occasionally become absorbed without suppuration. Such a resolution may occur even when lymphangitis, lymphadenitis and septicemia accompany the local cellulitis, though ordinarily these latter manifestations signify a more serious and complicated development of the infection.

2. *Suppuration* is one of the most common events resulting from the invasion of tissue by bacteria. It has been described in detail on p. 41. Suppuration is also frequently accompanied by lymphangitis, lymphadenitis, thrombophlebitis and septicemia.

3. *Local necrosis* may occur with or without actual pus formation, in which case replacement of the dead tissue by scar occurs, as described under healing. This is a rare but serious development, however, and occurs usually with the other

complications of infection and with special types of organisms (virulent strepto-cocci, gas bacilli, symbiotic bacteria, etc.).

4. *Death* is an ever-present danger in any infection when general invasion occurs. A fatal outcome may result rapidly within hours or days, due to the lack of resistance. So precipitate may the septicemia become that the French term *foudroyante* is sometimes used, which means fulminating or disastrous. More fre-

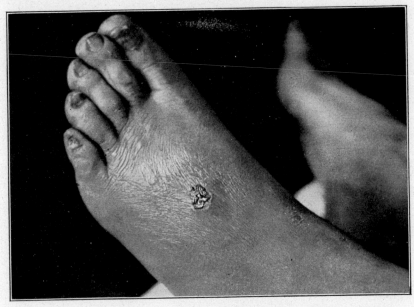

FIG. 20.—SUBSIDING CELLULITIS.

One week following an injury to the dorsum of the foot the patient developed a severe cellulitis which subsided without suppuration. Note the wrinkled appearance of the skin due to cessation of the swelling. The color was dusky red with a slight cyanotic tinge.

quently, the fatal outcome is delayed and preceded by prolonged evidence of pyemia and septic signs. This is due to the multiplicity of infective foci which are inaccessi-ble to surgical attack and thus maintain the septicemia. Cachexia, loss of morale, and anemia aggravate the other clinical signs after weeks have passed. Death may also be due to *local causes* such as hemorrhage from necrosis of a large vessel, an embolus to a vital center, and thrombosis of a vital vein such as the cavernous sinus or portal vein.

GENERAL PRINCIPLES OF TREATMENT

Preventive measures are most important in eradicating infection. Use of the measures described in Chapter III, under prophylaxis of infection minimizes the incidence in wounds made by the surgeon and also in contaminated wounds acci-dentally sustained. Such lesions should always be treated as soon after the accident as possible. Once the infection has invaded we are confronted in general with two therapeutic problems, *i.e.,* (1) the local lesions (cellulitis and suppuration) and (2) the general infection (septicemia).

Local Measures.—1. *Nonoperative Therapy.*—*Rest* of the affected part not only minimizes the pain which movement produces, but more important is the fact that immobilization reduces the danger of extension into lymphatics and adjacent tissue spaces, which might occur by muscular movements. Elevation of the part is advisable to promote the rapidity of the local circulation by aiding lymph and venous flow; swelling is also lessened and with it pain. An ordinary muslin sling is the simplest way to put the upper extremity at rest. With the patient in bed, elevation of the extremity on a pillow is just as effective. Splints are useful to immobilize fingers or hands and can be applied in addition to the use of the sling. Restriction of ordinary activities may be necessary to insure adequate local rest. With the lower extremities, confinement to a chair is almost mandatory; with lesions on the trunk rest in bed may be advisable. In no case, of course, should the

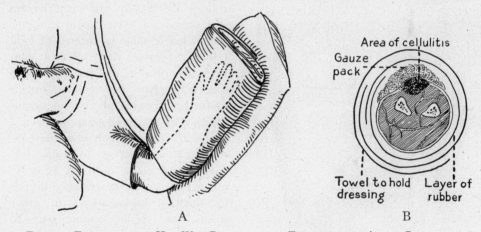

FIG. 21.—ELEVATION AND HOT WET PACKS IN THE TREATMENT OF ACUTE CELLULITIS.

A, proper angle of elevation on a pillow; *B,* diagram of the various layers constituting a wet pack.

sling or splint be applied so as to cause pressure sufficient to impair the local circulation. *Relief of pain* is achieved to a considerable degree by rest and immobilization; heat may add to the patient's comfort; cold sometimes does, but has its possible dangers (see p. 149). Drugs as aspirin, codein, and morphia are to be used freely as indicated during the few hours or days when the pain is most acute. *Local application of heat* aids in the favorable outcome of the inflammatory process whether it is abortion or localization with abscess formation. It increases the *active hyperemia* which means a greater blood flow, increased metabolism, and greater leukocytic activity, thereby aiding the reparative forces of the body. The use of heat thus makes the spontaneous response to injury more marked. It also relieves pain in many cases. It must be emphasized, however, that the degree of heat must not be excessive. As ordinarily applied, the effect is quite superficial. Penetration may be increased by diathermy or the infra-red ray. The methods of applying heat are described in Chapter VIII. Application of cold in acute infections has been recommended by many clinicians and is rather widely used. The authors do not use it. Cold has its definite dangers in the very young, the very old and over delicate tissues such as the scrotum, eye and ear (see p. 149). The use of *x-ray* therapy [4] over areas of acute cellulitis is often of great value. Though remarkable relief of pain, spontaneous resolution or rapid localization has been observed in certain cases, *x-ray* therapy is frequently ineffective. It should never be given except with the advice and under the supervision of a competent radiologist. *Antitoxin* for tetanus and gas bacilli is used prophylactically whenever the presence of these organisms in the wound is suspected (see Chapter X).

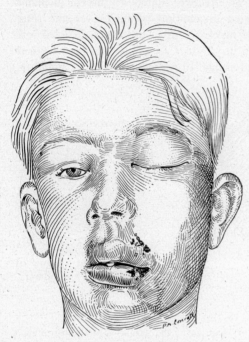

FIG. 22.—FATAL STAPHYLOCOCCUS SEPTICEMIA FOLLOWING AN ILL-ADVISED INCISION OF A CELLULITIS OF THE UPPER LIP.

The illustration shows the condition on admission five days after onset of a small "pimple" and two days after it had been incised.

2. *Operative therapy.*—As soon as pus has formed it should be evacuated by incision and drainage; this is a general principle in the treatment of acute surgical infections. A companion to this rule is the equally important dictum that operations, even simple incisions, should not be done in an area of local cellulitis because they offer a considerable danger of opening tissue spaces, lymphatic and venous channels to further invasion of virulent organisms. Rapidly developing septicemia frequently follows such ill-advised incisions. It is important to realize this danger and incise only on adequate indication, *i.e.,* in the presence of pus or localized suppuration; in other words, one should operate only to drain an abscess. To this general rule there are several notable but easily explained exceptions, *e.g.,* felon, acute tenosynovitis, acute pyogenic arthritis, acute appendicitis. These infections will be discussed separately; in each of them operation is carried out as soon as the diagnosis is made, without waiting for pus to form. The reason must be apparent, however, because in none of these infections is there a true diffuse cellulitis; in each of them the infection occurs in an already localized tissue or closed space and thus presents an entirely different problem of extension.

Incision and drainage is the operation of choice in the treatment of abscesses, though occasionally aspiration alone may be effective. In general, however, a well placed and sufficiently large incision is needed before rapid and complete healing can occur.

The time for operation is ordinarily not difficult to decide upon when suppuration is definite. Too early incision, *i.e.,* before definite pus is present, as just discussed, is apt to be dangerous due to opening new channels to extension of infection. Delay in drainage prolongs pain, lengthens the period of healing and aids in absorption and perhaps of extension of the infection. However, in infections of the face above the upper lip, *operation is practically always avoided* in favor of nature's method of spontaneous drainage, especially because of the danger of spreading the infection to the veins leading to the cranial sinuses (see Fig. 22). Moreover, in the face, spontaneous drainage is often prompt and effective.

The *incision* is best made with a sharp pointed bistoury knife in simple super-ficial abscesses such as furuncles. The point is inserted into the cavity gently and quickly, with the blade directed upward so that by carrying it outward it enlarges the point of entrance without causing any tension on the inflamed tissue. A single small slit is often sufficient, but in large abscesses it may be lengthened or a second

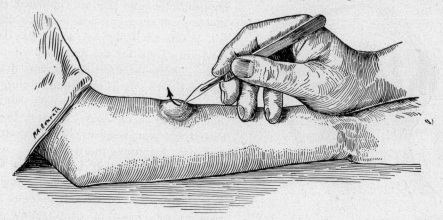

FIG. 23.—THE PROPER METHOD OF INCISING A SUPERFICIAL ABSCESS WITH A SHARP POINTED (BISTOURY) KNIFE.

The cutting edge of the blade faces upward.

incision made at right angles to it, the so-called cruciate or crossed incision. The opening in any case should be *large enough to open the cavity adequately.* In large abscesses the opening is made at the most dependent portion so that gravity may aid in drainage. When the cavity is large or irregular in extent, a second opening may be made for through and through drainage in order to avoid the trauma of a large incision. When multilocular cavities are present, the barriers must be gently broken. A drain is used to prevent the incision from closing before the cavity has emptied itself and become obliterated by healthy granulation tissue. Thus, its use depends on the size of the cavity. In small abscesses, drains may be omitted or perhaps confined to the first twenty-four hours, after which they are left out or are removed. Slips of rubber dam are usually used. The possibility of losing them in the cavity must always be guarded against by fastening a safety pin to the free end, or by leaving a large enough portion outside the skin so that it is impossible for the entire drain to enter the abscess cavity.

Anesthesia is often unnecessary when the skin over the abscess is already necrotic and insensitive, provided no pressure is made upon it during incision. If the overlying skin is inflamed but still too sensitive, it may be quickly frozen with an ethyl chloride spray just before inserting the bistoury knife. If the skin over the abscess is uninvolved by the infection, it may be anesthetized with novocain. In certain sensitive patients a short gas inhalation may be advisable. General anesthesia is particularly indicated in most infections of the hand, and in any large abscess when exploration of the cavity will be necessary. Usually nitrous oxide-oxygen is used.

Culture of the evacuated pus should always be carried out as a routine. Unsuspected organisms may thus be detected, the identification of which may prevent diagnostic and therapeutic errors. Culture at a later stage will be unreliable because secondary skin invaders soon overgrow the original bacteria.

Postoperative care is just as important as the operation itself. The measures already mentioned, *i.e.*, rest, elevation, immobilization and heat are continued. In simple small abscesses, heat may be omitted. When advisable, hot soaks may be used intensively for the first twenty-four hours. The moist dressing prevents drying, and thus aids in promoting drainage as well as mechanically loosening debris and necrotic tissue (see Fig. 21). Prolonged wet heat, however, is unnecessary and often macerates the tissues.

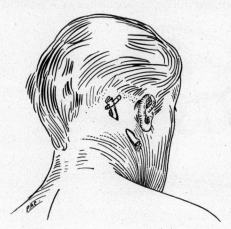

FIG. 24—A THROUGH AND THROUGH DRAIN.

The drain has been placed through two incisions because the use of a single large incision extending the entire length of the large abscess would have created an unnecessarily large wound. This is the most frequent indication for this type of drainage.

Early active motion is important in the extremities in order to restore function as quickly as possible. It is begun as soon as subsidence of pain permits it, and as soon as evidence of healing occurs. *Evidences of healing* are the diminution of such manifestations as pain, local tenderness, swelling, redness, etc. Wrinkling of the skin is a good indication of the subsidence of the inflammatory swelling.

General Measures.—These are important whenever a general septicemia is present because it is in these cases that the mortality is high.

1. *Rest in bed* is obviously important and with it we imply the proper comfort and care that go with adequate nursing. To bed rest is added local rest of the part involved in the local lesion.

2. *Large fluid intake* serves the purpose of preventing dehydration which is a deleterious and unfavorable feature of general sepsis. It also serves to increase urinary secretion, and with it presumably the excretion of bacterial toxins. Moreover, it serves to alleviate the unpleasant symptoms which are a part of fever in general. The actual amount of fluid which may be taken must be definitely prescribed. At least 3000 cubic centimeters per day in a normal adult should be given and as much as 4000 or 5000 cubic centimeters in hot weather or in the presence of high fever. When necessary, fluid by mouth may be augmented by rectal, subcutaneous or intravenous administration (see methods in Chapter VIII).

3. *General hygiene* is important, particularly in the long drawn-out cases lasting many weeks. Included here are adequate caloric, mineral and vitamin intake, catharsis, cleanliness and reassurance. A nourishing, ample, diversified diet is important in order to avoid wasting as much as possible. Loss of morale is a distressing symptom which the nurse and attending physician must combat as much as possible.

4. *Transfusions,* for reasons already mentioned (page 35) are considered by many surgeons an important aid in the treatment of general septicemia.

5. *Repeated search for metastatic foci* is urgent because each abscess becomes the site for further distribution of bacteria. It is, therefore, important to detect and drain each focus as rapidly as indicated. Areas of redness, swelling or pain, tenderness over bones and joints, etc., should be constantly looked for. Arthritis, empyema, osteomyelitis, as well as soft tissue foci, are common in septicemia and can be treated early only if recognized early.

6. *Chemotherapy* until recently has been the will-o'-the-wisp of treatment in bacterial infections ever since Paul Ehrlich discovered the silver bullet which kills the spirochete. Fortunately such agents are now available in the form of the sulfonamide drugs which have a remarkable and often life-saving efficacy in many pyogenic infections. They are discussed in detail on page 35 and elsewhere throughout the text.

7. *Antitoxins* are available for the treatment of staphylococcus, streptococcus and other severe pyogenic infections but their use is still in the experimental stage (see also page 34). Antitoxins for tetanus and gas bacillus infections, however, do have a definite therapeutic value (see Chapter VI). The use of vaccines in the treatment of severe pyogenic infections does not appear logical (see page 34).

SPECIAL TYPES OF SUPPURATION

Local suppuration takes a variety of forms dependent somewhat on the invading organism but largely on the anatomical structures at the portal of entry. Only suppuration occurring on the surface of the body will be described here. The lesions will not include suppurative wounds which are discussed in the chapter on wounds, nor hand infections to which a separate chapter is devoted. Most of the following infections seem to develop spontaneously.

1. **Simple abscess.**—A simple abscess may result from the introduction of bacteria through a puncture of the skin, although such a history is not always obtainable, or through a sweat gland. Simple abscesses may be metastatic, *i.e.,* result from an infected embolus being carried from another focus, or they may follow an acute lymphadenitis which has suppurated. Abscesses in the axilla, groin, and neck not infrequently are due to suppurative lymphadenitis. Treatment has already been outlined.

2. **Furuncle.**—The common boil is a special type of infection of the skin, because it has a definite anatomical location (hair follicle) and is always caused by the staphylococcus. Why this normal inhabitant of the skin suddenly invades the wall of the follicle is not always clear. In some cases mechanical irritation over the opening of a follicle from tight wearing apparel, ingrowing hair, etc., seems

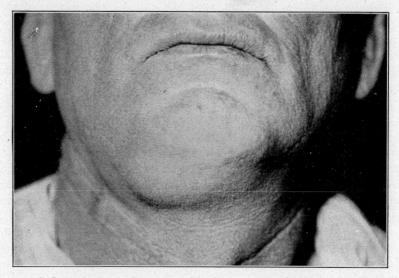

FIG. 25.—A SUBCUTANEOUS ABSCESS OF THE NECK BEFORE INCISION AND DRAINAGE.

This abscess resulted from an acute dento-alveolar abscess which ruptured through the tissue about the jaw, but did not enter the floor of the mouth or the deep cervical tissue.

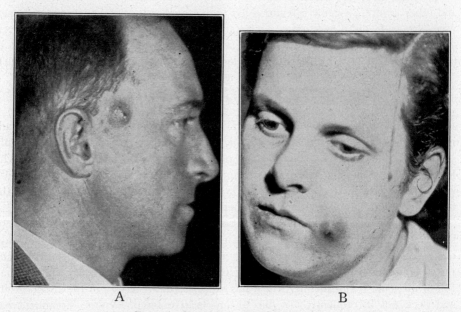

A   B

FIG. 26.—FURUNCLE; TWO EXAMPLES

A, large furuncle of the face near the hair line; B, an acute furuncle of three days' duration which, because of its location, represents a dangerous type of infection. Rest and local heat were applied with spontaneous drainage and rapid healing. Incision in this type of infection is hazardous (see Fig. 22).

to be a factor. In diabetics, who are especially subject to furuncles, lack of resistance seems to be an adequate explanation. Once the staphylococci get a foothold. the process extends beyond the wall of the follicle as an area of cellulitis which quickly softens into an abscess. The demarcated and necrotic remnant of the follicle in the center, however, resists digestion, and remains as a stout plug which is called the core, which is extruded or removed.

Though furuncles are often single, they sometimes exhibit a distressing tendency to recur often, like the fabled cat, having nine or even more lives. They usually follow one another in orderly sequence until, for no apparent reason, they stop. Such multiple lesions are called *furunculosis*.

In large furuncles the *treatment* is similar to that already described for abscesses in general. In small furuncles seen early, suppuration may often be prevented, and the infection aborted by covering the area with thick adhesive plaster. This simple procedure is probably effective because it prevents radiation of heat and thus maintains local hyperemia, and also because it insures local rest, since it prevents further irritation by clothing or by the patient's own fingers.

In furunculosis various forms of nonoperative treatment have been recommended to halt its development. Diabetes, of course, should always be suspected, and if present treated accordingly. The use of vaccines may be recommended in the protracted cases (see p. 34).

3. **Carbuncle.**—A carbuncle is an infection (deeper than a furuncle) consisting of extensive subcutaneous abscesses draining inadequately through many tiny openings in the skin. The infection may start as a simple boil which breaks into and extends along loose areolar and fatty subcutaneous tissue, coming to the surface here and there through tiny channels described by J. C. Warren [5] as columnae adiposae. The tough derma in the neck and back where they most frequently occur, resists digestion so effectively that the pus drains inadequately and suppuration persists often for weeks, involving more and more tissue and giving to the skin itself a necrotic appearance. One may describe a carbuncle also as multiple collar button abscesses (*vide infra*) whose deeper parts communicate with each other while the superficial lesions are separate.

The systemic manifestations vary considerably. Many patients have diabetes. Fever is usually moderate, pain may be absent or quite severe, local necrosis may be extensive or mild. Treatment consists of the establishment of adequate drainage by sufficient incisions preferably cruciate, through the tough derma into the subcutaneous abscesses. On rare occasions when the skin is necrotic beyond hope of recovery, actual excision of the area may be advisable, using the actual cautery followed later by skin grafting. When seen early, x-ray therapy is sometimes effective in hastening suppuration or even in aborting the infection (Firor [6]), but should be given only on the advice of and by a competent radiologist.

4. **Collar Button Abscess.**—This type of infection known also as a dumbbell abscess is a double abscess connected by a tiny communication which passes through some tough structure such as derma or fascia. One of the cavities is usually superficial and the other deep. The recognition of the deep abscess, and its evacuation is of course essential for adequate treatment. Collar button abscess occurs in the skin whenever a small abscess in the superficial layers of the epidermis

extends through a sweat gland or other opening into the subcutaneous tissue beneath the derma which may be so tough as to resist liquefaction and thereby conceal the abscess beneath it. Collar button abscess is also common in the hand where a deep palmar abscess may break through a tiny opening and present as a subcutaneous lesion in the web of the fingers on the dorsal aspect of the hand. Perirenal abscesses may also form a collar button abscess by rupture through the fascia and appear under the skin.

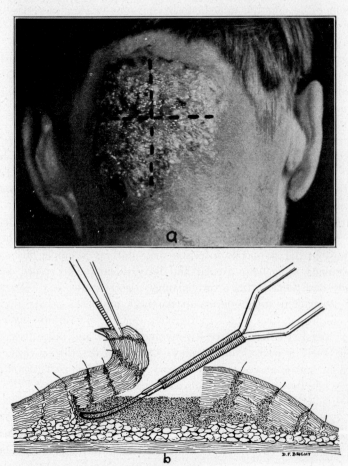

FIG. 27.—CARBUNCLE OF THE NECK.

a, The patient is a fifty-five-year-old machinist who first noted a tiny infection of a hair follicle two weeks previously which spread to its present size. The carbuncle is located higher in the neck in this patient than usual. The dotted lines indicate the lines of incision. Healing was complete after many weeks; *b*, Diagram of a cross section of a carbuncle showing the multiple "heads" and extension below the derma and involving the subcutaneous fat. The proper method of undermining the edges of the skin with a cautery in order to achieve adequate drainage is also indicated.

BIBLIOGRAPHY

1. McMaster, P. D. and Hudack, S. S.   The Participation of Skin Lymphatics in Repair of Lesions Due to Incisions and Burns, *Jour. Exper. Med.,* 60:479, 1934.
2. Whitby, L. E. H.   Septicemia: a Critical Review, *Brit. J. Surg.,* 28:124, 1940.
3. MacCallum, W. G.   *Textbook of Pathology,* W. B. Saunders Co., Phila., 1916, p. 155.
4. Desjardins, A. U.   Radiotherapy for Inflammatory Conditions, *J. Am. M. Ass.,* 96:401, 1931.
5. Warren, J. C.   Note on the Anatomy and Pathology of the Skin, *Boston M. & S. J.,* 96:453, 1877.
6. Firor, W. B.   Roentgen Treatment of Carbuncles, *Am. J. Roentgenol.,* 33:71, 1935.

CHAPTER V

ACUTE HAND INFECTIONS

Types of Infection
Operations on Hand Infections
Complications of Hand Infections

The increased liability of the fingers and hand to infection is not surprising, for their prehensile function places them constantly in contact with the outside world, particularly in individuals doing manual labor. An injury, though slight, is often sufficient to introduce the invading organism. Moreover, the folds and crevices of the hand may harbor many organisms which sometimes invade spontaneously or at least after trivial or nonapparent injury.

There are other special features which separate hand infections from other types. The manifold and delicate functions of motion in the hand are so essential in manual activity that any challenge to motor impairment becomes especially important. Infections are particularly serious because the fingers are composed largely of tendons, nerves, bone and tough connective tissue so that there is little room for swelling, little opportunity for increased blood flow, and small space for exudation and leukocytic invasion, all of which are so necessary in nature's response to injury. Probably because of this last factor, infections of the hand have a distressing tendency to spread, not only by direct extension into neighboring spaces and tendon sheaths, but particularly into lymphatics and into the general blood stream. General septicemia, therefore, is one of the dangers always to be feared in any severe hand infection. Finally, treatment exerts such profound influence in the final functional result, and the danger of ill-advised treatment is so great, that special study and care are essential for good results. Excellent detailed studies of hand infections have been reported by Auchincloss,[1] Kanavel,[2] Koch,[3] and Couch.[4]

Since many serious hand infections begin as trivial skin injuries, which serve as a portal of entry for virulent bacteria, it should be emphasized here that prompt and effective treatment of such lesions must be carried out in each case. Each scratch or break in the skin no matter how small, should be immediately cleansed, a surface antiseptic applied, the lesion protected with a sterile dressing, and the part immobilized for a day or two. This simple treatment *will prevent a large percentage of the severe infections* and cannot be too strongly urged as a routine, particularly in shops and factories where such injuries are common (see also p. 33).

TYPES OF INFECTION

Of the various types, perhaps the most serious are acute tenosynovitis and palmar and bursal infections, not only because they are more frequently associated with septicemia but also because the local manifestations are so intense. The entire hand becomes swollen, stiff and immobile in a position of slight flexion; such a condition is called *septic hand* or spade hand. Extreme disability frequently follows such infections even when the healing process is complete. A septic hand is not infrequently complicated by lymphangitis, lymphadenitis and thrombophlebitis. Other lesions may occur as later complications such as osteomyelitis, suppurative arthritis and gangrene.

1. **Superficial Infections.**—These infections of the hand are similar to those occurring elsewhere, and are caused by punctured wounds or other injuries. Only the skin, or at most the subcutaneous tissue, is involved. Although arising outside such structures as the closed space, tendon sheaths, or fascial spaces, they have a tendency to extend or penetrate into them. It is important, therefore, here as well as in any hand infection to repeatedly examine the structures for extension of swelling or tenderness. The treatment consists of drainage of the pus by an incision sufficiently shallow to avoid tendon sheaths and nerves.

Carbuncle of the hand is a term used to describe multiple abscesses of the furuncle type with a cellulitis affecting the dorsum of the hand. The infection is deeper, however, than in furunculosis. Treatment consists of adequate drainage, usually by cruciate incision.

2. **Paronychia.**—This is a less serious type of infection located under the eponychium and about the root of the nail, hence its name. It occurs as an acute or as a chronic (or recurring) paronychia. The infection is usually spontaneous, although a history of injury or "hang nail" is sometimes obtained. In the acute form the infection begins at one edge of the nail bed as a simple abscess. Because of its tendency to extend along the base of the nail to the other side it is often called a run-around. Treatment consists of a short incision in the abscess as soon as pus forms. Frequently, drainage may be established by elevating the cuticle and the adjacent reflected layer of eponychial epidermis. Often, most of the pus is trapped behind the nail (subungual abscess) so that a portion of the nail over the abscess may have to be excised to promote better drainage. A drain is rarely necessary.

In spite of adequate drainage, chronic suppuration occasionally occurs. Chronicity is frequently due to the fact that the base of the nail acts as a foreign body; in such a case removal of the loose portion of the nail is followed by cure. Occasionally, chronicity is due to a fungus infection, which is to be suspected when the therapeutic procedures just described have failed to effect a cure. In such instances the use of fungicides such as resorcinol lotion (containing resorcinol, alcohol and bichloride of mercury) will frequently result in healing. X-ray therapy is also useful.

3. **Felon.**—Felon (sometimes called whitlow) is a term which should be confined to infections involving the closed space of the terminal phalanx, although it is loosely applied to any serious finger infection, especially when the bone is involved. This closed space is located in the deeper portion of the pulp end of the finger, and contains fatty tissue supported by numerous fibrous strands radiating from the periosteum of the bone to the periphery. It has no communication with the joint or tendon sheaths, although the flexor tendon inserts nearby at the base of the bone. Infection develops whenever appropriate virulent organisms are introduced, usually by puncture of a sharp object, by direct extension from an overlying infection of the skin covering the finger pad, or by way of a sweat gland.

The exudation which is one of the first manifestations of infection, distends this closed space within a few hours, and since there is little room for swelling,

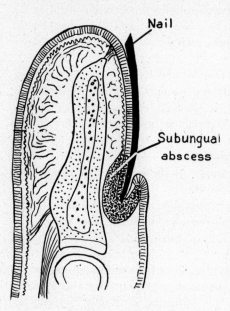

the tension becomes great and pain is exquisite. The pain is of a throbbing character and is much worse when the hand is carried in a dependent position. Tenderness is intense, but only slight redness is present. Yet the importance of diagnosis and treatment even at this early stage lies in its effect on the viability of the underlying bone, which is jeopardized because the nutrient artery supplying it is compressed by the increase of pressure within the closed space. In the severe and neglected cases this may lead to a massive necrosis of the entire phalangeal bone, which in the presence of infection causes an osteomyelitis. This complication may not be detected objectively until changes occur in the x-ray, which takes a week or two. Unless the pressure is relieved by early incision, the ultimate development of an osteomyelitis must be taken for granted. Eventually, dead bone (sequestrum) separates and may have to be removed, but even then the end result is a deformed, sometimes painful and often useless terminal phalanx (Dorrance [5]).

Treatment, as indicated, is urgent and de-

FIG. 28.—LONGITUDINAL SECTION THROUGH THE TERMINAL PHALANX WHICH IS THE SITE OF AN EXTENSIVE PARONYCHIA.

Note the superficial location of part of the abscess just beneath the cuticle, as well as the deeper (subungual) portion which is covered by the proximal part of the nail.

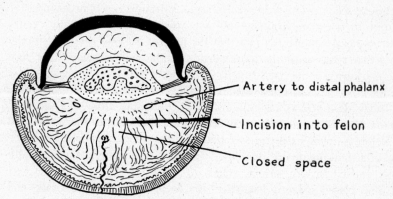

FIG. 29.—CROSS SECTION THROUGH THE TERMINAL PHALANX SHOWING THE RELATION OF THE CLOSED SPACE TO THE BONE AND THE ARTERIES SUPPLYING IT.

The sweat gland is shown to illustrate one method by which the closed space may be invaded without apparent trauma. The proper method of incision into the closed space for the drainage of a felon is also indicated.

mands early incision into the closed space on one or both sides of the finger, but never through the pad of fat on the palmar surface. This pad is a specialized end organ containing a great concentration of sensory endings. An incision through them, while theoretically the most direct approach to the closed space, often produces distressing symptoms of hyperesthesia or actual pain in the healed scar because of cicatricial contraction of the many delicate nerve endings in the pad of fat. The lateral incision just in front of the edge of the nail may be carried over the end of the finger (hockey stick incision), but in order to avoid entering the flexor tendon which is inserted at this point, should never reach the fold of the first joint. It is rarely necessary to carry the incision all the way around the end of the finger. Two lateral incisions with through and through drainage may be used but are rarely necessary.

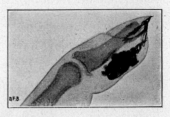

FIG. 30.—THE TERMINAL END OF THE FINGER HAS BEEN INJECTED WITH A RADIOPAQUE SUBSTANCE (RED LEAD) TO SHOW THE EXTENT OF THE CONNECTIVE TISSUE (CLOSED) SPACE.

(Redrawn from Dorrance.)

4. **Acute Tenosynovitis.**—This infection is limited to the flexor tendon sheaths of the fingers and usually follows trauma, frequently of a very minor character especially in the transverse creases. Moreover, it is not necessary that the injury penetrate the tendon sheath, since the infection may be carried to it by lymphatics or by direct extension through the sheath. It is a dangerous infection, first because it may lead to necrosis of the tendon with its resultant disability, and second because it may spread directly along the sheath into the hand and forearm. The danger of such an extension is much greater with tenosynovitis of the little finger and thumb. As can be seen from Figure 35 the flexor tendons of the middle, ring and index fingers are encased in a sheath terminating at the level of the distal metacarpal head by a thin fascial barrier. While this fascial barrier prevents further extension to a slight degree, rupture may occur across the barrier into the palmar or thenar space. On the other hand, infections of the tendon sheaths of the thumb and little finger are

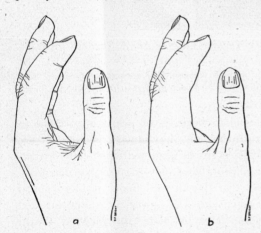

FIG. 31.—ACUTE TENOSYNOVITIS OF THE INDEX FINGER.

a, Early stage, showing merely the slight flexion and local swelling; this is the stage during which incision and drainage may be expected to result in complete return of function; b, Later stage, showing extension of infection with suppuration and rupture outside the sheath. The tendon is probably necrotic at this stage and severe disability may result even if the infection is controlled.

much more serious because the sheaths do not terminate but are continuous and communicate (in nearly all individuals) directly with the radial and ulnar bursae, respectively. These bursae frequently communicate with each other, or with other sheaths in the neighborhood of the proximal part of the palm. But of more serious importance is the fact that these sheaths or bursae extend under the annular ligament up into the forearm.

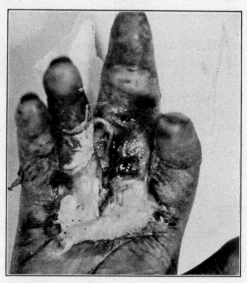

FIG. 32.—A NEGLECTED AND INADEQUATELY TREATED CASE OF ACUTE TENOSYNOVITIS.

The infection apparently ruptured into the subcutaneous tissue without extending into the fascial spaces; this abscess had been opened by a small incision. The necrotic tendon is visible. Healing was prolonged and resulted in a complete loss of power of flexion of the middle finger.

Early diagnosis of infection of the tendon sheath is of prime importance in order to institute immediate operative treatment, and thus prevent necrosis of the tendon and extension, both of which usually occur in neglected cases. The demonstration of a wound of entrance may be helpful, but is not essential for diagnosis. Important in the examination is the fact that the affected finger is more flexed than the rest and resists any attempt at extension. Any movement of the infected tendon provokes the most exquisite pain. Palpation along the infected sheath reveals extreme tenderness. Slight redness may be present, but the infection *must not be mistaken for acute lymphangitis,* which of course requires nonoperative treatment, whereas acute tenosynovitis requires prompt incision. Treatment is immediate operation as soon as the diagnosis is made. The sheath is opened for drainage by adequate lateral incisions; extreme care should be exercised in handling the tendon itself, particularly because of its poor blood supply. A drain is placed into the wound down to, but not into the sheath for the same reason. Because many of these infections are due to invasion by the streptococcus, the use of sulfanilamide is advisable and may prevent further spread. The sulfonamide drugs are discussed on p. 35.

5. **Palmar Abscess.**—Infections of this type involve the fascial spaces of the hand and develop from direct introduction of organisms through a palmar wound

or by extension from infections in the fingers or tendon sheaths; hence the importance in any hand infection for repeated investigation of these structures so as to detect their involvement as soon as possible. Two such spaces are described, the middle palmar and thenar spaces. (See Figure 35.) Though called spaces they are really only planes of loose areolar tissue lying beneath the flexor tendons of the palm.

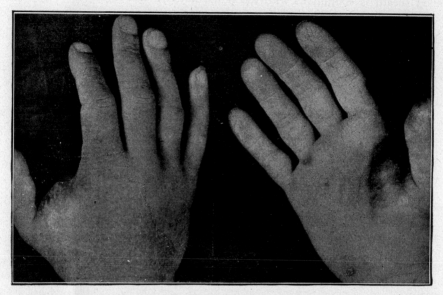

FIG. 33.—NEGLECTED THENAR-SPACE ABSCESS, SHOWING CHARACTERISTIC SWELLING IN WEB BETWEEN THUMB AND FIRST FINGER.

The infection developed after trauma due to rowing. There was no visible break in the skin. Operation was performed immediately after admission. (From Deryl Hart, *The Practitioners Library of Medicine and Surgery*, Volume V, D. Appleton-Century Co.)

(a) The *middle palmar space* lies in the ulnar side of the palm between the flexor tendons and the fascia covering the interosseus structures, and extends distally with prolongations along the lumbrical muscles to the base of the middle, ring and little fingers and is in close relation to the tendon sheaths of these fingers. Therefore, neglected tenosynovitis in any of these digits (except that of the little finger whose tendon sheath extends directly into the ulnar bursa) may rupture across the fascial barrier at the termination of the tendon sheath into the palmar space. When the palmar space is infected, the palmar concavity is more or less obliterated, although the paucity of soft tissue makes swelling less evident. Over the dorsum of the hand, however, there is a prominent swelling which is merely a lymphedema and not a true cellulitis. Excruciating tenderness over the space is a very diagnostic feature. Fever, prostration and severe pain usually accompany such infections. A midpalmar abscess lies next to the ulnar bursa and may rupture into it, thereby spreading directly under the annular ligament to the forearm. Not infrequently the abscess may break through the distal part of the deep aponeurosis of the hand and form a collar button abscess presenting dorsally at the web between the fingers. Any abscess at these sites should be suspected of communicating with the midpalmar space.

(b) The *thenar space* is on the radial side of the palm and partly covered by the thenar muscles. It extends distally as a prolongation along the lumbrical muscle to the base of the index finger. It becomes infected as an extension by rupture of a tenosynovitis of the index finger (but not of the thumb because its tendon sheath is continuous with the radial bursa). The infection usually breaks

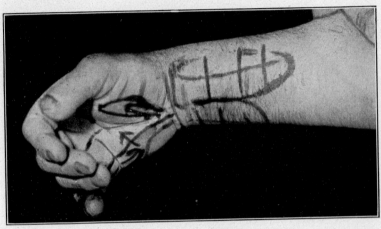

FIG. 34.—INFECTION OF ULNAR BURSA FROM AN ACUTE TENOSYNOVITIS OF THE LITTLE FINGER, SUSTAINED THREE DAYS BEFORE ADMISSION TO THE HOSPITAL FOLLOWING A SLIGHT SCRATCH.

Shortly after the rather trivial injury the patient, a fifty-five-year-old laborer had a severe chill lasting a half hour, followed by fever, local swelling and redness and general malaise. His doctor incised the finger twenty-four hours later with little relief. The extent of the process is outlined in the photograph. Operation revealed pus in both the ulnar and radial bursae, extending above the annular ligament and also in the thenar space. *Streptococcus hemolyticus* was isolated from the blood stream. The infection grew worse in spite of adequate drainage, tissue icterus developed and the patient died ten days after he was first seen. Note the small amount of swelling; this is characteristic of streptococcus infections of the hand. Since the introduction of sulfanilamide a fatal outcome can often be avoided in these cases.

through the boundaries of the thenar space, and points superficially in the web space between the thumb and index finger. Because of the proximity of the radial bursa, it may rupture into this space and in that manner spread into the wrist and forearm. Thenar abscesses are also prone to form collar button abscesses by burrowing and presenting dorsally into the web between the thumb and index finger producing obvious signs at this site.

The manifestations of abscess of the thenar space are thus similar to those produced by the palmar space except for the location of the swelling. Treatment is incision and drainage under precautions to be mentioned later.

6. **Infections of the Radial and Ulnar Bursae.**—As already indicated this type of infection is secondary to involvement of the tendon sheath of the thumb and little finger respectively, or of the palmar spaces. They are rarely involved primarily. The infection tends to spread rapidly up into the forearm and to produce necrosis of the flexor tendons. Infection of these bursae is accompanied by marked

local tenderness and swelling. Flexion and extension of the respective digits will be limited sharply because of pain. Fever is quite constant as in fascial space infection. Early incision is indicated (see Figure 36). Even if necrosis of the tendon is prevented by early incision, there may still be disability because of the adhesions between the tendon and its sheath.

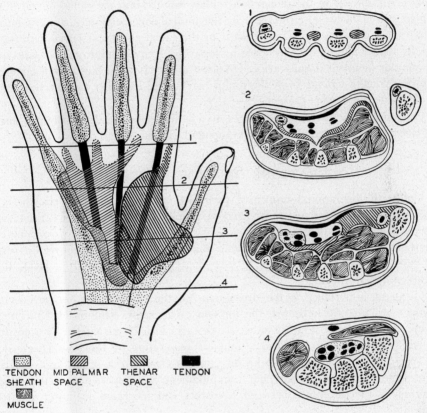

TENDON SHEATH MID PALMAR SPACE THENAR SPACE TENDON
MUSCLE

FIG. 35.—DIAGRAM ILLUSTRATING THE VARIOUS SPACES AND TENDON SHEATHS IN THE HAND WHICH ARE IMPORTANT IN TRACING THE PROBABLE PATHS OF EXTENSION OF INFECTION.

The four illustrations on the right represent cross sections taken from levels as indicated on the left. (Modified from Kanavel and from Eycleshymer and Schoemaker.)

Summary of Methods of Extension.—The mode and direction of extension of infection in the various spaces of the hand may be summarized as follows (modified from Homans) :

(a) Tenosynovitis of the thumb spreads readily to the radial bursa, and thence under the annular ligament into the forearm.

(b) Tenosynovitis of the index finger is limited slightly by the fascial barrier at the termination of the sheath, but ruptures (especially in neglected cases) readily into the thenar space, which is in close relation to the tendon sheath of the index finger.

(*c*) Tenosynovitis of the middle and ring finger is likewise limited slightly by the fascial barriers at the termination of the tendon sheaths, but ruptures readily into the midpalmar space. Occasionally, infection in the tendon sheath of the ring finger may rupture into the ulnar bursa.

(*d*) Tenosynovitis of the little finger extends readily into the ulnar bursa, and thence under the annular ligament into the forearm.

(*e*) An abscess in the thenar space may rupture into the radial bursa or mid-palmar space; likewise, an abscess in the midpalmar space may rupture into the thenar space or ulnar bursa; an abscess in the radial and ulnar bursa may rupture into the thenar and midpalmar space respectively. Extension into the forearm under the annular ligament usually arises from the ulnar or radial bursae, but apparently may occasionally extend from the midpalmar space. In either case such extension should be detected when present.

Obviously, any of the above spaces may be infected directly by wounds, including lacerations, punctured wounds, compound fractures, etc.

OPERATIONS ON HAND INFECTIONS

Unlike the operation for opening furuncles or simple abscesses elsewhere, the surgical treatment of the serious hand infections is often a major procedure requiring the utmost judgment and skill. With the exception of paronychia and superficial abscesses, all hand infections must be treated with the greatest respect and care. Unless one is prepared to treat these patients adequately it is far better to call in one who can.

Of great importance is the decision as to the proper time for incision and drainage. As already indicated, the incision of an acute cellulitis or lymphangitis is fraught with danger; on the other hand, early incision of a felon or acute tenosynovitis is essential to rapid and complete restoration of function. Diagnosis of the type and exact location of the infection is obviously a prime necessity. Frequent examinations may help, but the judgment and experience of the surgeon often spells the difference between a correct and incorrect diagnosis and treatment.

A general anesthesia (gas or pentothal sodium) should be used in operating upon the serious hand infections, not including the minor infections such as paronychia which necessitate only local or no anesthesia. By using a general anesthesia all pain is avoided, and the surgeon may carefully make his incision, explore the abscess or space without haste and make whatever counter or extended incisions are necessary. A tourniquet should be applied to prevent obscuring of the field with blood, and also to minimize the danger of infective material entering an open vein and gaining access to the general circulation. Before applying the dressing the tourniquet is removed and any bleeding points ligated. A knowledge of the finer anatomy of the hand is essential to avoid opening tendon sheaths when they are not involved, and to avoid nerve injury. The blood supply of the hand is so good that ligation of a major vessel results in no detrimental effects. Because of the free anastomosis between radial and ulnar arteries both ends of severed vessels must be tied.

The size and location of the incision or incisions depend on the type of infection. The locations of the various incisions advocated are indicated in the accompanying diagram (Fig. 36).

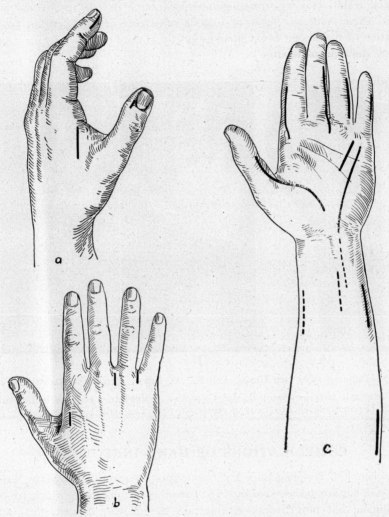

FIG. 36.—THE LOCATION OF THE VARIOUS TYPES OF INCISIONS USED IN INFECTIONS OF THE HAND.

a, The proper incisions for felon, thenar abscess and simple paronychia. In most instances, thenar abscesses need an additional incision on the palmar. side; *b,* The various incisions made upon the dorsum of the hand (redrawn from Kanavel) ; *c,* Possible incisions in case of infections of the tendon sheaths. The dotted lines indicate incisions made in exceptional cases (redrawn from Kanavel).

The incisions must be sufficiently long to adequately drain the abscess. On the other hand, it is essential that extension of the infections by incising uninvolved structures be avoided. Counter incisions on the hand, or rarely on the sides of the fingers may be necessary. When suppuration has extended into and beyond the wrist, the annular ligament should be divided. Boldness and accuracy should be the rule in the treatment of these patients.

The postoperative care is particularly important in order to achieve a perfect functional result. Hot wet dressings are used for a day or two to aid in drainage, and active motion is begun as soon as subsidence of pain permits. In this the coöperation of the patient is essential, especially in deep palmar infections and those involving the tendon sheaths.

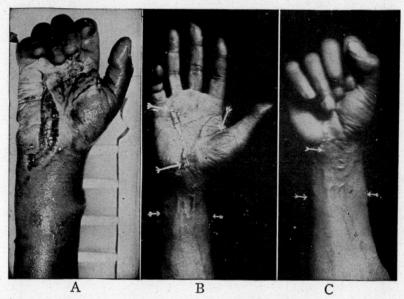

A   B   C

Fig. 37.—Incision into the Ulnar and Radial Bursa Extending above the Wrist.

A, photograph after incisions; *B,* and *C,* results obtained two and one half months after treatment. (From Kanavel, *Infections of the Hand,* 1933, Lea and Febiger, p. 420.)

COMPLICATIONS OF HAND INFECTIONS

Lymphangitis, lymphadenitis and septicemia frequently complicate infections of the hand, but are discussed elsewhere. The other complications which are perhaps less common, but nevertheless serious, are as follows: osteomyelitis, arthritis, gangrene and the disabled hand.

1. *Osteomyelitis* as a complication of hand infection is generally due to neglected or inadequate treatment. Its development in a felon has already been described. It also occurs in the metacarpal bones from severe and especially neglected fascial space infections. The phalanges are also infected occasionally from tenosynovitis and even from simple subcutaneous abscesses. Persistent drainage from a wound for more than two or three weeks suggests osteomyelitis, and an x-ray should be taken to verify the lesion.

2. *Suppurative arthritis* of the many joints of the hand is an infrequent complication and should not occur in promptly treated and effectively drained abscesses, unless, of course, a joint has been primarily infected at the time of the injury.

Diagnosis is difficult to make previous to destruction of the cartilage. After the cartilage is eroded, diagnosis is easily made by the grating sensation elicited in the joint upon movement of the finger. There may also be abnormal mobility of the digit due to destruction of the supporting ligaments. Early incision is indicated to prevent, as much as possible, the destruction of tissue (especially the cartilage).

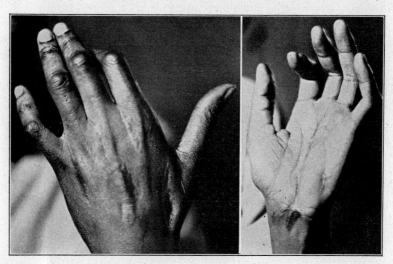

FIG. 38.—A PARTLY DISABLED HAND RESULTING FROM EXTENSIVE AND MULTIPLE INFECTIONS OF THE HAND IN A DIABETIC.

The infection started with a bruise which the patient opened with a pin; an infection developed, which was lanced three days later by her doctor. The thenar and mid-palmar spaces, as well as several dorsal abscesses had to be incised and drained before healing was complete. Present condition, one and one-half years later, represents only a partial return of function.

3. *Gangrene* of the fingers or entire hand is practically always due to special infections. Gas bacillus invasion is not the only cause. Human bites, because they introduce mixed organisms, are prone to cause symbiotic infections which may increase virulence to the point of producing gangrene. Human bites are discussed in more detail on the next page.

4. *The disabled hand* is a term used to describe the stiff atrophic useless hand which follows severe or inadequately treated infections. It is particularly prone to develop after acute tenosynovitis and infections of the bursal and palmar spaces. The tremendous scarring with adhesions between the tendons, their sheaths and adjacent tissues, is responsible in a large measure for the deformity and lack of mobility. To bring such a hand back to useful function presents a difficult therapeutic problem. Koch [7] has devoted special attention to rehabilitation in such disabilities. Undoubtedly many complications in hand infections are now prevented by the proper use of the sulfonamides which are discussed on page 35. Chemotherapy, it might be emphasized again, is most effective early in the stage of surgical infections before suppuration has occurred; it has no beneficial effect on pus which always requires drainage.

HUMAN BITES OF THE HAND.—These injuries deserve special mention because they present several unusual features. In the first place, the organisms introduced in such wounds often contain a variety of virulent bacteria which seem to invade much more rapidly than ordinary contaminants. For this reason, immediate cleansing treatment should be carried out, within an hour if possible, after the injury. Delay in primary treatment is much more apt to lead to serious results than in any other type of contaminated wound. A second feature of human bite infections is their tendency to produce infection of the joints, usually of the metacarpo-phalangeal joints at the knuckle. This is due to the fact that practically all of these injuries occur over the dorsum of the hand and fingers.

Treatment should be thorough and early and should consist of adequate cleansing of the entire hand and careful meticulous cleansing of the wound which must always be left open and the hand immobilized in a comfortable position. Should infection develop, and this occurs only in neglected cases, incision and drainage of abscesses, elevation and immobilization, heat and chemotherapy should be used. Because of the frequency of anaerobic organisms, the use of zinc peroxide paste is often indicated. The end result in the serious cases often involves ankylosis, destruction of tendon, and sometimes requires amputation of the digit. For further details, the reader is referred to other publications [6, 8].

BIBLIOGRAPHY

1. AUCHINCLOSS, H.   Surgery of the Hand, *Nelson's Surgery*, Vol. III, p. 459, 1927.
2. KANAVEL, A. B.   *Infections of the Hand,* Lea and Febiger, Phil., 7th ed., 1939.
3. KOCH, S. L. and KANAVEL, A. B.   The Diagnosis of Infections of the Hand, *Graham's Surgical Diagnosis,* Vol. I, p. 457, W. B. Saunders, 1930; also Felons, Acute Lymphangitis and Tendon Sheath Infections; Differential Diagnosis and Treatment, *J. Am. M. Ass.,* 92:1171, 1929.
4. COUCH, J. H.   Surgery of the Hand. *U. of Toronto Press,* 1939.
5. DORRANCE, G. M.   Felons, *Ann. Surg.,* 64:716, 1916.
6. MASON, M. L. and KOCH, S. L.   Human Bite Infections of the Hand, *Surg., Gynec. & Obst.,* 51:591, 1930.
7. KOCH, S. L.   Complicated Contractures of the Hand; Their Treatment by Freeing Fibrosed Tendons and Replacing Destroyed Tendons with Grafts, *Ann. Surg.,* 98:546, 1933.
8. MILLER, H. and WINFIELD, J. M. Human Bites of the Hand, *Surg., Gynec. & Obst.,* 74:153, 1942.

CHAPTER VI

MISCELLANEOUS INFECTIONS

Syphilis
Tuberculosis
Tetanus
Erysipelas
Gas Gangrene
Tularemia
Rabies
Vincent's Angina
Noma
Ludwig's Angina
Rat-bite Fever

Anthrax
Typhoid
Amebic Dysentery
Actinomycosis
Lymphogranuloma Inguinale
Echinococcus Disease
Granuloma Inguinale
Blastomycosis
Chancroid
Rarer Types of Miscellaneous
Surgical Infections

The miscellaneous infections described in this chapter differ greatly from the pyogenic infections already discussed. Most of them are caused by a variety of bacteria, some by viruses, and a few by agents still undiscovered. They are, in general, clinical entities however, although the clinical manifestations may be so obscure or puzzling as to create difficult diagnostic problems. Many of these miscellaneous infections are primarily of medical rather than surgical significance; all of them are important to the surgeon because they demand surgical treatment at one time or another or simulate diseases which do. The latter feature is undoubtedly of the most importance particularly because such surgical lesions as cancer may be simulated. In many instances these infections masquerade as acute and chronic pyogenic infections of the types already described. The diagnostic methods often necessary include most of the procedures used in other diseases although the principles involved in bacterial diagnosis are usually the most important. Besides direct examination and culture of purulent material, fresh, if possible, there are available the microscopic study of tissue removed as a biopsy, and the various immune reactions such as complement fixation, agglutination tests, skin tests, etc., to aid in diagnosis. In the difficult cases several or all of these various procedures may have to be used to arrive at an etiologic diagnosis, which of course should precede any hopeful method of therapy in all except the few infections which are self-limited and run their course without leaving any sequelae.

SYPHILIS

The history of the origin of syphilis is extremely interesting, chiefly because of the vast disagreement as to which nation was responsible for the epidemic which swept Europe during the last part of the fifteenth century. Previous to this time the disease cannot be identified with certainty in the medical writings. The Spanish soldiers of Columbus have been accused of bringing the disease back from America. It was not until 1905 that Schaudinn and Hoffmann [1] described the *Spirochaeta pallida* (*Treponema pallidum*) as the causative organism. The discovery of salvarsan by Ehrlich [2] a few years later is of epochal importance because the drug was one of the first synthetic specifics known to medicine. Its discovery started chemotherapy on its way.

The disease is of venereal origin and can be acquired in no other way except close contact, because the spirochete is delicate and only survives a very short time outside the body. Any organ of the body may be affected, and in such a variety of ways that the disease is of great surgical significance, especially from the standpoint of diagnosis. Numerous serological tests, including the Kahn, Wassermann, Kline, Kolmer, Hinton, etc., are in use and are extremely valuable in establishing the diagnosis.

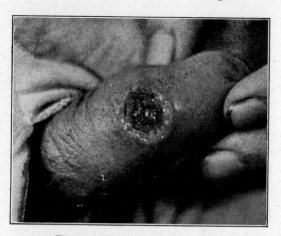

FIG. 39.—CHANCRE OF THE PENIS.

The *primary stage,* or chancre, appears usually on the genitals, sometimes on the lip, three to four weeks following exposure. The lesion is flat, indurated, button-like and after several days ulcerates over the surface. From this ulceration the spirochete is readily isolated and identified with the aid of dark field examination. The lesion is indolent and does not heal for several weeks unless active antiluetic treatment is instituted in the meantime. Regional lymph nodes may enlarge painlessly, but never break down unless secondarily infected with pyogenic organisms. Six to ten weeks after the primary lesion appears, the *secondary stage,* which is an expression of the systemic invasion of the spirochetes, manifests itself. The accompanying eruption which appears over the skin and mucous membranes has varied characteristics. At varying intervals, from a few months to several years, the *tertiary stage* develops. The gumma which typifies this stage is of variable size and may appear in any tissue or system of the body. Gummas are smooth and soft and because of associated arterial lesions such as thrombosis and endarteritis, are avascular and may break down, forming a necrotic mass. True suppuration, however, does not occur unless secondary pyogenic infection is implanted. Cutaneous tertiary lesions or syphilides may appear and produce stubborn ulcerations such as are commonly seen on the leg.

Syphilis is a prevalent disease, even at the present time, and its eradication presents a sharp challenge to the medical profession. Recognition of the disease should enlist every type of medical practitioner, public as well as private. It is of utmost importance to realize that the *adequate* treatment in the primary stage yields a far higher percentage of complete cures than therapy in the tertiary, or even in the secondary stage. Early recognition before the Wassermann or Kahn test becomes positive, is, therefore, an ideal to be constantly striven for. Identification of the spirochete by dark field illumination is a most positive diagnostic test and should be carried out on all primary lesions. In the later stages the search for syphilis should be intensified; it is made easier by the Wassermann reaction, which should become a routine procedure in all hospital patients. Thousands of unsuspected cases of syphilis are recognized each year by taking routine Wassermanns on all admissions, private or ward, in many general, obstetrical, and other hospitals. Its importance cannot be overemphasized. It is extremely important also that the treatment of syphilis be sufficiently intensive and prolonged; the physician must not be content with two or three injections of mercury and salvarsan.

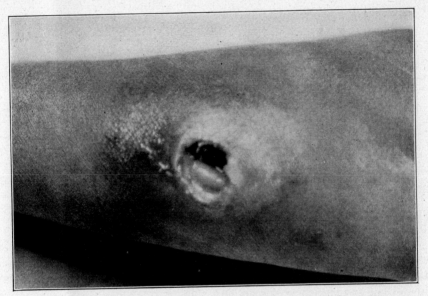

Fig. 40.—Gumma of Forearm in a Negro Woman Aged Forty-five.

Date of primary lesion unknown. The patient complained of a mass in the forearm which, under intensive antiluetic treatment, rapidly softened and sloughed, leaving a deep ulcer as shown in the photograph. Healing was complete in a few weeks.

Mouth.—Hutchinsonian teeth and scarring about the mouth are manifestations of congenital syphilis. Primary lesions may occur on the lips or tongue, and be occasionally mistaken for carcinoma, but gummas of the tongue are of much more surgical significance because of the enormous amount of destruction of tissue in some cases, and because of the frequent association with carcinoma. The differentiation between gumma and carcinoma of the tongue frequently cannot be made without a biopsy. Occasionally leukoplakia of syphilitic origin may simulate that associated with epithelioma (see page 302).

Nose and Throat.—Although redness and edema of the pharynx is a rather constant accompaniment of early syphilis, the rarer lesions (gummas) are of much more surgical significance. Gummas of the nasal septum may produce a perforation with a subsequent depression of the nasal bridge. Such deformities can only be corrected by plastic operations such as cartilage transplantation.

Gastro-intestinal Tract.—Gummatous ulceration of the stomach may produce symptoms of mild pain and dyspepsia associated with other clinical signs of a pyloric obstruction which are very similar indeed to carcinoma of the stomach. The roentgenological signs are also similar to those encountered in carcinoma of the stomach. The question of syphilis of the stomach always arises when manifestations of gastric ulcer or carcinoma occur in a patient with a positive Wassermann. Surgical excision of the ulcerated area is usually indicated, because the cicatricial obstruction which follows chemotherapeutic healing will probably make operation necessary anyway. For that reason differential diagnosis is somewhat academic, except that differentiation from carcinoma is helpful or even necessary, to aid in determination of the extent of resection.

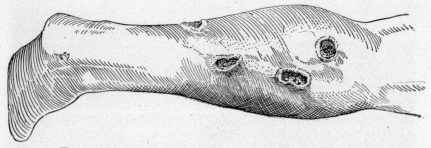

FIG. 41.—SYPHILITIC ULCERS (TERTIARY LESIONS) OF THE LEG.

Note the punched-out appearance. Such ulcers are usually multiple. Administration of antiluetic treatment is not always curative. Fever therapy usually results in complete healing, but recurrence is not uncommon.

Many years ago huge gummas of the liver were commonly seen, and presented considerable difficulty in differentiation from intra-abdominal cysts and benign tumors which might obviously be amenable to operation. During late years, because of the extent and efficiency of early antisyphilitic treatment, such lesions are rare. An acute syphilitic infiltration of the liver of the cirrhotic type, with the production of jaundice and other signs of portal obstruction is more common.

Gummas were formerly thought to occur frequently in the terminal portion of the rectum, and after the diffuse scarring which follows the massive destruction of tissue, to terminate in a stricture. However, it seems probable that most, if not all, of the cases of stricture of the rectum are really caused by lymphogranuloma inguinale (see page 101) and not syphilis.

Skin.—Reference has already been made to the primary and secondary lesions of the skin. More significant surgically are tertiary lesions (gummas) which appear in the subcutaneous tissues as indurated nodules, breaking down through the skin, forming ulcers. Such ulcers are usually punched out, occurring most commonly on the upper part of the leg, but may be encountered any place on the body (see Fig. 41).

Bones and Joints.—Infection of bones, especially the long bones, is common and manifests itself in one of three ways: (1) periosteal form, (2) hyperplastic or associated with overgrowth, and (3) destructive. Joints may become involved to such an extent that disability is pronounced (Charcot's joint). These features are discussed in detail in Chapter XIX.

Central Nervous System.—The most common types of syphilitic invasion of the central nervous system are tabes and paresis, but these conditions do not present the surgical problems that are encountered in gumma of the brain which is rare, but may present all the symptoms and signs of a brain tumor. Occasionally, visceral crises (in tabes) consisting of severe abdominal pain simulate an acute intra-abdominal surgical condition. In addition, however, to the presence of tabetic signs, a careful consideration will usually reveal a lack of muscle spasm, tenderness, leukocytosis, nausea, vomiting, etc., which would be present in an acute surgical process. Paretics are occasionally seen in the emergency room because of prostration and coma.

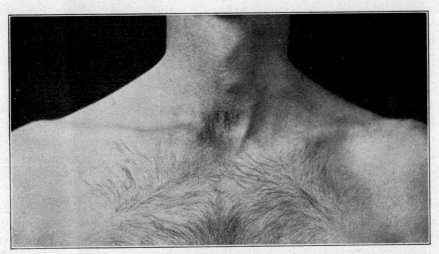

Fig. 42.—Gumma of the Right Sternoclavicular Joint in a Young Man, Aged Twenty-eight.

Within a few weeks after the onset of intensive antiluetic therapy the swelling disappeared completely (Washington University Clinic).

The tabetic bladder is commonly observed and presents disturbing symptoms such as incontinence, especially at night, and dribbling of urine. A varying amount of residual urine may be constantly present, but infection does not readily become implanted unless instrumentation is excessively or carelessly performed.

TUBERCULOSIS

In 1882 Koch[3] demonstrated the fact that tuberculosis was caused by an acid-fast organism which was given the name tubercle bacillus. He formulated a law relative to reproduction of the disease in animals. There are two important types of organisms (human and bovine) which differ considerably in virulence and method of invasion. The bovine strain was differentiated from the human strain by Theobald Smith.[4] Considerable evidence has accumulated to suggest that most of the primary infections of the lymph nodes, which were known years ago as scrofula, are caused by the bovine strain. The same may be said about tuberculous osteomyelitis of the long bones and hyperplastic tuberculosis of the cecum, which are commonly seen in the British Isles where pasteurization of milk is not universal, but rarely encountered in the United States where pasteurization is general. It is assumed that the bovine bacillus, present in contaminated milk, may penetrate the pharyngeal mucosa or tonsil, thereby infecting the cervical lymph nodes, and by ingestion into the alimentary tract give rise to certain types of alimentary tuberculosis. The fact that tuberculosis of the cervical nodes is decreasing as the practice of pasteurization of milk is becoming more prevalent, lends support to this theory.

Koch also originated the idea of using a preparation (tuberculin) obtained from the growing tubercle bacilli, as a diagnostic test of the disease. The von Pirquet test, which consisted of the introduction of a small quantity of tuberculin into the skin by scarification, is perhaps not so reliable as the intradermal injection with a hypodermic needle. The dose of 0.1 milligram should be decreased to 0.01 milligram if an active lesion is present. Since a positive reaction is obtained regardless of whether the lesion is healed or not, the test is obviously more valuable in children, because nearly all adults have healed lesions and will give a positive reaction. A negative test is of course valuable at any age.

Calmette, Guérin and associates [5] for years have been advocates of the efficacy of B.C.G. vaccine in the prevention of tuberculosis by immunization, especially in infancy and childhood. The vaccine consists of organisms which are attenuated by innumerable subcultures to the extent that they may be given orally or subcutaneously without instigating an active tuberculous infection. The method offers epochal possibilities, but as yet is not generally used or accepted.

Pulmonary Tuberculosis.—In unilateral tuberculosis, surgical procedures may be extremely efficient in arresting the disease and encouraging healing. Phrenicectomy (avulsion of the phrenic nerve) paralyzes the diaphragm on the side of the operation and obtains rest for the affected lung which is, of course, impossible if normal respiratory movements are allowed. Perhaps a more efficient method of obtaining rest and immobilization of the lung tissue is by means of extrapleural thoracoplasty. Frequently removal of the ribs over the apex (apical thoracoplasty) is sufficient to obtain the desired mechanical compression if the disease is confined to the apex. Tuberculous empyema is a stubborn and resistant disease (see Chapter XXIX).

Tuberculosis of the Lymph Nodes.—As stated, involvement of the lymph nodes is probably becoming less common in the United States. Onset is usually insidious without constitutional symptoms. Cervical and mediastinal nodes are commonly affected. The nodes in the axillary and inguinal region and in the intestinal mesentery are less commonly involved. For detailed description of tuberculosis of the lymph nodes see Chapter XXI.

Intestinal Tuberculosis.—Ulceration of the cecum may be produced by the tubercle bacillus and may clinically resemble carcinoma or idiopathic ulcerative colitis. However, roentgen examination with the barium meal will be of material aid in differentiation if lesions are demonstrable in the sigmoid, because tuberculosis rarely affects this part of the colon. The first symptoms of tuberculosis of the cecum are apt to consist of inconstantly cramping pain in the abdomen associated with diarrhea of varying degree and possibly nausea and vomiting. If the ulceration is present throughout the entire colon, the symptoms may vary but little from those produced by a localized tuberculosis. In either case blood should be found in the stool. Intestinal tuberculosis is apt to be associated with, or secondary to, pulmonary tuberculosis, thereby adding considerably to the seriousness of the condition.

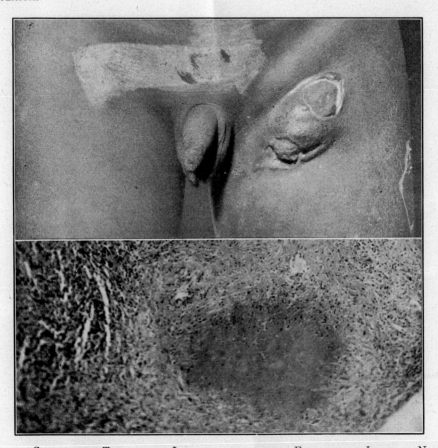

FIG. 43.—SUPPURATING TUBERCULOUS LYMPHADENITIS OF THE FEMORAL AND INGUINAL NODES.

Tuberculous lymphadenitis in this location is infrequent; the cervical and mediastinal nodes are involved most commonly. The patient is a Negro boy aged eleven, who noted a fluctuant swelling in the femoral region. Six months previously incision by a family physician resulted in the evacuation of an ounce or two of pus. The ulceration noted in the illustration developed since the incision. Total excision of the involved lymph nodes was carried out; complete healing occurred after two or three weeks. No other focus of tuberculosis was found at any time. Below the photo is a photomicrograph of the excised tissue, showing tubercle formation; note also the marked necrosis.

Occasionally, tuberculosis is demonstrable in fistulous tracts resulting from ischiorectal abscess and may be the primary etiological factor in the production of the abscess. In such instances there is usually an associated generalized tuberculous infection; it should be emphasized, however, that tuberculosis accounts for only a very small portion of the fistulas about the rectum and anus.

Tuberculous Peritonitis.—Invasion of the peritoneal cavity is, of course, a secondary infection, primary perhaps to tuberculosis of the mesenteric lymph nodes, intestine or Fallopian tube. The symptoms are extremely variable and diagnosis is frequently made only at laparotomy. The intestines and omentum are commonly studded with tubercles. On other occasions, ascites is more or less pro-

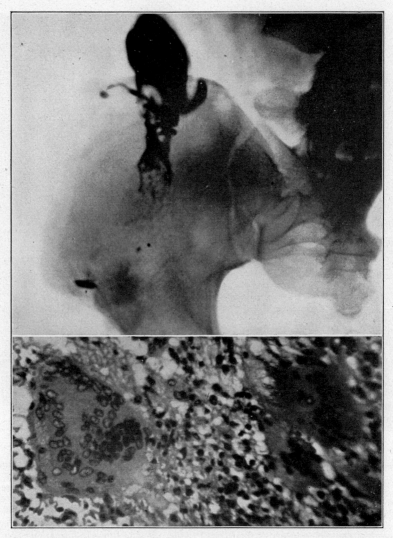

FIG. 44.—X-RAY OF PATIENT (NEGRO MAN, AGED THIRTY-FIVE) AFTER INJECTION OF A FISTULOUS TRACK IN THE RIGHT LOWER QUADRANT WITH LIPIODOL, MOST OF WHICH HAS PASSED INTO THE CECUM.

Twenty years previously the patient had an abscess of the right lower quadrant which was incised by a physician; the resultant sinus drained for two years, then closed, but reopened four months ago. At operation, a fistulous track connected with the cecum and surrounded by a large amount of fibrous tissue was excised. The opening in the cecum was closed by means of a purse-string suture. Below the x-ray film is a photomicrograph of the fistulous track showing two giant cells, indicative of tuberculosis.

nounced and the intestines may be matted together with adhesions which may likewise surround caseous areas. Not infrequently the disease may be much more acute and ushered in with symptoms suggestive of a subacute appendicitis. Treatment is unsatisfactory, but for some unexplainable reason laparotomy usually effects a definite improvement (see Chapter XXV).

Tuberculosis of the Bones and Joints.—As previously stated, the bovine bacillus is probably responsible for invasion of the bone and usually attacks children or young adults in preference to adults. Vertebrae are the bones most frequently affected, although the head of the femur is also commonly diseased. The joints are usually affected by extension from the bone. The most important feature in the treatment of tuberculosis of the bone or joint is rest and immobilization. A more detailed description of tuberculosis of bones and joints may be found in Chapter XIX.

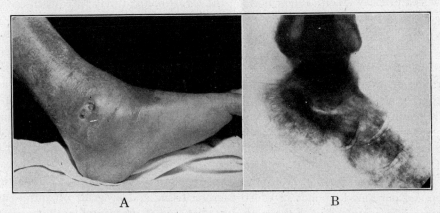

A   B

FIG. 45.—TUBERCULOSIS OF THE ANKLE.

Nine months previously, the patient, a man aged sixty-eight, sustained an injury to the ankle of sufficient severity to cause him to go to bed. Moderate disability persisted. Five months ago, his family physician incised an abscess about the ankle. There was roentgenological and auscultatory evidence of pulmonary tuberculosis, but there were no tubercle bacilli in the sputum. In view of disability, and poor prognosis as to healing of the process in the joint, amputation was performed. *A,* photo of the ankle and foot; *B,* the x-ray film reveals a suppurative process involving the tibia, fibula, and astragalus at the joint. Note the bone atrophy which is so common following prolonged disuse.

Genito-urinary Tuberculosis.—The most important organ of this system attacked by tuberculosis is the kidney. Destructive abscesses appear, but frequently with no significant symptoms until the disease is implanted in the bladder, at which time frequency and urgency of urination will be complained of. Red blood cells and pus cells, as well as tubercle bacilli, are found in the urine. Vague pains in the loin, mild fever and malaise are common symptoms as the disease progresses. If the disease is unilateral, as may be determined by pyelograms, nephrectomy is indicated. Elimination of the focus of infection practically always eradicates the infection in the bladder (see also Chapter XXXII).

In women the Fallopian tubes occasionally are infected. Tubercles first appear, but soon the fimbriated ends become sealed off and the walls thickened, but containing variable quantities of caseous thick pus. In the male, tuberculosis occasionally invades the epididymis, producing a mildly tender and painful organ which increases moderately in size and ultimately may break down and form a sinus extending through the scrotal wall. Removal of the epididymis yields satisfactory results. Occasionally the prostate and seminal vesicles are invaded.

Tuberculosis of the Central Nervous System.—Invasion of the nervous system may manifest itself either as a meningitis which, although of many weeks' duration, is universally fatal, or as a tuberculoma. The latter lesion may produce symptoms identical to those encountered in brain tumor.

There are innumerable other regions where tuberculosis may develop, but most of them are so rare as not to be of great importance. Tuberculosis of the *larynx* is a slowly developing, painful disease, usually terminating fatally. Invasion of the *skin* with the production of ulcers was common years ago, but is rarely encountered now as a primary lesion. Tuberculosis of the *breast* occurs rarely; it is discussed on page 823.

TETANUS

The etiological factor in this disease is the tetanus bacillus, an anaerobic spore-forming organism which was first described by Nicolaier [6] in 1884. The spores are extremely resistant to drying, and will survive boiling for one hour in plain water. It is regularly found in the intestinal tract of the horse, less frequently in many other domestic animals, and to a considerably less extent (20 to 30 per cent) in the intestinal tract of human beings. The bacillus is likewise widely distributed in soil which has been fertilized with manure.

Since the organism is anaerobic the disease is more apt to be contracted following deep and punctured wounds in which necrotic tissue and pyogenic organisms are present. The consumption of the oxygen in the tissue of the wound by the pyogenic bacteria creates the anaerobic conditions necessary for the growth of the tetanus bacillus and thus the production of the disease. Although the bacilli have been cultured from lymph nodes adjacent to infected wounds (Porter and Richardson [7]) they tend to remain locally in the wound. In the United States tetanus is more common in the South than in the North, being particularly prevalent in the states bordering the Gulf of Mexico (Moore and Singleton [8]). Confusion still exists as to the mechanism through which the toxin exerts its fatal effect. Meyer and Ransom [9] suggested that the toxin reached the spinal cord through the axis cylinders of the peripheral nerves. This was not confirmed by the experiments of Abel and associates,[10] who noted further that tetanus toxin is fixed by the tissues; only when more than a lethal dose was given could any be recovered from the circulating blood and lymph. Moreover, Firor and associates [11] found that the toxin does not travel up the spinal cord to the brain; they suggested also that "the toxin in the spinal cord is altered into or liberates a different lethal agent which is transported to and has its lethal effect on vital centers." Their experiments showed that this lethal agent was not neutralized by tetanus antitoxin.

Prophylaxis and Immunity.—Theoretically every patient sustaining a contaminated wound extending through the skin should have the benefit of a prophylactic injection of antitoxin. However, if careful judgment is exercised, a large percentage of patients with minor cuts or lacerations need not be given antitoxin. For example, a superficial laceration sustained by a housewife while washing glassware or dishes which are used and cleaned daily, is not apt to be contaminated with tetanus bacilli. Wounds sustained in the street, and punctured wounds produced by rusty nails or sharp objects lying in contact with filth or soil are apt to be contaminated with tetanus bacilli. In such instances an injection of 1500 units of tetanus antitoxin should be given. This dose may be reduced in children, but it *cannot safely be reduced in direct proportion to the weight.* It is also necessary to perform a débridement of the wound (except infected and punctured wounds) removing blood clots and foreign material and excising dead tissue (see Chapter X). When the wound is extensive, and contamination with tetanus bacilli seems

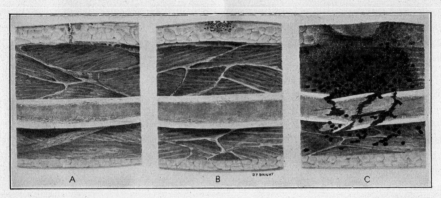

FIG. 46.—TYPES OF WOUNDS WHICH ARE PARTICULARLY PRONE TO RESULT IN TETANUS UNLESS ADEQUATE PROPHYLACTIC THERAPY IS INSTITUTED (see text).

A, punctured wound inflicted by a dirty nail; the anaërobic conditions resulting from this type of wound, along with the foreign bodies (rust, dirt, etc.) are conducive to the growth of tetanus bacilli; *B,* wound inflicted by blank cartridge pistol. Note the tiny but numerous perforations of the skin, and the implantation of such foreign bodies as burned powder, paper wadding and particles of clothing in the subcutaneous tissues; *C,* wound inflicted by shotgun at close range. Note the enormous destruction of tissue, including bone, and the large number of foreign bodies (shot). This type of wound is also very prone to result in the development of gas gangrene.

obvious (*e.g.,* gunshot wounds or injuries sustained in barnyards), the prophylactic dose should be increased to 3000 units. Since the *passive immunity conferred by the administration of antitoxin lasts only ten to fourteen days* it may also be advisable to repeat the injection in about ten days, especially if the wound was extensive and tissue destruction so great as to prevent rapid healing. Usually, however, the wound has healed so completely by the time the passive immunity has worn off that the local immunity of the tissue surrounding any remaining tetanus bacilli is sufficient to prevent the growth of the organism. It is a well-known fact that tetanus spores may survive in tissues for months without producing symptoms of tetanus. If this area containing the tetanus spores or bacilli is injured, as, for example, by a secondary operation for removal of a foreign body, the patient may then contract the disease. *For this reason, another prophylactic dose of antitoxin must be given at the time such secondary operations are performed, if more than ten days have elapsed since the initial prophylactic dose of antitoxin.* It is a well-known fact, however, that if tetanus develops even after the passive immunity produced by the initial prophylactic injection wears off, the disease will be mild, and with proper treatment the patient usually recovers.

Utilizing the injection of toxoid * as popularized by Ramon and associates,[12] it is now possible to produce an active immunization to tetanus lasting 2 or 3 years. The advantage of active over passive immunity would be appreciated most in military surgery or in trades where injuries are extremely frequent. The fact that injection of toxoid eliminates sensitization to horse serum is undoubtedly worthy of consideration. Favorable results have been obtained by Hall,[13] Gold,[14] and others. Very little immunity is conferred by the first dose. However, when a second dose is given four weeks later, definite immunity is conferred within four to six days following the second dose. A third dose produced a marked rise in antitoxin titer which is maintained over a longer period of time than after the second. Active immunization after this method is now being used in the U. S. Army and Navy.** The fact that no cases of tetanus were encountered following the Pearl Harbor attack (Halford [15]) is fairly good evidence of the efficacy of toxoid which had previously been given to practically all the casualties.

The great danger in administration of antitoxin is the development of *anaphylactic shock* (manifestations of which include marked tachycardia, laryngeal stridor, bronchial spasm, cyanosis and collapse) which if severe may result fatally within a very few minutes after the injection. Death occurs only in patients extremely sensitive to horse serum and is encountered rarely, indeed, except as an immediate reaction.

Before tetanus antitoxin is administered, inquiry should be made as to whether the patient has had any injections of serum within the past several years or is subject to asthma, hay fever or urticaria. If there is any possibility that the patient is sensitive to horse serum, it is preferable to inject a small drop of antitoxin, diluted several times with physiological saline solution, intradermally with a fine needle. If the patient is sensitive to horse serum, a large wheal surrounded by a hyperemic zone will develop within a few minutes. Desensitization can be fairly adequately accomplished by the frequent injection of graduated doses of serum. There are several methods of graduating these successive doses, but it is probably sufficient to start with the subcutaneous injection of .05 c.c. If no significant symptoms appear within thirty minutes the dose is doubled every thirty minutes until 1 c.c. is given. In twenty minutes 0.1 c.c. may be given intravenously and if no reaction is noted the intravenous dose is doubled every twenty minutes until the required amount of serum is given. Adrenalin should be given to combat any reaction sustained.

The term *serum sickness* has been assigned to the late allergic response of the body to the foreign serum and is fortunately encountered in only a small percentage of cases. This sensitivity may be due to a previous injection of serum or may be an inherited characteristic. In the latter instance, reactions are more apt to be anaphylactic in character. Symptoms appear four to ten days after the injection, and

---

* Toxoid is made by addition of formalin, agar, alum and other substances to tetanus toxin. The alum precipitated toxoid appears to be the most satisfactory.

** See note page 114.

are usually ushered in by a generalized itching, urticaria or erythematous rash of the skin, appearing first at the site of injection. Fever is not uncommon, especially in children; stiffness and pain about the joints is frequently complained of. Generalized enlargement of lymph nodes is common. Such nodes are usually tender to palpation, but of course do not suppurate. Treatment consists of the subcutaneous injection of adrenalin; serum sickness is practically never fatal. More recent reports (Foshay and Hagebusch [16]) suggest that histaminase may be much more effective in the treatment of the serum sickness.

Clinical Manifestations.—The incubation period of tetanus varies from four to ten days, but may be delayed several weeks by such mechanisms as insufficient prophylactic antitoxin, etc. In the acute cases death usually occurs within four or five days. It is an established fact that the longer a patient lives after the onset of symptoms, the better are his chances of recovery. It is likewise true that the severity of the disease decreases as the length of incubation time increases. On the other hand, the disease is much more serious when the wound is near the brain (*i.e.,* head, neck, etc.)

Usually the first symptom noted is limitation of movements of the jaw due to muscle spasm (lockjaw or trismus). It should be remembered, however, that lockjaw is most commonly produced by inflammatory lesions about the jaw. Stiffness of the neck, and cramps or stiffness of the muscles in the region of the wound soon follow. The muscles of deglutition are also affected, sometimes to the extent that it is impossible for the patient to swallow. Laryngeal spasm of sufficient severity to produce respiratory difficulty may also occur. Hesitancy in micturition caused by spasm of the sphincter is commonly encountered. In the more acute cases, spasm of the muscles of the back may be so marked as to produce a severe grade of opisthotonos. The eyes are usually fixed and staring. Spasm of the facial muscles produces the sardonic smile (risus sardonicus) which is notoriously known to accompany the disease. The rigidity of the muscles of the jaw may be so great as to demand feeding by means of a nasal catheter.

In addition to the tonic spasms described above, clonic spasms or convulsions develop later in the disease. The peripheral irritation producing these convulsions need be nothing more than a slight sound or light touch. The hideous facial expression of the patient in a convulsion is so impressive as not to be forgotten. The temperature may be normal or elevated, except that there is always a terminal hyperpyrexia. Tachycardia is not pronounced except shortly before death.

Treatment.—The treatment of tetanus is curative only when instituted early and in mild cases. As soon as the diagnosis is made, tetanus antitoxin should be administered in large quantities, assuming of course that proper attention is given to the possibility of sensitivity to horse serum. In many cases when the patient is first seen the diagnosis may be uncertain, but sufficiently suggestive to warrant administration of antitoxin. Recent investigations suggest that the intravenous method of administration is superior to others. The dose on the day of admission should obviously be larger than the succeeding days. As a routine 50,000 to 100,000 units should be given the first day. Additional serum should be given daily in smaller doses as indicated by progress of the disease. It is doubtful whether there is any advantage in the introduction of antitoxin intraspinally.

Cole and Spooner [17] have conducted observations on the rate of excretion of antitoxin and noted that seven days after the injection of 200,000 units there still remains slightly over 50,000 units of antitoxin in the circulating blood. On this basis they advise a single, massive, intravenous dose unless the focus of tetanus bacilli and spores in the wound and elsewhere has not been completely removed. However, since toxin in certain tissue (*e.g.,* nervous tissue) is neutralized slowly, it would appear necessary to maintain a high concentration of antitoxin in the blood at all times during the course of the disease.

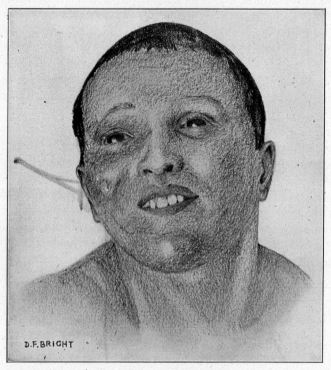

FIG. 47.—RISUS SARDONICUS AS OBSERVED IN A PATIENT WITH TETANUS.
Drawn from DeQuervain.

The patient must be kept in a quiet and dark room. Every possible effort should be exerted to *control the convulsions with heavy doses of narcotics and sedatives.* Gnagi [18] has called attention to the efficacy of sodium amytal, subcutaneously or intravenously, in controlling the convulsions. However, the rectal administration of avertin twice daily is probably superior. Prevention of convulsions is extremely important because the symptoms produced by the toxin are apparently more responsible for the patient's death than the toxin itself; all clinicians now agree on this point. Frequently the patient is unable to ingest or swallow food and fluids because of muscle spasm, thereby making it necessary to introduce them through a nasal catheter.

On many occasions the wound through which the infection was sustained will be healed; on a few occasions there will not even be a history of a wound. If the wound is healed, some surgeons advocate excising the area and not closing the resultant defect. On the other hand, there is a growing tendency (Spaeth[19]) to treat the wound in a case of tetanus as if the patient did not have the disease. However, if the wound is infected and sutures are in place they should be removed and the wound left open. Irrigation and *gentle* débridement may be carried out. The daily use of a creamy suspension of zinc peroxide (see page 123), especially in obviously infected wounds, is strongly indicated.

As stated, the prognosis of the fulminating case is poor. During the World War, Bruce[20] made a critical analysis of tetanus and noted that the mortality varied from 50 to 90 per cent, depending on the acuteness of the disease. However, if the adequately treated patient survives the first forty-eight to seventy-two hours recovery may be expected. The groups with the lower mortality possibly included patients who contracted the disease shortly after a prophylactic injection.

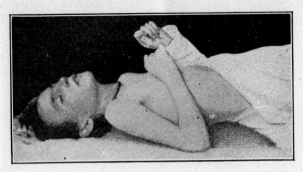

Fig. 48.—Opisthotonos in Third Day of Tetanus; Death Six Hours Later in Convulsions.

(From Ashurst, *Surgery*, 1931, 4th ed., Lea and Febiger, Philadelphia.)

These considerations suggest that tetanus antitoxin, although known to be very effective in preventing tetanus, may not be very effective in active treatment of the disease. This assumption is further borne out by the statistical data reported by Moore and Singleton[8] who studied their mortality rate year by year but noted no appreciable drop below their average mortality of 50 per cent, when the amount of antitoxin was increased. They have, however, noted a marked decline during recent years to a rate of 24 per cent for the last 25 cases, which they attribute to adequate sedation, tube feeding, parenteral fluids, radical treatment of the wound and better nursing care. In spite of the doubtful therapeutic value of antitoxin, it as yet appears advisable to administer it in large doses as already mentioned.

ERYSIPELAS

Erysipelas, which was commonly known years ago as St. Anthony's fire, is, at the present time at least, an acute, but only mildly contagious inflammation of the skin, especially of its capillary lymphatics, and is caused by the *Streptococcus erysipelatis* (Fehleisen[21]). Usually there is no visible lesion to explain the entrance of the organism into the skin. Presumably the invasion is made through tiny fissures or lesions microscopical in size. Although there is no doubt a contagious element to the disease, it seems probable that this phase of the disease has been exaggerated. Observation does not reveal many instances of contraction of the disease by contact, especially during recent years. Panton and Adams [22] analyzed the cases cared for in St. Thomas' Hospital from 1896 to 1905, during which time patients with erysipelas were not isolated. A review of the records after that time when isolation of the disease was instituted did not reveal any decrease in the number of cases occurring in the wards. Cooke [23] is of the opinion that the disease is contracted by auto-inoculation, that is, without coming in contact with an active case of erysipelas. The fact that the incidence of the disease shows equal distribution in males and females during infancy and childhood, but changes to 60 and 40 per cent respectively after the age of puberty when shaving is prevalent, appears to support the theory of auto-inoculation.

In his series of 1165 cases of erysipelas observed in various St. Louis hospitals, Cooke has also made an important observation regarding the pathogenesis and mortality of the disease. The analysis is so significant that Table 2 is reproduced from his report.

TABLE 2

Age Group	Number of Cases	Number of Deaths	Mortality, Per Cent
Under 1 year	98	54	55.1
1 year	23	6	26.1
2 to 14 years	116	2	1.7
15 to 29 years	130	4	3.1
30 to 49 years	343	25	7.3
50 to 64 years	306	44	14.4
65 and over	149	41	27.5
Total	1165	176	15.1

This series was compiled before the advent of the sulfonamides, but is reproduced because it shows so dramatically that the highest mortality rates are found in infants and in the aged. This difference in the mortality according to age of the patient no doubt accounts for much of the variation in mortality statistics as encountered in the medical literature.

The skin of the face is by far the site most commonly affected, but the skin of any portion of the body may be attacked. A red, edematous, tender and slightly raised area appears quite suddenly and usually shows a tendency to spread rapidly, but in no specific direction. Almost simultaneously with the appearance of the initial lesion, the patient develops fever and frequently a chill. Fever, however, may on rare occasions be absent. Pain and tenderness are extremely variable but may be absent. The border of the lesion is sharply defined and presents the most conspicuous evidence of inflammation. The reaction at the point of origin gradually fades and desquamation appears. Suppuration is uncommon, but occasionally is encountered as a localized superficial collection of thin pus, unless the area becomes contaminated with a staphylococcus, in which case the pus will be thicker and more profuse. The development of a dusky, cyanotic color usually indicates the onset of gangrene which, however, is rare.

Treatment.—In spite of the low degree of contagion, the patient should be isolated. Except in the very young and aged, the disease is self-limited and runs its course in about a week. Symtomatic treatment is usually all that is indicated in most instances. Adequate fluid and caloric intake should be maintained. Narcotics or sedatives may be necessary to permit sleep on account of pain. The older methods of therapy, *e.g.*, antitoxin (Symmers and Lewis [24]), x-ray and ultraviolet radiation

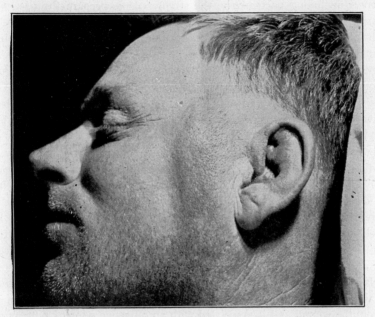

FIG. 49.—ERYSIPELAS OF THE FACE AFFECTING THE EAR.

Photograph taken twenty-four hours after onset which developed with a chill and fever. Note the edema. The raised precipitous edge which is so characteristic of erysipelas is present to a moderate degree in this patient (St. Louis City Hospital).

(Ude and Platou [25]), have been displaced by sulfanilamide. This drug (see p. 36) has resulted in a pronounced reduction in the mortality rate, for example, from 17.3 to 2.1 per cent in a series reported by Hoyne and associates.[26] As in the older reports most of the deaths occurred in the infants and the aged. Local applications of various kinds to the erysipelous lesions though long recommended and apparently useful on some occasions probably have no curative influence on the infection. Sulfadiazine is about as effective as sulfanilamide.

Erysipeloid is an infection of the skin which resembles erysipelas in appearance only. Often called "fish poisoning" it is acquired from handling fish and is really an occupational disease (Klauder [73]).

GAS GANGRENE

This disease has been of significance only during recent years, having first been encountered with any degree of frequency during World War I. The causative organism was originally thought to be specifically the *Bacillus aerogenes capsulatus* of Welch. It has since been demonstrated (Weinberg and Seguin [27]), however, that there are many other anaerobic organisms capable of producing gas gangrene. Perhaps the most important in addition to the Welch Bacillus already mentioned, are the Bacillus edematiens (Clostridium novyi), vibrion septique (Clostridium oedematis maligni), the Bacillus sordellii (Clostridium oldematoides) and the Bacillus histolyticus of Weinberg and Seguin. In many instances, colon bacilli and aerobic cocci, including particularly, the streptococcus, prepare the tissues for the development of the disease. Gas gangrene rarely occurs except in massive wounds in which considerable dirt has been deposited, and in which there has been considerable destruction of tissue, especially muscle. Compound fractures seem to encourage the development of the disease. Gas gangrene may occasionally be seen in which none of the so-called gas bacillus group of organisms is present. On these occasions very little gas may be noted in the tissues, but discoloration, edema, and destructive features are nevertheless present; the mortality rate in these lesions is not as high as in the typical gas gangrene.

Symptoms are apt to occur ten to twelve hours after the injury. Fever, tachycardia of an unusual degree, prostration and restlessness develop early and frequently progress in such a rapid fulminating manner as to cause death in two or three days. Swelling about the wound may occur so rapidly as to resemble a progressive hematoma. Crepitation produced by gas in the soft tissues, likewise, may be elicited as early as ten to twelve hours after injury. The crepitation produced by the forceful diffusion of air into the tissue by trauma may frequently resemble a gas gangrene in its incipiency, but observation over a period of a few hours relative to the progression of the crepitation should quickly differentiate between the two conditions. A profuse clear or slightly turbid brownish exudate drains from the wound and is associated with an offensive odor of putrefying flesh, which is so specific as to be almost pathognomonic of the disease. Gas bubbles may be seen in the discharge. Circulatory impairment, manifested by yellowish, bronze-colored or ecchymotic areas, which rapidly become cyanotic and then gangrenous, may appear in irregular patches in the skin surrounding the wound. From the onset the patient appears very ill, presenting many of the symptoms of shock. Delirium is frequently encountered. Pain is variable, but usually prominent. The causative organism may be found in the discharge from the wound a few hours after the accident, and usually before symptoms are manifested. Occasionally, however, gas-producing, anaerobic bacilli can be found in the wounds of patients who do not develop gas gangrene. Presumably, tissue immunity or efficient treatment has prevented the inception of the disease in such cases.

The infection primarily attacks the muscle, which early becomes cyanotic and edematous. It fails to bleed upon cut section, presumably because of vascular thrombosis or compression due to edema. Invasion may also take place between muscular sheaths or along fascial planes. A roentgenogram of the affected extremity may reveal collections of gas in the soft tissues which cannot be demonstrated by palpation. In spite of the brilliant work of Weinberg in isolating various strains of anaerobic organisms capable of producing the disease, it appears that the bacteriology of the disease is still not a closed subject. We are convinced, for example, that the amount of gas produced by the various strains of organisms is extremely variable and on many occasions, as stated previously, the disease may be present even in a severe form with the production of only a small amount of gas.

Treatment.—Prophylactic therapy consisting of early and thorough débridement (particularly with excision of devitalized muscle) minimizes development of the disease. Large doses of polyvalent antitoxin should also be given. Badly contaminated wounds in which gas gangrene is apt to develop should be left open after débridement, and packed gently with vaseline gauze and sulfathiazole (Reed and Orr[28]) or sulfadiazine (Dowdy and associates[28]). The drug should be continued orally or parenterally for several days. Either appears superior to sulfanilamide. Experimental studies by numerous workers suggests that penicillin may be still more effective prophylactically. Recent studies by Stewart[74] and others indicate that active immunity may be produced by administration of a toxoid as is now done for tetanus.

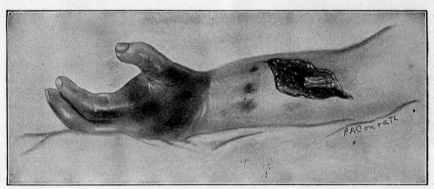

Fig. 50.—Gas Gangrene in a Patient Following a Compound Fracture of the Forearm.

When admitted to the hospital thirty hours after injury there already was marked swelling of the forearm with crepitation, patches of gangrenous skin and the typical offensive odor. Amputation was performed in the upper third of the arm several inches above the limits of crepitation. Within twenty-four hours the crepitation had involved the stump and shoulder. Patient was given massive doses of perfringens (anti-gas gangrene) antitoxin and made a miraculous recovery; sulfonamides were not yet available.

Once the disease has developed, active treatment must be begun immediately. (1) Intensive sulfonamide therapy should be instituted, preferably with sulfadiazine. (2) Likewise, in view of the favorable response obtained by Kelly[29] following x-ray therapy, this agent should also be utilized. It should be stated, however, that not all investigators utilizing x-ray therapy have had favorable results.[30] Preliminary information (Kelly[29], and Dowdy and associates[28]) suggests that x-ray therapy and sulfonamides should not be used in conjunction with each other. (3) Surgical treatment still remains important and no doubt is on many occasions the most important factor in therapy. If the disease is so far advanced that the extremity is enormously swollen and gangrenous, and toxicity severe, immediate amputation of the guillotine type will be necessary, and will frequently be a life-saving procedure. If the disease is detected early, multiple incisions and excision of devitalized tissue, particularly muscle, is usual'y indicated. Such wounds should be left open and packed with gauze saturated with a creamy suspension of zinc peroxide. (4) Opinions differ as to the value of antitoxin but the present authors recommend its use in large doses, *i.e.,* 100,000 to 150,000 units the first day and continuing as indicated, with smaller doses. The mortality should be less than 25 per cent.

TULAREMIA

This disease was first recognized by McCoy[31] in 1911, as a plague-like epidemic occurring in ground squirrels. A year later McCoy and Chapin isolated a bacillus which they called *Bacillus tularense,* after Tulare County, California, where the epidemic was investigated. The reports of a few cases in human beings appeared at sporadic intervals, but it was not until several years later that the disease was described in detail and the name tularemia given it by Francis.[32]

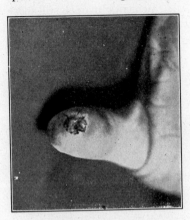

FIG. 51.—ULCER OF THUMB DUE
TO TULAREMIA.

The patient, a white woman aged thirty-six, suffered a punctured wound at this point five weeks previously while cleaning a rabbit. Three days later she had a chill and developed fever. A few days after this the ulcer on the thumb appeared. Fever persisted, accompanied by an occasional chill. Four weeks after onset the epitrochlear and axillary nodes enlarged and were incised later because of suppuration. The patient's serum agglutinated the *Bacillus tularense* in a dilution of 1 :160 (St. Louis City Hospital).

The disease is apparently prevalent in almost all the wild life of this country including especially the rabbit, squirrel, ground squirrel, woodchuck, fox and coyote. In animals transmission is by a parasite such as a tick, or by contamination of mouth lesions in carnivorous animals. The tick is the most common transmission factor in army recruits; in civilians nearly 95 per cent of the infections are contracted directly from rabbits, and nearly always while handling or dressing them. In most instances a history of sustaining a minor injury of the hands during the process of cleaning the animal can be obtained from the patient. The occurrence of the infection in laboratory workers suggests that the organism may invade the unbroken skin and produce the disease. The disease is not contracted by eating infected rabbits, providing the meat has been thoroughly cooked. The incubation time varies between extremely wide limits, but averages about six days. Natural immunity in human beings is apparently not common as is corroborated by the fact that numerous laboratory workers coming in contact with the bacillus have contracted the disease. It seems probable that tularemia is destined to become more frequent, but fortunately the mortality is comparatively low, approximately 4 per cent.

Clinical Manifestations.—The disease manifests itself clinically in four different ways. (1) The *ulceroglandular* type is by far the one most frequently recognized. The onset is abrupt with the typical features of an acute systemic infection including fever, chills, prostration, anorexia, headache, backache and occasionally delirium. The injury (usually on the hand) through which the disease was contracted, shows little tendency to heal and by the time clinical symptoms appear, begins to ulcerate. If the portal of entry is microscopical, a large indurated, only slightly tender papule appears at this time. As the disease progresses the central portion becomes necrotic and a superficial sinus or ulcer develops. Soon after the initial lesion reveals these signs of activation the lymph nodes draining that area become enlarged. These nodes, situated in the epitrochlear and axillary regions, are discrete and even during the process of suppuration cause little tenderness or pain. Suppuration of one or more of these nodes usually occurs at one time or another during the course of the disease. The period of febrile reaction is short, except in the serious and fatal cases, but returns intermittently after intervals of several days. Symptoms of this type may be encountered ten or twelve weeks after the onset of the disease. (2) In the *oculoglandular* type the primary lesion is in the conjunctiva, occasionally being found as a papule associated with edema, redness, lacrimation and photophobia. Ulcerations are not uncommon. The auricular, submaxillary and anterior cervical lymph nodes may enlarge and become moderately tender and painful. (3) A *glandular* type without evidence of a primary lesion is occasionally seen. In other respects, however, the symptoms and signs do not differ from those observed in the ulcero-glandular type. (4) A *typhoid type* producing fever without a visible primary lesion or lymphatic involvement is uncommon.

The diagnosis can be confirmed by agglutination of the bacterium tularense on addition of the suspected serum. However, a positive test is rarely encountered less than ten days after onset of the disease. More detailed data regarding pathogenesis, etc., may be found in Simpson's [33] monograph. The Foshay test, consisting of the intradermal injection of a B. tularense vaccine, is much more accurate and is positive from the second day of the disease up to about 18 months.

The most effective method of treatment is the administration of Foshay's antiserum.[34] Best results will be obtained if the serum is given early in the disease. Convalescent serum, as obtained from a patient who has recovered from the disease may be helpful if available. When suppuration appears at the site of infected lymph nodes, incision is indicated; drainage usually persists for many days or even weeks. Sulfonamides are occasionally effective.

RABIES

Rabies or hydrophobia is a spasmophilic or paralytic disease caused by a virus or micro-organism, and contracted by the bite of a rabid animal. The dog accounts for more than 90 per cent of the human cases, but wolves, cats, badgers, etc., may become infected and may also transfer the infection by their bite. Almost all animals, including horses, cows, etc., are susceptible and may contract the disease if bitten by rabid animals. Although the disease is less prevalent than fifty or one hundred years ago, it will probably always be a menace as long as misdirected human kindness allows the stray dog to roam the streets and countrysides. As an example of the constant prevalence of the disease over a period of eighteen months (1933 and 1934), the laboratories of the city of St. Louis gave preventive treatment (Harris [35]) to approximately 300 patients who had been bitten by presumably rabid dogs. It is quite certain that at least 80 or 90 per cent of these animals were rabid. The rest were doubtful. None of these patients developed rabies or any deleterious effects from the treatment. However, during this period there were at least four people who contracted rabies and died; none of these received the Pasteur treatment.

The greatest problem in rabies is determining whether or not the offending animal is rabid. This is usually not difficult. Healthy dogs are apt to bite, but usually are guilty of this offense only during the excitement of play or while being tormented. The actions of a rabid dog are rather typical. The usual story is that the dog, a stray animal, deliberately ran up to the patient, bit him, and rapidly disappeared. If an attempt is made to follow these animals, it will usually be learned that more people have been bitten by the same dog. It is of extreme importance, then, that any dog that bites a person without provocation should be caught and confined under observation for ten to fourteen days. However, if the animal is rabid, serious symptoms (*e.g.,* paralysis) will almost invariably develop within forty-eight hours. The onset of the disease in the animal is characterized by a restlessness and impulsive desire to run about aimlessly. He may become unusually affectionate, but with strangers is apt to be irritable. Within a day or two he shows a desire to leave home and it is during this period of two or three days, before paralyses set in, that he inflicts so much damage. The first group of muscles to become paralyzed are those controlling the lower jaw which then drops and reveals profuse salivation. Paralysis of the hind quarters is usually followed in twenty-four or thirty-six hours by death. The saliva of the animal is infective four to six days before symptoms develop. Due supposedly to a natural immunity, only 20 to 30 per cent of people bitten by rabid dogs will contract rabies if untreated.

Prevention.—Injection of attenuated virus (Pasteur treatment) is by far the most effective prophylactic therapy. If there is the slightest possibility that the animal was rabid the patient should be given this specific therapy. As first devised by Pasteur it consisted of the injection of an emulsion made from a diseased spinal cord which was attenuated by drying for 14 or 15 days. Modifications have been made in the preparation and in the treatment. Harris [37] has devised a method of maintaining the potency and immunizing power of rabies vaccine for at least 3 years by freezing and storing it at a temperature of $-1°$ C. Five daily doses of 25 mgm. of this attenuated virus are given and followed by five similar doses of less attenuated material. This procedure has been used in over 3,000 cases and has failed to prevent rabies in only one instance. The attenuated virus, ready for administration, can be obtained from most City Boards of Health. As to the wound, Harris recommends that it be cauterized with phenol and immediately wiped with alcohol; Gowen [36] favors the use of nitric acid. In any case the wound should not be closed but left open.

Clinical Manifestations.—The incubation period is variable, averaging fifty or sixty days, but may be as short as ten days or as long as two years (Harris). Because of the fact that the virus apparently attacks chiefly nerve tissue, and evidently makes its way to the spinal cord and brain through nerves, the *incubation time is shorter when the bite is inflicted on the face or trunk.* In man the disease is ushered in by an ungovernable restlessness and increased irritability and sensitivity to mild stimuli. He may suffer wild hallucinations and usually becomes maniacal soon after onset. Convulsions may be produced by the slightest stimulus, especially by draughts of air. As the disease progresses, hydrophobia is noted. The application of this term is quite suitable because of the fact that when the patient attempts to drink water he is seized with such severe pain and laryngeal spasm that respiration may be impossible; the mere sight of water may bring on these attacks of suffocation and pain. After two to four days generalized paralysis develops; death follows inevitably and rapidly.

Treatment.—After the development of the disease there is no known method of treatment which offers any hope of recovery. Symptoms are treated as they arise merely with the idea of making the patient comfortable. Convulsions and spasm should be controlled, if possible, by sedatives.

VINCENT'S ANGINA

This is a superficial, acute inflammatory disease of the mouth, gums or pharynx which is caused by a mixed infection of Vincent's fusiform bacilli and spirochetes. The lesion is really a form of stomatitis, may be multiple, and usually starts as a red edematous area, in the center of which a small patch or ulcer develops. These

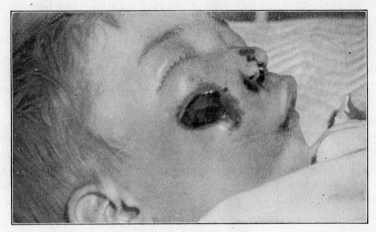

FIG. 52.—GANGRENOUS STOMATITIS (NOMA) EXTENDING THROUGH THE CHEEK IN A CHILD AGED FOUR.

Photograph taken four days after onset of "sore mouth"; the patient had contracted measles three weeks before development of stomatitis. Note the extensive area of gangrene, which was rapidly progressive. Only mild fever was present; leukocytosis 60,000. Death occurred seven weeks after onset of stomatitis. Autopsy revealed also generalized tuberculosis affecting particularly the lungs and liver (St. Louis Children's Hospital).

ulcers are covered with a grayish white membrane and vary tremendously in size and depth, although they are usually shallow and no greater than 0.5 centimeter in diameter. In its more severe form the disease is known as trench mouth. A moderate amount of tenderness and pain is present. The breath is foul. Secondary involvement of the cervical lymph nodes draining the area usually appears, but suppuration in the nodes is uncommon. The disease is usually of short duration, rarely presents a systemic reaction and usually terminates in eight to sixteen days. The local application of neosalvarsan or 10 per cent silver nitrate to the ulcer is effective in the mild cases. In the more severe cases with extensive invasion, neosalvarsan should be given intravenously. Occasionally the disease is resistant to therapy and persists for several weeks or months. Besides the specific drugs mentioned and oral hygiene, frequent irrigations with a 1 per cent solution of potassium permanganate or 3 per cent solution of chlorate of soda are useful.

NOMA

This is a rapidly spreading gangrenous process occurring usually in the gums, cheeks and mucous membranes of undernourished children between the ages of two and ten years. It is also known as cancrum oris or gangrenous stomatitis (see also page 651). Vincent's fusiform bacilli and spirochetes are frequently found in the tissue, but the exact causative organism is not known. In view of the convincing work of Meleney [38] on symbiosis it is possible that the process may be dependent upon a symbiotic growth of two or more organisms. The disease is fortunately becoming rarer than it was years ago. It is most often seen in debilitated children who are recovering from diseases such as measles, scarlet fever, diphtheria, typhoid, etc. It is not considered contagious, but on rare occasions has been reported as occurring in epidemics (Blumer and McFarlane [39]).

The disease begins as a sloughing ulcer which rapidly becomes surrounded by a red indurated and gangrenous margin and finally results in huge defects because of destructive loss of tissue. The odor given off by the gangrenous area is extremely offensive. Fever is usually present. The pulse rate is rapid, conforming to the profound seriousness of the disease which is fatal in at least 70 per cent of cases within four to seven days. As soon as the condition is recognized, probably the most effective means of treatment is wide excision by cautery. Plastic repair of the defect is performed later. The ulcerating area should be cleansed frequently by irrigation with a solution such as hypertonic saline, potassium permanganate (1:500), etc. Salvarsan or neosalvarsan should also be given intravenously. Sulfonamides should be tried.

LUDWIG'S ANGINA

In 1836, Ludwig of Stuttgart described an acute, deep-seated infection involving the floor of the mouth and upper portion of the neck. Blair and Brown,[40] however, have called attention to the fact that Gensoul had thoroughly described this unique type of infection six years previously (1830). Although the infection practically always remains localized in the floor of the mouth and upper part of the neck, constitutional symptoms, including fever, etc., usually are present and a mortality of fifteen or twenty per cent is experienced. The organism most frequently obtained on culture is the streptococcus, but other mouth organisms may be found sometimes singly, but at other times apparently growing in a symbiotic manner. Anaerobic organisms undoubtedly play an important role in the development of the disease. The most common source of the infection is an alveolar abscess which ruptures through the inner table of the mandible (Ivy). The infection may arise from dental caries, etc., but frequently no primary lesion can be discovered.

The induration and swelling of the floor of the mouth develop rapidly, are associated with pain, but with a variable amount of tenderness. As the swelling increases the tongue is pushed upwards and backward, thereby holding the mouth open and interfering with swallowing and breathing. Redness of the skin does not appear until late. Fever is usually present as are also constitutional symptoms such as prostration, tachycardia, etc., at least to a moderate degree. Edema of the glottis and bronchopneumonia are common and serious complications, especially in neglected or untreated cases.

Although fluctuation will rarely be detected, early and radical incision is indicated and in fact imperative. The incision recommended by Blair [41] is T-shaped, extending from the chin to the hyoid bone and penetrates into the depth of the indurated area by splitting the mylohyoid muscle. Even though very little, if any, pus may be formed, incision, nevertheless, appears to result in marked improvement. If at any time edema of the glottis or larynx is manifested, a tracheotomy

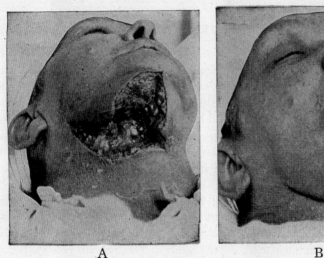
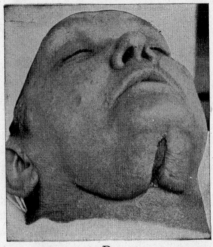

A   B

FIG. 53.—LUDWIG'S ANGINA.

A, note how the tissues open up after proper incision; *B*, same patient eight days after operation. As soon as the induration subsides, the flaps drop back in their normal positions. (From Blair and Ivy, *Essentials of Oral Surgery*, 1923, C. V. Mosby Co., pp. 263 and 264.)

should be performed without delay. Too often, tracheotomy is not performed in time to be the lifesaving procedure that it should be. William [42] found sulfanilamide efficacious, particularly when the streptococcus was evident on culture, as was noted in 72 per cent of his cases.

RAT-BITE FEVER

Although it has been known for many years that a prolonged illness with intermittent attacks of fever may develop in the human being ten to twenty-two days following a rat bite, it was not until 1916, that Futaki and associates [43] demonstrated a spirochete as the etiological factor. About the same time the fever and associated symptoms develop, the scar at the site of the bite breaks down, ulcerates and a regional lymphadenopathy develops. The symptoms, which may include fever, nausea, vomiting, pains in the joints and muscles, may be quite severe resulting even in delirium. Fatalities, however, are uncommon. During the attacks a rather typical erythematous, macular rash with lesions as large as 1 to 2 centimeters in diameter may develop. The attacks usually persist for two to three days, but recur again in four to six days over a period of several months unless treatment is instituted. The spirochete may frequently be found in the blood, skin lesion or lymph node of the patient, but is more consistently found in the blood of a mouse injected with the blood of the patient.

Treatment, consisting of the injection of salvarsan or neosalvarsan, is specific and is given in a manner similar to its use in syphilis, except that a few injections usually suffice to eradicate the spirochete causing rat-bite fever. The wound of entrance requires no special treatment.

ANTHRAX

A century or two ago anthrax was a miserable scourge in European countries, but during recent years it has become uncommon, especially in the United States. The causative organism, *Bacillus anthracis,* was isolated by Davaine[44] in 1850, although a year previously Pollender had discovered presumably the same organism in animals dying from "splenic fever." The disease is also known as malignant pustule or wool sorter's disease. Infection may be acquired by handling wool or hides from various animals, including sheep, cattle, horses, hogs, guinea-pigs and rabbits. In a few instances the source of infection has been found to be a newly acquired shaving brush.

There are three types of the disease: (1) the *cutaneous type,* which is associated with a low mortality, usually manifests itself as a furuncular-like lesion with a black necrotic center. (2) The *pulmonary* form of the disease is rare and presumably results from inhalation of the spores. The patient rapidly becomes very ill, develops chills, fever, prostration, tachycardia, cough and pulmonary edema and practically always dies within a few days after onset. (3) The *intestinal* form manifests itself by chills, fever, diarrhea and vomiting, and is associated with a high mortality.

The *treatment* of anthrax is apparently efficiently carried out by the administration of antitoxin. In the Sackville, Pennsylvania, epidemic of 1933, the first patient died, but the following six survived. The State Health Department reported that heavy doses of anthrax antitoxin were given in all except the first case which received a small amount. It has been known for a long time that attempts at surgical incision or excision of the lesions are poorly tolerated and tend to spread the infection.

TYPHOID

Fortunately, typhoid fever is now a rare disease. It is true that only its complications are of surgical interest, but these are so numerous as to demand consideration, especially in districts where the disease is prevalent. However, in many instances, the abdominal manifestations of typhoid may be so prominent as to simulate a low grade peritonitis, and thus be confused with other surgical diseases, particularly acute appendicitis.

Perforation of an ulcer in the ileum is the most important of the surgical complications, and accounts for approximately one-third of the deaths from typhoid. Because of the fact that the patient is already quite ill, has a moderate amount of abdominal pain and is distended, the diagnosis of a perforation may present a difficult problem. At the time of perforation there is almost always an accentuation of pain. Tenderness should be more marked and is usually more pronounced over the right lower quadrant because the perforation is apt to occur on the ileum a short distance above the ileocecal valve. Muscle spasm is not expected until the process has progressed to a point where recovery is unlikely. The characteristic slow pulse rate should show an appreciable rise. The polymorphonuclear count should be increased, although the total leukocytic count may not be appreciably elevated. Perhaps the most valuable diagnostic aid is a roentgenogram taken in a semi-sitting posture to determine the presence or absence of gas under the diaphragm. If a perforation is present, gas rarely fails to show up in at least a small quantity. As soon as the diagnosis is made, immediate operation, preferably under local anesthesia, should be performed and the site of perforation repaired.

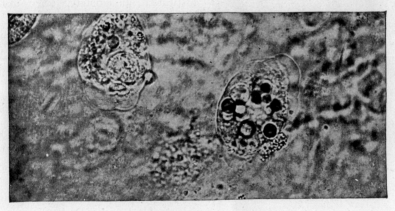

FIG. 54.—ENDAMEBA HISTOLYTICA.

Mobile forms showing ingested red cells, granules and clear actoplasm. (Army Medical School Collection, Washington, D. C.)

Because of the fact that typhoid bacilli are present in large numbers in the bile, *acute cholecystitis* is frequently encountered as a complication of typhoid. Rarely does it demand operative interference, however. On the other hand, operation may be indicated years later for *chronic cholecystitis* and *cholelithiasis,* whose pathogenesis was dependent upon an attack of typhoid fever contracted years previously. In most instances the source of infection in "typhoid carriers" is the gallbladder. Cholecystectomy will often eliminate the presence of the typhoid bacilli in the stool.

Typhoid *osteomyelitis* and *chondritis* are not uncommon when typhoid fever itself is prevalent. Invasion of bone or cartilage may appear before the patient recovers from the attack of typhoid, but is perhaps more often seen, at least during recent years, as an osteomyelitis of a rib or as a chondritis involving a costal cartilage years after the attack of typhoid fever. In this instance the process is insidious and resembles a tuberculous invasion of the rib or costal cartilage. Treatment consists of excision of the involved rib or cartilage.

AMEBIC DYSENTERY

There are several aspects of this disease which are of surgical interest, but one in particular is important, namely that the first symptoms of amebic dysentery usually consist of abdominal pain and cramps which in many instances will resemble the onset of acute appendicitis for which appendectomy may be performed. Such a mistake happened on numerous occasions throughout the country during the time when the Chicago epidemic of 1933 was at its peak. Submitting the patient to an operation during the onset of amebic dysentery will result in many fatalities even though the actual condition is recognized and emetine therapy instituted immediately. (See also page 685.)

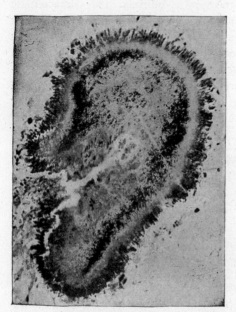

Fig. 55.—Sulphur Granule of Actinomyces.

Colony of actinomycosis with well-developed clubs at the periphery in a nodule in the peritoneal cavity of a guinea-pig inoculated with a culture from another guinea-pig. Paraffin section. Low magnification. (From Jordan, *General Bacteriology*, 1928, W. B. Saunders Co., p. 533.)

Abscess of the liver is a frequent complication of amebic dysentery, but usually occurs only in the untreated or inadequately treated cases. The typical symptoms and signs of abscess of the liver, including chills, daily intermittent fever, prostration, sweating, etc., are usually encountered. Drainage by operation is associated with a high mortality, whereas intensive treatment with emetine alone will often prove curative. Aspiration is permissible in the large abscesses (see page 602). Only on extremely rare occasions do amebic ulcerations of the intestine require operative interference because of perforation or obstruction due to stricture.

ACTINOMYCOSIS

The etiological factor in actinomycosis is the actinomyces or ray fungus, the most important bacteriological feature of which is the sulphur granule which is barely large enough to be recognized by the naked eye and consists of microscopic filaments, coccus-like bodies and clubs. Finding sulphur bodies in the pus from a lesion establishes the diagnosis, but it should be emphasized that they may be difficult to demonstrate, especially in sinuses of long duration; in a fresh abscess, however, they are numerous. There are numerous strains of the organism, most of which, as observed in man, are not the same strain that produces lumpy jaw in cattle. Some of the strains grow better culturally under aerobic conditions, whereas others grow better anaerobically. The fact that growth is not visible culturally for several days no doubt accounts for the failure to make the bacteriological diagnosis in many instances. The disease was first observed in man by Israel [45] in 1878, although the organism had been described previously. The portal of entry is usually by way of the mouth, but the original supposition that infection was produced by a foreign body such as a straw, etc., is probably erroneous. Wright [46] and Lord [47] have demonstrated clearly that the organism is prevalent in the human mouth and that infec-

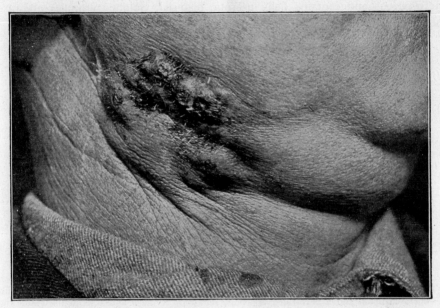

FIG. 56.—ACTINOMYCOSIS OF JAW. (From Wohl, M. A., *J. Am. M. Ass.,* 81:649, 1923.)

tion from that source may be spontaneous. The disease appears to be increasing rather than decreasing in incidence, at least in midwestern United States; it is of granulomatous nature, exhibits a strong tendency to invade with destructive characteristics, but *does not attack the lymph nodes.* There is scarcely any tissue other than the lymphatic system that is immune to invasion. This no doubt adds to the difficulty in establishing a clinical diagnosis. Bone is readily attacked and in one patient observed recently, the organism had perforated the base of the skull with the subsequent development of a meningitis.

Clinical Manifestations.—The disease manifests itself usually in one of three ways as indicated below. In a study of 680 cases, Sanford and Voelker [48] noted that the disease occurred in the head and neck in 60 per cent of cases, 14 per cent in the thorax (including lung) and 18 per cent in the abdomen. However, during recent years the incidence seems to have become reversed, the abdominal type being most common, at least in the author's experience. The disease occurs in children as well as adults, but in a series of 450 cases reported by Figi and Cutts [49] only 3 per cent occurred between the ages of two and fifteen years. The incubation period of the disease is not clearly established, but undoubtedly varies within very wide limits.

1. When the disease occurs in the *head* and *neck,* it usually begins as a hard superficial nodule which finally softens, breaks down, discharges pus and sulphur granules, and ultimately forms a sinus tract. Before the abscesses and sinuses form, however, a board-like induration surrounding the initial lesion usually develops; the lymph nodes, however, are not involved. Tenderness or pain is not significant, but may be pronounced when bone is involved. The sinuses may burrow deeply and form small abscesses or collections of pus, some of which may be secondarily infected if an external sinus is already present. The pus characteristically is thin, heterogeneous and contains flaky necrotic material. Sulphur granules are rarely demonstrable except in fresh abscesses. Fever may or may not be present.

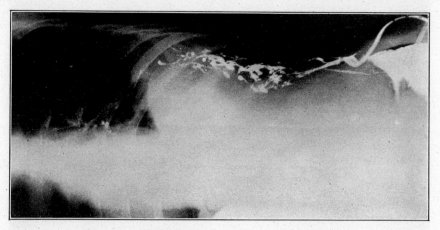

FIG. 57.—ABDOMINAL AND THORACIC ACTINOMYCOSIS.

The patient, a sixty-five-year-old housewife, first developed acute abdominal manifestations, was operated upon, and a perforated appendix removed. A mass appeared in the right lower quadrant three months later which was incised; pus was encountered in which the ray fungus was found. Later, abscesses formed in the lumbar region and thoracic cavity from which the actinomyces were identified and cultured. The x-ray photograph was taken after lipiodol had been injected into the sinus in the abdominal wall leading to the abscess; note the outline of the bronchi, and the shadow indicating the subphrenic and pleural abscess. Intensive radiotherapy and sodium iodide were used in addition to incision and drainage of abscesses; all incisions have remained healed and symptoms arrested for a period which is now ten years since onset.

2. The *abdominal* type of disease presumably is caused by implantation of swallowed organisms upon a small lesion or ulcer in the mucosa of the intestine, usually the cecum or appendix. In a series of abdominal cases reported by Good [50] he describes the initial lesion as appearing in the appendix in about 77 per cent of cases. In other reports, however, the cecum is stressed as being the most common initial site. The first symptoms of cecal actinomycosis may be acute and *may simulate appendicitis.* For some unexplainable reason many cases of actinomycosis of the cecum develop after the patient has been operated on for acute ruptured appendicitis. With the evidence available there is no way of determining whether or not the actinomyces were instrumental in the development of appendicitis in such instances. On other occasions, the onset is insidious with mild pain in the right lower

quadrant associated with the development of a mass in the cecal region. Sinuses may form anywhere about the abdomen and are frequently observed about the pelvis and back. In a review of subphrenic abscess of actinomycotic origin Graves and Ochsner [51] noted that most of them developed after appendectomy for acute appendicitis.

3. *Thoracic* actinomycosis usually results from invasion of an active initial lesion in the neck or abdomen. At times, however, it appears that aspiration of the or-

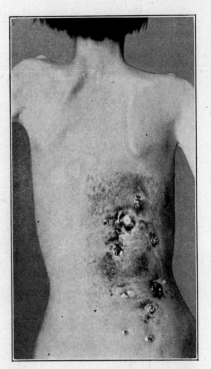

ganisms into the respiratory passages was responsible for the disease. The symptoms may simulate those of pulmonary suppuration (particularly tuberculosis), including cough, pain on respiration, fever, expectoration, sweating, loss of weight, etc. As the disease progresses, the pleura and finally the thoracic wall, including the ribs, are involved with the subsequent development of sinuses leading to the exterior.

Treatment.—Contrary to general belief a cure may be expected if the diagnosis is made early. Treatment should consist particularly of sulfanilamide (Walker,[52] Miller and Fell[53]) roentgen-ray therapy, aided by surgical incision of abscesses, excision of necrotic tissue and free drainage of the wound (Wangensteen [54]). The oral administration of 1 gram or more of thymol per day and packing of wounds with gauze saturated with 10 per cent thymol has been found efficacious (Myers,[55] Joyce [56]). It is to be emphasized, however, that when the disease is disseminated so that major organs, such as the liver, bones, etc., are involved, the chance of obtaining a cure is greatly diminished regardless of the type of therapy used.

FIG. 58.—MULTIPLE SINUSES OF THE BACK DUE TO ACTINOMYCOSIS IN A GIRL SIXTEEN YEARS OF AGE.

Onset two years previous with pain in chest, followed two weeks later by the development of a sinus under the right breast. Since that time numerous other sinuses appeared, particularly over the back. X-ray revealed a destructive process involving the 1st and 2nd lumbar vertebrae, and a thickening of lung markings; each process resembled tuberculosis but was undoubtedly due to actinomycosis. Sulphur granules were found in a fresh abscess on the back, but were absent in the discharge from the chronic sinuses.

VENEREAL LYMPHOGRANULOMA

Although venereal lymphogranuloma has been recognized in some form or other for several decades, it was not until the report of Durand, Nicolas and Favre [57] in 1913 that it was recognized as a specific disease. It is also known by such diagnoses as lymphogranuloma inguinale, esthiomene, tropical bubo, lymphopathia venereum, etc. The French investigators mentioned above recognized the disease as being of venereal origin and as being caused presumably by a virus which entered the body through a tiny unnoticed primary lesion on the genitals. The incubation time varies between five days and three weeks. In this country at least, the Negro race is affected much more commonly than the white. Manifestations of the disease are encountered much more commonly in females than males; this is particularly true of the Negro race.

The observations of Gray and associates [58] relative to incidence of the disease reveal the fact that lymphogranuloma is slightly more prevalent in the Negro race

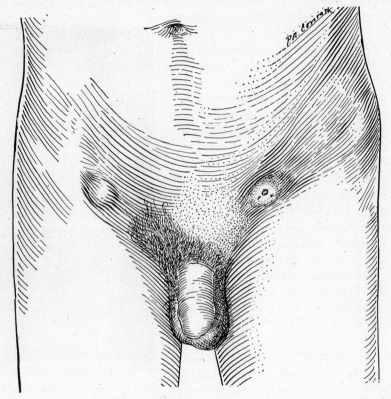

FIG. 59.—BILATERAL INGUINAL LYMPHADENITIS (IN A NEGRO MAN) DUE TO LYMPHOGRANULOMA INGUINALE.

The nodes on the patient's left have suppurated, resulting in the formation of a sinus as noted. The nodes on the right are enlarged, but did not suppurate although about five months were required for subsidence of the process on each side.

than is syphilis. They noted that in a series of nearly 500 Negro hospital patients, 40 per cent of the males and 40 per cent of the females had a positive Frei test. In a smaller series of white patients in the hospital they obtained a positive Frei test in only 3.4 per cent; again with an equal incidence in males and females. From these data it is apparent that many patients who contract the disease present few manifestations and recover, presumably without complications or sequelae. The pathogenesis, along with other data on the transmission of the disease described by various authorities, has been discussed in detail by Stannus,[59] H. N. Cole [60] and others. The disease is readily produced in various types of animals by local inoculation, particularly into the brain.

Clinical Manifestations.—The disease manifests itself in one of three ways. In men the most common feature is involvement of the (1) inguinal lymph nodes which frequently go on to suppuration. In women the most common complaint is referable to an (2) ulcerative proctitis which, at least in Negroes, frequently results in (3) stricture of the rectum. Occasionally inguinal lymphadenitis and ulcerative proctitis exist simultaneously.

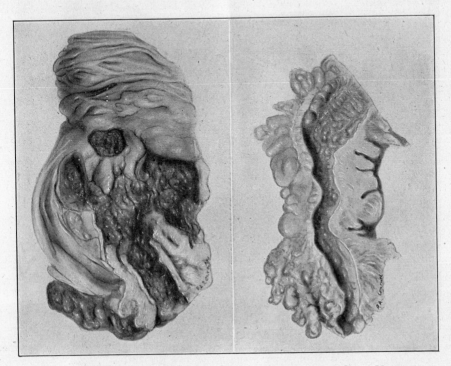

FIG. 60.—LONGITUDINAL SECTION OF STRICTURE OF RECTUM DUE TO VENEREAL LYMPHOGRANULOMA.

Each illustration represents specimen removed at operation. Note that the stricture extends not more than six to eight centimeters above the sphincter. Areas of ulceration are found scattered over the scarred mucosa. (Drawn from Gatellier and Weiss.)

The onset of the disease is frequently characterized by diffuse severe abdominal pain of a cramping nature. Fever, nausea and, rarely, vomiting may accompany the abdominal pain. Loss of weight is commonly observed and multiple arthritis is not uncommon. Severe systemic manifestations as described above usually occur, however, only in Negro women. They may occur at intervals for two or three years following the onset of the disease.

When the disease occurs in men the lymph nodes of one or both sides enlarge insidiously without the production of much pain. After a few weeks the pain and disability become more prominent and the nodes may suppurate. If the suppurating nodes are not incised they readily break through the skin spontaneously and form sinuses. Suppuration and the sinus formation may last for a variable length of time. In some instances healing has taken place in as short a time as three weeks. On other occasions the nodes have been known to exist for as long a time as two years.

When the disease manifests itself as an ulcerating proctitis the first symptoms experienced by the patient may be a mild tenesmus with the passage of blood, mucus and pus in the stool. These symptoms may persist for two or three years or longer.

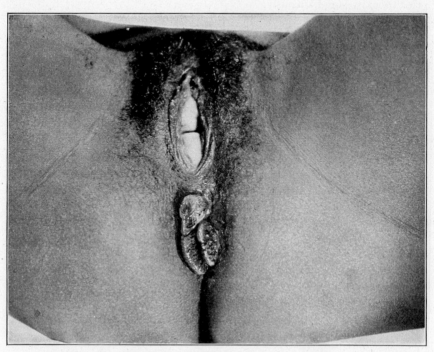

FIG. 61.—CONDYLOMAS, DUE TO VENEREAL LYMPHOGRANULOMA ABOUT THE ANUS IN A NEGRO WOMAN, WITH STRICTURE OF THE RECTUM.

The Kahn test was negative. Such lesions develop insidiously and may or may not be associated with ulceration. Previous to a few years ago almost all lesions of this type, as were also strictures of the rectum, were considered to be of syphilitic origin; by far the major portion of such lesions are due to venereal lymphogranuloma.

Most authorities are of the opinion that at least three-fourths, and perhaps all of the benign strictures of the rectum are caused by venereal lymphogranuloma, and are a sequel (two to three years later) to the ulcerative proctitis. Almost every patient with benign stricture of the rectum will have symptoms referable to the narrowing of the lumen, namely tenesmus and diarrhea with liquid or pencil stools. These benign strictures of the rectum persist indefinitely, but the patients frequently adjust themselves so that they have frequent liquid stools and suffer very little inconvenience from the stricture. Occasionally condylomatous lesions about the anus are observed in patients with lymphogranuloma. It is probable that many condylomas (particularly about the rectum) which in previous years were considered to be of syphilitic origin are in reality caused by lymphogranuloma. Elephantiasis of the genitals (particularly the vulva and penis) is not uncommon. Fistulas about the rectum are commonly observed in patients with lymphogranuloma.

The relative frequency of the various symptoms and signs as noted in a report of 40 cases from the Washington University Clinics by Rainey and Cole [61] are given in Table 3.

TABLE 3

CLINICAL MANIFESTATIONS OF LYMPHOGRANULOMA INGUINALE

Total 40 Cases (All had a Positive Frei Test)

Symptoms	Males, 3 White, 5 Negro	Females, 4 White, 28 Negro
Lymphadenitis	8	10
Ulcerative proctitis	2	7
Anal lesions	1	8
Rectal stricture	0	22
Rectal fistula	0	5
Systemic reaction	2	17

The systemic manifestations include: malaise, loss of weight, abdominal pain, fever, arthritis, anemia, vertigo, nausea and vomiting.

Diagnosis.—One of the most reliable features in the diagnosis is the Frei test. The Frei antigen is made from pus obtained from a suppurating lymph node of a known case of the disease. The pus is diluted 4 or 5 to 1 and heated at 60° C. for two hours, followed by similar exposure to heat forty-eight hours later. The antigen is injected intradermally in a dose of 0.1 c.c. A typical positive reaction appears in forty-eight hours and consists of induration at the site of injection with redness of the skin surrounding the induration. Positive tests have been obtained as long as twelve to fifteen years after the onset of the disease; the test is therefore remarkably valuable and accurate.

When the disease primarily affects the lymph nodes, it is often confused with lymphadenitis caused by a chancroid. The gradual enlargement of the lymph nodes, associated with a variable amount of pain, followed ultimately by suppuration, are identical in the two diseases. However, an important differential point lies in the size of the initial lesion; in lymphogranuloma, the initial lesion is small (seldom larger than ¼ centimeter in diameter), whereas the primary lesion in a chancroid is large (1 to 2 centimeters in diameter). The initial lesion in a chancroid is apt to be multiple; in lymphogranuloma it is usually single and even unnoticed in males, but is frequently multiple in women. Sensitivity tests will usually make a diagnosis, *i.e.*, the Frei test is specific for venereal lymphogranuloma, whereas the Dmelcos test is specific for chancroid.

When the disease is limited to the inguinal lymph nodes it may rarely simulate tuberculosis clinically, but it should be remembered that tuberculosis of the inguinal lymph nodes is extremely uncommon; microscopic section of the lymph nodes closely resembles tuberculosis. Giant cells are frequently observed in venereal lymphogranuloma. However, there is one feature which is apparently reasonably diagnostic, *viz.*, if the lymph node is removed in the proper stage of suppuration there will be seen tiny areas of caseation surrounded by a palisading of epithelioid cells. Such miliary abscesses may be round, but are usually star-shaped. Pus obtained by aspiration from these suppurating nodes reveals no growth on culture and will, of course, not produce tuberculosis when injected into a guinea-pig.

The disease may be confused with granuloma inguinale, but in reality only because of similarity in the terms. Granuloma inguinale is likewise a venereal disease, but is manifested by ulcerations about the perineum which are rather superficial, and do not attack the lymph nodes. Such ulcers, i.e., granuloma inguinale, may be located on the genitals or in the groin.

Previously, the majority of benign strictures of the rectum have been considered to be of syphilitic origin. Numerous observers have offered evidence to disprove the possibility of syphilitic origin. Out of a total of 22 cases of benign stricture of the rectum all of whom had a positive Frei test as observed by Rainey and Cole, only 5 (22.7 per cent) had a positive Wassermann or Kahn test, an incidence no greater than that present in another series of hospital patients with varied diagnoses.

Treatment.—The infection of the inguinal lymph nodes is treated as a low grade inflammatory lesion. When suppuration appears incision is recommended. On a few occasions merely aspiration of pus from the inguinal abscess has been sufficient to relieve symptoms and prevent further suppuration. Drainage of abscesses relieves the acute inflammatory manifestations but is by no means curative. Of the various medicinal agents sulfanilamide, as recommended by Knight and David,[62] promises to be the most efficacious. Apparently this drug is effective even in the treatment of rectal lesions so long as the lesion is still in the inflammatory stage. Tartar emetic has been used a great deal, but is not very effective. Fuadin and Frei antigen have also been used therapeutically.

ECHINOCOCCUS DISEASE

Hydatid or echinococcus disease is caused by one of the smallest of tapeworms, *Tenia echinococcus,* and is encountered occasionally in most regions throughout the world, but appears to be especially common in Australia and Iceland. Detailed accounts of the disease may be found in publications by Dew[63] and Arce.[64] The disease is contracted from dogs which are the tapeworm's host and excrete the eggs in their feces. After ingestion of the egg by the human being, the larva is freed by digestion of the shell and burrows into the intestinal wall. From there it may be carried in the portal blood stream to the liver, where it may lodge, or be carried to or through the lung and finally to such organs as the kidney, bone, brain, etc. After larvae have reached their destination hooklets disappear and a cyst develops, from the wall of which buds are developed; these are in turn converted into cysts identical to the original or mother cyst. Such daughter cysts also form grand-daughter cysts, which are contained within a thick outer mother cyst wall.

The cysts enlarge and develop insidiously without many clinical manifestations. Rarely are systemic symptoms encountered. When the cyst is located in the liver, a mild, rather constant pain, similar to that produced by chronic cholecystitis, but without much dyspepsia, is experienced. Sometimes the cyst is palpable upon abdominal examination. If the cyst is in the lung, symptoms of a benign tumor, such as cough, mild pain on respiration, dyspnea, etc., may develop. Bone is not infrequently the site of invasion. This feature of the disease has been described in detail by Ivanissevich.[65] Casoni's intradermal test * is usually considered the most important diagnostic procedure, although the echinococcus fixation test † of Weinberg is reliable. Both of these tests may give negative results when no absorption from the cysts is occurring. An eosinophilia is often present.

Unless inaccessible, the cysts should be removed as soon as discovered. If possible the entire outer cyst is removed, avoiding rupture if possible, because of the danger of implantation of the contents of the cysts. When in the liver it is usually impossible to remove the outer cyst wall because of the danger of hemorrhage. Under such circumstances, the contents should be removed without peritoneal contamination if possible, and 4 per cent formalin or tincture of iodine painted on the wall of the cyst to destroy the membrane. If all the cysts are removed and the lining of the mother cyst destroyed, recovery should be uneventful and permanent. (See Fig. 377.)

GRANULOMA INGUINALE

In 1905 Donovan described an intracellular micro-organism which, on a stained (Wright) smear obtained from the lesion, shows up as a small round pink body with a blue staining coccoid center. He associated the organism with granuloma

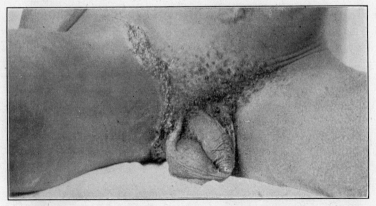

FIG. 62.—GRANULOMA INGUINALE AFFECTING THE GROIN AND BASE OF SCROTUM IN A COLORED MAN AGED FORTY-FIVE.

The lesion was cured by the administration of tartar emetic but recurred a few months later. The recurrent lesion was not as extensive as the original ulceration, but responded scarcely at all to tartar emetic and various other types of therapy.

inguinale, but it is not agreed that this is the etiological factor. The disease is of venereal origin, occurs more often among Negroes and was originally described as a tropical disease, but it is encountered occasionally in temperate zones as well. In males, the lesion usually starts on the penis or scrotum, but frequently the initial

---

* Casoni's intradermal test is dependent upon sensitivity, as is the tuberculin test. A small quantity of fluid obtained previously from a known cyst is injected into the skin. A local reaction results if the patient has echinococcus disease.

† The complement fixation test of Weinberg utilizes an antigen made from fresh hydatid fluid containing scolices. The test is performed on the patient's serum. The antigen required in this test may be obtained from some pharmaceutical houses.

lesion is in the groin. In females the lesion is first seen on the vulva, perineum or groin. The disease starts as an indurated papule which ulcerates and slowly involves the adjacent skin. The granulating tissue of the ulcer is elevated, especially at the edges, appears red and seldom reveals a necrotic base. Occasionally healing occurs in the center, either as a rough scar or combined with epthelization made possible by islands of epithelium which escaped destruction by the ulcer. At times the entire penis may be destroyed if treatment is not obtained. The lesion remains superficial and shows no tendency to develop sinuses or to invade the lymph nodes. The ulceration produces a thin milky secretion which at times has a characteristic sour fetid odor. Very little pain or tenderness is present. Occasionally the disease spreads toward the anus and produces a fungating, somewhat papillomatous lesion.

Treatment with intravenous tartar emetic is specific. A dose of 3 to 5 c.c. of a 1 per cent solution should be given every three or four days and increased to 8 or 10 c.c. as tolerated. Treatment should be continued until the patient has received 12 to 15 injections. Meticulous cleanliness is also important; hospitalization in stubborn cases for frequent irrigation is sometimes advisable.

BLASTOMYCOSIS

This disease was described independently in 1894 by Gilchrist [66] and Busse [67] as being caused by a yeast-like organism, blastomycete. These organisms multiply in the tissue by budding, but develop mycelial threads when growing in culture. They are about 8 to 10 microns in diameter and are readily identified by their

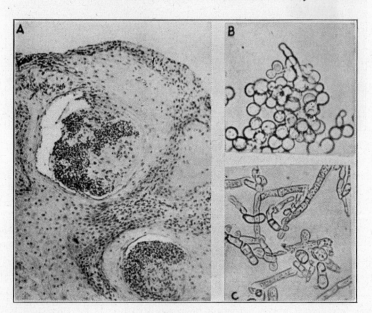

FIG. 63.—BLASTOMYCOSIS.

A, minute blastomycotic abscess (low power) in skin at border of lesion illustrated in Figure 113; *B*, appearance of blastomycetes suspended in saline after first culture (high power); *C*, after several subcultures; note the mycelial formation. (From Cole, *Ann. Surg.*, 80:124, 1924.)

double refractile capsule. They have no nucleus but the protoplasm contains coarsely granular material with refractile bodies. The organisms are most readily found by application of a small drop of 10 per cent sodium hydroxide to some pus under a cover slip in a fresh unstained preparation.

The lesion usually becomes implanted in the skin by a minor injury and manifests itself either primarily as an ulcer at the site of the inflicted wound or as a

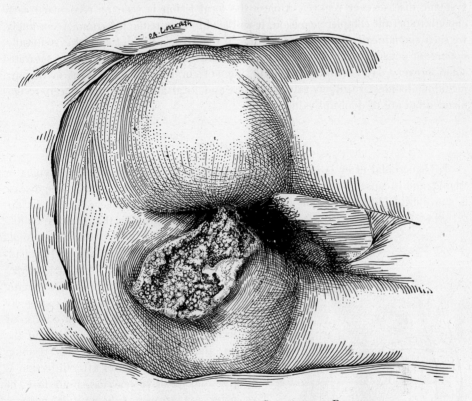

FIG. 64.—BLASTOMYCOSIS OF THE SKIN OF THE BUTTOCK.

Note the cauliflower-like surface. The patient, a young, white man, suffered an injury to a finger while working in a mine. This ulcer failed to heal. Several months later lesions developed in the skin at numerous places over the body. In spite of various types of therapy including administration of potassium iodide, x-ray therapy, local medicinal application, etc., patient slowly failed and died two and one-half years after onset. (Drawn from Cole, *Ann. Surg.*, 80:124, 1924.)

papule which breaks down and forms an ulcer. This ulcer starts originally as a local lesion and soon assumes characteristics which in appearance can be confused only with one other disease, lupus vulgaris (tuberculosis). The surface of the lesion is ulcerating, is raised above the adjacent skin and assumes a "cauliflower-like" or papillomatous appearance. Along the edges of the ulcers may be found tiny pinpoint abscesses which sometimes may be seen only with the aid of a lens. The organisms are most readily found in those tiny abscesses. This lesion may remain local for one to two years, but tends to become systemic partly because of autoinoculation, but more especially because of metastatic implantation by the organism.

The lungs are usually the first organs to become secondarily infected. Occasionally the infection is primary in the lung. From the clinical and radiological standpoint the infection in the lung cannot be distinguished from tuberculosis, but the organisms may be found in the sputum. Almost any organ in the body may become infected.

The treatment is so unsatisfactory that very few patients who develop the systemic disease ever recover. Unless the local lesion is seen or recognized early enough to permit complete excision, it will lead to a systemic infection. Accordingly, we then *emphatically recommend excision* if the disease has not spread systemically. Sodium or potassium iodide given in doses increasing to 150 to 200 drops of saturated solution every day is definitely helpful, but not curative. Various types of therapy, including iodides, roentgen ray, salvarsan and local antiseptics have been recommended but are of doubtful value.

CHANCROID

A chancroidal ulcer is of venereal origin, appears either on the penis, vulva or vagina, and is caused by the Ducrey bacillus which was isolated in 1889. The disease is auto-inoculable and for that reason may occur as multiple ulcers. Diagnosis can

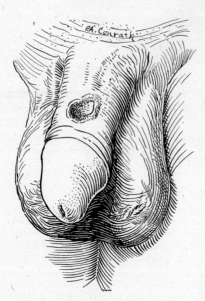

FIG. 65.—CHANCROID OF THE PENIS.

The ulceration may be widespread, multiple, and on rare occasions very destructive.

usually be made readily by the presence or history of a large primary ulcer on the genitals associated with a painful and tender lymphadenitis in the groin. The use of Dmelcos vaccine, which is a suspension of killed Ducrey bacilli, as a diagnostic test may be extremely helpful in doubtful cases. In this test 0.2 c.c. of the vaccine is injected intracutaneously in the forearm; the development of a local reaction (papule or pustule) 48 hours after injection is indicative of a positive reaction. Four to eight days after exposure a tiny pustule appears which develops into an ulcer several days later. From the ulcer, which may be slightly undermined and "punched-out," a foul profuse discharge is given off. The primary lesion heals within two to four weeks, but unilateral or bilateral inguinal lymphadenitis (bubo) usually develops. Differentiation from venereal lymphogranuloma has been discussed on page 104. The swelling in the groin is diffusely indurated, only mildly tender, but after a few weeks may suppurate. Frequently, secondary infection develops; an increase in the acute inflammatory reactions producing pyogenic bacteria will be obtained from the pus on culture. Culture of the causative organism from the ulcer is difficult and requires special technic. Frequently, aspiration of the pus in the suppurating lymph nodes is sufficient to allow the process to subside. At other times incision and drainage is necessary. Medicinal treatment of the primary ulcer is unsatisfactory, but cleanliness with frequent irrigation facilitates healing. Occasionally the intravenous injection of 3 to 6 c.c. of 1 per cent tartar emetic seems to be efficacious. Dmelcos vaccine has also been advocated in the treatment of chancroid, but is associated with considerable systemic reaction and commonly is ineffective. Good results have been obtained with sulfanilamide by numerous workers. Batchelor and Lees [68] recommend giving 8 grams per day in adult males for the first two days, and 6 grams daily for several days thereafter. Treatment may be ambulatory but strict supervision is necessary if large doses of sulfanilamide are used. Other sulfonamide compounds may be tried.

RARER TYPES OF MISCELLANEOUS SURGICAL INFECTIONS

Coccidioidal Granuloma.—This disease is caused by a yeast-like organism, but reproduces by sporulation contrasted to the blastomycete which reproduces by budding. When the sporozoites are mature they escape to the outside by bursting through the capsule. The disease was apparently first described by Wernicke in 1892. A short time later Rixford and Gilchrist [69] published a detailed account of it. On the skin (no specific localization) the organism produces nodules or a pustular, granulomatous eruption. Various organs of the body are invaded in a manner similar to blastomycosis, but perhaps with more resemblance to tuberculosis. It was originally thought that the disease was universally fatal, but it has been noted recently that cures or survival for many years are common. In this country most of the cases are seen in California and Texas.

Sporotrichosis.—The etiological factor is the sporothrix schencki which may readily be found in smears of pus obtained from the lesions. The characteristic feature of the disease is the formation of soft mildly inflamed nodules which appear in a chain-like fashion along the course of the lymphatics, particularly of the arms and legs. These nodules vary from ½ to 1 centimeter in diameter and may break down and suppurate. A primary lesion may be absent, but if present may readily be confused with tularemia. Few constitutional symptoms appear, but occasionally bone may be involved. The oral administration of potassium iodide, increasing the dose to 150 or 200 drops of saturated solution per day is very efficient in eliminating the disease.

Torula.—In 1916 Stoddard and Cutler [70] reported a group of patients with symptoms suggesting brain tumor, but in whom autopsy findings revealed an unusual type of meningitis caused by a yeast-like organism, *torula*. The organisms vary tremendously in size. Some are doubly contoured. The larger ones contain a dark staining chromatin-like substance which resembles a nucleus. Reproduction is by budding. The organism attacks the brain by producing a thickening of the pia-arachnoid associated with tiny vesicular nodules containing clear liquid material. Larger caseous nodules may often be found within the brain itself. In a survey of this disease, Watts [71] noted that the brain and meninges were the organs most often affected, but that many other organs, especially the lungs, were likewise involved. He was able to find only one instance when the skin was involved. In one of the three cases observed in Barnes Hospital, St. Louis, an ulcer of a toe had been present several weeks before development of the cranial symptoms and apparently was the primary lesion.

Yaws.—This is a disease with manifestations similar to syphilis and likewise causd by a spirochete (*Treponema pertenue*). The response to the serological tests is almost identical to syphilis. It is not a venereal disease, but infection usually occurs through a wound of the skin. The disease is common in Africa, India and parts of South America, but is rarely seen· in this country. Primary, secondary and tertiary stages are encountered with ultimate invasion of many organs, including

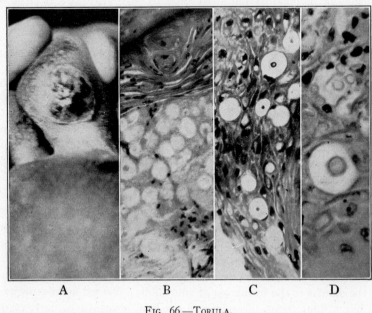

A   B   C   D

FIG. 66.—TORULA.

A, photograph of the under surface of the second toe, showing the ulcer due to torula. Patient died four months later, six months after the appearance of the ulcer and the development of symptoms typical of torular infection of the brain; *B, C* and *D*, microscopical section (high power) of the ulcer which was excised, revealed many torula organisms which characteristically vary considerably in size, staining qualities, etc. Insert *D* is slightly higher power than *B* and *C*, and shows the doubly contoured characteristic which is frequently noted, thereby simulating a blastomycete.

bone, unless treatment is instituted. Arsenic in the form of salvarsan or neosalvarsan is specific.

Leprosy.—This disease was a serious scourge centuries ago, but is rarely seen now except in the leper colonies. The most common lesion is a hyperemic nodule of the skin which may suppurate and produce prominent deformities because of cicatrization. On rare occasions, entire fingers or toes may be destroyed by the ulcerative process. Numerous internal organs may become affected. The disease resists treatment and may condemn the patient to isolation for the duration of his life. The victims usually live for years, but may die from intercurrent infection.

There are many chronic diseases of bacillary or parasitic origin which are commonly seen in foreign countries, especially the tropics, but are rarely encountered in this country. *Madura foot* is an inflammatory disease commonly seen in India, and is caused by the *Actinomyces streptothrix*. The characteristic lesion is a slowly forming nodule which occurs usually on the plantar surface of the foot. These nodes become soft and later form sinuses which penetrate so deeply as to involve any of the bony or soft tissues of the foot, and may require amputation. While madura foot (mycetoma) is encountered chiefly in the Orient, especially among poorly nourished Indians, it does occur in the temperate zones. The diagnosis may often be made by study of the discharge from the sinuses in the foot. In this country at least, the chief importance lies in its similarity to tuberculous and other chronic osteo-myelites of the foot. *Mycosis fungoides* is a chronic granulomatous disease possibly of parasitic origin which manifests itself as soft reddish nodules on the skin. These nodules may disappear or ulcerate with the production of fungoid tumors. Lymph nodes and internal organs may become involved. The mortality is high. *Leish-maniasis,* which is commonly called "oriental sore," is caused by a parasite known as *Leishmania tropica*. Painless multiple ulcers appear over the skin, but frequently the mucous membrane, especially of the mouth, is invaded. The ulcers usually appear as areas resulting from destruction of skin with an unhealthy granular base, but occasionally papillomatous surfaces are formed. *Tropical ulcer,* sometimes known as tropical phagedena, is caused by the *Spirocheta schaudinni* and fusiform bacilli in symbiosis and is rarely seen outside the tropics. The initial lesion is pain-ful, papillomatous in character, becomes necrotic and ulcerates. These ulcers may become multiple and enormous in size, but may heal with a deforming scar. The lesions apparently respond best to arsenicals and potassium iodide. The fusiform bacillus isolated in these instances is a strict anaerobe, whereas the spirochete may be cultured aerobically (Smith[72]).

BIBLIOGRAPHY

1. SCHAUDINN, F., and HOFFMANN, E. Vorläufiger Bericht uber das Vorkommen von Spirochaeten in Syphilitischen Krankheitsprodukten und bei Papillomen, *Arb. a.d.k. Gsndhtsamte,* Berlin, 22:527, 1905.
2. EHRLICH, P., and HATA, S. Die Exp. Chemetherapie der Spirilloson (Syphilis, rückfallfieber, etc.), Berlin, 1910.
3. KOCH, R. Die Aetiologie der Tuberculose, *Berl. klin. Wchnschr.,* 19:221, 1882.
4. SMITH, T. A Comparative Study of Bovine Tubercle Bacilli and of Human Bacilli from Sputum, *J. Exper. M.,* 3:451, 1898.
5. CALMETTE, et al. Essais de prémunition par le BCG contre l'infection tuberculeuse de l'homme et des animaux, *Bull. Acad. de méd.,* Paris, 93:681, 1925. Vaccina-tion Against Tuberculosis with BCG: The Present State of the Question, *Brit. J. Tuberc.,* 26:115, 1932.
6. NICOLAIER, ARTHUR. Ueber Infectiösen Tetanus, *Deutsche Med. Wchnschr.,* 10:842, 1884.
7. PORTER, C. A., and RICHARDSON, O. Two Cases of "Rusty Nail" Tetanus, with Tet-anus Bacilli in the Inguinal Glands, *Boston M. & S. J.,* 161:927, 1909.
8. MOORE, R. M. and SINGLETON, A. O. Tetanus at the John Sealy Hospital, *Surg. Gynec. & Obst.,* 69:146, 1939.
9. MEYER, H., and RANSOM, F. Untersuchungen über den Tetanus, *Arch. Exper. Path. u. Pharmakol,* 49:369, 1903.
10. ABEL, J. J., EVANS, E. A., HAMPIL, B. Researches on Tetanus, *Bull. Johns Hop-kins Hosp.,* 59:307, 1936.

11. FIROR, WM., LAMONT, A. and SCHUMACKER, H. B.　Studies on the Cause of Death in Tetanus, *Ann. Surg.,* 111:246, 1940.

12. ZOELLER, C., and RAMON, G.　Les Conditions Biologiques de la Vaccination. Antitétanique par l'anatoxine chez l'homme, *Bull. Acad. de med.,* Paris, 95:104, 1926.

13. HALL, W. W.　Active Immunization against Tetanus with Tetanus Toxoid, *Military Surgeon,* 80:104, 1937; Tetanus Toxoid Immunization in the U. S. Navy, *Ann. Int. Med.,* 14:565, 1940.

14. GOLD, H.　Active Immunization against Tetanus by Means of Tetanus Toxoid Alum—Precipitated Refined, *J. Lab. & Clin. Med.,* 23:903, 1938.

15. HALFORD, F. J.　Gas Gangrene and Tetanus, *Hawaii Med. J.,* 1:169, 1942.

16. FOSHAY, L., and HAGEBUSCH, O. E.　Histaminase in the Treatment of Serum Sickness, *J. Am. M. Ass.,* 112:2398, 1939.

17. COLE, LESLIE, and SPOONER, E. T. C.　The Treatment of Tetanus, with Observation on the Fate of Injected Antitoxin, *Quart. J. M.,* 4:295, 1935.

18. GNAGI, W. G., JR.　Personal communication, 1928.

19. SPAETH, R.　Therapy of Tetanus, *Arch. Int. Med.,* 68:1133, 1941.

20. BRUCE, D.　Analysis of Cases of Tetanus Treated in Home Military Hospitals, *Brit. M. J.,* 11:593, 1915.

21. FEHLEISEN.　Ueber die Züchtung der Erysipelkokken auf künstlichem Nährboden und ihre, Uebertragbarkeit auf den Menschen, *Deutsche Med. Wchnschr.,* 8:553, 1882.

22. PANTON, P. N., and ADAMS, J. E.　An Investigation into the Etiology of Erysipelas and Allied Infections, *Lancet,* 2:1065, 1909.

23. COOKE, J. V.　In Brennemans Practice of Pediatrics, W. F. Prior Company, Hagerstown, Maryland, 1937.

24. SYMMERS, DOUGLAS, and LEWIS, K. M.　Antitoxin Treatment of Erysipelas, *J. Am. M. Ass.,* 99:1082, 1932.

25. UDE, W. H., and PLATOU, E. S.　Erysipelas: a Comparative Study of the More Recent Methods of Treatment, *J. Am. M. Ass.,* 95:1, 1930.

26. HOYNE, A. H., WOLF, A. A., and PRIM, L.　Fatality Rates in the Treatment of 998 Erysipelas Patients, *J. Am. M. Ass.,* 113:2279, 1939.

27. WEINBERG, M., and SEGUIN, P.　La Gangrène Gazeuse, Masson et Cie, Paris, 1918.

28. REED, G. B., and ORR, J. H.　Local Chemotherapy of Experimental Gas Gangrene, *War Med.,* 2:58, 1942.
　　SEWELL, R. L., DOWDY, A. H., and VINCENT, J. G.　Chemotherapy and Roentgen Radiation in Clostridium Welchii Infections, *Surg., Gynec. & Obst.,* 74:361, 1942.

29. KELLY, J. F.　The X-ray as an Aid in the Treatment of Gas Gangrene. *Radiology,* 20:296, 1933; KELLY, J. F., and DOWELL, D. A. *The X-ray Treatment of Gas Gangrene, Acute Peritonitis and Other Infections,* C. C. Thomas, Springfield, 1940.

30. Editorial. *Lancet,* 1:885, 1940.

31. McCOY, G. W.　Studies upon Plague in Ground Squirrels, *Public Health Bulletin,* No. 43, 1911.

32. FRANCIS, E.　The Occurrence of Tularemia in Nature as a Disease of Man, *Public Health Report,* 34, 2061, 1919; 36, 1731, 1921. A Summary of Present Knowledge of Tularemia, Harvey Lectures, 1927-1928, Series 23, Page 25.

33. SIMPSON, W. M.　Tularemia, Paul Hoeber, New York, 1929.

34. FOSHAY, L.　Tularemia Treated by a New Specific Antiserum, *Am. J. Med. Sc.,* 187:235, 1934.

35. HARRIS, D. L.　Personal communication.

36. GOWEN, G. H.　Rabies in Illinois, 1936, *Ill. Med. J.,* 72:174, 1937.

37. HARRIS, D. L.　Antirabic Immunization with Desiccated Vaccine, *Am. J. Pub. Health,* 19:980, 1929.

38. MELENEY, F.　A Differential Diagnosis between Certain Types of Infectious Gangrene of the Skin, *Surg. Gynec. & Obst.,* 56:847, 1933.

39. BLUMER, G., and McFARLANE, A. An Epidemic of Noma, Report of Sixteen Cases, *Am. J. M. Sc.,* 122:527, 1901.

40. BLAIR, V. P., and BROWN, J. B. The septic phlegmon of the floor of the mouth (gensoul), *Internat. J. Orthod. & Oral Surg.,* 16:890, 1930.

41. BLAIR, V. P., MOORE, S., and BYARS, L. T. *Cancer of the Face and Mouth; Diagnosis, Treatment, Surgical Repair,* C. V. Mosby Co., St. Louis, Mo., 1941.

42. WILLIAMS, A. C. Ludwig's Angina, *Surg., Gynec. and Obst.,* 70:140, 1940.

43. FUTAKI, K., et al. The Cause of Rat Bite Fever, *J. Exper. M.,* 23:249, 1916. Spirochaeta Morsus Muris, n. sp., the Cause of Rat-Bite Fever, *J. Exper. M.,* 25:33, 1917.

44. DAVAINE, C. Quoted by Homan, *Textbook of Surgery,* Charles Thomas, Baltimore, Maryland. Page 147, 1931.

45. ISRAËL, JAMES. Neue Beobachtungen auf dem Gebiete der Mykosen des Menschen, *Virchow's Arch. f. path. Anat. u. Physiol.,* Berlin, 74:15, 1878.

46. WRIGHT, J. H. Quoted by Homan's Textbook of Surgery, Charles Thomas, Baltimore, Maryland. Page 144, 1931.

47. LORD, F. T. The Etiology of Actinomycosis, *J. Am. M. Ass.,* 55:1261, 1910. The Etiology, Pathogenesis, and Diagnosis of Actinomycosis, *Medical Clinics of N. Amer.,* 16:829, 1933.

48. SANFORD, A. H., and VOELKER, M. Actinomycosis in the United States, *Arch. Surg.,* 11:809, 1925.

49. FIGI, F. A., and CUTTS, R. E. Actinomycosis in Childhood, *Am. J. Dis. Child.,* 42:279, 1931.

50. GOOD, L. P. Actinomycosis of the Abdomen, *Arch. Surg.,* 22:307, 1931.

51. GRAVES, A. M., and OCHSNER, ALTON. Actinomycosis of the Subphrenic Space, *Am. J. Surg.,* 23:54, 1934.

52. WALKER, O. Sulfanilamide in Treatment of Actinomycosis, *Lancet,* 1:1219, 1938.

53. MILLER, EDWIN, and FELL, E. H. Sulfanilamide in Actinomycosis, *J. Am. M. Ass.,* 112:731, 1939.

54. WANGENSTEEN, OWEN. Role of Surgery in Treatment of Actinomycosis, *Ann. Surg.,* 104:752, 1936.

55. MYERS, H. B. Unappreciated Fungicidal Action of Certain Volatile Oils, *J. Am. M. Ass.,* 89:1834, 1927; Thymol Therapy in Actinomycosis, *J. Am. M. Ass.,* 108:1875, 1937.

56. JOYCE, T. M. Thymol Therapy in Actinomycosis, *Ann. Surg.,* 108:910, 1938.

57. DURAND, NICOLAS, J., and FAVRE. Lymphogranulomatose Inguinale Subaigue, *Bull. et mem. Soc. Med. d. hosp. de Paris,* 35:274, 1913.

58. GRAY, S. H., WHEELER, PAUL, HUNT, G., and BLASCHE, J. Lymphogranuloma Inguinale: Its Incidence in St. Louis, *J. Am. M. Ass.,* 106:919, 1936.

59. STANNUS, H. S. *A Sixth Veneral Disease,* Bailliere, Tindall and Cox, London, 1933.

60. COLE, H. N. Lymphogranuloma Inguinale, the Fourth Venereal Disease, *J. Am. M. Ass.,* 101:1069, 1933.

61. RAINEY, W., and COLE, W. H. Lymphogranuloma Inguinale: Its Relation to Stricture of the Rectum, *Arch. Surg.,* 30:820, 1935.

62. KNIGHT, H. A. and DAVID, V. C. The Treatment of Venereal Lymphogranuloma with Sulfanilamide, *J. Am. M. Ass.,* 112:527, 1939.

63. DEW, H. R. *Hydatid Disease.* Australian Med. Pub. Co., Sydney, Australia, 1928.

64. ARCE, JOSÉ. Hydatid Disease (Hydatidosis) Pathology and Treatment, *Arch Surg.,* 42:1, 1941.

65. IVANISSEVICH, OSCAR. Hidatidosis Osea, *Imprenta Amorrortu Ayacucho,* 774, Buenos Aires, 1934.

66. GILCHRIST, T. C. A Case of Blastomycetic Dermatitis in Man, Annual Meeting of Amer. Derm. Soc., June, 1894; *Johns Hopkins Reports,* 1:269, 1896.

67. BUSSE, O.   Ueber Parasitäre Zelleinschlusse und ihre Züchtung., *Centralbl. f. Bakt,* 16:175, 1894.

68. BATCHELOR, R. C. L. and LEES, R.   Treatment of Chancroid with Sulfanilamide, *Brit. Med. J.,* 1:1100, 1938.

69. RIXFORD, E., and GILCHRIST, T. C.   Two Cases of Protozoan (Coccidioidal), Infection of the Skin and Other Organs, *Johns Hopkins Reports,* 1:209, 1896.

70. STODDARD, J. L., and CUTLER, E. C.   *Torula Infection in Man,* Monographs of the Rockefeller Institute for Medical Research, No. 6, 1916.

71. WATTS, J. W.   Torula Infection, *Am. J. Pathol.,* 8:167, 1932.

72. SMITH, E. C.   Tropical Ulcer: The Distribution of Bacillus Fusiformis and Spirocheta schaudinni in the Lesion, *Proc. Roy. Soc. Med.,* 26:167, 1932.

73. KLAUDER, J. V.   Erysipeloid as an Occupational Disease, *J. Am. Med. Ass.,* 111:1345, 1938.

74. STEWART, S. E.   Active Immunization of Human Beings with Combined Clostridium Perfringens and Tetanus Toxoids, *War Med.,* 3:508, 1943.

** See page 80. The method authorized by the War Department (War Medicine 1:426, 1941) consists of three injections of 1 cc. given at intervals of 3 weeks. A "stimulating" often called "booster" dose (1 cc.) is given at time of injury or one year later.

CHAPTER VII

ULCER, GANGRENE, SINUS, FISTULA

Ulcer   *Sinus*
Gangrene   *Fistula*

ULCER

An ulcer is an open superficial defect of an external or internal body surface associated with retarded healing. Only the external body surface will be considered here. Most of these ulcers are in the lower extremity. The distinction between an ulcer and a superficial open wound is ill defined, although the duration of the lesion is usually the factor used in differentiating them, *e.g.,* a superficial wound which does not heal in a few weeks becomes known as an ulcer. Treatment will, of course, be haphazard unless the cause is known.

Etiologic Factors.—The diagnosis or identification of the various types of ulcers may be extremely difficult, chiefly because of the fact that so many of the types resemble each other clinically, but also because there are many in which the etiological factor is unknown. Moreover, many ulcers are frequently associated with *more than one etiologic factor.* For example, many patients with ulcers of the leg are afflicted with more than one circulatory lesion, or may have a nerve lesion, syphilis, etc., each of which may be of etiologic significance. In a few patients no plausible cause can be made out; in such cases treatment is obviously non-specific. One of the most helpful aids in the differential diagnosis of ulcers is the history. For example, the skin may have been destroyed by trauma, and chronicity result from inadequate or improper treatment such as lack of cleanliness, or application of irritating chemicals (the prolonged use of antiseptics). The patient's occupation may be indirectly responsible for his ulcer, because of continued trauma and irritation. The age of a patient is important, because ulcers due to such causes as vascular lesions, will rarely be encountered in children. In many cases a simple cause may be responsible for failure of the ulcer to heal, *i.e.,* too frequent changes in dressing without proper care may exert repeated mechanical trauma and interrupt normal epithelialization. Undoubtedly varicose veins are responsible for more chronic ulcers than any other single factor, even though they are encountered only on the leg. A posttraumatic scar in a dependent position may become the seat of an ulcer, especially if there is any irritation due to clothing, etc. Foreign bodies may be imbedded in the superficial tissue and be the cause of persistent ulcers. There are numerous *systemic diseases* such as syringomyelia, tuberculosis, diabetes, arteriosclerosis and syphilis (including tabes) which may be the instigating and sometimes the sole factor in the production of an ulcer.

Diagnosis.—Clinical characteristics are, of course, helpful in suggesting or excluding various etiologic factors, local or general. The location is important. As stated, varicose ulcers occur only on the leg and usually on the lower portion. If an ulcer is encountered on the abdominal wall, such etiologic factors as varicosities, arteriosclerosis, etc., could obviously be eliminated. Varicose, traumatic and malignant ulcers are apt to be single, but ulcers caused by infectious processes tend to be multiple. The base of an ulcer may be shallow or deep. Ulcers produced by electrical injury are apt to be deep and have a jagged necrotic base. The base may be shallow as in burns, or elevated as is usually noted in blastomycosis and granuloma inguinale. The base of many ulcers, including burns, etc., is usually smooth, but blastomycosis, malignant ulcer, etc., is characteristically irregular and possesses a "cauliflower" appearance. The edges of most ulcers are irregular except when the healing process is active, or in syphilis in which the characteristic "punched-out" appearance is noted. The edge may be undermined as is so characteristically noted in ulcers due to symbiotic infection, amebic ulceration, and tuberculosis. Raised edges imply the presence of an acute inflammatory reaction or malignancy. The discharge from ulcers such as those caused by syphilis and lymphatic stasis is serous, but may be purulent when secondary infection is pronounced. Occasionally small ulcers are in reality the superficial portion of a sinus or fistula.

On certain occasions the diagnosis can only be made by *laboratory procedures*. If the diagnosis is in doubt, smears and cultures of pus from the ulcer should be made. The pus should be taken from the surface of an active portion of the ulcer or from miliary abscesses along the edge if any are present. If one of the yeast-like organisms is suspected, the addition of a drop of weak solution of sodium hydroxide will aid in the detection of the organisms. Stained smears will be more useful if the ulcer is of bacterial origin. It should be remembered, however, that any superficial ulcer will in time become secondarily infected. Various types of cultures should be made, including anaerobic and aerobic. If the ulcer is thought to be caused by two or more organisms growing in symbiosis, a piece of tissue should be excised, ground up and cultured aerobically and anaerobically since one of the organisms is apt to be aerobic and the other anaerobic (Meleney). Inoculation of pus or ground tissue into animals may reproduce the disease. Advantage should be taken of the specificity of the various tests for syphilis. Agglutination tests (tularemia), sensitization tests (venereal lymphogranuloma, tuberculosis), etc., are valuable and are briefly described under the respective diseases in Chapter VI.

CLASSIFICATION OF CAUSES OF ULCER (EXTERNAL SURFACES ONLY)

1. Circulatory diseases
    (*a*) Varicose veins
    (*b*) Arteriolar disease
    (*c*) Lymphatic obstruction (lymphedema)
        with and without thrombophlebitis
    (*d*) Arteriosclerotic disease
    (*e*) Raynaud's disease
    (*f*) Buerger's disease

2. Produced by infections
   (a) Syphilis
   (b) Tuberculosis
   (c) Mycotic infection
       Actinomycosis
       Blastomycosis
       Sporotrichosis
   (d) Pyogenic infection
       Anaerobic and Symbiotic
3. Neurogenic (trophic)
   Tabes, syringomyelia, injury to spinal cord or nerves
4. Traumatic
   Physical, chemical, thermal
5. Malignant
   Basal and squamous cell carcinoma
6. Decubitus
7. Radium and x-ray
8. Miscellaneous causes
   Sickle-cell anemia and diabetes

Ulcers Due to Circulatory Disease.—(a) *Varicose ulcers* probably offer the least difficulty of all in diagnosis and comprise 55 to 65 per cent of the chronic ulcers of the leg as encountered in general practice outside the tropics. The ulcer usually occurs slightly above the internal malleolus, but may develop anywhere on the lower half of the leg. The size is extremely variable, but may progress if untreated until it encircles the leg. The ulcers are occasionally bilateral, but only rarely multiple. The ulcer is usually shallow with sloping irregular edges which are not undermined. The base is irregular and may present healthy or unhealthy granulations, depending upon the amount of stasis, treatment, etc. A moderate amount of purulent discharge is present, dependent, of course, upon secondary infection. Pain when severe is due to associated cellulitis. There is usually a moderate amount of edema present which is most pronounced at the end of the day and markedly diminished after a night's rest. The skin around the ulcer is usually pigmented, scaly and atrophic, and presents either a brown or a pitting edematous surface. Pigmentation and a scaly eczema usually precede the ulcer which commonly makes its appearance after a slight injury. There is seldom difficulty in demonstrating an abundant network of varicose veins, except that frequently large deep veins in the brawny skin near the ulcer may be discernible only as a linear area of softening in the skin. In the treatment of the ulcer, it is exceedingly important that these veins be discovered and obliterated. Rest is essential in preventing progression of the ulceration, but the most effective treatment is to obliterate the veins by some type of sclerosing agent. However, infection about the ulcer must be brought to a minimum before injections are made because of the danger of infective phlebitis and pulmonary embolism. Many surgeons, Ochsner and Mahorner,[1] Sarma,[2] and others, consider ligation of the saphenous vein contraindicated in the presence of an ulcer because of the increased incidence of complications. With an elastic stocking or bandage, the ulcer will frequently heal without injections, but recurrence is almost inevitable. Local medicinal therapy is not helpful. Contrast baths, application of heat, elevation of the leg, etc., may be helpful at times in accelerating the healing process. When scarring about the ulcer and its base is dense, it may be advisable to excise the entire area and resort to a skin graft, after preliminary treatment (bed rest and wet packs) to alleviate infection. The ulcers may resist treatment because of an associated lymphatic stasis, arteriolar disease, or other complicating diseases. Flamed adhesive or better still, elastic adhesive (elastoplast) may be applied directly

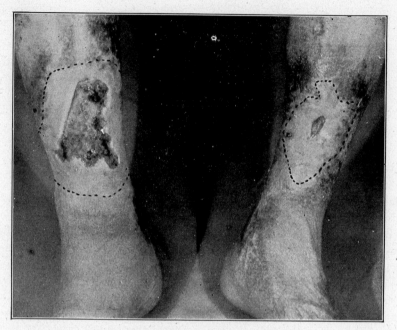

FIG. 67.—VARICOSE ULCERS OF THE LEGS.

The dotted lines illustrate the enormous size of the ulcers before treatment (injection of varicose veins) was begun. The ulcers healed rapidly, within six weeks, to the size depicted, but ultimate complete healing was sluggish and impaired because of a concomitant arterial disease.

over the ulcer in the absence of acute inflammation and will often promote rapid healing. An excellent study of the treatment and healing of varicose and other ulcers of the leg is that of Douglas [3] who studied especially the effect of elastic dressings.

(b) *Arteriolar disease* is a term applied by us to an arterial deficiency (see Chapter XX) frequently associated with ulcers, which, in our experience at least, cannot be satisfactorily explained without assuming the presence of vascular obstruction in the arterioles. Such ulcers are frequently seen in elderly people who are afflicted with arteriosclerosis, but are likewise common in young individuals. The dorsalis pedis and posterior tibial pulsation may be present and of normal volume. Frequently, however, one of these pulsations is absent. The fact that we have occasionally demonstrated a return of pulsation in these vessels (after spinal anesthesia, heat therapy, etc.) suggests that there is an angiospastic element present along with the anatomical obliteration.

The skin of the toes and distal part of the foot about the ulcer is usually flushed or slightly cyanotic when the patient is standing, but blanches when the foot is elevated. We have learned that such a finding, in the absence of edema, is practically pathognomonic of arterial obstruction, and since the obstruction is not in the major arteries (frequently, at least) it must be in the smaller ones (arterioles). In addition to the flushing, cyanosis and blanching as described above, the feet are usually cold and there is frequently a history that the feet become uncomfortably cold even in mild weather. The ulcers occur on the distal part of the leg, the plantar

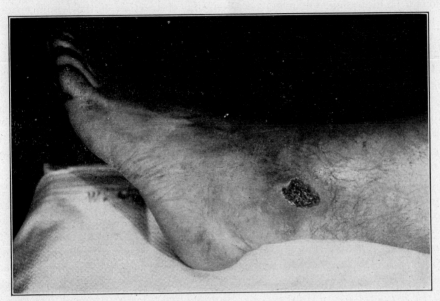

FIG. 68.—ULCER OF THE LEG DUE TO ARTERIAL (ARTERIOLAR) DEFICIENCY.

Ulceration at this point had appeared, healed and recurred at intervals for ten years and had been present for one year at the time the above photograph was taken. The patient was a woman, aged 34 years. A few varicose veins were found and obliterated by injection, but without any beneficial effect on the ulcer. Practically all the characteristics of ulcer due to arteriolar disease as described in the text were present in this patient. Healing was finally achieved by rest, heat, cleanliness and application of a pressure bandage to the leg.

surface of the foot or toes, and are occasionally of the perforating type, i.e., a small round, but deep ulcer. Originally these ulcers were considered purely neurogenic (trophic) i.e., secondary to a lesion of the nervous system such as tabes. However, they are seen so commonly in the absence of these diseases as well as arteriosclerosis, that arteriolar disease remains as the most logical explanation. Little tenderness or pain is present. Discharge is scanty and serous. When they are present on the plantar surface of the foot they may be preceded or surrounded by a callus. The blood supply in the neighborhood is obviously deficient, because it is difficult to produce bleeding by manipulation. The ulcers are relatively quiescent, but resistant to treatment because of the difficulty in reestablishing a circulation. From the above description a similarity to Raynaud's disease will be noted, but the lack of pain, the tendency for the ulceration to be unilateral, the location of the ulcers, and the absence of attacks of accentuation of symptoms, establishes it as a different disease.

Rarely the disease has been observed to develop into Buerger's disease. Cleanliness, heat, rest and Pavaex therapy (*i.e.*, alternate exposure to positive and negative pressure) may prove to be of value.

(*c*) Ulcers caused by *lymphatic obstruction* are exceedingly common, but frequently are complicated by thrombosis of a major vein and its tributaries. The lymphatic system is in reality a part of the circulatory system and the edema produced by chronic obstruction of lymphatic vessels obviously interferes with normal circulation and nutrition of the tissues and thus plays an important part in the etiology of ulceration. On many occasions the obstruction of the lymph channels is produced by spread of the inflammation accompanying thrombophlebitis femoris to the tissues outside the vein, especially the lymphatics. Although ligation of a major vein in itself produces only a mild transient edema, Zimmermann and de Takats [4] have shown that an extensive venous thrombosis, including tributary veins, will lead to severe lymphatic obstruction with accumulation in the tissues of fluid with a high protein content, followed by development of fibrosis. Occasionally there will be evidence of lymphatic obstruction with no demonstrable thrombophlebitis as, for example, in congenital anomalies and filariasis. Regardless of the cause of the obstruction, or the presence or absence of thrombophlebitis, the leg may be quite edematous, later becoming brawny. There is an associated pigmentation and scaling of the skin. Such edematous, unhealthy tissue is, of course, an ideal field for the production of ulcers, either spontaneous or secondary to mild injury. These ulcers are apt to be deep, have ragged edges with a dirty gray, unhealthy base and exude a profuse, serous discharge. Wearing an elastic bandage or stocking may reduce the edema and symptoms. It is important that general principles mentioned under the treatment for varicose ulcers be instituted. In protracted cases, the Kondoleon operation may so relieve the lymphatic obstruction as to allow healing to take place (Trout, see page 531). However, the skin and subcutaneous tissues of the leg of patients with ulcers caused by lymphatic obstruction frequently are not edematous, but brawny and the seat of deposition of considerable fibrous tissue.

(*d*) Ulcers due to *arteriosclerosis* are in reality preceded by superficial gangrene which in itself is considered in detail later in this chapter. However, there are numerous occasions when an ulcer has been produced primarily by trauma (frequently very slight) and it fails to heal because the degree of sclerosis in the artery is sufficient to create deficient circulation and prevent repair of the injured tissue.

(*e*) The ulcers occurring in *Raynaud's disease* are also secondary to gangrene which, however, is invariably superficial and usually bilateral. The diagnosis and treatment has been considered in Chapter XX.

(*f*) The lesion produced by *Buerger's disease* is likewise gangrene initially (see Chapter XX). The gangrenous tissue may separate or slough off, thereby leaving a sluggish ulcer which is usually located on the toes and on most occasions associated with severe pain in the foot and leg.

2. **Ulcers Produced by Infection.**—(*a*) Ulcers due to *syphilis* are so common in some localities that they have been considered second in frequency to varicose ulcers (Ochsner [5]), but for some reason they are rarely encountered by the authors. They are the result of a breaking down or necrosis of superficial gummas, and occur in the upper portion of the leg more often than the lower, but may develop on

various portions of the body. They are frequently multiple, but rarely are as large as varicose ulcers. They are round with smooth edges and usually present a "punched-out" appearance. Rarely are they painful. The base of the ulcer has been described as having a "washed leather" appearance. The discharge is profuse, serous and very offensive; bleeding is common. The Kahn or Wassermann test is almost always positive. Response to antisyphilitic treatment may be sluggish or absent, particularly if dense scarring exists. Fever therapy is effective but is apt to be followed by recurrence.

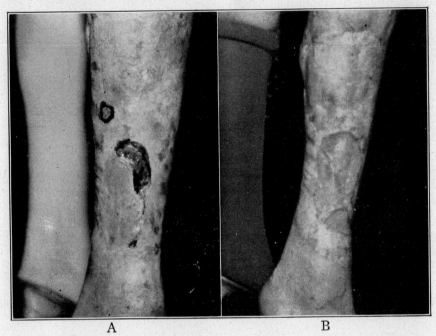

A   B

Fig. 69.—Syphilitic Ulcers of the Leg; Such Ulcers Are Usually Multiple.

A, note the smooth, punched-out appearance of the edge of the ulcer. As happens frequently, antiluetic treatment was ineffectual; *B,* appearance of leg three weeks after excision of the ulcer, and application of skin graft.

(*b*) *Tuberculous ulcers* are fortunately rather uncommon, but may appear in a variety of forms. Lupus vulgaris, which is the commonest form, starts as a reddish-brown patchy eruption usually on the skin of the face of children or young people. In most instances the eruption is secondary to a primary tuberculosis elsewhere. The lesion is extremely resistant to treatment and because of its presence over many years may result in unsightly scars. Bazin's disease (erythema induratum) manifests itself as multiple small soft nodules appearing on the skin of the legs of young girls who have a primary lesion elsewhere, *e.g.,* cervical lymphadenitis. The nodules tend to break down and form small superficial ulcers. They are not painful, but heal slowly. On rare occasions a deeper and larger ulcer forms, presumably over a mass of tubercles. The base of tuberculous ulcers presents a grayish, unhealthy appearance and the edges are characteristically undermined. The discharge may be profuse and rather thin, but contains considerable flaky material.

(c) *Mycotic ulcers* are described in detail in the preceding chapter. *Blasto-mycosis* typically produces an ulcer with a raised cauliflower-like base. *Actinomy-cosis* tends to produce sinuses, and any ulcers present are usually associated with sinuses. *Sporotrichosis* produces a small indolent primary ulcer, but multiple caseous nodules, which break down and form ulcers and are encountered along the lymphatic channels. Diagnosis in such instances is largely dependent upon the care and skill exercised in taking smears and examining them for mycelial threads, etc. The organisms associated etiologically with the three diseases mentioned can usually be grown on proper culture media.

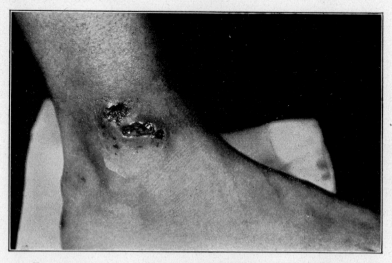

FIG. 70.—PYOGENIC ULCERS DUE TO A STREPTOCOCCUS INFECTION.

The above photograph was taken 5 weeks after onset at the site of minute abscesses which failed to heal presumably because of dependency and the virulence of the organism.

(d) Pyogenic ulcers are of little importance when they are a result of destruction of the skin by an abscess, furuncle, etc., because such lesions ordinarily heal rapidly. On many occasions, wounds of traumatic origin become pyogenic ulcers and heal very slowly, because of an unusual degree of infection associated perhaps with uncleanliness. Healing is frequently affected by such simple factors as dressings and cleanliness. Ulcers produced by *symbiotic* bacteria are associated with gangrene (see page 135).

The *chronic undermining ulcer* shown by Meleney [6] to be due to a micro-aerophilic hemolytic streptococcus, is much more serious because of its chronicity and progression, but fortunately is uncommon. It may occur on the torso or extremities, usually following an accidental or operative wound; the chief characteristic is undermining and thinning of the skin edges with increase in size, brought about by necrosis. Fever and pain are moderate, although the patient will become totally disabled because of the enormous size of the ulcer if it is allowed to progress; emaciation gradually takes place and the patient's morale sinks to a very low ebb. The most effective treatment consists of the local application of a 50 per cent suspension of zinc peroxide [6] in sterile distilled water applied once or twice per day.

With the aid of a syringe, the suspension is applied to all crevices and sinuses in the ulcerated area, and gauze or cotton soaked in the suspension placed in the ulcer. Vaseline strips are placed over the packs to prevent drying of the paste. The zinc peroxide must be of the active type and should be sterilized at 140° C. for 4 hours before using. The drug is tested for activity by making a 10 per cent (by weight) suspension and allowing it to stand. If active it should settle out rapidly, leaving a clear supernatant fluid; within an hour bubbles of oxygen begin to form in the sediment, and in 24 hours the mixture becomes flocculent and curdy, with evolution of more gas (Meleney and Johnson [6]). Either sulfanilamide or sulfa-

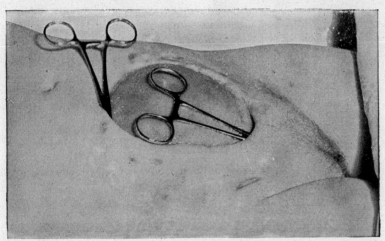

FIG. 71.—CHRONIC UNDERMINING ULCER OF MELENEY, PRODUCED BY A MICRO-AEROPHILIC HEMOLYTIC STREPTOCOCCUS.

The photo represents the ulcer on admission, one year after onset of illness. Note the extensive undermining extending into the vulva and into the flanks. The skin edges were rolled in. Counter incisions had been made in the groins. (From Meleney, *Ann. Surg.,* 101:1006, 1935.)

diazine are very effective. Strict cleanliness of the wound is essential; pus must not be allowed to pool in the undermined areas which should be packed open. Adequate incisions must be made to attain this. After the granulating base is healthy, and undermined areas are eliminated, skin grafts (Thiersch in preference to Reverdin) are applied.

A common type of pyogenic ulcer which heals slowly is that caused by *impetigo* which is a mildly contagious disease consisting of a vesicular-pustular eruption. It occurs more commonly in children than in adults; culture reveals a hemolytic staphylococcus. At times the ulcer produced by the pustule may attain a size equal to 1 centimeter or more in diameter and require three to five weeks for healing.

There are other kinds of pyogenic ulcers which in reality are the result of gangrenous processes; they are discussed under Gangrene later in the chapter.

3. **Neurogenic (Trophic) Ulcers.**—These lesions are usually secondary to diseases of the nervous system as *tabes* or *syringomyelia,* which produce a diminution of painful and thermal stimuli in the area containing the ulcer. This hypesthesia accounts for the numerous injuries (especially burns) sustained by these patients. Impairment of the nerve supply to the skin in some manner interferes seriously with the process of healing. An ulcer on the ball of the foot of the perforating type

may be present in tabes dorsalis, though no history of injury is obtained. Injuries of the *spinal cord* produce anesthesia of the skin; ulcers may develop as described above, because of the ease with which injury is inflicted in anesthetic areas. More important are the ulcers which are produced by pressure, even though slight, over bony prominences, *e.g.,* sacrum, trochanter, etc. Such ulcers develop more readily than the typical decubitus. The skin of extremities which is anesthetic because of

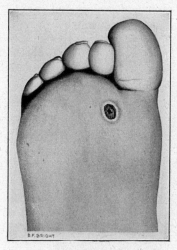

FIG. 72.—PERFORATING ULCER OF THE SOLE OF THE FOOT IN A MAN SEVENTY YEARS OLD WITH SEVERE ARTERIOSCLEROSIS.

Such ulcers are deep and are frequently associated with a large amount of callus. They may occur in patients with arterial as well as neurogenic lesions such as tabes dorsalis, etc.

injury to a major peripheral nerve is, of course, subject to the formation of ulcers in the same manner. It is not uncommon for ulcers also to appear spontaneously on any anesthetic skin, or at least to appear with little trauma or pressure. Neurogenic (or trophic) ulcers of the types described may be of variable size and appearance, but should offer no difficulty in identification because of the injury or disease associated with them. These ulcers respond slowly to treatment, but rest, elevation, bland dressing and cleansing of the wound, application of heat, etc., are useful. It is more important, however, that pressure over the ulcer be abolished; prophylactic avoidance of injury is obviously essential.

4. **Traumatic Ulcers.**—These ulcers may be due to continuous *mechanical irritation* or to injury inflicted by *chemicals* or *burns*. Occasionally an open wound due to direct violence will be delayed in healing because of persistent pressure or irritation caused by an ill-fitting shoe, etc., and thus be classified as a traumatic ulcer. There are many chemicals capable of producing ulcers. Various acids and alkalis, when coming in contact with the skin, will produce first a gangrene followed shortly by an ulcer which heals very sluggishly. More commonly, numerous irritating chemicals are often unwisely added to ointments (including the "carbolic salves") which when applied to simple wounds will prevent healing indefinitely, and even cause the resultant ulcer to increase in size. When the cause of delayed healing of an ulcer is obscure, we wish to emphasize the importance of inquiring diligently as to the application of salves, powders, etc., by the patient. Elimination of the irritating chemicals will often result in rapid healing. Thermal injury (burns and freezing) is considered in detail in Chapter XIV. The resultant ulcers are usually shallow, heal sluggishly, and in the case of burns may be so large as to require skin grafts.

The Thiersch graft will be preferable from the standpoint of adaptability and end results, although pinch grafts will take more readily.

5. **Malignant Ulcers.**—There are two major types of malignant ulcers (basal- and squamous-cell epithelioma). The basal-cell epithelioma or rodent ulcer is malignant only in so far as it invades tissue, but it does not metastasize to distant organs

or lymph nodes. The edges are raised, nodular, indurated and present a rather characteristic pearly appearance. Squamous-cell carcinoma is a malignant tumor which metastasizes readily to regional lymph nodes. The ulceration is not unlike the basal-cell ulcer except that the edge does not have the pearly appearance, and a greater invasive tendency is exhibited. The base of the ulcer is very irregular, presenting areas of necrosis as well as a fungating surface. These ulcers are described in detail on page 302. A *Marjolin ulcer* is a malignant ulcer (squamous-cell)

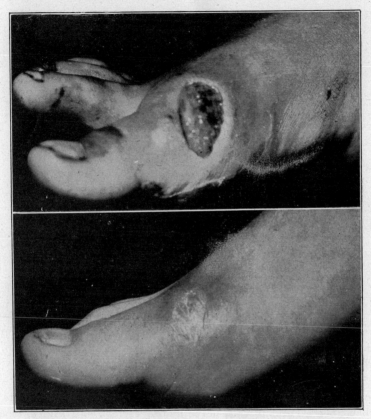

FIG. 73.—TRAUMATIC ULCER DUE TO REPEATED CHEMICAL INJURY.

The top figure shows an ulcer produced by daily application of carbolic ointment for four weeks following a small laceration of the foot in a girl eight years old. Below, within three weeks after elimination of the chemical irritation, the ulcer had healed.

developing in an ulcerating scar produced by injury such as a burn, excessive radium or x-ray radiation, or extensive mechanical injury involving loss of a large amount of skin. They may occur anywhere on the body. The malignant change usually occurs first on the edge of the ulcer as a raised cauliflower-like growth which slowly increases in size. The malignant growth may remain localized to one edge for several months or longer, or may spread to the entire ulcer presenting a raised, fungating hyperplastic base. They are not so malignant as the primary squamous-cell carcinomas and are less apt to recur following excision, providing the skin defect produced by the excision is eliminated by a skin graft.

6. Decubital Ulcers.—Any poorly nourished patient suffering from a prolonged and debilitating illness such as typhoid fever, tuberculosis, etc., may develop decubital ulcers or bed sores, unless adequate nursing care is exercised in turning the patient and protecting bony prominences. Local circulatory impairment plays an important role in the etiology of the decubital ulcers, and in many instances is the only factor producing the ulcer (*e.g.,* decubitus produced by plaster cast). The skin over the sacrum, iliac crest, trochanter, external malleolus and heel is especially

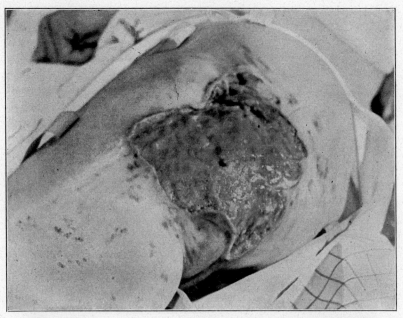

FIG. 74.—SQUAMOUS CELL CARCINOMA (MARJOLIN ULCER) OF THE THIGH AND BUTTOCK.

The patient had an old ulcer produced by a burn thirteen years previously which failed to heal. The hyperplastic changes at the edge of the ulcer were of recent origin, however. (Courtesy of Dr. J. W. Gale.)

susceptible on account of the continuous pressure sustained at these points against the underlying bone. Patients with nerve lesions (spinal cord injury, tabes, etc.) are more susceptible to decubital ulcers than others. The skin becomes slightly reddened, a blister forms and shortly thereafter the tissue becomes indurated and the skin acquires a cyanotic tint. By this time, however, it is too late to prevent the formation of the ulcer. The process of separation of necrotic tissue from living tissue may extend over a surprisingly long period of time (two to four weeks) and when completed may reveal an enormous destruction of tissue, sometimes exposing the bone. Repair and filling in of graulation tissue is even a slower process. Occasionally, in neglected cases, an infection spreads into the adjacent tissue. The added burden of the infection on the patient's physical condition may be sufficient to cause his death. The development of decubital ulcers is in reality a reflection on nursing care. They respond slowly to treatment. Attention should be directed to cleanliness, bland dressings and elimination of pressure over the ulcer; healing, however, is slow and requires weeks.

7. Ulcers Due to Radium and X-ray.—Shortly after the introduction of radium and x-ray in the treatment of malignant tumors, ulcerations resulting from excessive radiation were commonly encountered. Fortunately, however, because of a better understanding of dosage, etc., these ulcers are decreasing in number. The first evidence of injury is a hyperemia of the skin, which is the seat of most of the damage, because of the greater dose of radiation it receives, but more especially because of the sensitiveness of the skin to the rays. The ulceration does not occur

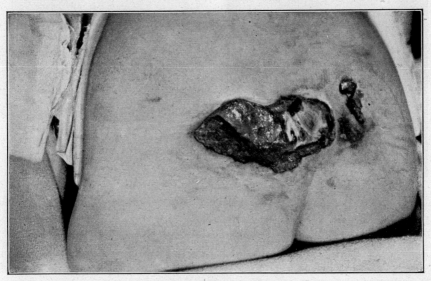

FIG. 75.—DECUBITAL ULCER.

The ulcer is in the sacral region of a patient with paralysis and anesthesia due to spinal cord injury and was produced by the pressure of a plaster cast applied for fixation of the fractured spine. Healing was eventually complete.

for some time after the burn (one to four weeks) and is in reality preceded by gangrene. The base is usually smooth and red. The skin surrounding the ulcer is hyperemic and pigmented. Considerable pain may be present. Healing takes place unusually slowly and the ulcer may be unchanged for years. Excision of the ulcer with application of a skin graft may result in a cure. Occasionally a squamous-cell carcinoma develops at the site of such a burn. This type of carcinoma is usually not very rapidly invasive and responds satisfactorily to thorough excision.

8. Ulcers Due to Miscellaneous Causes.—*Sickle-cell anemia* is a rare familial type of anemia occurring in the negro and may be accompanied by ulcers of the leg. According to Huck[7] these ulcers have the round, indurated, punched-out appearance of syphilitic ulcers. They are usually located in the region of the malleoli or on the dorsum of the foot or leg. The base is clear and not covered with necrotic material. Diagnosis is easy if a blood smear is made and examined. *Diabetes* may also be responsible for the production of ulcers on the extremities (especially the toes), but usually is preceded by gangrene as is described later in Chapter XII. On many occasions, however, ulcers of the perforating type, which have already been described, occur on the plantar surface of the toes or foot. When ulcers are present on the extremities of patients with diabetes, there is almost always a concomitant disease of the blood vessels (arteriosclerosis or arteriolar disease), which is no doubt a factor in the etiology of the ulcer.

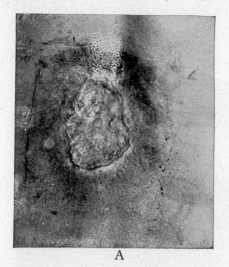
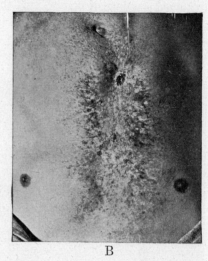

A   B

FIG. 76.—ULCERS DUE TO X-RAY BURN.

A, ulcer due to third degree radiodermatitis of the back, eight months' duration. Pain was severe at first, but decreased later. Eventually a plastic operation was necessary; *B,* chronic radiodermatitis, duration of many years. The area shows many sequelae—cicatrix, atrophy, hyperplasia, pigmentation, depigmentation, telangiectasia, keratoses and, at the lower pole, ulceration and early carcinoma. (From MacKee, G. M., in Christopher, *Textbook of Surgery,* W. B. Saunders Co.) See also, Fig. 156, page 282.

There are many other types of ulceration (granuloma inguinale, lymphogranuloma inguinale, etc.), most of which are of *infectious* etiology and have been discussed in the preceding chapter.

GANGRENE

The term *gangrene* is used to signify the death of tissue and implies that considerable degenerative changes have already taken place. It is the direct result, for the most part, of a loss of blood supply, but there may be a number of secondary factors, including infection, burns, chemicals, etc. Gangrene is in reality synonymous with *necrosis,* but the latter term is used to signify the death of small localized areas, whereas gangrene implies the death of tissue in mass. On many occasions the two terms are used indiscriminately, but clinically we allow location, extent and *discoloration* to influence us in the choice of terms. Necrotic tissue may or may not acquire the black discoloration so typical of gangrene, but usually is gray or white. The mechanism of production of the black discoloration may not seem clear, but is apparently dependent upon exposure to air and the extent of the process as well as the sequence of events in the development of the destructive lesion. *Dry gangrene* occurs when the death of tissue is due to arterial obstruction without an associated venous obstruction or infection. *Moist gangrene* develops if the gangrenous process begins when the tissue is edematous and filled with fluid, or in the presence of infection or venous obstruction.

Arteriosclerotic Gangrene (Senile Gangrene).—When gangrene results from arterial obstruction due to arteriosclerosis it is practically always of the dry type. It is relatively common and occurs in the aged as a result of narrowing of the lumen by the sclerotic process and may or may not be associated with an accompanying thrombosis of the artery. The development of gangrene is usually preceded by a history of pain in the extremity which is, in most instances, located in the calf of the leg. This pain may have been present for years, is dependent upon a decreased blood supply, and is most easily precipitated by extended exercise of the

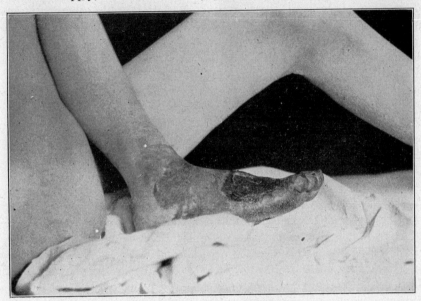

FIG. 77.—ARTERIOSCLEROTIC GANGRENE.
Amputation was advised, but the patient, a woman aged 67 years, refused and left the hospital.

extremity such as walking (*intermittent claudication*). The feet become cold very readily and a feeling of numbness is usually complained of. The actual gangrenous process may occur spontaneously or be started by a slight injury which precipitates inflammation thereby aggravating the effects of the vascular occlusion. Several toes or the entire foot may be included in the process. Before the line of demarcation forms, a moderate amount of burning pain is complained of. It is frequently relieved by elevation of the foot, especially after the line of demarcation is formed. There is usually a definite sequence of events as far as color reaction is concerned in the development of the gangrene. The tissue first becomes pale and white, and after varying periods of time turns red, later cyanotic and finally black.

Examination reveals the dried, shriveled and mummified characteristics of dry gangrene with a hyperemic zone intervening between it and normal appearing skin. Elevation of the foot causes a blanching of the hyperemic areas regardless of whether or not a gangrene is present. There will be no pulsation of the arteries below the obstruction. At times the entire artery from the femoral on down is involved so that even the pulsation of the femoral artery in the groin may be decreased or even absent. A roentgenogram will reveal calcification along the course of the artery, a finding, however, which is often noted in arteriosclerotic patients without circulatory disturbance. Fever is absent except on the occasions when the gangrenous area is extensive or associated with an infection. Since the gangrene is usually dry, the offensive odor of putrefaction is absent. The line of demarcation will usually not form until the gangrenous process has been present for ten to fourteen days. At first there is no break in the continuity of the skin, but a crack soon appears, deepens, and if the patient refuses operative treatment and survives, will result in a spontaneous amputation.

Treatment.—In general, the treatment of arteriosclerotic gangrene is amputation, at a level far above the line of demarcation, in tissue whose blood supply is not appreciably diminished. A more conservative attitude may be adopted in certain circumstances, but, as has been emphasized by Atlas,[8] should be confined to small local areas of gangrene, *e.g.*, gangrene of one toe. In such circumstances, a local amputation, that is, removal of the involved toe, may be permissible. However, if at any time during hospitalization the gangrenous process should spread upward or to other toes, a high amputation in the lower third of the thigh. (or rarely in the upper third of the leg) should be performed without further delay. The choice of level for amputation is determined by various tests, including the histamine flare test, etc., as described in Chapter XX. As already stated, an amputation is not urgent while the gangrene is of the dry type, but if infection develops, giving rise to the so-called wet type of gangrene, immediate amputation will be indicated. During the preoperative period the foot is protected with a cradle without electric bulbs, since heat is detrimental because of increased oxidation in the tissue, and other causes, as demonstrated in the experimental work of Brooks and Duncan.[9] Strict aseptic care, using sterile towels to protect the involved area against contamination from nonsterile bed clothing, etc., must be exercised at all times.

When amputation is performed in the presence of an infection, it is usually advisable to leave the stump wide open, resorting to reamputation at a later date when the stump is healed or the infection under control. Serious complications such as tetanus, gas bacillus infection and septicemia are very apt to develop in patients with moist gangrene, particularly following amputation. To combat these possibilities, it is, therefore, advisable to give sulfanilamide. Only rarely will such procedures as lumbar sympathectomy be advisable in these patients, since the lesion is primarily obstructive and not spastic in origin. Pavaex therapy as originated by Herrmann and Reid [10] may be used, but is contraindicated in the presence of infection, venous thrombosis or massive areas of gangrene. Transfusions and other supportive treatment are used as indicated. A detailed discussion of amputation may be found in Chapter XI.

Diabetic Gangrene.—This type of gangrene is similar to arteriosclerotic gangrene in so far as arteriosclerosis is frequent in diabetics and is the major factor in production of the lesion. However, diabetic gangrene is much more serious because of the higher incidence of infection which a diabetic patient is less able to withstand. Once gangrene of a significant degree develops in a diabetic patient, amputation is practically always indicated; delay is rarely justifiable except for the preoperative correction of acetonuria. It should be emphasized, however, that uncomplicated infections (as occur most commonly in the foot), can be treated by incision and drainage as in nondiabetic patients, but treatment must be most carefully executed. More details of diabetic gangrene will be found in Chapter XII.

Thrombo-Angiitis Obliterans (Buerger's Disease).—The obstruction in thrombo-angiitis obliterans is apparently due to a thickening of the vessel wall caused presumably by thrombosis with subsequent canalization or by a primary thickening of the wall of the blood vessel due to an inflammatory reaction of some kind. The feet are involved more often than the hands, but there is a tendency toward chronicity with involvement of first one extremity then another. Amputation is occasionally necessary, usually on account of the severe pain and not because of gangrene, since gangrene is rarely extensive. Ulcers of the toes are commonly present and are associated with redness, cyanosis and mild edema. The disease is described in detail in Chapter XX.

Gangrene Due to Embolism and Thrombosis.—The gangrene produced by an embolus is usually spectacular because of the suddenness and severity of the initial symptoms. The size of the clot is no doubt in most instances increased by an associated thrombosis extending back to the first major branch. The production of the embolus is dependent upon the presence of a primary site, *i.e.,* endocarditis, pneumonia, typhoid fever, septicemia, etc. The embolus may arise from a heart valve, the wall of the heart or the lung. Obviously, superficial gangrene will be produced only when the embolus lodges in one of the four extremities; the legs are more commonly involved than the arms. Frequently the patient is not aware of the primary lesion responsible for the embolus. Statistics reviewed by Pearse [11] showed that the femoral artery was the most common site of peripheral arterial embolism (39 per cent). Next in order of frequency were the common iliac artery (15 per cent), the brachial artery (11 per cent), aorta (10 per cent), and popliteal artery (9 per cent). Gangrene of the lower extremities is inevitable when the aorta is occluded, except when a partial obstruction of the distal portion of the abdominal aorta has been produced by a lesion such as an aneurysm, for a period sufficiently long to allow collaterals to develop. Ligation can then occasionally be performed successfully (Brooks, *J. A. M. A.,* 87:722, 1926). Utilizing such procedures as simultaneous ligation of the vein and novocain block of the sympathetics, the incidence of gangrene following ligation of smaller vessels would be approximately as follows: common iliac (45 per cent), popliteal (15 per cent), common femoral (15 per cent), and femoral below profunda (8 per cent). Gangrene is relatively uncommon (somewhat less than 10 per cent) when the major arteries of the upper extremity are occluded, occurring with about equal frequency in obstruction of the axillary and subclavian arteries, but is decreased to near zero when ligation is done between the thyrocervical trunk and the circumflex humeri arteries. In general, gangrene is more frequent in amputations in the lower than in the upper extremities.

The first symptom experienced is usually a sudden severe pain in the extremity (commonly the calf of the leg) associated with a complete disability including paralysis. The foot becomes white and cold and the muscles spastic. If the embolus has lodged at the bifurcation of the aorta, both legs will, of course, be involved.

After several hours the white, pallid color changes to a cyanotic blush, and after twenty-four to forty-eight hours, gangrenous patches will develop.

If the patient is seen within a few hours after the embolus has lodged in the artery, an attempt should be made to remove the clot (embolectomy). If this is done early and completely, gangrene will be prevented. Rarely is embolectomy indicated if more than 48 hours have elapsed since the embolism. The position of the embolus will be much higher than the external signs, but accurate localization is sometimes difficult. It is usually preferable to open the artery over the upper limits of the clot which is removed by suction and gentle traction. If the patient is seen after the early signs of gangrene are manifested, embolectomy will be of no value

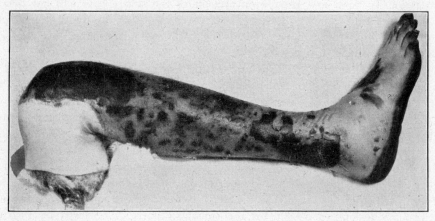

FIG. 78.—GANGRENE OF FOOT AND LEG RESULTING FROM EMBOLUS TO THE FEMORAL ARTERY, IN A YOUNG MAN, AGED TWENTY-SIX, WITH RHEUMATIC HEART DISEASE.

and it will be preferable to wait for the development of a line of demarcation between the gangrenous and viable tissue before performing amputation.

Regardless of whether or not embolectomy is performed, certain routine procedures are advisable. The use of vasodilating drugs such as papaverine (½ grain) or sodium nitrite (1 grain) is advisable (de Takats [12]). The extremity (e.g., foot) is protected with a cradle, but no external heat should be applied, since heat accelerates oxygen consumption in the affected extremity. The extremity should be kept in a slightly dependent position—not elevated.

Traumatic Gangrene.—Because of the increasing number of industrial and automobile accidents it is becoming necessary that traumatic gangrene be given more consideration than previously, especially when we consider that many amputations performed at the present time for crushed or injured extremities are in reality not necessary. Before the aseptic era, amputations for such injuries were indicated to prevent the universal development of serious infection. Such infection can at the present time be largely prevented by proper treatment of the wound (see Chapter X). Although a limb may be severely damaged, it is certainly worth while, with a very few exceptions, to postpone amputation with the hope that a sufficient blood supply will develop from the unsevered tissue to prevent gangrene. This is especially true if the bones of the extremity are not fractured. So often it will be discovered that the gangrene will be limited to the toes or fingers and that the important structures such as the joints can be preserved. It may require several weeks for collateral circulation to develop to the point where healing will progress, but if a portion of the hand or foot can be saved (even if it is partly disabled), it is usually of more value to the patient than an artificial limb. One of the strongest arguments for conservative treatment is that amputation may be safely performed at a later date, if it becomes evident that the extremity distal to the injury cannot survive. If the patient is watched carefully, only on rare occasions indeed will this delay jeopardize the patient's life. Débridement and primary repair of partially severed extremities should be done with as little manipulation as possible to prevent injury to what blood supply is remaining. It is surprising how often huge amounts

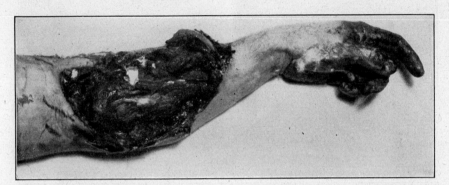

Fig. 79.—Traumatic Gangrene of Hand, Twenty-two Hours after Injury.

Note the crushed and lacerated tissues of the forearm; a severely comminuted fracture of the radius and ulna was also present. Amputation necessary because of the rapid progression of the gangrene. (St. Louis City Hospital.)

of soft tissue which are attached to the body by mere shreds will survive, especially if the patient is received immediately after the accident and the wound properly treated. The massive injuries of war are discussed in Chapter XXXIII.

Bacterial Gangrene.—Perhaps the most serious type of gangrene is that produced by a number of gas-producing anaerobic organisms, among which the *Welch bacillus, Bacillus oedematiens* and *vibrion septique* are the most important. It was an extremely common affliction during World War I, but is encountered only occasionally in civil life. For detailed description see Chapter VI.

In 1924, Meleney [13] described a particularly serious type of gangrene caused by the *hemolytic streptococcus,* which is definitely characteristic, and can readily be differentiated from the others. The initial lesion may or may not be associated with trauma. The skin over a large area becomes red, slightly swollen and hot. A moderate amount of pain and tenderness are present. After twenty-four to forty-eight hours this area of redness becomes cyanotic, and blisters form on the surface. A short time later the skin becomes definitely gangrenous and separation from the viable tissue begins. The base and edges of the defects left by this gangrenous process are dirty gray and necrotic. A small amount of seropurulent fluid collects under the gangrenous skin. Such areas may form elsewhere on the body in rapid succession. If treatment is not immediately and adequately carried out, the process becomes fulminating and the patient's condition critical. The prostration, tachycardia,

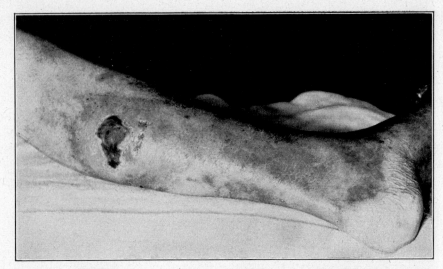

FIG. 80.—HEMOLYTIC STREPTOCOCCUS GANGRENE OF MELENEY.

Onset four days previously, in a healthy man twenty-six years of age, with swelling of leg, fever and other systemic manifestation of infection. This is an unusually mild case and subsided spontaneously.

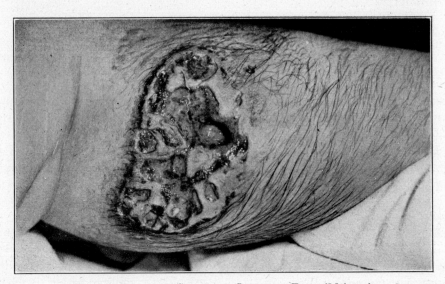

FIG. 81.—BACTERIAL GANGRENE, SYMBIOTIC TYPE (Meleney).

Onset 6 months previously in a woman aged 30 years. When first seen the edges of the ulcer were raised, reddened and very tender; a few patches of gangrenous skin were likewise present. Culture revealed a micro-aerophilic nonhemolytic streptococcus and a hemolytic staphylococcus. The photograph was taken after seven days' rest in bed with meticulous care of the wound. Epithelium is beginning to grow at the edges and likewise in certain areas over the base of the ulcer. Important therapeutic procedures are radical excision, local application of zinc peroxide, and oral administration of sulfanilamide.

fever, etc., clearly indicate the severity of the infection. The lack of a raised, indurated border differentiates the process from erysipelas even in its incipiency. Meleney originally advised radical incision but it is possible that sulfanilamide will adequately control the progress of the disease.

Meleney [13] has also described a *synergistic* or *symbiotic type* of bacterial gangrene which on culture yields in most instances a hemolytic *Staphylococcus aureus* and a micro-aerophilic nonhemolytic *streptococcus*. This lesion differs sharply from the one described above in many respects. It is apt to be a single lesion and commonly develops about the tenth postoperative day at the site of a stay suture following an abdominal operation. The lesion at first resembles a carbuncle with a wide area of inflammatory tissue and in reality produces gangrene of the skin

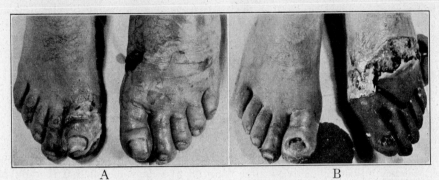

A   B

FIG. 82.—GANGRENE DUE TO FREEZING.

A, four days after freezing; *B,* five days later. Note that definite demarcation is beginning to show up on the left foot. Patient contracted tetanus on the fourteenth day and died. (St. Louis City Hospital.)

because of the undermining characteristics of the infection. The destructive effect is usually superficial and confined to the subcutaneous tissue immediately under the skin, but spreads rapidly in all directions. As the infection progresses, the skin becomes a bright pink in color for a distance of 1 to 3 centimeters from the edge of the ulcer, but after two or three days the margin of this pink area becomes raised, cyanotic and finally becomes necrotic, leaving an ulcerating base. The edges are extremely painful, are tender, and often have a tendency to bleed on the lightest touch. The advancing red or pink edge is sharp and serpiginous and leaves healing granulation in its wake which slowly epithelializes. Excision well beyond the red border is usually necessary to eliminate the disease; skin grafting is done at a later date. Because of its tendency to spread it is often called a phagedenic ulcer. Sulfonamides (preferably sulfadiazine) and active zinc peroxide (Meleney) are effective in this lesion, and may even be tried before resorting to excision.

Thermal Gangrene.—Either excessive heat or freezing will produce gangrene. The destruction of tissue in most burns is confined to the skin and subcutaneous tissue, because of the short exposure. On the contrary, the gangrenous process caused by freezing may include the entire digit or extremity if the member is exposed for hours as is frequently the case. See Chapter XIV for detailed discussion.

Miscellaneous Types of Gangrene.—A *chemical gangrene* may be produced by spilling corrosive substances (acids) on the skin, or by the intentional application of harmful medicinal agents. The most common example of the latter is the repeated and persistent application of "carbolized vaseline" (containing varying amounts of phenol) to lesions on the extremities. Since the phenol acts as a local anesthetic, its "soothing" local effect masks the tissue destruction which is only evident twenty-four to forty-eight hours later. The process of epithelialization progresses slowly following chemical burns. This is decisively illustrated by the slough and sluggish ulcer which develops following the accidental perivascular injections of sclerosing solutions (*e.g.*, sodium salicylate) for obliteration of varicose veins, or of calcium salts injected intravenously. If an acid or strong alkali is spilled on the skin it would appear advisable theoretically to treat it with an antidote or antagonistic chemical. Practically, it has been found that the use of large amounts of water is more effective, because the application of an antagonistic chemical may produce as much damage as the offending chemical, thereby more than offsetting the value of chemical neutralization.

Amebic gangrene of the skin is rare, but has been reported [14] in a few instances chiefly as a superficial gangrenous process complicating abdominal operations. The lesion is almost indistinguishable from that caused by the symbiotic growth of the staphylococcus and streptococcus (page 135). Although motile organisms were found in the pus from the wound of the case reported by Cole and Heideman, the wound did not respond to emetine therapy. Radical excision was necessary to effect a cure. On the other hand the ulcer of the first case described by Engman and Meleney [15] lost all activity after four or five days of emetine therapy and healed so rapidly that a skin graft was not even necessary. This might suggest that in some of these cases there may be a symbiotic relationship in which the amebae at times play a minor role.

In advanced cases of *Raynaud's disease* the fingers and toes may develop a gangrene which may or may not be associated with considerable pain. The gangrene, however, is always of a superficial type; never is an entire extremity involved. For detailed discussion see page 500.

Noma is a gangrenous process of infectious origin occurring about the mouth and cheeks of debilitated children, but which is fortunately becoming quite rare (see page 92.

Gangrene resulting from the poisonous effects of ingested *ergot* is extremely rare, but may occur in elderly people who have eaten large quantities of rye bread contaminated with the fungus, *Claviceps purpurea.* Young women who have taken large amounts of ergot to promote abortion may also suffer from the disease. The most frequent sites affected are the fingers and toes.

Gangrene resulting from *strangulation* is, of course, observed commonly in the intestine in strangulated hernias. Rarely it occurs in the gallbladder as a result of edema and thrombosis of vessels. Still more rarely is it encountered in extremities following injuries in which a plaster cast has been applied too tightly. Such an event is obviously a serious reflection on the surgeon responsible for the application of the cast.

Gangrene of the lung is a form of pulmonary infection in which several (probably symbiotic) organisms are involved and which is accompanied by foul expectoration and fulminating symptoms.

SINUS

A sinus is a track extending from the surface of the body into the deeper tissues, which frequently becomes the site of chronic discharge or suppuration. The superficial part of the lesion may appear to be a simple ulcer, but the history and examination will reveal its true nature. There are four main factors in the production of a sinus: (1) *Foreign bodies* such as metal, wood, unabsorbable sutures, necrotic bone (sequestrum), fecaliths, etc., in the presence of an infection, may lead to a sinus which may be permanent unless the foreign body is removed.

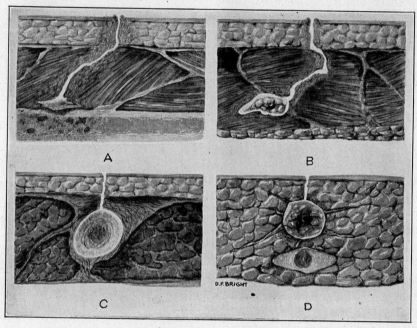

FIG. 83.—TYPES OF SINUSES.

A, sinus maintained by a foreign body (sequestrum); *B*, insufficient drainage of an abscess retards healing and may encourage spread of the infection; *C*, sinus communicating with a tuberculous lymph node; *D*, sinus connected with a pilonidal (epithelial lined) cyst which tends to become infected even before primary rupture of the sinus; strictly, this is a fistula.

(2) Perhaps the most common sinus encountered results from *insufficient drainage* of an ordinary pyogenic infection. The cause of the insufficient drainage may be due to inadequate incision of an abscess, or to tortuosity of the drainage track, or the presence of a collar button abscess, or to lack of a dependent opening. When an ordinary abscess heals there is usually an interval of a few days when a discharging inflammatory track is present after the walls of the cavity have approximated. Theoretically this should be called a sinus, but obviously does not possess the qualities of permanency or chronicity. (3) There are several *chronic infections,* including especially tuberculosis and actinomycosis, which form sinuses resulting from the rupture or incision of abscesses which fail to heal. (4) A sinus is often due to the presence of *epithelial cells* lining the track. These cells secrete more or

less constantly and prevent healing and closure of the sinus. A common example is the draining wound in the neck caused by a persistent thyroglossal duct. Another example is a pilonidal cyst which so commonly opens to the exterior and fails to heal.

Any *treatment* which aims to eliminate a sinus depends, of course, upon the etiologic factor. This must be determined if possible. Injection of the track with a radiopaque substance (lipiodal) followed by a roentgenogram often reveals the extent and relationships of the sinus. Examination by the roentgen ray will also aid in this differentiation if a radiopaque foreign body is present. Gentle probing of superficial sinuses occasionally reveals the presence of a foreign body. After removal of foreign bodies, sinuses usually close within a few days. A secreting epithelial lining must be completely removed by excision, or destroyed by chemical cauterization, preferably the former. A preliminary injection of the sinus track with methylene blue will so visualize its ramifications as to make complete excision easier. If inadequate drainage is the cause of the sinus a thorough incision should be performed. If tuberculosis or actinomycosis is the etiological factor, local treatment will usually be facilitated if the entire local process can be removed.

FISTULA

A fistula is an abnormal communication between epithelial or endothelial lined surfaces (usually hollow viscera) or a communication between a viscus and the exterior. They may be produced in several different ways: (1) Occasionally the communication may be *congenital,* that is, result from a defect in fetal development. Rectovaginal, rectovesical and rectal fistulas are often associated with an imperforate anus. (2) *Postoperative fistulas* may be divided into two types. In the first group (*a*) the fistula is produced intentionally, connecting one viscus with another for functional reasons, *e.g.,* cholecystogastrostomy, ileocolostomy, gastro-enterostomy, etc., (*b*) in a second group of cases, the fistula opens to the outside through accidental or intentional means, *e.g.,* urinary fistula, biliary fistula, etc. Pancreatic fistula and duodenal fistula likewise occur and develop most commonly following operation on the duodenum. A biliary fistula which persists is usually due to an obstruction distal to the opening. In a *fecal fistula* the intestinal content is diverted to the outside; it is frequently performed intentionally, *e.g.,* colostomy, preliminary to a resection of a carcinoma of the rectum. When a fecal fistula results accidentally it usually occurs because of a rupture of an intestinal suture line, which in most instances is caused by an obstruction distal to the operative site. (Frequently, such a leak of intestinal contents produces a fatal peritonitis, before a fecal fistula develops.) On most occasions, fistulas which develop in the absence of obstruction will close spontaneously; they may drain for months, however. If the fistula is located high in the intestine, it will usually not heal spontaneously; furthermore, it may result in the digestion of the skin or the walls of the wound. In addition to the methods of formation as described, a fecal fistula may also develop because of union of the skin with the intestinal mucosa. Treatment of fecal fistulas is considered below and elsewhere. (3) Fistulas caused by tissue destruction due to severe *infection* are extremely common, as clearly illustrated by the rectal fistula which forms as a complicating aftermath of a rectal abscess. (4) Fistulas may be of *mechanical origin*. A vesico-vaginal communication may develop as the result of pressure necrosis during childbirth. A cholecystenterostomy may be formed by the passage of a gallstone from the gallbladder into the intestine. (5) Occasionally a *malignant tumor* may be responsible for the development of a fistula. An intestinal operation performed through malignant tissue may produce a permanent fecal fistula leading to the exterior, if the patient does not first succumb to peritonitis caused by the leak in the suture line.

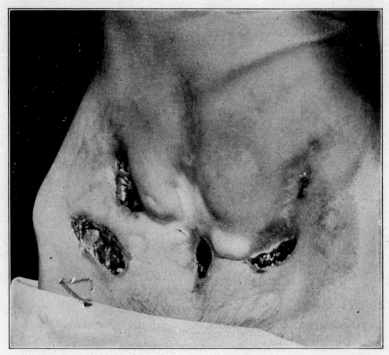

Fig. 84.—Multiple Sinuses and Fistulas of the Abdominal Wall.

Fecal material drains from only one of the openings. The lesions are of three years' duration and followed a pelvic operation.

The *treatment* of fistula depends upon its location and cause. If the communication has followed some type of infectious process, excision of the fistulous track and closure of the opening in the viscus will usually effect a cure. A fistulous communication between two loops of intestines may be cured by dissection of the walls from each other, excision of inflammatory edges, and closure of the openings. Resection of the affected loops followed by an anastomosis may be necessary. The edges of the opening in the intestine must be inverted since union will occur only when the peritoneal surfaces are approximated. A fistula produced by malignant tumors cannot be cured by closure with sutures, but may be eliminated if the growth can be completely excised and the resultant defect repaired.

As already stated, most fecal fistulas, with the exception of those high in the intestinal tract, will heal spontaneously unless there is an obstruction distal to the fistula. If such an obstruction is present, it will obviously have to be corrected by operative means before the fistula will close. If the fistula persists because of attachment of the intestinal mucosa to the skin, an operation consisting of division of the union between mucosa and skin with inversion of the intestinal mucosa should result in a cure. Occasionally, such a repair will produce so much narrowing of the intestinal lumen that either obstruction or a recurrence of the fistula will result. On such occasions, resection of the defect, with an anastomosis between the two loops (proximal and distal) of intestine is indicated.

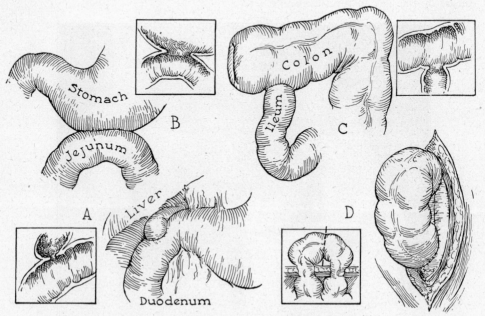

FIG. 85.—COMMON TYPES OF INTESTINAL FISTULA PRODUCED BY OPERATIVE MEANS.

A, cholecystoduodenostomy, performed usually for carcinoma of the pancreas or inoperable carcinoma of the ampulla of Vater; *B,* gastrojejunostomy, utilized in stenosis of the pylorus or duodenum; *C,* ileocolostomy, commonly performed in resection of the proximal colon for carcinoma; *D,* double-barreled colostomy, as performed to correct obstruction in inoperable carcinoma of the rectum, or in the Lockhart-Mummery type of resection of the rectum for carcinoma. On the second or third day the sigmoid is cut across, as shown by the dotted line in the insert.

As will be noted in the above paragraph, the suffix *"ostomy"* is commonly utilized to signify a fistulous communication between different organs of the body (especially intra-abdominal). The term implies the opening of an organ without closure, but establishment of communication with another organ or the exterior. The suffix *"otomy,"* however, implies the opening of the organ or viscus and closure without establishment of a fistulous tract. When the suffix *"ectomy"* is used in connection with an organ or tissue, excision of that organ or tissue is implied.

BIBLIOGRAPHY

1. OCHSNER, ALTON, and MAHORNER, H. R. The Modern Treatment of Varicose Veins, *Surgery,* 2:889, 1937.
2. SARMA, P. J. Saphenous Vein Ligation, *Surg. Cl. North Amer.,* 18:129, 1938.

3. Douglas, B.   Conservative and Radical Measures for the Treatment of Ulcers of Leg, *Arch. Surg.*, 32:756, 1936.

4. Zimmermann, L. M., and de Takats, G.   The Mechanism of Thrombophlebitic Edema, *Arch. Surg.*, 23:937, 1931.

5. Ochsner, A.   Chronic Leg Ulcer, *Internat. S. Digest.*, 11:259, 1931.

6. Meleney, F.   Zinc Peroxide in Treatment of Micro-aerophilic and Anaerobic Infections, with Special Reference to Group of Chronic Ulcerative, Burrowing, Non-Gangrenous Lesions of Abdominal Wall Apparently Due to Micro-aerophilic Haemolytic Streptococcus, *Ann. Surg.*, 101:997, 1935.
   Meleney, F., and Johnson, B. A.   Further Laboratory and Clinical Experiences in the Treatment of Chronic Undermining Burrowing Ulcers with Zinc Peroxide, *Surgery*, 1:169, 1937.

7. Huck, J. G.   Sickle Cell Anemia, *Bull. Johns Hopkins Hosp.*, 34:335, 1923.

8. Atlas, L. N.   Arteriosclerotic Gangrene—A Major Clinical Problem, *Am. J. Surg.*, 49:467, 1940.

9. Brooks, B., and Duncan, G. W.   Effects of Temperature on Survival of Anemic Tissue; Experimental Study, *Ann. Surg.*, 112:130, 1940.

10. Herrmann, L. G., and Reid, M. R.   Passive Vascular Exercises, *Arch. Surg.*, 29:697, 1934. Non-operative Treatment of Inadequate Peripheral Distribution of Blood, *J. Am. M. Ass.*, 105:1256, 1935.

11. Pearse, J. E.   Embolectomy for Arterial Embolism of the Extremities, *Ann. Surg.*, 98:17, 1933.

12. de Takats, G.   Vascular Accidents of the Extremities, *J. Am. M. Ass.*, 110:1075, 1938.

13. Meleney, F.   A Differential Diagnosis between Certain Types of Infectious Gangrene of the Skin, *Surg., Gynec. & Obst.*, 56:847, 1933.

14. Engman, M. F., Sr. and Heithaus, A. S.   Amebiasis Cutis, *J. Cutan. Dis.*, 37:715, 1919. Cole, W. H., and Heideman, M. L.   Amebic Ulcer of the Abdominal Wall Following Appendectomy with Drainage, *J. Am. M. Ass.*, 92:537, 1929.

15. Engman, M. F., Jr. and Meleney, F.   Amebiasis Cutis, *Arch. Dermat. and Syph.*, 24:1, 1931.

CHAPTER VIII

SURGICAL METHODS

Rest, General and Local
Bandaging
The Use of Heat and Cold
The Administration of Fluids
Transfusion

Resuscitation
The Use of the Hollow Needle
The Use of the Rubber Catheter
Preoperative and Postoperative Care

That principles are more important than details is nowhere more true than in the use of therapeutic agents.[1] An understanding of basic principles makes therapy easier, partly because remembering complicated details becomes unnecessary, and useless mental effort is avoided. Knowledge of biochemistry and physiology enables one to exclude many of the fads and fancies which always clutter up our therapeutic armamentarium. The methods advised and even recommended for various surgical diseases are legion, resembling somewhat the thousands of drugs in the pharmacopeia. Many of them are antiquated, some illogical, and a few are actually dangerous. It is axiomatic that the more therapy leans on established observations, whether pathological or physiological, clinical or experimental, the more effective and predictable will be its results. Blood letting, for example, remained such a universal panacea for centuries, because of lack of knowledge of the physiology of the blood and its circulation. The use of complicated dressing materials for wounds was banished as soon as asepsis and antisepsis were shown to control the healing process.

Therapeutic procedures reach their highest level of efficiency when their results are completely predictable. Such a high level has been reached in but few instances. It may be emphasized, therefore, that in so far as therapy remains unpredictable, procedures remain to that extent experimental efforts. It is important, therefore, to observe effects carefully and record the results in order to establish for future use their value or lack of value. In the following discussion an attempt will be made to emphasize the principles involved in order that such observations may be made, and in order that the most effective use may be made of the methods presented. As far as operations are concerned the simpler ones will be described as indicated from time to time. The more complicated ones will only be discussed briefly, particularly as they influence preoperative and postoperative care. The details of such procedures belong to the domain of larger works on operative surgery and will therefore not be described here.

REST, GENERAL AND LOCAL

Rest is probably the greatest single agent in the treatment of disease and, even though its use is almost axiomatic, full advantage of its benefits is not always taken. On the other hand, rest, if unduly prolonged may prove deleterious by inducing the atrophy of disuse and promoting invalidism.

1. *General rest* implies not only physical, but mental rest. The latter element is often overlooked or its significance minimized. Reassurance may be of paramount importance. We are apt to forget the influence of mind over matter, yet there is ample evidence that a patient whose mind is at ease, who sleeps well, has no pain, and who has implicit faith in his doctor will combat infection or injury much more effectively than one who is apprehensive, tired, worried or in pain. Bed rest is usually necessary to achieve this complete mental and physical effect. Unless the patient is very ill or too weak or has had a recent operation, bed rest may be modified in that bathroom privileges are allowed, or a commode provided to avoid using a bed pan and urinal which are always more or less annoying. Bed rest may be modified by elevating the head of the bed, and implies the availability of nursing care whether the patient is in a hospital or at home. Part of the mental and physical rest is the complete anticipation of the patient's needs so that he finds no necessity for thinking of or caring for those needs. Bed rest reduces to a minimum the circulatory and metabolic efforts so that all the bodily energy may be conserved for combating the disease. The disadvantage of prolonged bed rest lies in the possible promotion of atrophy of disuse which affects all the tissues and organs, but is particularly evident in the bones, joints and muscles. This will be discussed later. It may be minimized to some extent by nursing care, especially massage and gentle movements.

2. *Local rest* or rest of an individual part or system may be used either alone or in conjunction with general bed rest. The respiratory system may be rested by prescribing morphin or codein in order to minimize cough, or by a tight chest binder to limit chest movements when fractured ribs are causing pain. Wide adhesive strips or a cloth binder placed around the costal margin during expiration, and surrounding the entire chest are effective. The gastro-intestinal tract is put at rest by ordering "nothing by mouth" in order to limit the degree of intestinal movements. To prevent defecation while a rectal wound is healing, constipating drugs are given. Local rest is used chiefly when applied to local lesions such as infections, injuries, fractures, sprains, etc. Rest is best achieved by complete immobilization of the part, although lesser degrees of immobility are often sufficient. Such limitation of motion prevents pain directly and also relieves the apprehension which fear of pain often induces. Local rest thus aids in achieving mental rest. It likewise minimizes extension of infection, since movement tends to force the bacterial invaders into adjacent tissue. Nevertheless, if too prolonged, local rest may also lead to the atrophy of disuse.

Methods of Immobilization.—The various methods used to achieve immobilization in order of the degree of their completeness are: (*a*) slings and other bandages, (*b*) adhesive strips, (*c*) splints, and (*d*) plaster casts. Bandaging in general will be discussed separately.

(*a*) A sling, usually made of muslin, is the simplest agent with which to put the upper extremity at rest; it may be made to include the hand. With the corners

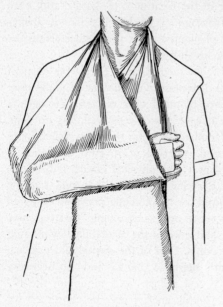

tied tightly behind the neck, the hand and forearm may be brought high up on the chest increasing the degree of immobilization and also producing elevation of the forearm. A useful modification of the sling is the so-called *collar and cuff* (Jones) *sling* which can easily be adjusted to any length allowing any degree of flexion of the elbow.

(*b*) Adhesive strips are used to immobilize the elbow in flexion, the ankle in either eversion or inversion, the patella (to a slight extent), the ribs, the pelvis and sacro-iliac joints. Adhesive is also used to hold dressings in place. Adhesive is not without its defects since it may act as a source of dermatitis in some patients.

(*c*) Splints are made of wood, metal or plaster. The wood boards are thin and cut to proper size and shape. Padding is added on the side next to the skin. Such rigid support prevents motion and is especially necessary in bone and joint injuries (see Chapter XVII). The danger of excessive pressure in fastening splints

FIG. 86.—THE PROPER METHOD OF APPLYING A SLING IN ORDER TO PRODUCE REST AND ELEVATION OF THE FOREARM IN AN AMBULATORY PATIENT.

More elevation of the hand may be obtained by tightening the sling.

in place is always to be avoided. On the other hand, when swelling is already present its subsidence may leave the splint too loose for adequate immobilization. The Thomas splint is an especially useful type for use in the upper and lower extremities and will be described later in discussing the care of fractures.

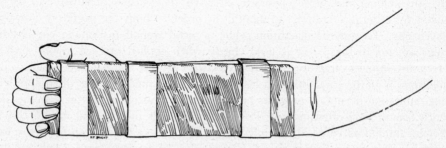

FIG. 87.—IMMOBILIZATION OF THE WRIST AND FOREARM BY MEANS OF A THIN BOARD SPLINT, HELD IN PLACE BY STRIPS OF ADHESIVE.

(*d*) Plaster casts are a fairly efficient means of immobilization. Rolls of gauze, impregnated with hemihydrated calcium sulfate (plaster of Paris) are soaked in water and applied as a bandage to the part which is first protected with cotton padding. In the so-called skin cast, padding is omitted so that the plaster fits more tightly and exerts more nearly perfect immobilization. After a few minutes the plaster hardens into a firm shell which serves to prevent motion. It is used not only over the extremities, but also for the pelvis, spine, head and neck. The term *spica* is used when the lower abdomen and leg are encased, thus immobilizing the hip. A shoulder spica is a similar arrangement about the upper arm and chest. A plaster cuirass is the name given to a body and neck cast used to immobilize the cervical spine, because it looks so much like the metal breast plates worn by the ancient knights. Plaster casts may soften from use or by soiling and may have to be replaced.

Plaster casts have a definite disadvantage in promoting the atrophy of disuse which may be minimized by splitting the cast in half (bivalving) thereby allowing motion under control for short periods between which immobilization continues. Splitting of the cast may be necessary occasionally because of circulatory impairment, *i.e.*, whenever swelling occurs after the cast has been applied. The toes or fingers distal to the cast must be observed for twenty-four hours. Coldness, tingling, numbness, blanching or cyanosis are manifestations of circulatory impairment.

Plaster splints are made of several thicknesses of impregnated gauze moulded over the part to be immobilized. A plaster splint, or slab, is especially convenient to maintain the elbow in flexion by applying it along the posterior surface of the arm, elbow and forearm.

BANDAGING

Bandaging, once a sort of minor art in surgery, now deserves no such designation. The technic of bandaging with the older roller gauze made of thick muslin required special training and courses in bandaging were given in most medical schools. With the advent of the thinner gauze bandage the situation has changed. Bandages used at present are applied with much greater ease and really require no special technic. A bandage serves the purpose not only of rest and immobilization, but also of holding the dressings in place and of protecting wounds against contamination. Bandages, over exposed parts of the body, also minimize heat radiation, thus inducing a higher local temperature which aids repair by increasing local blood flow. Bandages may be made of rolls of gauze, muslin, linen, etc. Wide strips (binders) are used around the chest and abdomen. A popular form of binder is the many-tailed or Scultetus binder. The sling has already been described.

There are many types of bandages which can be applied with a roll of gauze. The *circular or spiral bandage,* as its name implies, is used to cover the sides of an extremity or finger. If the tip of the finger is to be covered or an amputation stump dressed, recurrent layers are first placed over the end and the dressing called a *recurrent bandage*. The *figure-of-eight* is a widely used type which consists of two crossed circular loops of gauze. When used to immobilize a joint such as the knee, elbow or ankle, the loops are placed on either side of the joint. When the loops are passed around each shoulder crossing between the scapulae, traction is exerted on the clavicles. This is a useful bandage in fractures of the clavicle. A *gauntlet bandage* is really a figure-of-eight in which one or more fingers are embraced by one loop,

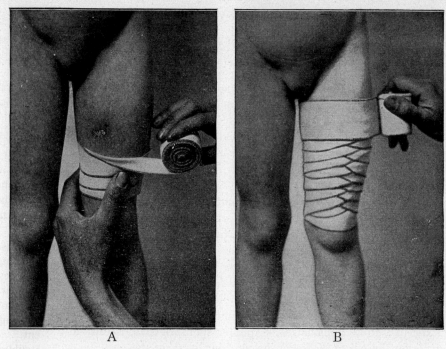

A   B

FIG. 88.—SPIRAL REVERSE BANDAGE OF THIGH.

A, introduction of the first reverse; *B,* completed.
(From Foote and Livingston, *Principles and Practice of Minor Surgery.*)

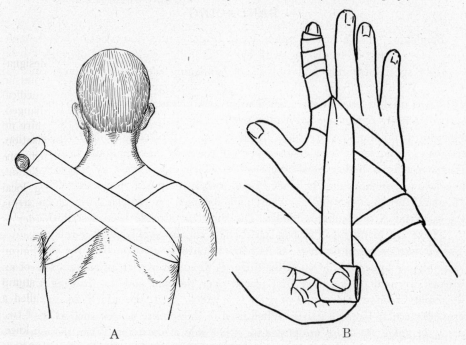

A   B

FIG. 89.—TWO TYPES OF FIGURE-OF-EIGHT BANDAGE.

A, around both shoulders it is useful in immobilization in case of fractured clavicle; *B,* this type is also called a gauntlet bandage. The finger is kept immobilized in extension, flexion being restricted or impossible.

and the wrist by the other, the bandage crossing over the dorsum of the hand. A *spica bandage* is applied in a manner similar to a plaster spica as already described, but gauze alone is used.

Special bandages go by the names of their inventors. Thus *Barton* described a head bandage in which the roll of gauze is made to form three loops, one encircling the head longitudinally in front of the ears, the second horizontally just below the lip including the chin and passing below the ear, the third obliquely joining the first

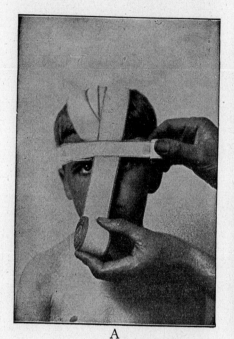 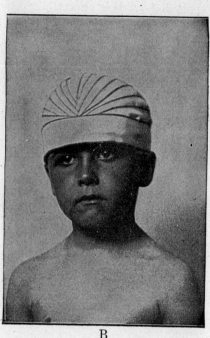

A   B

FIG. 90.—DOUBLE ROLLER BANDAGE OF THE HEAD.

A, each circular turn of the narrower bandage fixes the reverse of the wider one on the forehead and on the occiput; *B,* completed. The Barton bandage is also used for dressings about the head; it is a more extensive bandage since it passes beneath the jaw and around the occiput. (From Foote and Livingston, *Principles and Practice of Minor Surgery.*)

two and passing from the top of the head around the occiput. It is used in various head injuries. A *Velpeau bandage* serves to bind the arm to the chest and to elevate the arm. The hand is first placed on the opposite shoulder, the elbow resting against the chest wall. One turn of gauze passes around the shoulder and the flexed elbow, the other encircles the arm and the chest, binding them together. The hand is free in a Velpeau bandage. It is used in certain fractures of the humerus, shoulder and clavicle, but has lost popularity because of the pain frequently produced by it.

THE USE OF HEAT AND COLD

Disagreements as to the therapeutic indications for hot or cold applications, especially in surgical infections, are not only current now, but date back to the ancients. Esmarch, in 1861, wrote that the dispute even then was hardly modern for Hippocrates and Celsus favored cold applications to wounds while Galen used only warm water or oils. Through the centuries the ruling opinion swayed first one way and then another; enthusiasms waxed and waned. Esmarch himself extolled the so-called antiphlogistic or anti-inflammatory effects of cold; others denounced it as ineffective or dangerous. Such century-old differences of opinion are difficult to justify now for there is ample evidence that cold and heat both exert definite and well-known physiological effects. Disagreements must be due, therefore, to a lack of understanding of these effects.

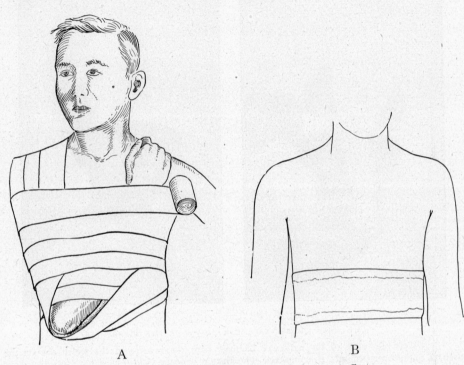

A   B

FIG. 91.—Two Types of Bandage Involving the Chest.

A, the well-known Velpeau bandage, named after the famous French surgeon. It is sometimes used in immobilizing the upper arm in certain types of injury; *B,* a simple chest binder to relieve pain and immobilize the ribs in fracture, as well as in acute pleurisy. The bandage consists of a wide strip of adhesive which firmly embraces the lower chest (while in forced expiration). A layer of thin gauze placed next the skin prevents irritation.

Physiological Effects.—To describe the physiological effects of heat and cold in detail would take us too far afield. For detailed discussion there are many publications [2], [3], [4], [5], [6], [7], [8] which may be consulted. Briefly one may say that heat, whether local or general, is beneficial up to 40° C. (104° F.) in increasing blood flow, exudation, cellular activity and in imparting a sense of warmth. Above this point injurious effects begin. However, when the circulation is impaired the increased tissue metabolism and blood flow produced by local heat may prove deleterious especially in shock (see p. 260). Cold, in general, has an effect opposite to that of heat, *i.e.,* blood flow, exudation and cell activity are slowed and a sense of cold is apparent. As the temperature decreases, anesthesia becomes more and more pronounced and is complete slightly above the freezing point. The process of exudation associated with inflammation also diminishes or may not occur at all under the influence of low temperatures. Cell activity becomes slower; at a point below the freezing point it ceases, and the cell dies. Blood flow also diminishes due to vasoconstriction, and the color of the skin becomes pale or cyanotic. This effect, however, may be replaced by intermittent waves of active vasodilatation, an increased blood flow, and a pink color of the skin as the freezing point is approached (Thomas Lewis[9]). Below the freezing point coagulation of the blood may occur, whereupon all blood flow ceases.

Of great importance in considering these effects of heat and cold is the question of penetration. Surface applications penetrate slowly and not very deeply, usually only a few millimeters. Certain kinds of heat do penetrate, however, i.e., infra-red rays, diathermy and radiothermy rays. Cold, on the other hand, unless excessive in degree cannot be made to penetrate by any special method. Another important factor in the use of heat and cold in bacterial inflammation is the effect they have on the various bacteria themselves. For example, the gonococcus cannot survive a rise in body temperature of more than a few degrees, as is proved by the beneficial effect of fever therapy. This factor is poorly understood and deserves much study.

Specific Uses.—A few of the commonly accepted uses for heat and cold may be mentioned. The application of wet, cold sheets, or immersion of the body in cold water is useful in reducing an abnormally high temperature, particularly in patients with thermic fever (sun stroke). An ice bag is of value in the relief of pain, and to limit or halt exudation. Its value in acute infections is disputed. The present authors feel that cold is apt to be injurious in severe bacterial inflammation. Certainly excessive cold is prone to damage delicate tissues, especially of the face, and is poorly tolerated by the very old and young. Its anesthetic effect is responsible for the absence of any warning stimuli before such damage is done. It finds its greatest value in relieving certain types of inflammatory edema, and in alleviating discomfort when applied locally, especially over deep seated lesions.

The frequent use of the ice bag in acute appendicitis is not only based on misconceptions, but may actually lead to danger. The frequent claim that cold aborts the inflammation, is based on fallacious reasoning for cold penetrates but a few millimeters below the skin surface. Moreover, its reputed inhibitory effect on intestinal peristalsis has not been substantiated by careful observation (Carlson and Orr[10]). Indeed, it has been shown that external cold actually stimulates gastrointestinal activity; inhibition is produced by application of heat (Bisgard and Nye[11]). A practical disadvantage of cold applications in acute abdominal disease is its effect on skin sensation at a time when the surgeon examines the abdomen. The chilling of the surface so interferes with the detection of tenderness, hyperesthesia and muscle spasm that the diagnostic difficulty is considerably increased. The most serious count against the use of an ice bag in acute appendicitis is the false sense of security it engenders. It is well known that, actually, there is no medical treatment for acute appendicitis because there is no sure method of preventing perforation with resultant peritonitis.

Heat is of value in a variety of surgical conditions. Induced elevation of body temperature (artificial fever) is finding increasing use in a variety of diseases. Local heat is useful because it imparts a sense of warmth which is appreciated in many painful lesions. Its greatest value, however, is the promotion of hyperemia and blood flow, exudation and cellular activity in inflammation, thus aiding in nature's defensive reactions. In any case the injurious effect of excessive heat must

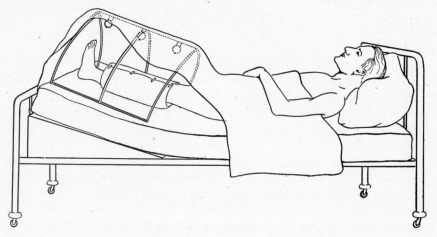

FIG. 92.—A METHOD OF APPLICATION OF LOCAL HEAT TO THE LOWER LEG BY MEANS OF A CRADLE CONTAINING ELECTRIC BULBS.

Rest and elevation of the limb is also achieved.

be avoided. Ordinarily the sense of pain is a safe guide, except in the unconscious patient and over anesthetic areas. Wet heat in the form of soaks or wet dressings is used especially in open wounds; it aids in promoting discharges and in mechanically loosening necrotic tissue. Wet dressings should rarely be used for more than twenty-four or forty-eight hours because they lead to maceration of tissue. Dry heat is applied by means of a hot water bottle, electric bulbs or pad, infra-red lamp, or poultices of various kinds, which are changed as frequently as they cool.

THE ADMINISTRATION OF FLUIDS

The administration of fluids is one of the most important therapeutic aids in surgery and is frequently a life-saving procedure; the surgeon, however, must realize that not only must the correct quantity of fluid be provided but also that the fluid be of the appropriate kind. In health, thirst and hunger ordinarily suffice to insure an adequate intake of fluid and nourishment. In the sick individual, particularly the surgical patient, such subjective sensations are usually depressed; as a result an inadequate amount of food and drink is ingested. Worse than this, many patients become depleted, i.e., they present a deficiency in one or more of the essential components of the body fluids. These components comprise in general the six nutritional elements: water, electrolyte (minerals), carbohydrate, protein, fat and vitamins. All but one (fat) may be considered essential for maintenance. Of the various deficiencies or combinations thereof many are associated with severe clinical manifestations and may even lead to death. Surgeons now realize that replacement of such deficient fluid or food elements is essential if the patient is to recover, especially if he requires an operation which in itself increases the body needs for fluid and food. Provocative discussions of this aspect of surgical therapy form the subject of papers by Holman [12] and Ravdin [13]. The problem confronting the surgeon is really a biochemical one but is easily solved by administration of fluid provided it is the right kind and is given in adequate amounts so as to restore the blood and body tissues toward normal.

KINDS OF FLUID.—While a great variety of substances may be given parenterally, the most important are the five nutritional elements just mentioned, *i.e.,* water, electrolyte, glucose, protein and vitamins. A nutritional approach to the administration of fluids emphasizes the evaluation and correction of biochemical deficiencies which are frequent in surgical patients and can often be remedied effectively only by appropriate parenteral therapy.

Water and electrolyte are given together, and glucose is frequently added thereto. Of these three, water is, of course, the most important, not only because it furnishes a vehicle for the administration of other substances, but because water itself is essential for life, comprising 70 per cent of the total body mass. Closely bound with the interchange of water and of about equal importance is the metabolism of electrolyte. Of the various electrolytes, sodium chloride is the most important.

Physiological sodium chloride or Ringer's solution is always necessary, but urgently needed, whenever electrolyte has been lost. The surgeon is constantly being confronted by conditions in which the electrolyte loss is abnormally great. Vomiting and diarrhea are frequent sources of such loss; various intestinal fistulas including enterostomy and biliary and pancreatic fistula are also important sources of abnormal electrolyte loss. Excessive perspiration also may play an important role. The exact magnitude of this daily loss cannot always be predicted and its actual measurement is laborious. Chemical analysis of the plasma for its base and chloride concentrations will give accurate information as to the existence or absence of electrolyte deficiency; however, because of the time required to make such determinations, there is a lag of several hours before the information can be used. Moreover, chemical analysis will not reflect the possibility of overtreatment; for example, too much saline may result in "salt edema," which is discussed below, yet the plasma chloride level will be normal or even slightly lowered. In general at least 5 to 10 grams of sodium chloride is a minimum daily requirement, provided urinary output is good. More will be needed at the beginning when depletion is severe. For example, Coller and associates [14] have calculated that ½ gram of sodium chloride per kilogram of body weight is required for every 100 mg. per cent that the plasma chloride is under the normal of 560 mg. per cent. Thus, in a 150 pound patient with chloride concentration of 360 mg. per cent (indicating severe deficiency) 70 grams of salt or about 8 liters of physiological salt solution should be given.

Clinical manifestations of electrolyte deficiency are usually striking and should often enable the surgeon and physician to make a bedside diagnosis, although such a condition should always be suspected whenever there has been an abnormal loss, as mentioned above. These manifestations are those of dehydration (see p. 758) and are often reflected in a general dryness of the body tissues, especially of the tongue and mucous membranes. Subjectively the patient first complains of weakness and anorexia with or without thirst. Sooner or later he becomes listless and may even go into coma. In severe cases the patient also complains of muscle cramps in the extremities and even of abdominal pain. Hemoconcentration is usually evident by sharp increases in the red cell count. Fortunately such patients respond remarkably to the administration of salt or Ringer's solution and this change from early shock to complete recovery may occur within the space of a few hours.

Glucose supplies calories and thus spares unnecessary tissue protein breakdown which would otherwise occur to supply (with metabolism of tissue fat) the energy requirements of the body. It must be emphasized, however, that the use of tissue fat is preferable because it is truly non-essential and insofar as it is used, the amount of glucose needed to supply calories is reduced. The utilization of intravenous glucose has been studied by Winslow [16] who found that 93 per cent or more of 5 or 10 per cent glucose was retained if the rate of flow did not exceed 500 c.c. per hour.

Protein nourishment is the most recent addition to parenteral fluid administration; its importance emerges from the increasing realization that protein deficiencies are prevalent in surgical patients and that their correction is extremely necessary. Much of this newer knowledge is based on extensive observations showing that a fall in plasma protein concentration (hypoproteinemia) is of frequent occurrence [17]. While hypoproteinemia may be due to actual loss as in hemorrhage and burns, or to deficient formation as in liver disease, many cases are due to an insufficient protein intake or to excessive tissue protein destruction, or to both. Such hypoproteinemia is often great enough to lead to nutritional edema, *i.e.,* edema which is not cardiac or nephritic, but which follows the lowered colloidal osmotic pressure of the plasma resulting from a sufficient fall in the level of plasma protein. Nutritional edema is apt to follow a drop in the serum protein below 5 grams per cent, particularly when the albumin fraction falls below 2 grams per cent. Nutritional edema is of particular importance to the surgeon, not only because its presence delays healing, but also because this edema may be present in the mucosa of the intestinal tract, producing symptoms of obstruction at gastrointestinal anastomoses (Ravdin [13]). The injection of plasma, which contains 6 to 7 grams per cent of protein, is one method of treating hypoproteinemia. Another is the injection of solutions of amino-acid mixtures, the latter being a method of physiologically short-circuiting the gastrointestinal tract as far as the digestion and absorption of protein nourishment is concerned. While plasma is of dramatic value in acute hypoproteinemia, for nutritional purposes it is more expensive, inconvenient, often ineffective, and theoretically not as satisfactory as amino-acid solutions. For example, one liter of plasma, which requires the bleeding of four donors, contains but 60 to 70 grams of protein which must be metabolized by being broken down to smaller units or even to amino-acids before it can be utilized by the tissues of the body outside the blood stream. Amino-acid solutions, on the other hand, are available in unlimited quantities because they can be made satisfactorily by properly hydrolyzing appropriate proteins. This new method of parenteral protein alimentation has already been used extensively, and may be considered as well beyond the experimental stage. Its use will increase as surgeons realize the importance of protein nutrition and necessity of supplying it parenterally whenever a patient has been or is unable to ingest any or enough protein by mouth [18]. In preparation for abdominal operations and during the postoperative period, amino-acid and peptide mixtures have already proved of great clinical benefit. Although larger amounts can be given by the intravenous route, such solutions have also been given by hypodermoclysis; because it must be isotonic, the latter method obviously requires more fluid for the same amount of nourishment.

Vitamins are now available as pure substances and many may also be given parenterally. The subcutaneous or intramuscular administration is preferable to the intravenous route because of the more rapid excretion in the urine with the latter. Vitamins C, B_1, B_2 and nicotinic acid are now commonly used parenterally; many more will become available. With the addition of vitamins and amino-acids the physician or surgeon is now able to give an almost complete diet intravenously, thus enabling the patient to clear temporary nutritional hurdles and allow healing to occur much more rapidly and with fewer complications.

VOLUME OF FLUID.—The actual volume of fluid required by surgical patients must be sufficient to keep the patient in *fluid balance, i.e.,* the total intake must equal or slightly exceed the total output including an adequate urinary excretion. According to the excellent balance studies of Coller and Maddock,[14] a urinary output of about 1000 c.c. per day in an adult is a fair assurance that fluid and electrolyte balance is being achieved. A rough estimate of the total intake required may thus be obtained by adding 2000 c.c., which is the insensible loss, to the entire fluid output including vomitus and urine. Thus the total intake should amount to between 3000 and 5000 c.c. per day. This amounts to about 40 to 70 c.c. per kg. of body weight. When the patient is dehydrated, more fluid, including especially electrolyte may be required. On the other hand, too much salt solution, particularly in the presence of hypoproteinemia, mey produce "salt edema." In such patients the urinary output is unusually small, the injected fluid accumulating in the tissues. Generalized edema of this type is best treated by the correction of the hypoproteinemia, although it may be helped by the substitution of 5 or 10 per cent glucose for saline. The elevation of the plasma protein concentration is important because the increased colloidal osmotic pressure produced attracts water from the tissues into the blood stream, once it is excreted in the urine. On rare occasions too much water without salt solution may be given, thus producing so-called "water intoxication". An excellent example of the severe manifestations thus produced is described by Helwig, Schurtz and Kuhn [15]: the patient absorbed in forty-two hours nine liters of tap water through proctolysis. Relief of symptoms was achieved and a fatality avoided by the prompt use of intravenous sodium chloride.

MODES OF ADMINISTRATION.—Fluids may be administered by way of the gastrointestinal tract or parenterally. In many cases, however, parenteral injections are used to supplement an inadequate oral intake.

The *gastrointestinal tract* may be used in a variety of ways. The oral administration of fluids and food, while the simplest, often requires constant nursing supervision; sometimes the patient can only be fed through a catheter introduced into the stomach (gavage). The latter is occasionally justifiable especially when the patient is unconscious or unable to swallow, or when it is necessary to put the esophagus at rest. A gastrostomy similarly permits full fluid and food intake in patients with esophageal obstruction. Fluids and predigested foods can also be given through an enterostomy tube when the obstruction is beyond the stomach. Finally, the rectum may also be used to administer fluids, which are then absorbed from the colon but only when the solution is hypotonic or isotonic (tap water, saline, 5 per cent glucose) ; such a procedure is called *proctoclysis* and because of its convenience is widely used to supplement or supplant the administration of fluid orally. Proctoclysis may be given in the form of a rectal tap (300 c.c. every four hours), or continuously by a Murphy drip. As much as 2,000 c.c. may be introduced to an adult in this way in 24 hours, but rarely for more than a few days because the rectal mucosa becomes irritated and expels the solution. In many cases, however, such evidence of irritation is due to a fecal impaction, which, if eliminated, will permit continuation of the proctoclysis. Proctoclysis is also useful for the administration of drugs which cannot be taken by mouth or given parenterally ; *e.g.,* chloral hydrate, a useful sedative, is readily absorbed from the rectum and is given preferably mixed with dilute starch solution, which is added to minimize mucosal irritation.

Parenteral administration of fluids must be used in patients when the gastrointestinal tract, for one reason or another, cannot or should not be used, or is inadequate. The indications for using the parenteral route may be summarized as follows:

1. *Hemorrhage or Surgical Shock.*—In such an emergency the need for fluid must be met rapidly and requires, therefore, the parenteral and especially the intravenous route.

2. *Vomiting.*—In any disease in which there is severe and repeated vomiting, the patient not only fails to assimilate what he ingests but in addition loses gastrointestinal secretions thereby leading rapidly to dehydration.

3. *Severe Diarrhea or a High Intestinal Fistula.*—The loss of gastro-intestinal secretions in such patients occurs because the intestine does not have time for absorption ; this may result in dehydration just as in those who have vomited profusely.

4. *Peritonitis and Gastro-intestinal Operations.*—Because the oral ingestion of fluid may prove injurious the surgeon wishes to put the gastro-intestinal tract at rest by ordering "nothing by mouth." Indeed, he may even introduce a catheter into the stomach for continuous aspiration in order to prevent even gastric juice from entering the intestines.

5. *Lack of Assimilation.*—This indication refers more to food rather than to water. Assimilation may be defective because of nutritional edema or faulty digestion ; it may, therefore, be necessary to resort to parenteral alimentation temporarily to overcome the nutritional depletion.

Parenteral fluids may be given subcutaneously or intravenously ; each has its advantages and disadvantages, and will be discussed separately. Long continued use of veins for intravenous injections often leads to phlebitis and thrombosis which, sooner or later, produces an obliteration of the vessel, precluding its use for further injections. This tendency toward phlebitis is greater with hypertonic solutions, when the period of injection is prolonged and when the needle fills the entire lumen of the vein. When all of the superficial veins have been used up fluid can still be introduced directly into the blood stream by means of an ingenious method described by Tocantis and O'Neill.[36] The procedure consists of injecting the fluid (including blood particularly) into the bone marrow with a special needle which perforates the sternum, or (in infants) the femur. In most cases this method is successful and achieves its results without untoward effects. The injection of fluids intraperitoneally though employed from time to time, has fallen into deserved disuse, owing largely to the dangers and to the irritation of the peritoneum associated with its use.

Subcutaneous fluid (hypodermoclysis) is administered through a needle inserted under the skin into loose subcutaneous tissue whence it is absorbed by the lymphatics.

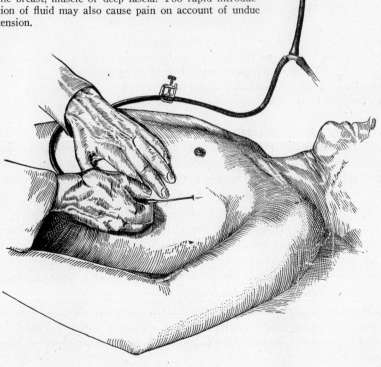

FIG. 93.—THE PROPER METHOD OF GIVING SUBCUTANEOUS SALINE SOLUTION.

Note that the needle is introduced below the lateral margin of the pectoralis major muscle and points upward toward the axilla. Aside from the momentary pain on piercing the skin, a properly administered hypodermoclysis should not cause much discomfort. Common causes of pain: insertion of the needle into the dense subcuticular tissue of the lateral chest wall, into the breast, muscle or deep fascia. Too rapid introduction of fluid may also cause pain on account of undue tension.

The best site is the axilla, because it accommodates large amounts of fluid without stretching the skin and because absorption is rapid due to the rich lymphatic supply. The groin may also be used and, if necessary, the thighs and lower abdominal wall. The fluid must be isotonic and neutral in reaction lest it produce inflammatory changes. Physiological saline or Ringer's solution are the most commonly used, although 5 per cent glucose has also been employed. About 1,500 c.c. can be given at one time and is usually absorbed in an hour or two after which the dose may be repeated. Absorption is most rapid in dehydrated patients needing fluid badly; in shock, on the other hand, the peripheral circulation may be so impaired that very little if any fluid will enter the blood stream in this way.

Intravenous fluid must be prepared with greater care than subcutaneous fluids in order to avoid untoward reactions which may follow intravenous therapy. Such

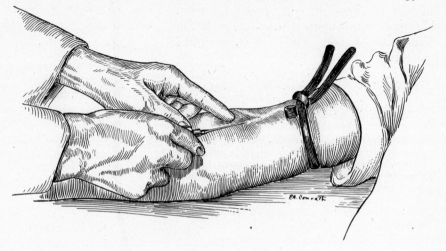

FIG. 94.—THE PROPER METHOD OF PERFORMING A VENIPUNCTURE FOR THE WITHDRAWAL OF BLOOD OR FOR INTRAVENOUS MEDICATION.

The tourniquet is placed to bring the veins into bold relief; it is removed as soon as the vein is entered, as indicated by the free flow of blood into the syringe.

reactions, chills and fever, are due largely to the presence of particulate matter, especially substances called pyrogens which are bacteria or products of bacteria. These bacteria are known to grow in distilled water which is not kept sterile. The first precaution, therefore, in making up solutions for intravenous injection is the use of freshly distilled water; passing all solutions through an efficient Berkfeld filter just before autoclaving is also an excellent way of removing particulate matter and bacteria. A second precaution is the absolute cleanliness of the apparatus including all its connections. Finally, the rate of injection must not be too rapid; usually 5 c.c. per kilo of body weight per hour is safe. Warming intravenous fluid before injection is probably unnecessary; it may be given at room temperature or even lower without deleterious results.

The intravenous route, though less convenient than hypodermoclysis, has the great advantage of rapidity, and in the fact that a greater variety of fluids can be given. These have already been discussed in considerable detail beginning on page 151.

TRANSFUSION

The removal of blood from the veins of one individual followed by its introduction into the veins of another was advocated as early as the 16th century but really lacked any physiological basis until the discovery of the circulation of the blood by Harvey in 1616. Richard Lower in 1665 is credited with being the first to carry out the procedure, which he did successfully in dogs. Two years later lamb's blood was injected into the vein of a human for the first time; the patient recovered but was observed to pass urine "as black as soot" soon after, obviously hemoglobinuria due to hemolysis. Further similar experiences were recorded until a fatality followed a transfusion, whereupon the method was prohibited by law. One hundred fifty years passed before transfusions were tried again. Extensive use of the procedure, however, awaited the discovery of the blood groups by Landsteiner at the turn of the last century. Further details will be found in the excellent book by Wiener [19].

The surgical indications for transfusions are many. In severe septicemia their value has already been discussed on page 35. In surgical shock, especially when there has been considerable hemorrhage, transfusion is particularly indicated and may be life-saving. Its value is enhanced when used prophylactically, for example, when given during the course of a severe operation which is expected to result in shock. Although red cells are important in many conditions in which whole blood is transfused, it is really the plasma portion of the blood which exerts the greatest therapeutic effect. This, as discussed on page 263, is because the protein content of the plasma exerts a colloidal osmotic pressure upon which the circulation and interchange of fluid depends. Thus one c.c. of plasma exerts twice as much colloidal osmotic pressure as one c.c. of whole blood; red cells occupy space but contribute no colloidal effect. This is one of the reasons plasma is greatly displacing the use of whole blood except where there is a severe anemia. Anemia, of course, does follow severe hemorrhage and whole blood is preferable if available. The English learned this fact early in World War II, and in the Libian campaign used huge quantities of whole blood, which was donated by civilians and shipped in by plane (with refrigeration) or was obtained from convalescent soldiers. In the early treatment of burns, on the other hand, plasma is preferable because plasma is actually lost into the burned area and there is a high red cell count (see page 273). The urgent need for plasma to treat shock in severe burns just as in severe hemorrhage is really due to the fact that the body cannot restore the lost plasma rapidly enough. There is an acute hypoproteinemia which may be considered as one of the decisive factors leading to a fatal outcome.[37]

Plasma rather than whole blood transfusions has other advantages of a practical nature. As mentioned later, typing is obviated when plasma is used instead of whole blood particularly when plasma from a large number of donors is pooled. Moreover, plasma may be stored indefinitely, particularly when frozen or dried, unlike whole blood which even with the addition of glucose must be used within a short period of time. Although as generally used plasma is processed from whole blood which has been kept liquid by the addition of sodium citrate, this addition may be avoided by using heparinized plasma or serum. Sodium citrate may indeed provoke toxic manifestations if injected rapidly and in large amounts [20, 21]; such deleterious effects are possible when large citrated blood or plasma transfusions are given rapidly.

The use of whole blood requires careful and special precautions (1) in order to prevent clotting and (2) to insure the injection of compatible blood, *i.e.,* blood from a donor which mixes with the patient's blood without agglutination or hemolysis. Prevention of clotting is achieved by one of two methods. In the first, the transfer of blood from the donor to recipient is so rapid that clotting does not have time to occur. This is called direct transfusion and in the early days was done by joining the artery of the donor to the vein of the recipient. Later, clotting was prevented by using paraffin lined containers (Kimpton Brown tubes). Both of these methods have now been abandoned. At the present time *direct transfusions* may be given by one of several types of special apparatus by which, through a three-way valve and syringe, one draws blood from the donor and injects it into the recipient (Unger, Scannell). The successful use of this type of apparatus may be jeopardized by blood clotting in the valve or tubing. More laborious, but more trustworthy is the multiple syringe cannula (Lindeman) method in which a syringe of blood is withdrawn from the donor and injected immediately into the recipient. A nurse disconnects the syringe and washes it out for use again. This procedure is, of course, carried out under aseptic technic. In the second or *indirect method* clotting is prevented by the addition of an anti-coagulant (sodium citrate) to the blood obtained from the donor (10 c.c. of 2 to 3 per cent sodium citrate solution to each 100 cubic centimeters of blood). The solution must be carefully prepared of pure citrate and distilled water. The advantages of the indirect method are that blood may be obtained and carried wherever needed, and that all need not be given at once, for such sterile citrated blood may be kept in the ice box for several days.

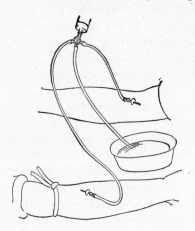

FIG. 95.—A METHOD OF DIRECT TRANSFUSION BY MEANS OF THE SCANNEL APPARATUS.

The Unger method is similar in so far as a three-way stopcock is also used.

"Blood banks" have been established in many hospitals throughout the country for the storage of citrated blood of all groups. The advantages are obvious : transfusions can be given as soon as the patient's blood is typed and cross matched. Stored blood up to a week old can be safely given but after 9 to 10 days is apt to produce reactions, unless the blood is drawn into a flask containing glucose in addition to citrate. Detailed observations and a discussion of the use of preserved blood are excellently presented in the papers of DeGowin, Harris and Plass [22] and in the monograph of Wiener.[19] The use of plasma instead of whole blood is discussed on p. 263.

Compatible blood must be used in whole blood transfusions in order to avoid serious reactions which may even be fatal. Such an accident is due to the agglutination, hemolysis, etc., of the donor's red cells by the patient's serum. The immediate effect is the development of profound dyspnea and cyanosis, accompanied by smothering sensations and severe pain in the chest. A chill and high fever usually follow. Death may result immediately or several hours later. Obviously, should any of these manifestations develop during transfusion, the procedure must be stopped at once. Evidence of severe hemolysis may occur as revealed by hemoglobinuria, anemia and icterus. The donor's and recipient's blood are considered compatible when they belong to the same group or type, and show no agglutination on cross matching. These two prerequisites should be met before a transfusion is undertaken. There are exceptions which will be mentioned below. Needless to say, the Wassermann or Kahn reaction of the donor's blood must be negative.

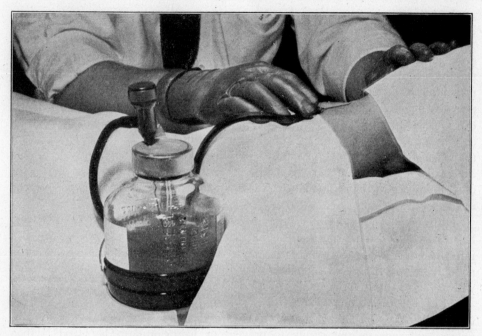

FIG. 96.—A METHOD FOR OBTAINING BLOOD FROM DONOR.

Note that this is a closed system. The airtight flask contains the proper amount of citrate solution (50 cc. of 2.5 per cent for 500 cc. of blood) and is sealed with a partial vacuum so that the flow of blood is automatic and does not depend on gravity or a positive venous pressure.

It should be emphasized that the usual transfusion is about 500 cc. only because it represents the volume which can be safely drawn from the average adult donor. Actually most patients require much more, often two to four times as much.

The four groups into which human blood falls are designated (according to the Jansky classification) as I, II, III and IV. Moss who discovered these groups independently used the same numeration but in a different order, i.e., a Moss I is a Jansky IV and vice versa, although groups II and III are the same (see Table 4). A less commonly used but more scientific designation is that which goes by the name of Landsteiner, who in 1901 discovered [23] the existence of three of the four groups and later did so much to elucidate the nature of the groups. He calls the four groups, AB, A, B and O (see Table 4). The behavior of these blood groups when cross matched, i.e., when red blood cells of one group are mixed with serum of another, is measured by the presence of agglutination.

TABLE 4

Various Designations

Jansky	Moss	Landsteiner
I	IV	O
II	II	A
III	III	B
IV	I	AB

It has been found that reactions rarely occur even when blood from a different group is given, *provided* that the donor's cells are compatible with the patient's plasma. The donor's plasma under these conditions, even though it agglutinates the patient's cells *in vitro* does not do so *in vivo* because it is rapidly diluted by the patient's blood and never is concentrated enough to do so. It is for this reason that plasma transfusions can be given if necessary without typing. For this reason also Group O blood may be given to anyone because the cells of this blood group are not agglutinated by the plasma of any other group. A Group O donor is thus said to be a universal donor. It should be emphasized, however, that the use of universal donors without preliminary cross matching is not advisable except in case of emergency.

Refusion is another term for autotransfusion. When intra-abdominal hemorrhage has occurred, it is sometimes possible at laparotomy to save the spilled blood and inject it into the patient's veins. If the injury is a gunshot or stab wound which has not only severed a large vessel, but also perforated a viscus so that the blood is mixed with urine or intestinal contents, refusion should not be done.

The procedure of refusion consists of dipping out the spilled blood (suction has the disadvantage of breaking up the red blood cells) and collecting it in a basin containing sufficient sodium citrate to prevent or halt clotting. The blood is then given intravenously by the gravity method after filtering through gauze. Physiological saline and glucose may be added to augment the volume of fluid. Gum acacia solution, however, *cannot be used simultaneously with citrated blood* because of chemical incompatibility.

RESUSCITATION

Resuscitation may be necessary in case of sudden respiratory failure (asphyxia) or circulatory failure (heart stoppage) and is often successful if done within a very few minutes, and if no irremediable organic basis for the accident is present. There is in the United States a Society for the Prevention of Asphyxial Death whose publications have an especial interest.[24] A brief discussion of methods of resuscitation may be found in an excellent report by Waters.[25] Respiratory and cardiac emergencies are also discussed in Chapter IX.

1. *Artificial respiration* is instituted when breathing stops suddenly, whether from drowning or other causes. In order for interchange between the lungs and outside air to occur, the upper airway must be patent. To insure this the tongue and jaw must often be drawn forward in order to prevent obstruction of the pharynx

by the base of the tongue. Interchange is brought about by (*a*) forcing air intermittently into the lungs and allowing the elasticity of the chest wall to expel it on the
release of pressure. This is the principle involved in the use of a pulmotor, or a gas
anesthesia machine. (*b*) Forcing air out by external compression of the chest wall

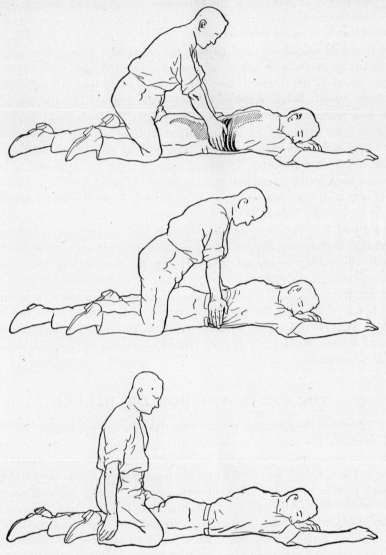

FIG. 97.—THE SCHÄFER METHOD OF RESUSCITATION.
(From Homans, *Textbook of Surgery,* 1931, C. S. Thomas, p. 141.)

is a simpler method; air will then enter on release of pressure owing to the elastic
recoil of the thoracic cage. The greatest expansion of the chest is produced by extending the arms overhead. Expiration is then effected by bringing the arms down and
compressing them against the chest. The patient is usually in a supine position
(on his back) when the accident occurs during an ordinary operation. When pos-

sible, however, the prone position (face down) as in the Schäfer method is preferable inasmuch as it allows the tongue to drop forward, thus keeping the air passage open. This position also aids in the expulsion of vomitus which might otherwise be aspirated, especially on comatose patients in whom also the tongue falls back, producing obstruction. It also aids in the expulsion of water from the lungs in drowning. Artificial respiration is obviously useless when an organic obstruction is present. This is evident by forceful attempts on the part of the patient to breathe. Tracheotomy or laryngeal intubation must be resorted to in such a case. The use of drugs such as caffeine and lobelin are of no proved value, although there is no harm in their use, especially the former. There is no evidence that they can start respirations which have ceased. When respirations are weak and shallow the use of carbon dioxide as a respiratory stimulant (Y. Henderson [26]) is advisable, particularly in carbon monoxide poisoning. It is given mixed with a high concentration of oxygen.

2. After sudden cardiac cessation, *puncture of the heart* with injection of adrenalin has been responsible for saving many lives. Cardiac puncture is usually done with a long needle introduced at the apex of the heart into the ventricle. When blood is obtained, one cubic centimeter of 1:1000 adrenalin solution is injected. A clinical analysis by Hyman,[27] who has studied the question at some length, seems to indicate that it is not the adrenalin which is the effective agent, but rather the mechanical stimulus of the needle. It is true that digital massage of the heart is often successful in starting a stopped heart. It can be done during the course of a laparotomy through the diaphragm or by means of an intercostal incision over the precordium. According to Hyman, the most effective site for mechanical stimulus is not the left ventricle, but the tip of the right auricle which can be reached most easily by a long curved needle introduced just to the right of the sternum. Other features of rescuscitation more directly related to anesthetic complications are discussed in Chapter IX.

THE USE OF THE HOLLOW NEEDLE

It is interesting to speculate on the role that the hollow needle has played in medical advance. Its origin is clouded in the dim mists of antiquity, though it is probable that goose quills were used by savages, and bronze tubes by the ancients as trocars. Thus, Celsus wrote of a cannula for draining ascitic fluid. Hippocrates employed a tube in empyema and mentioned beveling its edge, although an incision was first made. The syringe is not of such ancient lineage. Abulcasis, an Arabian physician of about A.D. 1000, is credited with the first description of a "cannula" which contained a plunger of copper armed with cotton and was used to irrigate the external auditory canal. A goose quill attached to a bladder was used in 1658 to inject medicaments into the vein of a dog for the first time by no less a person than Sir Christopher Wren, the famous English architect and astronomer. The modern hypodermic to introduce drugs is said to have been developed only as recently as 1834 by a Dr. Alexander Wood of Edinburgh. In its present form the needle is made of stainless steel with a sharp beveled edge to permit easy introduction.

The hollow needle may be used either to introduce or withdraw fluid or air. The injection of fluid may be intradermal, subcutaneous, intramuscular, intravenous, intraperitoneal or intraspinal. Withdrawal of fluid is spoken of as aspiration and sometimes as tapping. Needles are used to aspirate fluid from the vein, peritoneal cavity, spinal subarachnoid space, the cerebral ventricles, cisterna magna, pleural space, joints, etc. Often a needle is used to obtain fluid from abscesses or cysts and in large solid tumors of doubtful nature large needles are often useful in actually aspirating enough tissue for microscopic diagnosis.

1. Intradermal injections are made with a fine hypodermic needle to introduce novocaine for local anesthesia or biological materials such as tuberculin, scarlet fever antigen, etc., for diagnostic purposes. A raised wheal is formed when the material is injected into the derma.

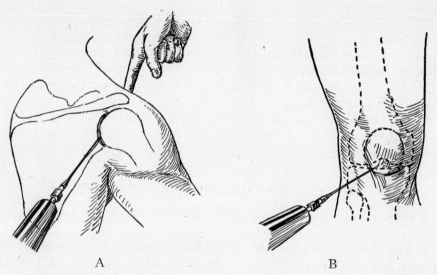

A   B

FIG. 98.—THE USE OF THE HOLLOW NEEDLE IN ASPIRATING FLUID FROM JOINTS.

A, from the shoulder joint (posterior approach); *B,* from the knee joint (just lateral to the patella).

2. Subcutaneous injections are made for the administration of most drugs (morphine, atropine, etc.), a small hypodermic needle being used. When large amounts of fluid (saline) are injected a larger and longer needle is employed.

3. Intramuscular injections are absorbed more rapidly than those into sub-cutaneous tissue, but may be used only when the amount of fluid is small (up to 5 cubic centimeters). The deltoid and gluteal muscles are the usual sites, care being taken to avoid nerves and large vessels.

4. The intravenous route is used both for aspiration of blood as well as for the injection of fluids directly into the blood stream. Venipuncture should be done with a fairly large needle for the former, with a smaller one for the latter purpose. The vein selected is usually at the fold of the elbow (the antecubital space), though veins over the wrist and dorsum of the hand and about the angle are often large enough to be used. Occasionally the external jugular vein may have to be used. In infants the superior sagittal sinus may be the only venous channel large enough. When no vein is apparent, the skin may have to be incised in order to expose a vein. When

the upper or lower extremity is used a tourniquet is first applied to bring the veins into bold relief. It is removed as soon as the vein is entered as shown by the free flow of blood.

5. Peritoneal puncture has been used for diagnostic purposes in infants. As a means of introducing parenteral fluids it is rarely used because of the dangers associated therewith. More commonly it is done to remove ascitic fluid in cases of heart disease, cirrhosis of the liver, and tuberculosis or carcinomatosis of the peritoneal surfaces. Such a procedure is called tapping (paracentesis abdominis) and a large hollow needle (trocar) is used with a stilet in its lumen. Air is sometimes introduced into the peritoneal cavity preparatory to x-ray studies of the viscera (diagnostic pneumoperitoneum).

6. The intraspinal (lumbar subarachnoid) space is often entered to obtain spinal fluid for diagnosis. Spinal puncture is also used to introduce novocaine for spinal anesthesia, air for diagnosis by x-ray (encephalography) and serum in spinal meningitis. Suboccipital (cisterna) puncture has also been used. The epidural space may be entered at the sacral notch to introduce novocaine for the production of so-called sacral anesthesia.

7. The pleural space is entered for aspiration of fluid for diagnosis and treatment (paracentesis thoracis) and for the aspiration or injection of air (artificial pneumothorax).

THE USE OF THE RUBBER CATHETER

A catheter is a rubber tube in which one end is closed, but with an opening near the closed end.

1. *The stomach tube,* for introducing fluid (gavage) or for removing fluid (lavage), is ordinarily used in one of two sizes. The large, more or less rigid, stomach tube can be made to enter the stomach rapidly without the necessity of the patient's swallowing. It is hence of value in uncoöperative or unconscious patients, especially where rapid evacuation and lavage of the stomach is necessary, notably after the taking of poison. The large tube also enables removal of thick or tenacious material in cases of pyloric obstruction with a high degree of retention. The large tube should not be used in patients suspected of having an ulcerated lesion of the esophagus or in individuals with heart disease.

The small tube is used more frequently. It is available in two forms: one with a perforated metal bulb at one end (Rehfuss tube), the other with an opening near the end, as in a catheter. The choice of tube depends upon circumstances. In surgical patients the rigid bulbless nasal tube is commonly used. The tube, cooled by immersion in ice water and lubricated with oil, is passed into one nostril, enters the pharynx, esophagus and stomach. Continuous drainage as popularized by Wangensteen for intestinal obstruction may be carried out by fastening the end of the tube to the face or nose with adhesive. Double lumened tubes are also used particularly for intestinal intubation (see Miller-Abbott tube, p. 767).

2. *The rectal tube* is of the same caliber as a large stomach tube, but much shorter and is used (a) to permit evacuation of gas and (b) to introduce solutions for absorption or as enemas to stimulate bowel movements. Rectal tubes do not go

above the rectum unless introduced higher by means of a proctoscope. Fluid in small amounts (200 cubic centimeters) merely fills the rectum; larger amounts up to one liter may reach the cecum. To stimulate defecation various solutions are used and the procedure is described as a low or high enema, dependent on the amount of fluid employed. Ordinarily a small or low enema is sufficient, for it is merely necessary to chemically stimulate the rectal mucosa. When the amount of fluid given is large stimulation is partly due to the distention produced.

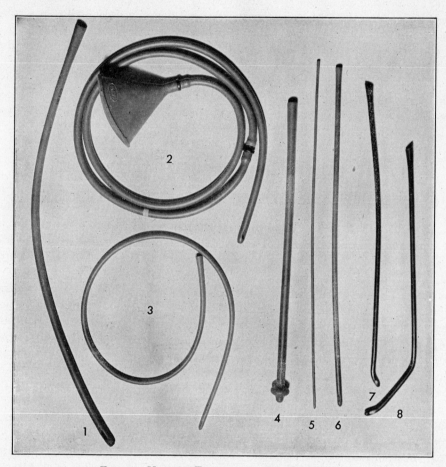

FIG. 99.—VARIOUS TYPES OF RUBBER CATHETERS.

1, Rectal tube (size 28 F.). 2, Stomach tube. 3, Nasal catheter for adults (size 16 F.). 4, Pezzar (mushroom) catheter. 5, Nasal catheter for infants (size 10 F.). 6, Soft rubber urethral catheter (size 20 F.). 7, Urethral catheter (coudé). 8, Urethral catheter (bicoudé).

There are many different kinds of enemas, but the most common are the following:

(a) *Soap suds* (*S.S.*) enema consists of one liter (30 ounces) of warm tap water to which sufficient soap has been added to produce a light suds. It is given slowly and administration is stopped at the first evidence of discomfort. If defecation does not follow and the enema is retained it is necessary to siphon off the solution.

(*b*) *Magnesium sulphate, glycerine and water* (*M.G. and W.*) enema is smaller in amount but more irritating to the mucosa and hence more efficient than an S.S. enema. It ordinarily contains 60 cubic centimeters of a 50 per cent solution of magnesium sulphate, 60 cubic centimeters of glycerine and 60 cubic centimeters of water.

(*c*) *Oil enema* consists of 100 to 200 cubic centimeters (3 to 6 ounces) of warm olive or vegetable oil which is retained for several hours in order to soften a mass of impacted feces. It is then followed by an ordinary S.S. or M.G. and W. enema.

(*d*) *Other enemas* such as milk and molasses and ox-gall solutions are also used by many surgeons.

3. *Catheterization* of the bladder is necessary in many conditions such as prostatic obstruction, postoperative retention, etc. In spite of aseptic precautions there is a danger of introducing bacteria. Careful technic must be observed in any case to minimize this danger.

PREOPERATIVE AND POSTOPERATIVE CARE

Although the description of the actual performance of an operation belongs to special works on operative surgery, the preparations for and after care of operative cases should be part of the knowledge of every physician, and an essential part of the duties of the surgical intern. Actually the diagnosis and indications for operation are decided on by the surgeon in charge, who should also in all cases direct preoperative and postoperative care. It is the resident house officer, however, who sees the patient most often, and is in a favorable position to note and observe signs and symptoms as well as institute prompt treatment for the many untoward events which may occur in surgical patients. An ever watchful and alert resident staff frequently spells the difference between a so-called "smooth" and "stormy" postoperative course. A detailed report on preoperative and postoperative care, prepared for the American College of Surgeons, has been published by Kanavel and Koch.[28] The excellent monograph of Blalock is also recommended.[29]

Preoperative Care.—This includes not only the proper rest for the patient the night before the operation, but also thorough examinations and preoperative preparations, both routine and special.

1. *Rest,* mental and physical, plays an especially important part in the preparation for operation. Apprehension is present to a greater or less degree in all patients before operation, and it may be either banished or aggravated by various contacts after entering the hospital. Courteous, considerate and sympathetic service, quiet and restful surroundings and prompt efficient attention to a definite routine all serve almost at once to put the patient's mind at rest and to engender that sense of security which constitutes mental rest. Cheerfulness and reassurance on the part of the nursing and intern staff achieve the same end. It is continued during the entire stay of the patient, but is particularly important just before and after operation. Sedatives, ordinarily a barbiturate, should also be used to combat restlessness and insure a good night's rest. Catharsis as a preoperative preparation is to be *con-*

demned because it is apt to increase the postoperative nausea, gas pains, vomiting and distention (ileus).

2. *Thorough physical and laboratory examinations* are particularly important in surgical patients about to be operated on, in order to prevent the tragedy of an ill advised procedure and to detect physical defects which may contraindicate it or demand special preparation. Diagnosis, while the responsibility of the surgeon in charge, is often affected decisively by the intern's observations. His history, physical and laboratory examinations may reveal details of significant bearing on the case. Thus an early pregnancy may be detected in a patient about to have an appendectomy for supposed sub-acute appendicitis. Finding amebae in the stool may contraindicate a laparotomy for an acute surgical condition of the abdomen; herpes zoster may be noted in a patient with a diagnosis of acute cholecystitis; neurological changes may indicate that a gastric (tabetic) crisis rather than a perforated ulcer is the disease present. On the other hand, the intern may detect a sore throat, or a furuncle or other beginning infection near the operative field which may demand postponement of an operation of choice. He may find a carcinomatous lump in the breast of which the patient has been completely unaware. The blood pressure should always be reported when abnormally high. In special cases vital capacity measurements should be made.

3. *Immediate preoperative orders* in major operations usually include the following routine: (*a*) Preliminary medication alleviates apprehension and aids in the induction of anesthesia (morphine) and minimizes pharyngeal secretions so inconvenient in giving inhalation anesthesia (atropine). Other hypnotic or soporific drugs are often used, *i.e.,* barbiturates by mouth and avertin by rectum. (*b*) An enema is usually given before operation because the bowels are generally inactive for several days afterwards; catharsis, as already mentioned, is never permitted. (*c*) Gastric lavage is important when a gastric operation is contemplated, particularly when considerable gastric retention is present. (*d*) The field of operation must be adequately prepared by shaving and cleansing the skin widely. Antiseptics are also used to aid in surface sterilization. In operations on the hands or feet this process should be especially thorough and should be repeated, for the exposed horny skin harbors many more bacteria than other areas. Before bone operations the skin is similarly prepared. (*e*) Parenteral fluids are essential to any patient who is dehydrated from vomiting, severe diarrhea, etc. Even if the operation is urgent the delay due to administration of fluid is not great, and is often as necessary for a favorable outcome as the operation itself, since any major operation on a severely dehydrated patient is associated with a very high mortality. Intravenous glucose is important in patients with hepatic disease.

Postoperative (and Post-traumatic) Care.—This period often represents the most crucial time of the surgical patient's illness. Avoidance of accidents, their prompt detection and treatment, and the promotion of rapid and complete healing depend in large measure on efficient and adequate postoperative care. The most important details will be discussed somewhat in order of their frequency and importance.

1. *An accurate record* of frequent and careful observations including pulse, respirations, blood pressure, etc., is a *sine qua non* of good postoperative care. The

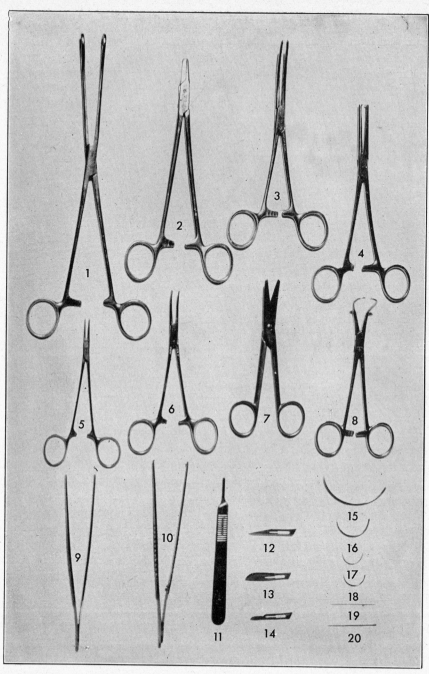

FIG. 100.—VARIOUS INSTRUMENTS USED COMMONLY IN SIMPLE SURGICAL OPERATIONS.

1, Sponge forceps. 2, Needle holder. 3, Rochester curved Pean (old Kelly) clamp. 4, Ochsner clamp (with teeth). 5, Halsted straight mosquito clamp. 6, Curved Kelly (small hemostat). 7, Mayo curved scissors. 8, Towel clip. 9, Thumb forceps (without teeth). 10, Tissue forceps (with teeth). 11, Bard Parker knife handle. 12, Straight bistoury blade. 13, Scalpel blade (med. size). 14, Scalpel blade (small size). 15, Surgeon's cutting needle (full curved). 16, Mayo needle. 17, Ferguson needle. 18, Murphy intestinal needle. 19, Milliner's needle. 20, Keith cutting needle.

first indication of shock may be a progressive increase in pulse rate; pneumonia may be suggested by an increased respiratory rate, etc. These observations must be detailed and begin immediately after the patient leaves the operating room. In special cases other examinations such as repeated blood counts may be indicated.

2. *Pain* may be an early complaint, caused by the wound itself, abdominal cramps (gas pains), pulmonary accidents, urinary retention, etc. Investigation of the nature of the pain should always precede treatment. That due to the wound lasts only a few days and is relieved by analgesics (morphine, etc.). Morphine is said to aggravate abdominal distention, but is the most efficient drug for relief of pain.

3. *Gas pain* is usually associated with *abdominal distention* and is similar to that caused by intestinal obstruction (see page 762), being due to waves of hyperperistalsis which produce cramping. When the pain occurs several days after operation, the problem of differentiation of paralysis of the intestine (ileus) from actual mechanical occlusion may be difficult especially if vomiting is present. Ordinarily, gas pains and distention yield to simple measures such as change of position, loosening of dressings, gastric lavage, passing a rectal tube, and enemas. Heat applied to the abdomen may help. Cathartics are severely to be condemned. Indeed everything by mouth may have to be withheld in order to put the bowel at rest for a short time. Pituitrin is frequently used, but is a drastic means of whipping paralyzed bowel into action. If an occlusion is present it aggravates the lesion. We do not advise its employment.

Acute dilatation of the stomach is really a form of distention occurring not infrequently in peritonitis; repeated regurgitation of small amounts of fluid is very suggestive of this condition. It is accompanied not so much by pain as by vomiting. Its mechanism has been investigated and discussed admirably by Dragstedt.[30] Treatment consists of evacuation of the stomach contents through a nasal catheter or stomach tube as frequently as necessary or by an indwelling tube provided with continuous mild suction. Such gastric decompression may even be started immediately after operation as a prophylactic measure; it also serves to prevent a good deal of nausea and vomiting associated with mild degrees of gastric dilatation.

4. *General rest* and sleep obviously play an important part in achieving complete and satisfactory care. Good nursing, change of position, absence of noise and excitement and reassurance are frequently all that are necessary. Relief of pain is axiomatic. Hypnotics may be used to combat sleeplessness which is due to simple apprehension or restlessness, when physical means are insufficient. Morphine may be used as a last resort when rest cannot be achieved in any other way, though barbiturates by mouth, or chloral hydrate by rectum usually suffice.

5. *Nausea and vomiting* are to the patient the most distressing of postoperative symptoms and are due ordinarily to the effects of the anesthetic, and to the peritoneal irritation in laparotomies. They are frequently entirely absent. If continued for several days other more serious causes are to be considered, such as intestinal obstruction, acute dilatation of the stomach, general peritonitis, and nephritis.

In sensitive patients the problem of postoperative nausea and vomiting may be an especially difficult one. Gastric lavage is effective, especially when much gastric retention is present, and if followed by an adequate sedative may effect relief. A period of twenty-four hours or more of "nothing by mouth" may be indicated before beginning ingestion of fluid. Then one may start with crushed ice or unsweetened carbonated beverages. In some patients solid food such as crackers or toast, etc. will

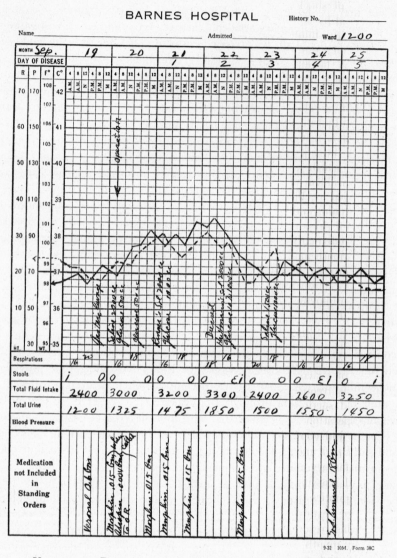

CHART 2.—UNEVENTFUL POSTOPERATIVE COURSE FOLLOWING A GASTRIC RESECTION IN A FIFTY-SIX-YEAR-OLD MAN WITH CARCINOMA OF THE STOMACH.

The elevation of temperature and pulse shown in this case is undesirable but was of no significance.

be less apt to provoke vomiting. Anything very much desired by the patient is less apt to produce nausea and vomiting except that food rich in fat or carbohydrates should not be given. Tea, coffee, sometimes milk mixed with carbonated water and unsweetened lemonade are useful. Reassurance, sympathy and psychotherapy in general are of extreme importance; they sometimes spell the difference between a rapid and prolonged convalescence.

When vomiting results in the loss of much fluid, dehydration of the blood and tissues inevitably occurs. Large amounts of parenteral fluid must be given early to prevent it and to maintain an adequate intake in spite of loss of fluid through vomiting. An accurate record of intake and output is useful in estimating the development of dehydration; the secretion of a small amount of concentrated urine is also suggestive.

6. *Fluid intake* after operations must be high because of the necessity of replacing the large amounts of fluid lost during operation, and because of its value as a prophylactic measure in shock. See detailed discussion on the administration of fluid as previously described in this chapter.

7. *The position of the patient* after operation should be with the head low in order to minimize cerebral anemia and the danger of aspirating vomitus. As soon as consciousness returns this is no longer necessary, and the comfort of the patient is to be considered. Turning the patient frequently is necessary in order to care properly for the skin and to minimize hypostatic pulmonary congestion. Elevation of the back rest of the bed a notch or two relieves much abdominal discomfort about the wound. Frequent movements of the legs aids in the circulation of the lower extremities, tends to avoid phlebitis and embolism from the femoral or iliac veins.

8. *Urinary retention* is a not infrequent cause of pain, often without the patient's knowledge of its cause, for he may attribute it to the wound or to the abdominal distention. A record of urination is therefore important, and percussion of bladder dullness essential to make a diagnosis and to estimate the degree of retention. The mechanism is a spasm of the bladder sphincters of reflex origin, and is particularly prone to occur after pelvic and rectal operations. Simple measures to encourage voiding should be used early and are usually effective. Warmth, applied as a hot water bottle over the bladder, as a Sitz bath, or as a perineal douche will often start urination. A warm tap water enema or vaginal douche is sometimes effective. Allowing the patient to sit up or stand up (when possible) may be effective. A warm urinal and bed pan must be used, since cold increases the reflex spasm. Catheterization is used only as a last resort for it has the danger of introducing infection into the bladder even when performed under careful aseptic precautions. In performing a catheterization the external parts are cleansed as for a sterile operation, sterile rubber gloves are worn, and strict aseptic technic observed. Gentleness and meticulous avoidance of trauma are obviously of extreme importance.

9. *Anuria* is occasionally the cause of the failure to void and is to be suspected when there is no pain or distention, and when bladder dullness is absent. Anuria is probably present when catheterization yields no urine. Anuria may be due to actual disease of the kidney, to functional obstruction (ureteral spasm), to organic obstruction, or to suppression of secretion. In the last case, dehydration is the usual cause, which can be removed by giving adequate amounts of appropriate fluids which include saline, glucose (especially 20 to 50 per cent glucose which is a better diuretic), and, in patients with hypoproteinemia, large amounts of plasma (see p. 150).

10. *Hiccough* (hiccup, singultus) is an annoying, but infrequent post-operative complication. It is supposed to be due to diaphragmatic spasm. When persistent it may be associated with serious complications such as general peritonitis or sub-diaphragmatic abscess. Commonly it is transient and responds to ordinary sedatives. The most effective treatment, however, is inhalation of carbon dioxide in high concentration. The simple procedure of rebreathing into and out of a paper bag for several minutes may be effective. The exhaled carbon dioxide rapidly accumulates and acts as a respiratory stimulant and the hiccough stops. The procedure may have to be repeated several times. In more severe cases nitrous oxide gas may be effective. Rarely, this phenomenon is of hysterical origin.

11. *Cardiac failure,* a fortunately rare postoperative event, is manifested first by dyspnea, cyanosis and then by the signs of pulmonary edema. The pulse becomes fast and thready. Oxygen therapy (by nasal tube, mask, or tent) is perhaps the most important feature in treatment. Digitalis may be helpful. The use of a small dose (50 cubic centimeters) of hypertonic glucose (50 per cent) into the vein will often relieve pulmonary edema promptly and allow a circulatory recovery to take place.

12. *Pulmonary complications* comprise pneumonias (usually lobular), pleurisy, bronchitis, pulmonary infarcts, and massive collapse (or atelectasis) of the lung. As to etiology of the various pulmonary complications, much has been written, particularly in regard to the role of embolic factors, aspirated material, and more recently the effect of bronchial obstruction. Complete discussion of those factors can be found in the excellent résumé by Cutler and Scott.[31] Following early after operation is a type of pneumonia due to actual aspiration of regurgitated gastric contents into the lungs. It is called aspiration pneumonia and should, of course, be prevented by pre-operative gastric lavage in all necessary cases. Aspiration pneumonia is nevertheless a not infrequent cause of death as shown by the excellent postmortem studies of Irons and Apfelbach.[32] The incidence of postoperative pulmonary complications varies between one per cent and four per cent. While, in general, laparotomies and other serious operations are much more apt to be followed by pulmonary complications, the factors of increasing age and recent upper respiratory infections greatly aggravate the patient's susceptibility. Perhaps the most frequent of pulmonary complications, but fortunately least serious (if treated promptly) is atelectasis. Symptoms include fever, severe tachycardia, cyanosis, dyspnea and slight cough which is nonproductive at first but later becomes productive. Signs include absent breath sounds on the affected side, shift of the mediastinum, etc. When following abdominal operations, treatment consists of rolling the patient on his unaffected side, and supporting the abdominal wound while the patient coughs, thereby helping to evacuate mucus from the bronchi.

Roentgenograms will be very helpful in differentiating the various lesions; further details in the differential diagnosis may be found in the report already referred to.[31] Treatment is largely medical. The use of carbon dioxide inhalations as a routine postoperative measure has resulted in the prevention of many cases although there is evidence to refute its efficacy as a prophylactic measure (King[33]); as a form of treatment in atelectasis, it is often effective. Oxygen therapy is useful in practically all pulmonary complications; occasionally it is so beneficial as actually to be life-saving. Papaverine gr. ½ and atropine gr. ⅟₁₅₀ has been found of much value by deTakats and Jesser[34] in pulmonary embolism.

13. *Fat embolism* is a remarkable postoperative and post-traumatic complication which, though rare, is a dangerous event and is associated with a high mortality. It is due to the appearance of microscopic fat droplets in the blood which plug pulmonary and cerebral capillaries especially, and produce symptoms of shock or of pulmonary distress. It occurs after fractures and operations, particularly the former,

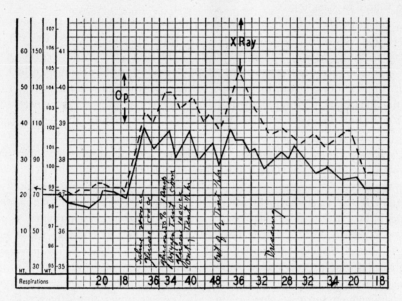

CHART 3.—POSTOPERATIVE PULMONARY COMPLICATION (BRONCHOPNEUMONIA).

The patient was a young girl, the operation a simple appendectomy. Note the sharp increase in the respiratory rate, temperature and pulse; recovery was uneventful but would now be more rapid with chemotherapy.

and was originally thought to be due to the entrance of fat from the traumatized bone marrow or from the injured adiposus panniculus into the blood stream. Lehman and Moore,[35] however, have presented evidence to show that the fat in the blood is indigenous, being formed by a change in the physical character of the blood lipoids. Symptoms are of two types, one circulatory, the other pulmonary. In the former, signs and symptoms of shock develop indistinguishable from those due to trauma in general, except that the blood from a vein may show visible fat; cerebral symptoms such as hemiplegia, convulsion, aphasia, and Cheyne-Stokes respirations may also be present. Ophthalmoscopic examination may show retinal vessels filled with fat. In the pulmonary form the signs are apt to be cyanosis, dyspnea, cough and pulmonary edema. In the more severe cases there are many petechial hemorrhages in the skin. Treatment is that of shock and pulmonary complications in general.

14. *Air embolism* occurs occasionally, but is usually serious only after operations involving the pleural cavity, because of the access of air into the pulmonary vein which carries it to the left heart and thence to the brain, thereby producing signs of cerebral embolism. Air entering the right heart through operations involving the

large veins of the neck is less serious, but may give rise to signs of pulmonary embolism. To produce death a much larger amount of air must be introduced into a systemic than into a pulmonary vein.

15. *Infection* of the operative wound represents one of the serious postoperative complications, especially in large incisions. Such infections are often ushered in by an unexplained increase in the temperature, an increased local tenderness, redness or swelling of the wound, or in some cases may be present silently. Further details will be found in Chapter X.

16. *Surgical shock* following operation presents more or less the same clinical manifestations as shock occuring after any other trauma, except for the added influence of the anesthetic which, if ether, is apt to aggravate the degree of shock and in any case affect the sensorium, so as to make clinical diagnosis a little more difficult. On the other hand, knowledge of the operative procedure helps to decide as to the likelihood of internal hemorrhage, which, if present, may necessitate a second operation to ligate the bleeding vessel. Treatment of shock is considered in Chapter XIII.

17. *Acute rupture of abdominal incisions* does occur occasionally, particularly if the patient coughs or vomits persistently and severely during the first few days of convalescence. Vitamin C deficiency is undoubtedly a frequent cause of wound disruption. To a fresh surgical intern the sight of coils of intestine under the dressing is one of his most tragic experiences. Its seriousness, however, is not as great as it seems. Peritonitis or herniation is not apt to occur if the wound is promptly closed. This is done under local or general anesthesia by means of several through and through sutures which embrace all the layers of the abdominal wall.

More commonly, rupture is incomplete and is confined to the deeper layers of the incision which separate slowly; this also occurs under the influence of a persistent cough and may lead to the formation of postoperative hernia.

18. *Care of the bowels,* after operation, if neglected, may lead to fecal impaction. To prevent this many surgeons as a routine give postoperative abdominal cases a small M.G. and W. enema about forty-eight hours after operation, to be followed in forty-eight hours or sooner with a milder (S.S.) but large enema (see page 163). Mild intestinal lubricants such as mineral oil should then be used. *Fecal impaction* is apt to occur in elderly patients and children and in most cases is readily diagnosed by rectal examination, but will be overlooked unless such an examination is made. A fecal impaction will not necessarily result in absence of bowel movements; many of these patients indeed have frequent but small liquid stools. Considerable rectal pain and tenesmus may be present particularly at each attempt to move the bowels. A severe grade of fecal impaction may be associated with so much abdominal pain and distention that a diagnosis of intestinal obstruction may be made. These manifestations are so readily relieved by removal of the impaction that a rectal examination should not be delayed whenever the condition is suspected. An oil enema followed in several hours by a soap-suds enema is occasionally effective in softening and expelling the fecal mass aided especially by digital manipulation. In some cases instrumental removal may be necessary.

19. *Dressings* in clean (aseptic) wounds are ordinarily not changed for a week unless some indication develops. However, change of dressing before then is often

appreciated by the patient. The presence of drains necessitates earlier and more frequent dressings to care for the discharge. They should be loosened perhaps, but should not be shortened or removed except on advice of the surgeon in charge. Sutures in the skin are removed in abdominal wounds in a week, but when cosmetic results are more important, in a few days. In the latter case the skin edges are protected from possible separation by adhesive strips or pieces of gauze held in place with collodion. Stay sutures are left in place ten to fourteen days. When infected wounds are dressed, instruments or rubber gloves are used in order to avoid contaminating the fingers of the surgeon and to prevent additional infection of the patient.

20. *Termination of bed rest* following uncomplicated abdominal operations is begun on about the tenth postoperative day when the patient is allowed to sit up out of bed. This should be preceded by a few days of graded muscular exercise. Walking is permitted on the eleventh or twelfth day and increased steadily. The duration of bed rest in other surgical conditions varies greatly, depending upon the individual case.

BIBLIOGRAPHY

1. GRAHAM, E. A. and BERCK, M. Principles *vs.* Details in the Treatment of Acute Empyema, *Ann. Surg.,* 98:520, 1933.
2. BAZET, H. C. The Physiological Basis for the Use of Heat, Vol. I, Chapter 4, of *Principles and Practice of Physical Therapy,* edited by H. E. Mock, *et al.,* W. B. Prior, Hagerstown, 1932.
3. LEWIS, THOMAS and LOVE, W. S. Vascular Reactions of the Skin to Injury. Part III. Some Effects of Freezing, of Cooling, and of Warming, *Heart,* 13:28, 1926.
4. GOLDSCHMIDT, S. and LIGHT, A. B. The Effect of Local Temperature Upon the Peripheral Circulation and Metabolism of Tissues as Revealed by the Gaseous Content of Venous Blood, *Am. J. Physiol.,* 73:146, 1925.
5. SONNE, C. The Mode of Action of the Universal Light Bath, *Acta Scand. Med.,* 54:384, 1921.
6. LAKE, N. C. An Investigation Into the Effects of Cold Upon the Body, *Lancet,* 2:557, 1917.
7. McCUTCHEON, M. The Effect of Temperature on the Rate of Locomotion of Human Neutrophilic Leucocytes in Vitro, *Am. J. Physiol.,* 66:185, 1923.
8. SPECIAL ARTICLE: What Can the General Practitioner Expect from Infra-Red Therapy, *J. Am. M. Ass.,* 103:27, 1934.
9. LEWIS, THOMAS. Observations upon the Reactions of the Vessels of the Human Skin to Cold, *Heart,* 15:177, 1930.
10. CARLSON, H. E. and ORR, T. G. Penetration of Moist Heat Applied to the Abdomen and Its Effect on Intestinal Movements, *Arch. Surg.,* 30:1036, 1935.
11. BISGARD, J. D. and NYE, D. Influence of Hot and Cold Applications upon Gastric and Intestinal Motor Activity, *Surg., Gynec. & Obst.,* 71:172, 1940.
12. HOLMAN, E. Vitamin and Protein Factors in Pre- and Postoperative Care of Surgical Patients, *Surg., Gynec. & Obst.,* 70:261, 1940.
13. RAVDIN, I. S., STENGEL, A., JR. and PRUSHANKIN, M. Control of Hypoproteinemia in Surgical Patients, *J. Am. M. Ass.,* 114:107, 1940.
14. COLLER, F. A. and MADDOCK, W. G. Water and Electrolyte Balance, *Surg., Gynec., & Obst.,* 70:340, 1940. See also *Surg.,* 12:192, 1942.
15. HELWIG, F. C., SCHURTZ, C. B. and KUHN, H. P. Water Intoxication, *J. Am. M. Ass.,* 110:645, 1938.
16. WINSLOW, S. B. Dextrose Utilization in Surgical Patients, *Surgery,* 4:867, 1940.

17. ELMAN, R. and LISCHER, C. The Occurrence and Correction of Hyproproteinemia (hypoalbuminemia) in Surgical Patients; Collective Review, *Surg., Gynec. & Obst.*, 76:503, 1943.

18. ELMAN, ROBERT and WEINER, D. O. Intravenous Alimentation with Special Reference to Protein (Aminoacid) Metabolism, *J. Am. M. Ass.*, 112:716, 1939, *Ann. Surg.*, 112:594, 1940.
ELMAN, R., WEINER, D. O. and BRADLEY, E. Intravenous injections of Amino-acids (Hydrolyzed Casein) in Postoperative Patients, *Ann. Surg.*, 115:1160, 1942.
ELMAN, R. Parenteral Replacement of Protein with the Amino-acids of Hydrolyzed Casein, *Ann. Surg.*, 112:594, 1940.

19. WIENER, A. S. Blood Groups and Blood Transfusions, 3rd Ed. Thomas, Springfield, Ill., 1943.

20. IVY, A. C. et al. Effect of Various Blood Substitutes in Resuscitation after otherwise Fatal Hemorrhage, *Surg., Gynec. & Obst.*, 76:85, 1943.

21. BRUNEAU, J. and GRAHAM, E. A. A Caution Against Too Liberal Use of Citrated Blood in Transfusions, *Arch. Surg.*, 47:319, 1943.

22. DeGOWIN, E. L., HARRIS, J. E. and PLASS, E. D. Studies on Preserved Blood, *J. Am. M. Ass.*, 114:850, 1940.

23. LANDSTEINER, KARL. Ueber Agglutinationserscheinungen normalen menschlichen Blutes, *Wien. klin. Wchnschr.*, 14:1132, 1901.

24. SOCIETY PROCEEDINGS, *J. Am. M. Ass.*, 102:1795, 1934.

25. WATERS, R. M. Methods of Resuscitation, *J. Lab. & Clin. Med.*, 26:272, 1940.

26. HENDERSON, Y. The Dangers of Carbon Monoxide Poisoning and Measures to Lessen These Dangers, *J. Am. M. Ass.*, 94:179, 1930.

27. HYMAN, A. S. Resuscitation of Stopped Heart by Intracardiac Therapy, *Arch. Int. Med.*, 46:553, 1930.

28. KANAVEL, A. B. and KOCH, S. L. Pre-operative Preparation and Post-operative Care of Surgical Patients, *Bull. Am. Coll. Surgeons*, 11:14, 1927.

29. BLALOCK, A. Surgical Care; Shock and Allied Problems, C. V. Mosby, St. Louis, 1940.

30. DRAGSTEDT, L. R., MONTGOMERY, M. L., ELLIS, J. C., and MATTHEWS, W. B. The Pathogenesis of Acute Dilatation of the Stomach, *Surg., Gynec. & Obst.*, 52:1075, 1931.

31. CUTLER, E. C. and SCOTT, W. J. M. Postoperative Complications, *Surgical Diagnosis*, edited by E. A. Graham, W. B. Saunders, Philadelphia, 1930, Vol. I.

32. IRONS, E. E. and APFELBACH, C. W. Aspiration Pneumonia, *J. Am. M. Ass.*, 115:584, 1940.

33. KING, D. S. Postoperative Pulmonary Complications. II. Carbon Dioxide as a Preventive in a Controlled Series, *J. Am. M. Ass.*, 100:21, 1933.

34. DeTAKATS, G. and JESSER, J. H. Pulmonary Embolism; Suggestions for Its Diagnosis, Prevention and Management, *J. Am. M. Ass.*, 114:1415, 1940.

35. LEHMAN, E. P. and MOORE, R. M. Fat Embolism—Including Experimental Production Without Trauma, *Arch. Surg.*, 14:621, 1927.

36. TOCANTIS, L. M. and O'NEILL, J. F. Infusion of Blood and other Fluids into the Circulation via the Bone Marrow; Technic and Results, *Surg., Gynec. & Obst.*, 73:287, 1941. *J. Am. M. Ass.*, 117:1229, 1941.

37. ELMAN, R. Acute Protein Deficiency (Hypoproteinemia) in Surgical Shock, *J. Am. M. Ass.*, 120:1176, 1942.

CHAPTER IX

ANESTHESIA

General Anesthesia
Agents Used in General Anesthesia
Local Anesthesia

GENERAL ANESTHESIA

General anesthesia shares with antisepsis the distinction of being largely responsible for the great advance made in surgery during the past century. It should be noted, however, that although ether and chloroform were introduced nearly 100 years ago the greatest development in operative procedures did not occur until infection was overcome nearly fifty years later. Instead of anesthetic agents, various analgesic and soporific drugs were used by the ancients for the relief of pain during operations, which, however, were largely confined to amputations. Even when they used large doses of opium to deaden sensation, and alcohol to produce an actual intoxication, the performance of a surgical operation was a terrifying affair. Just as the old surgical wards overwhelmed the sense of smell with the odor of putrefying wounds, so did the operating rooms of the preanesthetic era assail the ears with the shrieks of their unfortunate victims. Many strong-armed assistants were needed to hold the struggling patient in place. Whenever the patient fainted, as he occasionally did, such restraint obviously became unnecessary, to the great relief of all concerned. Speed, naturally, became the prime attribute of the successful surgeon. Indeed, the eager medical students of those days watching an operation were admonished, "Do not blink your eyes!" for fear of missing the sweeping stroke with which the useless limb was dismembered. It is surprising that excessive speed in the performance of an operation is occasionally the boast of some surgeons even at the present time.

General anesthesia implies the use of an agent which not only produces analgesia, *i.e.*, loss of pain sensation but also loss of consciousness, *i.e.*, loss of all sensation. In addition to this loss of sensation, anesthetic agents possess the power of eliminating motor nerve impulses which results in more or less complete muscular relaxation. This property is possessed by the agents in varying degrees, and determines in part the choice of anesthetic, depending, of course, on the degree of muscular relaxation required for the particular operation to be carried out.

No anesthetic is quite ideal; the advantages and disadvantages of the various agents can only be appreciated if there is close cooperation between the surgeon and anesthetist as recommended by Waters and Schmidt.[1] Attempt should be made to choose the anesthetic or combination of anesthetic agents which is best suited for the patient. An excellent monograph on anesthesia has been published by Guedel.[2] Since anesthesia is fast becoming a specialty of its own, only the general principles will be discussed here.

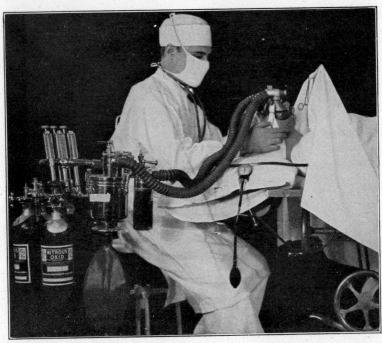

FIG. 101.—METHOD OF INTRODUCING ANESTHESIA UTILIZING A "CIRCLE FILTER" TYPE OF APPARATUS.

Jaw can be held forward by either the left hand holding the mask, or by the right hand pushing the ramus forward. A blood pressure cuff and stethoscope on the arm permit constant observation regarding the blood pressure level.

Preanesthetic Medication.—Legitimately regarded as part of the anesthetic procedure is the administration of preparatory drugs. A sedative drug, such as morphine or nembutal, will allay apprehension, reduce the amount of anesthetic agent required, and make the anesthesia smoother. Atropine will minimize pharyngeal secretions reducing the tendency to obstruction and aspiration. Similarly, scopolamine will dry secretions, and has the advantage over atropine in that it also produces some psychic sedation and amnesia. The dosage of these drugs should be carefully individualized. The aged can tolerate much less sedation than the young adult; factors which alter the metabolic rate will correspondingly increase or decrease the dosage required. Sthenicity, fever, pain, excitement and hyperthyroidism will all increase the amount of premedication required. The anesthetic agent to be used and the degree of relaxation to be achieved must also modify the dosage. Nitrous oxide and ethylene call for heavy sedation, ether for moderate sedation, and cyclopropane for very light sedation to avoid respiratory depression. Paradoxically, the deeper the anesthesia required, the lighter should be the preliminary sedation, because heavy sedation causes respiratory depression which may lead to anoxia and slows or prevents the administration of enough inhalation agent to produce deep anesthesia.

Stages and Signs of General Anesthesia.—General anesthesia is divided into four stages. The first is the stage of *analgesia* in which there is a progressive loss of sensation but not of consciousness. The second is the stage of *excitement* during which the patient, though already unconscious, tends to exhibit a hyperactivity which occasionally requires forcible restraint. The third is the stage of *surgical anesthesia* during which operations may be carried out. There may be certain reflex responses to stimuli but these diminish and relaxation increases as anesthesia deepens. This stage is divided into four planes. Entry into the first plane is indicated by loss of the eyelid reflex; into the second plane by cessation of eyeball movement; into the third plane by beginning intercostal paralysis; and into the fourth plane by complete intercostal paralysis, breathing being entirely diaphragmatic. The fourth stage is that of *complete respiratory paralysis*. This should be regarded as dangerous and usually constitutes a respiratory emergency.

Respiration may be irregular in the second stage but becomes full and regular in the first plane of the third stage. As anesthesia deepens the depth of respiration decreases and in the deep third stage, respiratory exchange may be inadequate although not completely abolished. The depth and nature of respiration therefore are among the most valuable signs of the depth of anesthesia. The pupil may be dilated during excitement but contracts in the first planes of the third stage. As anesthesia deepens the pupil tends to dilate, but this varies with the agent and with the preliminary medication. The patient's reaction is, in all cases, the guide as to the amount of anesthetic required. Deep anesthesia in one patient may be produced by a low concentration of the drug, while it may require an unusually high concentration in another. The anesthetist must therefore think in terms of the patient's response rather than in terms of percentages. Obviously, when complete abdominal relaxation is needed a deep plane of anesthesia will be required; for a circumcision in an infant a light anesthesia is adequate.

The immediate postoperative period is of great importance, inasmuch as several hours may elapse before consciousness is regained. During this time the upper air passages must be kept open. Constant attendance by a nurse is essential.

The Air Passages.—Of primary importance in giving any anesthetic is the patency of the air passages. After relaxation occurs the tongue tends to drop back and, aided by the accumulation of mucus, a partial obstruction of the pharynx may thus occur. This is avoided to a large extent by elevation of the patient's chin and by holding the head back, the fingers of the anesthetist grasping the under surface of the mandible for this purpose. If difficulty in the free passage of air is still present as shown by the forcible respiratory efforts of the patient, a curved flattened metal tube (called an airway) is inserted between the teeth above and behind the tongue to overcome the obstruction.

For the relief of upper respiratory obstruction which will not yield to simpler methods, or as an assurance that such obstruction will not ensue, an endotracheal tube may be used. A specially constructed catheter, large enough to almost fill the glottis, is passed through the larynx into the upper trachea. This method facilitates the use of positive pressure and is invaluable for certain operations on the widely opened pleural space and operations about the head and neck where anesthetic apparatus would otherwise encroach on the surgical field.

Technics of Inhalation Anesthesia.—The simplest method for the administration of volatile agents such as ether and chloroform is the *open drop* technic. The drug is dropped on a gauze covered wire mask where it vaporizes and permeates the atmosphere which is being inhaled by the patient. Another relatively simple method used for maintenance of anesthesia in some cases is that of *insufflation* in which air, laden with ether or some other agent, is blown into the mouth of the patient. Other methods applicable for the administration of anesthetic gases, or oxygen laden with ether or chloroform vapor are used much more commonly,

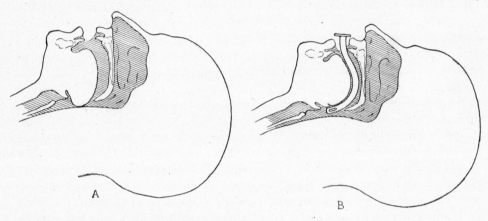

A

B

FIG. 102.—DIAGRAM ILLUSTRATING THE USE OF A PHARYNGEAL AIRWAY.

A, obstruction caused by apposition of the tongue to the posterior wall of the pharynx; *B*, obstruction relieved by insertion of metal airway.

and utilize a gas machine. The classification suggested below is based largely on the amount and type of rebreathing:

(1) The *closed* method (carbon dioxide not removed) in which the anesthetic agent and oxygen are inhaled from a bag and closely fitting mask is a type of mechanism in which the gases are completely rebreathed. Owing to the rapid accumulation of carbon dioxide this method is not physiologic and cannot safely be used except for very short periods.

(2) The *semi-closed* method involves the use of a bag and mask, but the flow of gases is maintained at a sufficient rate to eliminate much of the exhaled carbon dioxide. Some excess carbon dioxide usually develops. The flow of gases required proves quite expensive.

(3) An *open* technic can be used if the exhaled gases are prevented by a valve from being rebreathed, and on each inhalation the patient receives a fresh mixture. Accumulation of carbon dioxide is avoided but the expense is much greater.

(4) In the *carbon dioxide absorption* technic complete rebreathing of the anesthetic agent plus oxygen occurs but the exhaled carbon dioxide is removed by passage of the mixture through soda lime which combines with the carbon dioxide. Oxygen is added constantly to replace that used by the patient and the anesthetic

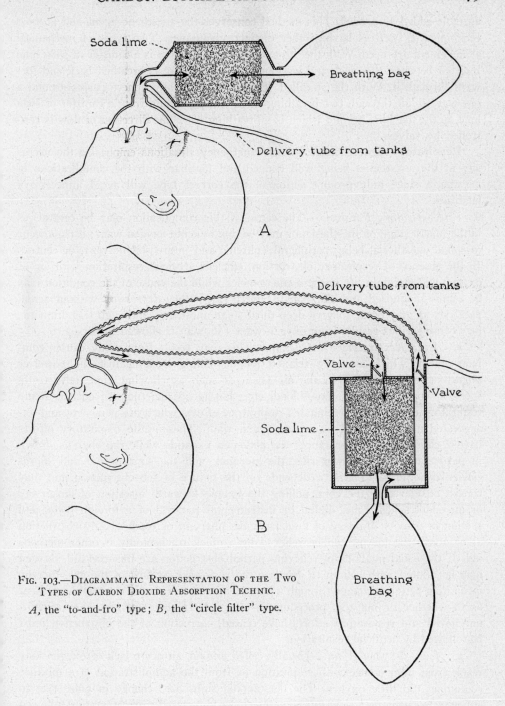

Fig. 103.—Diagrammatic Representation of the Two
Types of Carbon Dioxide Absorption Technic.

A, the "to-and-fro" type; B, the "circle filter" type.

agent is added as needed. This method conserves the anesthetic agent and is most economical as well as having other distinct advantages. Two types of mechanical arrangement are used. With the "to-and-fro" system there is a canister of soda lime inserted between the mask and bag, and the atmosphere is breathed back and forward through it. With the so-called "circle filter" the atmosphere passes around a one-way circuit through two breathing tubes leading to and from a canister of soda lime on the machine beyond which is a breathing bag. The direction of flow is controlled by valves.

Respiratory Emergencies.—Such emergency situations emphasize the necessity of the anesthetist being well trained and familiar with the complications of anesthesia since only prompt action of the correct type will avoid unnecessary fatalities.

1. *Respiratory Paralysis.*—The cause of this complication may be central, as in the fourth stage of anesthesia, or may be due to acute oxygen want; it may occur in spinal anesthesia, being peripheral (phrenic and intercostal nerves), or central. In the absence of respiratory obstruction, efficient artificial respiration with air or oxygen will maintain life in these emergencies while the cause of the condition may be calmly diagnosed and eliminated. Severe *respiratory depression* without actual paralysis as may occur in very deep third stage anesthesia, although less dramatic, may cause serious results from oxygen want (anoxia) if allowed to persist.

2. *Acute Respiratory Obstruction.*—This may result from many causes common among which are: the relaxed tongue falling back against the posterior pharynx; foreign bodies in the air passages such as chewing gum, false teeth, sponges, vomitus, mucus, pus, blood, etc.; laryngospasm; tumors; edema. Acute respiratory obstruction precipitates respiratory efforts which are persistent and exaggerated until abolished by acute oxygen want. These futile respiratory efforts have a characteristic appearance; the abdomen expands while the chest is drawn in particularly at the lower ribs, the sternum, and the suprasternal and supraclavicular regions. Treatment depends on the nature of the obstruction and may consist of, elevating the chin, pulling the tongue forward, insertion of an airway or an endotracheal tube, digital or instrumental removal of a foreign body, and suction or gravity drainage of fluid from the pharynx or trachea. Any obstruction at or above the larynx can be relieved by a quick tracheotomy if other methods fail. If the usual methods of relieving partial obstruction are unsuccessful, oxygen may be diluted with helium to decrease the resistance to flow of the gas, thereby facilitating better exchange through a narrow aperture. There is not total agreement as to whether or not this procedure is effective. If acute oxygen want remains unrelieved and respiratory efforts have ceased, correction of the obstruction must be followed by artificial respiration.

3. *Acute Oxygen Want.*—Usually called *anoxia,* an acute lack of oxygen may result from interference with respiration or from the administration of a mixture containing too little oxygen. The outstanding signs are: change in pulse rate to either tachycardia or a slow full bounding pulse; increased respiratory rate followed by respiratory arrest; muscular spasms resulting in movement of the limbs, vomiting, phonation, rigidity, or severe tonic convulsions. Cyanosis sometimes but not always occurs since the appearance of cyanosis depends upon many factors includ-

ing the amount of hemoglobin, the texture and color of the skin, and the distribution of the blood. The treatment is obviously to remove the cause and administer oxygen or air. It should be emphasized here that anoxia is to be meticulously avoided, regardless of the type of anesthesia used. Much harm is wrought by anoxia especially in poor risk patients and in those with circulatory shock (see p. 250). The anesthetist's point of view in anoxia has been well discussed by Waters.[3]

In the treatment of acute respiratory emergencies stimulant drugs or carbon dioxide are of little use particularly in the presence of obstruction. The essential thing is to supply adequate oxygen without delay, and to remove the cause, as for example by providing free escape of an overdose of an inhalation agent.

Cardiac Emergencies.—Cessation of cardiac activity due to acute cardiac failure, ventricular fibrillation or autonomic reflex stimulation is fortunately much less common than cessation of respiration, but on the other hand is much less likely to respond to treatment. Its causes should be avoided, particularly severe oxygen want, stimulation during light chloroform or ethyl chloride anesthesia, or the administration of adrenalin during inhalation anesthesia. If the heart stops, artificial respiration with oxygen along with cardiac massage offers the best hope of recovery (see also p. 160). By cardiac massage is meant intermittent squeezing of the heart about 60 times per minute to produce artificial circulation. It is done through an upper abdominal incision, and the hand inserted under the diaphragm and behind the heart so that the heart can be squeezed between the hand and the anterior thoracic wall. Time is important, but an effort must be made to maintain as aseptic a technic as possible. In the presence of efficient artificial respiration and artificial circulation, oxygenation of the tissues is maintained. Return of spontaneous cardiac action has occurred as long as twenty minutes after such treatment was instituted, ultimate recovery of the patient being complete.

AGENTS USED IN GENERAL ANESTHESIA

Although ether was one of the first anesthetic agents discovered, it is still used, and perhaps more commonly than any other. However, numerous other agents have been introduced in the past two or three decades, many of which have specific advantages for certain types of anesthesia.

Ether.—Diethyl-oxide ($C_2H_5OC_2H_5$) was first used as a surgical anesthetic in Jefferson, Georgia, by Dr. Crawford W. Long, who in 1842 painlessly removed a tumor from the neck of a patient. Its widespread use followed an independent demonstration of its value at the Massachusetts General Hospital in Boston in 1846. Ether (also called sulphuric ether) is a volatile liquid which is administered by inhalation of the vapor, which, in a warm atmosphere, is rapidly given off by the liquid. If the temperature is low it is necessary to warm the ether in order to insure sufficient vaporization.

Advantages of Ether.—It is probably the most widely used general anesthetic for the performance of operations requiring good muscular relaxation. It is also used extensively for children. It has a wide margin of safety, *i.e.*, there is a considerable range between the amount of ether which produces anesthesia, and the amount which is toxic. Very few fatalities have resulted from the hundreds of thousands of ether anesthesias given each year. Ether is one of the most convenient of inhalation anesthetics since it requires only a simple gauze mask for its administration.

Disadvantages of Ether.—The slight though definitely deleterious action of the drug itself on liver cells makes it somewhat dangerous in patients suffering from a severe degree of hepatic disease. In surgical shock it is especially disadvantageous since it has an unfavorable effect on a falling or low blood pressure. Its irritant action on the mucous membranes of the respiratory tract renders ether a poor agent in patients with any type of pulmonary lesion. It does not act as rapidly as other anesthetics and is not therefore advisable for short operations. Ether is undoubtedly a mild emetic and is also prone to increase the postoperative nausea and vomiting. Its inflammable property makes it dangerous when a hot cautery or flame is being used in or near the operating room.

Nitrous Oxide.—Though known long before as an interesting gas, nitrous oxide as an anesthetic agent was first used in 1844 by Dr. Horace Wells, a dentist of Hartford, Connecticut, for the extraction of teeth. Nitrous oxide (N_2O) was originally called "laughing gas" because of the hilarious mood it often invoked in patients. It is always given mixed with oxygen in varying percentages, and being a gas is, of course, administered with a gas machine.

Advantages and Disadvantages.—Nitrous oxide acts very quickly, requiring only a few deep inhalations, and in most cases does not exhibit an excitement stage. Its effect is over just as quickly, and there is no disagreeable odor as is true of ether. The rapidity of its anesthetic action and recovery is due to the diffusibility of the gas which enters and leaves the blood rapidly. On the other hand it produces very little muscular relaxation since at best it can produce only first plane anesthesia (of the third stage) and in some individuals not more than second stage anesthesia without severe oxygen want. Its margin of safety is not very wide even though the gas is in itself not toxic, because its effectiveness depends on a rather high concentration of the gas. In many patients the concentration required to achieve anesthesia is 90 per cent or more, thus leaving less than 10 per cent of oxygen to carry the respiratory function. Asphyxia, therefore, is the dangerous feature in nitrous oxide administration, and requires expertness to avoid it. It is thus a more difficult anesthetic to give than ether. The rise of blood pressure and slowing of the pulse rate by nitrous oxide are apparently due to its asphyxial effect on the blood.

Nitrous oxide oxygen inhalation finds an ideal application for short operations when relaxation is not essential. It is used most commonly in the extraction of teeth, incision and drainage of abscesses, skin grafting, removal of superficial tumors, etc. It may be given after any of the basal anesthetics mentioned and with their aid may achieve sufficient relaxation to permit certain pelvic and abdominal operations.

Ethylene.—This gas (C_2H_4) is a relatively recent addition to our anesthetic agents. It has a slightly pungent odor and has been advocated as a substitute for nitrous oxide because (1) it requires a smaller concentration to induce anesthesia and hence permits a greater degree of aeration and (2) it induces moderate muscular relaxation, second plane of third stage. Ethylene possesses explosive properties which nitrous oxide does not have, and hence cannot be used in the presence of a flame or of diathermic or other cauteries. Otherwise its advantages, disadvantages and method of administration are somewhat similar to those of nitrous oxide as already described.

Cyclopropane.—The use of this gas as an anesthetic was introduced by Henderson and Lucas[4] and developed clinically by Waters and Schmidt.[1] It is a more powerful anesthetic, produces greater relaxation and allows the use of a much higher concentration of oxygen than does ethylene. It is thus a particularly useful agent when respiratory disease is present. Since it is explosive it cannot be used in the presence of a cautery.

Divinyl Ether.—One of the newer general anesthetics, this volatile liquid is inflammable and deteriorates on exposure to air. It has a narrow margin of safety. Divinyl ether has a rapid action with a short induction period and quick recovery. Its use has been limited largely to operations requiring but a short period of anesthesia. It may be used as an induction agent to be followed by open drop ether.

Chloroform.—Chloroform ($CHCl_3$) was first used in Scotland by Sir James Y. Simpson in 1847 and thus was really introduced contemporaneously with ether. Chloroform is a volatile liquid and is administered by inhalation of its vapor just as in the case of ether. It produces rapid anesthesia, induces excellent relaxation and is not inflammable. But for its toxic effects on the liver and its narrow margin of safety, it might well be the perfect anesthetic it was originally proclaimed to be. Even short periods of chloroform inhalation produce demonstrable necrosis of hepatic cells, and deaths occurring several days after its prolonged administration are occasionally due primarily to hepatic insufficiency. This danger may be greatly minimized by the ingestion of large quantities of carbohydrate preparatory to operation, and by the administration of a high concentration of oxygen along with the chloroform. Even then it has been found too toxic, and now is scarcely used in this country except for short anesthetics or when a cautery is to be used about the mouth. The narrow margin of safety possessed by chloroform also accounts for the high incidence of fatalities following its use. Ventricular fibrillation due to excitement or stimulation during light anesthesia, or to injection of adrenalin is a serious hazard with chloroform.

Allied to chloroform is ethyl chloride, a still more volatile liquid which indeed evaporates so rapidly that it is used as a local anesthetic by freezing the sensitive skin over an abscess. Sprayed over or dropped upon a gauze mask as an inhalation anesthetic, it produces a rapid anesthesia but has such a narrow margin of safety it cannot safely be used for operations which last more than a few minutes.

Barbiturates.—Evipal and pentothal sodium are very short-acting derivatives of barbituric acid and lend themselves to the production of anesthesia by intravenous administration. They produce an immediate though short-lasting anesthesia, i.e., 10 to 20 minutes with excellent relaxation. The duration of the anesthesia may be extended by giving subsequent intermittent injections as required. Respiratory depression must be guarded against. The anesthetist must watch the patient's respiration and maintain a free airway. An assistant should make the injections. These drugs have the advantage of being safe in the presence of cautery. They are used for short operations, for operations which do not require deep anesthesia, or for operations on patients in whom a gas-oxygen or other inhalation anesthetic is inconvenient or inadvisable. Though relatively new agents they give promise of being very useful anesthetics.

Avertin.—This drug is usually considered a basal anesthetic agent and is widely used. It is a white crystalline solid, tribromethanol, which is available in a solution of amylene hydrate (avertin fluid) each cubic centimeter of which contains one gram of the drug. The fluid is dissolved in water and then given per rectum one half hour before the operation, in the patient's room, if desired. The dose (per kilogram of body weight) ordinarily given for adults is 70 to 100 milligrams of the drug (.07 to .1 cubic centimeters of the fluid) dissolved in enough distilled water to produce a 3 per cent solution. It produces a complete unconsciousness which lasts several hours. Though total anesthesia is not desirable the amount of ether or gas necessary becomes considerably diminished after its use.

REGIONAL ANESTHESIA

A common misconception about local anesthesia is that it involves no danger. Actually the hazards are far from negligible; although they are uncommon, one should be thoroughly familiar with them before undertaking to administer a local anesthetic. The *toxic effects of local anesthetic drugs* are too often regarded as mere nervousness. Actually they consist of both circulatory and neurologic manifestations, *e.g.,* there may be nervousness, talkativeness, excitability, delirium, convulsions, weakness, faintness, palpitation, nausea, vomiting, pallor, falling blood pressure, slow or fast pulse, loss of consciousness, complete circulatory collapse, and death. Toxic effects may be minimized by noting any history of idiosyncrasy, and by use of the smallest volume and lowest concentration required, by the use of adrenalin to minimize the rate of absorption when used for infiltration, by slow injection, and by avoidance of intravascular injection. Neurologic reactions may be minimized by preliminary administration of a barbiturate, but this has no prophylactic effect on circulatory reactions. The most important element of treatment is the maintenance of respiration by artificial respiration if necessary. Administration of a barbiturate intravenously may be employed to control convulsions; if a circulatory collapse (low blood pressure, bradycardia, or less commonly tachycardia) is present, adrenalin may be given cautiously if an adrenalin reaction can be ruled out. Since the potency and toxicity of the various drugs differ considerably it is not safe to substitute one for another without being thoroughly acquainted with its peculiarities. It is also important always to use similar technic, particularly in spinal anesthesia, because injudicious variations from the procedure with which one is familiar may result in disaster.

1. *Cocaine* is useful in solution (5 to 10 per cent) to anesthetize mucous membranes, notably in the oral and pharyngeal cavities. It need not be injected for this purpose, but merely swabbed over or applied to the area with a pledget of cotton. It is also used to anesthetize the conjunctiva, urethra and bladder. In preventing the gag reflex during the passage of a stomach tube or especially duodenal or nasal tube, it finds a useful place. It has the disadvantage of being toxic and habit forming, and for hypodermic use has been superseded by a related drug,

novocaine. In addition to novocaine, there are many other related drugs with local anesthetic action. Nupercaine, while much more active even than cocaine, is also much more toxic. It is used in ointments and for prolonged spinal anesthesia. Pontocaine is similar to novocaine but is much more effective on mucous membranes; it is also used in spinal anesthesia. Metycaine is also used for spinal anesthesia, its action being slightly longer than that of novocaine.

2. *Novocaine* (*procaine*) is the most widely used local anesthetic for hypodermic use. It is used in a variety of ways as described below.

(*a*) *Infiltration* is begun by forming a wheal in the skin, using a hypodermic needle which is introduced into the derma. A one-half to one per cent solution is usually used. Anesthesia is due in part to the pressure of the nerve endings destroying their sensitivity, and thus may be achieved with plain water which, however, loses its effect as soon as the wheal disappears (5 to 10 minutes). Novocaine has in addition an anesthetic effect on the nerves themselves and hence its effect lasts longer (30 minutes). Adrenalin (5 drops of 1 to 1000 solution to each

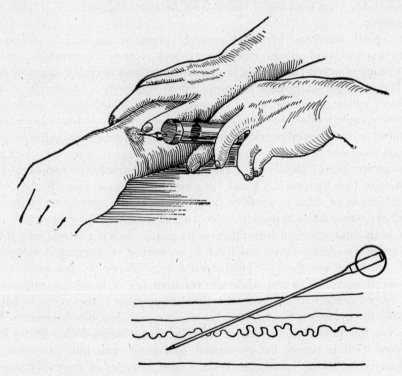

FIG. 104.—THE LOCAL INFILTRATION OF NOVOCAINE.

Note the formation of a wheal in the skin. This is produced by injecting the agent into the derma as shown in the lower insert. This wheal establishes a painless portal of entry for the further injection of novocaine.

100 cubic centimeters) causes vasoconstriction and thus prolongs anesthesia by diminishing absorption. Once this anesthetic portal of entry is made, the rest of the process is painless and simply consists of completing the infiltration of the skin and operative field.

Novocaine may also be injected into the hematoma at the site of fractures (10 to 30 cubic centimeters of 1 per cent solution) and often achieves sufficient anesthesia to enable satisfactory reduction, especially of the small bones, such as the radius and ulna. This use of local anesthesia has been particularly emphasized by the Viennese surgeon Lorenz Böhler.

(*b*) *Block anesthesia or nerve-blocking* is used in operations about the mouth, head and in the extremities. A solution of one to two per cent novocaine is usually used in adults, a few cubic centimeters are injected in direct proximity to the nerve supplying the area to be anesthetized. Brachial plexus block is particularly useful in certain patients with fractures and other injuries of the upper extremity. This important application of local anesthesia was discovered by W. S. Halsted according to an award made to him by the American Dental Society in 1922. Bilateral block of the intercostal nerves will give fair relaxation for laparotomies. Splanchnic anesthesia, obtained by infiltration of the prevertebral tissues of the upper abdomen (by the anterior or posterior route) so that the splanchnic fibers and coeliac plexus are blocked, has been used but is losing favor because of superiority of other types of anesthesia.

(*c*) *Spinal anesthesia* by being properly given in appropriate patients has achieved a widespread use in recent years, and competes successfully with the various forms of general anesthesia in certain clinics and in certain types of operations. The great advantage of a successful spinal anesthesia is the flaccid paralysis it produces which, in robust, muscular and often obese individuals, produces an even more complete relaxation of the abdominal muscles than does ether narcosis. For difficult intraperitoneal operative procedures this is particularly valuable. Spinal anesthesia moreover does not produce a loss of consciousness, a feature which many patients prefer. Spinal anesthesia is also useful diagnostically in peripheral circulatory disease (see Chapter XX) and Hirschsprung's disease (see Chapter XXII) and is said to be of value in paralytic ileus because of the stimulation of intestinal tone and peristalsis which results from blocking of the sympathetic innervation.

One of its most serious disadvantages is its relative lack of control; once the full dose is given its effect follows, and there is no method of stopping it as one may do with inhalation anesthetics. Spinal anesthesia paralyzes the autonomic as well as the spinal nerve fibers and while the resultant fall of blood pressure may be minimized, its deleterious action on the circulation makes it dangerous in patients susceptible to circulatory insults, namely, patients with low blood pressure, heart disease, late low intestinal obstruction, etc. The danger of producing injury to the spinal cord itself is remote but permanent neurologic signs and symptoms have been observed following spinal anesthesia. Listed in order of increasing duration of effect the drugs commonly used are novocaine, metycaine, pontocaine and nupercaine. With the exception of nupercaine the effect of the drug nearly always wears off in from one to two hours. The effect of nupercaine is much longer. A great advance is the so-called continuous spinal anesthesia. This method of using repeated injections of procaine to prolong spinal anesthesia has been described by Lemmon.[5]

Many methods of administration have been reported but the one commonly used consists of the removal of 2 to 5 cubic centimeters of spinal fluid by lumbar puncture, dissolving in it 50 to 250 milligrams of specially pure novocaine crystals, and reinjecting the fluid after solution is complete. The amount of fluid injected, the dose of drug and the rapidity and force with which the fluid is reinjected, the specific gravity of the fluid, and the slope of the patient's spine determine the level and somewhat the duration of the anesthesia. The dose of metycaine is slightly less than that of novocaine. The dose of pontocaine is from about 8 to 20 milligrams. Nupercaine is used in a 1:1500 solution of which 8 to 20 c.c. is given.

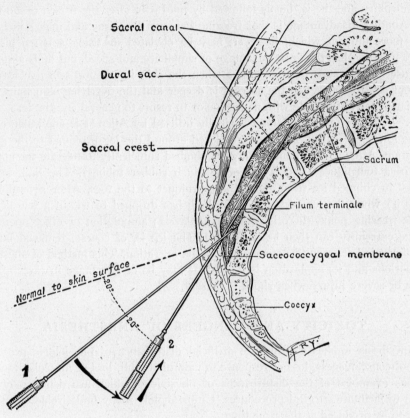

FIG. 105.—LONGITUDINAL SECTION OF THE LOWER VERTEBRAL COLUMN, SHOWING THE MANNER BY WHICH NOVOCAINE IS INTRODUCED IN PERFORMING A CAUDAL BLOCK.

After piercing the sacrococcygeal membrane, the needle impinges on the anterior wall of the sacral canal and passes from position 1 to position 2 in direction of the arrow. (From Labat, *Regional Anesthesia,* 1924, W. B. Saunders Co., p. 278.)

(*d*) *Caudal (sacral) anesthesia* is useful in operations about the external genitalia and anus. It is administered by inserting a needle into the sacrococcygeal notch through the skin and ligament into the epidural space. About 30 to 40 cubic centimeters of 1 per cent novocaine solution can be injected at this site. This bathes the emerging sacral nerves and in most instances produces a satisfactory anesthesia of the saddle type. The anesthesia is more certain if several of the sacral foramina, particularly the second, are also injected with about 5 cubic centimeters of 1 per cent novocaine. Such procedures as hemorrhoidectomy and cystoscopy can be performed with this type of anesthesia.

(e) *Therapeutic nerve block* should be included under local or regional anesthesia and has many applications as discussed in other parts of the text. Indeed, use of alcohol instead of novocaine often leads to permanent interruption of pains, spasm, etc.; one disadvantage is that occasionally a painful neuritis results. A brief discussion will be found in the paper of Rovenstine and Wertheim.[6]

3. *Freezing* the part to be incised, by means of an ethyl chloride spray, causes a momentary anesthesia, but is followed by mild pain after the frozen tissue thaws out. Another disadvantage is that freezing hardens the tissue and makes incision a little more difficult which, however, may be obviated by using a sharp bistoury knife. Freezing has the great advantage of simplicity and speed, but finds almost its sole use in very superficial abscesses when the skin is still too sensitive to incise without anesthesia. When the abscess is deeper and the overlying skin uninvolved it is far better to infiltrate with novocaine or to resort to general anesthesia.

4. *Refrigeration anesthesia* (originally utilized by Allen [7]) is applicable chiefly to the lower extremity. Ice bags are placed around the leg proximal to the site of operation. After half an hour the area is numbed sufficiently to tolerate the application of a tourniquet (two layers of half-inch rubber tubing). The limb is then packed in chipped ice from above the tourniquet to the toes. After several hours (2 to 4) when the temperature of the limb has dropped to within a few degrees of the freezing point, there is complete analgesia; amputation or other operations on the extremity can then be performed. The ice is, of course, removed but the tourniquet is left on until near the end of the operation. This method of anesthesia is laborious and its application is limited. It may be of advantage in cases of gangrene or severe injury when shock is present.

TOXICITY AND DANGERS OF ANESTHESIA

Anesthesia implies a deliberate artificial disturbance of physiologic processes. Loss of consciousness, loss of response to painful stimuli, loss of muscular tone are obvious examples of the disturbances of physiology which are deliberately produced to facilitate surgical procedures. Unfortunately many undesirable effects are likely to be produced at the same time.

Respiratory disturbances include depression, obstruction, obtundation of protective cough reflex, increased secretion, etc. The gastro-intestinal system may be affected with resultant nausea, vomiting (with the possibility of aspiration of vomitus), increased salivation, altered intestinal motility, etc. If vomiting persists in the post-operative period, it interferes with normal feedings, results in loss of fluids and chlorides and may seriously affect the patient's convalescence.

Serious *circulatory disturbances* may result from anesthesia. There may be circulatory depression contributing to shock, changes in pulse rate, changes in the distribution of blood, sudden cardiac arrest, etc.

Besides the obvious effects on the *nervous system* (loss of consciousness, loss of reflexes) there may be other serious disturbances. Excitement may result in injury to the patient or others. Convulsions may occur. These are usually associated with increased body temperature (hot weather, heavy drapes) and carbon dioxide excess. The autonomic nervous system is also affected. Some agents stimulate the sympathetics while others stimulate the parasympathetics. The size of the spleen, an important consideration in splenectomy, may be altered. Ether contracts the spleen and is, therefore, the agent of choice for splenectomy.

The *acid-base balance* is disturbed usually towards the acid side. Not only do some agents cause an acidosis, but also respiratory depression and the probability of some rebreathing of the expired atmosphere result in accumulation of carbon dioxide and further acidosis.

Liver function is depressed by most anesthetic agents, particularly chloroform, and by oxygen want. Recovery is usually rapid, but in cases with preoperative liver damage the additional impairment may be serious. The damage may be minimized by preoperative preparation of the patient designed to increase the carbohydrate and protein and reduce the fat in the liver. Also, the use of a high oxygen atmosphere during anesthesia is helpful. Based upon a study of liver function tests, Boyce[8] noted that there was a depression of liver function following practically all anesthetics. Of the various agents tested by him, this depression was noted following chloroform, spinal anesthesia, ether and ethylene with a degree equivalent to the order named. He explained the serious depression following spinal anesthesia on the basis of the fall in blood pressure resulting in a decreased oxygen supply to the liver. Although cyclopropane was not tested, Boyce was of the opinion that it would be followed by a minimal amount of hepatic depression because of the high oxygen content of the gaseous mixture used. Maddock and associates[9] approximated the degree of hepatic injury following anesthesia by determining the glycogen content of the liver. In these experiments, the average glycogen content for the normal liver was 3.96 per cent, whereas it was 3.15 per cent following spinal anesthesia. The glycogen content in patients with normal livers was raised to an average of 5.03 per cent by supplementary glucose feedings for 12 hours preceding operation. However, the operation itself will naturally be a factor in depressing liver function.

Kidney function is also depressed by anesthetics. Coller and associates[10] noted a decrease in glomerular filtration (persisting for a few hours to a week) following anesthesia induced by ether, cyclopropane and avertin. They considered the decreased function to be related to the amount of blood lost and the severity of the blood pressure fall. Serious acidosis may result from renal impairment.

Another disturbance of physiology under anesthesia which is too often overlooked is the *impairment of heat regulation.* In hot weather the patient may develop a pyrexia which may contribute to shock, disturbed metabolism, increased oxygen demand, and in some cases to the development of convulsions. This is particularly true of operations upon patients with hyperthyroidism. In general, such operation should be performed in hot weather only when an air conditioned room is available for the operation and during the post operative course. In hot weather the amount of sterile drapes should be held to a minimum; in fact, if the patient appears warm, his legs should be uncovered and cold wet packs applied.

Many of these disturbances of physiology may result from local or spinal anesthetics. Convulsions, circulatory collapse, and oxygen want may be cited as examples.

Only the well trained physician anesthetist collaborating with the rest of the surgical team can appreciate all these disturbances of physiology and by the judicious choice of anesthetic agents and technics minimize their seriousness.

BIBLIOGRAPHY

1. WATERS, R. M. and SCHMIDT, E. R. Anesthesia and Surgery, *Ann. Surg.*, 106:788, 1937; Cyclopropane Anesthesia, *J. Am. M. Ass.*, 103:975, 1934.
2. GUEDEL, A. E. *Inhalation Anesthesia—A Fundamental Guide.* The Macmillan Co., New York, 1937.
3. WATERS, R. M. Anoxia—The Anesthetist's Point of View, *J. Am. M. Ass.*, 115:1687, 1940.
4. LUCAS, G. H. W., and HENDERSON, V. E. New Anesthetic Gas: Cyclopropane, *Canad. M. A. J.*, 21:173, 1929.
5. LEMMON, W. T. A Method of Continuous Spinal Anesthesia, *Ann. Surg.*, 111:141, 1940.
6. ROVENSTINE, E. A. and WERTHEIM, H. M. Therapeutic Nerve Block, *J. Am. M. Ass.*, 117:1599, 1941.
7. ALLEN, F. M. Refrigeration Anesthesia, *Am. J. Anes.*, 45:459, 1939.
8. BOYCE, F. M. *The Role of the Liver in Surgery*, Charles C. Thomas, Springfield, Ill., 1941.
9. MacINTYRE, D. S., PEDERSEN, S., and MADDOCK, W. G. The Glycogen Content of the Human Liver, *Surgery*, 10:716, 1941.
10. COLLER, F. A., MOYER, C. A., CAMPBELL, K. N., and REES, V. L. The Parenteral Administration of Fluids during the Operation and the Immediate Postoperative Period in the Light of Additional Knowledge of the Effects of Surgical Anesthesia (ether, cyclopropane and avertin), Upon Renal Function in Man, Presented at the *Annual Meeting of the Amer. Surg. Assn.*, Cincinnati, Ohio, 1943.

CHAPTER X

WOUNDS

Contused Wounds	*Infected Wounds*
Open Wounds	*Wounds Inflicted by Animals*
Crushed Wounds	*and Insects*

A *wound* may be defined as a solution of the continuity of the external or deep tissues of the body due to violence. Ordinarily, the term is restricted to open lesions of the surface of the body or to lacerations of internal organs, but the trauma to subcutaneous tissue in such minor injuries as contusions should likewise be classified as wounds. The latter are called closed wounds since the skin remains intact.

The *Healing of Wounds* is discussed in Chapter II but important points should be reviewed here. The type and rate of healing is determined by the type of treatment and presence or absence of infection. Under optimum conditions in the absence of infection, healing is rapid and firm. However, Howes and associates [1] have shown that there is really no healing during the first four days, the tensile strength being contributed only by the sutures and slight adhesion of the wound surfaces by fibrin. After four days, healing per primam, as indicated by its tensile strength, mounts rapidly, reaching a maximum on the twelfth or fourteenth day. The primary factor in the development of tensile strength of the wound is regeneration of fibrous tissue and might, therefore, be termed fibroplasia. The first step in the healing of the wound is the filling in of the space between the wound edges by an exudate consisting of serum, fibrin, leukocytes and erythrocytes. Proliferation of epithelial and connective tissue cells on the edge of the wound begins early. Shortly after this, regeneration of capillaries takes place, and penetrates the exudate; at this stage the reparative tissue is spoken of as granulation tissue. Following this the young connective tissue undergoes shrinkage, the cells become spindle-shaped, the newly formed intercellular collagen fibers contract and squeeze the capillary loops into atrophy. The principles of wound healing should be well understood by all surgeons; they have been discussed in detail by Whipple,[2] Mason,[3] Reid and Stevenson,[4] Harvey,[5] and others.

The *clinical manifestations* produced by wounds vary considerably, depending upon the extent and type of wound inflicted. Pain is experienced immediately unless it is masked by excitement, traumatic shock, unconsciousness, etc. Swelling, tenderness and ecchymosis are almost constant features of wounds except in minor ones. The pain usually subsides and disappears within twenty-four hours, except that movements of the injured part may create pain for seven to ten days, until

189

the time when healing of the tissues takes place. However, there are many complicating features of wounds such as those produced by fracture, injuries of ligaments (sprains), tendons, etc., in which pain upon motion may be prolonged for weeks. Open wounds, of course, are associated with a variable amount of bleeding. Manifestations consisting of hemorrhage, tenderness, pain, disability, etc., are discussed in greater detail under the specific types of wounds.

In the following pages wounds will be classified arbitrarily into five general groups, *i.e.*, contused, open, crushed, infected, and wounds inflicted by animals and insects.

CONTUSED WOUNDS

A *contusion* or bruise is an injury of the subcutaneous tissue inflicted usually by a blunt object. There is frequently a laceration of the soft tissues beneath the skin, but it may be of a microscopical character. The injury to the overlying skin

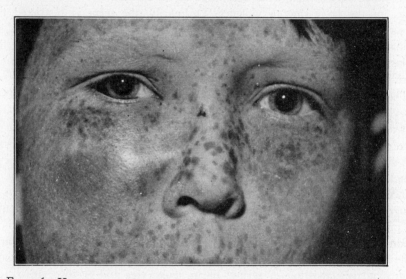

FIG. 106.—HEMATOMA OF FACE SUSTAINED BY A BLOW TWO DAYS PREVIOUSLY.

X-ray revealed no fracture of the facial bones. Frequently, such injuries produce marked swelling with ecchymosis about the eye, so that the eye becomes "swollen shut." This is particularly apt to occur when the injury is near the eye or the base of the nose.

or mucous membrane is usually trivial and insufficient to allow the entrance of bacteria. Blood vessels are invariably severed except in the minor injuries and give rise to subcutaneous hemorrhage. If the hemorrhage arises from small vessels the blood will infiltrate the tissues, perhaps becoming visible as a "black and blue" spot of the skin and is known as *ecchymosis*. If the blood does not infiltrate the tissue, but remains localized in a circumscribed manner, it is known as a *hematoma*. A hematoma may be palpated as an indurated or fluctuant area which frequently is absorbed very slowly. The blood may clot, but usually remains liquid, day by day becoming darker and more viscid until after several days it is so thick that it cannot be aspirated through a needle of the type used in venipuncture (*i.e.*, Nos. 19

and 20). If the blood is not absorbed satisfactorily and it cannot be removed by aspiration, healing may be hastened by making a small incision to evacuate it. An adequate pressure bandage must be applied to eliminate the resulting dead space; otherwise, a brownish discharge may drain from the wound for many days. When a subaponeurotic hematoma forms in the scalp, the edges become raised and indurated, and the injury is frequently erroneously diagnosed as a depressed fracture of the skull. Occasionally a hematoma becomes infected, producing an abscess, but usually only when associated with a punctured wound; infection, however, may on rare occasions arise from blood-borne bacteria, as illustrated in Figure 107.

The *treatment* of contusions, if seen immediately, consists primarily of the application of pressure, and cold packs to stop the hemorrhage and extravasation. Rest of the injured part is essential to obtain optimum healing. After twenty-four hours the application of heat will facilitate healing, because it produces an increased blood supply, etc. (see Chapter VIII). When the laceration of subcutaneous tissue has been extensive, such as is encountered in crushing injuries, extensive contracture due to scar or atrophy of important structures may develop. Wisely supervised active and passive motion may be useful in preventing these complications. When an injury is of the crushing type and severe, the patient should be examined for shock which, if present, should receive the proper treatment (see Chapter XIII).

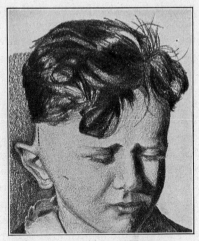

FIG. 107.—INFECTED HEMATOMA.

This boy sustained an injury to the side of the head in a fall, resulting in a hematoma above the ear. Pain and tenderness decreased, but in two or three days became mildly intensified; doubtful fluctuation but no redness was present. Aspiration of the swollen area yielded pus; incision was carried out as indicated by the dotted line. Culture revealed streptococcus. Infection may develop in hematomas anywhere on the body, but is relatively uncommon; the organisms may gain entrance spontaneously (*via* blood stream) or through microscopic punctured wounds or lacerations.

OPEN WOUNDS

There are many types of open wounds. An *abrasion* consists of a tearing or cutting of the superficial layers of the epithelium and is associated with an effusion of serum or slight amount of capillary bleeding. *Punctured wounds* are made by sharp objects and may be comparatively deep, although the surface wound may be very small. *Lacerated wounds* are produced by dull objects and present torn and uneven edges. An *incised wound* is produced by a sharp object and presents smooth, even edges. A wound is considered *penetrating* when it enters a body cavity. A *contaminated* wound is one which contains organisms, but in which sufficient time has not elapsed for the body tissues to kill the bacteria, or for an infection to develop. Practically all open wounds sustained outside the operating wounds are contaminated. An *infected* wound implies previous contamination, but sufficient time has elapsed since injury to allow the invasion of the tissue by the bacteria and the development of the manifestation of infection. *Avulsions* are wounds in which a portion of the body has been torn away. The scalp and extremities are most often involved. The edges of such wounds are practically always uneven and jagged, due to the tearing of tissue. When an extremity such as the arm is avulsed, shock may be considerable, but fatal hemorrhage does not always ensue, because of the rapidity of clotting in torn vessels. Chemical and thermal agents may also produce wounds which, because of their specific nature, are discussed elsewhere (Chapter XIV). Wounds may be classified as superficial or deep.

Superficial Wounds.—Under this heading are included only those wounds which involve the skin and subcutaneous tissue to such a slight extent that suture is not required. Even though all layers of the skin may not be penetrated, a serious and even fatal infection may develop usually due to a streptococcus and beginning as a lymphangitis or cellulitis. Therefore, the most important element in the treatment is the prevention of serious infections.

Treatment.—Because of the danger of serious infection all superficial wounds should be treated immediately after the injury and as many of the contaminating organisms eradicated as is possible. Abrasions should be washed gently with soap and water if the injured area is dirty. Local application of antiseptics is not encouraged because of possible damage to tissue cells, but of the vast list available, a 2 per cent aqueous solution of iodine † (U.S.P.) is to be preferred. Work reported during the past several years (Browning,[12] Albert and associates [13]) indicates that some of the acridine compounds, particularly proflavine (in a 1-1000 solution), are not irritating to tissue cells and are effective antiseptics (see also page 25). The proflavine compounds are much less irritating than acriflavine, but some are somewhat unstable on exposure to light; solutions are therefore stored in brown bottles. Sulfonamide powders are likewise safe and effective locally. A dry sterile dressing should be applied, and the part immobilized for a day or two.

If a wound bleeds, the blood tends to wash out clumps of bacteria and foreign particles, and is therefore an aid to aseptic healing. In punctured wounds dirt and foreign bodies may be retained because of the small opening and lack of bleeding. These wounds are, therefore, more apt to become infected. Although on certain occasions it might appear wise to open and cleanse them, this is not advised as a routine. Such additional injury adds to the inflammatory reaction and may also spread the bacteria. Moreover, it is known that after infliction of such a wound, bacteria are taken up by the lymphatics quite rapidly and travel far beyond reach of any antiseptic within a very short time following the puncture. It is *very important that rest be obtained* to combat infection and encourage healing. A punctured wound on the sole of the foot produced by a rusty nail,* for example, is much more apt to become infected if the patient is allowed to walk. Punctured wounds in general are most prone to produce tetanus (see Chapter VI); for that reason it is more necessary to give a prophylactic dose of antitetanic serum, at least 1500

† If a solution resistant to freezing is desired, it may be prepared in a 30 to 50 per cent solution of propylene glycol.
* It should be emphasized that it is not the rust itself, but the foreign bodies and bacteria on the rusty nail which are responsible for the infection.

units. If the wound is known to contain a significant amount of foreign material it is often essential that it be opened and the debris removed. When cinders, etc. are imbedded in a superficial abrasion, they may be removed advantageously by scrubbing with a brush after an anesthetic has been administered. This is particularly important when the wound is over the face because it will preclude subsequent cosmetic blemishes. Superficial and short lacerations may conveniently be closed and the edges approximated by the application of a strip of adhesive tape which has been "flamed." If such a wound occurs on the face, however, it may be advisable to apply sutures since less scar will result from the better approximation.

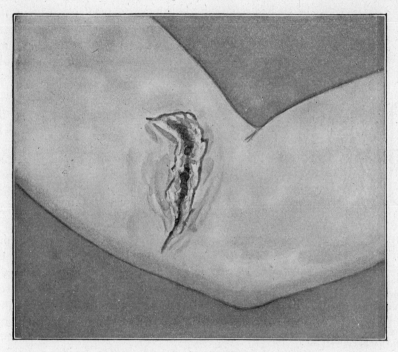

Fig. 108.—Deep Lacerated Wounds of This Type Are Sustained by Relatively Blunt Objects.

Because of the jagged edges, traumatized tissue and contamination, débridement is an important feature in their treatment.

Deep Wounds.—The most important symptoms and signs of wounds have been discussed earlier in this chapter. The manifestations of a more specific nature can be considered more adequately under the various steps in the treatment which are taken up below, as far as possible in a chronological order. Before the local wound is repaired, the patient must be *thoroughly examined* for other injuries, some of which may prove much more serious than the local wound. War wounds are discussed in detail in Chapter XXXIII.

Treatment.—(*a*) *Control of hemorrhage,* if present, is obviously the first step in the treatment of any wound, superficial or deep. Usually, all that is necessary is to apply pressure, or to insert a gauze pack and apply a tight dressing over it

This pressure may have to be maintained for several minutes to allow the development of a clot in the lumina of the severed vessels. If the bleeding is an ooze from innumerable points, the application of hot moist packs may be a more efficient way of controlling it. On the other hand, if a large artery has been severed, it will be necessary to isolate the vessel, clamp, and ligate it. Under some conditions it may be impracticable or impossible to find the bleeding vessel; in such a case a tourniquet must be applied if the wound is located on an extremity, at least during the transportation of the patient to a place suitable for proper treatment (see Figs. 121 and 138). The tourniquet should be released for a moment every twenty or thirty minutes to allow flushing of the extremity and prevent gangrene. It must not

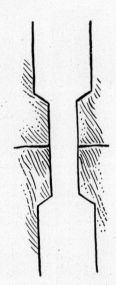

FIG. 109.—THE EDGES OF SHORT AND SUPERFICIAL WOUNDS MAY CONVENIENTLY BE APPROXIMATED BY FLAMED ADHESIVE AS ILLUSTRATED, THEREBY ELIMINATING THE INCONVENIENCE OF SUTURES.

be applied too tightly lest the nerve trunks be injured, thereby resulting in a subsequent paralysis. Whenever convenient, a blood pressure cuff should be used as the tourniquet since the amount of pressure can in that way be controlled accurately. However, it must be remembered that tourniquets are potentially dangerous (see also page 259). When it is difficult to isolate the bleeding vessel in the depth of the wound, it may be desirable to isolate and ligate the artery proximal to the wound.

(b) *Shock* and *syncope* should be treated almost simultaneously with the control of hemorrhage. If shock is present, therapeutic measures such as lowering the head of the bed, administration of physiological saline, glucose and acacia intravenously, as well as transfusion of blood, may be instituted (see Chapter XIII). However, the patient may present many of the symptoms and signs of shock, including pallor, cold sweat, vertigo, weak pulse, etc., but may actually be suffering merely from a "fainting attack." It will rarely be difficult to differentiate a syncope of this type from true shock if one considers the severity of injury and the physical findings. Lowering the head, and inhalation of aromatic spirits of ammonia will be sufficient to combat syncope.

(c) *Examination of the wound* should be carried out soon after the bleeding has been controlled and shock and syncope treated. The wound is inspected for the possible presence of foreign bodies, unless the history obviates this necessity. Injury to the nerves and tendons is determined by inspection of the wound for cut ends, but a more reliable method of examining for severed nerves or tendons is to examine the part of the extremity distal to the wound. A *careful sensory examination must be made*. Disability in the movement of parts distal to the wound may be due to severed nerves, tendons, ligaments, or muscles. Identification of the structure damaged is determined by the location of the wound, the type of disability, and inspection of the depth of the wound. Examination should also be made for the possibility of fracture of bones (see Chapter XVII). Occasionally roentgenograms may be advisable. If the wound is located over the torso the possibility of internal injuries must be considered; if it is present over the skull, intracranial trauma and fracture of the skull are to be suspected and appropriate examinations carried out.

(d) *Antisepsis* is actually best promoted by mechanical cleansing, which is the most effective method of eliminating contamination. Cleansing of the skin around the wound is of preliminary importance in order to prevent further contamination therefrom during the subsequent procedures. There is probably no better method of cleansing the skin than the proper gentle yet thorough use of soap and warm water. A fat solvent such as benzene or ether may be needed if considerable grease is present on the skin. After the skin is dry it may be sterilized by the application of some antiseptic such as weak tincture of iodine, removed in a minute or two with alcohol to prevent blistering. Through this relatively sterile area of skin novocaine can be readily injected to provide anesthesia, thus enabling the surgeon to then thoroughly cleanse, debride, and suture the wound itself. When general anesthesia is used, the cleansing of both the skin and wound is done after the production of anesthesia. The mechanical cleansing is aided by *gentle irrigation with physiologic saline solution* which is particularly important if the wound contains dirt or foreign material, even in small amounts.

The importance of antiseptics in the treatment of wounds has been greatly exaggerated, particularly because it is only a matter of a few minutes or an hour following injury until the organisms will penetrate the tissues deeply enough to prevent their destruction by the local application of an antiseptic. Most antiseptics also inflict severe damage to the tissue cells of an open wound and in that way interfere with healing as discussed on pages 25 and 26. Moreover, in punctured wounds, the antiseptic cannot reach the depths of the wound, and its use therefore is limited to the prevention of a secondary infection; this, however, is of considerably less importance than the danger of an infection resulting from the initial contamination.

In war wounds adequate and prompt antisepsis by débridement, cleansing, irrigation, and the use of antiseptics is sometimes impossible because so much time elapses between the infliction of the wound and the time when the soldier is evacuated to a station where surgical·care can be carried out. In such situations the use of the sulfonamides has been found effective (often dramatically so) in the prevention and control of infection (see page 200 and Chapter XXXIII).

(e) *Closure of the wound,* under ideal conditions, can be carried out with full expectation of primary healing. Unfortunately this is not always possible. For example, in massive war wounds primary closure is unsafe (see Chapter XXXIII). The decision as to whether a wound is (1) to be closed by primary suture, (2) to be closed around a drain, (3) to be closed later by secondary suture, or (4) to be allowed to heal by granulation without suture depends to a large extent on the presence or likelihood of infection, which is governed by many factors. The most important factor is the *length of time which has elapsed between the injury and treatment.* In general, wounds over twenty-four hours old are considered too deeply invaded by bacteria to permit primary closure; those under eight hours are nearly always suitable for immediate suture. In wounds between eight and twenty-four hours old, the appearance and type of the wound, the probable amount of contamination, the extent of the inflammatory signs, as well as the factors mentioned below, determine the question of closure and drainage. Another important factor is the amount of traumatized tissues, dirt and debris in the wound. In wounds treated early and effectively, however, the relation of these factors to infection and delayed healing can be eliminated in most instances by *débridement*. This consists of the excision of all badly contaminated, devitalized, or jagged tissue, and the removal of all foreign bodies by careful and painstaking exploration of the injured tissue. To be properly done, débridement of the deeper portions of the wound should be done with a second set of sterile instruments. Before actual closure with sutures is begun, the wound should again be irrigated with physiologic saline solution. In general débridement, however, *should not be done* on wounds over eight hours old, because the bacteria have already invaded the tissue, producing a cellulitis which would be aggravated by the mechanical trauma incident to the operation. However, if the wound shows no evidence of infection, and particularly if sulfanilamide had been placed in the wound at the time of injury, débridement may still be done even though twelve hours or more have elapsed since injury. The term débridement, originally French and meaning literally "de bridle," is now defined in a far wider sense as the excision of traumatized non-viable parts of the wound and removal of foreign material. The treatment of infected wounds is described later in the chapter.

After débridement is completed, the walls of the wound are approximated by interrupted sutures as described later, so as to obliterate dead space, but only if necessary. Based on the epochal work of Halsted [6] and the experience of many surgeons during recent years, it is being recognized that buried sutures should be cotton or silk instead of catgut because the incidence of infection will be thereby greatly reduced. It is well known, however, that when the silk technic is used in the repair of wounds, the utmost care including gentleness, etc., must be utilized in the handling of tissues. Traction should be gentle, utilizing a flat bladed retractor or the blade of an instrument and not the bite of a hemostat. Only sterile instruments, and not one's finger, should be used when working in the depth of the wound, except when actual exploration with the hand or fingers is necessary. The operating team should be masked. Drapes of sterile towels or sheets about the wound should be adequate. Sponges should be applied gently to the bleeding point and not wiped across the wound. It is true that if infection develops in the presence of buried cotton or silk there is more likelihood of prolonged drainage. Fine catgut may be used in wounds which are repaired more than four to six hours after injury. If the wound is properly treated and not of the massive type it will rarely become infected if closed less than four hours after infliction. This is explainable on the basis that bacteria as emphasized by Mason [3] and substantiated by clinical experience and the experiments of Friedrich,[7] do not begin to penetrate immediately upon implantation into a wound, but require an interval of four to six hours before they multiply and invade.

During closure the bleeding points are searched for and ligated, in order to avoid the danger of the formation of a hematoma. Effort should be made to apply artery forceps (with narrow blades) on the vessel itself and not take huge bites with resultant necrosis of considerable tissue, because these necrotic areas encourage the development of infection. If the bleeding point cannot be ligated with inclusion of a minimal amount of tissue, a transfixing suture should be inserted with a needle, and the ligature tied just tightly enough to stop the bleeding. The presence of a blood clot in a wound not only delays union, but invites infection. When sutures are applied, tension must be avoided at all costs, since necrosis of tissue will most certainly result from the consequent impairment of the blood supply. Avoidance of tension is especially important when a flap of skin is partly avulsed with consequent impairment of blood supply. One can usually determine the effect of tension at operation by noting the color of the involved skin. A suture which is too tight is apt to cut through the tissue, and approximation will thereby be lost. When repairing tendons or muscles, flexion of the joints aids in relieving tension.

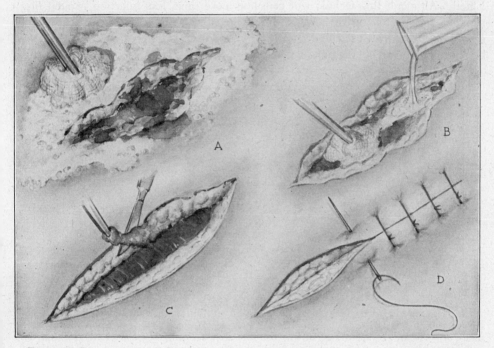

FIG. 110.—STEPS IN THE CLOSURE OF A WOUND INFLICTED OUTSIDE THE OPERATING ROOM.

A, the area surrounding the wound is cleansed with soap and water; *B,* the wound is irrigated with physiologic saline solution; *C,* débridement is performed excising all traumatized and contaminated tissue. Subcutaneous interrupted sutures (usually silk) may be necessary to obtain approximation and eliminate dead space; *D,* the skin is closed with interrupted or continuous silk or horsehair sutures. Interrupted sutures of horsehair are commonly used on the face.

In the repair of wounds it should be emphasized that only mesothelial surfaces will grow together. Muscle unites to muscle only by union of the fibrous tissue strands about the muscle bundles. Fatty tissue likewise unites only by union of the fibrous tissue contained in it. The best closure of a wound is obtained, therefore, when fibrous structures can be approximated. A drain is rarely indicated unless hemostasis has been unsatisfactory or a dead space could not be obliterated; in such a case it may be removed in 24 hours. For closing the skin, interrupted or continuous sutures of fine cotton or silk are usually used, but on the face, where a minimal scar is desired, some type of suture whose surface is impermeable to moisture (*e.g.* horsehair, dermal, nylon, etc.) will be superior, because less reaction is produced in the tissue about them. Interrupted sutures are usually used on the face. Details of suture material, drains, infections, etc., are discussed elsewhere in this chapter.

The principles just discussed in the treatment of accidental wounds can be applied to a great extent to operative wounds, the most important of which are *abdominal incisions.* Most surgeons utilize a longitudinal incision but many surgeons favor a transverse type of incision because postoperative strain is less likely to lead to disruption. The advantages of closing abdominal wounds with deep interrupted nonabsorbable sutures have recently been summarized by Whipple and Elliott.[8] Although this technic will consume more time, less infection, wound disruption, and postoperative hernias will ensue. The skin adjacent to the wound should be covered with sterile drapes. The wound itself is by no means sterile as has been demonstrated by Ives and Hirschfeld [9] who took cultures of clean operative

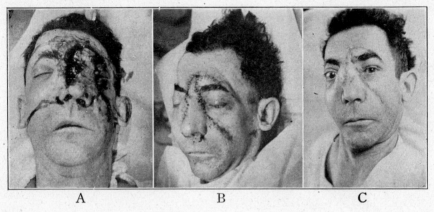

A   B   C

FIG. III.—SEVERE LACERATION OF THE FACE.

A, photo on admission. The wound is associated with an unusual amount of trauma to the subcutaneous tissue; *B,* appearance of wound after débridement and closure with interrupted suture of horsehair; *C,* appearance of scar ten days after accident. The mass to the right of the nose represents an enchondroma, present before the accident and not associated with the trauma (St. Louis City Hospital).

wounds at various stages throughout the operation and found positive cultures in practically 100 per cent of cases. This is explained by the fact that the skin, air, improper masking, etc., are serious sources of contamination. Hart [10] has been an advocate of the use of ultraviolet light in an operating-room to kill circulating air bacteria which might be an important source of infection in prolonged operations. Blalock [11] and others have emphaszed the importance of keeping tissues (particularly intestines) moist during prolonged operations, because drying of tissue results in its death. Most surgeons who advocate nonabsorbable sutures prefer not to bury catgut in the same wound on the assumption that the possibility of infection is thereby increased. Stay sutures are rarely necessary when abdominal wounds are closed with silk. To combat the development of infection in abdominal wounds contaminated by spillage during colonic resections, etc., gentle irrigation with physiologic saline may be instituted at the end of the operation. The local application of four to six grams of sulfanilamide, or smaller doses of sulfathiazole or sulfadiazine, in the wound is still more effective in preventing postoperative wound infection (see page 200). However, it must be emphasized that no drug can take the place of careful surgery in the prevention of postoperative infections. Although peritonitis of a serious degree rarely results from the contamination of a well performed resection of intestine (unless a leak in the suture line develops), infection of the wound in the abdominal wall is common. Proper draping of the wound, careful and gentle handling of tissue, etc., as already discussed, must not be neglected, regardless of the type of wound.

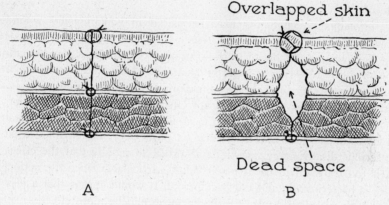

Overlapped skin

Dead space

A   B

FIG. 112.—SUTURE OF A WOUND IN LAYERS.

A, correct way to close a wound; *B,* incorrect way to close a wound; note the dead space in the subcutaneous tissue, and the overlapping of skin edges.

(*f*) *Tetanus antitoxin* (*A.T.S.*) need not be given if the wound is small, superficial, and inflicted by a clean sharp object. In deep punctured wounds antitoxin is specially indicated, unless the wound has been caused by an instrument such as a clean, smooth needle. In localities where tetanus is prevalent because of such factors as extensive use of fertilizer, etc., administration of tetanus antitoxin as a routine may be indicated even in small wounds. It should always be given when the wound is extensive or contaminated with dirt and foreign bodies. A dose of 1500 units, subcutaneously or intramuscularly, should be sufficient except perhaps in destructive gunshot wounds, or in massive wounds inflicted in barnyards or the streets; in these instances the dose should be doubled (see Chapter VI). Since the immunity conferred by the administration of a dose of tetanus antitoxin *lasts no longer than ten to fourteen days,* it will be necessary to *repeat the prophylactic dose* if operative procedures about the original wound are contemplated more than two weeks after administration of tetanus antitoxin. If there is massive destruction of tissue with excessive contamination, a prophylactic dose of gas bacillus antitoxin should be given as well as tetanus antitoxin.

(*g*) *Anesthesia* is nearly always necessary. The facility of closure and débridement depends to a certain extent on the presence of good anesthesia. The choice of an anesthetic is important. Good anesthesia allows a more thorough exploration of the wound for foreign bodies, severed tendons, nerves, etc., and a more careful approximation of tissues. If the patient is composed and the wound small, a local anesthetic (novocaine, one-half per cent) may be used; otherwise a general anesthetic will be preferable, unless the patient has eaten a significant amount of food less than two or three hours previously. A preliminary dose of morphine hypodermatically, is usually advisable regardless of whether a local or general anesthetic is used. When a general anesthetic such as ether is to be given, it is advisable to add atropine to the morphine in order to dry up the respiratory secretion stimulated by the anesthesia. If intracranial or intrathoracic injuries are also present, it may be imperative to use a local anesthetic even for the repair of an extensive wound, because of the damage which might be inflicted on the circulation and the respiration by a general anesthesia.

(*h*) *Sulfonamide compounds* may be placed in contaminated wounds after débridement and just before closure. Needless to say, sulfonamides need not be placed in fresh wounds produced in the operating room, unless contamination such as that incurred by resection of intestine has taken place. Recent work reported by Meleney [14] suggests that local use of sulfanilamide in the treatment of wounds sustained in automobile accidents, etc., is not effective in minimizing infection. However, most surgeons still believe that local use of sulfonamides in contaminated wounds is justifiable (see also discussion on page 35). Sulfanilamide used locally has one serious disadvantage, *viz.*, it is absorbed so rapidly that the effect on the bacteria is too transient to be of much value, particularly since the action of sulfonamides is bacteriostatic and not bactericidal. It would appear that a less soluble compound such as sulfathiazole or sulfadiazine would be more effective since they would not be absorbed for 48 hours or thereabouts. However, if these relatively insoluble compounds are used, they must be used in moderate doses (no more than 3 grams for a laparotomy wound), because an excess of the drug might result in persistence of the drug in the wound longer than 48 hours, consequently giving rise to a foreign body reaction. Sulfadiazine has an added advantage in so far as it has a wide specificity of action, being effective against a large variety of bacteria. When contamination has been profuse, parenteral administration (see page 35) of one of the sulfonamides will also be indicated for a few days until danger of infection is past; sulfadiazine is the drug of choice for this purpose. All workers agree that use of sulfonamides markedly decreases the incidence of systemic infection as well as the mortality rate, although as mentioned above there may be lack of agreement that the incidence of infection itself is decreased by local sulfonamides. The use of sulfonamides in war wounds is discussed in Chapter XXXIII.

Suture of Special Structures.—When a major *nerve* has been severed it should be repaired. Before approximation, the severed ends if jagged, should be cut across cleanly with a sharp knife. Two sutures of fine silk should be sufficient to maintain end to end approximation. The stitch should be of the mattress type and be taken deep enough to include only the epineurium. Care should be exercised in approximating the ends in order to avoid rotation which would delay or prevent regeneration. In massive war wounds which are debrided and packed open (not closed), divided peripheral nerves should be approximated with chromic catgut in order to prevent retraction, thereby facilitating second stage repair later.

When *tendons* of the wrist or hand are severed primary suture is advisable only when aseptic healing is certain. A severe infection in the presence of the repaired tendons usually results in a failure of maintenance of approximation and the development of a contracture. It is for this reason that Koch [16] has suggested that if there is a strong probability of a wound infection because of the long period intervening between injury and repair, it is better to close the wound and perform the tenorrhaphy at a later date. Koch emphasizes the fact that infection of the wound following repair of a tendon surrounded by a sheath is much more apt to result in a permanent contracture (because of the spread of the infection throughout the sheath) than when the sheath is absent. He remarks further that, as a rule, if more than four hours have elapsed since injury to a palmar tendon, it is wiser to close the wound and perform the. tenorrhaphy after the wound' has healed. The decision as to repair of the tendons must be made by the surgeon, depending upon the type of wound, because in many instances if the wound has been made by a clean, sharp object and properly cared for, repair of tendons may be successful when six to eight hours have elapsed since injury. The slow rate of healing of injured tendons, which is probably dependent upon inadequate blood supply, demands secure fixation and approximation of the cut ends over a period of seven to twelve days. Therefore fine silk is the suture of choice because catgut may be absorbed too soon. There are innumerable variations in the technic of suturing tendons. Three or four interrupted mattress sutures usually will suffice, but since a single mattress suture may tear out, many surgeons, including Koch,[16] Bunnell,[17] and others advise more complete fixation (see Fig. 113); the latter uses fine wire for sutures. The cut ends should be freshened by cutting them off cleanly with a sharp knife. Knots must not be allowed to interpose between the cut ends of the tendon. When several adjacent tendons are involved, extreme care must be exercised in identifying the tendons and attaching the correct central to the correct distal end. When the wound is in the palm of the hand or the wrist, it may be necessary to make an incision one and one-fourth to one and three-fourths inches proximal to the wound so that the retracted stumps may be found. This additional incision may be obviated by the application of an Esmarch (elastic) bandage starting at the elbow. This compresses the muscles, and forces the tendons downward into the wound. The hand must be immobilized for at least fifteen days in a position which relaxes the sutured tendons and, except in occasional instances, no active or passive motion should be instituted for the same period. The atraumatic technic of repairing tendons, utilizing small instruments, fine needles and fine silk sutures has been admirably summarized by Mason.[18]

Any wound sustained over a *joint* should be closely inspected for possible laceration of the joint capsule. If an opening is found, it is imperative that the joint be inspected for foreign bodies and dirt, and if present these must be removed. Removal of débris is facilitated by irrigation with a solution such a physiological saline. The' wound in the joint capsule should then be closed by interrupted sutures of fine silk. The rest of the wound is closed in the routine fashion. It should be inspected daily and the patient's temperature observed closely for the possible occurrence of infection within the joint. The presence or absence of pain about the joint is usually helpful in determining whether or not an infection has occurred. It is imperative to discover the infection as soon as it occurs, so that the joint may be reopened and the chance of destruction of the cartilage minimized (see Chapter XIX).

The treatment of a wound associated with a compound fracture is discussed in Chapter XVII.

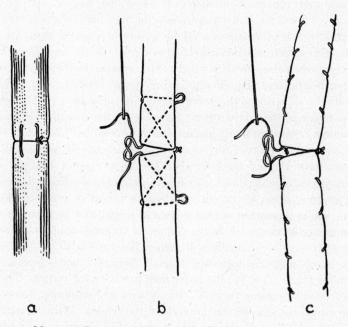

a   b   c

FIG. 113.—METHODS COMMONLY USED IN THE REPAIR OF LACERATED TENDONS.

a, Fixation by three or four interrupted subcutaneous sutures; *b*, Insertion of the suture through the entire tendon and back again to prevent the suture from tearing out; *c*, Extensive transfixation after the Bunnell technic.

Sutures.—There are numerous varieties of suture material in use at the present time. Many of them are merely substitutes for each other without obvious advantages or disadvantages. However, on certain occasions one type of suture will be superior, whereas on other occasions a distinctly different type of suture will have obvious advantages.

Types of Suture Material.—Sutures are classified as absorbable and nonabsorbable. The latter type are not affected by the digestive action of body fluids and leukocytes, and remain indefinitely, unless cast off or removed. Nonabsorbable sutures most commonly consist of silk, but linen, nylon, cotton, silver wire, silkworm gut, and varieties of vegetable fiber (dermal) are also used under special conditions. Silk may be used in a variety of sizes from the finest split strands to thick braided cords. The advantages of silk lie in the fact that it does not lose its tensile strength, except to a slight degree, and holds the approximated structures together almost indefinitely. Silk provokes a minimum of tissue reaction in the absence of infection, and healing therefore is accompanied by very little scar tissue. Silk, more-over, has such intrinsic tensile strength that very fine strands are adequate to hold most structures in place. The *disadvantage of silk* is confined to its action in the presence of infection, for under such conditions it acts as a foreign body and as already mentioned will prevent healing until it is discharged. However, it should be emphasized, as has been shown by Shambaugh and Dunphy,[19] that wounds closed with interrupted silk will tolerate contamination better than wounds closed with catgut. Since the onset of World War II cotton is displacing silk to a great extent, although its tensile strength is not as constant as silk; it invokes perhaps even less reaction in tissues than does silk (Meade and Ochsner [23]). Practically all the other remarks just made about silk apply likewise to cotton. Other nonabsorbable suture material such as horsehair, linen, metal clips, dermal (vegetable fiber), and nylon sutures are available, but are used largely in the skin. During recent years two or three types of fine, pliable, strong metallic sutures made of stainless steel, aluminum, etc., have been introduced. They are, of course, nonabsorbable, are strong and from initial reports appear to be tolerated well by tissues, even in the presence of infection. More experience with them will be required before it can be determined how exten-sively they may be used.

Absorbable sutures are those which are digested by the tissue juices and leukocytes, and replaced by scar. Catgut is the commonest representative of ab-sorbable suture but kangaroo tendon is sometimes used. Catgut is of animal origin, being prepared from the submucosa or fibrous layer of the terminal ileum of sheep. It is prepared in a variety of sizes, the finest being designated by 00000 and increasing in caliber to No. 2 or larger which is quite stout. They are also prepared in a variety of ways which affect the speed with which they are absorbed in the tissues. Thus, 10 day (plain), 20 day and 30 day catgut are supposed to re-tain their tensile strength during these periods, but as has been demonstrated by Howes and Harvey,[20] Jenkins [21] and others, actually do not. Slow absorbability is achieved by treating the material with various chemicals, usually potassium bichromate; hence the 20-day variety is often called "chromic catgut." Potassium mercuric iodide, tannic acid and other chemicals are likewise used to decrease the absorbability. The *advantages* of catgut lie in the fact that it is absorbed, but as absorption takes place scar tissue becomes deposited which binds the ap-proximated structures together. Since it is absorbed, it does not act as a foreign body and in grossly infected wounds does not lead to persistent drainage, as would be the case with nonabsorbable sutures. The *disadvantages* of catgut are that it can be sterilized less readily than silk and that a reaction in the tissue with a tendency toward development of infection follows its use; in a study of 2360 inguinal herniotomies, Shambaugh [22] noted that the incidence of suppuration was twice as great in those repaired by catgut as it was in those repaired with silk. Moreover, in the presence of infection its tensile strength decreases rapidly even though chromicized gut is used (see Fig. 115). In the presence of infection catgut delays healing. Moreover, it is widely known that, until perhaps recently, numerous infections have been produced by unsterile catgut.

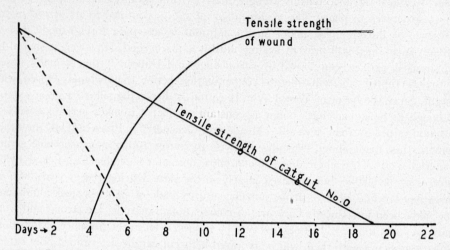

FIG. 114.—RELATION OF DECREASING TENSILE STRENGTH OF CATGUT TO INCREASING TENSILE STRENGTH OF WOUND (HEALING UNDER ASEPTIC CONDITIONS).

The broken line illustrates the rapid loss in tensile strength of even large catgut (No. 2) in an infected wound. (Modified from Howes and Harvey, *N. Eng. J. M.,* 1929, 200:1289.)

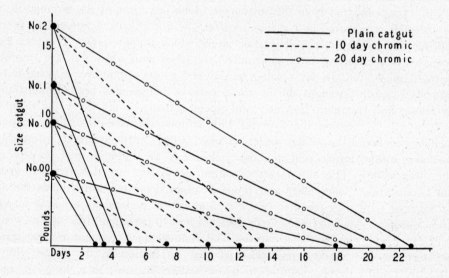

FIG. 115.—DECREASE IN TENSILE STRENGTH OF VARIOUS SIZES OF CATGUT BURIED IN A NONINFECTED WOUND.

Note that regardless of size, plain catgut (indicated by solid line) loses its tensile strength within five days, whereas, twenty-day chromic catgut (indicated by line with circle) loses its tensile strength only after eighteen days even in the finest (oo) size. (From Howes and Harvey, *N. Eng. J. M.,* 1929, 200:1288.)

Application and Choice of Sutures.—When a wound is superficial and the subcutaneous tissue is not gaping, closure of the skin with a continuous or inter-rupted suture of fine cotton or silk will suffice. Black silk may have a slight advantage over white because it can be seen so readily, except perhaps in Negroes. For approximation of the skin other nonabsorbable material may be used, including cotton, linen, metal clips, nylon and dermal sutures. If the wound is on the face, interrupted sutures of fine horsehair should be used, since this type of suture encourages healing with the least amount of scar tissue. Because of the need for good cosmetic results in wounds of the face or scalp, these sutures may be removed on the third or fourth day. If an operation must be conducted through a frankly infected field, catgut will be the suture of choice because it is absorbed, therefore not tend-

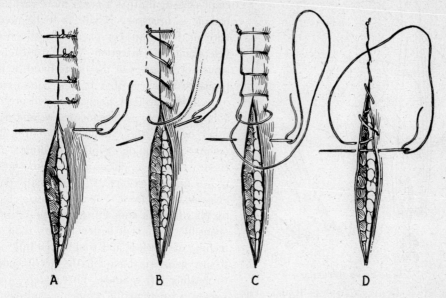

FIG. 116.—COMMONLY USED METHODS OF SUTURING SKIN.

A, interrupted; *B,* continuous; *C,* blanket; and *D,* epithelial stitch. In the last method the suture is placed so near the edge of the skin that it will drop out, or be removed merely by traction on one end.

ing to produce persistent drainage through foreign body action, as might be the case with nonabsorbable sutures. However, Cutler and Dunphy (*New England J. Med.,* 224:101, 1941), although they do not advise routine use of silk in infected wounds, obtained fairly good results and concluded that the supposed incompatibility is greatly exaggerated.

When catgut is used for closure of abdominal wounds the chromic type is indicated since it maintains tensile strength longer than plain gut. On certain other occasions (*e.g.,* fixation of bone fragments in a fracture) it may be desirable to use a still more slowly absorbable suture, and one which has more tensile strength than catgut, *e.g.,* kangaroo tendon. Metallic sutures made of silver, stainless steel, and aluminum may also be used in such instances, particularly if fixation can be obtained with comparatively few short sutures, which may or may not be removed later. To guard against the possible rupture of an abdominal wound with resultant gaping of the edges, it is desirable frequently to insert through and through dermal or braided silk stay sutures which may be left in place eight to twelve days. Silver wire has also been found to be relatively nonirritating and is occasionally used for stay sutures when considerable strain may be exerted upon the sutures. Stay sutures are placed deeply through all layers of the abdominal wall but are not necessary if the fascia has been closed by cotton or a similar nonabsorbable suture.

The advantages of silk over catgut in clean wounds, as being appreciated during recent years, have already been discussed in this chapter, and are particularly valued and demonstrable in thyroidectomies and herniotomies. However, it is important to emphasize again that a much more careful technic is necessary if silk is to be used without the serious complication of the development of infection with persistent sinus formation. On the other hand, it is probably also true that if this same care in technic is utilized, fine catgut will probably give nearly as satisfactory results. In other words, the "philosophy" of silk technic (including gentle handling of tissue, careful application of hemostats, use of fine sutures, etc.), as originally developed by Halsted [6] should be mastered by all surgeons and will no doubt be responsible for much better results than a technic of careless and rough handling of tissue, which is bound to be detrimental to healing of wounds. Fortunately, the reason a great many competent surgeons still use catgut and are not inclined to change to silk lies in the fact that they are using silk "philosophy" in the use of catgut, and are, therefore, obtaining such good results that they see no reason to change. Unfortunately, this is not true in all instances.

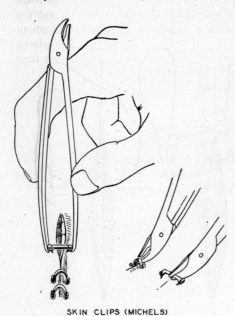

SKIN CLIPS (MICHELS)

FIG. 117.—MICHELS CLIPS, AS ILLUSTRATED, ARE PREFERRED BY MANY SURGEONS FOR CLOSING THE SKIN.

They may be applied and removed by any of several different types of instruments.

Drains.—Although drains are distinctly contraindicated when aseptic healing is expected, there are occasions when the closure of the wound around a drain is advisable. The use of drains in the repair of accidental (*i.e.*, grossly contaminated) wounds is confined chiefly to two types: (1) in wounds where hemostasis could not be satisfactorily attained (under such circumstances the drain is removed in 12 to 24 hours when all bleeding has stopped) ; and (2) in wounds where dead space could not be effectively eliminated. Opinions differ considerably as to whether or not a drain should be left in wounds which are closed eight hours or more after the injury. Some surgeons are of the opinion that if infection develops, the presence of a drain will help to keep the process localized and to produce fewer systemic or local manifestations. This is no doubt true, but it is likewise true that on numerous occasions the drain will act as a foreign body and aid in the development of an infection, whereas the wound would not have become infected if it had been closed without drainage. The argument can scarcely be settled because it is impossible to predict which wound would or would not become infected. In general, wounds closed with cotton or silk should *not* be drained because the drain exerts a foreign body action, and permits skin bacteria to travel along its course, thereby encouraging development of infection, which is particularly undesirable in a wound closed with silk. The question of insertion of drains after opening abscesses is a separate one and is discussed elsewhere.

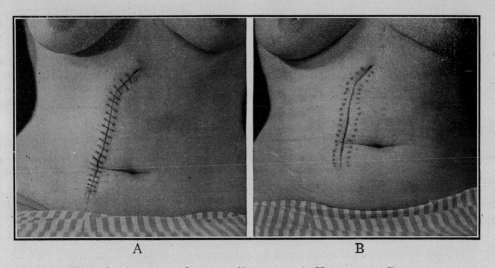

A   B

Fig. 118.—Abdominal Incision (Laparotomy) Healing per Primam.

A, five days after closure of skin with continuous cotton suture. *B,* ten days after operation. The sutures were removed on the seventh postoperative day.

A small strip of rubber dam is superior to almost any other type of drain and in most instances should be anchored with a suture to *prevent losing the drain* in the depth of the wound. The loss of the drain in the wound may also be prevented by attaching a safety pin to that portion outside the wound or by using such a large piece that it is impossible for the entire drain to be lost in the wound. When draining small wounds a wick made of doubling several strands of catgut or silkworm gut may be adequate. When a penetrating and very extensive wound needs drainage a large drain will, of course, be needed. Rubber dam may be rolled up to the size desired and is particularly satisfactory as a drain because it is soft and pliable, thereby causing no pressure necrosis.

In most instances a drain left in a wound at time of closure may be removed in twenty-four or forty-eight hours. If a definite infection develops it may be advisable to keep a drain in the wound for several days. The length of time is dependent upon the severity of the infection, size of the cavity, efficiency of the drainage, etc. Gauze wicks or packs are very useful in stopping hemorrhage from the edges of the wound, but the mesh becomes plugged with fibrin so rapidly that they do not serve as drains, and should be removed in twelve to eighteen hours, and a rubber drain inserted if drainage is desired for a longer period of time.

The use of large rubber tubing for drainage of wounds, as so often recommended, is in reality to be condemned, except for drainage of large cavities (empyema, etc.).

Postoperative Care.—On many occasions healing by primary or secondary union is determined largely, if not entirely, by the postoperative care of the wound. If the wound is large this treatment can best be carried out in a hospital. Hospitalization is likewise strongly indicated when a large vessel has been severed and secondary hemorrhage is likely.

Types of Dressing.—When the wound has been closed without drainage, nothing more than a sterile dry gauze dressing need be applied. If the wound is deep, or hemorrhage likely, it is usually advisable to apply a firm dressing so as to minimize the possibility of bleeding and the formation of a hematoma. Dry dressings have an obvious advantage over others in so far as the secretions which escape from the wound edges are rapidly absorbed by the gauze, and bacteria which may be present in the secretion are killed by drying. A dry dressing, likewise, allows the edges of the wound to adhere fairly firmly in thirty-six to forty-eight hours with the formation of a crust which seals the wound, thereby minimizing the possibility of infection from the exterior. Silver foil, partly because of its antiseptic qualities, is an excellent dressing and is used extensively over craniotomy wounds. Ointments are disadvantageous because they prevent drying and the formation of the protective crust, thereby encouraging the development of secondary infection. However, if the gauze sticks to the wound it will be necessary to apply a small amount of bland ointment (*e.g.,* boric acid), to prevent pain and injury to the epithelial edge at subsequent dressings.

Gauze dressings may be anchored by adhesive or a bandage. A bandage is apt to be more comfortable and will assist in absorbing wound secretions, but cannot be applied conveniently on the torso. On certain occasions when it is necessary to apply a small dressing (as on the scalp) the dressing may be anchored by collodion or liquid adhesive, which must be applied only on the edges of the dressing so as not to seal over the wound edge. It has been learned from experience that sealing the sutured wound with collodion may be quite harmful by increasing the danger of infection.

It is necessary to change dressings frequently only to insure cleanliness and comfort for the patient, or to detect infection so that treatment may be instituted for it as early as possible. A clean wound which is not draining and not infected need not be dressed for four or five days following its repair. Frequent dressings in such instances may even be harmful, especially if the physician resorts to such unwise procedures as probing the depth of the wound and removing crusts or scabs. If a drain is placed in the wound chiefly for prophylactic reasons, it is usually still permissible to apply a dry dressing. As stated previously, such drains may be removed in twenty-four to forty-eight hours. However, if at time of closure a drain is inserted into a wound which is probably infected, it may be desirable to keep the drainage tract from healing over, by the application of a wet dressing or a liberal quantity of a bland ointment. In such instances, daily dressings will probably be necessary, especially if infection seems imminent or the discharge saturates the dressings. If the discharge from the wound, or the application of too much ointment produces a maceration of the skin, it may be advisable to remove all dressings and expose the wound to the air, taking care to protect it from insects and other contaminants.

At each dressing the wound must be carefully examined for the possible presence of a hematoma, collection of fluid in a dead space, or infection, and possible fluctuation. If there is a collection of fluid within a dead space there will be no local swelling, but a soft spot with fluctuation may be detectable. As soon as discovered, the contents of a hematoma or dead space should be evacuated through a small opening made into the cavity by separation of the wound edges. On some occasions it may be advisable to keep this opening patent with an ointment or a small drain for a day or two in order to prevent reaccumulation of fluid. If the cavity is large it may be desirable to apply a pressure dressing, using a small sea sponge so as to obliterate it. If dead spaces or hematomas are unnoticed they may break through the wound and evacuate to the exterior.

Immobilization.—One of the most important features in the postoperative treatment of wounds is *immobilization of the injured part.* Any movements which allow the wound edges to become detached and traumatized will, of course, delay

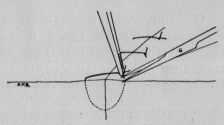

FIG. 119.—TECHNIC OF REMOVING SUTURES.

The suture is grasped by the forceps and lifted up, so that when pulled out, no extraneous material such as crusts, etc., are dragged into the track occupied by the suture.

healing, but more important than that, will encourage the development of infection. If the wound is on the upper extremity, a sling may be sufficient to obtain this immobilization. If the wound is on the lower extremity, it may be necessary to confine the patient to bed for two or three days. For obvious reasons, it is important to immobilize the extremity, including the joint, when the wound is located over the extensor surface of a joint. If the wound involves the joint capsule complete immobilization is indicated until such a time when the possibility of infection has been eliminated (four to eight days).

Removal of Sutures.—The time for the removal of sutures depends in general on the rapidity of the fibroblastic reaction. As expressed by Harvey[1] "tensile strength of a healing wound is a function of multiplication and maturation of the fibroblasts. There is a latent period of approximately four days before growth becomes appreciable in terms of function." It is only after ten to fourteen days that this process reaches a level. Skin sutures, however, may be removed much earlier than this, *i.e.,* five or six days after injury, depending upon the location of the wound. In an area as vascular as the scalp, and regions where little movement is present, sutures can be removed at the end of forty-eight hours, especially if subcutaneous interrupted stitches have been applied. On the face, which is likewise quite vascular, wounds also heal rapidly; some of the sutures (perhaps every other one) may be removed on the second day and the rest on the third or fourth day, depending upon the condition of the wound. If left in place longer the amount of scar formation is increased. Skin sutures should not be removed from a wound in a dependent position such as the leg, earlier than the eighth postoperative day unless it is a very superficial wound. The dependent position and the movements associated with walking delay healing, and the wound is apt to separate if stitches are removed earlier than the eighth day.

Symptomatic Treatment.—Under this heading may be included numerous miscellaneous therapeutic measures, the chief ones of which are medicinal. On many occasions it may be advisable to prescribe a sedative (aspirin, codeine) for pain or discomfort, especially if the patient is "nervous" and easily excitable. If a local anesthetic (novocaine) has been used, there may be considerable burning for an hour or two while the effect of the anesthetic is wearing off. This may be relieved by a hot water bottle.

CRUSHED WOUNDS

Obviously, crushed wounds of varying severity may be produced with or without destruction of the skin. One of the most frequent types of crushed wounds encountered at the present time is that inflicted by the electric wringer on the upper extremity (usually in children). However, fractures are rarely produced by this type of injury. The enormous amount of pressure exerted by the wringers produces a varying amount of permanent damage to the skin, subcutaneous tissue and muscles. Most of the damage to the skin is inflicted usually on the forearm at the point where the wringer stops (or perhaps spins). Not infrequently the skin is damaged so much that ultimately (after a few days) it becomes gangrenous. Rarely is the defect large enough to demand skin graft. A variable amount of swelling, produced by edema and hemorrhage, develops shortly after the injury. Such injuries are usually very painful. A surprisingly large amount of disability (fingers and hands) is associated with the injury. Only rarely is there sufficient scar deposited in or about the muscles and tendons to produce a permanent contracture. Treatment consists of immobilization, followed by active and passive exercise.

Occasionally, crushing injuries of the extremities as sustained in railroad accidents, etc., may be of sufficient magnitude to demand amputation. Laceration and tearing of the skin and deep tissue usually exist. Large vessels may be torn, resulting in severe hemorrhage which may be internal or external, depending upon whether or not the skin is broken. Crush injuries are often accompanied by severe shock which is not always helped by transfusions of blood or plasma. Formerly it was assumed that the loss of serum and blood was the major factor in the production of shock. At present considerable evidence has been adduced that a special entity called Crush Syndrome (see page 1059) is responsible and is associated with the absorption of myohemoglobin released from the crushed muscle and which acts as a toxin on the kidney (Bywaters and Popjak [15]). The extravasation of fluid, and hemorrhage from smaller vessels may be sufficient to compress the larger vessels and produce gangrene *per se*. Fracture of the bones obviously adds to the severity of any crushing injury. Treatment of such crushing injuries should be undertaken with extreme conservatism. Years ago, before the aseptic era, amputation was frequently necessary because of the likelihood of severe infection. Although the prevention of infection by careful aseptic technic in dressings,

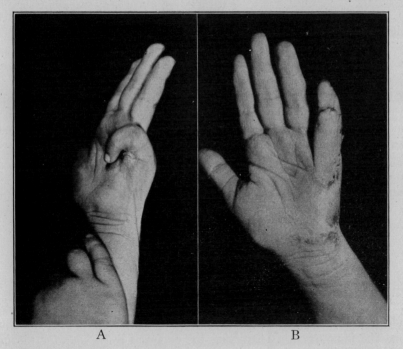

A   B

FIG. 120.—CRUSHED WOUND PRODUCING FLEXION CONTRACTURE OF FINGER.

A, two months after crushing of hand by an electric wringer; no open wound was sustained. *B,* the scar was excised, the finger released, and the resultant defect repaired by a "flap" skin graft removed from the inguinal region. (St. Louis City Hospital.)

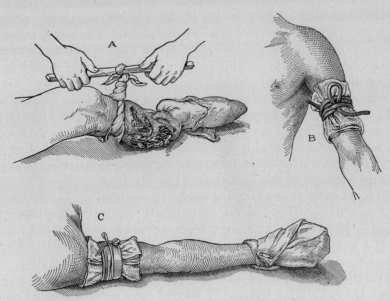

FIG. 121.—USE OF THE TOURNIQUET.

A, a crushed leg with a cloth tourniquet applied and twisted tight with a stick; *B,* rubber tubing applied as a tourniquet for temporary purposes; *C,* an Esmarch bandage used as a tourniquet for an operation upon the forearm. (From Homans, *Text Book of Surgery,* 1931, Charles C. Thomas, p. 136.) (See also Fig. 184.)

etc., has decreased the number of amputations tremendously, there is no doubt that amputation is still being performed more often than necessary. Even in partially avulsed extremities, it is surprising how little tissue is necessary for the maintenance of viability in a hand or foot. An obvious advantage in delay of amputation lies in the fact that the line of demarcation between viable and gangrenous tissue almost always forms farther distally than is suspected at the time of injury. If the bones are intact, the demand for conservatism becomes even more strongly indicated. Conservative treatment should include careful aseptic technic in the care of the wound, removal of dead tissue, application of heat (wet or dry as indicated), immobilization, and efficient nursing care. Occasionally amputation will be a life saving procedure in late cases because of the presence of gangrene or infection. However, delay will rarely jeopardize a patient's life because of infection or gangrene, in civilian injuries, if the patient is watched *carefully* from day to day.

INFECTED WOUNDS

The discussion of infected wounds may be conveniently divided into a consideration of (1) infection present in open wounds, *i.e.,* old untreated accidental wounds, and (2) infection sustained after operation, *i.e.,* postoperative wound infection. The importance of identifying the organism responsible for the infection cannot be too strongly emphasized. Infected material should be examined at once both directly and by culture whenever possible.

Infection Developing in Open Wounds.—Most of these wounds will have been accidentally inflicted, occurring in patients presenting themselves for treatment of a wound some time after the injury, and after infection is already present. The common manifestations of infection as already described, including redness, pain, tenderness, swelling, and local heat will be present, but in addition, an induration about the wound edges is practically always made out. From the wound an exudate is being discharged, the thickness and amount of which is determined by the age of the wound and the types of organisms present. Usually many types of pyogenic as well as nonpathogenic organisms may be found on culture. Fever may be present. Radiating proximally from the wound, there may be red streaks in the skin, indicative of lymphangitis. Regional lymphadenitis with or without visible lymphangitis, is much more common, however. Because of the danger of activating and spreading the infection, wounds of this type *must not be subjected to operative repair,* particularly if the infection is severe and producing constitutional manifestations. The affected part should be *put at rest* and slightly elevated; if the manifestations, including tenderness, pain, induration, fever, etc., are pronounced, bed rest is indicated. Hot wet dressings, irrigation of the wound, frequent change of dressings, sulfanilamide therapy and many other procedures described under the treatment of postoperative infection are of value in therapy.

There are many other features of infected open wounds, which are common also to infection in closed wounds. They are described below, and need not be repeated here.

Infection Developing in Wounds Repaired by Suture (Postoperative Wound Infection).—In general these wounds consist of two groups: (1) those inflicted by accident and repaired perhaps hours afterwards; and, (2) those made intentionally by the surgeon and repaired immediately. The manifestations and treatment of infection in these two types of wounds will, for the most part, be the same.

As stated in Chapter III, the organisms most commonly responsible for acute infection of wounds are the *Staphylococcus aureus* and *Streptococcus*. Most of the serious infections with rapid invasion and systemic symptoms are caused by the streptococcus, although the hemolytic type of staphylococcus may also produce fulminating infections. Less commonly the anaerobic gas producing organisms will be the offenders. The colon bacillus is capable of producing a serious infection of a wound, but usually only by contamination from a ruptured viscus. Other organisms,

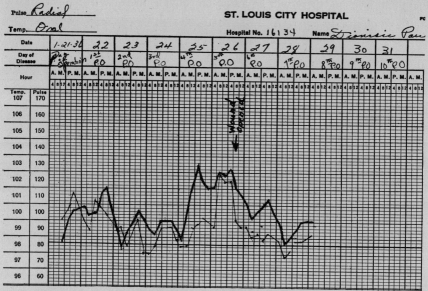

CHART 4.—POSTOPERATIVE WOUND INFECTION IN A TWENTY-FIVE-YEAR-OLD MAN FOLLOWING A HERNIOTOMY.

Note the fall in temperature following the opening of the wound. The organisms cultured from the pus were streptococci and staphylococci. The infection was traced to a respiratory infection in one of the operating room personnel. Recovery was uneventful.

such as the pneumococcus, influenza bacillus, etc., which are also capable of producing abscesses rarely act as the etiological factor in an infected wound. Obviously, the chief source of infection in accidental wounds is the contamination sustained at time of injury. This is not the chief source of infection in wounds made in the operating room under aseptic technic. Sources, including the nose and throat of the operating room personnel, bacteria in the air and patient's skin, and contamination by instruments as well as surgeon's hands are more common sources of infection, except in operations on the intestine on which occasions the infection usually arises from local contamination. Meleney[24] has reviewed these features in an article in which he emphasizes the use of silk as a prophylactic factor in minimizing the development of wound infection.

The *manifestations* of postoperative wound infection are similar to the manifestations of infection developing spontaneously. One of the earliest symptoms of the development of infection in a wound may be pain, aggravated especially by movement. Frequently, however, infection may progress to the stage of formation of an abscess with the production of very little pain. If the wound is large and the infection very severe, fever will always be present. Fever and pain may be manifested in twenty-four hours with a streptococcus infection, but when the staphylococcus is the offending organism, may not be present for forty-eight hours or more. By this time swelling and redness of the wound will be demonstrable. Redness of the skin is more apt to be present if the wound is superficial and if the infection is severe, such as that caused by a streptococcus. Associated with the redness and swelling there will be an accompanying increase in temperature of the

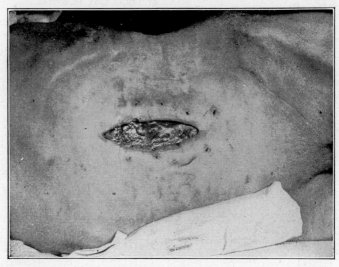

Fig. 122.—Postoperative Wound Infection.

A few days after laparotomy the entire wound became swollen, reddened and tender, and was therefore opened for drainage by removal of all skin sutures. Healing is now (two weeks after operation) taking place by the process of granulation.

skin about the wound. The most constant positive finding is *local tenderness* over the wound. When a wound heals without the development of an infection, only very slight tenderness is elicited by pressure after the first twenty-four hours. As the infection progresses, the local tenderness increases until by the time pus accumulates (three to six days) the tenderness is quite acute. Fluctuation is a late sign which is usually demonstrable if the infection proceeds on to suppuration. There are many more manifestations of infection, including headache, backache, malaise, anorexia, nausea, etc., which are of a systemic nature and are described in detail in Chapter IV.

If an infection develops in a wound closed with a drain, the evidences of infection are apt to be much less severe. Within twenty-four hours there will be an increase in the amount of serous drainage escaping from the wound over that expelled by a wound healing without infection. This increased drainage must not be confused with the profuse discharge associated with a wound containing a dead space. The fluid draining from a dead space is more apt to be thinner and frequently is stained brown because of the presence of old blood. If the infection is due to a staphylococcus, the exudate at first is turbid, but thickens rapidly to form frank pus after three or four days. The pus is apt to be thinner and less profuse if a streptococcus is the cause of the infection.

Healing is delayed considerably by infection, and the slightest strain may cause a separation of the entire wound, particularly after the sutures have been removed, even though the skin may appear to have healed solidly. As mentioned in earlier chapters, the reparative process in an infected wound takes place by second intention; that is, by filling in with granulation tissue and the deposition of scar tissue. As the infection subsides, the cavity in the depth of the wound and the drainage openings made in the skin become smaller. Occasionally the sinus in the skin will heal over before the cavity has been obliterated, especially if the openings for drainage have been inadequate. This must be prevented by dilation of the sinus, or insertion of a small drain, because premature closure of the sinus in the skin will lead to retention of pus and perhaps a renewed spread of the infection particularly if the drainage opening was small in comparison to the size of the abscess cavity.

Treatment.—The *importance of rest* of the affected part in the treatment of infected wounds should again be emphasized. If the wound is on an upper extremity, a sling may furnish sufficient immobilization; if on a lower extremity, bed rest may be required. Treatment varies considerably, depending upon the type and severity of infection. In the absence of suppuration drainage is unnecessary, but if there is any question about the presence of pus, a blunt instrument may safely be inserted between the edges of the wound under sterile precautions to determine whether or not pus is present. If a few drops of turbid fluid or pus are found, the insertion of a small rubber drain will do no harm and may prevent spreading of infection into the adjacent tissue. When a wound becomes infected (even though no abscess is present) skin sutures must be left in longer than the regulation time of five or six days because of the delayed healing and consequent danger of separation of the wound edges.

If an abscess develops in the wound, it should of course be opened as soon as detected. Two or three sutures may be removed, the wound spread, and the pus evacuated. If the cavity is not large, such an opening should be adequate, especially if a rubber dam drain is inserted. As mentioned previously, such drains must be anchored in some way to prevent them from slipping into the depth of the wound. If the entire wound is infected and the symptoms are fulminating, it may be advisable to remove all the sutures and open the wound in its entire extent for adequate drainage. Such radical treatment is frequently necessary when the causative organism is a virulent streptococcus. On most occasions drainage, as mentioned above, may be instituted without an anesthetic simply by separating the wound edges. Counter incisions of course require an anesthetic, local or general.

Except in mild infections, hot wet dressings are beneficial and usually advisable for twenty-four to forty-eight hours. If the wound is extensive and considerable necrosis of tissue is present, Carrel tubes may be inserted and the wound irrigated with Dakin's solution. After the infection has subsided and the cavity obliterated, the edges of the wound, if small, may be approximated by means of adhesive. On rare occasions it may be advisable to do a secondary suture.

Medicinal therapy including the sulfonamide compounds, and zinc peroxide, may at times be extremely helpful (even curative), depending upon the type of organism present. As has been mentioned previously sulfanilamide is most active against the streptococcus, sulfathiazole against the staphylococcus, and zinc peroxide (applied locally in the wound) against anaerobic organisms. This selectivity of action emphasizes the importance of identifying the causative organism or organisms immediately. Nevertheless, sulfonamide therapy, on many occasions, must not be delayed for the return of the culture report. Thus, if a severe streptococcic infection is suspected it will be necessary to give sulfanilamide by mouth or parenterally immediately. On the other hand, if a mixed infection is present sulfadiazine or sulfathiazole is considered superior. These drugs are given orally or parenterally as indicated. Although the prophylactic dose of a sulfonamide such as sulfadiazine need not be greater than 60 grains per day, the dose is usually increased to 90 or 100 grains per day in the presence of an active infection.

The efficacy of ointments and other medicinal agents, except the two groups mentioned above, in the treatment of infection has been greatly exaggerated. Boric acid ointment (10 per cent) is used extensively, but chiefly to prevent the dressing from sticking to the wound, and to prevent closure of a sinus because of dried secretions. It is only mildly antiseptic. Zinc oxide ointment (20 per cent) is very useful in protecting the skin from irritating exudate or medicinal agents, because it adheres to the skin and is impervious to liquids, etc. Xeroform (5 to 10 per cent) apparently does have moderate antiseptic qualities, and when applied over the skin about a wound will minimize the spread of infection over the surface. Scarlet red ointment (10 per cent) is said to stimulate the growth of epithelium and granulation tissue because of its slight irritating quality. Balsam of Peru, likewise, is said to exert a stimulating effect on the growth of granulations, but is more important as a deodorant. The application of chemicals such as iodine, acriflavine, etc., to wounds is not recommended because of the damage inflicted upon the tissues and also because any bactericidal action is necessarily confined to the surface organisms. The frequent irrigation of wounds with bland solutions is an advisable procedure because of the mechanical cleansing effect. Dakin's solution for use in irrigations has an added advantage in that it is apparently capable of dissolving necrotic tissue, at least to a slight degree, and in this manner aids in the cleansing process. Any local or general discomfort resulting from the infection is treated by the proper dosage of such drugs as aspirin, codeine, morphine, etc.

As already stated, adequate drainage is obviously of great importance in the treatment of infected wounds. This implies not only a sufficiently large opening but also that the opening be made in a position as dependent as possible, so that gravity may aid in drainage.

In *summarizing* the treatment of infected wounds, the importance of obtaining early and adequate drainage of the wound should be emphasized. If the infection is mild, a simple separation of the wound edges, with the insertion of a small rubber drain may be sufficient. If an abscess cavity has formed, the wound must be opened adequately and, if necessary, counter incisions be made so that there are no undrained undermining pockets. Rest of the affected part is extremely important in preventing the invasion of new tissue by infection. Cleansing of the wound by daily dressings are known from experience to encourage healthy granulations and healing. Aseptic technic in dressing is, of course, essential in order to prevent secondary infection, especially during the time before a wall of granulation tissue has formed in the wound (five to six days). It is known that after a dense bed of granulation tissue has formed, infection will rarely penetrate beyond the surface. The organisms with which the wound may come in contact may even be killed by the secretions, but a more certain and important feature is the fact that organisms will not penetrate a healthy layer of granulation tissue. The latter may of course be penetrated by instruments or rough handling, and reinfection may occur in this way. The sulfonamides, given orally or parenterally, are particularly useful if the infection seems to be invasive. These drugs may also be used locally in infected wounds and there is evidence that they are absorbed when given this way; the wounds are "frosted" with sulfanilamide after cleansing at the time of dressings.

CAUSES OF DELAYED HEALING

1. **Infection.**—Of the many instigating factors, the most important cause of delayed union, at least from the standpoint of frequency, is infection. In the presence of infection the incised tissues of the wound fail to adhere to each other and pus accumulates between them. This failure of union is usually more marked in the subcutaneous tissue than in the skin itself. The presence of an infection in a wound, even though it is adequately drained, may delay solid healing with complete closure from the average time of about ten days to several weeks.

Occasionally a chronic infection, such as blastomycosis, actinomycosis, tularemia, tuberculosis, etc., is implanted into the wound at the time of injury and results in the formation of a chronic ulcer or sinus. The various peculiarities of these infections should lead to a correct diagnosis; in general, however, they are very rare.

Practically all the conditions listed below as factors in the causation of delayed healing are, likewise, important because of the tendency to encourage the development of infection. In many instances a wound becoming infected and healing by secondary intention would have healed *per primam* if that factor had been eradicated.

2. **Incorrect Closure.**—If the subcutaneous tissue of the wound is closed inadequately so that a dead space is formed, fluid will accumulate within it and will remain for many days before it is absorbed and the cavity filled with granulation tissue. If the skin edges are overlapped during approximation, they will separate and expose subcutaneous tissue when the sutures are removed (see Fig. 112).

Not infrequently a hematoma will form within the depth of the wound because of failure to ligate all bleeding points at time of closure of the wound. Occasionally a vessel which is cut or torn at the time of injury is not bleeding during closure of the wound, but the clot in its lumen becomes dislodged, and hemorrhage ensues after closure. It is prone to occur when a low blood pressure develops during the operation, and returns to normal after closure of the wound.

3. **Excessive Trauma during Operation.**—As stated previously, careful surgical technic aids asepsis. Careless technic, including rough handling of tissue and excessive trauma results in delayed healing, not only because of the increased tendency to infection, but also because of the excessive amount of necrotic tissue produced (see Fig. 123).

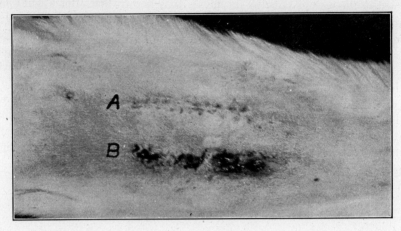

FIG. 123.—PHOTOGRAPH ILLUSTRATING THE VALUE OF CAREFUL OPERATIVE TECHNIC.

Both incisions were made on the animal's abdomen seven days previously. Wound *A* was made and closed with careful technic whereas in wound *B,* the tissues were handled roughly, with crushing of tissue, etc.

Incisions should be made with a sharp scalpel, which should likewise be used in dissection except when sharp dissection becomes dangerous. Scissors may be used for blunt dissection but should not be used to cut tissues. Artery forceps should be placed on the bleeding point avoiding large bites. Retraction must be gentle and other precautions taken as previously described in this chapter. A few years ago when the diathermy or electrosurgical knife was introduced, it was thought that less trauma would be inflicted on the wound because very few ligatures were required. However, even the slight charring of the skin induced by the electric knife resulted in damage to tissue which as was shown by Ellis,[25] delayed healing to such an extent that primary healing was obtained in only 60 per cent of instances versus 97 per cent following incision by a sharp scalpel.

4. **Lack of Immobility.**—Movement of the portion of the body about the wound, such as would be produced by active use of an injured extremity, is not conducive to rapid healing. This is, of course, exemplified most sharply in the treatment of fractures. Lack of rest for the affected part is therefore very detrimental to healing and in the case of freshly closed wounds may result in infection, hemorrhage, etc., but perhaps more frequently delays healing by breaking down the newly regenerated tissue, which is very friable and nonresistant to stresses when only a day or two old.

5. **Mechanical and Chemical Trauma.**—The constant irritation of portions of clothing, appliances, etc., likewise, interferes with healing to the extent that removal of sutures in the routine time (five to six days) may allow the wound

edges to fall apart, even though infection is absent or not demonstrable. Obviously, any severe trauma such as a blow inflicted over the wound may destroy the repair which has taken place since the injury, by disrupting the adhesion of the edges and sides of the wound. The application of ointments containing irritating chemicals (phenol, particularly) will also interfere with healing. One of the most frequent causes of delayed healing of an abdominal wound, even to the point of actual rupture, is the development of a persistent cough during the first days of convalescence. Active measures must be undertaken to eradicate cough, retching, vomiting, hiccups, excessive movements of the patient, and other causes of strain on the healing

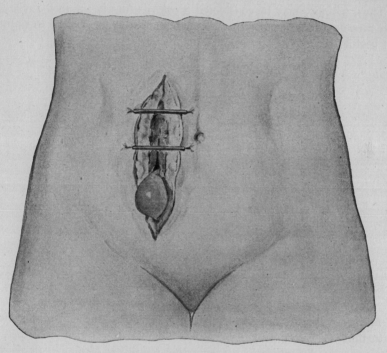

FIG. 124.—RUPTURE OF ABDOMINAL WOUND.

Ileocolostomy was performed at the original operation for an inoperable carcinoma of the cecum. The patient developed a persistent cough and on the fourth day the wound suddenly ruptured, with a loop of intestine exposed as illustrated. Closure was immediately instituted, using several stay sutures traversing all layers of the abdominal wall. Peritonitis follows in a surprisingly small percentage of such cases, in spite of obvious contamination.

wound. Added support to the abdomen may be secured by the application of a tight binder.

6. **Foreign Body.**—Any wound tolerates the presence of a foreign body poorly. Although certain objects (for example, Lane plates, silver wire, braided silk sutures, etc.) sometimes remain innocuous in aseptic wounds, they should be used only when necessary, because of the tendency to convert a minimal contamination into a severe infection with the development of a *persistent sinus*. Obviously, the more "dirt" that is imbedded with the foreign body, the more likely is the possibility of development of infection. A clean object, such as a piece of glass from

a broken tumbler, on the other hand, may be buried in a wound, which heals without the subsequent production of any difficulty except pain and local tenderness over the object.

7. **Impaired Circulation.**—An example of the deleterious effect of impaired circulation on the healing of a wound is encountered when a patient is allowed to walk around as usual with a wound on one of the lower extremities. This delayed healing may be manifested by a slight amount of redness and edema, due presumably to the inadequate circulation created by the dependent position. Removal of sutures under eight days in such instances may result in separation of the wound edges. Thus, mobility may be considered a contributing factor to the delayed healing. On rare occasions, bandages, casts or splints may be applied so tightly as to prevent healing because of impaired circulation resulting therefrom.

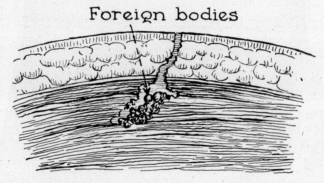

FIG. 125.—CROSS SECTION OF A WOUND CARELESSLY CLOSED.

Foreign bodies (*F.B.*) (gravel) still embedded in the subcutaneous tissue. Healing is impaired or prevented because of the consequent chronic suppuration.

8. **Malignancy.**—A wound inflicted in malignant tissue will very seldom heal. This situation will rarely be encountered in wounds sustained in accidents, but is a frequent cause of difficulties in the operative treatment of malignant disease. For example, if the anastomosis following the excision of a carcinoma of the intestine is performed through malignant tissue, there will very likely be a leak at that point because of lack of healing. Such a complication is, of course, very serious.

9. **Miscellaneous Causes of Delayed Healing.**—There are numerous local diseases which may be responsible for lack of healing, especially when the wound is located on one of the lower extremities. The most important of these are varicose veins, ischemia due to arteriosclerosis or Buerger's disease, and lymphedema due to femoral thrombosis, etc. Wounds inflicted on the lower extremities of patients with diabetes usually heal slowly. On rare occasions delayed healing will be caused by systemic diseases such as syphilis and tuberculosis. Wounds sustained by patients suffering from a severe grade of malnutrition and dehydration usually heal very slowly. Severe anemia may delay healing. More important are the plasma proteins in the proper healing of wounds as emphasized years ago by Clark,[26] Harvey and Howes [27] and others. Another important cause of delayed healing and wound disruption lies in a low vitamin C blood level. Proof of this relationship was

first offered by Lanman and Ingalls [29] who showed in animal experiments (guinea pigs), that when the vitamin C content in the blood was near the scorbutic level delayed healing and wound disruption was common. A low vitamin C reserve is comparatively frequent in charity patients with intestinal diseases such as carcinoma of the stomach, etc. For example, 40 per cent of a series of 90 patients with intestinal lesions (chosen consecutively) at the Illinois Research Hospital had a blood cevitamic acid level below 0.40 mgm. per 100 cubic centimeters of blood (normal 0.70 to 1.0). This high incidence emphasizes the importance of giving fruit juices or cevitamic acid to such patients. Moreover, Lund [30] has shown that laparotomies deplete this level still further, at least for a period of four to six days. The relationship of various vitamins to wound healing and various surgical complications has been discussed in detail by Holman.[31]

WOUNDS INFLICTED BY ANIMALS AND INSECTS

Dogs and cats are responsible for most of the wounds inflicted by animals. The possibility of contraction of rabies from these and other animals is discussed in Chapter VI. Moreover, there is a strong possibility of the development of local pyogenic infection, because of the myriads of pathogenic organisms constantly present in the mouths of such animals and because of the penetrating nature of the wound made by the teeth. Wounds caused by the bite of a cat are much more prone to become infected than those caused by a dog, but neither are as likely to result in infection as a bite inflicted by human teeth. If the wound is superficial (for example, a cat scratch) and seen within a few minutes following the injury, thorough cleansing with soap and water, or the application of an antiseptic such as 2 per cent aqueous solution of iodine (U.S.P.) may be very helpful in preventing the development of infection; sulfanilamide may also be used. A sterile dressing will, of course, serve as a protection and prevent secondary infection.

Rat bites are not uncommon and are most commonly sustained at night while the patient is asleep. A surprisingly large number of rats, at least the ones guilty of attacking the human being while asleep, are infected with the spirochete (*Spirillum minus*) which is responsible for rat-bite fever (see Chapter VI).

Snake bites are dreaded, perhaps, more than the bites of any other animal, but fortunately, of the various kinds of snakes found in North America only four are poisonous. The rattlesnake, copperhead, cotton-mouth moccasin and coral snake comprise this group. At the present time several reputable pharmaceutical companies make an antivenene which contains antitoxin for the toxin contained in the venom of the first three snakes mentioned above and if given in time (up to eight or ten hours) and in large quantities, may prevent a fatal outcome. Unfortunately, antivenene is rarely available at the time of injury and it is necessary to resort to other measures while this is being procured. If the bite is inflicted by one of the four snakes mentioned above and on an extremity, it is advisable to apply a tourniquet which is tight enough to obstruct the lymphatics, part of the venous flow, but *must not* block the arterial supply. Cross incisions are then made with a sharp knife through the fang marks. Suction is very effective in draining toxin out of the incised area, providing the incisions have been made adequately. The best method to apply suction is to use a regular cupping apparatus; if not available, one may be made by taking a large rubber bulb and inserting the end of a small funnel into the open end of the bulb. In absence of such apparatus suction may be achieved by the mouth although the resultant infection is a serious disadvantage. There need be no fear of being poisoned by the absorption of venom through the mouth or intestinal tract, since the venom is destroyed by the digestive ferments. Absolute rest of the patient is essential. One of the most serious mistakes that can be made is to give the patient large doses of alcohol, since the depressant effect of the alcohol accentuates the depressant effect of the venom on the medullary centers and thereby hastens death. The seriousness of snake bites is considerably exaggerated since not over 15 to 18 per cent of untreated rattlesnake bites in adults are fatal. The bite of the cobra, encountered in the Eastern Hemisphere, is by far the most fatal of all snake bites. About 40 per cent of people bitten by the cobra will die unless treatment is given instantly and adequately.

There are numerous insects whose bites are poisonous but very few, indeed, are fatal. The most common of the poisonous bites are those inflicted by the black widow spider and the scorpion. The condition produced by the bite of poisonous spiders is called arachnoidism. The black widow spider is probably the most poisonous of all the members of the Arachnida class of insects and may be recognized by its large size (2 to 3 cm.) and by a reddish brown area shaped like an hourglass on its abdomen. Important to the surgeon is the fact that the bite of a black widow spider may be soon followed by severe abdominal pain; examination may reveal a hard "board-like" abdomen which simulates that observed in perforated peptic ulcer. There is, however, little associated tenderness and within a few hours the signs and symptoms gradually disappear although distention may be present and persist for several days. The bite is associated with a fatality of less than one per cent (Kirby-Smith [28]).

BIBLIOGRAPHY

1. Howes, E. L., Harvey, S. C. and Hewitt, C. Rate of Fibroplasia and Differentiation in the Healing of Cutaneous Wounds in Different Species of Animals, *Arch. Surg.*, 38:934, 1939.
2. Whipple, A. O. The Essential Principles in Clean Wound Healing, *Surg., Gynec. & Obst.*, 70:257, 1940.
3. Mason, Michael. Wound Healing, *Surg., Gynec. & Obst.*, 69:303, 1939. Int. Abst.
4. Reid, M. R. and Stevenson, J. The Treatment of Fresh Wounds, *Surg., Gynec. & Obst.*, 66:313, 1938. Int. Abst.
5. Harvey, S. C. The Velocity of the Growth of Fibroblasts in the Healing Wound, *Arch. Surg.*, 18:1227, 1929.
6. Halsted, W. S. The Employment of Fine Silk in Preference to Catgut and the Advantages of Transfixing Tissues and Vessels in Controlling Hemorrhage.
7. Friedrich, P. L. Die aseptische Versorgung frischer Wunden, unter Mittheilung von Thier-Versuchen über die Auskeinungszeit von Infectionserregern in frischen Wunden, *Arch. f. klin. Chir.*, 57:288, 1898.
8. Whipple, A. O. and Elliott, R. H. The Repair of Abdominal Incisions, *Ann. Surg.*, 108:741, 1938.
9. Ives, H. R. and Hirschfeld, J. W. The Bacterial Flora of Clean Surgical Wounds, *Ann. Surg.*, 107:607, 1938.

10. HART, D. Sterilization of an Operating-room by Special Bactericidal Radiant Energy: Result of its Use in Extrapleural Thoracoplasties, *J. Thoracic Surg.*, 6:45, 1936; HART, D. and SANGER, P. W. Effect on Wound Healing of Bactericidal Ultraviolet Radiation from Special Unit: Experimental Study, *Arch. Surg.*, 38:797, 1939.

11. BLALOCK, Alfred. *Principles of Surgical Care, Shock and Other Problems*, C. V. Mosby Co., St. Louis, Mo., 1940.

12. BROWNING, C. H. The Present Status of Aminoacridine Compounds (Flavines) as Surface Antiseptics, *Brit. Med. J.*, 1:341, 1943.

13. ALBERT, A., DYER, F. J., and LINNELL, W. H. Chemotherapeutic Studies in Acridine Series, *Quar. J. Pharm. & Pharmacol.*, 10:649, 1937.

14. MELENEY, F. Prevention of Infection in Accidental Wounds and Burns, Presented at the Annual Meeting of the Amer. Surg. Assoc., Cincinnati, May 14, 1943.

15. BYWATER, E. G. L. and POPJAK, G. Experimental Crushing Injury, *Surg., Gynec. & Obst.*, 75:612, 1942.

16. KOCH, S. L. The Immediate Treatment of Injuries of the Hand, *Surg., Gynec. & Obst.*, 52:594, 1931.

17. BUNNELL, S. Contractures of the Hand from Infections and Injuries, idem., 14:27, 1932; BUNNELL, S. Contractures of the Hand from Infections and Injuries, *J. Bone & Joint Surg.*, 14:27, 1932; Treatment of Tendons in Compound Injuries of the Hand, *idem.*, 23:240, 1941.

18. MASON, M. L. Primary and Secondary Tendon Suture, *Surg., Gynec. & Obst.*, 70:392, 1940.

19. SHAMBAUGH, P. and DUNPHY, J. E. Postoperative Wound Infections and Use of Silk, Experimental Study, *Surgery*, 1:379, 1937.

20. HOWES, E. L. and HARVEY, S. C. Strength of Healing Wound in Relation to Holding Strength of Catgut Suture, *New England J. Med.*, 200:1288, 1929.

21. JENKINS, H. P. A Clinical Study of Catgut in Relation to Abdominal Wound Disruption with a Test of Its Tensile Strength in Patients, *Surg., Gynec. & Obst.*, 64:648, 1937.

22. SHAMBAUGH, P. Postoperative Wound Complications. A Clinical Study with Special Reference to the Use of Silk, *Surg., Gynec. & Obst.*, 64:765, 1937.

23. MEADE, W. H. and OCHSNER, ALTON. The Relative Value of Catgut, Silk, Linen and Cotton as Suture Material, *Surgery*, 7:485, 1940.

24. MELENEY, F. Infection in Clean Operative Wounds. A Nine-Year Study, *Surg., Gynec. & Obst.*, 60:264, 1935.

25. ELLIS, J. O. The Rate of Healing of Electrosurgical Wounds as Expressed by Tensile Strength, *J. Am. M. Ass.*, 96:16, 1931.

26. CLARK, H. H. The Effect of Diet on the Healing of Wounds, *Bull. Johns Hopkins Hosp.*, 30:117, 1919.

27. HARVEY, S. C. and HOWES, E. L. Effect of High Protein Diet on the Velocity of Growth of Fibroblasts in the Healing Wound, *Ann. Surg.*, 91:641, 1930.

28. KIRBY-SMITH, H. T. Black Widow Spider Bite, *Ann. Surg.*, 115:249, 1942.

29. LANMAN, T. H. and INGALLS, T. H. Vitamin C Deficiency and Wound Healing. An Experimental and Clinical Study, *Ann. Surg.*, 105:616, 1937.

30. LUND, C. C. The Effect of Surgical Operations on the Level of Cevitamic Acid in the Blood Plasma, *New England J. Med.*, 221:123, 1939.

31. HOLMAN, E. Vitamin and Protein Factors in Pre-Operative and Post-Operative Care of the Surgical Patient, *Surg., Gynec. & Obst.*, 70:261, 1940.

CHAPTER XI

AMPUTATIONS

Indications for Amputation *Operative Considerations*
Determination of Extent of Amputa-
tion

The impact of modern methods and concepts on the status of surgery is perhaps nowhere more dramatically illustrated than in the case of amputations. Up until a century ago, amputation was probably the most frequently performed operation. By far the most common indication was trauma to an extremity, especially the presence of a compound fracture. Indeed, surgeons would even amputate following relatively trivial wounds because such wounds were known to be frequently followed by serious infection and often by death from a generalized septicemia. Unfortunately, the operation itself was also apt to be followed by the same train of events. An eminent writer in London about 1782 said that amputation "is an operation terrible to bear, horrid to see, and must leave the person on whom it has been performed in a mutilated, imperfect state." A surgeon who observed personally 46 amputations stated that of these, ten died, one of locked (sic) jaw, two of hemorrhage, four of hectic fever, and three from spreading gangrene. In 18, severe hemorrhage occurred and all suffered from violent "symptomatic" fever. Of those who survived many had painful stumps or wounds which failed to heal, probably because of osteomyelitis.[1] The absence of anesthesia made the actual performance of the amputation a terrifying affair and many are the weird tales of the slashing brutal methods incident to the operation. Time became the most important factor in the technic; the reputation of the surgeon depended almost entirely on the number of seconds he needed to dismember the affected limb. It was a shameful distinction for a surgeon to require as much as three or four minutes for the operation.

This tradition of speed has unfortunately been handed down far too literally even to the present time. Many surgeons still use the time factor as a measuring rod of surgical excellence because they fail to realize that in the average amputation at the present time other factors are of equal or greater significance. Thus, far less harm is sustained by the patient if the procedure is done with proper care and respect for tissues (though requiring twenty to thirty minutes) than if performed in seven or eight minutes in a dramatic but needlessly traumatic fashion, necessitating mass ligatures and gross mauling of tissues. Needless to say, the operating time must be reduced to a minimum and there will be in each case a time limit which will permit careful work. Nevertheless the blind worship of speed alone is an anachronism in the present century, and when cultivated, deserves universal adverse criticism.

During the last decade or two the relative number of amputations has increased considerably, largely because the life span has increased so that more people are attaining the age when arteriosclerosis and other vascular lesions become prevalent, thereby increasing the incidence of gangrene from various causes, for which amputation is so often indicated.

INDICATIONS FOR AMPUTATION

The two major factors determining the necessity of amputation are dependent upon the degree to which the blood supply is impaired and upon the existence of certain types of infection, such as that produced by the gas bacillus. The following conditions are capable either alone or in combination, of leading to such changes to the degree that amputation will be necessary:

1. *Trauma.*—Extensive trauma may of itself result in total dismemberment or destruction of so much tissue as to destroy the blood supply to the distal portion. However, experience has taught us that when only a portion of the limb is severed, amputation should be withheld, particularly if the bone is not fractured. So often, extremities, which at first appeared doomed to gangrene, recover with conservative care, so that perhaps only toes or portions of them are eventually lost. Naturally, if infection develops the indication for amputation is greatly increased. Fortunately, great strides in combating infection have been made and many limbs which might otherwise be sacrificed can now be saved. The measures which minimize the incidence of infection in wounds have been discussed in Chapter X. Important ones are complete immobilization of the part, sulfonamide therapy, adequate irrigation, zinc peroxide, and gas gangrene antitoxin. The incidence of amputation in war wounds involving the extremities is apt to be much higher than in injuries sustained in civil life, partly because of more severe trauma and the presence of foreign bodies (shell fragments, dirt, clothing, etc.) but particularly because infection is much more likely, due to the fact that many hours frequently elapse between injury and of therapy. For details of amputations under war conditions see Chapter XXXIII.

2. *Arteriosclerosis.*—Amputation performed because of arteriosclerotic gangrene is comparatively frequent and naturally is limited to patients in the latter decades of life. The gangrene may be extensive involving the entire foot and part of the leg. Fortunately, it is usually of the dry type, with a minimum amount of infection, thereby permitting conservatism in regard to the time of operation. Such delay is frequently advisable because spontaneous demarcation of the extent of gangrene usually occurs with a consequent preservation of a maximum amount of tissue. On the other hand conservative therapy is often inadvisable because of increased disability, expense of prolonged hospitalization, and particularly because of the danger of infection. When infection develops immediate amputation may be indicated.

3. *Diabetic Gangrene.*—The gangrenous process occurring in diabetes is usually not very extensive, but is directly secondary to occlusive arteriosclerotic changes which are so common in diabetes. The gangrene is usually associated with infection, thereby making amputation urgent. If the process is primarily of infectious origin with little or no gangrene, conservative therapy including incision and drainage will usually suffice, particularly if there is relatively little evidence of occlusion of the major arteries (see Chapter XII).

4. *Buerger's Disease.*—The gangrene incident to Buerger's disease is relatively superficial and is not commonly associated with severe infection. For these reasons amputation will rarely be necessary, and usually need be no more extensive than removal of a toe.

5. *Infection.*—The type of infection most commonly demanding amputation is that produced by the *gas producing organisms*. When the gangrene is beyond the limits of local care, amputation will be urgent and should be performed high, particularly if there is evidence of arterial obstruction. The guillotine type of operation should be utilized along with other measures as discussed later in this chapter.

There are other types of infections which may act as indications for amputation but practically only when significant arterial obstruction is also present. This point should be kept in mind, *lest amputations be performed needlessly* when incision and drainage together with other conservative measures will suffice. As already stated, any type of infection superimposed upon a gangrene may make amputation urgent. Meleney[2] has called attention to the importance of making cultures on all such lesions, so that the etiologic organism or organisms may be identified and treatment varied accordingly. If a gas bacillus is cultured from the lesion before amputation, even with no clinical manifestations, the wound should be left wide open. Even if the material for bacterial examination is obtained for the first time at the operating table, the information may still be of great aid. Thus, even if a gas bacillus is identified twenty-four to forty-eight hours after operation, the wound, if closed, should be opened widely and zinc peroxide applied and antitoxin injected.

Occasionally, amputation will be indicated for tuberculous or pyogenic osteomyelitis of the tarsal bones of the foot, because either type rarely heals and usually is so painful as to be totally disabling.

6. *Embolism.*—When an embolus lodges in a major artery, the clot should be removed, with few exceptions, if the patient is seen within eight to ten hours after the embolism occurs. In late cases, or in unsuccessful embolectomy, amputation may be necessary. However, since infection is usually absent in these cases amputation may be delayed in order to wait for the development of a line of demarcation, thereby saving a maximum portion of the extremity. If the patient is young, delay is advisable because it permits the collateral circulation to reach its maximum. Not infrequently, the patient may then suffer only the loss of perhaps not more than a part of one or two digits, whereas the loss of a major part of the extremity might have seemed imminent earlier in the disease.

Of the major vessels to the extremities, obstruction of the common iliac is most apt to lead to gangrene. Embolism to the major arteries of the upper extremity results in such limited gangrene that amputation is rarely indicated, although embolectomy may be advisable to minimize the effects. (See also p. 131.)

7. *Malignant Neoplasms.*—Sarcoma of bone is the most important neoplasm for which amputation is sometimes indicated, although there is considerable dispute as to whether amputation is advisable in certain types of bone tumors (see also page 311). Occasionally, neglected squamous cell carcinomas (most common in the upper extremity) may invade so deeply that amputation is justified.

8. *Deformity.*—Occasionally amputation is advisable for deformity, but usually only when part of an extremity is involved. For example a severe injury or infec-

tion in a finger might result in a total loss of function. If the patient makes his living in a vocation or trade requiring deft movements of the fingers, the deformed finger might be a tremendous handicap in carrying out his duties; amputation of the deformed digit will frequently increase his efficiency. Injuries of the foot, with

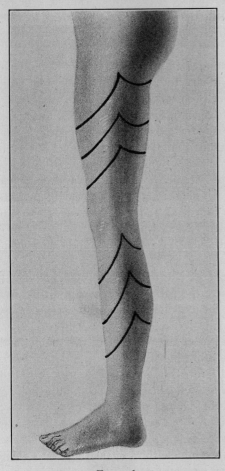
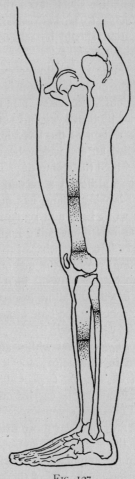

FIG. 126

FIG. 127

FIG. 126.—LINES OF SKIN INCISIONS FOR LEG AND THIGH AMPUTATIONS.
(Redrawn from Orr's Modern Methods of Amputations, 1926, C. V. Mosby Co.)

FIG. 127.—THE SHADED AREAS OF THE BONES REPRESENT PREFERENTIAL LOCATIONS FOR AMPUTATION; THE OPTIMUM LEVEL IS INDICATED BY THE MOST DENSE SHADING.

preservation of a part of the foot (for example, the Pirogoff and Chopart amputation) with or without deformity, may result in a painful or inefficient stump as far as function with a prosthesis is concerned; amputation at a higher level may be the procedure of choice in such instances.

Optimum Levels.—Not always does the surgeon have the opportunity of performing the amputation at the ideal level as a primary operation. This is particularly true in serious infections in very ill patients; in such a case a guillotine type of amputation may have to be performed, followed later by a reamputation at a higher level when the infection has subsided. Likewise in a seriously injured patient an imperfect amputation may have to be performed through the injured part to minimize shock, even though it is obvious that reamputation at a higher level will have to be performed later. With these exceptions, the ideal location for amputation should be selected and carried out in practically all cases; these levels are now discussed.

Amputations in the lower extremity present entirely different problems from those in the arm. If the patient is to walk without crutches an artificial limb of some type is obviously necessary. For this reason, close coöperation is essential between the artificial limb makers and surgeons. In general, two types of limbs are made. In one the weight of the body is transmitted to the end of the stump, which thus may be called an end-weight-bearing stump. In the other type a conical bucket is made into which the stump fits so that the weight is transmitted largely to the sides of the stump although a certain amount of pressure is carried by the end. The end-weight-bearing stump has qualities of durability and is employed in patients who must work hard and remain on their feet all day; its disadvantages are that the prosthesis is often bulky and that walking is far from normal, in appearance at least, partaking somewhat of the gait of the well-known peg-leg. The side-weight-bearing stump permits the use of a prosthesis which is cosmetically excellent and enables the wearer to walk in a manner almost like that of a normal individual. However, it will not allow heavy labor where the patient must remain on his feet all day. In choosing the type of amputation the individual needs of the patient must obviously be considered.

In the *thigh* a level within an inch or two of the junction of the middle and distal third is satisfactory for a side-weight-bearing (conical) stump. For end-weight-bearing stumps (*e.g.*, Callender and Gritti-Stokes amputation, as described later) operation may be carried out at a lower level. The end of the stump resulting from the Callender operation is usually fitted against the bottom of the socket; although it may not bear more than 20 per cent of the weight (most being borne on the side of the stump) the end-bearing feature adds a great deal to stability of the limb. When the amputation is performed in the middle third of the thigh or higher, weight bearing on the end of the stump is not possible; most of the weight is borne by the ischium. Up until recently short amputations of the thigh could not be fitted with efficient artificial limbs, but since the introduction of the hip control limb, fair control can be obtained with a two or three inch stump. The original type of artificial limb which was held in place by shoulder straps, tends, with certain movements, to fall away from the stump when it is short. When it is necessary to extend the amputation upward so that a disarticulation at the *hip* is necessary, the modern pelvic socket type of prosthesis will be surprisingly satisfactory. All muscles except those of the buttock should be removed.

Amputation through the *knee, i.e.*, disarticulation, has two disadvantages: (1) the level is so low that the joint and lower leg control of the prosthesis must be on the outside of the limb, thereby constituting an obvious disadvantage; and, (2) the skin over the irregular condylar surface will permit no weight-bearing.

Moreover, the condyles make a bulbous end which is difficult to fit with a prosthesis, and usually requires a limb larger than the natural extremity.

In the *leg* a stump about seven inches long is considered ideal. However, it should be emphasized that a stump of but one and a half inches is preferable to a knee joint disarticulation, because the patient's own knee joint can then be utilized even with such a short stump. Excision of the fibula is advisable when possible in short leg stumps, because it yields a rounder and more conical stump. Amputations in the lower third of the leg are unsatisfactory for several reasons. This area has a poor circulation, is composed of little soft tissue, and becomes so tender and sensitive that it tolerates pressure poorly. Moreover, the long stump offers no increased aid in leverage for an artificial limb and indeed may interfere with the ankle mechanism of the prosthesis. Of amputations at the ankle, the Syme (½ inch above the tibio-astragaloid joint), being end bearing, is extremely serviceable. Of the amputations through the foot, the Lisfranc (through the metatarsotarsal joint) is so superior to the Chopart or Pirogoff (see Fig. 132) that the latter two are only of historic interest. Amputation of toes or the distal portion of the phalanges will, of course, leave a serviceable stump and is a perfectly justifiable procedure.

In amputations through the *arm* it is desirable to make the stump as long as possible, particularly in the upper portion. Although prostheses can be fitted to stumps only two or three inches long they are of little functional value and are worn chiefly for cosmetic purposes, *i.e.,* to fill out the shirt or coat sleeve. There is little difference, from the standpoint of efficiency of the stump, between an amputation just above the condyles, and a disarticulation at the elbow. In the latter instance, the prosthesis can be held more securely with a minimum amount of apparatus, but the artificial joint will have to be put on the outside, thereby making the limb more cumbersome. In the *forearm* the ideal level is at the junction of the middle and lower thirds. In amputations above this level the minimal length of the stump, for functional value in fitting the prosthesis, is two and one-half inches. Amputations in the distal third are less satisfactory because of poor blood supply and paucity of soft tissue. Amputation through the *wrist* is difficult to fit with a prosthesis since the artificial joints will usually have to be on the outside and the forearm will have to be longer or the hand shorter than its fellow. Moreover, amputations through the wrist are bulbous, unsightly, and complicated by a poor blood supply. In amputations of the *hand,* save as much as possible. One functioning finger is usually of more service than an artificial limb, although it is of course more desirable to have two fingers, so that the function associated with apposition may be maintained. The thumb is usually the most important since, even in the absence of all the other fingers, objects may be grasped between the thumb and stump of the hand.

DETERMINATION OF EXTENT OF AMPUTATION

Although the optimum level for amputation in each segment of the upper and lower extremity as just described, is fairly well agreed upon, the decision must be made as to how much of the limb needs to be sacrificed, *e.g.,* shall the lower extremity be removed at the thigh or leg? This problem usually develops because of uncertainty as to the status of the blood supply to the lower leg, and is complicated also by the presence of infection and gangrene. In many instances (particularly in diabetic gangrene and infection) the amputation should be done through the thigh, because the blood supply is so much more adequate than in the leg. In

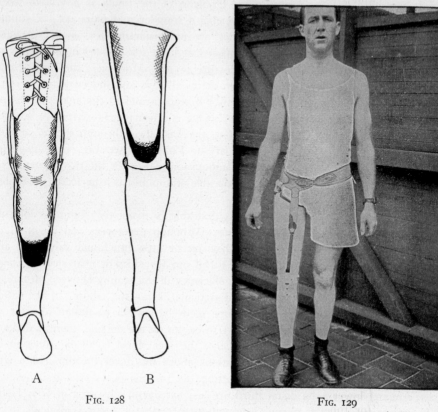

A   B
Fig. 128   Fig. 129

Fig. 128.—Longitudinal Section of the "Buckets" of Artificial Limbs.

A, weight-bearing on the sides of the leg stump. Occasionally it is necessary to remove the entire fibula before the limb can be worn with comfort; B, the soft tissues of the thigh serve admirably to sustain the weight of the body. Many artificial limbs are designed so that considerable weight is borne on the ischial spine, but there is a growing tendency to have the weight borne entirely on the sides of the stump.

Fig. 129.—Simplified Type of Artificial Limb for Thigh Amputation.
Note absence of shoulder straps. (Courtesy Hanger Artificial Limb Co.)

selected cases, when the blood supply appears good, the Maes amputation through upper leg is very satisfactory. On other occasions, particularly in very ill patients with serious infection, a rapid guillotine amputation through the leg may be admirable as a primary operation with the intention of doing a reamputation through the thigh after the infection has subsided. This decision is based on the assumption that the exposed and cut ends of thigh muscles are poorly resistant to infection, whereas the structures in the knee are traversed relatively slowly by infection;

however, there is some dispute about this assumption. In doubtful cases valuable information as to the status of the circulation may be gained by making an exploratory incision through the leg to determine the actual condition of the blood vessels. Since numerous tests are available, which are of valuable assistance in determining the status of the circulation, such an exploratory incision should rarely be necessary. These tests may be described as follows:

1. *Temperature of the Skin.*—One of the simplest, and yet not least valuable, of the tests is the determination of skin temperature, and particularly of a line of temperature demarcation. This may be done by thermocouple or thermometer, but the hand is fairly accurate in determining differences between warm and cool areas over the extremity. Frequently the gradation from warm to cold will be abrupt, thus indicating sharply the site where serious arterial deficiency begins; usually it is fairly gradual. The borderline can usually be accentuated by exposing the patient's extremities for fifteen or twenty minutes to room temperature and then covering them with warm blankets for a similar period. Upon exposure, the area with deficient blood supply will become quite cold and when covered, will fail to become warm with the rest of the extremity. These features will be more noticeable by contrast, if one extremity is reasonably normal. With few exceptions, the amputation should not be performed below the line of temperature demarcation.

2. *Color.*—The color of the skin may be of considerable aid in determining the status of the circulation and thus the appropriate level of amputation. Although the skin of the patient may be pale over the entire body, the area deficient in arterial supply will usually have a cadaveric pallor. Any doubt about a true deficiency pallor can be cleared to some extent by pressing the patient's skin firmly with the finger tip of the examiner. If the blood supply is efficient the pallor produced by the pressure will be replaced by the normal color in two or three seconds; if the blood supply is deficient the color may not return for many seconds. Upon elevation of the extremity, the foot will become extremely pale, if arterial deficiency exists, and upon dependency will become red or purplish. If this deep blush extends very far past the foot, amputation below the knee will rarely be advisable. The skin over the involved extremity is usually atrophic and shiny. The Moszkowicz [3] test which is dependent upon color change following application of a rubber tourniquet, should not be carried out on arteriosclerotic patients because of the danger of injury to the sclerotic vessel walls.

3. *Condition of Major Arteries.*—Practically all tests devised to aid in determination of the optimum level of amputation are obviously concerned with measuring the blood supply to the distal portion of the extremity. Many of them, however, are concerned primarily with estimating the extent and efficiency of collateral vessels rather than the presence or absence of pulsations of a major artery inasmuch as the latter might not be as accurate in determining healing power for a given area, as the status of collateral circulation. It is, nevertheless, important to palpate for the dorsalis pedis and posterior tibial pulse; extensive gangrene would not be apt to develop if both pulses were present. The presence or absence of the two pulses would also be important in deciding upon the advisability of a conservative course of therapy in a diabetic infection with doubtful areas of early gangrene. The popliteal pulse is usually valuable in a negative way; *e.g.,* amputation below the

knee is seldom safe in the absence of a popliteal pulse. Kirk [4] obtains additional data concerning the blood flow through the popliteal artery by taking a blood pressure reading over the lower femoral region. Normally, it should be fifteen or twenty millimeters higher than the brachial pressure. If it is lower or no higher than the brachial, he considers the circulation impaired and amputation below the knee unsafe. A roentgenogram of the leg will determine the amount of calcification in the wall of the major arteries and thereby furnish accessory data as to the vessels themselves. Additional roentgen studies two to three minutes after the injection of thorium dioxide into the vessel above the suspected lesion may reveal obstructive lesions and the condition of the arterial wall.

4. *Histamine Flare Test.*—This test as suggested by Lewis consists of the injection of 0.1 cc. of 1 to 1000 solution of histamine in 0.5 per cent procaine intradermally at various levels on the extremity. With a normal circulation there will be a hyperemic flare surrounding the point of injection, constituting a positive reaction. De Takats and Reynolds [5] are of the opinion that a positive reaction indicates that primary healing of a skin flap will follow amputation at that level, but that a negative reaction does not exclude the possibility that healing of the stump at that point will take place.

5. *McClure-Aldrich [6] Test.*—Intracutaneous injection of 0.2 cc. of 0.85 per cent saline at various levels may be of value. The wheal should disappear normally in 60 minutes; in the presence of abnormal circulation, particularly in the presence of edema the wheal disappears more rapidly.

6. *Freezing Test.*—To gain information regarding the circulation, Nyström [7] resorts to freezing of the skin by holding a cylinder of packed carbon dioxide snow on the skin for three seconds at various levels on the extremity, and observes the reaction. With a normal circulation, the area will thaw and form a hyperemic area in about two minutes. The blanching produced by pressure of the finger over the area returns to a hyperemic color in one or two seconds. If the arterial supply is inadequate the return of the hyperemic color may be delayed fifteen seconds or more.

7. *Oscillometric Readings.*—Various types of oscillometers for recording the amount of pulsation (diffuse—not over the arterial trunk) at a given level are available. Many of them record very accurately the amount of pulsation at that point. By comparing these records with normal curves, an estimation of arterial damage may be made, except that it is not possible to ascertain the proportion of pulsation which is due to collateral flow. This latter feature constitutes the major criticism of the oscillometer, since the amount of collateral vessels and the rapidity of development of new ones are of vital importance in the indications for, and site of amputation.

OPERATIVE CONSIDERATIONS

Immediate Preparation of Patient.—In traumatic cases attention must be directed to the presence of shock, and treatment such as transfusions and intravenous glucose administered before amputation is performed. In badly crushed and contaminated extremities, tetanus and gas bacillus antitoxin, in doses at least double the usual prophylactic dose * should be given. In neglected patients dehydration is apt to be present and must be corrected. In diabetic patients (see Chapter XII), acidosis should at least be corrected and the urine be made as nearly sugar-free as possible in the time available. Because of the high postoperative incidence of gas bacillus infection in amputations for gangrene, regardless of the type, perfringens antitoxin should be given as just described, when severe trauma is present. If cultures reveal gas bacilli, it is particularly important that antitoxin be given in more than a prophylactic dose; it perhaps should be continued for a few days after the amputation.

The night before operation (if this much time is available) the amputation site should be shaved and washed gently but thoroughly with soap and water and covered with a sterile towel. The next morning in the operating room this cleansing should be repeated and after the skin is dried, prepared with iodine and alcohol.

Anesthesia.—The most satisfactory anesthetic is a small dose of procaine given intraspinously (75 to 120 mg. dissolved in a few cubic centimeters of the patient's spinal fluid). The advantage of spinal anesthesia lies in the fact that with the small dose there is little or no drop in blood pressure. It is preferable, nevertheless, to inject a small amount of neosynephrin or ephedrine just before the spinal puncture is done. Ethylene, nitrous oxide, or intravenous pentothal sodium may be used as alternates. Refrigeration anesthesia, as discussed on page 188, is satisfactory, and is particularly indicated in patients who are poor operative risks.

Operative Principles.—After the important decision is made as to whether the amputation should be performed above or below the knee, or elbow, the exact site is determined as already discussed. Since a *closed stump* has the advantages of rapid healing and good scar line, this type of amputation should be utilized when possible. Some surgeons prefer to close the wound around a small rubber tissue drain, but there is a growing tendency to either close the stump tightly or leave it entirely open.

If it appears that a bilateral amputation will be required on the lower extremities, one knee should be preserved if possible because it is extremely difficult for the patient to learn to manipulate two artificial knee joints. Naturally, the surgeon should not allow this fact to cloud his judgment when an amputation below the knee may be dangerous to life.

Orr [8] has effectively summarized the types of incisions for the various sites by recommending (1) long anterior and short posterior flaps for the thigh and leg; (2) flaps of equal length for the forearms; (3) long palmar and short dorsal flaps for the hand and fingers; and (4) long plantar and short dorsal flaps for the foot and toes. Since infection is so apt to develop in amputation stumps, the utmost care and gentleness must be exercised in handling the tissues: traction must be gentle, no mass ligation is permitted, and the minimum amount of hemostasic forceps applied.

Conservation of blood is extremely important since these patients are so often precarious surgical risks. The application of an Esmarch bandage from below upward would obviously conserve blood, but is practically always *contraindicated*

---

* The prophylactic dose of gas gangrene antitoxin contains 1500 units tetanus antitoxin, 2000 units perfringens antitoxin and 2000 units vibrion septique.

because of the tissue damage resulting therefrom. However, elevation of the limb before applying the tourniquet will result in conservation of considerable blood, particularly if a high thigh amputation is being done. Very frequently indeed, even the application of a tourniquet will be contraindicated because of the damage inflicted on arteriosclerotic vessels by the pressure of the tourniquet. In such cases, however, the need for a tourniquet will not be so acute.

The bone should be cut across far enough above the level of the skin so that the wound can be closed without tension. The periosteum must carefully be scraped from the end of the bone for a distance of one centimeter to prevent periostitis and spur formation; the edges of bone are then rounded off with a rasp or ronguer. In amputation of the leg, it is essential that the fibula be cut off at least an inch shorter than the tibia. Because the fibula is commonly a source of discomfort in spite of proper care at operation, some surgeons prefer to remove it completely at the time of the amputation, particularly in short stumps. It is not necessary in the function of the artificial limb. The anterior and posterior fascial layers should be approximated so that a thin layer of muscle overlies the bone; a thick layer of muscle overlying the bone is undesirable. During the process of exposing the bone and suturing the fascial and muscle layers, care must be taken lest the various planes unnecessarily be separated from each other. It is particularly important not to detach the fascia from the skin because of danger of destruction of blood supply to the skin with consequent gangrene and perhaps severe infection. Blood vessels may be tied with catgut when infection appears obvious; otherwise cotton, silk, or nylon is preferable. Nerves are pulled down gently and cut with a sharp knife. Opinions differ as to whether or not they should be injected with alcohol. However, ligature of the nerve as recommended by Wheeler [11] and others appears to offer a possibility toward minimizing the formation of neuromas.

The *open or guillotine* type of amputation is done with a circular incision and is especially indicated in cases where infection seems so imminent that closure of the stump would be dangerous. Although the skin is retracted somewhat by slight proximal tension before the muscle and fascia layer is cut, no attempt is made to divide the deep structures (especially the bone) high enough to be covered with skin; instead, a second operation, *i.e.,* reamputation, is always anticipated. On certain occasions, flaps may be designed with the guillotine type of operation. The bone is then cut sufficiently high so that it may be covered later by approximating the skin flaps when danger of infection has passed. (See also Chapter XXXIII.)

Postoperative Care.—Patients with amputations require more than the average post operative care because of the danger of infection and its seriousness when present. If the stump has been closed, the wound need not be dressed every day, but the temperature and pulse chart must be observed closely for an elevation which might be indicative of development of infection. Likewise, if the patient complains of pain in the stump the dressings should be changed and the stump inspected. If there is sufficient redness, edema and tenderness to indicate the presence of infection, a number of sutures must be removed to allow drainage. Frequently it will be advisable to open the wound completely. In the presence of infection, the wound should be dressed and irrigated daily. Carrel Dakin treatment or application of zinc peroxide may be utilized. Wound secretions should be cultured as soon as infection is suspected so that immediate therapy for the gas bacillus (antitoxin, sulfathiazole, and x-ray therapy) and streptococcus (sulfanilamide) may be instituted. When such a wound has been opened the skin flaps tend to retract. After the infection has subsided it is, therefore, usually necessary to exert some type of traction on the skin to bring it down into its former position so that the stump will be covered adequately with soft tissue. This is readily accomplished by placing adhesive strips on each of the four sides of the stump and attaching them with the aid of a Thomas splint to a ring or pulley at the foot of the bed. Sufficient traction (5 to 10 lbs.) is applied to bring the flaps down. The stump should be placed in a comfortable position. For the thigh and knee a slight amount of flexion is preferable. Arms should be placed in moderate abduction. Pillows for elevation are utilized as indicated.

If the wound heals per primam it should be ready for the fitting of a prosthesis in four to six weeks. However, for several days previous to this a tight fitting bandage or laced leather cuff must be applied to decrease the edema, and shape the stump for the artificial limb. It is essential that the fitting of the limb should not be postponed lest sufficient muscle and bone atrophy take place to *seriously delay walking*. Such delay in starting function with the artificial limb is particularly *serious in the aged* and may even be the primary factor in inability of the patient to learn to use a prosthesis.

When a guillotine operation has been performed, there is frequently a temptation, when infection begins to subside, to perform some type of plastic operation on the stump, such as amputation of the bone an inch or two higher to obtain a properly padded stump. Such procedures are rarely indicated because they are apt to cause a serious flare-up of infection. It is usually preferable to adhere to the original plan of waiting until the wound has healed.

Reamputation is occasionally indicated when not originally planned. For example, osteomyelitis of the end of the bone or tender bone spurs in the absence of infection may develop, thereby making reamputation necessary. Not infrequently tender scars are so troublesome that a prosthesis cannot be worn comfortably. In such an instance, simple excision of the scar with interposition of some soft tissue, preferably a thin layer of muscle and fascia (if the scar was adherent to the bone or directly overlying it) will suffice. The tenderness associated with a neuroma will require excision of the end of the nerve, but not reamputation. Occasionally an ulcer develops at the end of the stump and stubbornly refuses to heal, frequently because the bone is too long. Excision of a few centimeters of bone together with scar tissue or reamputation at a higher level will be indicated depending upon the circulation in the stump. If the bone has adequate coverage with soft tissue, simple excision of the ulcer and scar tissue may suffice. In any case, these secondary procedures *must not be performed until all evidence of infection* such as induration, redness, edema, etc., *has disappeared*.

Individual Types of Amputation.—A *disarticulation* of the knee or shoulder implies amputation at the respective joint. Many different types of skin flaps have been described for *amputation of the shoulder, e.g.,* Kocher, Larrey, Dupuytren, etc. A shoulder girdle amputation includes removal of the entire upper extremity with the scapula and most of the clavicle. The most conservative *amputation of the* *foot* is performed by disarticulation of the tarsometatarsal joint as first described by *Lisfranc*. It is a satisfactory amputation, although amputation through the metatarsophalangeal joints is still more satisfactory since more weight-bearing surface is preserved. Disarticulation through the midtarsal region was described by *Chopart* but has never been popular because of poor results obtained. A *Syme* amputation is performed by disarticulation of the tibialastragaloid joint and removal of malleoli, using a posterior heel flap. Gallie [12] has been an ardent advocate of the *Syme* amputation, claiming that it results in a very serviceable stump which will allow weight bearing hour after hour. Gallie claims that most of the poor results following the *Syme* operations are due to (1) improper relationship of weight-bearing heel pad

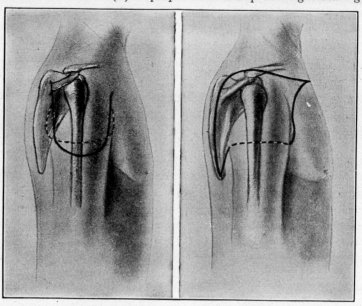

FIG. 130   FIG. 131

FIG. 130.—LINES OF INCISION FOR DISARTICULATION AT THE SHOULDER OR AMPUTATION HIGH THROUGH THE SURGICAL NECK OF THE HUMERUS.
(Redrawn from Orr, Modern Methods of Amputations, C. V. Mosby Co., St. Louis).

FIG. 131.—LINES OF INCISION FOR INTERSCAPULOTHORACIC AMPUTATION BY THE METHOD OF BERGER.
(Redrawn from Orr, Modern Methods of Amputations, C. V. Mosby Co., St. Louis).

to the bones of the leg, (2) looseness of the pad, and (3) pain from irregular bony points, etc. Care must be exercised in the dissection on the inner side of the ankle lest the posterior tibial artery be injured, thereby resulting in an ischemic flap. About two to three centimeters of the ends of the tibia and fibula are removed with the saw so that a flat weight-bearing stump is obtained. Needless to say, even though the *Syme* operation may be superior to an amputation through the upper tibia, it will not be possible if the foot and lower leg are destroyed (see also page 228). *Amputation through the upper tibia,* leaving a stump about seven inches long, has been briefly discussed under the heading of Optimum Levels. Amputation at this level is considered optimum from the standpoints of ease of fitting an artificial limb and preservation of the knee joint with an adequate stump for leverage. However, one disadvantage of this type of stump is the irritation frequently produced on the weight-bearing surfaces of the sides of the leg by prolonged usage of an artificial limb. The skin chafes and blisters, and hair follicle infections are common. In women who do not need to be on their feet hours at a time, it is particularly adaptable, because of the good cosmetic appearance. The *Gritti-Stokes amputation* is performed at the knee joint; the lower end of the femur, and posterior part of the patella are removed with the saw so that the patella can be rotated and approximated

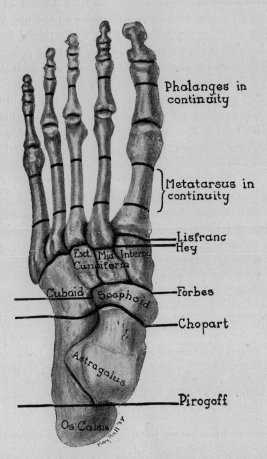

Phalanges in continuity

Metatarsus in continuity

Lisfranc
Hey

Ext. Mid. Intern
Cuneiform

Cuboid   Scaphoid   Forbes

Chopart

Astragalus

Pirogoff

Os Calcis

FIG. 132.—SKELETAL LINES OF INCISION IN SEVERAL OF THE WELL-KNOWN FOOT AMPUTATIONS. (Redrawn from Orr, Modern Methods of Amputations, C. V. Mosby Co., St. Louis).

against the end of the femur. This procedure has been modified by *Callander*[9] who makes long anterior and posterior flaps, saws across the lower end of the femur above the condyles, just proximal to the abductor tubercle, removing the patella, so that the stump of the femur may fit into the tendinous patellar socket and thus allow weight-bearing. This amputation is becoming quite popular and can be fitted very satisfactorily with an artificial limb, utilizing a small amount of end-bearing, the chief advantage of which is stabilization of the artificial limb.

The Callander, Gritti-Stokes and Syme amputations represent types of procedures which should yield the most satisfactory weight-bearing stumps. A detailed discussion of amputations may be found in the monograph by Orr.[8] It should be emphasized that very few of the amputations described under this heading, *i.e.,* Individual Types of Amputations, are utilizable in war as the initial operative procedure at the front. The *Syme, Gritti-Stokes,* and *Callander* operations are reserved as secondary procedures performed at a base or general hospital. The guillotine operation as discussed on page 234 and in Chapter XXXIII remains as the one major type permissible as an initial amputation in war injuries.

Cineplastic Amputations.—This term may be defined as being any type of plastic operation on an amputation stump (usually on the upper extremity) which allows transmission of voluntary movement to the artificial limb. The procedure was first utilized by Vanghetti, an Italian, in 1898. At the present time the method is relatively unsatisfactory, but the principle is sound, and with skill and experience, as well as cooperation between the surgeon and limb manufacturer, results should improve. A tube flap of skin is made over the muscle to be utilized and threaded through a hole made in the body of the muscle whose function is to be utilized. The defect made by raising the tube skin flap is closed with or without a skin graft as indicated. After healing has taken place a peg is placed through the opening and the ends of the peg attached to levers on the prosthesis so that when the muscle contracts, the hand, for example, will open or close. Obviously, delicate movements of fingers cannot be duplicated. However, the function of grasping and releasing objects with the mechanical hand should be possible if sufficient arm stump is available, and the operative procedures are successful. The points of attachment on the extremity are called "motors." To be effective they should have at least a two or three centimeter range in motion induced by contraction of the muscle. A report by Kessler [10] gives details of the procedure and its application.

BIBLIOGRAPHY

1. ALANSON, E. *Practical Observations on Amputations,* London, 1782, 2nd Edition.
2. MELENEY, F. Bacteriology of Amputations, *Surg. Clin. N. Am.,* 18:321, 1938.
3. MOSZKOWICZ, Ludwig. Die Diagnose des Arterienverschlusses bei Gangraena pedis, Mitt. a. d. *Grenzgeb. d. Med. u. Chir.,* 17:217, 1907.
4. KIRK, N. T. *Dean Lewis' Practice of Surgery,* Vol. 3, W. F. Prior Co., Hagerstown, Md., 1929.
5. DE TAKATS, Geza and REYNOLDS, J. Amputation for Peripheral Vascular Disease, *Arch. Surg.,* 40:253, 1940.
6. McCLURE, W. B. and ALDRICH, C. A. The McClure-Aldrich Test—the Salt Solution Wheal, *J. Am. M. Ass.,* 81:293, 1923.
7. NYSTRÖM, Gunnar. A Method of Testing the Superficial Blood Circulation for Considering the Indication and the Proper Level of Amputation, *Surgery,* 1:487, 1937.
8. ORR, Thomas. *Modern Methods of Amputation,* C. V. Mosby Co., St. Louis, 1926.
9. CALLANDER, C. L. A New Amputation in the Lower Third of the Thigh, *J. Am. M. Ass.,* 105:1746, 1935.
10. KESSLER, H. H. The Cineplastic Amputation, *Surg., Gynec. & Obst.,* 68:554, 1939.
11. WHEELER, W. I. DE C., in *Bailey's Surgery of Modern Warfare,* The Williams and Wilkins Co., Baltimore, 2nd Ed., 1942.
12. GALLIE, W. E. Some Lessons Learned in the Great War, *Surg., Gynec. & Obst.,* 74:370, 1942; The Experience of the Canadian Army and Pension Board with Amputations of the Lower Extremity, *Ann. Surg.,* 113:925, 1941.

CHAPTER XII

SURGERY IN DIABETES

Surgical Diseases Unrelated to Diabetes   Surgical Diseases Secondary to Diabetes

Because of the use of insulin, life has been lengthened in diabetic patients; indeed, a large proportion enjoy a normal life expectancy and die of other causes. The resultant increase in the number of diabetics made the need for surgery in diabetes more frequent and important.

There are a number of surgical lesions (particularly infections) which increase the severity of diabetes. This fact must be appreciated, and the dosage of insulin increased lest diabetic coma develop as a result of the infection. Conversely, it is likewise true that diabetic patients are prone to develop infections, particularly about the toes and feet, as will be discussed later.

In many ways diabetics, particularly adults, appear much older than their true age. This is explained in part by the fact that they are much more prone to develop arteriosclerosis than the average nondiabetic individual. Joslin has made the statement that a diabetic patient is as old as his real age plus the number of years he has had diabetes. The arteriosclerosis which develops is generalized in character, affecting the coronary and renal vessels, as well as those of the extremities.

In the absence of complicating factors, wounds in diabetic patients heal as readily as wounds in nondiabetics, but because the former have a lowered resistance to bacteria, their wounds are more apt to become infected. DaCosta and Beardsley [1] have demonstrated that the blood serum of diabetics has a lower opsonic index toward tubercle bacilli, staphylococci, and streptococci than the serum of normal people.

For purposes of clarity, the discussion of surgical conditions in diabetes should be divided into a consideration of lesions unrelated to diabetes and lesions secondary to diabetes. Another reason for dividing the discussion into these two groups lies in the fact that the latter group of conditions (*i.e.,* lesions secondary to diabetes) is much more serious than the former, requires a different type of therapy, and is associated with a much higher mortality.

SURGICAL DISEASES UNRELATED TO DIABETES

As previously intimated, operations for such conditions as benign tumors, hernias, etc., can be carried out with comparative safety, so long as the diabetes is under control. Some surgeons have such fortunate results in this group of patients that they do not consider diabetes as a contraindication for surgery. However, Smith [2] has very appropriately emphasized that even a controlled diabetic patient is distinctly not as safe a risk as a nondiabetic patient, *e.g.*, the incidence of pneumonia in abdominal operations is greater than in nondiabetic patients. The mortality following operations for carcinoma is considerably higher when there is a coincident diabetes.

In many acute surgical conditions, particularly those within the abdomen, the manifestations are milder when they develop in diabetics, *e.g.*, an acutely inflamed appendix may proceed to the point of perforation with comparatively few symptoms. For that reason delay is very unsafe when acute abdominal manifestations suggestive of appendicitis develop in a diabetic patient. Moreover, acute lesions such as appendicitis, acute cholecystitis, etc., are less apt to subside and are more prone to progress on to perforation than in nondiabetic patients.

It is not generally appreciated that patients in diabetic acidosis or impending coma may develop acute abdominal symptoms not unlike those of acute appendicitis, acute pancreatitis, etc. All of the manifestations of appendicitis, including nausea, vomiting, abdominal pain and rigidity, leukocytosis, etc., may be simulated by diabetic acidosis. The importance of this may be appreciated when we realize what a serious error it would be to submit a diabetic patient with impending coma to operation. Usually, however, the differentiation can be made by the sequence of development of vomiting and pain. In diabetic acidosis the vomiting is apt to precede the pain, whereas in appendicitis the pain precedes the vomiting. Routine examination of the urine for sugar reveals the existence of diabetes which of course should lead to the true explanation of the symptoms.

Diabetic patients must be treated with unusual care when subjected to trauma. In *fractures,* particularly, the insulin requirements will have to be raised considerably. For example, a diabetic remaining sugar-free on 20 to 30 units daily may require 70 to 100 units daily for many days or weeks following a severe fracture such as one involving the hip or shaft of the femur.

In addition to surgical infections, there are a great many diseases including hyperthyroidism, cholecystitis, etc., which increase the intensity of diabetes. Naturally the presence of the two diseases will complicate the therapy and require more skilful care. On the other hand, it must be borne in mind that eradication of the accompanying disease such as would be attained by thyroidectomy, cholecystectomy, etc., may result in a marked reduction in insulin requirements. If this tendency is not appreciated postoperatively, and the insulin reduced as indicated, a severe hypoglycemia may result.

Preoperative Treatment.—The marked diminution in the operative mortality on diabetics since the introduction of insulin is shown in a survey of the literature by John [3] who noted that in 2023 operations on diabetic patients before the advent of insulin, the mortality was 24.2 per cent, whereas in 14,251 operations performed with preoperative insulin therapy, the mortality was only 5 per cent. Other factors are, of course, important in maintaining a low mortality. For example, it is particularly important that the liver be prevented from reaching a state of low glycogen reserve. Satisfactory glycogen reserve can be attained only by the administration of a diet containing adequate amounts of carbohydrate, protein, vitamins, fluids, etc., along with proper insulin therapy.

Since arteriosclerosis is frequent in diabetics, it is important that these patients be submitted to thorough examination, paying particular attention to the heart and kidneys, organs which are apt to be seriously affected by arteriosclerosis of the advanced type. Generally speaking, because of the features just mentioned, the best results in diabetic surgery will be attainable only by utilization of the utmost degree of cooperation between the internist and the surgeon. Lack of such joint effort will perhaps account in part for the large variation in the mortality of operations (5 to 50 per cent) in diabetic patients in the various clinics throughout the country.

When the operation is not an emergency, it is highly desirable that the operation be preceded by a preliminary period of preparation and study so that the insulin requirements may be fully understood. Though protamine insulin has been of considerable value in the treatment of the surgical diabetic patient, its prolonged action may serve as a disadvantage, making it necessary sometimes to resort to feedings at bed-time and between meals. In general, it is more difficult to use protamine insulin in children. The amount of carbohydrate, protein and fat in the diet will naturally depend on the severity of the diabetes, and will vary from 175 to 250, 75 to 80, and 70 and 90 grams respectively.

On the morning of operation McKittrick and Root[4] advise giving one-half to two-thirds the usual dose of insulin and no nourishing liquids for twelve hours preceding operation. Protamine insulin is very satisfactory as the preoperative dose because of the excellent protection during the operation, but should not be given if it has not been used in the routine care of the patient previously. Hypodermoclysis or intravenous fluids are not given on the morning of operation unless there are specific indications. The dose of drugs, preoperative and otherwise, should be decreased slightly under the average dose because diabetic patients are slightly less tolerant to drugs than are nondiabetic patients.

If the operation under consideration is an *emergency,* there will obviously not be sufficient time to make the urine sugar-free. The administration of such massive doses as to attain this effect in a few hours would be unsafe because of the danger of severe hypoglycemia. However, if possible, the urine should be free from diacetic acid.

Anesthesia.—There is no single anesthetic agent which can be used effectively and safely as a routine in diabetic patients. Certain of the gases, including nitrous oxide, ethylene, and cyclopropane are relatively innocuous. As Hale and Tovell[5] have emphasized, one of the greatest anesthetic dangers in diabetic patients lies in the production of acidosis. Unlike the three agents mentioned above prolonged administration of ether has a distinct tendency to produce acidosis. Furthermore, ether results in the production of hyperglycemia, either through defective utilization of carbohydrates, prevention of conversion of dextrose to glycogen, or by depletion of hepatic glycogen. Asphyxiation of tissues may be partly responsible for these changes. At any rate it is obvious that anoxia should be avoided, regardless of the agent used. Chloroform should never be used on account of the severe damage inflicted by it upon the liver. Avertin should not be used because of its deleterious effect on the liver (Coleman, F. P., *Surgery,* 3:87, 1938), which, however, is obviously not as pronounced as that produced by chloroform.

In general, local anesthesia is one of the safest and should be used whenever feasible. For amputations, spinal anesthesia (50 to 75 mg. procaine) will probably be as free from deleterious effects as any other type. However, in doses large enough to permit abdominal operations spinal anesthesia is probably no less toxic than a general anesthetic. For abdominal operations gas-ether anesthesia (utilizing nitrous oxide or perhaps ethylene) will be as safe as any other. Intravenous anesthesia (*e.g.*, sodium pentothal) may be used when relaxation need not be complete or prolonged, but must be given with considerable caution.

Postoperative Treatment.—The maintenance of proper fluid intake is an especially important obligation in the care of diabetic patients following operation. If the operation is a major laparotomy and oral intake is limited to insignificant quantities during the first 24 to 48 hours, the fluid (3000 cubic centimeters or more in 24 hours) will have to be given subcutaneously or intravenously. Since most controlled diabetic patients will have an elevated blood sugar immediately following operation, it will usually be preferable to give physiologic saline subcutaneously up to 1500 cubic centimeters, at least until the results of a blood sugar determination are available. To prevent the possible development of insulin shock, relatively small doses of insulin at frequent intervals are preferable. The interval between doses for a day or two following operation should be shorter than preoperatively because the duration of its effect is shortened. Later in the day the remainder of the fluid may be given in the form of 5 per cent glucose intravenously. Authorities differ as to the necessity of covering this glucose solution with an extra amount of insulin. It is agreed, however, that if insulin is given to cover it, the dose should be small (not more than 15 to 20 units for 75 grams of glucose). If an error is made in the amount of insulin it is preferable to err on the side of giving too little. Blood sugar determinations are supposedly more accurate than urine analyses in determining the amount of insulin to adminster, but each should be made at intervals of 4 to 8 hours during the first day or two. It should be remembered that slight glycosuria does little harm whereas insulin coma may give rise to serious or even fatal consequences, even though recognized early and treated. For this reason little or no attempt is made to make the urine sugar-free during the first 3 or 4 days postoperatively. However, the urine must be watched for acetone, and insulin with ample fluids be given as indicated.

McKittrick and Root [4] suggest a very simple and practical method of determining the amount of insulin required during the first few postoperative days; namely, "(1) test the urine (Benedict's test) every four hours and (2) give insulin (crystalline), 15 units if the reaction is red, 10 units if it is yellow, and 5 units if it is yellow-green." Such procedure is obviously only an approximate method of determining the amount of insulin needed but since a definite mathematical method is unavailable, this simple rule will be found useful.

Oral feedings, including fruit juice, ginger ale, etc., are administered as soon as tolerated, followed, on the second or third day, by portions of solid food more readily tolerated. Attempt should be made, particularly after the first 24 hours, to reach a daily carbohydrate intake of 100 to 150 grams. If the oral intake falls short of this amount, the remainder may be given as 5 per cent glucose intravenously or as 2.5 per cent glucose in physiologic sodium chloride solution subcutaneously.

All nurses and physicians attending the diabetic patient should be trained in observation for the manifestations of insulin shock. Such symptoms as weakness, sweating, pallor, hunger and mental confusion demand consideration of such a diagnosis. The problem can be settled by a blood sugar determination. However, the condition is so serious that it should be recognized and proper therapy (intravenous glucose) instituted at once.

SURGICAL DISEASES SECONDARY TO DIABETES

Many of the features related to insulin requirements, etc., as discussed in the preceding pages, apply to the lesions which are spoken of as being complications of, or secondary to diabetes. The physician must be aware of the need of an increased amount of insulin during an infection, and a decrease in the needs when that infection is relieved. The most significant complications of diabetes are carbuncles, infections and gangrene of the lower extremity.

Carbuncles.—It is important to emphasize that carbuncles are much more serious in diabetic patients than in nondiabetics, and therefore require more care in therapy. They are usually located on the back of the neck and commonly occur when the diabetes is out of control. They are so definitely related to diabetes that all patients with carbuncles should at once have a urine examination. Carbuncles, like other infections, increase the severity of diabetes, making it necessary to watch the urine and blood sugar daily. It will be necessary to increase the amount of insulin while the infection increases in intensity, and decrease it as drainage is established. To prevent development of carbuncles, diabetic patients should not shave their necks, and should under no circumstances squeeze or irritate hair follicle infections.

Opinions differ somewhat as to the treatment of carbuncles in diabetic patients, some surgeons choosing to treat the infection conservatively with x-ray therapy, whereas others recommend surgical drainage, as do the authors. It is frequently difficult to determine when drainage should be established. Ordinarily, if the carbuncle is producing no fever or pain, and still remains relatively small in size, treatment may remain conservative, utilizing x-ray therapy. The development of local tenderness, fever, and especially fluctuation are usually indications for incision to establish drainage. The patient should be confined to bed and instructed to eliminate activity which would result in movement of the neck. Since the offending organism is a staphylococcus, sulfathiazole may be given.

Gangrene.—Diabetic gangrene is a serious condition because of its frequency and serious outcome. In a large series of cases collected from the literature, John[9] noticed an incidence of 5 per cent in diabetic patients, with a mortality of about 18 per cent. The high mortality has a direct relationship to the age of the patients which averaged 64 to 15 years. The development of gangrene is determined by the degree of vascular occlusion (arteriosclerosis) and bears little relationship to the severity of the diabetes. The gangrene may be "dry," *i.e.*, of the type usually seen in arteriosclerosis, but is more apt to be "wet" because of the high incidence of infection.

Diabetic gangrene may occur anywhere on the body, but is usually located on the toes or feet, where it starts as a small gangrenous area. Occasionally the process is superimposed upon an infectious process because of the interference to circulation by the edema, etc., incident to the infection.

Pain at the site of the gangrene, or of the intermittent claudication type in the leg, is apt to be minor in character. Besides the area of gangrene, examination will reveal a variable degree of impairment of blood supply. The skin is apt to be dry, thin and parchment-like, and the nails dry and brittle. Other manifestations of damage to the blood supply may include pallor of the foot upon elevation and a slowly developing rubor or cyanosis upon dependency. The dorsalis pedis, posterior tibial, and frequently the popliteal pulses on the affected side are apt to be absent.

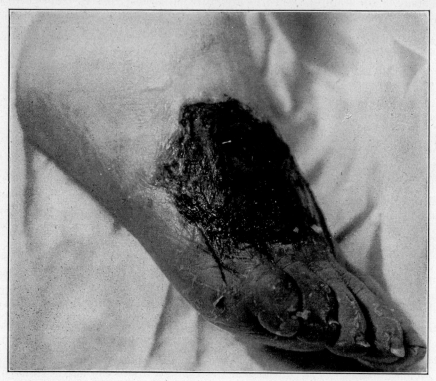

Fig. 133.—Diabetic Gangrene in a Woman Aged Forty-five.

A moderate amount of infection was present as is commonly noted in diabetic gangrene, thereby making amputation more urgent than in arteriosclerotic gangrene as illustrated in Figure 77. Note the cyanosis with impending gangrene of the toes.

If infection is present there will be edema, redness, etc., as described later in this chapter.

Treatment.—A very important feature in the therapy of diabetic gangrene is *prophylactic treatment.* Since gangrene or infection is so apt to follow trivial injuries in diabetes, it is essential that diabetic patients avoid trauma to their feet. Epidermophytosis should be watched for at all times and treated in its incipiency. Hot water bottles, cold weather, new shoes, wrinkles in hosiery, electric pads, etc., may result in trivial injuries which may serve as the instigator of serious trouble. The care of nails, corns, etc., should be entrusted to someone careful and experienced.

In the active therapy of diabetic gangrene rest in bed is of course imperative; the leg should be put in a position where blanching of the foot is minimal and precautions taken lest decubital ulcers develop. If the gangrenous area is dry and not infected, dry sterile dressings should be applied to prevent contamination and subsequent infection. If infection is present, wet dressings, consisting of equal parts of saturated boric acid solution and 50 per cent alcohol, or some other weak antiseptic should be applied. In either case the foot should be protected with a cradle. Pavaex therapy is contraindicated because infection is so prevalent.

Local superficial areas of gangrene rarely require any operative therapy. With conservative measures, the gangrenous portion will usually separate from viable tissue and healing will result. On certain occasions, however, the gangrene may extend and involve an entire toe. In this case there is no urgency about operation but removal will ultimately be necessary. Delay may allow the development of a superimposed infection. Occasionally, a dry gangrene of the toe may be treated by simple amputation of the toe if the popliteal pulsation is strong and the physical condition otherwise seems excellent. With slightly less favorable conditions, amputation may be performed below the knee (i.e., through the upper third of the leg). However, patients upon whom these conservative types of amputation are performed must be well chosen. The skin below the knee must be in good condition and there must not be any color or temperature change above the ankle. Infection beyond the base of the toe also contraindicates amputation below the knee. In spite of precautions postoperative infection is very common (McLaughlin [12]).

Amputation through the knee, of the Gritti-Stokes or Callander type, may give a serviceable end-beading stump but should not be performed in diabetics except by one experienced in this type of amputation. These two types of amputation have about the same indications as amputation through the upper third of the leg.

Amputation above the knee (supracondylar) is usually the simplest of the various types of amputations and in general the safest. In a large series of personal cases McKittrick [7] noted an operative mortality of 7.1 per cent in amputation of the toe, 5.4 per cent in the leg, 13.6 per cent through the knee and 11.7 per cent in thigh amputations. Obviously, these figures do not indicate the severity of the various types of amputations. In the presence of severe infection accompanying gangrene, McKittrick [6] and others advise a two stage operation, i.e., first a low guillotine amputation, followed in a few days (after subsidence of the infection) by a closed amputation at the supracondylar level.

Spinal anesthesia is the anesthesia of choice, although refrigeration anesthesia (see page 188) is likewise satisfactory. The dose of preanesthetic drugs should be small, since these patients seem to be somewhat insensitive to discomfort and pain, and frequently sleep through their operation.

Drainage of amputation stumps is becoming less popular during recent years; usually the stump should either be closed tight without drains or left wide open. The latter procedure (guillotine amputation) is reserved for emergency amputations when the infection is so serious and widespread that it may burrow upward into the stump if it is closed. McKittrick and Root [8] have very correctly emphasized the fact that tourniquets should not be used in amputations for diabetic gangrene.

More details regarding indications for the level of amputation as related to the vascular deficiency may be found in Chapter XI. Postoperative care as already discussed in this chapter and in Chapter XI should be meticulous.

Infections.—As mentioned in the discussion of gangrene, infection is a frequent complication of gangrene and is much to be feared. Overnight it may change a condition from one allowing conservative treatment to one demanding immediate amputation. However, it is well known that amputation for gangrene in the presence of a severe acute infection of the foot is associated with a very high mortality rate. This fact has led certain surgeons (Zierold,[9] Pearse and Ziegler [10]) to treat such patients conservatively until the acute infection has subsided before resorting to amputation. By this procedure Zierold was able to reduce the mortality rate from 50 to 10 per cent.

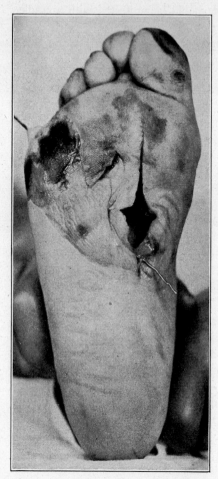

FIG. 134.—DEEP PLANTAR ABSCESS IN FOOT OF A DIABETIC.

Large patches of gangrene are also present. In this case amputation was necessary. Without the development of gangrene this abscess would have been treated by incision as in a nondiabetic.

Frequently a serious infection may develop in the foot and leg of a diabetic patient in the complete absence of any gangrene. This condition has so many features different from those in gangrene that the two conditions should be discussed separately. In the first place, infection is not dependent upon arterial deficiency; gangrene though dependent upon arterial deficiency may be increased by the edema and inflammatory reactions incident to infection. Infections may start spontaneously, or following slight trauma as already described. Commonly the infection spreads rapidly without producing any significant local manifestations, e.g., from a toe into the entire plantar space with no pain or redness and only slight tenderness. The only dependable indication of the spread may be the swelling accompanying the advance of the infection. The amount of fever is extremely variable as is also leukocytosis. The increase in severity of diabetes by infection has already been discussed; this feature and the tendency toward rapid spread of the infection constitute reasons why the infection should receive prompt attention and treatment.

In the *treatment* of infections, amputation need rarely be considered, but incision with adequate drainage is urgently indicated when pus is present. The differentiation between a cellulitis and an abscess cavity is frequently very difficult to make because of the absence of the usual signs of cellulitis. Moreover, the infection burrows so rapidly and readily along fascial planes and tendons that any pus present will not be under enough tension to produce fluctuation. Olmsted and Olch [11] have emphasized the fact that such infection should be treated in about the same manner as identical infections in nondiabetics. It is nevertheless more important that incision not be delayed when pus is present. Moreover, the incision for drainage must be adequate and must extend upward as far as the infection has burrowed: if the infection is extensive, counter incisions may be used instead of one long incision. Rubber drains are used as indicated.

Amputation may be indicated if gangrene develops, if osteomyelitis of major bones of the foot is present, or on rare occasions, when the infection becomes so extensive that incision and drainage seems inadequate or proves ineffective in controlling spread. Cultures should be made and sulfonamide therapy instituted.

Although infections in diabetic patients are usually encountered in the lower extremity, they may occur anywhere over the body. When occurring in the hand they are likewise serious because of the rapidity with which they spread along the sheaths and fascial spaces, and even subcutaneous tissue.

Miscellaneous Complications.—*Furuncles.* Furuncles are also prevalent in diabetic patients and commonly become multiple (furunculosis). All patients with furunculosis should have their urine examined for sugar. Treatment is usually conservative, incising the larger ones as indicated (see also page 51). *Cholecystitis* cannot be classified as a true complication of diabetes but it is true that the incidence of gall bladder disease is higher in diabetics than in nondiabetic patients. Some observers go so far as to state that in certain instances cholecystectomy will prevent the development of diabetes; it is well known that removal of a diseased gallbladder almost invariably results in a decrease in severity of the diabetes.

BIBLIOGRAPHY

1. DaCosta, J. C., and Beardsley. Quoted by DaCosta, *Modern Surgery*, W. B. Saunders Co., 1931, Phila.
2. Smith, B. C. The Therapy of Surgical Complications of Diabetes Mellitus at Presbyterian Hospital in New York City, 1930-1935, *Surgery*, 2:509, 1937.
3. John, H. J. Surgery and Diabetes, *Ann. Surg.*, 108-1052, 1938.
4. McKittrick, L. S., and Root, H. F. Preoperative and Postoperative Treatment of the Patient with Diabetes, *Arch. Surg.*, 40:1057, 1940.
5. Hale, D. E., and Tovell, R. M. Choice of Anesthetic Agents and Methods of Their Administration for Diabetic Patients, *Surgery*, 3:100, 1938.
6. McKittrick, L. S. Surgical Procedures in the Presence of Diabetes Mellitus, *Surg., Gynec. & Obst.*, 68:508, 1939.
7. McKittrick, L. S. Diabetic Gangrene—A Clinical Problem, *Am. J. Surg.*, 44:46, 1939.
8. McKittrick, L. S., and Root, H. F. *Diabetic Surgery*, Lea and Febiger, Philadelphia, 1928.
9. Zierold, A. A. Gangrene of the Extremity in the Diabetic, *Ann. Surg.*, 110:723, 1939.
10. Pearse, H. E., and Ziegler, H. P. Is the Conservative Treatment of Infection or Gangrene in Diabetic Patients Worth While? *Surgery*, 8:72, 1940.
11. Olmsted, W. H., and Olch, I. Y. Arteriosclerosis of the Lower Extremities with Special Reference to Treatment in Diabetic Gangrene, *J. Missouri M. A.*, 30:427, 1933.
12. McLaughlin, C. W. Problems in the Surgical Management of Diabetic Gangrene, *Surgery*, 13:423, 1943.

CHAPTER XIII

SHOCK AND HEMORRHAGE

The clinical picture of shock may be produced in a number of ways, *e.g.*, after severe accidental injury and is, in such an instance, called traumatic shock. But the same signs and symptoms may develop after an intentional trauma such as an operation, or following an extensive burn, or in a patient after a serious but non-traumatic hemorrhage as from a gastric ulcer. In describing shock it will be useful to separate the clinical causes and manifestations from its pathogenesis. About the former there is considerable, though not entire agreement; about the latter there is still a great deal of dispute. A concise and complete discussion of the literature on surgical shock may be found in a monograph by Blalock[1] and in two reviews by Wiggers[30] and by Harkins.[31]

Hemorrhage is usually discussed with shock because bleeding frequently accompanies the various factors, usually traumatic, which individually or together initiate the condition of shock. Moreover, hemorrhage alone, even without other factors, if severe enough, will produce the same clinical manifestations. Ordinarily, however, a hemorrhage alone, particularly when it is not severe enough to induce manifestations of shock, results in certain characteristic signs and symptoms which are described separately because they are often of diagnostic value.

Shock may be defined as a condition of collapse or prostration accompanied by a fall in blood volume and flow, and evidence of peripheral circulatory impairment or failure. Because shock also depresses the sensorium, the term is used in other conditions where only the nervous system is affected without involvement of the circulation. Thus "nervous shock" may occur after hearing tragic news, after seeing anything intensely disagreeable or frightful, or experiencing profound fear and excruciating pain. The depression of the psyche may be so profound in such instances as to be followed by actual unconsciousness (fainting, syncope). Such attacks of fainting may also occur in hysteria. However, in all these situations the circulation is only temporarily impaired, and recovery is prompt. In other conditions the word shock is used to describe phenomena entirely different in nature. Thus insulin shock is due to hypoglycemia (see Chapter XXX) and may be severe enough to result in complete loss of consciousness. Anaphylactic shock is a complex affair due to the reaction of the body to foreign proteins, though it may be accompanied by circulatory impairment. On the other hand, coma, a term used to describe the most complete sensorial depression, may be due to cerebral edema or uremia with little or no circulatory change. Heart failure in myocardial disease, however, results in both sensorial and circulatory changes and may be a possible source of confusion to the novice. The profound prostration which occurs in severe infections such as virulent pneumonias, meningitis, etc., is another type. Patients exhibiting shock with intestinal obstruction are superficially similar in clinical appearance to those suffering from surgical or traumatic shock, but present entirely different therapeutic problems which are discussed in detail in Chapter XXVI particularly in regard to their differential diagnosis. It should be emphasized, however, that the circumstances and history accompanying these types of shock are so different that there is ordinarily no difficulty in differentiating them from true surgical shock.

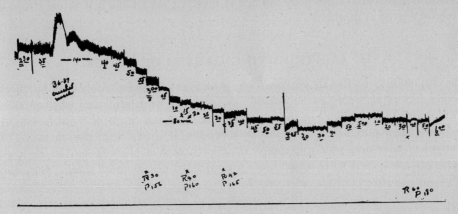

FIG. 135.—TYPICAL FALL OF ARTERIAL BLOOD PRESSURE AFTER CRUSHING MUSCLES OF THE THIGH IN AN EXPERIMENTAL ANIMAL.

(From Cannon, W. B., *Traumatic Shock,* D. Appleton-Century Co.)

The terms primary and secondary shock, though sometimes used, are often a source of confusion. Primary shock usually occurs immediately after the injury and if due entirely to nervous factors is transient and rapidly disappears. Secondary shock develops a little later and is due to the organic lesions associated with physical trauma. Only the shock due to the organic effects of trauma, regardless of the time interval, is considered herein.

I. FREQUENT CLINICAL CAUSES OF SHOCK

The picture of surgical shock is met with in a variety of conditions of which the following are the most important:

1. *Severe hemorrhage* will bring about shock without any other cause although in traumatic cases other factors are frequently present. The amount of hemorrhage (without other factors) necessary to produce shock varies with the individual and especially with the sex, the male being far more susceptible. Ordinarily, loss of blood equal to 2 or 3 per cent of the body weight in normal adults will bring on the picture of severe shock. This represents about 25 to 40 per cent (about 1500 to 2000 cc.) of the total circulating blood.

According to experiments reported by Freeman [2] the condition of shock is produced by any hemorrhage which is severe enough to induce severe vasoconstriction. The role of vasoconstriction in producing many of the manifestations of shock will be discussed under pathogenesis.

2. *Severe trauma* without hemorrhage may produce shock although the presence of bleeding is an important accessory cause. Extensive crushing injuries are particularly prone to be followed by shock; in such an event the incidence of tissue necrosis may play an important part in the pathogenesis. (See Crush Syndrome, page 1059.) Surgical operations are included in the traumatic cause of shock.

3. *Severe burns* are frequently followed by shock as soon as there has been sufficient loss of plasma to lower blood volume significantly. This is especially true when a large part of the body surface is involved even though it is only first or second degree in depth.

II. CONTRIBUTING CAUSES OF SHOCK

In addition to the above conditions which are frequently followed by shock, other factors also play an important role, not only in determining whether shock will occur, but especially in the severity of the process. Some of these factors are of extreme importance also in the pathogenesis of shock since they increase the output of adrenalin which promotes vasoconstriction, a phenomenon which if excessive is supposed to be responsible for many of the signs of shock. They have thus an important bearing on treatment.

1. *Cold and exposure,* while themselves an occasional primary cause of shock when extreme, always aggravate an existing shock or cause it to appear after relatively mild trauma or moderate hemorrhage. The presence of wet clothing adds to the seriousness of exposure to cold.

2. *Severe pain* alone is said to be able to initiate shock, but such a shock is usually temporary even when the patient faints. When accompanied by hemorrhage, burns, severe trauma, etc., any degree of pain increases the liability to shock and aggravates its severity to a remarkable degree, probably by increasing vasoconstriction through sympathetic stimulation.

3. *Duration* of the factors producing shock without treatment is of extreme importance in determining not only the development and severity of shock, but also its prognosis. Indeed, when a patient has been left in a condition of shock for a long time (twelve to twenty-four hours) no form of treatment can save him; the vital processes have reached an irreparable stage, and death is inevitable.

4. *Anoxia,* or lack of oxygen, from any cause, always contributes to the severity of shock. Indeed, many of the tissue changes found at autopsy are due to the effects of anoxia. They are thus much more pronounced, the longer the patient has lived after the onset of shock; very little change will be found when death has occurred rapidly. The lack of oxygen is due, of course, primarily to the failure of the circulation, but other factors may contribute to the degree of anoxia. Very important are depression and obstruction to normal respiratory exchange, *e.g.,* inadequate oxygenation during general anesthesia.

5. *General anesthesia,* particularly ether, when administered to an injured patient, promotes the development and severity of shock. The depressing influence of

ether on the blood pressure in shock has been demonstrated experimentally by Cattell.[3] Although nitrous oxide and oxygen do not have the depressing effects of ether, their use may be deleterious in shock because of the anoxia (see p. 180) which so often occurs. A further disadvantage of nitrous oxide is its failure to induce relaxation which frequently produces excessive respiratory excursions. For these and other reasons, ether-oxygen, or one of the other gases is usually preferable. The important principle is the fact that any anesthesia which may lead to anoxia by depressing or obstructing respiratory exchange is distinctly to be avoided. If local anesthesia (*i.e.,* some form of regional or block anesthesia) will meet the requirements, it is by all odds the safest.

6. *General factors* are important contributing agents. Sex has already been mentioned; females are able to stand much greater losses of blood than men, probably because their inherited immunity from menstrual and parturient hemorrhage is greater than that of males from the blood losses during warfare and injury. Even in shock without hemorrhage females are more resistant. Other conditions, such as advanced age, the presence of other disease, general lowered vitality, etc., have an obvious bearing on the development and severity of shock.

III. THE CLINICAL MANIFESTATIONS OF SHOCK

The clinical manifestations of traumatic or surgical shock as about to be described are those which, in general, are common to shock, regardless of the cause. Differences do exist, for example, in severe hemorrhage, which often produces manifestations so characteristic as to be of diagnostic importance. For this reason, the signs and symptoms of severe hemorrhage are discussed separately. It should be emphasized, however, that the following description does not apply to reflex declines in blood pressure, in which general vasodilatation is present and in which the extremities are warm.

1. The *general appearance* of the patient is frequently characteristic and indicative of the seriousness of the condition. The facies is that of a person very ill, the features pinched, eyes sunken, pupils dilated, beads of perspiration standing out on the forehead, the lips pale or ashen in color; the skin is cold and clammy, particularly of the extremities. There is a pronounced grayish pallor of the skin over the entire body—most noticeable, however, over the face. Many of these manifestations, such as pallor, coldness and perspiration, are the same as those produced by intense sympathetic stimulation.

2. The *sensorium* is depressed but the degree of mental dullness and apathy varies considerably. When shock is severe or critical, the patient lies as if unconscious so that if one raises an arm it falls to the bed at once as if lifeless. He really is not *unconscious,* however, for he will answer questions and complain of symptoms if urged to do so. Painful stimuli will evoke a groan or slight defensive movements. In the milder cases, the patient will be listless, apathetic and extremely weak. On the other hand, in certain patients, the sensorium may be so clear that nurses and interns may not suspect the presence of shock without careful examination. In patients suffering from severe hemorrhage, restlessness is apt to be a prominent manifestation which is often of diagnostic value.

3. The *circulatory depression,* which is the most important clinical manifestation, is usually evident on inspection, *i.e.,* the hands and feet are cold and the color of the skin pale or slightly ashen, indicating peripheral anemia and circulatory stasis. The pulse is often absent at the wrist, but may be felt over the carotids. It is in any case rapid, 120 to 160 in rate, of poor quality, soft, compressible and thready in character and thus promptly reflects the reduced blood flow and cardiac output. These evidences of circulatory impairment occur early and often precede the fall in blood pressure which sometimes remains unchanged or varies considerably. The experimental studies of Wiggers[4] and the clinical example illustrated in Chart 5, page 263, indicate that the diastolic falls before the systolic blood pressure. Other observations, however, have shown that the earliest change is a slight rise in diastolic and a slight fall in systolic pressure. The *shock level* of blood pressure varies from one individual to another and depends somewhat on the patient's normal pressure. Undoubtedly a fall in systolic pressure from 150 to 70 millimeters of mercury in one patient will be more likely to be accompanied by shock than a fall from 90 to 60 in another. The *critical level* of blood pressure is that point, usually about 85 millimeters of mercury, at which a slight additional loss of blood or trauma will result in a disastrous decline in pressure. Extensive investigations of the critical level in falling blood pressure have been reported by Cannon and Cattell.[5] The rapidity with which the pressure falls is important as is also the duration of the lowered pressure. A *low venous pressure* is present in shock and is evident clinically by the collapse of the superficial veins particularly in the hand.

4. The *temperature and respiration* exhibit moderate changes. A depression of one to two degrees centigrade or more in rectal temperature is not infrequent and is probably a reflection of the lowered blood flow and reduced metabolic rate. The respirations may be unchanged, but are usually shallow and rapid, except in severe hemorrhage when "air hunger" may be present. This is probably a compensatory mechanism to overcome the greatly impaired gaseous metabolism resulting from the loss of oxygen carriers, the erythrocytes.

5. *Subjective symptoms* when elicited on urgent questioning include coldness, faintness and "deadness" of the extremities. In mild cases dizziness may be the only symptoms; this may be of diagnostic value, in that it implies cerebral anemia, which, however, is more frequent after severe hemorrhage.

6. *Laboratory examination* may reveal distinctive features. (*a*) Secretion of urine is sharply decreased; the urine obtained is highly concentrated, but contains no abnormal elements. (*b*) The red blood count of capillary blood may show no changes, but often an increased value. Cannon[6] found in 16 out of 27 cases of severe shock, a count of six million or more. In shock due to burns the erythrocyte count may be high, accompanied by a tremendous increase in the hemoglobin of the blood which in some cases reported by Underhill[7] reached 200 per cent. In hemorrhage the erythrocyte count ordinarily falls, but if severe shock is present this reduction may be less noticeable. (*c*) The white cell count is usually increased within a few hours after injury, particularly if the injury is accompanied by hemorrhage. The leukocytosis usually disappears in uncomplicated cases within forty-eight hours. The change has been called traumatic leukocytosis. (*d*) Blood volume in shock is lowered, often profoundly. In 27 of 29 cases examined by

Keith [8] the estimated blood volumes ranged from 52 to 85 per cent of the normal. This reduction of blood volume has been confirmed in many experimental studies and is apparently the most characteristic finding in shock; it is, moreover, easy to see how a serious fall in blood volume alone could lead to circulatory impairment. (e) Blood chemistry studies have shown a reduction of the alkali reserve (as measured by the CO_2 capacity). Values as low as 21 volumes per cent (normal 55 to 60) were found by Cannon,[9] the degree of reduction being roughly proportional to the reduction in blood pressure. Whether this fall is due to excessive production of acid or as a consequence of overbreathing was not determined. The blood sugar is not changed, but occasionally may be higher than normal. The

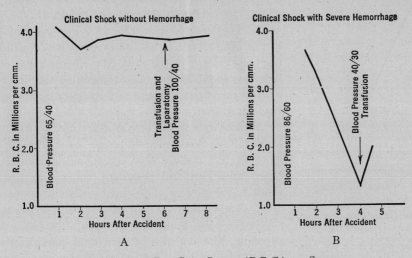

FIG. 136.—THE RED CELL COUNT (R.B.C.) IN SHOCK.

A, this patient was shot in several places, including the abdomen, but suffered very little loss of blood; he had all the clinical manifestations of shock. Note the absence of any fall in the erythrocyte count even though parenteral fluids were administered. B, this patient was struck by a street car which crushed and severed both lower extremities, the loss of blood was considerable. Note the rapid fall in the erythrocyte count indicating a dilution of the circulating blood. Parenteral fluids were given while the transfusion was being prepared.

nonprotein nitrogen of the blood is increased to about 50 per cent above the normal, a reflection perhaps of concentration of the blood. An extensive review of the blood changes in shock including his own experimental and clinical observations, especially determinations of specific gravity and of potassium, has been published by Scudder.[28] This work points to the diagnostic value of specific gravity determinations of whole blood and of plasma, the former being a measure of hemoconcentration, the latter of plasma protein content. The falling drop method is used and well described. The finding of high potassium values in certain types of shock suggested the use of adrenal cortical extract in treatment. Injection of the extract seemed to have a beneficial effect in several cases. These latter studies await confirmation by others. (f) Blood viscosity is obviously increased except, of course, when dilution following hemorrhage has occurred. The increased concentration of the blood is probably responsible for this change, but the fall in body temperature may also play a role.

IV. CLINICAL MANIFESTATIONS OF HEMORRHAGE

Occasionally a single severe hemorrhage occurs without producing true surgical shock. The clinical manifestations, nevertheless, include a degree of collapse which is fairly distinctive and enable one ordinarily to suspect the cause. This is of especial diagnostic importance when there is no external bleeding (*e.g.,* bleeding ectopic pregnancy, hemorrhage from a peptic ulcer or esophageal varix, hemangioma, etc.). Nevertheless it should be emphasized that if the hemorrhage is severe and *persistent* the clinical manifestations will be more nearly like those just described for shock.

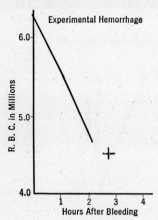

This is true because a sufficiently large and continuous loss of blood can produce the same serious impairment of the circulation so characteristic of shock.

1. The *general appearance* of a patient after a severe hemorrhage is one of extreme pallor which is not only evident in the skin everywhere, but particularly in the blanched appearance of the lips and mucous membranes. There is frequently an apprehensive expression.

2. The *sensorium* is not depressed as in shock. Indeed the patient may show no apathy at all, but more or less evident restlessness, unless the hemorrhage is severe and persistent enough to produce shock.

Fig. 137.—The Red Blood Count (R.B.C.) in Experimental Hemorrhage.

A dog was bled 4 per cent of its body weight, a fatal outcome occurring two and one-half hours later. Note the almost immediate drop in the erythrocyte count indicating dilution. No parenteral fluids were given in this experiment.

3. The *circulatory depression* is similar to that in shock, the pulse being fast and weak, the blood pressure low. The evidence of peripheral stasis as shown by an ashen color is not so apt to be present as in shock.

4. The *temperature* is usually subnormal as it is in shock, but the respirations are apt to be deep and rapid (air hunger), unlike the shallow respiration in shock.

5. Although patients suffering from shock of any type may complain of *thirst,* it is apt to be encountered more frequently in patients suffering a severe hemorrhage, particularly if it is sudden and massive.

6. *Laboratory examinations* have been somewhat contradictory, but the present authors have noted that findings which are characteristic of hemorrhage without shock include the lowered erythrocyte count and hemoglobin content which occur promptly after the loss of blood. It is undoubtedly due to dilution, *i.e.,* the passage of fluid into the blood stream from the tissue spaces through the capillary walls. This is in contrast to the normal or high count in shock which is associated with a concentration of the blood. Doubtless the greater pallor after hemorrhage as compared with shock is due to the dilution of blood. Leukocytosis is much more marked in hemorrhage than in shock. The concentration of serum protein, as might be expected, falls; according to experimental observations (Elman [10]), this fall is not rapidly restored, at least in the fasting state. Clinical observations by Scudder [28]

have also shown a low serum protein in hemorrhage which was difficult to restore even with transfusions.

It should be emphasized again that the above manifestations of hemorrhage are present usually only when the bleeding is not severe enough to produce surgical shock. If the loss of blood is severe, a shock of the type first described may ensue. Under these circumstances the manifestations presented by the patient will not be those of hemorrhage alone, but will be so complicated by the symptoms of shock that differentiation may be impossible. Very important is the fact that the dilution of blood as revealed by the erythrocyte count and hemoglobin reading, may be completely inhibited when the hemorrhage is so severe as to be accompanied by shock.

V. PATHOGENESIS OF SHOCK

Thus far only the known features of shock have been presented without definitely stating what their mechanisms are. What produces the profound impairment of the circulation? What causes the depression of the sensorium? Why do patients die of shock? These questions have evoked endless discussion and have been responsible for a number of theories of shock. A toxic theory, an anemia theory, an acapnia theory, a neurogenic theory, are but a few of those propounded; all have had their proponents. A complete and critical review of these theories has already been referred to.[1] Here an attempt will be made to answer the above questions with reference less to theories than to general physiologic mechanisms, particularly as they may be useful in outlining treatment.

1. **Depression of the Circulation.**—A circulatory impairment may be caused by failure in one of the three main factors which maintain it, *i.e.,* the force of the heart beat, the size of the vascular bed and the blood volume.

(*a*) The heart may fail as the terminal feature of heart disease and pressure fall just as a pump may fail. This is not the case in ordinary shock, however, for it has been found that the heart function is normal (Burton-Opitz [11]). In heart failure, moreover, the venous pressure is high, whereas in shock it is low. Nevertheless heart failure may be mistaken by the novice for surgical shock, particularly when it is sudden as in coronary occlusion.

(*b*) A second possible cause is an increase in the size of the vascular tree. This may occur either by a widening of the capillary bed, especially by the opening of collapsed channels, or by dilatation of the arteries and veins, or both. Vasomotor paralysis is a glib term which describes such an increase in the blood bed (confined ordinarily to arterial and venous channels) and is the basis of Crile's neurogenic theory of shock (reflex vasomotor paralysis from painful stimuli in the wound and elsewhere). Convincing evidence that vasomotor paralysis may produce surgical shock has not been adduced. Indeed, Wiggers [12] has shown that peripheral vasodilatation produced by inhaling amyl nitrite induces a fall of blood pressure which is scarcely perceptible. In spinal anesthesia, on the other hand, the nerve paralysis is often associated with a definite fall of blood pressure yet the pulse is usually slow and the extremities are warm and dry in contrast to the cold and moist skin in surgical shock. This and other differences suggest that the mechanisms producing the fall in blood pressure in spinal anesthesia and surgical shock are different.

The greatest argument against the theory of vasomotor paralysis in shock is the fact that actual and often marked vasoconstriction rather than vasodilatation is observed during severe surgical shock. This important observation was first made in 1909 by Seelig and Lyon.[13] These workers found no evidence of vasodilatation in the limb or in the retinal vessels after severe experimental shock even just before death; marked vasoconstriction was the rule. Other investigators have since confirmed this phenomenon which is discussed at some length in a provocative book by Cannon.[14] While it undoubtedly is true that such vasoconstriction is a normal defense reaction against loss of blood in hemorrhage in order to maintain blood pressure by diminishing the size of the blood bed, it is probable that, like other purposeful reactions, vasoconstriction may become too pronounced and lead to deleterious results. Experimental studies reported by Freeman[2] have shown, in fact, that vasoconstriction is apparently able to produce many of the manifestations of shock. This does not mean that vasoconstriction is not useful, because it has also been shown that totally sympathectomized animals withstand less loss of blood than those with an intact sympathetic system.

Because the capillary circulation may thus be impaired by excessive arteriolar spasm, changes thereby occur in the normal interchange of fluid between the tissue spaces and blood through the capillary walls (see p. 257). The capillaries thus play an important part in any discussion of vasomotor reactions. Moreover, the capillaries constitute an obviously important part of the vascular tree whenever any increase or decrease in the size of the circulatory bed occurs. They are also intimately connected with changes in blood volume.

(c) Reduction of blood volume in itself may cause a fall of blood pressure and probably is the most important mechanism in the pathogenesis of surgical shock. In hemorrhage the immediate reduction in blood volume is obviously equal to the amount of the lost blood. Difficult to understand is the fact that in the absence of obvious blood loss there is nevertheless a lessened total blood volume, a finding which has been confirmed by many observations both clinical and experimental. In the absence of hemorrhage, what causes this reduction? In some cases the location of the lost fluid is known. Thus, in extensive crushing lesions much serum and blood may be lost by extravasation into the tissues without overt hemorrhage. The loss may be great enough to produce shock without resorting to theories of toxic absorption or vasomotor paralysis. These important observations have been made by Parsons and Phemiser,[15] by Blalock,[16] and by Freedlander and Lenhart.[17] The handling of intestines during abdominal operations may result in traumatic outpouring of plasma, imperceptible perhaps, but which actually may be sufficient as shown by Blalock[18] to lower the blood volume. In burns the extensive inflammatory exudation may cause the loss of a large amount of blood serum which pours out through the dilated capillaries into and from the injured area.[19]

Convincing as these observations are, they do not explain the reduction of blood volume which occurs when there is no hemorrhage or no loss of fluid into traumatized or burned areas. Moreover, in many patients the depth of the shock seems out of proportion to the relatively slight tissue damage. To explain the marked drop in blood volume which nevertheless occurs in such cases it has been assumed that plasma is lost through the intact but obviously damaged capillaries all over the body. Objective evidence of increased capillary permeability is the observation in certain types of shock that there is a greater increase in the erythrocyte count (hemoconcentration) than can be explained by the amount of plasma lost. Extravasation of plasma and even blood into undamaged tissues particularly of the splanchnic area is added evidence, although this finding is probably terminal. If there is an increased capillary permeability it may be limited to shock associated with a possible "toxic" factor produced by serious tissue damage (see Crush Syndrome, page 1059). On the other hand, vasoconstriction itself may so reduce capillary blood flow as to lead to a local asphyxia which, according to Landis [22], increases permeability and thus allows plasma to pass into the tissue spaces, a process which could be so diffuse as to produce no perceptible evidence of edema. Indeed, Freeman [21] has produced a decrease in blood volume by experimental vasoconstriction alone. It should be emphasized, however, that many experimental observations deny the existence of a general increase in capillary permeability even in the advanced stages of traumatic shock.

It might appear that vasoconstriction is incompatible with the existence of low blood pressure. However, the presence of a diminished blood volume prevents the rise of blood pressure, which might be otherwise expected from the vasoconstriction. The diminished blood volume, of course, in itself provokes a compensatory vasoconstriction. Under these circumstances the stage is set for the establishment of a vicious circle; i.e., the factors (trauma and hemorrhage) responsible for the initial loss of fluid, incite vasoconstriction, which, when excessive, produces capillary asphyxia and exudation of plasma. This loss of plasma, in turn, leads to a further lowering in blood volume which again stimulates vasoconstriction.

2. **Depression of the Sensorium.**—The dizziness, the prostration and the slight to moderate impairment of consciousness in shock are due undoubtedly to the cerebral anemia which results, of course, from any significantly severe fall of blood pressure. It is well known, of course, that nervous tissue is extremely sensitive to reduction in its blood supply. The blood to a limb, for example, may be shut off entirely for an hour or more and the cells suffer no permanent injury or at most a transient one. The brain cells, however, are easily damaged by complete arrest of the circulation of even a few minutes duration. This fact emphasizes the importance of lowering the head in shock so that gravity may aid the cerebral circulation as much as possible.

3. **The Cause of Death.**—The cause of death in shock, though perhaps apparent from what has already been said, may be described as a peripheral circulatory failure due to the body's inability to maintain the blood pressure and blood volume above the critical level. When the shock is due to a single severe hemorrage death will result if the power of the body to restore the blood volume by dilution is inadequate. This dilution occurs through the capillary walls from the tissue spaces, particularly of the spleen, muscles, skin and intestines; anything which aids this process minimizes, and anything which inhibits it, magnifies the danger of death. Treatment which augments the body supply of fluids, especially fluids containing colloids, obviously is of greatest importance.

More commonly a lethal outcome occurs because the blood volume continues to diminish due to the fact that the lesion responsible for shock is not eradicated, *e.g.,* when an intermittently bleeding blood vessel is not controlled. An extensively injured mass of tissue often leads to continued loss of plasma; if the loss is severe enough and not replaced a lethal outcome is also probable. In still other cases the blood volume is supposed to fall because fluid is lost through uninjured capillaries which contain stagnant blood due to excessive vasoconstriction or because the capillaries are damaged by a toxin or other substance (see p. 257). Since such factors as fear, pain, exposure and cold are known to stimulate the sympathetic nerves and result in an outpouring of adrenalin thus promoting excessive and, therefore, deleterious vasoconstriction, their presence increases the liability of a fatal issue. Failure to remove the cause, whatever it may be, may obviously lead to a fall of blood pressure below the critical level. In any case, anoxia is particularly important because it leads to an increase in capillary permeability, and thus to general loss of plasma from the blood stream and to death. Treatment, therefore, is directed toward removal of the primary cause when possible and particularly the elimination of all the contributory causes of shock. If this is done and the natural reparative processes of nature are directly aided, blood volume and blood pressure will be raised to a safe level.

VI. TREATMENT OF SHOCK (AND HEMORRHAGE)

While the treatment of shock depends to some extent on the nature of the clinical cause preceding its development, certain features of treatment may be applied to all cases regardless of etiology. Removal of the primary cause is, of course, obviously indicated whenever possible.

It should be emphasized that nonsurgical shock, particularly that due to heart failure, must obviously be excluded from most of the following therapy. For example, deleterious results will occur if a patient in collapse from an acute cardiac failure is given large quantities of intravenous fluids; actually in such cases bleeding is what may be required. The differential diagnosis of the various conditions which produce prostration are discussed in Chapter XV.

1. **Prophylaxis or Prevention of Shock.**—This is, of course, chiefly applicable to the trauma intentionally inflicted during operations. This includes careful preoperative preparation. It implies the gentle handling of tissues, complete hemostasis, a minimum of exposure of viscera to the air, the control of the patient's apprehension and pain, careful anesthesia and finally, proper postoperative care. These details are all described elsewhere. It is important here to emphasize their role in preventing postoperative shock.

Avoidance of delay in the treatment of injured patients in general is extremely important in minimizing the incidence of shock. Even when shock is not present undue delay in treatment may permit it to develop. When shock is already present prompt therapy will halt its progress and promote its disappearance.

2. **Control of Hemorrhage.**—To check hemorrhage when possible is obviously indicated in order to prevent further loss of blood. Often, however, when the patient is seen by the surgeon, bleeding has already stopped. The various methods of controlling hemorrhage are described in Chapter X.

Cessation of bleeding is aided by several natural forces which develop spontaneously. The drop in blood pressure itself frequently is sufficient to stop further blood loss even in moderate hemorrhage when the vessel is not too large. Thus a drop of blood pressure to a point well above the critical level, and not maintained too long, serves a useful purpose. Secondly, the local factors such as contraction of the severed vessel, the development of thrombokinase from torn tissue (especially in parenchymatous organs) to promote clotting and the development of a hematoma which by its pressure compresses the bleeding point, all act to stop further loss of blood. Finally, there is a delicately adjusted mechanism which increases the

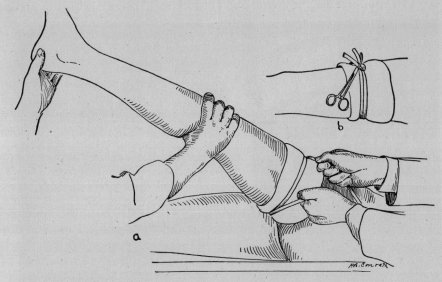

FIG. 138.—THE PROPER METHOD OF APPLYING A TOURNIQUET TO THE UPPER THIGH IN SEVERE HEMORRHAGE FROM THE LOWER EXTREMITY.

a, Application of the rubber tubing with sufficient force to obliterate the femoral *artery*. A counter force against the knee is exerted by an assistant. The limb is elevated during this procedure. *b*, Tourniquet in place with a clamp to insure against its becoming loose. Note the towel beneath the tourniquet to insure against injury to soft tissue. This is especially important in the arm where the nerves are less completely protected by overlying muscle, and hence are injured more readily. (See also Fig. 121.)

clotting power of the blood as hemorrhage continues (Gray and Lunt [23]). This spontaneous decrease in clotting time has as its purpose obviously the stopping of the leak with a thrombus.

A tourniquet is probably one of the oldest methods of controlling hemorrhage over an extremity. Unfortunately, it is now known that severe systemic effects are likely to follow the release of a tourniquet which has been left in place for several hours (see Crush Syndrome, page 1059). For this and other reasons a tourniquet should be employed for the control of bleeding only if other available methods do not suffice, but should be left on for only short intervals, or if possible the temperature of the part distal to the constriction should be reduced by artificial means in order to minimize the development of deleterious metabolic changes from autolysis.

In occult hemorrhage the question of operation to stop the leak is discussed on p. 264. The efficacy of so-called hemostatic agents (fibrinogen, horse serum, etc.)

to stop internal bleeding is claimed but unsupported by convincing evidence.

3. Conservation of Body Heat.—This is important in shock when there has been exposure to cold which unnecessarily increases the already excessive peripheral vasoconstriction. Thus, cold, wet clothing should be removed at once and warm blankets applied not only under but over the patient, particularly when the environmental temperature is low. Body warmth also may be maintained by the administration of warm drinks (provided no intra-abdominal injury is present), which has the added advantage of slaking thirst and supplying needed fluids. On the other hand, the application of heat may be *deleterious* (Blalock and Mason [33]). This is particu-

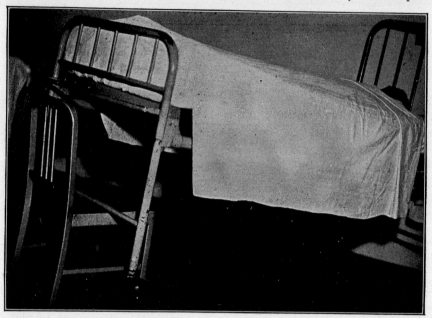

FIG. 139.—BED IN THE "SHOCK POSITION"; INSTEAD OF SHOCK BLOCKS UNDER THE FEET OF THE BED, A CHAIR HAS BEEN USED.

larly true if such application is sufficient to produce cutaneous vasodilatation which is harmful because it withdraws blood from vital tissues needing it urgently. Moreover, local heat increases tissue metabolism in the skin unnecessarily, with production of deleterious catabolic products. Finally, in profoundly depressed patients, there is danger of producing burns with hot water bottles. Although the shocked patient complains of being cold, it is much safer and just as effective to wrap him in blankets, thus conserving his own body heat, than to apply external heat.

4. General and Local Rest.—Immobilization of the injured part, and rest in bed are obvious requirements. Moving any severely injured patient from his bed to a stretcher, *e.g.*, to take an x-ray, may have to be postponed because such movement may increase the severity of the shock.

The posture with feet elevated and head lowered is so universally used that it is called the *shock position* and is usually achieved by placing blocks of wood (shock blocks) under the foot of the bed. The value of the shock position in raising blood pressure is probably due to the conservation by gravity of blood otherwise stagnant in the extremities; it, moreover, allows gravity to help in overcoming the cerebral anemia produced by the general circulatory impairment (see Fig. 139).

5. Relief of Pain.—Relief of pain is of great importance, for pain is one of the contributing factors in the causation of shock. The pain in fractures is severe, and is best treated by immediate immobilization. In the extremities this is best achieved with a Thomas splint. During World War I Thomas splints were applied on the field. British surgeons noted that the use of the Thomas splint was a most important agent in reducing the incidence of traumatic shock (Cannon).

Morphine is used for the same reason when indicated. It is also important in patients with severe hemorrhage to allay restlessness and control apprehension. Effective sedation prevents movements which might increase bleeding by dislodging clots or interfering with their formation. Morphine has also been shown to have a favorable effect in conserving blood pressure (Cannon and Cattell[5]). Morphine is not given, however, in any patient with a head injury or an intra-abdominal lesion, for it may so mask symptoms as to interfere with diagnosis and treatment.

6. Improvement of Peripheral Circulation.—The important basic aim in the treatment of shock is to improve the peripheral circulation by increasing blood flow, particularly by means which increase blood volume. In many instances, of course, such improvement will be evident as a result of the methods already mentioned. The increase of blood pressure is, of course, quite urgent whenever the systolic measurement is near the critical level, that is, whenever the shock is profound. In the presence of an inaccessible or uncontrollable source of hemorrhage, however, it may be dangerous to elevate a moderately low blood pressure because it may start up bleeding which has ceased as a result of its fall.

There are two possible methods which are useful in increasing the blood pressure. They are, first, the elevation of the blood volume, and second, the reduction in the blood bed; the former is by far the more important.

An *increase in blood volume* may occur spontaneously, especially after hemorrhage, by a mobilization of the body's stores of fluids, such as lymph and various tissue juices which, under favorable conditions pass the capillary wall from the interstitial spaces and enter the blood stream. To aid in this process the patient must obviously maintain a good fluid intake. During World War I it was often noted that shock was much less likely to occur in soldiers having access to plenty of water than in those deprived of water, other conditions being the same. Oral administration of fluids is, therefore, extremely important in the treatment of shock, except, of course, when the parenteral route is indicated instead (see administration of fluid, p. 150). In shock the choice between the subcutaneous and intravenous route is sometimes important. In severe shock hypodermoclysis may be useless when the peripheral circulation is so poor that absorption occurs slowly if at all. The intravenous method, on the other hand, while the more direct, rapid and certain, has a possible disadvantage in patients suffering an occult hemorrhage, because of the danger of raising the pressure too rapidly, dislodging a clot, and provoking, thereby, a recurrent hemorrhage.

Many kinds of fluids have been injected intravenously in shock in the attempt to increase blood volume and with it blood pressure. These fluids have been used instead of blood itself largely as a matter of convenience and speed, because of the difficulties and delay often associated with the giving of a blood transfusion. Such fluids, really therefore blood substitutes, have included isotonic and hypertonic saline and glucose, solutions of gelatin, gum acacia and hemoglobin; an excellent and interesting summary of the use of the various blood substitutes may be found in the paper of Amberson.[24] Of these, saline and glucose were the most widely used. It was soon found, unfortunately, that though the results were usually beneficial, the effect was *temporary, i.e.,* the rise in blood pressure lasted at most an hour or two. Obviously the injected fluid did not remain in the blood stream but rapidly filtered through the capillary wall into the tissue spaces. This diffusion was partly due, undoubtedly, to the increased capillary permeability which has already been mentioned. In the presence of gross capillary damage, there is a loss not only of

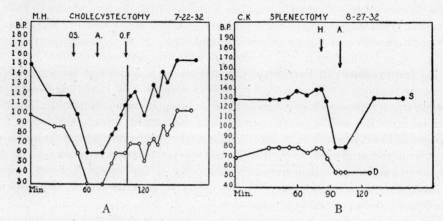

FIG. 140.—RECOVERY OF BLOOD PRESSURE IN SHOCK FOLLOWING THE INTRAVENOUS INJECTION OF GUM ACACIA IN GLUCOSE AT POINTS MARKED *A*.

A, in this patient the fall of blood pressure occurred soon after the operation was started (*O.S.*) but was continued and the gallbladder removed without further difficulty; *O.F.* indicates completion of operation. Recovery was uneventful. *B*, in this patient, the fall of blood pressure was due to hemorrhage (*H*) from a large vessel during the course of a splenectomy which was being performed because of Banti's disease. Recovery was uneventful. *S*, indicates systolic; *D*, diastolic pressure.

most of the injected saline or glucose solution but of plasma protein as well, with a resulting dilution of the protein remaining in the blood stream. In other words, the injection of large quantities of solutions of crystalloids may result in harm rather than in benefit. More important is the fact that glucose and saline do not form colloidal solutions. Only colloidal solutions are able to remain within the capillaries, whose walls act as semipermeable membranes through which crystalloids such as sodium chloride can readily pass. Indeed, the normal function of the protein of the plasma is largely embodied in its colloidal property enabling plasma to remain within the capillary lumen. These facts form the basis for Starling's hypothesis, first announced fifty years ago, but now known to be extremely important in the treatment of shock.

To effectively maintain blood volume and pressure, therefore, a solution capable of maintaining its osmotic pressure inside the capillaries should be used; the most perfect is, of course, blood itself. A solution of gum acacia, because of its colloidal properties, is much superior to glucose or saline alone and has perhaps been the most extensively used of the various blood substitutes (others: pectin, gelatin). As a single injection they may be advisable when blood is not available or is being prepared. However, acacia and pectin, unlike blood and plasma, are foreign substances and are not metabolized by the body.

Although whole blood contains red cells which are helpful in hemorrhage, it is really the plasma which is the most active component as far as improving the circulation is concerned, for reasons just discussed. Plasma transfusions rather than whole blood have, indeed, proved quite effective in the treatment of shock of various kinds. Plasma, moreover, has advantages over whole blood: first, typing is not required, second, it can be stored with less deterioration than whole blood, and finally can be concentrated even to dryness and stored in a powder form for future use. Serum also may be used and has many advantages if precautions are exerted to avoid reactions. The amount of plasma needed to effectively combat shock is relatively large; between 10 and 20 cc. per kilo of body weight will be required in many patients.

Adrenal cortical extract has been used with disappointing results, particularly in shock due to hemorrhage. However, experiments by Swingle, Parkins and Remington [32] suggest that desoxycorticosterone, one of the active principles, improves capillary permeability.

Another possible method of increasing blood pressure is the *reduction of size of the vascular bed*. This may be done by bandaging the extremities, but the clinical results are apt to be disappointing. Vasoconstrictor drugs, such as pituitrin, adrenalin and ephedrine, used to be popular in the treatment of shock, but it is now realized that while a transient increase of blood pressure does occur, the reaction is deleterious because the pressure promptly falls to a still lower level after the initial effect of the drug wears off. Moreover, as pointed out above, the deleterious effects of shock to a great extent may be due to excessive vasoconstriction. The use of such drugs therefore is contraindicated. Ephedrine has a more prolonged effect than adrenalin and finds a useful place in *preventing* drop of blood pressure occurring after induction of spinal anesthesia.

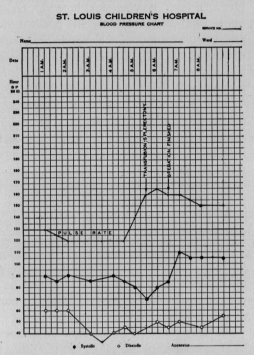

CHART 5.—SEVERE INTRA-ABDOMINAL HEMORRHAGE FOLLOWING A TRAUMATIC LACERATION OF THE SPLEEN IN A FOUR-YEAR-OLD GIRL.

Note the early fall of diastolic pressure; a recurrent hemorrhage apparently began at about 2 A.M. There was a further drop in the red cell count of nearly a million between this time and the time of operation. Note the prompt rise of systolic blood pressure following transfusion. The spleen at laparotomy was completely torn across; it was removed. Recovery was uneventful.

7. Operations in the Presence of Shock.—In general, operation is usually contraindicated at least until the shock is partially relieved, because the added trauma of the operation and the effects of the anesthesia will add greatly to the severity of the shock. Nevertheless, operation is sometimes necessary to stop hemorrhage which threatens life. Thus, immediate operation is often indicated to stop occult bleeding which has failed, or we know will fail, to cease spontaneously or following the use of conservative measures, and when death from shock is threatened by further delay. The operation, however, must offer some assurance that the bleeding can be controlled; this is usually possible in certain lesions such as ruptured ectopic pregnancy, postoperative hemorrhage, gunshot or stab wounds of the abdomen and rupture of the spleen. The possibility of actually using some or all of the escaped blood by collecting it and re-introducing it into the circulation (refusion, autotransfusion) adds to the advantages of the operation. The danger of operation as a factor in increasing shock may be minimized by choosing an anesthetic which will not increase anoxia (see page 250); intravenous therapy should be instituted before and during the operation. Spinal anesthesia, because it produces a fall of blood pressure itself, is generally contraindicated in shock. Delay in operation is indicated when there is likelihood of spontaneous cessation of the hemorrhage. When the site of the hemorrhage is such as to make control of the bleeding point difficult or impossible, operation is rarely advisable. Moreover, with adequate conservative treatment many patients bleeding from occult sources (*e.g.,* peptic ulcer, esophageal varices) will recover without operation. On the other hand, if an emergency operation is indicated for a perforated viscus, delay of more than an hour or two is rarely justified. Although amputation of a severely crushed limb was formerly performed to prevent shock, it has been shown to be unjustifiable for this reason except in unusual instances (see Chapter XI). In most cases conservatism will conserve life as well as limb.

8. Oxygen.—In so far as anoxia occurs in shock, inhalation of oxygen may be of some therapeutic value. On the other hand the arterial blood is usually saturated normally in surgical shock. Nevertheless, in certain cases oxygen inhalations have proved beneficial whether respiratory difficulties are present or not. The gas is given in high concentration (95 per cent with 5 per cent CO_2) under a tight tent or through a mask. The effect of oxygen inhalations in experimental shock has been well studied by Wood, Mason and Blalock.[29]

BIBLIOGRAPHY

1. BLALOCK, A. *Principles of Surgical Care; Shock and Other Problems,* C. V. Mosby Co., St. Louis, 1940.
2. FREEMAN, N. E. Hemorrhage in Relation to Shock: Experimental Effect of Intravenous Injections of Saline, Gum Acacia, and Blood on the Rate of Adrenal Secretion Resulting from Hemorrhage, *Ann. Surg.,* 101:484, 1935.
3. CATTELL, M. The Action of Ether on the Circulation in Traumatic Shock, *Arch. Surg.,* 6:41, 1923.
4. WIGGERS, C. F. The Pathologic Physiology of the Circulation During Hemorrhage, *Arch. Int. Med.,* 14:33, 1914.
5. CANNON, W. B., and CATTELL, M. Studies in Experimental Traumatic Shock: The Critical Level in a Falling Blood Pressure, *Arch. Surg.,* 4:301, 1922.
6. CANNON, W. B. *Traumatic Shock,* D. Appleton & Co., New York, 1923, p. 41.

7. UNDERHILL, F. P., *et al.* Blood Concentration Changes in Extensive Superficial Burns, and Their Significance for Systemic Treatment, *Arch. Int. Med.*, 32:31, 1923.

8. KEITH. Quoted by Cannon, *loc. cit.*, p. 35.

9. CANNON, W. B. *Loc. cit.*, p. 54.

10. ELMAN, R. Acute Hypoproteinemia Following a Single Severe Hemorrhage in the Fasting Dog, *Am. J. Physiol.*, 128:332, 1940.

11. BURTON-OPITZ, R. The Functional Capacity of the Heart During Hemorrhage, *J. Am. M. Ass.*, 78:1377, 1922.

12. WIGGERS, C. F. *Loc. cit.*

13. SEELIG, M. G., and LYON, E. P. The Condition of the Peripheral Blood Vessels in Shock, *J. Am. M. Ass.*, 52:45, 1909.

14. CANNON, W. B. *The Wisdom of the Body*, Chapter 2, The Safe-guarding of an Effective Fluid Matrix, W. W. Norton Co., New York, 1932.

15. PARSONS, E., and PHEMISTER, D. B. Hemorrhage and Shock in Traumatized Limbs, *Surg., Gynec. & Obst.*, 51:196, 1930.

16. BLALOCK, A. Experimental Shock: Cause of Low Blood Pressure Produced by Muscle Injury, *Arch. Surg.*, 20:959, 1930.

17. FREEDLANDER, S. O., and LENHART, C. H. Traumatic Shock, *Arch. Surg.*, 25:693, 1932.

18. BLALOCK, A. Trauma to the Intestine, *Arch. Surg.*, 22:314, 1931.

19. BLALOCK, A. Experimental Shock: the Importance of the Local Loss of Fluid in the Production of the Low Blood Pressure after Burns, *Arch. Surg.*, 22:610, 1931.

20. CANNON, W. B. *Traumatic Shock*, D. Appleton & Co., New York, 1923, p. 137.

21. FREEMAN, N. E. Decrease in Blood Volume after Prolonged Hyperactivity of the Sympathetic Nervous System, *Am. J. Physiol.*, 103:185, 1933.

22. LANDIS, E. M. The Effect of Lack of Oxygen on the Permeability of the Capillary Wall to Fluid and to the Plasma Proteins, *Am. J. Physiol.*, 83:528, 1928.

23. GRAY, H., and LUNT, L. K. Factors Affecting the Coagulation Time of the Blood: Effects of Hemorrhage before and after Exclusion of Abdominal Circulation, Adrenals or Intestines, *Am. J. Physiol.*, 34:332, 1914.

24. AMBERSON, W. R. Blood Substitutes, *Biological Rev.*, 12:48, 1937.

25. STRUMIA, M. M., WAGNER, J. A., and MONAGHAN, J. F. Intravenous Use of Serum and Plasma, Fresh and Preserved, *Ann. Surg.*, 111:623, 1940.

26. MUDD, S., *et al.* Preservation and Concentration of Human Serum for Clinical Use, *J. Am. M. Ass.*, 107:956, 1936.

27. FLOSDORF, E. W., STOKES, F. J., and MUDD, S. The Desivac Process for Drying from the Frozen State, *J. Am. M. Ass.*, 115:1095, 1940.

28. SCUDDER, John. *Shock; Blood Studies as a Guide to Therapy*, J. B. Lippincott Co., Phila., 1940.

29. WOOD, G. O., MASON, M. F., and BLALOCK, A. Studies on Effects of Inhalation of High Concentration of Oxygen in Experimental Shock, *Surgery*, 8:247, 1940.

30. WIGGERS, C. J. The Present Status of the Shock Problem, *Physiol. Rev.*, 22:74, 1942.

31. HARKINS, H. N. Recent Advances in the Study and Management of Traumatic Shock, *Surg.*, 9:231, 1941.

32. SWINGLE, W. W., PARKINS, W. and REMINGTON, J. W. *Am. J. Physiol.*, 134:503, 1941.

33. BLALOCK, A., and MASON, M. F. A Comparison of the Effects of Heat and Those of Cold in the Prevention and Treatment of Shock, *Arch. Surg.*, 42:1054, 1941.

CHAPTER XIV

THERMAL, CHEMICAL AND ELECTRICAL TRAUMA

Thermal Burns
Chemical Burns
Heat Stroke and Heat Exhaustion

Injuries due to Cold
X-ray and Radium Burns
The Effects of Electricity

THERMAL BURNS

There are many kinds of burns including those due to the sun (sunburn), hot water, oil and steam (scalds), mechanical friction and flames. Sunburn, unless a very large area of the body is involved, is of clinical importance only in that it is frequently very painful and in some cases may be associated with sunstroke as discussed on page 280. Though blistering may occur, the sun rarely provokes necrosis or infection. Its treatment, therefore, consists of the local application of soothing lotions, powders or ointments to ease the pain which, however, is rarely of more than two or three days' duration. Burns resulting from hot water, oil, flames and steam, on the other hand, are usually serious because they produce necrosis of tissue. Their seriousness depends also upon the extent and depth of the burn.

Pathology of Burns.—The changes in the body induced by burns are local and systemic and depend, of course, on their severity.

1. *Local effects of burns* are described according to their depth and the extent of the body surface involved. In estimating the area involved it is useful to remember that the lower extremities comprise 38 per cent, the trunk and neck 38 per cent, the upper extremities 18 per cent and the head 6 per cent of the entire body surface (Berkow [1]). The extent of skin involved should be recorded if possible; prognosis as to life depends to a large degree on the proportion of the body involved. It is generally considered that a burn involving over 50 per cent of the body surface, even though superficial, is incompatible with life. With deeper burns a fatal outcome may result even if only one-third or less of the body is affected. As to the depth and degree of injury to the skin, burns are classified into three groups. (In parts of Europe the six groups of Dupuytren are used.) *First degree* burns show merely a hyperemia of the skin, *i.e.,* injury but no necrosis. The inflammatory reaction, while intense, is mild and rapidly subsides producing at most a desquamation of the outer skin layer, and some pigmentation. However, if a large part of the body is affected (over one-half), systemic effects are almost sure to follow promptly. *Second degree* burns are evident by actual blister formation and more or less necrosis of the outer layers. The inflammatory reaction is, of course, more marked and is frequently followed by infection of the necrotic tissue. Although the

germinative layer of the skin is destroyed, new epithelium rapidly grows out from the cells lining the many hair follicles and sweat glands, producing a blemish but no real scar. *Third degree* burns produce unmistakable necrosis of all layers of the skin and frequently involve underlying structures. This is usually evident by the gray coagulated appearance of the burned skin which in some cases may even be black or charred. The inflammatory reaction which follows is, of course, more marked and may be associated with severe suppuration. Ultimately the dead tissue loosens and is sloughed off, leaving a defect which fills in with granulations, and slowly becomes covered with new epithelium which, as mentioned before, does not

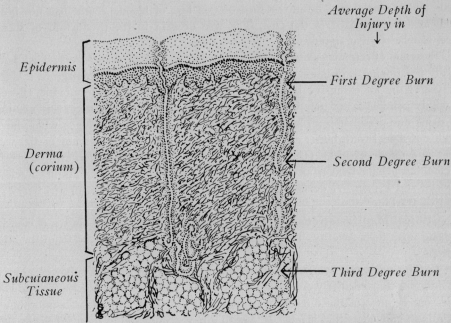

FIG. 141.—DIAGRAM OF A CROSS SECTION OF NORMAL SKIN SHOWING THE LAYERS INJURED IN THE VARIOUS TYPES OF BURNS.

have the resistance of normal skin. The granulation tissue, moreover, is always excessive, so that healing is followed by a prominent scar.

2. *The systemic effects* of burns are always prominent and serious when much skin is involved, and is often the direct primary cause of death in the fatal cases. These effects develop within a few hours and may persist for several days; their clinical manifestations are described below.

There is considerable dispute as to the pathogenesis of these systemic effects. Two general theories are current, one physical, the other chemical; the former concerns the loss of plasma into the burned area producing shock, the latter postulates the existence of a toxin in the burned area which is absorbed producing toxemia. The present authors are convinced that the early systemic effects of burns are in most instances due to the physical changes due to fluid losses, although they admit that "toxic" manifestations may be produced by absorption from autolyzed or infected moist necrotic skin. In contrast to the toxic theory, the changes due to fluid loss rest on well confirmed observations. The fluid loss leads to hemo-concentration and fall in blood volume; peripheral circulatory impairment (shock) then occurs. The mechanism of shock has been discussed in the preceding chapter. It is probable that the fluid lost into the extensive burned area is almost pure plasma. The composition of the blister fluid in burns is approximately that of blood plasma (McIver [2]) and is similar to that lost in mechanically traumatized tissue (Beard and Blalock [3]), *i.e.,* the fluid part of whole blood. Evidence of such loss of plasma is indicated by the relatively normal content of blood protein in spite of the extreme concentration of the blood as shown by the very high values for the red cells and hemoglobin. The importance of this loss of blood protein has not been sufficiently emphasized in the past. The role of pain in the production of shock may also be of great significance.

Systemic effects may possibly be due in part to loss of skin *per se*. That normally functioning skin is essential to life has long been known. Damage to a large part of it by an extensive burn may of itself result in serious systemic effects. Another possible factor may be the production of adrenal insufficiency. Suppression of urine due presumably to kidney damage also occurs. Other changes which have been noted in severe burns are splanchnic congestion, cloudy swelling of the viscera and duodenal ulcer (Curling's ulcer). The changes which occur in experimental burns have been reported by Underhill, Kapsinow and Fisk,[4] and by Keeley, Gibson and Pijoan.[5] A detailed and extensive review of the literature in burns is that of Harkins.[6]

Clinical Manifestations.—Clinical manifestations produced by burns obviously depend upon their severity. They may be divided arbitrarily into the following five groups:

1. *The subjective symptoms* are relatively few in number. *Pain,* however, may be prominent particularly in first degree burns. In the severe cases the patient cries out because of the intense pain, until relieved by a large dose of morphine. Pain is so immediate that it must be due to direct stimulation of the pain fibers and not to inflammation. A second symptom of importance in many patients is intense *thirst* which remains a prominent manifestation for some time even when vomiting occurs. *Vomiting* is not a primary symptom in most cases but usually develops on the second day; it is not always relieved by administration of saline as has been often stated.

2. *The systemic manifestations* of burns may be surprisingly few at the onset of the disease, particularly after pain is relieved. The blood pressure may be low but is frequently unchanged; the pulse, while fast, subsides rapidly after the injection of morphine. The temperature is usually elevated. In the severe burns in which death occurs within twelve to twenty-four hours the patient develops rapidly increasing coma, often with irrational behavior and a sharp increase in pulse and temperature. Abnormal respirations may also occur in such severe burns. If extensive infection occurs, the patient will exhibit many of the manifestations of septicemia.

Complete anuria may occur after extensive burns, but usually only after several days; it is accompanied by the usual manifestations of uremia and a fatal outcome may be expected. Even when true uremia does not develop there is nearly always a marked diminution in the urinary output, in spite of a large fluid intake. This may be due to the loss of plasma protein (see p. 271) since it is often associated with a superficial edema, which is benefited by intravenous injections of gum acacia or plasma. Indeed, urinary output often increases sharply following a large plasma transfusion.

3. *The local lesions* of burns have already been described. The extent as well as the depth of the burn is often difficult to estimate from mere inspection. Unless there is an actual coagulation of tissue or charring, it may be impossible to tell which part of the skin will actually become necrotic. The history is of some value in that burns due to the actual flame, especially when the clothes have caught fire, are nearly always deeper than scalds. Since blistering in itself may be produced by superficial injury its presence cannot be used as an indication of the depth of the necrosis. Doubtless much of the variability observed in the clinical outcome of apparently equally serious and similarly treated burns, is due to this fact. In a few days, of course, a line of demarcation forms between the viable and necrotic skin, and eventually the thickness of the slough reveals the depth of the burn. It should be stated, however, that application of tannic acid frequently indicates the line of demarcation between living and dead skin, since the viable tissue will not take the tan (see p. 272). Regardless, however, of the degree of injury, signs of inflammation are soon observed, unless they have been minimized or obviated by the therapeutic measures instituted. Later the dead skin sloughs or is removed. In third degree burns in which all the derma has ben destroyed a granulating defect remains presenting the usual features of an ulcer.

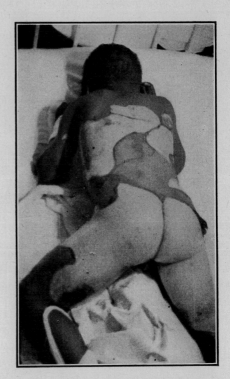

FIG. 142.—SEVERE ACUTE BURNS.

Photograph taken immediately after the patient, aged 8, entered the hospital. The burn was extensive, involving over 60 per cent of the body and was sustained by scalding hot water. The local treatment consisted of moderate cleansing and a compression bandage. In spite of the administration of 750 c.c. of plasma and a fall in the red blood count from 6.7 to 4.8 million, this patient died 36 hours after admission.

4. *Laboratory study* has shown, as already suggested, a number of important changes in extensive burns. A complete study was reported by McIver [2]. He found increases in the erythrocyte count as high as 7,000,000 per c.mm.; the present authors have noted counts above 8,000,000. A leukocytosis is also present, usually as high as 20,000, but even higher in the fatal cases, *i.e.*, 70,000 cells per c.mm. The higher white cell counts, particularly those above 25,000, are in general a bad

prognostic sign. Early plasma protein values may be normal, which, in the presence of hemoconcentration really means an actual loss of plasma, inasmuch as high values follow hemoconcentration from loss of water alone. Nevertheless, hypoproteinemia soon develops (see Fig. 144) usually affecting the albumin fraction (see Fig. 143). The nonprotein nitrogen of the blood may exhibit a transient rise, but increases progressively with persistent anemia.

5. *Later manifestations* are serious, but fortunately occur only in fairly extensive full thickness burns in which there is a complete loss of skin. To a certain extent many of these later manifestations are due to extensive suppuration and the

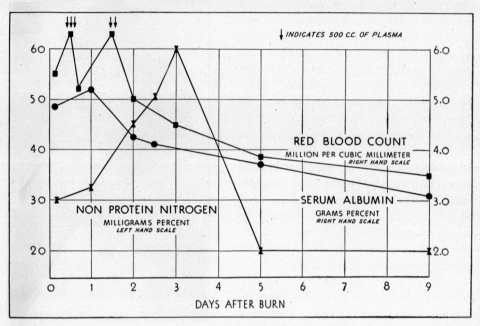

FIG. 143.—BLOOD CHANGES IN A SEVERE BURN.

The patient was a 45 year old female whose clothes caught fire; she sustained a third degree burn of about 40% of the body. Note the complete correction of hemoconcentration following transfusion of 2500 c.c. of plasma and the fall below normal, in spite of this, of the serum albumin. Note also the rise and fall of the non-protein nitrogen.

clinical manifestations are similar to those produced by suppuration from any other cause. Sooner or later, however, with adequate local treatment, necrotic tissue separates and the patient is prepared for skin grafting.

Too often skin grafting is delayed for weeks and months because of the poor general condition of the patient; yet with the passage of time the general condition may deteriorate rather than improve. In many instances this deterioration is based on extreme malnutrition due to a combination of anorexia and increased nitrogen loss from the excessive tissue protein destruction [27, 28]. These manifestations may be prevented to a large extent by special and early attention to the caloric and particularly the protein intake. As much as 2 or 3 grams of protein per kilogram of body weight a day may be required to avoid or minimize the severe protein deficiency which is sure to occur otherwise (see also page 152).

Treatment.—Treatment of burns, regardless of variations in local applications is based on the same fundamental principles which aim, first, to lower mortality, second, to avoid infection, and third, to shorten disability and healing. Systemic therapy, because it is designed to lower mortality, rightly demands rigid priority.

1. *Systemic treatment* aims to combat shock and hemoconcentration particularly with plasma transfusions and to control pain, when present, particularly with morphine. If pain is severe, one-half grain of morphine may be required (part intravenous) except in the presence of pulmonary complications (see page 1041).

In order to reduce early mortality in severe burns the prompt use of large plasma transfusions is essential. Intravenous injections of water, electrolyte and glucose alone are inadequate and indeed may even prove deleterious, unless urinary output is sufficient, because generalized edema may be produced thereby. This is similar to "salt edema" and emphasizes the importance of loss of plasma into the burned area as described on page 268, producing hypoproteinemia, which requires plasma for its correction (Elman [7]).

Plasma transfusions in burns must be adequate in amount, must have rigid priority over local therapy, and must often be given rapidly, with a syringe if necessary. As much as 4000 c.c. of whole plasma may be required in an extensive burn, *i.e.*, 25 c.c. per pound of body weight. The amount depends on the degree of the burn and of hemoconcentration. A rough though liberal rule is 1000 c.c. for each 10 per cent of the body surface burned above 5 per cent. Actually in most severe burns a liter is used to start with and repeated as

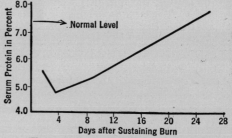

FIG. 144.—SERUM PROTEIN IN A SEVERE BURN.

Note the low value which developed during the first few days, and the slow increase back to normal, requiring nearly four weeks.

indicated by the clinical response. Improvement of the sensorium, of the circulation, and of the urinary output are favorable signs. On the other hand, anuria, a rise in the red cell count, etc., call for more plasma. Whole blood may be used in the absence of plasma and, when anemia is present, is, of course, preferable. Reassurance and psychotherapy are especially necessary in order to sustain the patient's morale in large third degree burns; the importance of a high protein and caloric diet must also be re-emphasized. Adrenal cortical extracts have been used [26].

2. *Immediate local treatment* in small first degree burns consists merely of the relief of pain by some bland ointment, as protection against air. First aid consists of sedation plus protection of the burned area with a sterile dressing preferably over a water-soluble jelly. The dead skin over blisters is not removed.

In the local treatment of burned skin the general principles for the care of any traumatic wound should apply. Although burns, because of the heat, are sterile at the time of injury, they usually become rapidly contaminated, in many cases by the application of some bacteriologically dirty home remedy. Unless a burn is seen at once, therefore, it must be considered contaminated. If seen after 24 hours or if infection is obvious, burned skin should be treated as an open infected wound.

In severe burns seen within a few hours after the accident, a variety of local treatments are available, dependent somewhat on the extent of the burn. (*a*) Cleansing, especially when charred clothing, etc., is adherent to the burned skin, is performed so carefully and painlessly that a general anesthetic should rarely be required. If it is, intravenous pentothal sodium is preferable. Scrubbing is avoided; gentleness is extremely important. (*b*) Tannic acid has been used extensively ever since it was advocated by E. C. Davidson in 1925. As used at the present time it is applied, after thorough cleansing, in a spray with an atomizer as a 10 per cent solution alternating with 10 per cent silver nitrate solution; a dry, black crust forms almost at once. This method is rapid and convenient; pain, after the initial application, is relieved promptly, and frequent dressings become unnecessary. This treatment has no effect on normal skin and thus indicates rather clearly the line of demarkation of the burn. As to infection, dry coagulated tissue apparently is less easily invaded by bacteria; although suppuration may occur even when preceded by adequate cleansing, it is usually confined to the edges of the burned skin along areas which have not been adequately tanned. Rapid coagulation also has the advantage of halting the loss of plasma from weeping surfaces and may also minimize

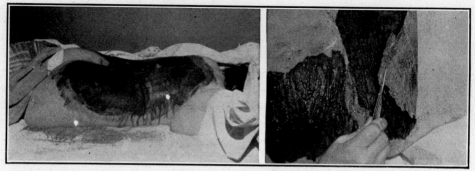

FIG. 145.—SECOND DEGREE (PART THICKNESS) BURN.

The patient, a 28 year old woman, 7 months pregnant, sustained a burn of her back when her clothes caught fire. The burned area was cleansed and coagulated rapidly with tannic acid and silver nitrate. The photograph on the left was taken just as she returned from the operating room; note the line of demarkation over the right buttock. The photograph on the right was taken 15 days later when most of the crust was removed.

absorption of toxic material from moist, necrotic skin, the latter being the original basis upon which Davidson recommended this treatment. Rapid coagulation with tannic acid and silver nitrate is particularly valuable in burns of the torso. However, slow methods of tanning, especially with tannic acid jelly, are not recommended. Aldrich [9] has introduced solutions of gentian violet and other aniline dyes which also produce a dry crust over the burned skin. (*c*) If the burned areas are not tanned but bandaged, elastic compression should be applied to minimize edema and loss of plasma into the tissues [30]. Vaseline gauze, saline compresses or a sulfonamide cream is usually applied under the dressings. This method is particularly convenient in burns of the extremities; a plaster splint in addition achieves excellent immobilization. It must be emphasized, however, that *infrequent dressing* is an important principle in order to avoid the danger of secondary contamination which may occur whenever a large open wound is exposed. Once an efficient dressing is applied, it should not be changed for a week or more except when definitely indicated. (*d*) The sulfonamides (see page 35) have been used widely in the treatment of burns both locally and systemically. Because of the danger of absorption from large burned surfaces, the amount of drug applied locally must not exceed 10 grams. The internal use is advisable and in doses of 4 to 6 grams a day. (*e*) Although exposure to dry heat is an old accepted procedure, usually by means of a cradle equipped with electric light bulbs, this procedure may do more harm than good [29] (see also discussion on p. 260). A tent to protect dressings is permissible. (*f*) Immersion in a bath of warm physiological saline is a time-honored method for the treatment of burns and is undoubtedly an effective procedure in certain deep third degree burns or more superficial extensive burns which have, for one reason or another, developed considerable infection.

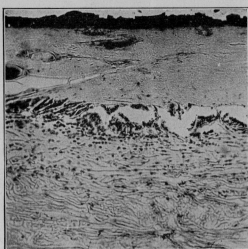

Tannic Acid Crust

Depth of Derma Killed by the Burn

Inflammatory Zone Demarcating Viable and Killed Derma

Viable Derma

FIG. 146.—PHOTOMICROGRAPH OF A SECOND DEGREE BURN IN A YOUNG WOMAN, WHO DIED FORTY-EIGHT HOURS AFTER THE ACCIDENT.

Note the superficial extent of the tannic crust and the thickness of the dead but uncoagulated derma.

Such immersion is often gratefully enjoyed by the patient, eases removal of adherent dressings and serves to wash away purulent discharge and débris, thereby aiding epithelialization and healing. Immersion is alternated with periods during which the wound is exposed to air under a tent without dressing (Blair, Brown and Hamm [10]). This method requires much nursing care; it is used after the acute stage is over, especially in preparation for skin grafting.

3. *Treatment of defects* produced by third degree burns presents a special problem in therapy because nature's spontaneous efforts are often faulty. This is due to the fact that the scar which replaces the lost dermis contains no elastic fibers, no sebaceous or sweat glands and that the new epithelium produces little keratin. Moreover, scar is deposited so densely under the new epithelium that contraction frequently results. Deformities due to contraction of scar tissue *cannot* be prevented by holding the part in a natural position forcibly with splints, traction, etc. If it is apparent that natural healing will produce such an end result, skin grafting should be carried out as soon as healthy clean granulations have formed, and the

general condition of the patient permits. Once the defect has healed completely, any deformity, including cosmetic blemishes, may be corrected by excision of the scar and application of a skin graft, the type of which is determined by various indications which are discussed below. Another disadvantage in the spontaneous

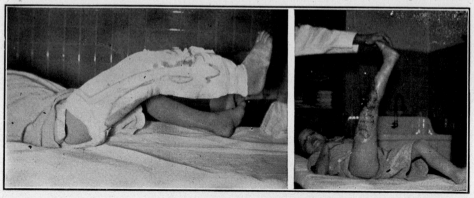

FIG. 147.—MODERATE SECOND AND THIRD DEGREE BURN OF THE RIGHT LEG.

The patient, aged 6, sustained a burn of the right leg when his clothing caught fire. After cleansing, a bulky compression bandage was applied and the leg immobilized with a plaster splint. The photograph on the left shows the dressing on the 10th day; note evidence of exudation, which has soaked through to the outside. On the right is the leg after removal of dressing; the burned area is clean and uninfected, and eventually healed without skin grafting.

healing of deep burns without the use of skin grafts is the long period required for final healing. Healing may be delayed because of the large granulating area to be covered by new epithelium, but it may also be partly due to an actual slowing

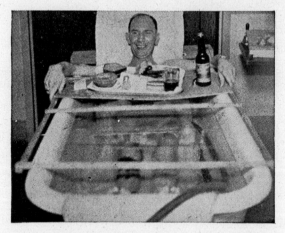

FIG. 148.—PATIENT IN A DAILY SALINE BATH.
(From Brown and Blair, *Surg., Gynec., & Obst.,* 1935; 60:380.)

up of the healing process due to a slight injury to the adjacent, though viable, epithelium from which regeneration occurs. Regardless of the reason for such delayed healing, application of skin grafts to the granulating area is frequently advisable in order to shorten the period of disability. It should be mentioned, however, that grafts applied to such a granulating defect should be of the split thickness type, since a full thickness graft will not "take" in the presence of even slight infection.

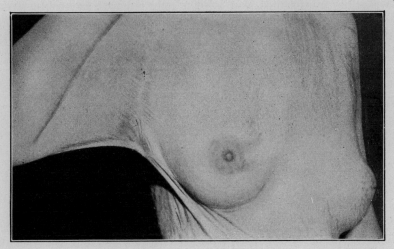

FIG. 149.—CONTRACTURE OF AXILLARY SKIN FOLLOWING THE HEALING OF AN EXTENSIVE BURN IN A NINETEEN-YEAR-OLD GIRL.

The burn was sustained ten years previously. Limitation of abduction of the arm is shown; complete mobility resulted after a plastic repair with skin graft.

Skin Grafting.—Transplantation of skin is one of the most widely used procedures in plastic surgery. As indicated above, it is particularly important in third-

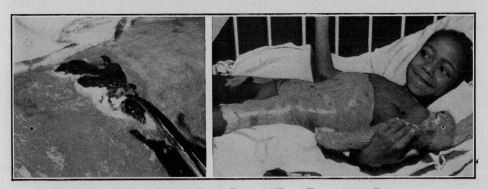

FIG. 150.—EXTENSIVE THIRD-DEGREE (FULL THICKNESS) BURN.

The patient, aged 6, was burned when her clothes caught fire. She received over 1000 c.c. of plasma during the first 3 days; the burned skin was cleansed and coagulated by tannic acid and silver nitrate. Note in the close-up photograph on the left, taken at 4 weeks, the remaining islands of necrotic skin; the clamp is lifting the thin, black, coagulated surface from the thick layer of white necrotic skin beneath. Note also the vaselined fine mesh gauze used to cover granulations. In the photograph on the right, six days later, i.e., 34 days after the accident, the dead skin had all come away, showing relatively healthy granulations.

degree burns. While belonging to a special branch of surgery, some of the simpler methods can be performed without great difficulty. Skin transferred from one part of the body to another part is called an autoplastic or homoplastic graft. Skin transferred from one individual to another of the same species is an isoplastic graft; it is not permanently successful except in identical twins.[11] A *free graft* is one in which the transplanted skin is completely removed and transferred to its new location. If the graft, though attached to its new bed, still retains a connection with its original site, the transplant is called a *pedicle graft* or *flap*. As soon as the flap establishes vascular connections with the new bed, the pedicle is cut and the transplantation is complete. This method of transplantation was used 400 years ago by Tagliacozzi.[12] It is used now in more difficult cases when thick or massive grafts are needed. The various types of free grafts may be classified as follows:

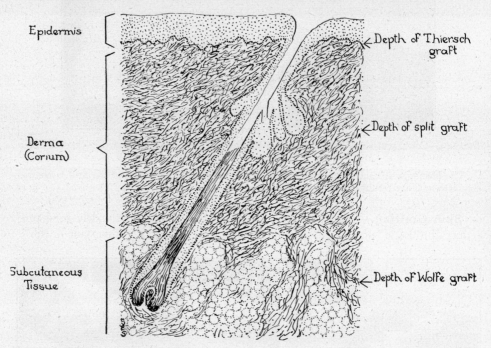

Epidermis

← Depth of Thiersch graft

Derma (Corium)

← Depth of split graft

Subcutaneous Tissue

← Depth of Wolfe graft

FIG. 151.—DIAGRAM OF A CROSS SECTION OF NORMAL SKIN SHOWING THE APPROXIMATE DEPTH AT WHICH THE VARIOUS TYPES OF SKIN GRAFT ARE CUT.

1. REVERDIN (PINCH) GRAFT.—Free transplantation of skin was first performed by Reverdin,[13] a Swiss surgeon who removed tiny pieces of skin (2 to 4 millimeters in diameter) from one part of the body and placed them over the granulating defect. The method is still in wide use and can be easily and simply done. This method, however, is cosmetically imperfect and in many clinics has been replaced by the grafting of larger areas of skin. Another name associated with skin grafting is that of Ollier,[14] who increased the size of the graft to many centimeters (as much as 8 centimeters in diameter) and advocated using a thicker layer of skin. The "small deep graft" as described by J. S. Davis [15] is similar to, but deeper than a pinch graft.

2. THIERSCH GRAFT.—This term, now infrequently used, is of historical interest because Thiersch [16] was a pioneer in skin grafting and described the use of the razor to remove large thin sheets of skin which he said included only part of the

germinative layer, but left enough for regeneration to occur. It is probable, however, that all of the papillae and some derma were removed.

3. THE SPLIT GRAFT.—As described and used by Blair and Brown [17] this is a modification of the Thiersch graft and represents a great improvement, because the greater thickness results in a graft which is not only more resistant to injury, but presents a more normal appearance. This graft is cut deep enough (with a long sharp knife) to include all the epithelial layers and part of the derma. The regeneration which occurs so readily at the site of the removed skin takes place by growth of the epithelial cells in the hair follicles and sweat glands just as it

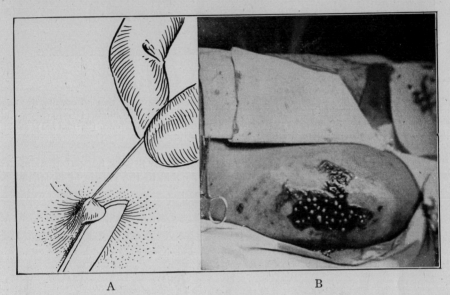

A   B

FIG. 152.—PINCH OR REVERDIN GRAFTS.

A, method of removing the graft; a portion of derma is obviously included at the center of the removed skin; *B*, appearance of wound after the grafts are placed. Pinch grafts have the advantage of simplicity and ease of performance but lack the perfection of the other types.

does in the case of second degree burns. The grafts are cut slightly larger than the defect and overlapped. The edges are anchored by a continuous stitch and numerous perforations are made in the graft in order to prevent accumulation of fluid under it. Firm pressure must be maintained (preferably with a marine sponge) over the graft for several days. The split graft is especially applicable in the treatment of ulcers produced by burns or any destructive process (traumatic or infective) as soon as the infection has been converted to a minimum. Grafts of consistent and any desired thickness may be cut with a calibrated dermatome (Padgett [18]).

4. WOLFE [12] GRAFT.—This is a full thickness graft including all of the derma, but the graft is cut carefully (with a scalpel) so that no fatty or areolar tissue remains on the under surface. Such a graft will not live when transplanted to a base where any significant infection is present. It cannot, therefore, be applied to a chronic ulcer, but is especially useful in covering raw surfaces produced by excision of healed scars. It is especially useful in correcting facial deformities due to contrac-

ture. The scarred area must be thoroughly healed and all procedures, including the excision of the cicatrix, and transplantation of the graft must be done aseptically.

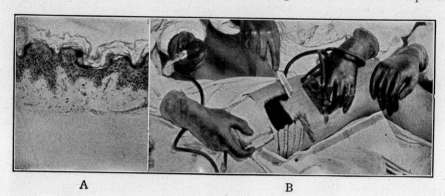

A   B

FIG. 153.—REMOVING A SPLIT SKIN GRAFT.

A, the thickness of the graft is shown in the photomicrograph; this represents the depth included in a split graft. *B,* technic of cutting skin graft from the thigh. (From Brown and Blair, *Surg., Gynec. & Obst.,* 1935; 60, 383.) A calibrated machine (dermatone) for the removal of split grafts has been invented by Padgett.[18]

The full thickness graft produces a skin surface more nearly normal than any of the other grafts and for this reason is very applicable in the repair of facial defects

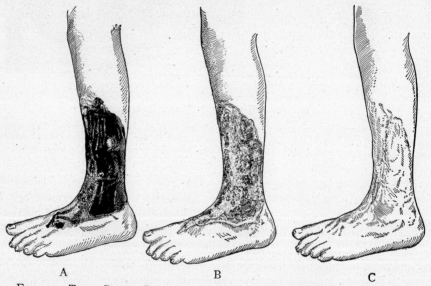

A   B   C

FIG. 154.—THIRD DEGREE BURN OF THE LEG IN A THIRTY-EIGHT-YEAR-OLD MAN.

A, condition after the application of silver nitrate and tannic acid; *B,* several weeks later after all the slough had separated, leaving healthy granulation tissue; *C,* three weeks later after application of a split graft.

where the color and appearance of the graft is an important feature. It is especially necessary that the graft be perforated and a pressure dressing applied, since greater care must be exercised in obtaining a "take" than with any other type of graft.

CHEMICAL BURNS

The accidental spilling of caustic alkali, acid, liquid bromine, etc., produces but a superficial injury of the skin provided the contact is momentary. However, the degree of necrosis may be severe if the corrosive chemical is not promptly removed. Once the tissues are killed the process of demarcation begins, and is often accompanied by infection. Ultimately a granulating ulcer is produced which gradually heals. Regeneration after chemical burns is slow and the spontaneous repair is apt to be considerably delayed.

Treatment.—The emergency measures are important, and if effective will minimize the degree of necrosis. Prompt application of large amounts of water to the affected skin in order to dilute the chemical is probably better than any attempt at neutralization by the application of antagonistic substance. Thus Davidson,[19] who has investigated the problem experimentally, found much less damage to the skin following the use of plain water than by any other material. The ready availability of water, moreover, also insures its prompt use.

Once the damage is done the care of the injured area is the same as that due to destruction of tissue by any other cause (see under Thermal Burns).

HEAT STROKE AND HEAT EXHAUSTION

Though associated with thermal trauma, these two diseases are chiefly of medical rather than surgical interest, except that patients (and also personnel) may develop serious symptoms due to the effects of heat during operations performed during hot weather. All patients should be observed carefully for evidence of heat exhaustion as well as heat stroke during severely hot weather; preventive measures such as insuring adequate fluid and sodium chloride intake, as well as special nursing care, should be provided. Of even more importance *in hot weather is the care of the patient in the operating room* during the operation itself; fatalities have been observed, due undoubtedly to the effects of excessive heat. It should be emphasized that during very hot weather particular care should be taken that no more sterile sheets be used over the patient than is absolutely necessary. Moreover, the patient must be watched with more than the usual care during the course of the operation, particularly for the development of tachycardia and other evidences of circulatory changes. If such changes are noted, the patient's temperature should be taken, and if it is unduly high, immediate measures must be instituted for its reduction. Such measures include the use of an electric fan which is made to blow over wet towels which cover as much of the body surface as is available (see p. 280). Air-conditioning in the operating room which is becoming fairly prevalent, solves this problem.

Patients with heat stroke are also of surgical interest because they are often brought into an emergency room and may, indeed, present a problem of differential diagnosis. Heat stroke and heat exhaustion are really quite different, though occasionally both may be present in the same patient. Ordinarily they are encountered under entirely different circumstances.

1. *Heat stroke* (thermic fever, sunstroke) is seen during hot summer months, especially when the temperature exceeds 100° F. (38° C.). The victims may lose consciousness, present a hot flushed skin, full rapid pulse and a high fever which may reach 110° F. (43.3° C.). There is obviously a disturbance of the heat regulating mechanism. Studies of the blood chemistry showed no marked changes in the patients treated at the St. Louis City Hospital during the hot summer of 1934. Treatment is urgent and consists of rapid, but careful, reduction of the fever. Immersion in an ice water bath is effective. The body temperature is carefully taken every few minutes and the patient removed when it has dropped to 102° F. (39° C.) ; the fall continues for some minutes. An efficient but slower method consists of covering the nude patient with wet sheets over which air from an electric fan is blowing.

2. *Heat exhaustion,* which in reality consists of severe dehydration and sodium chloride depletion, is met with ordinarily only in workmen confined to hot boiler rooms and in heavily clad marching soldiers, *i.e.,* when excessive perspiration occurs and when more fluid and salts are lost than are ingested. Under such conditions, McCord and Ferenbaugh,[20] state that "in 24 hours the loss from the body of chlorides approximates 20 grams—an amount that certainly may not be replaced by chlorides normally in food and drinks." Victims of heat exhaustion at the Boulder Dam construction were studied by Talbott and Michelsen [21] who found a pronounced reduction in the blood chlorides of these patients.

Clinically the symptoms come on gradually and include fatigue, cramps of muscles, and only in the worst cases severe prostration. Even then the picture is entirely different from heat stroke, *i.e.,* the temperature is normal or subnormal, although slight elevations were noted. The skin is moist, pale and cool and the pulse normal. Treatment consisting of administration of saline solution is specific. Heat exhaustion may be prevented by supplying sufficient water and sodium chloride (in the form of tablets) to individuals working under conditions producing excessive loss of body fluids through perspiration.

INJURIES DUE TO COLD

The systemic reactions to cold are those of profound shock and are produced only under conditions of extreme exposure which are relatively rare. More common are the local effects, usually on the extremities, nose and ears. These vary in degree from slight injury to gangrene. Permanent effects are also seen and are of great importance. A description of the diseases produced by cold is the classic monograph by Marchand.[22]

Tissue injury, short of actual necrosis, is probably the most frequent effect of cold. Nevertheless, such injury may by secondary factors lead to necrosis of tissue. The key to an understanding of those secondary factors is the vascular as well as cellular response to cold, particularly when the exposed part is brought into a warm atmosphere. The primary response to the injury produced by cold is, of course, the usual inflammatory changes already described. These changes, however, cannot occur at once because of the cellular paralysis and vasoconstriction which results from cold. Inflammation due to injury from cold can occur only when the temperature returns to normal, *i.e.*, when the chilled part is warmed. Vasodilatation and exudation then take place and may become so marked that vesicles appear in the skin just as if the part were burned. Much more serious may be the effect of cold on the veins and lymphatics (*i.e.*, thrombosis) which thus interferes with rapid drainage of fluid. Exudation thus leads to tremendous pressure and swelling in the inflamed area which may finally become great enough to occlude the arterial supply. As a final event actual gangrene may develop.

The various clinical types of injury due to cold are as follows: *chilblains* or pernio is a mild inflammatory reaction which develops after exposure to cold, especially damp cold, even when slight in degree. In its severe form, scaling of the skin may follow, and even a local patch of gangrene appear which finally heals.

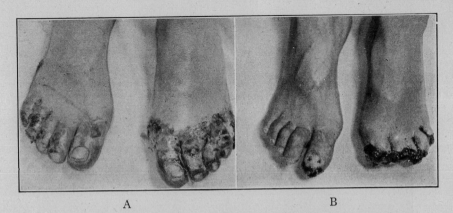

A   B

FIG. 155.—FROST-BITE OF THE TOES IN A THIRTY-YEAR-OLD MALE.

A, three days after exposure; note the marked inflammatory reaction. *B*, one month later, after spontaneous amputation of the dead tissue. The clean granulating surfaces rapidly epithelialized. Conservative therapy was used, *i.e.*, elevation, rest and heat.

Certain patients are particularly susceptible to chilblains after previous injury by cold. This may be due to the production of permanent alterations, vascular or neurogenic. *Trench foot* is a form of chilblains which was seen in soldiers whose feet are exposed to damp cold for many days. It is similar to "immersion foot" which is described on page 1066. Blistering, edema and areas of gangrene occur. Healing of these lesions was often prolonged. Such feet often showed more or less permanent disability due to inadequate blood supply and were especially susceptible to further injury from cold. *Frost-bite* is a term often applied to any injury due to cold. As used herein it refers to actual necrosis of tissue. Edema, blistering and (later) evidence of infection may precede the necrosis or gangrene which not infrequently develops; following this a line of demarcation forms and the dead part eventually sloughs off.

Treatment.—Of greatest importance is the prevention of necrosis by thawing out all frozen tissue *slowly*. While this may be achieved by the ancient and still popular practice of rubbing the part with snow or cold water such a procedure is *dangerous* because it frequently leads to mechanical injury of the frozen tissue which is friable and easily broken. Rapid and excessive vasodilation has been combated by the use of vasoconstrictive drugs (Lake [23]). Thomas Lewis suggested the use of a tourniquet or pneumatic cuff in patients with frozen extremities. If this is done the patient can be brought into a warm room and the pressure loosened from time to time to permit gradual return of the circulation without allowing it to produce excessive hyperemia and exudation. Of great prophylactic importance, too, is adequate protection against damp and cold, especially in susceptible individuals. The anesthetic effect of cold always makes it a treacherous injurious agent in that warning is thus impossible. Necrotic tissue is treated as if it were due to any other cause. Amputation is not ordinarily advisable early in the process unless severe infection supervenes; ordinarily the dead area sloughs off spontaneously. After the line of demarcation forms the rapidity with which the dead tissue is cast off may be accelerated by gentle operative procedures.

X-RAY AND RADIUM BURNS

Injurious effects of x-rays and radium are used therapeutically to destroy malignant or other neoplasms. Sometimes normal tissue is intentionally injured in order to achieve this end. Accidental or unintentional burns or injuries to skin by x-ray

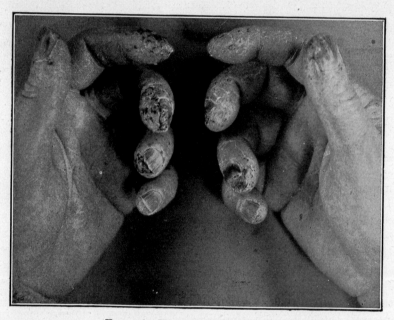

FIG. 156.—X-RAY BURN OF HANDS.

This lesion was produced by exposure to x-ray frequently and over a long period of time. Even though exposure is stopped the lesion may progress and go on to malignant degeneration. (From Deryl Hart in *Practitioners Library*, D. Appleton-Century Co.)

and radium did occur in the early days of radiotherapy and are still encountered after its inexpert use. The effects of x-ray injury are not evident immediately, but are manifested in about a week or ten days and consist of hyperemia, tanning and exfoliation. When serious lesions occur they develop later and consist of indolent ulcerations which do not heal, but tend to become malignant and lead finally to death. General effects of x-ray therapy also occur within a few hours following a treatment and produce a syndrome which is called roentgen sickness. Nausea and vomiting, asthenia and headache are complained of.

Treatment of the ulcerated lesion consists of excision and application of a skin graft. Obviously prophylaxis is most important; use of x-ray and radium should be confined to expert radiologists.

THE EFFECTS OF ELECTRICITY

An electric current which comes in contact with the skin produces reactions which vary widely, depending upon its method of introduction into the body, the voltage, amperage and kind of current (alternating or direct) and on the variety of alternation. Obviously, not all electric currents are damaging; many of them have beneficial therapeutic effects and are used in a variety of ways. In general the high voltage currents are the most deleterious.

Accidental electrical injuries may be local or general. The *local effects* occur at the site of entrance and exit of the current, and, depending on various factors, produce a superficial localized burn or a deep and extensive coagulation of tissue. The necrosis of tissue may be due to the heat generated by the passage of the current or to a direct effect of the current itself. Undoubtedly both factors play a role, for even if the local lesion is charred and resembles an ordinary burn it is apt to become indolent and heal very slowly, suggesting neurotrophic injury. The local lesions are treated as are burns due to any other cause. The extent of necrosis usually is apparent from the grayish color of the damaged skin.

The *general effects* of electricity are apt to occur only if the current passes through the central nervous system or heart. Langworthy [24] has studied two electrocuted criminals and found marked changes in the cells of the medullary center concerned with respiration. The clinical manifestations of electrical shock are in most cases due to respiratory paralysis. Unconsciousness and circulatory impairment may also be present (Wright [25]). Treatment is that of shock in general but in addition should include persistent artificial respiration, which should be continued for hours if the circulation is maintained. Obviously, if the medullary cells are merely injured, recovery is possible; if killed beyond repair, death is inevitable. Since evidence of cerebral edema has been noted, some recommend lumbar puncture and the intravenous injection of hypertonic solutions.

BIBLIOGRAPHY

1. BERKOW, S. G.   Method of Estimating Extensiveness of Lesions (Burns and Scalds) Based on Surface Area Proportions, *Arch. Surg.*, 8:138, 1924.
2. McIVER, M. A.   Study in Extensive Cutaneous Burns, *Ann. Surg.*, 97:670, 1933.
3. BEARD, J. W., and BLALOCK, A.   Experimental Shock: The Composition of the Fluid that Escapes from the Blood Stream after Mild Trauma to an Extremity, after Trauma to the Intestines, and after Burns, *Arch. Surg.*, 22:617, 1931.
4. UNDERHILL, F. P., KAPSINOW, R., and FISK, M. E.   Studies on the Mechanism of Water Exchange in the Animal Organism: The Nature and Effects of Superficial Burns, *Am. J. Physiol.*, 95:302, 1930.

5. KEELEY, J. L., GIBSON, J. G., and PIJOAN, M.   Effect of Thermal Trauma on Blood Volume, Serum Protein and Certain Blood Electrolytes, *Surgery*, 5:872, 1939.

6. HARKINS, H. N.   *The Treatment of Burns*, Chas. C. Thomas Co., 1942.

7. ELMAN, R.   The Therapeutic Significance of Plasma Protein Replacement in Severe Burns, *J. Am. M. Ass.*, 116:213, 1941. WEINER, D. O., ROWLETTE, A. P., and ELMAN, R. Significance of Loss of Serum Protein in Therapy of Severe Burns, *Proc. Soc. Exp. Biol. & Med.*, 34:484, 1936.

8. DAVIDSON, E. C.   Tannic Acid in the Treatment of Burns, *Surg., Gynec. & Obst.*, 41:202, 1925.

9. ALDRICH, R. H.   Treatment of Burns with Compounds of Aniline Dyes, *New England J. Med.*, 217:911, 1937.

10. BLAIR, V. P., BROWN, J. B., and HAMM, W. G.   The Early Care of Burns and the Repair of Their Defects, *J. Am. M. Ass.*, 98:1355, 1932.

11. BROWN, J. B.   Homografting of Skin: with Report of Success in Identical Twins, *Surgery*, 1:558, 1937.

12. TAGLIACOZZI, Quoted by WOLFE, J. R.   A New Method of Performing Plastic Operations, *Brit. M. J.*, 2:360, 1875.

13. REVERDIN, J. R.   De la Greffe Epidermique, *Arch. Gen. de Med.*, 129:276, 1872.

14. OLLIER, M.   Greffes Cutanées ou Autoplastiques, *Bull. de l'Acad. M.*, 1:243, 1872.

15. DAVIS, J. S.   *Plastic Surgery*, Blakiston, Philadelphia, 1919.

16. THIERSCH.   Ueber die feineren Anatomischen Veränderungen bei Aufheilung von Haut auf Granulationen, *Arch. f. Klin. Chir.*, 17:318, 1874.

17. BLAIR, V. P., and BROWN, J. B.   The Use and Uses of Large Split Skin Grafts of Intermediate Thickness, *Surg., Gynec. & Obst.*, 49:82, 1929.

18. PADGETT, E. C.   Calibrated Intermediate Skin Grafts, *Surg., Gynec. & Obst.*, 69:779, 1939.

19. DAVIDSON, E. C.   Treatment of Acid and Alkali Burns; Experimental Study, *Ann. Surg.*, 85:481, 1927.

20. McCORD, C. P., and FERENBAUGH, T. L.   Fatigue in Soldiers due to Chloride Losses: Replacement through the Use of Sodium Chloride in Drinking Water, *Milit. Surg.*, 69:608, 1931.

21. TALBOT, J. H., and MICHELSEN, J.   Heat Cramps, A Clinical and Chemical Study, *J. Clin. Invest.*, 12:533, 1933.

22. MARCHAND.   Die Kalte als Krankheitsurache, *Khehl u. Marchand's Handbook der Allg. Path.*, Vol. 1, 1908.

23. LAKE, N. C.   An Investigation into the Effects of Cold Upon the Body, *Lancet*, 2:557, 1917.

24. LANGWORTHY, O. R.   Nerve Cell Injury in Cases of Human Electrocution, *J. Am. M. Ass.*, 95:107, 1930.

25. WRIGHT, W.   *Cecil's Textbook of Medicine*, 3rd ed., W. B. Saunders, Philadelphia, 1927, p. 546.

26. RHOADS, J. E., WOLFF, W. A., and LEE, W. E.   The Use of Adrenal Cortical Extract in the Treatment of Traumatic Shock of Burns, *Ann. Surg.*, 113:955, 1941.

27. LUCIDO, J.   Metabolic and Blood Chemical Changes in a Severe Burn, *Ann. Surg.*, 111:640, 1940.

28. TAYLOR, F. H. L. et al.   Abnormal Nitrogen Metabolism in Burns, *Science*, 97:423, 1943.

29. ELMAN, R., COX, W. M., JR., LISCHER, C., and MUELLER, A. J.   Mortality in Severe Experimental Burns as Affected by Environmental Temperature, *Proc. Soc. Exper. Biol. & Med.*, 51:350, 1942.

30. ALLEN, H. S. and KOCH, S. L.   The Treatment of Patients with Severe Burns, *Surg., Gynec. & Obst.*, 74:914, 1942.

CHAPTER XV

THE EMERGENCY PROSTRATE PATIENT: COMA, UNCONSCIOUSNESS, DELIRIUM AND CONVULSIONS

General Consideration in the Examination
Intracranial Lesions
Physiochemical Coma

Prostration is a clinical manifestation of many different diseases although it is often incorrectly used to describe a specific pathologic state. The term is, in fact, a general one meaning merely a degree of illness which is so severe that it requires the patient, often involuntarily, to assume the prostrate or horizontal position. Prostration and collapse are often used to mean the same clinical state; neither term indicates the cause but merely the effect, indeed the most dramatic effect, of the illness. Thus a patient may be prostrated without being in surgical shock, although nearly all patients suffering from surgical shock are prostrated. Moreover, prostration is obviously produced by a host of diseases which are associated with sensorial dysfunction and especially with varying degrees of unconsciousness.

On admission to the emergency room the prostrate, more or less unconscious patient always presents a complicated diagnostic problem, the solution of which is often urgent, because of the necessity of instituting life-saving treatment. Superficially such a patient may present a similar clinical appearance whether he is suffering from traumatic shock, alcoholism, diabetic coma, concussion of the brain, uremia, etc. The absence of an adequate history and the inability of the patient to speak for himself, of course, add to the difficulty. Yet, though extended examinations are impossible, it is surprising how much information can be obtained by a few rapid, but systematic observations which in many cases will solve the mystery at once.

Great variations occur in the degree of sensorial depression manifested by these patients. There may be but slight impairment of consciousness, the patient lying prostrated and weak, but able to answer questions. More severe degrees of insensibility occur in which the patient will not respond to questions, but will react to ordinary painful stimuli. When there is no response to any sensory stimulation the term coma is ordinarily used. A comatose patient, while ordinarily quiet and immobile, may at the same time be restless or even exhibit convulsive movements. Delirium, too, may be a part of the clinical picture in this group of severely prostrated individuals. Detailed clinical studies of the differential diagnosis and care of comatose patients have been reported by Solomon and Aring [1] and by Greene [7].

Important in the diagnosis and treatment of such patients is the knowledge of the various diseases which are capable of producing more or less complete loss of consciousness and other evidence of sensorial dysfunction. While such an enumeration includes a great variety of conditions they can be classified, in general, into the following ten groups:

1. Cerebral damage: trauma, apoplexy, embolism, tumor, infection (meningitis and encephalitis), thermic fever.
2. Poisoning (by ingestion or inhalation) : alcohol (by far the most frequent cause), carbon monoxide, morphine, chloral, veronal, lead, mercury, ether, etc.
3. Uremia: Bright's disease, urinary obstruction (enlarged prostate, stone, etc.), pyelonephritis
4. Hyperglycemia (diabetes) or hypoglycemia
5. Circulatory shock: burns, hemorrhage, trauma, exposure, heart failure, cardiac tamponade
6. Psychosis: manic-depressive insanity, dementia praecox, senile dementia, epilepsy, hysteria, dementia paralytica
7. Asphyxia: drowning, respiratory obstruction, electricity, etc.
8. Dehydration: severe loss of fluid in vomiting, diarrhea or starvation, heat exhaustion
9. Toxemia: septicemia, late low intestinal obstruction, extensive gangrene, malignant malaria
10. Hepatic disease: severe jaundice, acute hepatic necrosis including acute yellow atrophy

Study of the many diseases and conditions listed above might suggest a division into traumatic and nontraumatic or surgical and medical groups. However, such a division is far from mutually exclusive. Thus a patient under medical treatment for gastric ulcer may have a sudden hemorrhage and present all the signs and symptoms of surgical shock such as that due to severe bleeding from a wound. On the other hand, an old man may have an apoplectic stroke and fall, yet be suspected of having a fractured skull. An accurate diagnosis as to the actual condition present is obviously important.

Based on etiology, it seems simpler to classify the above-mentioned causes of prostration into three groups:

1. *Circulatory shock* produces severe prostration; it may also cause cerebral symptoms which are not striking and are caused by the partial cerebral anemia due to the general circulatory impairment. This group has already been discussed in Chapter XIII.

2. *Intracranial lesions* produce more evident sensorial depression, often coma and convulsions, and sometimes restlessness or delirium. Such disturbances are due either to actual cerebral injury or more commonly to increased intracranial pressure from edema, hemorrhage, tumor or obstruction to outflow of cerebrospinal fluid.

3. *Physiochemical coma* comprises a group in which the mechanism is not circulatory, but due to physiological (functional) or chemical action on the cerebral

TABLE 5

The Emergency Prostrate Patient: Types and Differentiation *

	Shock	Intracranial Lesions	Physiochemical Diseases

Etiology	Primary
	  Hemorrhage
	  Trauma
	  Burns
	Contributory
	  Exposure, pain
	  General anesthesia, etc.
		Trauma to brain tissue and increased intracranial pressure; i.e., injury, hemorrhage, edema, tumor; infections	Poisoning, uremia, profound infections and toxemia, dehydration, hypo- and hyperglycemia, psychosis, asphyxia, hepatic disease

Pathogenesis	Low blood pressure due to low blood volume	Direct brain damage; cerebral anemia due to increased intracranial pressure	Toxic action on brain; abnormal cerebral function
Clinical Picture	1. Low blood pressure 2. Fast thready pulse 3. Respirations may be shallow; air hunger in hemorrhage 4. Subnormal temperature 5. Slight to moderate sensorial depression 6. Restlessness and thirst in hemorrhage 7. Pallor 8. Collapsed veins	1. Varied blood pressure 2. Full pulse; may be slow 3. Irregular respirations 4. Normal or elevated temperature 5. Coma, hyperactivity, convulsions 6. Pathologic neurological signs 7. Choked disk 8. If traumatic: scalp lacerations, fractured skull, etc. 9. Abnormal spinal fluid	1. Normal or high blood pressure 2. Full pulse; may be fast 3. Variable respirations (Cheyne-Stokes, air hunger, etc.) 4. Normal or elevated temperature 5. Deep coma, convulsions, delirium 6. Special signs as revealed by odor of breath, bladder dullness and rectal examination, urine and blood examination, etc.
Emergency Treatment	Control of hemorrhage, rest, warmth, sedatives, fluids, transfusion	Conservative reduction of increased pressure; operation (for middle meningeal hemorrhage, depressed fracture)	Gastric lavage, insulin, glucose, catheterization, fluids, artificial respiration, lumbar puncture, etc.

* It should be emphasized that the features listed above represent average data and must not be interpreted dogmatically.

cells by poisons introduced from the outside or intrinsically by perverted metabolism.

Further details concerning these three groups will be found in Table 5, which lists many of their pathologic and clinical differences. A more complete description of the second and third groups will be furnished after considering some general points in the physical examination of these prostrate patients.

GENERAL CONSIDERATIONS IN THE EXAMINATION

Delirium may be present alone or with a state resembling coma. Convulsions are not infrequent in certain comatose patients. Such hyperactivity is generally due to psychiatric or neurological diseases, but in alcoholics is frequently encountered after accidents which necessitate confinement to bed (delirium tremens). Severe infections of many types, especially when accompanied by high fever, are also a not infrequent cause of delirium and convulsions, especially in children.

It should be emphasized also that multiple lesions are often present in these patients. Thus an epileptic may fall during a fit and sustain a fractured skull, an alcoholic may also have nephritis, a nephritic with hypertension may have an apoplectic stroke, a tabetic may have an enlarged prostate, and psychiatric patients may swallow poison or injure themselves. As might be expected from the variety of diseases which may be present, adequate diagnosis implies rather complete clinical study. If treatment is not urgent this is often possible. The following description aims to include the most important clinical observations.

1. **General Appearance.**—Superficial observation should reveal first of all the presence of shock or asphyxia, since each requires prompt emergency treatment. Evidence of trauma such as torn clothes, lacerations (with or without active hemorrhage), blood clots and stains are noted; inquiry should be made of those who brought the patient, so as to obtain all the information possible. Frequently such information makes possible an immediate diagnosis. The presence of vomitus about the mouth, burns about the lips and face are looked for. Evidence of poisoning should be searched for by examining the patient's pockets, noting empty bottles or boxes. The facial expression may suggest severe pain, long-continued illness and dehydration. The skin, if pale and cold, of course indicates shock; if cyanotic, suggests respiratory or cardiac disease; if grayish and pale, lead poisoning. The breath is frequently a great source of information. The sweet odor of acetone, the fetid breath of uremia, the fecal odor in late intestinal obstruction, or the putrefactive smell in gangrene of the lung often suggests the correct diagnosis at once.

2. **Circulatory Change.**—This is often apparent from the general appearance, especially of the skin; a fast thready pulse and low blood pressure both indicate shock. The veins are collapsed in shock, but stand out and are distended when circulatory collapse is due to heart disease. Blood pressure on the other hand is high in Bright's disease, essential hypertension and in the active stage of extradural hemorrhage. A normal circulation rules out shock. Examination of the heart is obviously important.

3. **Changes in the Sensorium.**—Sensorial changes indicate the degree of coma and can be determined by the response elicited by such stimuli as pressure over

the supra-orbital nerve, the corneal reflex, and dilatation of the rectal sphincter. Hysterical patients, for example, will seldom fail to react to one or the other of these stimuli. In shock, unconsciousness is slight and ordinarily the patient will respond to simple stimuli such as pinching the skin. Deep coma with no response may indicate profound shock, but is more commonly due to cerebral injury, uremia or poisoning. Delirium or convulsive movements (especially in children) may accompany coma in severe infections, intoxication or disease of the brain. In psychoses the coma will be inconstant and often accompanied by peculiar behavior. In head injuries an uncontrollable hyperactivity sometimes amounting to an actual mania may be present. It is also seen in psychoses. In most instances the depth of the coma, however, has been of little diagnostic aid (Solomon and Aring[1]). Increased intrapericardial pressure (cardiac tamponade) due to hemorrhage from wounds of the heart usually produces a delirium with muscular hyperactivity.

4. **Changes in Respiration.**—Abnormal breathing sometimes gives a clue as to the diagnosis. A very slow rate, five or ten per minute, suggests morphine poisoning. Rapid, shallow respirations are common in shock; when deep and eager (air hunger) it may indicate serious hemorrhage, but is most notable in diabetic coma as a symptom of acidosis. Irregular breathing, such as Biot's or Cheyne-Stokes', indicates a cerebral lesion, either traumatic or secondary (cerebral edema) to an infection or uremia. When respirations are forced and accompanied by exaggerated use of all the accessory muscles of respiration, a physical obstruction is probably present in the larynx or trachea (exudate, spasm, edema, foreign body or tumor), and explains the cause of cyanosis. Cyanosis and increased respiratory rate may be the manifestations of cardiac disease; dyspnea and orthopnea may give the clue. Pulmonary edema or pneumonia also cause an increased respiratory rate; pulmonary signs may be present on examination of the chest.

5. **Changes in Temperature.**—A body temperature below normal points to shock. It is elevated, of course, in most severe infections, although in sepsis the low point may be subnormal, usually in the morning. A high temperature is found in sunstroke and occasionally in intracranial lesions, particularly in the terminal stages.

6. **Miscellaneous Signs.**—Numerous miscellaneous signs may be of much diagnostic value. Argyll Robertson pupils (lost reaction to light with retention of accommodation) point to tabes; pinpoint pupils to morphinism. In deep coma, however, examination of the eyes is not apt to be helpful, since the pupils are so often abnormal regardless of the cause (Solomon and Aring[1]). This is true also of the reflexes. Ophthalmoscopic examination may reveal choked disk indicative of increased intracranial pressure; retinal hemorrhages are present in nephritis, diabetes, etc. Hemorrhage from the ears or nose, especially the former, suggests basal fracture of the skull. Scalp lacerations may accompany or reveal a fracture of the skull; there may be an escape of cerebrospinal fluid or actual brain tissue in the wound. Cerebrospinal fluid draining from the nose or ear indicates a serious injury to bone and meninges, because of the location at the base of the skull. Mouth burns indicate the swallowing of caustic poisons; spasm of the masseter muscle, laryngeal spasm and risus sardonicus point to tetanus. Stippling along the gums (lead lines) are diagnostic of lead poisoning. Percussion of bladder dulness may

indicate prostatic obstruction. This is made more plausible by the palpation of an enlarged prostate per rectum. Catheterization may yield a liter or more of urine in such cases. Gastric lavage may reveal contents indicative of poison. Neurological signs indicative of disease of the brain and spinal cord should be looked for in questionable cases. Important are the sensory and motor disturbances when obtainable.

7. **Laboratory Tests.**—Frequently, laboratory tests are the only means of making a diagnosis. Examination of urine, usually obtained by catheter, may reveal sugar (diabetes), casts, albumin (nephritis), pus (infection), or blood (bichloride poisoning). The usual routine blood examinations are carried out and may show a high red cell count in dehydration, shock and polycythemia, or a low count in hemorrhage. Stippling of the red cells indicates lead poisoning; plasmodia are diagnostic of malaria. Leukocytosis is present in serious infections and leukemia. Blood may also be examined for its sugar content to determine whether hypo- or hyperglycemia is present. In uremia there will be an increased nonprotein nitrogen of the blood. The blood chlorides are low in dehydration from excessive loss of intestinal secretion from vomiting, diarrhea, etc.

Lumbar puncture is often indicated in comatose patients and may reveal clear fluid under increased pressure in syphilis of the central nervous system, tuberculous meningitis or cerebral edema from tumor, alcoholism or uremia. The presence of mononuclear cells indicates chronic infection, *i.e.,* syphilis, tuberculosis or encephalitis. Turbid fluid usually means pyogenic meningitis. Evidence of increased intracranial pressure may be shown by the force with which the fluid escapes; it can actually be measured by connecting a manometer to the needle. Bloody fluid usually means intracranial trauma.

INTRACRANIAL LESIONS

Most of the important intracranial lesions seen in an emergency room are traumatic. When severe symptoms are produced immediately, direct damage to the brain is usually present. Not infrequently, however, symptoms develop more slowly because they are due to a secondary rise in intracranial pressure. It is useful, though not always possible, to distinguish between the effects of direct injury to the brain and the effects of increased intracranial pressure (see Chapter XXII).

Increased intracranial pressure produces symptoms not only because of the direct effect of pressure on nerve centers or tracts, but also because of the associated cerebral anemia which it produces. Convulsions, when they occur, are probably due to cortical stimulation, usually by the same lesion causing the increased pressure. Uncontrollable hyperactivity is also seen in head injuries and is presumably due to the same cause.

Etiological Factors.—The traumatic and nontraumatic causes of increased intracranial pressure are listed below. Much of our present knowledge of the physiological reactions to increased intracranial pressure is based on the early observations of Harvey Cushing.[2]

1. Trauma, *i.e.,* head injury involving brain damage (concussion or laceration), with or without skull fracture, is frequently followed by increased intra-

cranial pressure because of active bleeding, (intracranial or extradural), because of subdural escape of cerebrospinal fluid, or because of cerebral edema which often follows trauma to brain tissue.

2. Apoplexy or spontaneous intracranial hemorrhage is an obvious cause of increased intracranial pressure. When a small vessel within the substance of the brain bleeds, the hemorrhage is not great and recovery of consciousness may be rapid. On the other hand, the outcome in severe cases is rapidly fatal.

3. Infections, *i.e.,* meningitis (pyogenic, tuberculous, syphilitic), encephalitis and tetanus may produce increased intracranial pressure by (*a*) inducing an edema of the brain tissue itself or by (*b*) obstructing the flow of cerebrospinal fluid by exudate or adhesions.

4. Neoplasms increase intracranial pressure by their actual growth within the rigid cranial cavity or by interfering with the flow of cerebrospinal fluid. When cerebral neoplasm is the cause of sudden unconsciousness, hemorrhage into the tumor is usually the primary factor in its production.

Clinical Manifestations.—In head injuries a history of trauma is usually obtained. Evidences thereof are lacerations and contusions of the scalp, crepitus or depressions of the skull itself (a hematoma, however, may simulate a depressed fracture), bleeding from the ears or nose, or escape of cerebrospinal fluid. A roentgenogram may be necessary to detect fracture. Further examination is directed toward eliciting positive neurological signs. Depth of coma is determined by noting the effect of stimuli of varying intensity. The circulation is observed at intervals, for although unchanged at the onset of the injury, it may undergo alterations which are frequently diagnostic of a steadily increasing intracranial pressure. Thus a slowly bleeding middle meningeal artery produces an extradural hematoma which increases the intracranial pressure progressively. The resulting cerebral anemia stimulates a reflex increase in the general blood pressure designed presumably to force more blood into the anemic brain. However, this leads to further extradural bleeding. As the general blood pressure rises, the pulse rate falls and may become quite slow (40 to the minute). Such an increase in blood pressure apparently occurs only from localized arterial bleeding of this type. Another sign of middle meningeal hemorrhage is the so-called "lucid interval." This period represents a temporary restoration of consciousness occurring between the initial unconsciousness due to the accident and that produced by the slowly forming hematoma. Eventually the circulation fails and death ensues unless operation relieves the situation.

Lumbar puncture in the presence of increased intracranial pressure is condemned by many surgeons because of the danger of medullary compression at the foramen magnum. It is, nevertheless, widely used in traumatic cases and serves a diagnostic purpose by revealing the presence of bloody fluid. This may be of medicolegal importance when the x-ray of the skull is negative. It also serves to decrease intracranial pressure. The authors, however, do not recommend lumbar puncture as a routine procedure. Its danger can be lessened or eliminated by using a manometer and avoiding the loss of cerebrospinal fluid.

The relation of skull fracture to intracranial injury is an inconstant one, *i.e.,* fracture may be present without evidence of brain damage, or it may be absent with serious injury to the cerebrum. A demonstrable skull fracture is of great importance medicolegally. The various aspects of intracranial injury are discussed under skull fractures in Chapter XXII.

Not infrequently comatose patients with meningitis of one kind or another are brought into an emergency receiving room. There may be an elevation of temperature and leukocytosis to suggest the presence of infection, and a rigid neck or positive Kernig sign to point to meningeal irritation. A lumbar puncture usually reveals abnormal fluid. The eyegrounds may show a swelling of the disks.

In slowly increasing intracranial pressure such as occurs typically in a brain tumor, three cardinal symptoms occur, i.e., headache, vomiting and choked disk. Convulsions may occur. Localizing symptoms of neurological nature depend on the location and type of tumor and a discussion of them belongs to special works on brain tumors (Sachs [3]) (See also page 569).

Treatment.—In general, therapy is directed toward the cause of the brain injury or of the increased pressure. In traumatic cases the detection of middle meningeal hemorrhage demands immediate craniotomy in order to evacuate the clot and ligate the artery. When a depressed fracture is present, operation is also indicated, but rarely is a decompression advisable. Usually, however, the treatment is conservative and is directed toward reduction of the intracranial pressure by intravenous hypertonic saline or glucose and lumbar puncture. Morphine is not to be given since it masks cerebral symptoms, and depresses respiration. If persistent convulsions or hyperactivity are too intense, chloral hydrate, paraldehyde or sodium amytal are given. Wechsler [4] has reported that severe convulsions which fail to respond by other means will often cease following the intravenous injection of 1 cc. of paraldehyde. If lumbar puncture reveals cloudy fluid the patient is presumably suffering from a pyogenic meningococcus meningitis and antimeningococcus serum is usually given, even before the organism is identified. In other infections the treatment is nonspecific. Apoplexy is treated symptomatically; the increased intracranial pressure, though difficult to control, requires no special treatment. In brain tumor the treatment is neurosurgical.

PHYSIOCHEMICAL COMA

The diseases in this heterogeneous group have in common the fact that the sensorial depression (or hyperactivity such as delirium and convulsions) is produced by a disturbed cerebral physiology, as occurs in the psychiatric diseases, poisoning, uremia, etc. The classification is not exact, however, because the coma in uremia is sometimes due as much to an associated cerebral edema as to direct toxic injury to the brain itself, as shown by the occasional though transient improvement following lumbar puncture (Christian and O'Hare [5]). The wet edematous brain is a well-known lesion in alcoholism; in very acute cases, lumbar puncture has also been used therapeutically (Williams [6]).

Diagnosis and treatment are urgent, of course, in patients who have ingested poison or are suffering from carbon monoxide poisoning. In the former case gastric lavage is instituted at once to rid the stomach of as much of the poison as possible. A large tube is necessary in order to effect rapid evacuation and to allow the use of large volumes of fluid; this cannot be done efficiently with a small tube. In carbon monoxide poisoning, artificial respiration with a gas containing a high percentage of oxygen and also carbon dioxide is indicated. The former is necessary because of the need to displace CO from the hemoglobin molecule as rapidly as possible, so that gaseous metabolism can occur normally. Carbon dioxide acts as a respiratory stimulus which also aids in overcoming the deficiency in oxyhemoglobin in these cases. The treatment of asphyxia has already been described. If a laryngeal obstruction is present intubation or tracheotomy is life-saving. Comatose patients are particularly liable to asphyxia due to relaxation of their pharangeal muscles and obstruction due to the tongue falling back over the larynx; aspiration of vomitus is likely for the same reason. The prone position is therefore safer in comatose patients, or care must be exerted to pull the tongue forward and to apply suction to the throat. In diabetics the prompt use of insulin and intravenous alkali (in the form of sodium lactate and Ringer's solution with or without glucose) may be life-saving in the most severe cases. On the other hand, in hypoglycemia intravenous glucose is specific. Severe dehydration requires the adequate administration of appropriate fluids parenterally which will relieve many of the symptoms rapidly.

BIBLIOGRAPHY

1. SOLOMON, P., and ARING, C. D. The Differential Diagnosis in Patients Entering the Hospital in Coma, *J. Am. M. Ass.*, 105:7, 1935.
2. CUSHING, HARVEY. Some Experimental and Clinical Observations Concerning States of Increased Intracranial Tension, *Am. J. M. Sc.*, 124:375, 1902.
3. SACHS, ERNEST. *The Diagnosis and Treatment of Brain Tumors*, C. V. Mosby Co., St. Louis, 1931.
4. WECHSLER, I. S. Intravenous Injection of Paraldehyde for the Control of Convulsions, *J. Am. M. Ass.*, 114:2198, 1940.
5. CHRISTIAN, H. A., and O'HARE, J. P. *Nephritis*, in Oxford Medicine, Oxford University Press, New York, 1920, Vol. III, Part II, p. 618.
6. WILLIAMS, I. D. The Emergency Treatment of the Alcoholic, *J. Nerv. & Ment. Dis.*, 74:171, 1931.
7. GREENE, B. A. Recent Advances in the Care of the Comatose Patient, *Arch. Int. Med.*, 16:727, 1942.

CHAPTER XVI

NEOPLASMS AND CYSTS

Malignant Neoplasms
Benign Neoplasms
Cysts

For practical purposes, a swelling or tumor may be classified into one of two general groups, inflammatory or neoplastic. The term tumor, however, is commonly used synonymously with neoplasm. The terminology, moreover, is not exact, because a neoplasm such as keloid may actually follow an injury. Certain cancers, too, follow chronic irritation and there is some theoretical and experimental evidence that neoplasms are in reality expressions of repair, exaggerated or gone wrong. Nevertheless, the division into inflammatory and neoplastic tumors serves a useful purpose in diagnosis when one is confronted with a swelling of unknown etiology. Inflammatory tumors are discussed under their respective causes. A few congenital tumors which are not neoplastic, such as meningocele and spina bifida, are considered under cysts. (See Table 7, page 543.)

Neoplastic tumors may be divided into the two great groups of malignant and benign growths, but some tumors have characteristics which are not consistent with either group. Both groups, moreover, have this feature in common, *i.e.,* they are formed by the abnormal and purposeless multiplication of previously normal cells. In the benign neoplasm the new growth resembles closely the tissue it originated from; the cells are arranged in orderly fashion and though the tumor may attain great size it never jeopardizes the life of the host except that it may involve vital functions by pressure and occasionally by functional activity. Malignant neoplasms, on the other hand, consist of abnormal cells which tend more or less to approach the undifferentiated embryonic type; they are not orderly in growth, but invade and destroy adjacent tissues or spread to distant parts of the body and lead finally to the death of the individual. Complete description of theoretical and practical knowledge of the various neoplasms may be found in Ewing's classic text.[1] The following classification, though in some cases imperfect or arbitrary, will be used in this text:

CLASSIFICATION

A. MALIGNANT NEOPLASMS. Etiology, clinical characteristics, microscopic features and types (carcinoma and sarcoma)
    I. Carcinoma (epithelial)
        1. *Carcinoma of skin and squamous mucous membrane*
           (*a*) squamous-cell, (*b*) basal-cell, (*c*) malignant melanoma, (*d*) Paget's disease of the nipple

      2. *Carcinoma of glandular origin* (breast, urinary and genital tract, and other internal organs)

      3. *Miscellaneous carcinoma*

  II. Sarcoma (mesodermal)

      1. *Fibrosarcoma* (spindle cell or fibroblastic sarcoma)

      2. *Bone sarcoma,* classification, general features and types, *i.e.,* osteogenic and nonosseous (or miscellaneous) sarcoma

      3. *Sarcoma of lymphoid tissue*
        (a) simple lymphoma, (b) leukemia, (c) Hodgkin's disease, (d) lymphosarcoma

      4. *Miscellaneous sarcoma* (liposarcoma, rhabdomyosarcoma, thymoma)

  III. Brain tumors
      Neurocytoma

B. BENIGN NEOPLASMS. Etiology, clinical characteristics and types (based on cell of origin)

  I. Connective tissue origin

      1. *Fibrous tissue,* (a) keloid, (b) simple fibroma, (c) epulis, (d) giant cell tumor

      2. *Fatty tissue,* (a) lipoma, (b) xanthoma

      3. *Bone and cartilage,* (a) osteochondroma, (b) chondroma, (c) bone cyst, (d) benign giant cell tumor, (e) multiple cystic disease

  II. Nervous tissue origin

  III. Blood vessel origin

      1. *Capillary hemangioma*

      2. *Hypertrophic hemangioma*

      3. *Cavernous hemangioma*

  IV. Lymphatic origin

      1. *Lymphangioma*

      2. *Thymoma*

  V. Muscle tissue origin

  VI. Mixed tissue origin

      1. *Mixed tumor*

      2. *Teratoma*

  VII. Epithelial cell origin

      1. *Adenoma*

      2. *Skin tumors,* (a) wart, (b) cutaneous horn, (c) mole (benign melanoma)

      3. *Jaw tumors,* (a) adamantinoma, (b) dentigerous cyst, (c) odontoma, (d) fibrous osteoma

C. CYSTS

  I. Retention cysts (galactocele, pancreatic cyst, ranula, wen)

  II. Inflammatory cysts (abscesses, bursae)

  III. Degeneration cysts

  IV. Neoplastic cysts (ovarian, bone)

  V. Dermoid cysts

  VI. Congenital cysts (branchial, thyroglossal, meningocele, spina bifida, polycystic disease)

A. MALIGNANT NEOPLASMS

Etiology.—There are many theories as to the etiology of malignant neoplasms, but it is generally admitted that the cause is still unknown. One of these theories is the *embryonal theory,* usually associated with the name of Cohnheim, who assumed that the tumor originated from an embryonic rest and that its malignant quality is simply the fetal power of growth carried into adult life. This undoubtedly applies to some congenital kidney tumors in childhood and perhaps to teratomas which become malignant. Another theory is that of *cell autonomy* which offers a conception of tissue tension which restrains growth. According to this theory chronic irritation is one of the factors which enables certain cells to overcome this balance or restraint and allow rapid growth. Still another belief is that a malignant tumor is in reality an *infection*. For example, at least one type of experimental tumor, the Rous chicken sarcoma, is transmissible by a filterable agent, and is possibly an inflammatory lesion. Various bacteria have been isolated from human cancerous tissue from time to time; they probably have no etiological significance. The theory of an *inherited tendency* is now subject to intensive experimental and clinical study. In mice its importance is amply demonstrated but in man its significance is as yet not completely understood. The greatest recent advance in research as to the cause of cancer is the discovery that certain chemicals (*e.g.,* hydrocarbons and sterols) will produce cancer when injected into rats and mice [2]. Many of them, not normally present in the body, are therefore called exogenous carcinogens. Some of these compounds are normally present in the human; they are therefore called endogenous carcinogens.[33]. This important line of investigation furnishes a definite basis for a *chemical-metabolic theory* for the cause of cancer. Of practical importance is the theory that *acute trauma* may cause cancer. The evidence is conflicting, but the question arises more often in sarcoma, particularly bone sarcoma, than carcinoma (Knox [3]). A history of trauma is so frequently given in various diseases that its relationship is always open to suspicion. Nevertheless, the matter has medicolegal importance, for courts have on occasion recognized such a relationship even though scientific evidence in its favor is not all convincing and have awarded large compensation claims.

Malignant disease is serious because it is a frequent cause of death (ranking second to fourth), and cure is impossible without early diagnosis and adequate treatment. Another serious feature is that the recorded incidence of malignant disease is apparently on the increase, having doubled during the past forty years. This increased frequency may not be a cause for alarm since part of this is undoubtedly due to improvement in diagnostic accuracy. Moreover, greater numbers of people now attain the age when cancer is prevalent. In the United States 60 per cent of cancer deaths are in patients over forty-five. In Prussia, for example, the average span of life is twenty-five years longer than it was in 1860. In New York City the proportion of persons over forty-five is one-third greater than a generation ago.

A very important and excellent monograph devoted to the entire problem of human cancer is that of Stout.[4]

Clinical Characteristics.—The earlier the lesion the more difficult it is to make a diagnosis of cancer. It should be emphasized, however, that with thorough general and perhaps special examinations, the detection of cancer in its early stages is possible. The clinical manifestations of malignant disease depend of course on its site. Certain general characteristics, however, may be described, although most of them are obvious only in the visible (*i.e.,* external) types of cancer.

(*a*) Continued or progressive growth, as well as progression of symptoms, is an important feature. Malignant tumors in most instances grow without interruption, whereas benign tumors stop growing after attaining a certain size.

(*b*) Local recurrence following incomplete removal of a tumor always happens if the lesion is malignant. It should be remembered, however, that this feature is also manifested by some of the benign tumors.

(*c*) Metastasis is the most characteristic clinical manifestation and is perhaps the most important factor in the fatal outcome. Metastasis is the spread of the growth usually by way of the lymphatics or blood vessels to regional lymph nodes and distant organs (liver, lung, brain, etc.); however, it should be emphasized that enlargement of lymph nodes adjacent to an ulcerating carcinoma may be due entirely to secondary infection and not to metastasis. Although metastasis is usually assumed to occur only by way of the lymphatics and the systemic and portal veins,

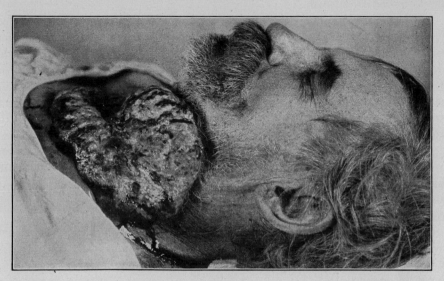

FIG. 157.—EXTENSIVE ULCERATION AND BLEEDING IN A FAR ADVANCED FUNGATING CARCINOMA OF THE NECK.

an additional mode of spread has been postulated by Batson,[5] who has presented evidence that the system of vertebral veins (overlying the lumbar and thoracic vertebrae) play an important role in metastasis. Such channels would explain, for example, how metastasis to a vertebra might develop secondary to an abdominal cancer without involvement of the lung and without transmission through the lung. According to Batson, the cancer cells are forced into the involved areas through the vertebral veins and collaterals by sudden changes in pressure.

(*d*) Local invasion of tissue by contiguity is another manifestation of most malignant tumors and may be very destructive. This invasive property resembles that exhibited by certain types of infection.

(*e*) Hardness or firmness is an important diagnostic feature of most types of cancer, but is obviously of value only when the tumor can be felt, as in the breast, prostate or skin. This hardness is usually produced by excessive fibrous tissue which, however, varies greatly in different tumors. A sarcoma, for example, is apt to be so cellular and vascular that it will have a soft consistency; scirrhous cancer, on the other hand, contains so much fibrous tissue that it is often stony hard.

(*f*) Carcinoma in general is a disease of later adult life though not infrequent below the age of forty. Sarcoma, on the other hand, respects no age group.

(*g*) Ulceration is of frequent occurrence in cancer of epithelial surfaces and, moreover, does not heal and tends to progress. In the skin, the edges of the ulcer are elevated, hard and firmly elastic. Cancer of the mucous surfaces is especially prone to ulcerate, *e.g.*, carcinoma of the stomach, colon, cervix, bronchus, lip and tongue.

(*h*) Bleeding is only occasionally encountered in the superficial malignant lesions of the skin, but is frequent in carcinoma of the colon, stomach, cervix and bladder. The hemorrhage, though slight, is apt to persist and on many occasions leads to secondary anemia.

(*i*) Disability as a characteristic of cancer is not of diagnostic importance since it occurs late and may be caused by any tumor or any type of inflammation. Cachexia and asthenia are present only in the terminal stage of cancer and are due at least in part to the effects of ulceration such as bleeding and secondary infection. This is of practical importance because in some instances removal of an ulcerating cancer for its symptomatic relief may be justified even though the tumor has already metastasized, and there is no hope of complete removal and cure. Cachexia and weakness when present without ulceration, indicate that the cancer may act as a true parasite, growing within and ultimately destroying its host. Pain as a symptom of cancer is present only in the terminal stages of the disease, except when the tumor irritates nerve endings by pressure or invasion, or is growing rapidly in dense structures such as bone. Because it detracts from early diagnosis, this painless feature of malignant disease is particularly unfortunate.

(*j*) A fatal outcome of cancer is inevitable unless the entire tumor is completely removed or destroyed. Although spontaneous cures have undoubtedly occurred they are too rare to be of significance in diagnosis and treatment. Variations in duration are not uncommon.

(*k*) Sensitivity to x-ray and radium is a characteristic of malignant disease which is very important in therapy; however, certain benign neoplasms share this sensitivity.

Microscopic Features.—Because clinical diagnosis is often so difficult it frequently becomes necessary to resort to microscopic examination of the suspected lesion. Such a procedure is called a biopsy; the tissue removed may consist of a part of the primary neoplasm or of a metastatic nodule. Biopsy of the original lesion should include normal as well as abnormal tissue in one piece so that the transition between the two can be studied. Serous effusions due to malignant disease may contain a sediment which will reveal cancer cells. Aspiration biopsy which requires only a large needle is an alternative method and may be used in certain patients (see Pack and Livingston,[6] p. 72, Vol. 1).

The histological evidences of malignancy are as follows:

(*a*) *Abnormal cells,* more or less undifferentiated, even though growing in a form somewhat characteristic of the original tissue, are present. Nuclei stain more deeply and cytoplasm is more abundant.

(*b*) The growth is characteristically *invasive,* breaking through the normal tissue boundaries and extending into adjacent structures.

(c) Rapid growth is often evinced by *numerous mitotic figures* and abnormally formed cells.

(d) The *fibrous tissue reaction* of the body to the tumor is sometimes very marked, especially in the so-called scirrhous type in which the intense fibrous tissue wall is formed presumably in an attempt to envelop and destroy the malignant cells. In rare instances this seems to have been achieved, since thorough search of the fibrosed tissue reveals few if any cancer cells. Such observations suggest the existence of a resistance on the part of the body to cancer.

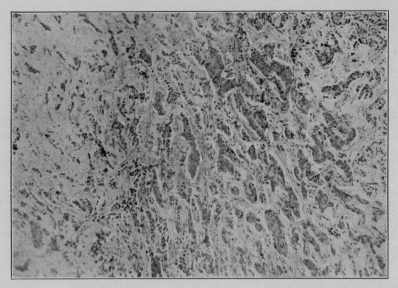

FIG. 158.—PHOTOMICROGRAPH SHOWING THE INVASIVE CHARACTER OF MALIGNANT DISEASE.

The section was taken from a carcinoma of the breast which had been removed surgically. Note the penetration of the strands of cancer cells through the fibrous stroma with no evidence of encapsulation or limitation.

(e) Attempts have been made to estimate the degree of malignancy by studying more or less quantitatively the above features of the cancer cells. Thus Broders [7] has divided cancer into four arbitrary groups of malignancy, Type I, II, III and IV, depending upon their histological features. While helpful in prognosis in certain cases, such histologic predictions are often inaccurate. The degree of malignancy is estimated with accuracy only by observing the clinical behavior of the growth.

Types of Malignant Disease.—Malignant neoplasms are customarily divided into two groups, depending upon whether they originate from connective (mesodermal) or epithelial (ectodermal) tissue, although, as will be seen, this division is not absolute, for some tumors contain both types of cells. Occasionally it may be difficult to determine whether a neoplasm has originated from mesoderm or ectoderm. Ordinarily, however, this classification is fairly exact. The term *sarcoma* is applied to malignant tumors arising from mesoderm, *i.e.,* fibrous tissue, cartilage, bone, fat, blood vessels, lymph tissue and muscle, whereas *carcinoma* includes tumors of ectodermal or epithelial origin, *i.e.,* skin, mucous membrane, liver, kidney, pancreas, thyroid, etc. There are certain other distinguishing features which separate sarcoma from carcinoma. Sarcoma in general is bulky and soft, tends to remain demarcated, but grows rapidly along a vascular framework, often to great

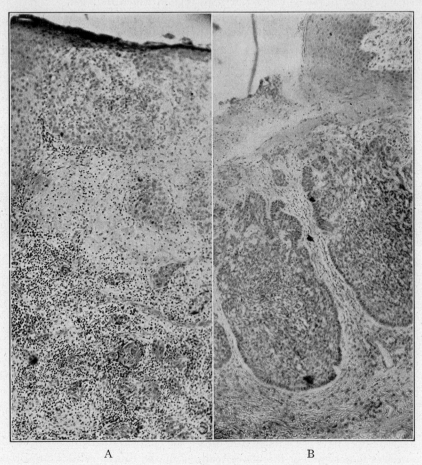

A   B

FIG. 159.—PHOTOMICROGRAPH OF THE TWO COMMON CARCINOMAS OF THE SKIN, SOMETIMES CALLED EPITHELIOMAS.

Both sections were taken at the edge of the lesion and both show the same depth of skin. *A*, squamous cell carcinoma. This section shows the edge of a small ulcer removed from the back of the neck. For two years the patient, a sixty-five-year-old man, noted an area of eczema which failed to heal. The gross appearance of the lesion did not suggest cancer but because of the history and the age and sex of the patient the ulcer was excised. Note the invasive character of the growth and the lack of limitation as the neoplasm penetrates the deeper layers of the skin far beyond the photomicrograph. Note also the extensive lymphocytic infiltration; *B*, basal cell carcinoma. This section is from the lesion illustrated in Figure 165. Note the sharp limitation in the deepest extent of the growth at a point well above the bottom of the photomicrograph. One of the characteristic features of this lesion is the palisading of the cells around the periphery of the growth, which is clearly shown.

size and is locally destructive. Notable exceptions are the hard osteosarcoma and some fibrosarcomas. Areas of hemorrhage, degeneration and necrosis within the tumor are common. Sarcoma tends to break into blood vessels and metastasizes first to the lungs and later to other organs. Carcinoma in general, grows more slowly, but may metastasize when the tumor is small, first to the regional lymph nodes, then to the liver, lungs, bone, etc. Originating from epithelial surfaces it is of course much more susceptible to ulceration and infection than sarcoma.

Treatment.—Although discussed in more detail under each type of cancer, it should be emphasized that the general principles of cancer therapy are always the

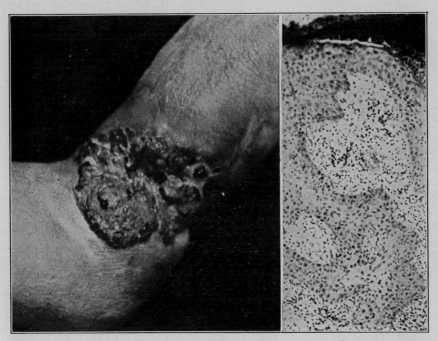

FIG. 160.—SQUAMOUS CELL CARCINOMA OF THE ARM; THE GROWTH FORMED IN AN OLD ULCER WHICH PERSISTED FOLLOWING AN INJURY TO THE ARM FIFTY-SEVEN YEARS PREVIOUSLY (MARJOLIN'S ULCER).

One year before admission, the patient, an eighty-year-old farmer, noted a fungating growth at the site of the ulcer which grew steadily to the size shown in the illustration. Pain also developed and grew steadily worse. This represents the hypertrophic type of squamous cell carcinoma and is of a relatively low degree of malignancy. The photomicrograph is from a biopsy specimen; note the extensive growth of squamous epithelium and the lymphocytic infiltration. Treatment in this type of tumor consists of wide local excision and the application of a skin graft to cover the defect; regional lymph nodes are also excised; occasionally amputation is indicated.

same. At the present time eradication of *all* malignant cells is the only known manner of cure. This eradication may be achieved (1) by surgical excision, (2) by destruction with x-ray, radium, or radium emanation, (3) by a combination of both. The details of therapy vary tremendously and are often a matter of considerable difference of opinion. An extensive treatise on therapy of cancer is that of Pack and Livingston.[6]

I. Carcinoma.—Malignant tumors of epithelial origin may arise from the skin or mucous membranes or from glandular tissue such as the breast, stomach, colon, ovary, thyroid, etc. The term adenocarcinoma is used when the growth assumes an acinose form or originates from glandular tissue. When the tumor takes the form of a polyp or papilloma it may be called papillary carcinoma. The hard center of breast carcinoma with its lateral invading extensions suggested to Galen the appearance of a crab, hence its Latin equivalent, cancer.

1. *Carcinoma of the Skin and Squamous Mucous Membranes.*—These comprise (*a*) squamous-cell, (*b*) basal-cell and (*c*) malignant melanoma. A fourth type

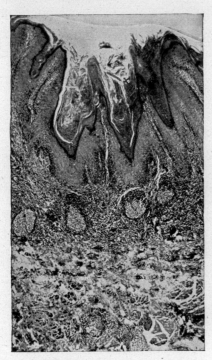

FIG. 161.—LEUKOPLAKIA.

Photomicrograph from a section of a small white elevated area removed from the inner side of the patient's cheek. Note the hyperplasia of the keratin layer and the characteristic lymphoid infiltration and follicle formation just beneath the epidermis. This lesion is definitely a precursor of squamous cell carcinoma, and total removal is generally indicated.

(*d*) Paget's disease of the nipple is also included here because it starts as a skin lesion though its malignant development is that of adenocarcinoma of the breast. The term epithelioma is commonly applied to either the squamous- or basal-cell tumors of the skin, or collectively to both.

(*a*) *Squamous-cell carcinoma* occurs not only in the skin, but also in mucous membranes composed of squamous cells (buccal and genito-urinary orifices). It also occurs at times by metaplasia from mucous membranes not normally composed of squamous cells, *i.e.*, bronchus and gallbladder.

In the *skin* it is rare except in the head and neck, but is prone to develop at the site of an old scar following a burn or extensive trauma (Marjolin's ulcer). Indeed, a previous lesion of some kind or a source of chronic irritation seems a common precursor of squamous-cell carcinoma wherever its site. Males are more frequently affected than females (2:1). The growth takes one of two general forms, the papillary or ulcerating type. The former is much less malignant and grows slowly as a cauliflower projection from the skin and metastasizes late. The ulcerating form is invasive, spreads rapidly and metastasizes to the neighboring lymph nodes early. The edge is raised and indurated; the base is deep and bleeds easily. The ulcerative type is to be distinguished, however, from basal-cell carcinoma which is described later.

In the *buccal cavity* squamous-cell carcinoma attacks the lip, jaws, tongue or pharynx. It affects males predominantly (5:1), but is not a common lesion, accounting (with the skin) for but 6 per cent of malignant disease. As in the skin, previous lesions or chronic irritation in the buccal mucosa are frequent precursors of cancer. *Leukoplakia* is a common predisposing lesion which is said in turn to be associated with excessive use of tobacco and with syphilis. Leukoplakia is manifested as a whitish area in the mucosa of the borders of the tongue or lip, of tough leathery consistency, having a tendency in its later stages to become the site of fissures or ulceration. Microscopically the lesion consists of a proliferation of the outer squamous-cell layers. Other predisposing lesions are fissures of the lip, herpetic ulcers which do not heal, ulcers at the site of sharp teeth or dental

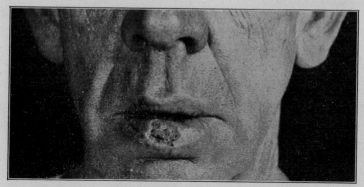

FIG. 162.—SQUAMOUS CELL CARCINOMA IN THE LOWER LIP.
Verified by microscopic examination of a biopsy removed from the edge of the lesion.

appliances, inflammation due to the prolonged use of pipes, etc. Years ago syphilis was said to be associated etiologically with carcinoma of the mouth, but, apart from causing leukoplakia, such a theory is not tenable. As in the skin, two broad forms are distinguished clinically, the hard ulcerating type and the soft cauliflower or

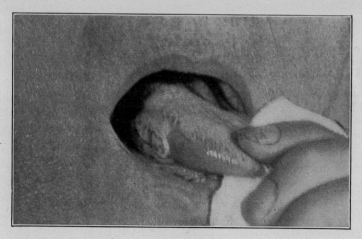

FIG. 163.—SQUAMOUS CELL CARCINOMA OF THE TONGUE.
Diagnosis was verified by microscopic examination of a biopsy specimen. The lesion, apparently of one year's duration in a forty-five-year-old male, disappeared after local radium treatment; a regional lymph node (neck) dissection was also carried out. Some surgeons prefer to completely excise the primary lesion when feasible.

papillary type. In the lip, squamous-cell cancer commonly attacks the lower lip. The ulcer is characteristic with a raised indurated edge, but may be flat and grow slowly, and seem to heal over in its less malignant form. Metastases occur to the cervical nodes which become enlarged; enlarged nodes, however, may be due to infection and not to cancerous invasion. Chancre of the lip may be mistaken for carcinoma, although the history, its short duration, early involvement of lymph nodes should point to chancre. The finding of spirochetes in the discharge by dark field illumination will establish the diagnosis of chancre.

In the *tongue, jaws and pharynx,* carcinoma also presents a characteristic appearance, but occasionally is detected only by careful search. Patients are usually aware of lesions in the mouth regardless of their characteristics. If in the cancer age they should be taught to have such lesions investigated. Pain, salivation and hemorrhage are generally present only in the later stages. Dentists frequently see

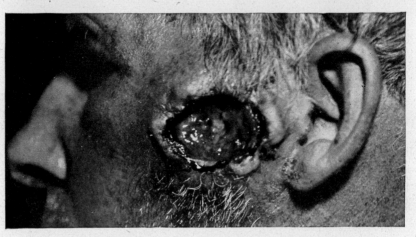

FIG. 164.—BASAL-CELL CARCINOMA OF THE FACE AFTER IMPROPER TREATMENT BY THE APPLICA-CATION OF A "CANCER PASTE," SEVERAL WEEKS PREVIOUSLY.

Note that the central portion of the lesion was destroyed at least in part, but the tumor at the edges is growing very actively. Radiotherapy is now being used.

such lesions first. In the deeper recesses of the buccal cavity, especially the larynx, carcinoma is frequently unsuspected until such symptoms as hoarseness, bleeding or, in some instances, cervical metastases occur. In the antrum carcinoma is rare.

Treatment of squamous-cell carcinoma of the skin and buccal mucosa first of all should be directed at the detection and treatment of the predisposing lesions which have been already mentioned. If doubt exists as to the nature of a chronic lesion, excision and microscopic section should be made. Destruction of such lesions is less advisable since it eliminates the opportunity for histologic study. There are two accepted methods of treating carcinoma of the buccal cavity. Many surgeons prefer wide excision of the lesion with bloc (neck) dissection of the regional lymph nodes. Other surgeons favor x-ray or radium therapy; combination of surgery and radiation may be used.

In the other orifices containing squamous cells, namely the genital and urinary openings, cancer is also relatively easy to detect early, because the surface involved can be inspected and the lesion seen. In the bladder this requires a cystoscope, but in the cervix merely a speculum. Very important is cancer of the female generative organs, since carcinoma of the cervix and uterus alone constitute 14 per cent of all malignant disease. The symptoms which should direct attention to such lesions are few. Abnormal bleeding, even though slight in amount, should always warrant an examination. Further discussion will be found in later chapters.

(*b*) *Basal-cell carcinoma* (rodent or Jacob's ulcer) occurs in most instances in the skin of the face and neck where it slowly invades the adjacent skin and underlying structures, although it practically never metastasizes. In rare instances it may arise in the skin of other regions such as the legs, perineum, and upper chest wall. Basal-cell carcinoma is a common disease in older persons and is frequently seen

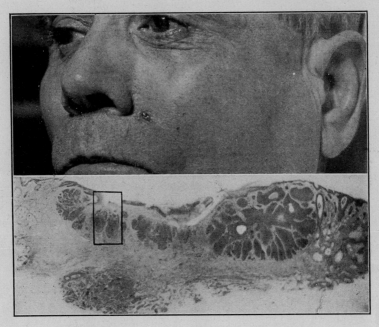

FIG. 165.—BASAL-CELL CARCINOMA.

The lesion, shown in the top photograph, started as a tiny "pimple" several months previously; the patient was a sixty-five-year-old male. Entire lesion was excised and the wound closed by primary suture; healing was prompt and permanent. A low power photomicrograph of the entire specimen is also shown. Note the transition in the epithelium where the lesion begins and the sharply limited extent of the growth. A higher power photomicrograph of the area indicated is presented in Figure 159B.

at a site of chronic irritation. Chronic exposure to the elements predisposes to its occurrence, hence its frequency in farmers. Blondes are especially susceptible to the disease and preëxisting lesions, such as hyperkeratosis, often precede the ulceration. In the early stage one sees merely a smooth nodule in the skin which grows in size and eventually breaks down in the center giving rise to an ulcer whose edges are elevated, indurated, nodular and present a characteristic pearly appearance. The base is apt to be shallow, fibrotic and covered with pale granulations. The ulcer progresses in size, but advanced cases with extensive destruction of tissue are rarely seen at the present time because adequate early treatment is so generally used and effective. Radiation (these are among the most radiosensitive tumors), excision or local destruction by cautery is curative. However, unless completely removed or destroyed the growth recurs at an increased rate.

(c) *Malignant melanoma* (melanoblastoma, chromatophoroma) is a special form of malignant tumor of the skin arising in a mole. The term melanoma is applied to tumors containing melanin, a brownish black pigment; melanomas may

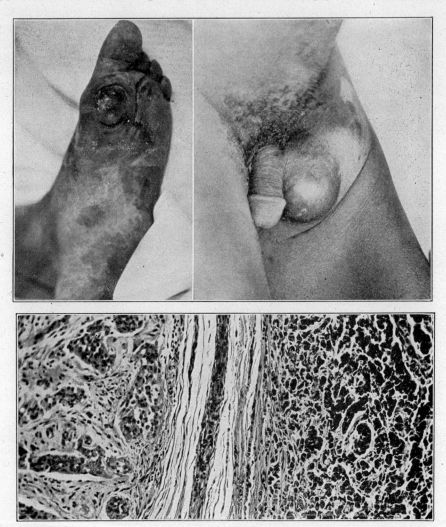

FIG. 166.—MALIGNANT MELANOMA.

The course was rapidly fatal. The patient was a forty-five-year-old Negro; however, this type of cancer is relatively rare in the Negro race. The lesion started under the ball of the foot as a callus which the patient pared repeatedly. Rapid growth occurred during the past six months and a mass appeared in the groin. The photos show the primary lesion in the foot and the metastasis in the regional (femoral) nodes. Death occurred one week later; autopsy revealed widespread metastases. The photomicrograph shows malignant cells both with and without the melanin pigment.

be malignant or benign. The benign type is discussed on page 338. Opinions differ as to whether malignant melanomas are of ectodermal or mesodermal origin, and hence the term melanosarcoma, as well as melanocarcinoma is often used.

The retina of the eye, which contains the pigmented cells, is also a source of the neoplasm. The disease is often very malignant, but in some cases a number of years may elapse between apparent successful removal of a primary growth and

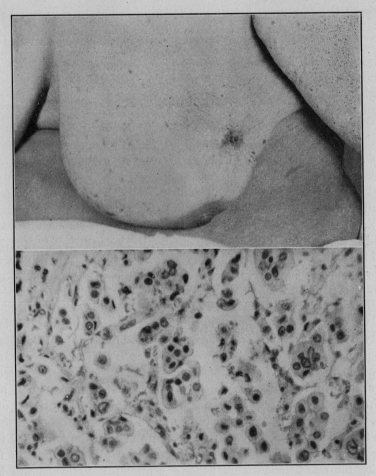

FIG. 167.—CARCINOMA OF THE BREAST IN AN EIGHTY-FOUR-YEAR-OLD WOMAN.

Note the retraction or puckered appearance of the skin over the lesion which was observed during a routine examination. The patient had been admitted to the medical ward because of severe hypertension; she claimed that the breast tumor had been present for ten years. It was observed for three more years without any appreciable change. The photomicrograph was obtained from the specimen which was removed at autopsy when the patient died of cardiac disease. This represents a very slowly growing, almost benign, type of carcinoma and is, of course, unusual; it is of importance to note, however, that the microscopic appearance of the lesion gives very little indication of this characteristic.

death from distant metastases which are rapid and widespread. The factors responsible for the prolonged inhibition of spread in such cases are unknown.

Metastasis may occur by way of the lymphatics or the blood stream. These tumors may be encountered at any age, but most of them occur in young adults. After malignant characteristics have developed, cure is rarely effected. It is important, therefore, to remove moles which have a tendency to become malignant. It is obviously impracticable to remove all moles, but those subject to continued irritation should be excised since irritation is prone to provoke the malignant change. It is important especially to remove moles on the head and feet since those areas are the most frequent sites of the initial lesion of malignant melanoma. Any mole which exhibits sudden growth or bleeds without sufficient provocation should also be excised. If the mole shows microscopic evidence of malignancy the regional lymph nodes should be removed. Fortunately, malignant melanoma is a rare disease. One type which occurs in the nail bed is called Hutchinson's melanotic whitlow (Womack [8]). It should be mentioned that occasionally nonpigmented moles undergo malignant change.

(d) *Paget's disease* of the nipple is a specific disease of the epithelium of and surrounding the nipple of the breast which ultimately develops into carcinoma. It starts as an exfoliating dermatitis or eczema which does not heal. The carcinoma is a typical adenocarcinoma of the breast whose histologic relation to the changes in the skin remains unestablished, though clinically the one seems to follow the other rather definitely. As a matter of clinical practice any chronic dermatitis of the nipple should be examined at frequent intervals; if it responds to local treatment and heals, as most cases of dermatitis do, the lesion is benign. If it does not heal and the patient is in the cancer age, operation is indicated (see also p. 821).

2. *Carcinoma of Glandular Origin.*—This group is by far the largest and comprises most of the other epithelial malignant tumors. The malignant cells usually assume the form of acini, rosets or alveoli. Occasionally they are arranged in cords of cells. Other variations are also described. *Scirrhus* is a term which is applied to that type of cancer which is marked by fibrosis in and around the tumor as if the defense mechanisms of the body were trying to strangle the cancer. *Medullary (encephaloid) carcinoma* is a term applied to a soft bulky tumor composed largely of cancer cells with very little associated fibrosis. *Colloid carcinoma* refers to tumors arising from mucous glands or to the growths which produce a great deal of mucoid material, visible grossly or microscopically. Colloid is found in cancer of the breast, stomach and colon. When the cells take the form of acini the term used is *adenocarcinoma* which may arise from either the secreting glandular cells or from the cells lining the ducts. Detailed discussions of glandular carcinoma will be found under the descriptions of diseases of the individual organs.

3. *Miscellaneous Carcinomas.*—There are other carcinomas of miscellaneous types which are difficult to classify under a single designation. These tumors include hypernephroma, metaplastic neoplasms of the lung, malignant teratomas, etc., and will be discussed under the various organs affected.

II. Sarcoma.—Sarcoma is less common than carcinoma, comprising but 3.5 per cent of all malignant tumors. It may develop wherever mesodermal tissue cells are present or grow from preëxisting benign tumors which are thus said to undergo "sarcomatous degeneration." The terms spindle-cell, round-cell and giant-cell sarcoma are histologically descriptive, but they do not indicate from which mesodermal element the tumor arises. To designate the exact tissue of origin the terms fibro-, lipo-, and osteo-sarcoma are used. In some instances the histological appearance of the tumor indicates its cell of origin. In many, however, this may be impossible to detect, especially when the growth is composed entirely of small or large round cells, although round-cell sarcoma is ordinarily of lymphoid origin. Regardless of their microscopic appearance, the gross clinical manifestations as mentioned previously are fairly distinctive. The tumor when soft is often mistaken for a hematoma, an abscess (tenderness may be present) aneurysm, lipoma or fibroma. With a large

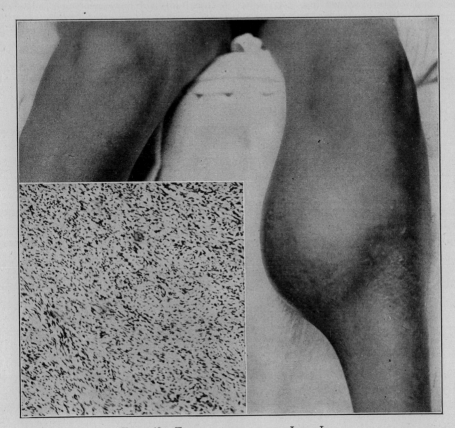

FIG. 168.—FIBROSARCOMA OF THE LEFT LEG.

The patient, a nineteen-year-old Negro girl, first noted a swelling a year before admission; growth was rapid. In spite of amputation, pulmonary metastases occurred and the patient died six months later. The insert is a photomicrograph of the tumor and shows the undifferentiated spindle-cell growth; there is less intercellular material than occurs in the more benign type of fibrosarcoma shown in Figure 169A.

aspirating needle one is sometimes able to obtain a sufficient amount of tissue for microscopical study (see p. 299), although an actual biopsy is usually preferable.

Although no classification is entirely satisfactory, the various kinds of sarcoma may be most simply divided into (1) spindle-cell (fibroblastic) sarcoma, (2) sarcoma of bone, (3) round-cell (lymphogenous) sarcoma. To this may be added (4) a small group of miscellaneous sarcomas, most of which are very rare.

1. *Fibrosarcoma (Fibroblastic or Spindle-cell Sarcoma).*—This tumor represents the commonest type of sarcoma and is encountered chiefly in the subcutaneous and submucous tissue, the fascia, intermuscular septums, periosteum and also in

parenchymatous organs. The size, consistency and rate of growth vary greatly. Histologically the cells are arranged in whorls of spindle cells which resemble fusiform fibroblasts and which may be either large or small. Because of their arrangement around the arteries they often seem to arise from the adventitial cells of the blood vessels. When they are present in the thigh, which is a frequent site, the tumor is bulky and has a tendency to local mucoid degeneration. When the entire tumor contains mucoid material it may be spoken of as *myxosarcoma* which

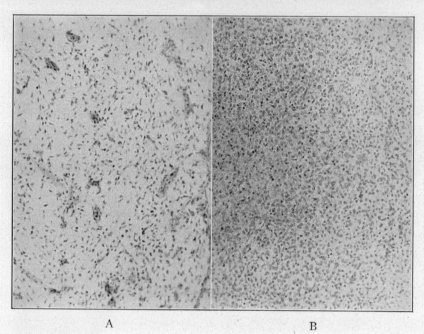

A   B

Fig. 169.—Myxosarcoma, a More Benign Type of Fibrosarcoma in a Male, Aged Fifty.

A slowly growing tumor of the thigh was excised three times during the course of six years because of recurrence. The photomicrographs are both from the tumor removed at the last operation; a fatal outcome several months later, was due to widespread metastases. *A*, histologic appearance of a typical myxosarcoma, quite similar to that noted in the original tumor; *B*, this appearance was noted but a few millimeters away on the same slide as that of *A;* it shows a more cellular phase of tumor growth which is characteristic of this lesion whenever it develops increased malignant tendencies.

grows slowly, is prone to recur after excision, is not apt to metastasize, but is nevertheless usually fatal.

When the growth is small, it may be impossible to differentiate fibrosarcoma from a fibroma, even on histological study. The sarcoma usually grows rapidly, but produces few symptoms until a large size is attained. Clinical manifestations are due to pressure of the tumor on adjacent structures. More often its size alone is the only complaint. Treatment consists of complete excision, removing all of the malignant tissue. Recurrence, however, is common; in the relatively benign myxosarcoma careful excision of the recurrent tumors will be all that is justified. However, amputation may be indicated in the more malignant types of myxoscarcoma when the tumor is in an extremity. Occasionally the tumor grows so rapidly that death occurs from metastases, particularly to the lungs regardless of therapy. Other types of sarcomas, fibroblastic in origin, are occasionally found in the esophagus, stomach, intestine, uterus, ovary, etc., where they produce special symptoms dependent upon their location and may exhibit special and unusual microscopic features.

2. *Sarcoma of Bone.*—Though in general a rather rare tumor (1 per cent of all malignant lesions), bone sarcoma has long been a source of confusion because

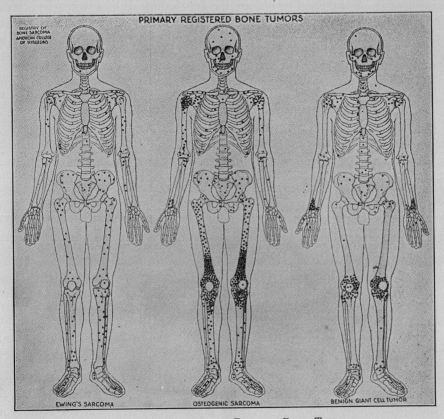

FIG. 170.—DISTRIBUTION OF PRIMARY BONE TUMORS.

Note that the region of the knee is the most frequent site for osteogenic sarcoma (from the *Bull. Am. Coll. Surg.*, 1935; 20:148).

it produces a great variety of clinical, roentgenological and histological manifestations. In recognition of this a Registry of Bone Sarcoma was formed by the American College of Surgeons. A clinical study of this material was made and published by Kolodny.[9] Another extensive study has also been made by Geschickter and Copeland[10] who analyzed 1500 cases of bone tumors, both malignant and benign. In order to recognize primary sarcoma of bone it is useful to realize that there are other bone lesions which simulate it. In surveying these various bone diseases one must distinguish first of all the malignant neoplasms which are not primary, *i.e.*, carcinomas which have metastasized to bone from a focus elsewhere; second are the group of true neoplasms of bone which are benign, particularly the giant cell tumor; third are the other diseases, inflammatory and metabolic, which simulate bone tumors.

Metastatic carcinoma to bone, the first group, is statistically important because of its frequency. Of the 1500 cases studied by Geschickter and Copeland [10] 40 per cent fell into this group. The primary tumor may be located anywhere but is more common in the breast, kidney (hypernephroma), lung, prostate and thyroid. Common clinical manifestations are pain, swelling and spontaneous ("pathological") fractures. Occasionally these lesions are the first intimation of disease, the primary focus remaining occult. The roentgenogram reveals bone destruction often described as a "moth-eaten" appearance, although in other instances there are areas of in-

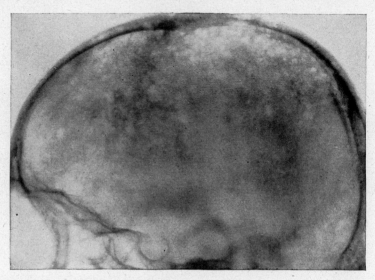

FIG. 171.–METASTATIC CARCINOMA IN THE SKULL ARISING FROM A PRIMARY (BRONCHIOGENIC) CARCINOMA OF THE LUNG.

creased density simulating new bone formation. Of the *benign bone neoplasms* giant cell tumor is most frequently a source of difficulty in diagnosis; these lesions are discussed further on page 323. Of the *inflammatory and metabolic diseases* of bone which are confusing, osteomyelitis is perhaps the most important especially in differentiating from Ewing's tumor. These lesions have been described in Chapter XIX.

The classification within the group of true primary bone sarcoma also offers considerable difficulty particularly in regard to the histologic appearance and pathogenesis of the various types. For this reason no attempt will be made to distinguish, for example, between those arising from cartilage and from bone, those which destroy or form bone, or those which are central, subperiosteal or periosteal.

The four groups described below are those finally adopted by Kolodny on the basis of cases comprising the Registry of Bone Sarcoma.[9]

(*a*) OSTEOGENIC SARCOMA.—This term, first used by Ewing, refers only to sarcoma originating in bone and must not be confused with the same term used to imply a sarcoma which forms bone (in contrast to osteolytic sarcoma which destroys

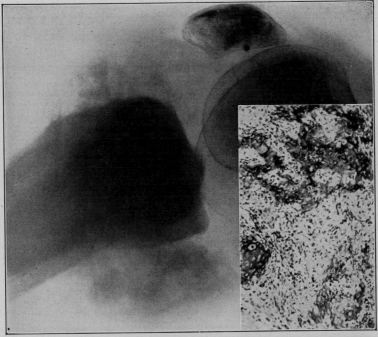

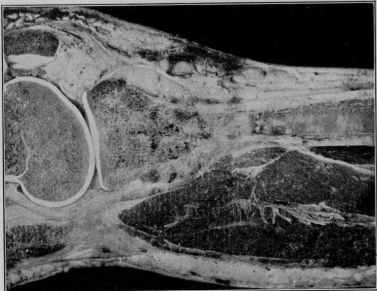

FIG. 172.—OSTEOGENIC SARCOMA OF THE TIBIA IN AN EIGHTEEN-YEAR-OLD BOY.

There was a history of trauma several weeks before the onset of a continuous ache which antedated the appearance of the swelling by two weeks. Swelling increased rapidly for six weeks before operation; a mid-thigh amputation was performed. The x-ray film shows a suggestive "sun-ray" effect; the lower photograph represents a longitudinal section of the amputated leg and shows the destructive process in the upper end of the tibia. The insert is a photomicrograph which shows malignant cells forming bone.

bone). Actually both bone destruction and bone formation may occur and is, of course, extremely important roentgenologically. As pointed out by Kolodny a better term for malignant bone forming tumors would be osteoblastoma. In European literature the term osteosarcoma is widely employed. In the Bone Sarcoma Registry [9] osteogenic sarcoma is further subdivided into four groups, *i.e.*, periosteal, medullary and subperiosteal, sclerosing and telangiectatic; these subgroups will not be discussed herein.

Clinical features of osteogenic sarcoma are usually distinctive. It is a tumor of adolescence, 50 per cent occurring in the second decade of life during which normal bone growth is most active. Moreover, 72 per cent occur in the lower extremity and of these 82 per cent are about the knee. They start at the end of the bone near the epiphysis. The most important manifestation is pain, which precedes the appearance of the tumor and is severe and persistent. Such pain when it develops in the long bones of the young adult should always arouse the suspicion of bone sarcoma. The significance of trauma, though of great medicolegal importance, is questionable clinically, although such a history is frequently obtained (see p. 296). The swelling is slight at first but in neglected cases is characteristic, exhibiting a dusky hyperemia and often numerous dilated veins in the overlying skin. Local tenderness may be present but on palpation the tumor will be hard and firm. Systemic manifestations are usually absent in this tumor. In some instances, where the tumor is near a joint, the signs and symptoms suggest a clinical diagnosis of arthritis and treatment for this condition is erroneously instituted.

Diagnosis is often aided by two procedures: x-ray and biopsy. The roentgenogram may be characteristic but is often equivocal. Both lytic and blastic processes are evident though one or the other predominates. The so-called "sun-ray" picture is usually pathognomonic but is not frequently observed, appearing in only 18 per cent of the Bone Registry cases. Adequate biopsy should be performed wherever possible to establish the correct diagnosis. This procedure is not easy in the case of malignant bone tumors as the surgeon only too frequently removes overlying compressed tissue about the tumor and not portions of the neoplasm itself.

Treatment consists of operation or radiotherapy or a combination of both. Surgery may be either conservative (resection) or radical (amputation). Although "cure" is obtained only in a minority of cases (15 to 20 per cent), the surgeon aims to prolong life as much as possible and to insure the comfort of the patient. When the tumor appears relatively small and has not perforated the overlying periosteum, Phemister [11] raises the question of whether conservative therapy, *i.e.*, resection and bone graft with radiotherapy, might not offer as good results as the more mutilating high amputations; otherwise, high amputation remains the treatment of choice. While rarely curative, radiotherapy may afford excellent palliation lasting for prolonged periods (Brunschwig).

(*b*) EWING'S SARCOMA.—This neoplasm is relatively rare, comprising less than 10 per cent of all bone sarcomas; more than half are seen in children between the ages of 6 and 15 years.[9] It originates as a small round cell tumor resembling lymphosarcoma, probably from lymphatic channels within the cortex, but produces pronounced bone changes. Unlike osteogenic sarcoma it attacks the shaft rather than the end of the bone. Another characteristic of Ewing's sarcoma is that it metastasizes to the other bones as well as to the lungs. Clinically, pain is apt to occur in attacks and is usually preceded by trauma. Systemic manifestations of fever and leukocytosis as well as local tenderness often lead to a suspicion of osteomyelitis. Roentgenograms are often diagnostic because the tumor is located in the intracortical part of the shaft and also because the so-called "onion-peel" and "sun-burst" appearance is sometimes present. Treatment is that of osteogenic sarcoma. Immediate response to x-ray therapy characterizes this group of neoplasms.

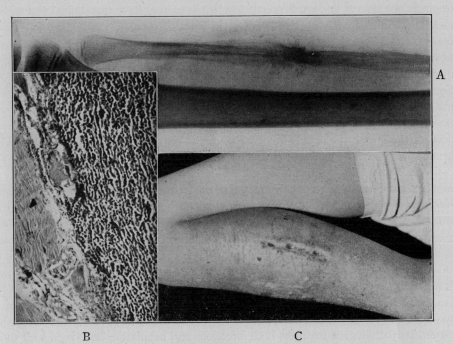

A

B   C

FIG. 173.—EWING TUMOR OF THE FIBULA IN A TWELVE-YEAR-OLD BOY.

There was a history of swelling of the calf, and pain of four months' duration. *A*, x-ray on admission; note the location of the lesion in the center of the shaft and the "onion peel" appearance above and below the central portion of the tumor. *B*, photomicrograph of biopsy which confirmed the x-ray diagnosis; note the lymphoid character of the tumor invading the adjacent stroma. *C*, photograph of the leg one month later, following radiotherapy. Death followed within a year.

(*c*) MYELOMA.—This is even more rare, occurs mostly in middle and advanced age and is manifested by rheumatic pain and skeletal deformities in advanced stages. Spontaneous fractures, most often in the ribs, are frequent. The common histologic type is characterized by large plasma cells; less frequently the type cell consists of a myeloblast. Roentgenograms show multiple "punched-out" areas; between one-half and three-fourths show Bence-Jones proteinuria. All cases are fatal in about two years. Treatment is symptomatic, x-ray often alleviating the pain.

(*d*) UNCLASSIFIED SARCOMA.—In this final group are placed two tumors—angio-endothelioma and extraperiosteal sarcoma of bone. The first is extremely rare and presents the same diagnostic and therapeutic problem as osteogenic sarcoma; it is described separately largely because of its peculiar histologic appearance.

The second tumor is in reality no bone sarcoma at all but a fibrosarcoma of the periosteum or adjacent fascial planes and behaves and is treated as other fascial sarcoma (see p. 309). It may produce bone changes but only by pressure from without.

3. *Sarcoma of Lymphoid Tissue (Malignant Lymphomatosis)*.—Though essentially a round-cell tumor, this type may be classified according to Ewing into at least four groups. This division is largely arbitrary, however, since the cell of origin is not always known. Nevertheless, these tumors have the clinical features of malignancy and seems to arise from, or at least to involve, the lymph nodes primarily. (*a*) *Simple lymphoma* (lymphadenoma, hyperplastic lymphadenitis) though histologically a benign and usually inflammatory enlargement of lymph nodes, is mentioned here because it sometimes presents difficulty in microscopic diagnosis. Some cases persist, grow and eventually cause death (Ewing). Subsequent study may show that they bear a relation to the other obvious malignant tumors of lymph nodes. (*b*) *Leukemia,* though a neoplasm of the blood forming cells, is included here because the lymph nodes are involved in the disease whether lymphatic or myelogenous in type. The nodes are usually discrete, although when large they soon coalesce. The spleen is often enlarged. Blood examinations make the diagnosis, except in some cases when there may be no leukocytosis (aleukemic leukemia). Excision of a node reveals a microscopic picture which is characteristic. Deposits of lymphogenous or myelogenous cells are sometimes seen at other sites including the skin (leukemia cutis). A greenish tumor of a leukemic type may occur in the skull, vertebrae and ribs, is called *chloroma* and, curiously enough, appears now to have become almost extinct. (*c*) *Hodgkin's disease* (Hodgkin's granuloma, lymphogranuloma) is classified as a malignant disease because it is manifested by enlargement of the lymph nodes and is fatal. There is some suggestion, however, that it is an infection (fever, leukocytosis), hence the use of the term granuloma in its designation. Its pathological features, both infectious and neoplastic, have been well summarized by Krumbhaar.[12] Its cause, like cancer, in general is still unknown. In some of the early cases described by Sternberg, he claimed to have found tubercle bacilli in the lymph nodes. Though never confirmed there is still a dispute as to the relationship of the disease to tuberculosis; an excellent discussion is that by Stewart and Doan.[13] Hodgkin's disease is manifested by progressive enlargement of the lymph nodes most frequently in the cervical region, but also in the mediastinum and elsewhere; the disease is often associated with fever, anemia and other blood changes. The enlarged nodes on microscopic section show a fairly characteristic hyperplastic picture upon which the diagnosis frequently depends. Fibrosis of a diffuse nature is a constant finding, but can be differentiated from that encountered in tuberculosis by the absence of necrosis and tubercles. Other features include the presence of numerous eosinophils and large multinucleated reticulum (Dorothy Reed) cells. The genetic neoplastic relationship of Hodgkin's disease to other malignant lymph node neoplasms has been discussed by Warthin.[14] The disease is subject to much clinical variation; it is to some extent dependent upon the chain of nodes involved. In superficial locations, usually the cervical region, the individual nodes are palpable as discrete elastic masses, variable in size and not tender. The spleen is enlarged in over half the cases. X-ray may reveal enlargement of the mediastinal nodes;

bone and skin involvement have been described. Generalized pruritis is said to be a frequent symptom at an early stage of the disease, the itching being due presumably to infiltration of the skin with lymphoid cells. Systemic symptoms may be absent; in some patients, on the other hand, high fever of the Pel-Epstein intermittent type and prostration develop. Changes in the white blood cells have been described, but are frequently absent; eosinophilia and increase in the mononuclear cells of the blood, however, are often present and may be of diagnostic value. X-ray

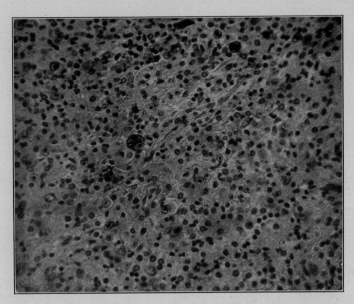

FIG. 174.—HODGKIN'S DISEASE IN A THIRTY-SEVEN-YEAR-OLD MALE.

Enlarged cervical nodes were observed three months before admission. The photomicrograph is from a section of one of them which was excised for diagnosis. Note the characteristic multinucleated (Dorothy Reed) cell in the center of the field; many eosinophiles are also present. Death occurred one and one-half years later with enlargement of the spleen, mediastinal and mesenteric nodes. Radiotherapy was refused by the family because the patient was a mental defective.

or radium therapy will cause temporary but usually rapid and complete regression of the enlarged nodes, although the course is eventually downhill and death occurs after months or years from cachexia and anemia. (d) *Lymphosarcoma* (lymphoblastoma, lymphocytoma) is a true primary neoplasm of the lymphoid tissue. Lymphoid tissue is, of course, distributed more or less throughout the human body but is especially concentrated in the lymph nodes. At the present time it seems probable that this lymphoid tissue has its origin in a syncytial type of undifferentiated supporting cell which has the power of producing the so-called lymphocyte as well as the reticulo-endothelial cell. Tumors arising from these two cell types may sometimes resemble each other and make classification extremely difficult. As a rule, however, they differ in microscopic and clinical characteristics just as normally they differ as to structure and function. For purposes of classification, therefore, we have two types of lymphosarcoma, the lymphocytic and the reticular cell. (1) Lymphocytic lymphosarcoma is a primary tumor the type cell of which tends to

resemble the lymphocyte. The chief symptoms are those produced by the local enlargement of groups of discrete nodes, without local tenderness or general symptoms, although a low grade fever and weakness may at times be present. Cachexia

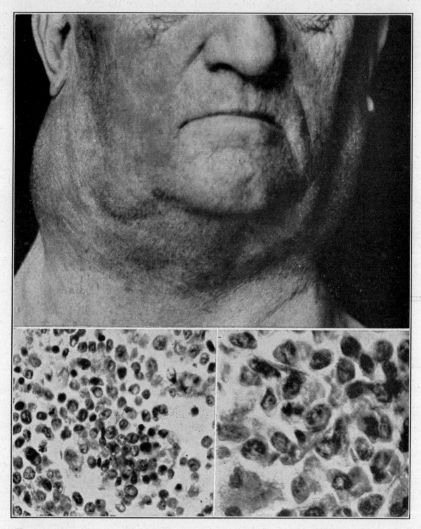

Fig. 175.—Lymphosarcoma, Rapidly Fatal, in a Sixty-six-year-old Man.

The onset was only two and one-half months previously with a gradually increasing swelling
of the neck and groin. At autopsy the nodes in the mediastinum and abdominal mesentery were
also enlarged. Metastatic nodules were found in the lungs, kidney and spleen. The low and
high power photomicrographs show the histologic appearance of the cells.

is absent. Microscopically the lymph node loses its normal architecture and in its
place one sees masses of abnormal lymphocytes growing at random with a minimum of reticulum and usually no germinal centers. While this cell is extremely
sensitive to irradiation at first, it eventually becomes resistant and the life expectancy in this disease is rarely over two years except in unusual cases. In the later

stages of this type of lymphosarcoma, fixed lymphoid tissue in many parts of the body may become involved or the tumor may metastasize as does any other sarcoma. At such times the lungs and heart are frequently involved. (2) Reticulum cell sarcoma is a primary tumor the cell type of which tends to resemble the reticulo-endothelial cell. It involves most frequently the lymph nodes of the neck, axilla, mediastinum and abdomen. As this same cell type is dominant in Hodgkin's disease the lymph node enlargement may often resemble this condition. In fact there are some authorities who prefer not to separate the two diseases but rather to consider them as manifestations of the same fundamental disturbance. While at the onset the glands are generally discrete, there is a tendency toward coalescence during the later stages giving clinical features not unlike those seen in certain types of exudative tuberculous lymphadenitis. The nodes are hard and not tender and tend to remain local for a much longer period of time than does the lymphocytic type. Because of this fact local excision has at times been advocated and we have seen cases free from recurrence for a long period of time following this procedure. Recurrence does generally take place, however, along with involvement of other nodes and tissues. At this time loss of weight is often seen and the picture becomes one of sarcomatous invasion. Microscopically the picture is that of cells growing with an effort to form reticulum. The nucleus is large and vesicular and the cytoplasm abundant. Phagocytosis may even be observed in the slower growing types. Silver stains show a massive amount of reticulum.

4. *Miscellaneous Sarcomas.*—Included under this heading are the following malignant growths of mesodermal origin: (*a*) *liposarcoma,* while rare, is a very malignant tumor with a rapidly fatal course, producing local and general metastases, especially to the lung. It is important to remove completely all lipomas, for they may, on rare occasions, contain sarcomatous areas recognizable grossly as being very cellular and on section containing cells with only traces of fat. (*b*) *Rhabdomyo-sarcoma* are tumors of striated muscle which have become malignant. They are so rare that diagnosis may not be suspected even after microscopic section. (*c*) *Thymoma* is a rather loosely used term to indicate a neoplasm involving the thymus. Many tumors in this region are really mediastinal lymphosarcoma. Tumors which involve the thymus primarily are quite rare; moreover there is considerable dispute as to the histological evidence of their origin.

III. Brain Tumors.—Brain tumors are special neoplasms which are really difficult to classify. Many of them (gliomas) are of ectodermal origin; many, however, are really of uncertain origin. In many instances they produce death not by the usual means, *i.e.,* metastasis, ulceration, cachexia, wasting, etc., but by virtue of their local effects on brain function and intracranial pressure. Some are benign in that they can be removed and the patient cured; others are malignant in the sense that they recur after removal, and invade the brain tissue. Other brain tumors are metastatic from distant primary sites, especially from carcinoma of the lung. Consideration of these tumors belongs to the special field of brain surgery, the details of which may be found in special publications [15] (some of these details will be found in Chapter XXII).

Neurocytoma.—This neurogenic tumor has general surgical interest because it occurs outside the brain and cord in the rich autonomic network of the posterior abdominal wall producing a retroperitoneal tumor which causes symptoms by its size and by pressure on adjacent structures. Though malignant, and sometimes rapidly so, this neoplasm often responds dramatically to radiotherapy. It is rather rare and simulates even on microscopic section other abdominal growths. Other terms for neurocytoma are neuroblastoma, sympathicoblastoma, etc. A group of 16 such cases have been described by H. K. Ransom.[16]

B. BENIGN NEOPLASMS

Benign neoplasms, unlike cancer, grow to a limited size, do not metastasize, and in general are not fatal. A few are really not true neoplasms in so far as they result directly from irritative or inflammatory stimuli (keloid, clavus, cutaneous

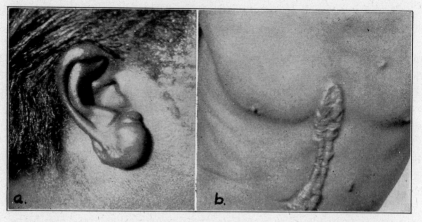

FIG. 176.—KELOIDS OF TYPICAL APPEARANCE, BOTH IN NEGROES.

a, Keloid at the site of a puncture for earrings; there was a history of considerable suppuration at the time the puncture was performed several months previously. *b,* This keloid formed at the site of a razor slash of the abdomen which had become infected and healed slowly.

horn, etc.). The etiology of most benign tumors, however, is unknown except that some cellular stimulus to useless growth of this type must be present. Occasionally the stimulus appears to be due to abnormal endocrine activity, particularly in the development of certain adenomas. The neoplastic change though apparently different from that seen in cancer may be of the same kind, but merely different in degree. Some benign tumors, moreover, have a malignant tendency in so far as they *recur* unless entirely removed. On rare occasions benign tumors undergo spontaneous malignant changes, metastasize and finally result in the death of the patient. It is possible, therefore, that when the cause of cancer is discovered one may also learn why benign tumors develop.

Benign tumors may be classified as were the malignant growths, into those arising from mesodermal and those arising from epithelial cells. However, it is clinically more useful, to divide the benign neoplasms into seven groups depending upon the tissue of origin, regardless of its embryonic type.

I. **Connective Tissue Origin.**—These tumors may be further classified into three sub-groups: fibrous, fatty, and bone (and cartilage) tumors.

1. *Fibrous Tissue Tumors.*—These neoplasms are various in form and appearance, but have in common a predominance of fibrous tissue on microscopic section. It will be recalled that this is in fact the microscopic characteristic of the end stage of repair; scar tissue is nothing more than a mass of fibrous tissue. However, scar is distinguished from tumor by its inconspicuous size, *i.e.,* though composed of the same tissue as a fibrous tissue tumor (fibroma), it is not large enough to be called

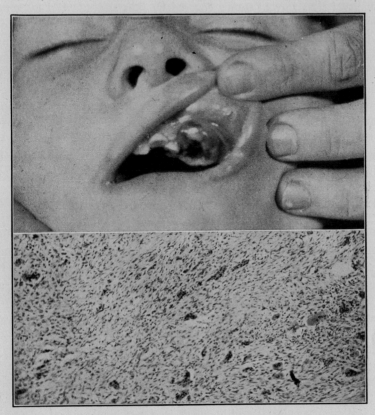

FIG. 177.—EPULIS IN A TEN-YEAR-OLD GIRL.

There was a history of an injury to the jaw before the onset of the tumor which was of two months' duration, growing slowly and bleeding occasionally. The insert is a photomicrograph of the excised tumor; note the numerous giant cells throughout the fibrous tissue stroma.

a tumor. Sometimes, however, the deposition of scar is sufficiently large and conspicuous to be called a tumor; it is then called a keloid. (*a*) *Keloid* is in reality a fibroma which grows, however, only after a stimulus of injury which may be trivial, such as the puncture of an ear lobe for wearing earrings. The demarcation between a normal scar and a keloid is inexact but depends largely on size. Other features of keloids are their tendency to form in the Negro race, their predilection for large granulating areas in which burns and severe suppuration have occurred, and their relative absence in clean aseptic wounds which have healed without irritation. Though of considerable theoretical interest in wound healing and in their relation to neoplastic growth, keloids have a practical importance only when they become large or painful or when they are present over the face, neck and arms, especially in young women. Excision is the treatment of choice, plus skin graft when the keloid is extensive. Radiotherapy has been disappointing. (b) *Simple fibroma* is a circumscribed tumor arising spontaneously, anywhere in the body, but usually in the skin or subcutaneous tissue. When it occurs in the form of a papilloma it is an ovoid tumor covered by skin and attached by a thin stalk or pedicle. Fibroma, though it may consist entirely of fibrous tissue, is commonly associated with other mesodermal or epithelial elements and is therefore called lipofibroma, neurofibroma, adenofibroma, myofibroma, etc. Neurofibroma occurs in Recklinghausen's disease which will be considered on page 328. When the cells in a fibroma have mucoid material between them the tumor may be spoken of as a *myxoma* or fibromyxoma. Many fibrous tumors which are soft contain myxomatous material. Certain small fibromas occur in the skin and become painful to the touch because of the presence of nerve fibers, though they are not true neurofibromas. Treatment consists of excision when indicated. *Desmoid tumor* is a rare type of fibroma which originates from the fascial structures of the anterior abdominal wall, nearly always in women and in those who have borne children. While the tumor may sometimes contain cellular or myxomatous areas it is really a benign tumor, in spite of its tendency to recur after removal. Treatment consists of wide excision followed by adequate repair of the defect in the abdominal wall. (c) *Epulis* is the name given to a fibroma (which often contains giant cells on microscopic section) arising from the portion of the gum which lines the submerged surface of the tooth (peridental membrane). It grows sometimes as a papilloma with the stalk attached to the gum at this point, but usually has a broad base and is expansile in its growth. It rarely grows to a large size, but recurs unless removed completely with a margin of normal gum tissue. It is usually necessary to extract one or two teeth. In some instances sarcomatous changes have been observed. (d) *Giant-cell tumor* of tendon sheaths and aponeuroses is a small fibroblastic neoplasm which contains giant cells and occurs usually in the hands and feet. It is easily removed, but tends to recur if not completely excised. Clinically it has no malignant tendencies, although it is occasionally spoken of as giant-cell sarcoma largely because of its histological appearance.

2. *Fatty Tissue.*—There are but two representatives in the group of fatty tissue tumors: the lipoma which is common, and the xanthoma which is rare. (a) The *lipoma* is composed of normal fat cells, or at most, cells larger than normal, arranged in the form of lobules which may be large and few in number, or so multiple as to resemble a cluster of grapes. True lipomas are definitely delimited by the surrounding fibrous tissue which fits tightly around each of those lobules. Its most common site is the subcutaneous tissue of the shoulders, back, upper arm and buttocks, more frequently in obese individuals. It has been found, however, in nearly every part of the body including the pelvis, kidney, bone and spinal cord. The tumor varies in size from a pea to a person's head. Its softness is a source of confusion to the novice, for it gives a sense of fluctuation which may lead to the diagnosis of a cyst or cold abscess. It may cause symptoms because of its size or cause pain by pressure on nerves. Treatment consists of excision which

must be complete in order to prevent recurrence. A rare disease in obese individuals with multiple painful fatty tumors has been described by Dercum (adiposis dolorosa). (*b*) Xanthoma, a rare tumor, may be single or multiple (xanthomatosis) and in the gross is yellow, hence the name. When the tumor is superficial the color can be seen through the skin. Microscopically it consists of foamy cells and frequently giant cells. The fat in the cells is composed of cholesterol, and is supposed by some to represent a defect in cholesterol metabolism. These tumors may develop about the eyelids, joints or in tendon sheaths and are usually small. On rare occasions they are found in the ribs and cranium; when they are associated with diabetes and exophthalmos the condition is called Christian's syndrome.

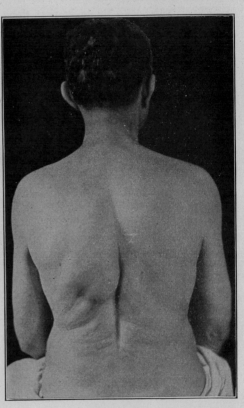

FIG. 178.—LIPOMA OF BACK, A COMMON LOCATION.

Tumor is subcutaneous and lies between the skin and underlying fascia.

3. *Bone and Cartilage.*—These tissues are conveniently considered together since they are frequently associated in the development of benign bone tumors. The classification and much of the data recorded by Geschickter and Copeland [10] will be used in this discussion. The tumors comprise five types. (*a*) *Osteochondroma or exostosis (osteoma)* is a common tumor, sometimes multiple, occurring most frequently near the ends of long bones, particularly at the distal end of the femur. It arises presumably from misplaced cartilaginous tissue, but consists primarily of bone. It produces no symptoms, often being noted accidentally in an x-ray film taken for another purpose. However, sometimes a mass is noticed; pain, when present, is more of an ache or discomfort. Occasionally a bursa forms over the tip of the tumor and may produce symptoms of bursitis when injured. Malignant changes may occur, but only after the age of thirty. Osteochondroma is most frequent between the age of ten and twenty. Roentgenologically the tumor has a base of normal bone protruding through the periosteum, the tip of which is covered more or less completely by cartilage. If symptoms are present, excision, including a cuff of normal bone, is indicated. When noted after the age of thirty the possibility of malignant change should be borne in mind. *Subungual exostosis* is a special variety of osteochondroma which grows under the nail of the fingers or toes where it may cause considerable pain and by breaking through the skin, lead to secondary infection. Excision is usually indicated after in-

fection, if present, has subsided. (*b*) *Chondroma* (*enchondroma*) *or chondromyxoma* is a fairly common tumor and while it resembles the exostosis microscopically, it is a central tumor in contrast to osteochondroma which is periosteal. It is most frequently present in the phalanges of the hand or foot, but also is seen in the long bones, sternum and spine. It is only rarely multiple. The symptoms are those of swelling, tenderness and pain. The larger tumors in the sternum and spine are prone to malignant change in that they are apt to recur, unlike those appearing in the phalanges which are more benign. Microscopically the tumor contains fairly normal adult cartilage, but grossly shows much gelatinous or myxomatous material. Roentgenologically there is a translucent central area with thinning and expansion of the cortex. Unlike the osteochondroma, it contains no bone. It is the commonest

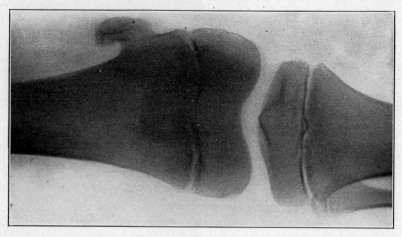

FIG. 179.—OSTEOCHONDROMA IN A CHARACTERISTIC LOCATION AT THE ADDUCTOR TUBERCLE OF THE FEMUR IN A NINE-YEAR-OLD BOY.

There was a history of injury to the knee which became "black and blue" at the site of a swelling noted by the mother. Operative excision was carried out; the diagnosis was confirmed microscopically.

cause of central bone destruction in the phalanges (see Fig. 180, p. 325). Though rare in the long bones its x-ray appearance is similar to bone cyst or benign giant-cell tumor. Treatment when indicated because of pain or swelling consists of thorough excision. (*c*) *Bone cyst* is different from osteitis fibrosa cystica in that it is solitary, whereas the latter term implies multiple lesions (see page 327). Bone cyst is most frequent in the upper humerus, tibia and femur. It is most common in children under fifteen years of age, occasionally produces pain and evident swelling, but more commonly is noted in the x-ray because it becomes the site of fracture which may be of the "spontaneous" type, *i.e.,* occurs following normal movements or with very slight trauma. The x-ray shows an expanding central defect with thinning of the cortex. The cavity contains clear or straw-colored fluid and is lined by cells showing fibrous tissue and some new bone formation. Phemister [17] has presented evidence that the lesion is inflammatory in origin. Treatment in case of fracture is the same as if the cyst were not present; complete union and disappearance of the lesion is the rule. If operated on because of swelling or pain the cavity is opened and swabbed with an antiseptic such as alcohol and the wound closed. Some surgeons fill the cavity with bone chips to

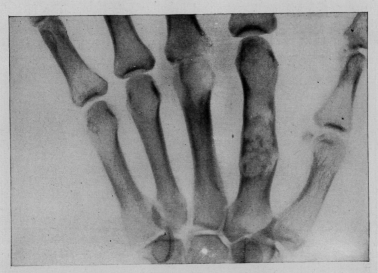

Fig. 180.—Enchondroma of the Second Metacarpal in a Twenty-five-year-old Machinist.

The tumor produced no symptoms but was noted in the x-ray which was taken because the patient had a serious hand infection; a pyogenic arthritis with destruction of the articular cartilage of the third metacarpophalangeal joint can be clearly noted.

promote osteogenesis. Lack of healing points to the existence of general disease such as Paget's disease of bone, generalized osteitis fibrosa, or bone lesions due to

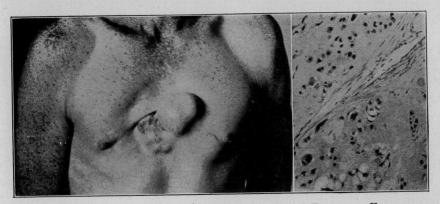

Fig. 181.—Enchondroma of the Sternum; Recurrent Tumor Following Excision of the Original Tumor Six Months Previously.

Though histologically similar to the tumor illustrated in Figure 180 this type is quite different in its clinical behavior. The photomicrograph is from a section of the original tumor and shows typical chondroblasts.

parathyroid tumor. (d) *Benign giant-cell tumor* occurs in many bones, but is most common in the epiphysis of the lower femur, upper tibia and distal radius. It produces pain, is often preceded by a history of trauma and may be the site of fracture, thus resembling the symptoms produced by a bone cyst. X-ray reveals a central translucent trabeculated osteolytic lesion which has expanded and thinned out the cortex, perforating it often and invading soft tissue. The fact that it involves the epiphysis is often of diagnostic value. At operation the tumor often appears hemorrhagic, bleeds when touched, and is soft and friable. Histologically

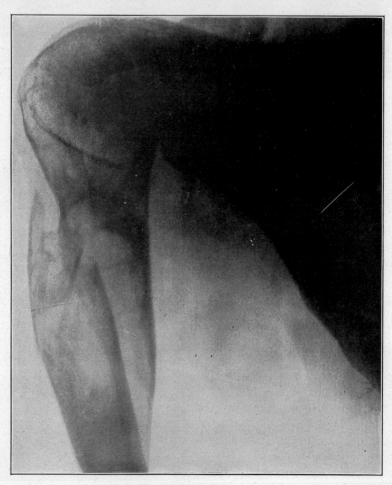

FIG. 182.—BONE CYST.

This is a solitary lesion as was shown by x-rays taken of many other bones. The lesion was noted because of the fracture which was sustained while the patient, a healthy twenty-one-year-old male, was pitching a base ball. The fracture was treated just as if no cyst were present, and healed normally.

it contains many giant cells in contrast to malignant bone tumors which contain only a few such cells. Treatment is essentially conservative and includes radiotherapy, operation or both. Surgical procedures include curettage and chemical or thermal cauterization. Recurrence may take place, but healing and disappearance of the tumor is the rule. The changes occurring in giant-cell tumors following radiotherapy with or without operation have been studied by Brunschwig[18] in an excellent detailed follow-up of nine cases. On the basis of his findings he prefers conservative surgical therapy alone to radiotherapy alone, but recommends as best, an operation followed by accurately administered radiotherapy. Among other things operation yields tissue for histologic study which is diagnostically important. *Tumors containing giant cells* comprise a variety of lesions. There are certain types of malignant bone tumors which, though containing giant cells, have obviously an entirely different clinical significance. But there occur giant-cell tumors of the jaw, subperiosteal giant-cell tumors, spindle cell variants and types of giant-cell

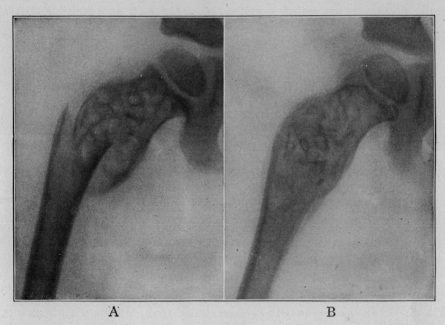

A   B

Fig. 183.—Benign Giant Cell Tumor in a Four-year-old Boy (Unverified by Microscopic Section).

The lesion was noted only because of a fracture which followed a fall. *A,* x-ray taken at time of injury; note the trabeculated nature of the shadow as well as the expansion of the cortex. *B,* x-ray taken three months later; the fracture was treated by reduction and immobilization in a plaster cast. This patient, now eight years old, is normal in every way.

variants in osteitis fibrosa which present special features (Ewing). Many giant-cell tumors of bone are manifestations of hyperparathyroidism (see p. 919). The extraskeletal giant-cell tumors include epulis, xanthoma and giant-cell tumor of the tendon sheath. (*e*) *Multiple cystic disease of bone* was described in 1891 by von Recklinghausen and is sometimes called von Recklinghausen's disease; this designation, however, has no connection with the more commonly known disease which also goes by his name, *i.e.,* neurofibromatosis which he described in 1882. The bone disease is often called osteitis fibrosa cystica or osteoplastica, but as described by von Recklinghausen was not a well-defined clinical entity. Adams, Compere, and Jerome [19] have described ten cases in detail under the name of regional fibrocystic disease and emphasize in therapy the need merely for preservation of function and correction of deformities.

On the other hand, it should be emphasized that the bone defects in many of these cases have been shown to be one of the manifestations of hyperparathyroidism and the lesions have disappeared on removal of the parathyroid adenoma. Chievitz and Olsen [20] collected 31 such instances in 1932 and Churchill and Cope [21] reported 11 cases in 1934. The discussion of hyperparathyroidism in general will be found in Chapter XXX.

II. Nervous Tissue Origin.—True neural tumors are rare except those in the brain (glioma); those which arise from the sympathetic nervous system are usually malignant, are called a variety of names such as sympathicoblastoma,

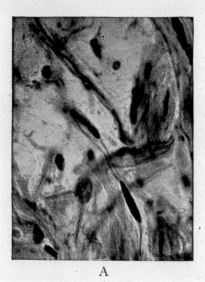
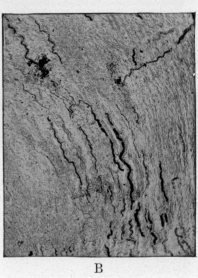

A   B

Fig. 184.—Photomicrographs of a Neurofibroma, Stained to Show Nerve Elements.

A, nonmyelinated nerve fibers intermingling with collagen in a peripheral neurofibroma; *B*, myelinated nerve fibers entering a neurofibroma (Morgan myelin sheath stain). (From Penfield, *Cytology and Cellular Pathology of the Nervous System*, 1932, P. B. Hoeber, p. 977.)

ganglioneuroma, etc., and are discussed on page 319. Spina bifida and meningocele are not really neoplasms and are described elsewhere. In the peripheral nerves traumatic *neuroma* may result following injury or division of nerves, but are discussed in detail in Chapter XXII. *Glomus tumors* are rare, tiny neoplasms which, however, contain vascular and epithelial as well as nerve tissue. They occur most frequently in the nail bed and about the fingers and toes, elbow, knee and leg. The tumors are characteristically painful, either spontaneously or to the touch (Lewis and Geschickter [22]).

An easily recognized type is *Recklinghausen's disease (neurofibromatosis)*, a rare but disfiguring affliction due to extensive multiple tumors of the skin and rarely the deeper tissues. They originate from the neurilemmal sheath of peripheral nerves and contain definite nerve filaments which, while diagnostic of the disease, are demonstrable only with special stains.[23] While the disease has been named after the German physician who reported instances of the disease in 1882, a Dublin surgeon, Robert W. Smith, first described the condition in 1849 in a monograph which was privately printed and apparently lost to medical records. Fulton[24] in 1929 called attention to this communication. The eponymic term applied to the disease should possibly be that of Robert W. Smith, whose description was accurate and included microscopic observations and carefully executed plates illustrating the lesion.

Clinical manifestations are generally due only to the appearance of tumors themselves. Pain, though generally absent, may be present in some cases. Because the tumors are often white, soft and pedunculated, the term *fibroma molluscum* is also used. Areas of skin pigmentation are so frequently encountered as to be of diagnostic value. In addition to the skin lesions which vary in size from a pea to a grapefruit, tumors are also found in the bone (Brooks and Lehman[25]), central nervous system and pelvis where they may cause severe symptoms of pain and disability merely by their pressure. Malignant (sarcomatous) changes are occasionally encountered, and unless the growth is removed early, recovery may be impossible. There is no treatment for the multiple skin tumors since they are usually too numerous for complete excision. When large and causing symptoms by pressure, removal may be urgently indicated. *Perineurial fibroblastoma* occurs in the same locations as Recklinghausen's disease but is usually single. Histologically it is differentiated from neurofibroma by the fact that the nerve fibers do not pass through the tumor nodule. They are common only along the eighth nerve (acoustic neuroma). Their treatment belongs to the domain of neurosurgery.

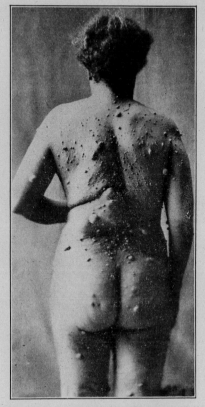

Fig. 185.—Multiple Neurofibromatosis in a Forty-five-year-old Negress.

No symptoms were present, except for moderate disability due to a tumor in the right axilla. This was excised for that reason.

III. Blood Vessel Origin.—Many of the various tumors arising from blood vessels are of neoplastic nature. Lesions such as aneurysms and arteriovenous fistulas are described in detail in Chapter XX. The blood vessel neoplasms are called angiomas and hemangiomas in contrast to lymphangiomas which are somewhat similar in structure, but contain lymph instead of blood. The angiomas are new growths containing vascular tissue of capillary, venous or arterial origin, with a variable amount of connective tissue stroma. The vascular spaces are lined by endothelium and may be very large. Though congenital and present at birth, they sometimes have a power of growth which develops later or they may remain occult until adult life when symptoms may be produced. They occur in practically all tissues of the body and assume a great variety of clinical forms to which many terms have been applied. Of those located in the deeper structures, most are of the cavernous type (see p. 332) and usually produce symptoms by pressure or by abnormal bleeding. They occur in the brain, orbit, intestines, pelvic organs, muscle, and especially in the liver where they may be a rare cause of intraperitoneal hemorrhage. Symptoms depend on their location and size. True malignant change, including metastasis, has been described in angiomatous tumors, but is extremely rare.

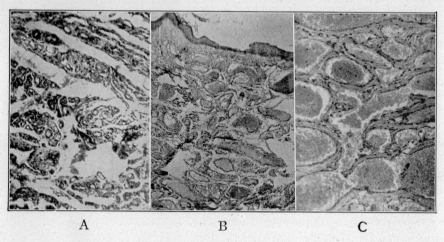

A   B   C

FIG. 186.—PHOTOMICROGRAPHS OF THE THREE TYPES OF BLOOD VESSEL NEOPLASMS DESCRIBED IN THE TEXT.

A, capillary hemangioma; section is from a small port-wine stain excised from the neck of a two-month-old infant. Note the numerous small capillaries in the midst of many angioblasts; all of the channels contained blood. *B, hypertrophic hemangioma;* section is from a small red tumor with roughened surface, removed from the arm of a six-year-old girl. Note the dilated thin-walled channels filled with blood. *C, cavernous hemangioma;* section is from a tumor, about 3 centimeters in diameter, over the elbow of a twelve-year-old boy. A small tumor was present at birth but it began to grow markedly in the past three weeks. The skin may not be involved in this type of hemangioma. Note the thick-walled large sinuses filled with blood. This cavernous appearance is possessed by most of the hemangiomas encountered in the deeper structures of the body.

The visible hemangiomas, *i.e.,* those which occur in or under the skin and mucous membranes are perhaps the most common. In spite of the large and confusing terminology often applied to these lesions, the following classification of skin angiomas (modified after Zeisler [26]) has been adopted.

1. *Capillary hemangioma,* or flat vascular nevus, is well known as the *port wine stain* and is sometimes called nevus flammeus or vinosus. Though a neoplasm, it is manifested not as a tumor at all, but as a disfiguring red or purple discoloration due to a plexus of newly formed, but normally sized capillaries in the corium of the skin. Its origin is probably due to some accident of maldevelopment during embryonic life, though popular belief ascribes its etiology to some profound nervous shock to the mother while pregnant. Port wine stains ordinarily maintain a constant size and rarely increase in extent. The problem of treatment is a real one in the large areas which occur on the face or head. The use of radium has caused satisfactory blanching in some cases although it may be followed by a dis-

figuring scar. Skilled dermatologists sometimes achieve excellent results with carbon dioxide snow.

2. *Hypertrophic hemangioma* also called *angioma simplex* or angioma plexiforme, differs from the capillary nevus in being a true tumor, raised above the surface of the skin, though composed similarly of newly formed capillaries which, however, are dilated. The tumor varies in size from a millimeter to several centimeters in size; it shades gradually into the larger ones which are generally called

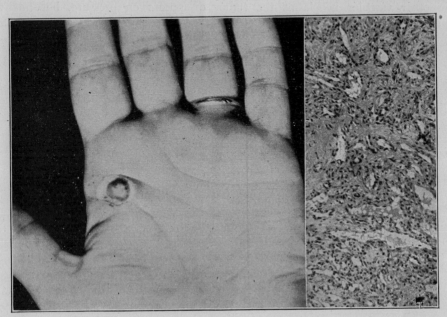

Fig. 187.—Infected Hemangioma of the Hand, in a Twenty-two-year-old Housewife.

This is a not uncommon type but the true diagnosis is often masked by the secondary inflammation which gives to the lesion the appearance of exuberant granulation tissue. This tumor was in the form of a papilloma and was easily excised. The photomicrograph reveals the true nature of the tumor; the dilated blood spaces resemble those shown in Figure 186B.

cavernous angioma and have different histologic characteristics (see p. 332). In color the hypertrophic hemangioma varies from a bright red to a dull purple. The large red tumor is often called a strawberry mark. Over three-fourths of these tumors are on the head, commonly over the forehead, occiput, scalp, lip, but may occur over any part of the body. The clinical course of this small angioma varies. A few seem to shrink and disappear. In some instances they ulcerate, become infected, slough and heal, leaving only a tiny scar. Most of them remain stationary or merely grow with the growth of the child and are presented for treatment in childhood or adult life because they act as a cosmetic blemish. Of great importance, however, is the tendency of some of those tumors to exhibit rapid active growth, particularly in infants. If this occurs, a tiny birth mark of apparently no significance may finally involve an entire eyelid, nose or lip or spread over half of the face or scalp and finally become a true cavernous angioma. It must be emphasized, therefore, that every angioma in infants, regardless of its size, should be watched carefully and be removed even in the first weeks of life if any growth occurs. The treatment of the small lesions is relatively simple. Electrotherapy or irradiation of various types and other means have been used, but should be carried out only by those expert in their use. Surgical excision is sometimes possible when the lesion is superficial.

3. *Cavernous hemangioma* is a disfiguring vascular tumor usually involving a large part of the scalp, face, tongue or other part of the superficial surfaces. Like the other vascular neoplasms the tumor disappears on pressure, but fills up

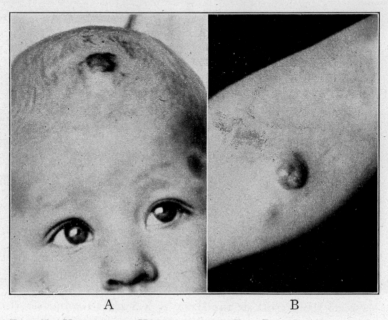

A   B

FIG. 188.—HYPERTROPHIC HEMANGIOMAS IN TWO DIFFERENT LOCATIONS.

A, the patient is a three-months-old infant; the tumor has been growing slowly since birth. Obliteration of the tumor was achieved by the use of radium. *B*, the patient is a five-year-old girl and the tumor of the leg has been growing slowly for several months. This tumor was excised. Section revealed a microscopic appearance approximately midway between that shown in *B* and *C* of Figure 186.

rapidly. It differs from the other two types because of its size and because it contains true vascular channels (venous and arterial) which resemble the structure of the corpora cavernosa of the penis, hence its name. Cavernous hemangiomas present a grave problem in treatment, especially when they involve the face, for they are not only extensive superficially, but often penetrate deeply and bleed profusely if any part of the mass is incised, thus making hemostasis during excision difficult. Because of the difficulties of surgical excision, other methods of treatment, such as diathermy, radiotherapy and injection of various substances, have been tried from time to time and in some instances gratifying results have been achieved. The choice of method depends on the size and location of the tumor.

Other forms of congenital vascular tumors of the skin are described, but are rather rare. *Angioma racemosum* or cirsoid aneurysm is composed of both arteries and veins which form large serpentine swellings which pulsate visibly and give rise to an audible bruit due to the presence of many communications between the venous and arterial channels. They are in reality not neoplasms, but congenital abnormalities of blood vessels (arteriovenous fistula) and are described in Chapter XX.

IV. Lymphatic Origin.—Lymph channels are frequently involved by obstructive and inflammatory, but only rarely by neoplastic, disease. (1) *Lymphangioma* is an actual neoplasm of the lymphatic channels which occurs in a great many clinical forms, usually, however, as a boggy tumor of the skin and sub-

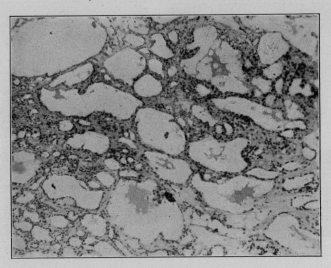

FIG. 189.—LYMPHANGIOMA OF THE TONGUE.

Photomicrograph of a tumor removed from the tongue of a twenty-five-year-old woman. Note the dilated, thin-walled channels, which are, however, filled with lymph and not red blood cells. Another differential feature is the frequent presence of nests of lymphocytes which are seen only in lymphangiomas and not in hemangiomas. However, this tumor did not possess this differentiating feature.

cutaneous tissue more particularly where the lymphatics are abundant. It may occur in the form of a pedunculated mass. Lymphangioma may be a diffuse, slowly growing tumor involving the tongue or lip giving rise to *macroglossia* or *macrolabia* (*microcheilia*) respectively. The tumor may be so disfiguring or result in such disability as to require excision and plastic repair. Lymphangioma often occurs concomitantly with cavernous hemangioma which is occasionally associated with a type of varicose veins. Lymphanigoma frequently contains islands of lymph cells in addition to lymphatic vessels. The channels themselves vary in size and when large present a cystic appearance (hygroma or lymphangiocysticum). When it occurs in the neck (usually in infants), it is called *Cystic hygroma* and consists of multilocular lymph filled sacs arising in the tissue beneath the deep fascia. The large cystic mass frequently produces serious obstruction to the trachea and esophagus and occasionally becomes infected, necessitating drainage. Excision is often difficult or impossible. Injections of sclerosing solutions are often useful. Lymph nodes themselves do not give rise to benign tumors of neoplastic origin except as a part of lymphangioma. When enlargement of lymph nodes occurs it is due either to inflammatory causes or to malignant diseases. (2) *Thymoma* is a loose term applied to tumors originating from the thymus gland. Actually there are various types of growths, mostly malignant, which cause symptoms by increased mediastinal pressure. Thymic enlargement is physiologic in infants, but when excessive is known as *status thymolymphaticus,* a condition which is also associated with general lymphoid hyperplasia and is supposed to be a cause of sudden death in children.

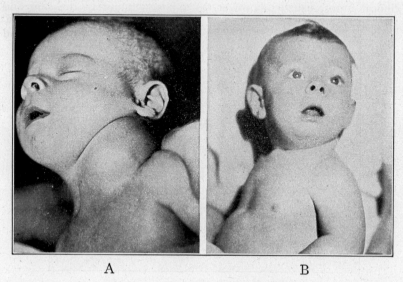

A   B

FIG. 190.—CYSTIC HYGROMA OF NECK.

A, photograph of infant on admission at the age of one month. Note the enlargement in the left side of the neck which was cystic to palpation; *B,* photograph of patient five months later after several procedures including partial excision as well as the use of sodium morrhuate as a sclerosing agent. The patient also had a similar swelling in the left axilla which was successfully treated in the same way. Microscopic sections of tissue removed showed dilated lymph channels as well as lymphocytic infiltration.

V. Muscle Tissue Origin.—Muscle has but one common representative in benign tumors, and that is the myoma of the uterus, often called fibromyoma because it contains fibrous as well as smooth muscle tissue. It often grows to huge size and produces many local symptoms and signs (see Chapter XXXI). Though benign tumors of striated muscle (rhabdomyoma) also occur they are so rare that they are recognized usually only after microscopic examination.

VI. Mixed Tissue Origin.—1. *Mixed tumors* occur most frequently in and upon the salivary glands, most commonly the parotid. Microscopic section reveals not only mesodermal cells such as cartilage and fibrous tissue, but also epithelial elements and other tissue unrecognizable as to origin. There is usually a history of a small quiescent tumor for several years preceding active growth. When growth is rapid it is frequently indicative of malignant change. The typical tumor is firm, limited, and presents a nodular surface, later becoming cystic. These tumors recur unless completely and carefully removed together with their surrounding capsule. Benign teratomas are also composed of mixed tissue, but are more obviously embryonic rests and are described below.

2. *Teratoma* represents, according to most authorities, an absorbed or partly grown twin which stopped development at some early stage and became encapsulated by the other normal fetus. Thus it contains as already mentioned mixed or diverse structures, which are epithelial and mesodermal, *e.g.,* muscle, hair, teeth, intestine, etc. Great variations in size and development occur. A teratoma usually develops in the midline but is found most frequently in the testicle, ovary,

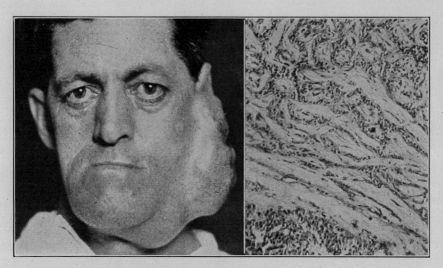

FIG. 191.—MIXED TUMOR OF THE PAROTID IN A FORTY-SEVEN-YEAR-OLD MALE.

The tumor was first noted eighteen years previously; after excision it recurred and grew more rapidly for four years when it was excised a second time. The present tumor is the second recurrence which has been growing slowly for fourteen years. An extensive dissection was necessary before the tumor could be completely removed. The photomicrograph shows cords of epithelial cells which seem to form intercellular myxomatous material; this is one of the features of this type of neoplasm.

sacrococcygeal region and in the mediastinum. It causes symptoms by pressure or by undergoing malignant degeneration or both. It is, of course, present at birth, but often remains occult until symptoms develop in later life. It is described in detail in later chapters. When a teratoma contains skin elements only (hair and sebaceous material), it is often called a dermoid.

VII. Epithelial Cell Origin.—The various benign tumors of epithelial origin are a rather heterogeneous group and although a few are common, they represent in general rather rare types of benign tumors. They comprise three arbitrary groups: adenomas, skin tumors and tumors of the jaw.

1. *Adenoma.*—This tumor is a benign collection of epithelial cells originating from glandular tissue. When in endocrine glands the tumor may actually function as secretory tissue as noted in the hypoglycemia produced by adenoma of the islets of Langerhans of the pancreas (see pp. 927 to 929). In other endocrine glands, such as the thyroid, adenomas may also cause symptoms, but frequently occur "silently" without producing any manifestations of functional activity. In

the pituitary an adenoma may lead to abnormalities in growth; in the adrenal it may produce peculiar sex development. Adenoma of the parathyroid may result in abnormal calcium metabolism and the formation of multiple bone lesions. When adenomas form in glands with external secretions they rarely cause symptoms from functional activity since they rarely function as normal tissue. Thus an adenoma of the breast (usually fibro-adenoma or intracanalicular fibromyxoma dependent on its microscopic features) does not produce milk, but merely manifests itself as a circumscribed lump which is sometimes painful. Other circum-

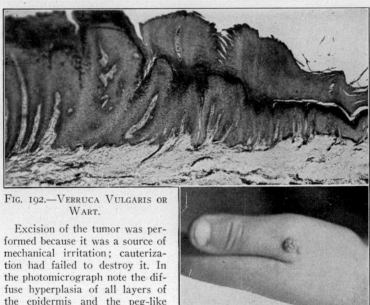

FIG. 192.—VERRUCA VULGARIS OR WART.

Excision of the tumor was performed because it was a source of mechanical irritation; cauterization had failed to destroy it. In the photomicrograph note the diffuse hyperplasia of all layers of the epidermis and the peg-like arrangement of the growth which gives to the surface its cauliflower appearance.

scribed adenomas include the sebaceous adenoma which, though rare, may be the site of squamous or basal-cell epithelioma. Treatment of adenoma consists of excision. *Rhinophyma* is a peculiar enlargement of the nose due to hypertrophy rather than actual neoplasm of the sebaceous glands and skin. Plastic repair is often indicated.

Attention should be called to adenomatous hyperplasia which may result in papillomatous formation, especially in the stomach and colon (polyposis). Other examples of adenomatous hyperplasia are fungous or glandular endometriosis in the uterus, and prostatic hypertrophy.

2. *Epithelial Benign Tumors of The Skin.*—Prominent among the benign skin tumors are (a) *warts* (*verruca vulgaris*) which are epithelial neoplasms originating from the germinative epithelium of the skin. They sometimes are papillomatous, but usually are manifested as a cone-shaped elevation with a flat top whose surface exhibits a characteristic cauliflower-like appearance and numerous tiny black dots. Warts have a tendency to become irritated, painful and occa-

sionally infected. Ordinarily, however, they produce no symptoms, or at the most, a slight "sticking" sensation. Nevertheless, when the warts are located under the nail, on the cuticle or the sole of the foot, pain may be pronounced. The tumor occasionally disappears spontaneously, sometimes within a short time after its development. This feature undoubtedly accounts for the reputed efficacy of the many home remedies, some mixed with the use of magic formulas which have been used from time immemorial for their removal. The wart has considerable theoretical interest because, although possessing all the characteristics of a true neo-

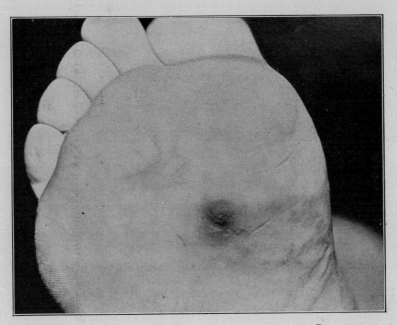

FIG. 193.—PLANTAR WART IN A SIXTEEN-YEAR-OLD GIRL.

Symptoms of pain and disability were marked. Note the slight redness, indicative of a mild degree of inflammation. Radiotherapy was curative in this case; it is obviously a very convenient form of therapy. Unfortunately it is not always effective.

plasm, evidence indicates that it is in reality an infection due to a filtrable virus. This probably explains why warts may appear and disappear suddenly without apparent reason, and why they may spread by contact as from one finger to a comparable point on the next digit or directly from a distal point to one proximal to it. If the tumor is excised aseptically and ground up and passed through a Berkefeld filter the clear filtrate upon injection into the skin will give rise to a new wart. It has been said that if we knew the pathogenesis of the common wart we would know something about the etiology of cancer.

Treatment is rarely indicated for cosmetic reasons because warts ordinarily grow on the hands and feet. When infection is present it should be treated first. The tumor may be either destroyed or excised. Destruction of the wart may be achieved with (1) the x-ray, (2) by some form of cautery, e.g., electrical, thermal, or by chemicals (fuming nitric acid, trichloracetic acid, salicylic acid), or (3) surgical excision. Palmar and plantar warts are often the most difficult to eradicate. Irradiation is often effective in treating plantar warts but must be used with great care and only for one trial; if the lesion does not respond, surgical excision should be used. When the wart is more superficial and in soft thin skin, chemical cauterization is the simplest method and consists simply of applying a drop of the acid over the plateau of the wart (not involving the adjacent skin) and letting it seep in. When it has reached the base of the growth a burning sensation is noted by the patient. The excess acid is then wiped off. The process may be repeated in forty-eight hours. After several days the wart drops out leaving a shallow insignificant ulcer which heals readily. If a tiny recurrence occurs it can be treated similarly later. (*b*) *Cutaneous horn* (*cornu cutaneum*) is a form of cutaneous wart in which the horny layer (cornified epithelium) gives rise to the actual tumor. It may consist of a small area of hyperkeratosis, but fair-sized hard projecting growths may form, chiefly on the scalp. (*c*) *Moles or pigmented nevi* occur commonly in the skin and are usually congenital. A much better term is *benign melanoma*. There has been considerable dispute as to the actual cell of origin. Although the evidence that melanomas arise from epithelial cells seem convincing, the most recent work points to the chromatophores which are mesoblastic, as the cells of origin. Their designation, whether under epithelial or mesothelial tumors, thus is still uncertain. Clinically, benign melanomas are small raised areas which occasionally take the form of a papilloma and often have hairs growing out of them. Their importance lies largely in the fact that certain types give rise occasionally to the highly malignant melanoma (see page 306). Excision is generally advisable if moles become chronically irritated or bleed, if sudden enlargement occurs, or if they are present on the feet. They may also be destroyed by the electrical cautery. Occasionally they are removed for cosmetic reasons when present in an exposed part of the body, particularly in young women.

3. *Jaw Tumors.*—Though largely of ectodermal origin, jaw tumors comprise a great variety of neoplasms. Blair and Ivy [27] have considered most of them as varieties of odontomas or tumors derived from special cells concerned with the development of teeth. The following groups are described, modified from their classification: (*a*) *Adamantinoma* is a solid or often multilocular cystic tumor which develops within the alveolar bodies of the maxilla, but more frequently in the mandible. Microscopically it contains cells of squamous epithelium, or fibrous tissue and even of the enamel organ. Clinically it is slowly growing, is present most commonly in the molar region and produces no pain. When large it may present a lobulated surface and upon pressure the thin walls of the cyst may produce a sensation such as the crackling of parchment or celluloid. Excision is the only form of treatment, but must be complete in order to avoid recurrence. (*b*) *Dentigerous cysts* (odontocele, corodental cyst, periosteal cyst) is probably the most common tumor of the jaw and is a benign hollow cyst lined with epithelium containing viscid straw-colored fluid with a partly or fully developed tooth projecting into the cavity. Symptoms arise only when they reach a sufficient size to be noticed. When large the cyst may give a sensation of "celluloid crackling." Treatment consists of complete removal of the cyst and its capsule, and extraction of the tooth. A *dental root cyst* is another type of jaw tumor and results from irritation of the dental epithelial cell rests in the peridental membrane of a

tooth that has undergone eruption, usually a pulpless tooth (Blair and Ivy). (c) *Composite odontoma* is a calcified tooth tumor composed of varying elements which often demands excision. (d) *Osseous tumors* also occur in the jaw. In addition to the various types of benign bone tumors which may develop in the jaw, the so-called *fibrous osteoma* is a characteristic growth of the mandible.

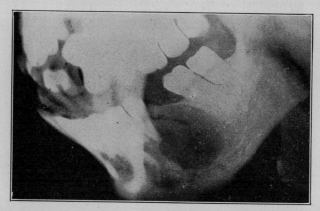

FIG. 194.—DENTIGEROUS CYST IN A TWENTY-FIVE-YEAR-OLD MALE.

This lesion produced no symptoms and was first noted in the roentgenogram which was taken because of an injury to the jaw. Note the fracture line extending into the cyst (St. Louis City Hospital).

All jaw tumors may become infected and the true nature of the tumor may thus be obscured. The roentgenogram is usually characteristic and enables an accurate diagnosis in most cases.

C. CYSTS

Cysts form a special group of tumors which owe their swelling to the presence of fluid rather than cellular elements. However, the designation is far from absolute for many solid tumors contain cystic areas and many cysts harbor solid cellular areas. The clinical designation may also be difficult in that some sarcomas are soft and fluctuant as if they contained fluid, whereas some cysts contain fluid under such high tension that on palpation they resemble a hard solid mass. Such difficulties, however, may usually be overcome by aspiration of the tumor. Cysts are much more difficult to classify than other tumors. The following groups, therefore, represent a purely arbitrary classification.

I. **Retention Cysts.**—These tumors form because the duct of a gland becomes occluded, usually by inflammation, so that the secretion of the gland accumulates as a cyst.

Galactocele is a type of retention cyst in the breast which occurs during lactation and will be discussed in Chapter XXVIII. Mucoceles are tiny cysts commonly in the mouth which are due to the occlusion of the opening of a tiny mucous gland. *Ranula* is a retention cyst located in the floor of the mouth under the tongue, is first confined to one side, later projecting across the midline. It is caused by an obstruction of one of the tiny, sublingual ducts which becomes distended with clear mucoid material and often attains a large size.

The most common representative of the retention cyst is the so-called *wen* or *sebaceous cyst*. In its simplest form it manifests itself as the ordinary comedo in which the retained sebaceous material is visible under the skin. In its most pronounced form it presents a semispherical elevation in the skin to which it is

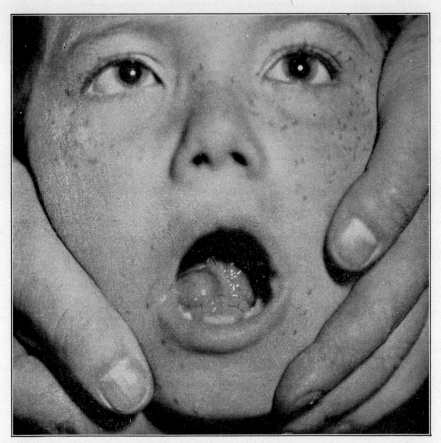

FIG. 195.—RANULA IN A FOUR-YEAR-OLD BOY.

The smooth cystic tumor was noted by the mother accidentally. It increased in size steadily. Note that it is confined to one side of the floor of the mouth and does not cross the midline. Treatment consisted of complete excision of the cyst.

attached. The tiny opening of the obstructed gland can often be seen at the pole of the tumor. It occurs most commonly in the scalp, back and neck and may be multiple. It is soft and fluctuant, containing characteristic greasy, thick, grayish paste. The contents sometimes escape spontaneously or on pressure through a tiny opening, only to refill again. Complete excision of the sac is curative. Sometimes the cyst becomes infected, whereupon it presents the signs of an abscess which should be incised. The infection may destroy the secreting cells so that after inflammation subsides, recurrence may not occur. If it does fill up, excision can then be done. Malignant degeneration (carcinoma of a sebaceous gland) is rare but should be suspected if a draining sinus persists and fails to heal after incision of any superficial abscess of the skin.

II. Degeneration Cysts.—This term applies to cysts which sometimes form at the site of large hematomas which, instead of becoming absorbed and replaced with fibrous tissue, liquefy and remain as permanent tumors. They may be present in the abdomen after an intraperitoneal hemorrhage, in the chest or in the brain. Ordinarily the fluid is first brownish, but later it undergoes changes which convert it into hematoidin which is the same as bilirubin (Rich and Bumstead [28]) and

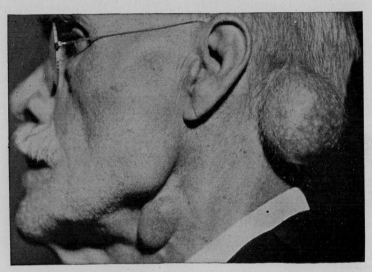

Fig. 196.—Sebaceous Cysts.

Two of these tumors are present in this patient; they are of many years' duration and have been increasing slowly in size. The one at the back of the head, though unusually large, is in a characteristic location above the hairline; it was excised under local anesthesia and contained typical grayish greasy sebaceous material.

colors the fluid yellow. Occasionally cholesterol crystals are found in such degeneration cysts.

III. Neoplastic Cysts.—Neoplastic cysts generally include those which depend for their formation on a new growth, although in most cases the new cells are in reality abnormalities, congenital in origin. Ovarian cysts of various types have been described and belong in this group. Bone cysts have been described under bone tumors.

IV. Dermoids or Dermoid Cysts.—These terms should in reality include only cysts dependent for their formation on an inclusion of squamous epithelium under the skin. In some instances the cells continue to function as normal skin, and a cyst containing hair, sebaceous material and cellular débris is formed. The small cysts, however, only contain clear fluid. The inclusion is usually congenital and occurs around the orbits, temple, mastoid and neck or floor of the mouth. When a similar cyst is encountered in the ovary or mediastinum it should in reality be classified as a teratoma containing only epithelial elements. Dermoids of the skin, moreover, unlike ovarian and mediastinal dermoids, practically never undergo malignant change. Excision of the dermoids of the skin is indicated chiefly for cosmetic reasons. Those in the floor of the mouth are in the midline and may cause pressure symptoms; they are very rare, but should not be confused with ranula, which is unilateral. Those over the forehead should be distinguished from meningoceles which communicate with the brain; they may also be confused with lipomas and sebaceous cysts. Dermoids which occur in the sacral region are called pilonidal cysts or sinuses, and are seen frequently.

A pilonidal cyst is a derivative of skin ectoderm which becomes invaginated during embryonic life and remains only as a vestigial skin appendage, which de-

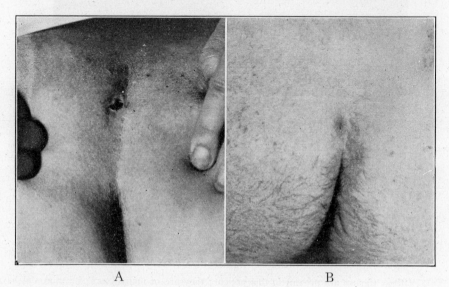

A   B

Fig. 197.—Two Examples of Pilonidal Sinus.

A, in a twenty-year-old girl; symptoms started at puberty with the appearance of a tender coccygeal mass which opened and drained pus only to heal and recur at intervals of many months. The photograph was taken a few days after the last abscess had opened and drained. Excision of the entire track was performed later after the acute inflammation had subsided. *B,* a more characteristic appearance in a twenty-five-year-old male with a similar history. The acute infection has long since subsided and now exhibits only a tiny, chronically draining opening; the track itself, however, extends upward and medially for several centimeters.

velops at puberty, thereby explaining its age distribution (Fox [29]). Thus it rarely produces clinical manifestations until young adult life (twenty to twenty-five years), and then only because the cyst becomes infected and forms an abscess which usually opens spontaneously and gives rise to a chronic draining sinus. This sinus may close, fill up, break down and discharge intermittently. Occasionally the infection undermines the subcutaneous tissue over the coccyx and results in an extensive abscess. Even if drainage is adequate healing will not occur, presumably because of the presence of living and therefore secreting epithelium in the lining of the tortuous sinus.

Inspection in the sacral region will nearly always reveal one or more tiny dimples in the midline over the coccyx. They resemble in appearance the pre-

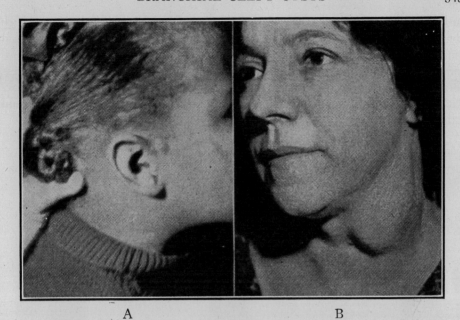

A   B

FIG. 198.—BRANCHIAL CLEFT CYSTS AT TWO DIFFERENT CLEFTS.

A, cyst of the first branchial cleft; note the pre-auricular dimple which is associated with the cyst but is often present alone; *B*, cyst of a lower cleft. Excision was performed in both cases; the lining of the cyst consisted of squamous epithelium and also contained nests of lymphoid cells.

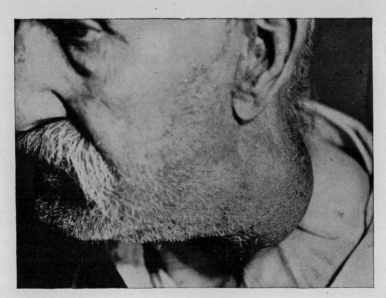

FIG. 199.—BRANCHIAL CLEFT CYST WHICH HAS UNDERGONE CARCINOMATOUS CHANGE IN A SEVENTY-YEAR-OLD MAN.

The tumor was of steady growth, apparently of only six months' duration. Aspiration of a cystic area yielded sufficient tissue to make a diagnosis of malignant disease. Complete excision was performed under local anesthesia.

auricular dimple seen in a branchial cyst at the first cleft (see p. 345). Such dimples are common, and may on rare occasions be associated with severe local pain in absence of infection. Ordinarily, however, the superimposed infection contributes nearly all the local signs and symptoms. The location of the abscess or sinus opening over the coccyx plus the midline dimples are sufficiently characteristic to easily differentiate pilonidal infections from ischiorectal abscess and fistula-in-ano.

Treatment consists of complete excision of the diseased tissue after allowing acute infection to subside. All cells lining the tract must be removed, else recurrence is inevitable. This requires in most cases, a rather extensive dissection;

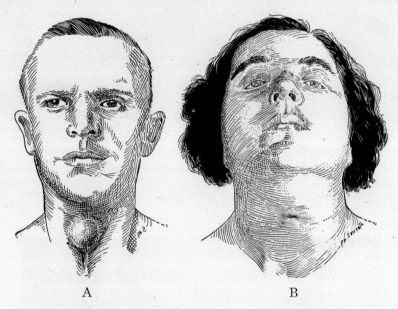

A   B

FIG. 200.—TWO EXAMPLES OF THYROGLOSSAL DUCT CYSTS.

A, the cyst has not been opened. Note its position in the midline. It has been present for many years with very little increase in size; *B,* in this patient the cyst had been incised some years previously and the depressed scar is the site of a chronic draining sinus. The entire track was excised; as is usually the case, an extensive dissection almost to the base of the tongue was necessary.

preliminary injection of the track with methylene blue will aid in complete excision. The wound is ordinarily left open and packed gently with vaseline or iodoform gauze, healing then occurring by granulation. Gage [30] has reported a low recurrence rate following closure of the wound with the aid of a pressure dressing. Rogers and Hall [31] have found their lowest rate of recurrence with a many-stage, simpler procedure which does not require hospitalization.

Epidermoid cysts are similar in pathogenesis to dermoids except that they are due to traumatic inclusion of epithelial cells, often after a trivial wound, in which the cyst later develops. They are smaller than dermoid cysts, contain only clear fluid and are common in the hands (fingers) and feet. Treatment consists of simple excision.

V. Congenital Cysts.—This group includes several types:

1. *Branchial cleft cysts* originate from the embryonic branchial clefts, and hence occur in the lateral aspect of the head or neck along a line extending from the ear to the midclavicle. The most common location is at the site of the first branchial cleft; the presence of a pre-auricular dimple is frequently seen and is often associated with a cyst just below and anterior to it (Becker and Brunsch- wig[32]). The cysts of the upper clefts are usually small, but those lower in the neck may attain considerable size. If they open or are incised they become the site of a chronic draining sinus. The cells lining the cyst in most instances are

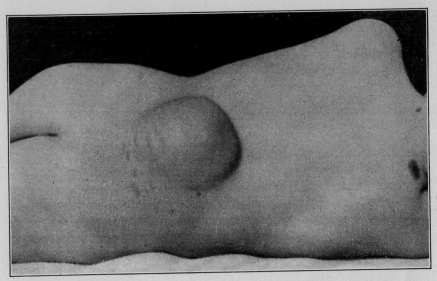

Fig. 201.—Spina Bifida and Meningocele in a Three-year-old Girl.

The mass was first noted at birth; the child had no use of either leg but was not incontinent. The defect in the spine could be felt clearly; transillumination showed a clear sac. Operative excision of the sac and plastic repair were performed; recovery was uneventful. Four years later the reflexes were still absent but the child was going to school, her grades being above normal. (Courtesy of Dr. Ernest Sachs.)

squamous in type, and the wall also shows many collections of lymphoid cells. Because of their similarity in structure, branchial cleft cysts are often classified with dermoids. Branchial cleft cysts which are deeper may communicate with the oral or pharyngeal cavity and exhibit columnar rather than squamous epithelium. On rare occasions carcinomatous change develops. Their treatment consists of complete excision.

2. *Thyroglossal duct cyst* is always in the midline of the neck and is a remnant of the thyroglossal duct which in embryonic life extends from the base of the tongue (foramen cecum) beneath the hyoid bone to form the thyroid gland. Any portion of this track may be left and give rise to a cyst in later life. It often opens spontaneously after which it may manifest itself as a chronic draining sinus or as a cyst which opens, drains, closes and fills up intermittently. Treatment consists of complete excision which may be difficult and necessitate a dissection up to the

base of the tongue. If any epithelial cells remain recurrence follows. It is an operation which should not be undertaken lightly.

3. *Meningocele and spina bifida* are forms of congenital cysts due to failure in development of the central nervous system and its meninges and bony covering. Spina bifida is most common over the lumbar region as a cystic mass and may be associated with motor and sensory disturbances. X-ray will reveal a bony defect, nearly always a bifid spine. Meningocele is really a herniation of the spinal or cerebral meninges through any bony defect which, however, is generally insignificant in size. It is seen commonly in the lumbar region and less frequently in the midline over the forehead or occiput. Treatment belongs to the domain of neurosurgery.

4. *Polycystic disease* occurs in the lungs, kidneys, liver and spleen, this is a rare form of congenital cyst, but usually manifests itself in adult life.

BIBLIOGRAPHY

1. Ewing, J. *Neoplastic Diseases,* 4th ed., W. B. Saunders, Philadelphia, 1940.
2. Cook, J. W., Kennaway, E. S., et al. Chemical Compounds as Carcinogenic Agents. *Am. J. Cancer,* 29:219, 1937; 33:50, 1938; 39:381, 1940.
3. Knox, L. C. Trauma and Tumors, *Arch. Path.,* 7:274, 1929; *Am. J. Surg.,* 26:66, 1934.
4. Stout, A. P. *Human Cancer,* Lea and Febiger, Philadelphia, 1932.
5. Batson, O. V. Function of the Vertebral Veins and their Role in the Spread of Metastasis. *Ann. Surg.,* 112:138, 1940.
6. Pack, G. T. and Livingston, E. M. *Treatment of Cancer and Allied Diseases,* P. B. Hoeber, N. Y., 1940.
7. Broders, A. C. Squamous Cell Epithelioma of the Lip, *J. Am. M. Ass.,* 74:656, 1920.
8. Womack, N. A. Subungual Melanoma, *Arch. Surg.,* 15:667, 1927.
9. Kolodny, A. Bone Sarcoma, *Surg., Gynec. & Obst.,* 44:1 (April, Part 2), 1927.
10. Geschickter, C. F., and Copeland, M. M. Tumors of Bone, *Am J. Cancer,* New York, 1931. A shorter description by the same authors may be found in Lewis's System of Surgery, *Int. Surg. Digest,* 10:323, 1930.
11. Phemister, D. B. Conservative Surgery in the Treatment of Bone Tumors, *Surg., Gynec. and Obst.,* 70:355, 1940.
12. Krumbhaar, E. B. Is Typical Hodgkin's Disease an Infection or a Neoplasm? *Am. J. M. Sc.,* 188:597, 1934.
13. Stewart, F. W., and Doan, C. A. An Analysis of the Lymphadenopathy Question with Special Reference to Hodgkin's Disease and Tuberculosis, *Ann. Surg.,* 93:141, 1931.
14. Warthin, A. S. The Genetic Neoplastic Relationships of Hodgkin's Disease, Aleukaemic and Leukaemic Lymphoblastoma, and Mycosis Fungoides, *Ann. Surg.,* 93:153, 1931.
15. Sachs, Ernest. *The Diagnosis and Treatment of Brain Tumors.* C. V. Mosby Co., St. Louis, 1931.
    Penfield, W. *Cytology and Cellular Pathology of the Nervous System,* Paul Hoeber, Inc., New York, 1932.
    Davis, Loyal. *Intracranial Tumors,* Paul Hoeber, Inc., New York, 1933.
    Bailey, P. *Intracranial Tumors,* C. Thomas, Springfield, Illinois.
16. Ransom, H. K. Abdominal Neoplasms of Neurogenic Origin, *Tr. Am. S. A.,* May, 1940.

17. PHEMISTER, D. B., and GORDON, J. E. The Etiology of Solitary Bone Cyst, *J. Am. M. Ass.*, 87:1429, 1926.

18. BRUNSCHWIG, A. Observations on the Changes Occurring at Benign Giant Cell Tumor Sites Several Years Following Treatment by Conservative Measures, *Am. J. Roentgenol.*, 40:817, 1938.

19. ADAMS, C. O., COMPERE, E. J., and JEROME, J. Regional Fibrocystic Disease, *Surg., Gynec., & Obst.*, 71:22, 1940.

20. CHIEVITZ, O., and OLSEN, H. C. A Case of Generalized Osteitis Fibrosa Improved after Removal of a Parathyroid Tumor, *Acta Chir. Scand.*, 71:172, 1932.

21. CHURCHILL, E. D., and COPE, O. Parathyroid Tumors Associated with Hyperparathyroidism, *Surg., Gynec. & Obst.*, 58:255, 1934.

22. LEWIS, D., and GESCHICKTER, C. F. Glomus Tumors, *J. Am. M. Ass.*, 105:775, 1935.

23. PENFIELD, W. *Loc. cit.*, Vol. III, p. 974.

24. FULTON, J. F. Robert W. Smith's Description of Generalized Neurofibromatosis (1849), *N. Eng. M. J.*, 200:1315, 1929.

25. BROOKS, B., and LEHMAN, E. P. The Bone Changes in Recklinghausen's Neurofibromatosis, *Surg., Gynec. & Obst.*, 38:587, 1924.

26. ZEISLER, E. P. *Abt's Pediatrics*, Vol. VIII, p. 23, W. B. Saunders, Philadelphia, 1926.

27. BLAIR, V. P., and IVY, R. H. *Essentials of Oral Surgery*, C. V. Mosby, St. Louis, 2nd ed., 1936.

28. RICH, A. R., and BUMSTEAD, J. H. On the Identity of Hematoidin and Bilirubin, *Bull. Johns Hopkins Hosp.*, 36:225, 1925.

29. FOX, S. L. The Origin of Pilonidal Sinus, *Surg., Gynec. & Obst.*, 60:137, 1935.

30. GAGE, Mims. Pilonidal Sinus, *Ann Surg.*, 109:291, 1939.

31. ROGERS, H., and HALL, M. G. Pilonidal Sinus; Surgical Treatment and Pathological Structure, *Arch. Surg.*, 31:742, 1935. See also Rogers and Dwight, *Ann. Surg.*, 107:400, 1938; and Rogers, *New England J. Med.*, 222:79, 1940.

32. BECKER, S. W., and BRUNSCHWIG, A. Sinus Preauricularis, *Am. J. Surg.*, 24:174, 1934.

33. STEINER, P. E. Cancer-Producing Agents from Human Sources, *Surg., Gynec. & Obst.*, 76:105, 1943.

CHAPTER XVII

FRACTURES, DISLOCATIONS AND SPRAINS:
GENERAL CONSIDERATIONS

Fractures
Dislocations
Sprains

The injuries suffered by the body which involve the bony skeleton and its attachments present many special problems, not only in diagnosis, but particularly in treatment. Movement in general, and particularly weight-bearing, depends to a large extent upon the integrity of the various bones. When they are broken or even slightly injured these functions are seriously impaired. Moreover, nature unaided is frequently a poor healer and will produce an end result which is accompanied by serious and often permanent disability. The responsibility of the surgeon in the care of the injured is, therefore, nowhere greater than when the bony skeleton is involved.

The diagnosis and treatment of bone injuries has been revolutionized since the days of the old time bone-setter, largely because of the use of the x-ray. With its aid the presence of bone injury may be established or ruled out and the type and extent of the injury accurately determined and permanently recorded. For this reason the x-ray film has achieved tremendous medicolegal significance. Indeed, the obligation of the physician to have an x-ray film taken whenever a broken bone is present or suspected is recognized by most legal authorities and neglect to do so may constitute malpractice. Moreover, there is no better method of measuring the progress of healing than x-ray films taken regularly. In the reduction of broken bones the fluoroscope may be invaluable in enabling an accurate approximation under direct vision. In the reduction of fractures by suspension and traction, as described later, portable x-ray films form an indispensable feature of the treatment. It should be emphasized that a single view in the x-ray is often misleading; in most fractures at least two views are essential (see Fig. 202).

So great is the importance of the x-ray in bone injuries that much of the older art of diagnosis based on simple clinical examination is gradually being lost. This is a deplorable tendency for several reasons. The ability to estimate bone injury by inspection and palpation alone is, of course, essential when no x-ray is available, a condition which still remains in rural sections, in spite of the extension of modern hospital facilities. Moreover, it may be inadvisable to subject severely injured patients to the manipulations and movements necessary to obtain x-ray films in the first hours or days after an accident, particularly in the presence of shock. In such an instance a bedside examination will be necessary to diagnose the degree of injury. Then, in most patients, it is important to limit the number of x-ray films to the regions of the body which seem to be injured. In order to avoid undue expense, finally, it is important that the physician know enough about the clinical manifestations of bone injury to judge which bones require x-ray films.

For these reasons it should be a part of every physician's training to acquaint himself with the simple clinical manifestations of injury to bones, joints and

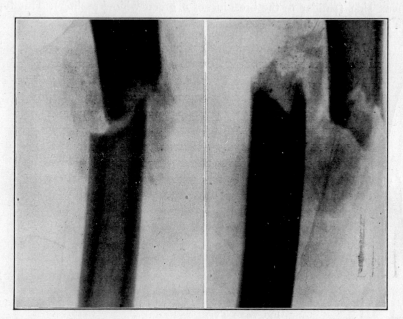

Fig. 202.—Roentgenograms Illustrating the Importance of Obtaining More Than One View.

One of the x-rays shown above is an anteroposterior view, whereas the other is a lateral view of a fractured femur. It is obvious that without both views, an accurate estimation of the type and amount of displacement of fragments is not possible.

ligaments, even though the x-ray will make the more important and accurate estimate of the extent of the lesion. In the following discussion these simple features will be considered. In this chapter only general principles will be discussed. In the next chapter the individual types of injury will be considered. More complete details may be found in special textbooks. [1, 2, 3, 4, 5, 27].

FRACTURES

Definitions.—A *fracture* may be defined as a break in the continuity of a bone. It may be complete, with or without displacement of the broken ends, or incomplete without displacement. Deformity nearly always depends on the existence of displacement; however, angulation without displacement frequently occurs.

A *simple fracture* is one in which there is no connection between the site of fracture and the surface of the body.

A fracture is *compound* when there is a break in the skin or mucous membrane which communicates with the site of fracture, thereby producing a possible source of infection.

A fracture is said to be *comminuted* when there is considerable fragmentation of bone.

A *greenstick fracture* consists of a bending of the bone with crushing of the cortex on the concave side and a tearing with a variable amount of separation on the convex side (similar to the breaking of a green willow sapling). This type of fracture is observed, with few exceptions, only in children.

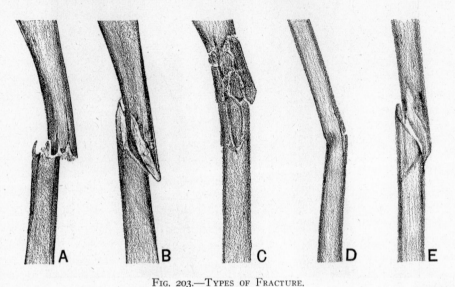

FIG. 203.—TYPES OF FRACTURE.

A, transverse; *B*, oblique; *C*, comminuted; *D*, greenstick; *E*, spiral.

When one fragment is driven into the other and remains in a fixed position the fracture is spoken of as being *impacted*.

An *epiphyseal separation* involves a break in continuity through the epiphyseal line of the bone.

A *spontaneous* ("*pathological*") *fracture* is a fracture through a diseased portion of bone and may be sustained after injury of the most trivial character, or spontaneously after normal movements.

Delayed union is said to exist when the deposition of callus or fixation of the ends of the bone is considerably less than that normally present for such a fracture at a given time.

Nonunion exists when the reparative process has come to an end without union of the fragments.

Malunion represents healing of the bone with deformity, usually shortening or angulation.

Some of the more common fractures have been named after the men who originally described them; *e.g.*, a *Colles' fracture* is one consisting of a transverse fracture of the radius about an inch proximal to the articular margin at the wrist, with the distal fragment displaced dorsally, thus creating the "silver fork" deformity. There are, of course, many variations of this fracture which are loosely called Colles' fractures. A *Pott's fracture,* as originally described, consists of a fracture of the fibula 2 to 4 centimeters above the external malleolus. It is often associated with a fracture of a small portion of the medial malleolus of the tibia.

Etiology and Mechanism.—Although trauma is ordinarily looked upon as the one decisive factor in the production of fractures, there are, nevertheless, many predisposing or indirect factors which are of importance. For example, in senile persons osteoporosis, which affects the upper end of the femur and humerus, and the distal end of the radius especially, may be responsible for a fracture of these sites when the same amount of violence would not produce a fracture in a young person. The position, as well as the exposure, of the extremities to direct violence is also important in the incidence of fracture. This factor is perhaps best exemplified by the fact that a trained athlete can enter into much more violent athletic combat than an untrained athlete without sustaining a fracture. This may be explained by the fact that the trained athlete has stronger bones, but there is another explanation perhaps more important, namely, that he has learned how to fall without exposing his bones to the type of violence which will produce a fracture.

The mechanism involved in the production of fractures is classified as direct and indirect. When a blow over a bone is sufficient to cause a fracture at that point the fracture is said to be produced by *direct violence.* When a fracture is produced by *indirect violence* the force is transmitted as a leverage action resulting in a fracture at or near the fixed point which may be at a considerable distance from the point where the violence was exerted. The fixed point may be produced by some object associated with the injury or accident, but is probably most frequently produced by the attachment of muscles and ligaments. The mechanism of production of the violence determines to a great extent the type of fracture produced, but since bone is somewhat brittle the type of fracture is apt to vary considerably for the same type of injury (see Figure 203). The violence sustained by an extremity is frequently of a rotary type, thereby resulting in a spiral fracture.

As an example of the effect of indirect violence, let us consider the type of injury sustained by the common accident of catching the weight of the body with the outstretched hand when falling to the ground. Perhaps the most common fracture sustained by such a fall is a Colles' fracture. The force transmitted to the lower end of the radius through the carpal bones at the time of impact may be sufficient in itself to cause a fracture at this point. However, the compression of the radius by hyperextension of the wrist adds considerably to this force, and in many instances is also an important mechanism. If the elbow is held in partial flexion as the hand strikes the ground the impact is transmitted to the lower end of the humerus which in children frequently results in a supracondylar fracture of the humerus. Occasionally a supracondylar fracture is sustained by falling with the elbow extended; by hyperextension the pull of the lateral ligaments attached to the lower end of the humerus aided by the fulcrum action of the olecranon in its fossa may be the important feature in the production of the fracture. However, in the presence of hyperextension of the elbow, the fall is more likely to result in a posterior dislocation or a fracture of the coronoid. If the arm is held in the position of abduction at the time of impact, the force, which is likewise transmitted to the shoulder, may result in a dislocation of the head of the humerus. In such a case the impact ruptures the ligaments of the inferior border of the capsule of the shoulder joint where bony support is weakest. On other occasions a fracture of the surgical neck may result from the fixation of the head of the humerus by the muscles and ligaments, creating severe tensile stress at their point of attachment.

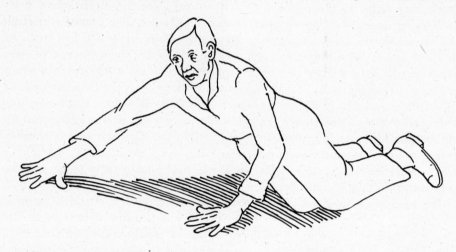

FIG. 204.—ILLUSTRATION TO SHOW MECHANISMS OF FRACTURE, FOLLOWING A FALL.

When the patient falls to the ground sustaining body weight with a dorsiflexed wrist and partially flexed elbow as noted on the patient's left, a number of important injuries, including particularly Colles' fracture, fracture of the coronoid process (with or without dislocation of the elbow), supracondylar fracture of the humerus, or even a fracture of the neck of the humerus may occur. If the arm is extended and abducted as on the right, a dislocation of the shoulder may be produced; if the elbow is hyperextended, a posterior dislocation may be sustained, usually without fracture of the coronoid.

On some occasions the fixation of one end of a long bone by muscular attachments may actually increase the tendency toward production of a fracture distal to the point of fixation when violence is sustained. Moreover, this muscular pull is responsible in many instances for the type of deformity encountered in fractures at certain points. For example, when the surgical neck of the humerus is fractured, the muscles attached at the greater tuberosity tend to rotate the head of the humerus outward in abduction, whereas the pectoralis major and teres major tend to pull the distal fragment upward and inward.

Repair of Fractures.—The healing of fractures does not take place by an actual union of the ends of the fragments, but in reality by a solidification (calcification) of the new tissue laid down around and between the ends of the fragments. At the time of the injury there is always a certain amount of bleeding from the fractured bone and adjacent tissue. This blood clots and it is in this clot that the new bone formation takes place. At first the clot becomes organized as it does in other tissues of the body by the ingrowth of capillaries and fibroblasts. Macrophages (wandering phagocytic cells) make their way into the blood clot and are largely responsible for the removal of the extravasated red cells and débris. The resolving blood clot, which ultimately becomes converted into bone, is in reality granulation tissue, containing fibrin, fibroblasts and newly formed blood vessels. There are two features of bone formation known to be actual facts, namely that there is a diffuse deposition of calcium throughout the callus (confirmed by x-ray) and that there is a gradual resorption of most of this callus after many weeks or months.

When the deposition of lime salts begins, the tissue is designated as callus, but there is considerable argument as to the actual mechanism in the formation of the new bone. According to one theory (Hamm [6] and Rhode [6]) new bone is formed by proliferation of osteogenic cells growing out from the broken ends of the bone. It should be emphasized that the adult bone cell is incapable of reproducing bone. Microscopical examination of the site of a recent fracture reveals a marked thickening of the osteogenic layer of the periosteum near the injury with active mitoses of the osteogenic cells. The cells resulting from this proliferation apparently have the power of differentiating into either cartilage or bone cells. If lime salts are available and an adequate blood supply is present, bone is formed. This differentiation depends somewhat upon the availability of lime salts, but primarily upon the blood supply. The portion of the callus not directly adjacent to the periosteum has a poor blood supply and for that reason transformation into cartilage instead of bone takes place. As the vascularity increases, thereby increasing the supply of lime salts, the cartilage is converted into bone. On the other hand, the portion of the callus near the exterior, although it acquires a blood supply early, is transformed into cartilage instead of bone because of the great distance from the local depot of calcium salts, i.e., the bone. The osteogenic cells of the endosteum also have the power of forming bone, but ordinarily seem to play an insignificant role.

In contrast to the above theory, many authorities believe that the osteogenic cells are created by metaplasia of fibroblasts diffusely throughout the callus, bone being thus formed directly or through the intermediary production of cartilage. This theory seems plausible in that it explains the generalized deposition of calcium which occurs normally during the early weeks of repair. Moreover, it seems unlikely that osteogenic cells originating only from the periosteum could assume such an even distribution throughout the callus.

It is apparent from this brief description of the two theories of bone formation that neither explains all of the known features of bone healing. The authors are of the opinion that both processes take place, but that each serves its own purpose, i.e., true bone of a permanent nature is produced by the osteogenic cells (sometimes designated as osteoblasts) adjacent to the periosteum, whereas bone of a temporary nature is formed by metaplastic fibroblasts throughout the callus. Thus, we may designate the bone produced at the central portion of the callus as true bone since it is made up of identifying components, lacunae and trabeculations. This type of bone is probably not produced to any extent for three weeks or more following the fracture, whereas the deposition of calcium salts throughout the callus occurs earlier. This latter phenomenon is undoubtedly nature's attempt to give early support while true bone is being formed. The fact that the greater part of this early callus is absorbed at a later date supports the theory that it is not true bone, but exerts merely a temporary function early in the healing process. That this explanation is hardly original can be seen from the following quotation from Dupuytren [7] writing over a century ago "... nature never accomplishes union of fractures save by the formation of two successive deposits of callus ... one provisional and the other permanent. The former of these, which is usually perfected in about 30 or 40 days ... has not always strength enough. .... The second (permanent) callus, formed by the reunion of the surfaces of the fracture, possesses a solidity superior even to that of the bone itself. .... The production and organization of the permanent callus is never completed under 8, 10, or 12 months, a period which is further marked by the disappearance of the provisional callus and the renewed continuity of the medullary canal."

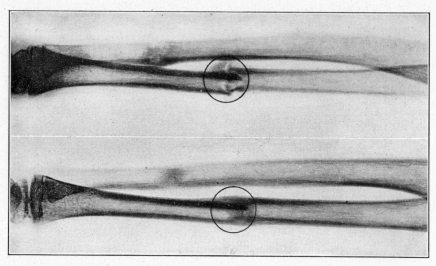

FIG. 205.—CHANGES IN THE CALLUS DURING THE HEALING OF A FRACTURE.

The top picture was taken six weeks after fracture (radius and ulna). The lower picture shows the same view of same fracture six months after injury. Note that as time passes the width of the dense callus surrounding the fracture becomes narrower because of absorption of calcium at its periphery; the callus between the ends of the bone, on the other hand, is not visible at six weeks but is demonstrable at six months (this is even more evident in larger bones). This early deposition and eventual resorption of callus surrounding the bone in contrast to the slow deposition of a dense callus between the bone ends supports the theory, stated in the text, that the callus deposited at these two sites may be of a different type.

Clinical Manifestations.—The clinical evidence of fracture may be so obvious in some instances, because of deformity, that the diagnosis may be made by the patient himself. More frequently, however, especially when there is no displacement of fragments, a careful examination by a competent physician is required to determine the presence or absence of a fracture. On a few occasions it will be impossible to come to a definite decision without the aid of the x-ray which, moreover, for reasons already mentioned, must always be taken in doubtful cases.

1. *Pain.*—Unless the accident results in unconsciousness, pain is universally experienced when a fracture is sustained, except that the shock and excitement inflicted upon the patient may minimize, or even completely obliterate, the sensation of pain for a short time following the accident. This pain tends to decrease rapidly if the fragments are immobilized. As soon as the fragments are moved a severe

exacerbation of pain is experienced. Pressing one end of the bone toward the other, or rotation of the portion of the extremity distal to the injured part will almost always produce pain if a fracture is present. If impaction is present this pain will, of course, be less. Manipulations should be performed carefully in such a way that movement can immediately be stopped on account of the severe pain which may be produced. Occasionally in senile people the pain associated with fracture may seem trivial. The absence of pain should ordinarily lead one to eliminate the possibility of fracture or, if a fracture is present, to make a tentative diagnosis of "pathological fracture" which at times is accompanied by very little pain. After the fracture is reduced and properly immobilized, pain usually disappears within twenty-four hours.

2. *Disability.*—The disability or loss of function produced by a fracture may result either from the pain produced by attempt to use the injured part or from the

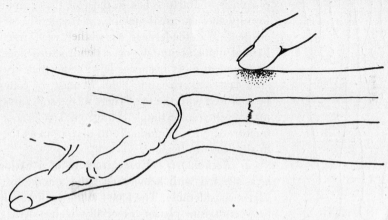

FIG. 206.—LOCAL OR POINT TENDERNESS IS ONE OF THE MOST USEFUL SIGNS OF FRACTURE. The shaded area illustrates the relation of the local tenderness to the fracture site.

loss of support of the bony framework. On rare occasions when the bone is solidly impacted, or when the fracture is incomplete, this disability may be insignificant. Likewise, a robust individual may be able to stand pain so well that he may be capable of walking with an incomplete fracture of one of the bones in the lower extremity. A contusion of a part of the lower extremity rarely results in the inability to walk as is so constantly observed with a fracture. Although a severe sprain of the knee or ankle may be so painful as to make walking impossible, as a rule the ability or inability to walk is a fairly good index as to differentiation between fractures and sprains of the lower extremity (see also page 448). Refusal to use the hand or arm after injury is usually most suggestive of the presence of a fracture, especially in children or infants.

There are certain fractures, however, which, although affecting important bones, create surprisingly little loss of function. In this group fractures of the vertebrae should be mentioned especially, because on many occasions patients with such fractures (even with compression or displacement) are able to walk about, at least for several days following their accident, with no more complaint than a mild backache.

The impaction which is so constantly present in vertebral fractures is the chief factor in the prevention of much more serious disability. For this reason any patient who has been injured in a serious accident should have a careful examination of his vertebral column and roentgenograms (lateral view especially) if any suspicious areas are found.

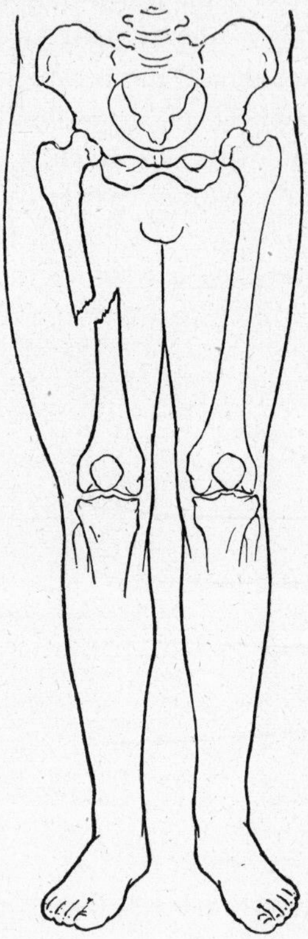

3. *Local Tenderness over the Fracture.*—This is perhaps the most constant sign elicited in fractures and for that reason, from the standpoint of usefulness, is certainly the *most valuable* of the various manifestations of fracture, although it of course does not have the diagnostic value that crepitus, deformity and abnormal mobility have. The reason that local tenderness is of so much more importance to the physician in diagnosis of fracture lies in the fact that crepitus, deformity and abnormal mobility so frequently cannot be elicited. The tenderness associated with fracture is located quite accurately over the fracture line in the bone and in most instances is so acute that firm pressure causes excruciating pain. It must, of course, not be confused with the tenderness of the soft parts which may result from a simple contusion. Tenderness at the fracture site tends gradually to disappear as the callus finally leads to healing.

4. *Ecchymosis.*—Every fracture of a major bone is associated with hemorrhage, the amount of which varies considerably. The blood tends to dissect its way between tissue planes, especially if hemorrhage has been sufficient to create tension in the tissues. When it reaches the skin a bluish color is noted which is known as ecchymosis. This ecchymosis may not be manifested for several hours and in the course of a few days fades gradually to a greenish, then to a brownish or yellowish hue on account of the destruction of hemoglobin to hemosiderin, bilirubin, etc. As these pigments are absorbed the color fades entirely. If the bone is covered deeply with muscles or if fascial layers intervene between the bone and skin, ecchymosis may be delayed for a day or two or be entirely absent. Ecchymosis is not diagnostic of fracture, however, since it occurs in other injuries, particularly sprains.

FIG. 207.—SWELLING IS FREQUENTLY SO MARKED AS TO COMPLETELY CONCEAL THE BONY DEFORMITY EXISTING IN A FRACTURE.

This is particularly true of bones surrounded by considerable soft tissue.

5. *Swelling.*—Swelling is a constant accompaniment of a fracture, but may, of course, be encountered in almost any other type of injury and is therefore not a valuable sign of fracture. The hemorrhage and extravasation of serum, which are the factors responsible for the swelling, are manifested within a few hours after the fracture and may remain in decreasing amount for several days. Ordinarily the degree of swelling is dependent upon the severity of the trauma associated with the fracture.

6. *Deformity.*—Displacement of the fractured ends of bone or angulation without displacement will ordinarily produce a visible deformity. On many occasions the deformity will be so prominent that the patient is able to make the diagnosis of fracture himself. Care must be exercised lest a localized swelling of the soft parts be confused with deformity due to fracture. On the other hand, deformity is often obscured by the swelling about the site of fracture. Palpation will usually reveal

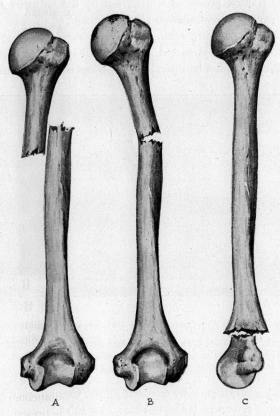

FIG. 208.—THREE GENERAL TYPES OF DEFORMITY WHICH MAY BE PRODUCED BY FRACTURE.

A, displacement with overriding of fragments. *B*, angulation. *C*, rotation. The deformity of rotation can be shown in the x-ray only if the entire bone is shown, *e.g.*, the proximal end of the humerus as shown above represents an anteroposterior view, whereas the distal end is rotated 90° to a lateral view.

bony prominences which can be identified as the fractured ends of bone. Obviously a deformity which is not present in the opposite extremity lends valuable support to the diagnosis of fracture. Occasionally the patient will have had a previous injury with mal-union, thereby minimizing the importance of deformity. Many fractures, however, are sustained without displacement of fragments, or without deformity.

There are three possible types of deformity, corresponding to the three planes of space. (1) When the fragments are completely displaced the "muscle pull" produces an overriding and consequent *shortening*. (2) *Angulation* may occur in any direction, depending upon the direction of the impact and the force exerted by the muscles attached to the bone; it may be present with or without displacement of the fragments. (3) The direction of the impact and the pull exerted by the attachment of various muscles may produce a *rotation of fragments*. On some occasions, forces tending to create rotation at time of injury are sufficient to produce a spiral fracture (see Figure 203E).

7. *Crepitus.*—When the two ends of a broken bone are moved against each other, the grating friction produced will be felt by the palpating fingers and may be audible to the ear as a crepitant sound. On account of the severe pain produced by this procedure an attempt to elicit this sign is rarely justifiable. Obviously, if the fracture is incomplete or impacted, crepitus will be absent. Crepitus is pathognomonic of fracture, but must be differentiated from the soft grating which is pro-

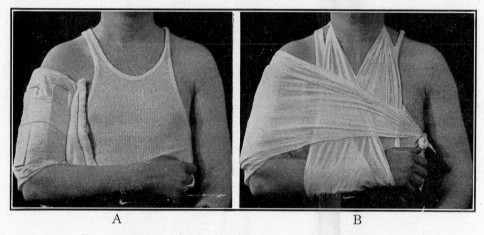

A   B

FIG. 209.—FIRST AID DRESSING FOR FRACTURE OF THE HUMERUS.

A. A pad is placed between the arm and chest, and coaptation splints applied after the arm is well padded. *B.* The wrist and distal forearm are suspended in a sling; fixation of the arm against the chest is achieved by using a sling or circular bandage.

duced by epiphyseal separation or by diseased joints. Crepitus of a similar type may also be due to chronic synovitis, tenosynovitis and a subcutaneous emphysema.

8. *Abnormal Mobility.*—When a complete fracture is present, abnormal mobility or a "false joint" may be elicited at the site of fracture. If a complete fracture of the shaft of the femur is present, rotation of the leg will not cause a rotation of the greater trochonter. Likewise, when a complete fracture of the humerus exists, rotation of the elbow will not cause rotation of the head of the humerus. Demonstration of this sign is of great value diagnostically, but on account of the pain produced in eliciting it, great care should be exercised during manipulation so as to minimize the pain.

General Principles in Treatment.—There are certain principles in the treatment of fractures which must be strictly adhered to if satisfactory results are expected, but the details, including the type of immobilization and the method of reduction, vary considerably among different surgeons.

The presence or absence of displacement is important, because reduction will obviously be unnecessary when no displacement is present. Certain displacements are more serious and require more accurate correction than others. For example, a Colles fracture should be reduced accurately, whereas a deformity in a fractured clavicle is of little significance as far as function is concerned, but may be important cosmetically. Occasionally the surgeon will be forced to try one method after another before he achieves a satisfactory result. The two types of procedures which are important in the local treatment of fractures are (1) reduction of deformity or displacement, and (2) immobilization (fixation) until sufficient healing has occurred. As stated above, reduction is not always indicated; many fractures have no displacement or exhibit such slight deformity as to require no manipulation or

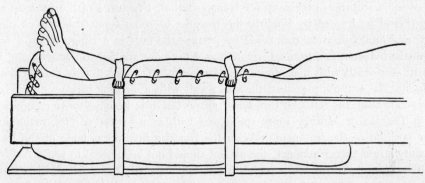

FIG. 210.—THE PILLOW SPLINT IS A COMFORTABLE FIRST AID APPLIANCE FOR THE CARE OF FRACTURES OF THE LEG.

The leg is encased in a soft feather pillow and fixation attained by wooden slabs anchored on each side and the bottom.

other method of reduction. The second procedure (*i.e.*, fixation) is always necessary, although the degree and duration of immobilization varies considerably among

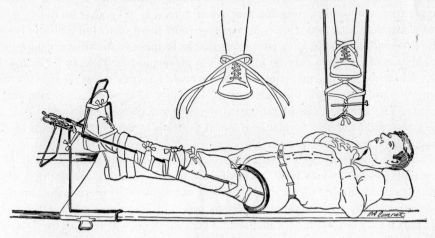

FIG. 211.— THE USE OF THE THOMAS SPLINT IN THE FIRST AID TREATMENT OF FRACTURES.

For transportation of patients with fracture of the shaft of the femur as well as about the knee and upper tibia, the Thomas splint, which enables traction to be exerted at the same time, is perhaps the most satisfactory. The efficacy of this procedure was fully demonstrated during World War I. Inserts show how traction may be applied to the foot with the shoe on.

the various types of injury. Of almost equal importance, however, is the first aid treatment of fractures, which will be considered first.

1. *First Aid Treatment.*—First aid procedures should be carried out at the scene of the accident with the idea in mind of obtaining the best immobilization available, and of transporting the patient as quickly as possible to a place where x-rays may be taken, and where reduction and permanent immobilization may be instituted. On rare occasions it may be possible to reduce the fracture by a simple painless maneuver and to apply temporary splints. For such simple fractures as those involving the clavicle and bones of the hand, a sling is probably the only type of immobilization necessary for transportation. Fractures of the forearm and wrist should be treated by binding the forearm to some type of board or metal splint, and immobilization completed by putting the arm in a sling. When a fracture of the humerus is sustained, coaptation splints are applied to the arm, and the forearm suspended with a narrow sling (see Fig. 209) ; fixation is then achieved by binding the extremity against the chest wall with a circular bandage. This type of immobilization for first aid care and transportation is perhaps more comfortable than a Thomas or Murray-Jones splint and will, as a matter of fact, maintain a better position of the fragments. When the fracture involves a bone of the lower extremity larger than phalanges, the patient should not be allowed to walk. A Pott's fracture may not need much immobilization, but if pain is severe should be treated by binding the ankle and leg to a padded board on the medial side of the leg with the foot in an inverted position. By so doing, the slight jarring incident to transportation will tend to reduce the fracture. The application of a pillow splint is a comfortable and convenient way of applying fixation to fractures of the leg and foot (see Figure 210). For fractured femur, the Thomas splint, as emphasized in World War I, is ideal, combining immobilization and traction. The U. S. Army is now using the Keller splint, a modified Thomas, having but half a ring, thus enabling its application without inserting the ring over the foot. If a Thomas or Keller splint is not available a long board or pole reaching from the foot to the axilla is bound to the extremity and body after adequate padding is applied. Additional data on the first aid care of fractures may be found in the publication by Cole and Puestow [31].

2. *Reduction.*—This procedure is nearly always necessary when the fracture is complete and significant displacement or deformity is apparent or demonstrable by x-ray. The primary consideration is, of course, a perfect functional result ; a perfect restoration of the normal anatomical position is the best assurance of obtaining such a result, but in certain fractures (*e.g.,* clavicle) good function is possible without obtaining perfect reduction of fragments. Even the end result in a fracture of a bone so important as the femur may be entirely satisfactory when reduction was incomplete. As a rule, alignment of fragments is more important than the actual reduction of fragments. Certain types of fractures, particularly those about joints, may heal with poor end results because of persistent pain, even though good reduction of fragments is obtained. The above features make it essential that the surgeon know what types of fractures demand perfect reduction and in what types of fractures he may be content with only fair reduction of fragments.

Reduction of displaced fractures (and dislocations) is effected by two general types of maneuver ; *i.e.,* manipulation and traction. Each may be applied individually or together in one of three ways. (*a*) The simplest and most convenient method, when possible, is *primary manual reduction* under local or general anesthesia. This is the oldest method and one which was used from time immemorial by the old bone-setters, many of whom possessed remarkable skill considering the fact that they had no x-rays and were unaided by anesthesia. Traction is exerted manually, but may be aided by various apparatus, including the insertion of pins or wire through one or both fragments. (*b*) The second method of reduction consists of *continuous traction* and does not ordinarily require any anesthesia. The reduction

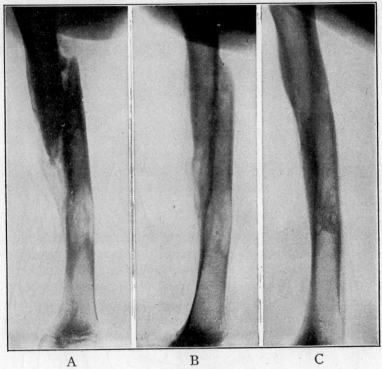

A   B   C

FIG. 212.—THESE ROENTGENOGRAMS WHICH ARE LATERAL VIEWS OF THE FEMUR IN THE SAME PATIENT, TAKEN AT DIFFERENT INTERVALS, ILLUSTRATE WOLFF'S LAW.

A, fracture of the femur with malposition of the fragments, three months after injury, in a boy aged eight; *B*, five months after fracture; *C*, fourteen months after fracture. Note that the extreme thickness of the newly formed shaft produced by the markd displacement of fragments, is diminishing. Within a year or two the shaft will be reduced still further in size and roentgenologically will not be much unlike the opposite femur. Note also the bone cyst beyond the fracture site; its gradual disappearance by ossification is clearly shown.

is gradual, but correction of the displacement must be achieved within a few days before significant callus has formed. This method produces fixation and immobilization as well as reduction and thus completes the essential requirements for treatment. Obviously, it will be necessary to note the effect of the traction on the position of the fragments by the use of a portable x-ray machine. (*c*) The third method consists of *open reduction* in contrast to the first two methods, which are closed. Strict asepsis must be observed during such an operative procedure, because the bone is prone to become infected readily. Ordinarily, open reduction is resorted to only when closed reduction has failed or when the fracture is compound and a débridement necessary. Displaced fractures of the patella, olecranon, neck of femur, and head of the radius, however, are nearly always treated best by primary open operation.

As stated previously, an attempt should be made to obtain reduction and permanent splinting immediately, unless contraindicated by the general condition of the patient. There are several reasons for this. In the first place, reduction will be easier if it is carried out before the swelling is manifested to any great degree. Immediate reduction eliminates the continuous trauma and pain which is inflicted by an unreduced fracture. Moreover, a delay of a day or two in a child may allow the deposition of sufficient callus to interfere with reduction. With few exceptions, some type of anesthesia, local' (novocaine injected into the hematoma and between

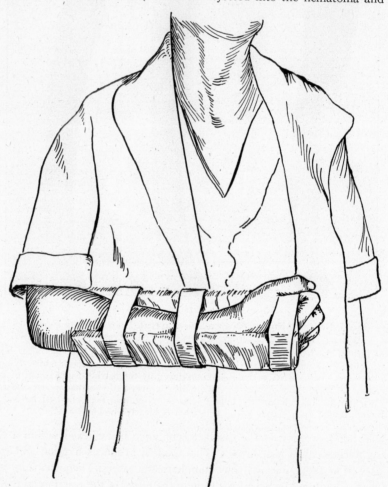

FIG. 213.—WOODEN SPLINTS ARE WIDELY USED FOR OBTAINING IMMOBILIZATION IN FRACTURES, BUT THEIR USEFULNESS IS CONFINED CHIEFLY TO FRACTURES OF THE DISTAL RADIUS AND ULNA.

The splint is padded with cotton and wrapped with gauze; for complete fixation an anterior as well as posterior splint should be applied. The adhesive straps binding the splints against the forearm may be tightened as indicated. The forearm is then suspended in a sling.

the bone fragments), intravenous (evipal or pentothal sodium), nitrous oxide, or ether, is used to eradicate pain and obtain relaxation of muscles. Before attempting reduction the exact position of the fragments should be determined by x-ray so that as far as possible the manipulation necessary for reduction can be planned in advance. Reduction is aided further if carried out under a fluoroscope, or at least in the x-ray department where a fluoroscope is available to determine the results of manipulation before the splints are applied. Roentgenograms should be made at intervals during the healing of the fracture in order to detect any shifting of fragments which may occur at times in almost any type of fixation apparatus. The amount of callus noted on the x-ray film will also be of assistance in determining when function may be resumed.

On rare occasions, especially in children, radical treatment to correct certain deformities will not be advisable, because of the spontaneous tendency for healing bone to correct deformity. This is accomplished by the deposition of bone where it

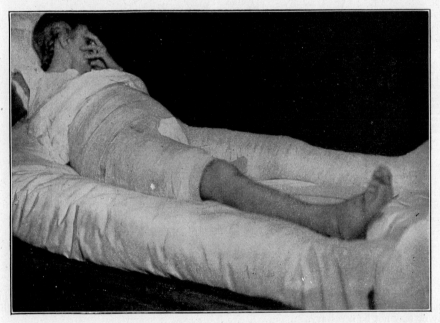

FIG. 214.—MANY FRACTURES ARE PARTICULARLY AMENABLE TO TREATMENT WITH THE PLASTER CAST, WHICH PERHAPS OFFERS THE MOST COMPLETE IMMOBILIZATION OF ANY FORM OF FIXATION.

The patient in the above illustration had sustained a fracture through the trochanters of the femur but without displacement of fragments.

is most needed, and by the absorption of bone where it is excessive. This tendency for the natural correction of deformity of bone is known as Wolff's law [8] (see Fig. 212).

3. *Immobilization (Splints, Traction, etc.).*—The procedure of immobilization or fixation may be internal or external, the former consisting of sutures, plates, wires, screws, pegs, etc., which are attached directly to the fragments and hold them fixed. Some form of external fixation is nearly always used with internal

fixation. Internal fixation is carried out usually by an open operation. In certain instances internal fixation is achieved by inserting a steel pin, Smith-Petersen nail, etc., through a small incision in the sterilized skin into the bone, as in fractures of the neck of the femur, thus avoiding an extensive open operation. Venable and Stuck [28] have called attention to the advisability of using the alloy vitallium for plates, pins, etc., because this alloy is inert in the tissues, *i.e.,* free from harmful electrolytic effects. On certain occasions two pins are passed through the broken bone, one on each side of the fracture, the fragments reduced and the pins incorporated in the plaster cast which is applied after reduction is achieved. This is an example of combined internal and external fixation. Stader [29] has modified the

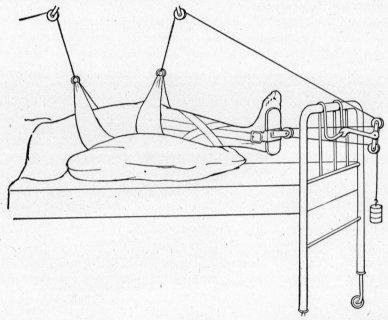

FIG. 215.—RUSSELL TRACTION, AS UTILIZED FREQUENTLY FOR FRACTURES OF THE SHAFT OF THE FEMUR.

Traction is obtained by use of adhesive strips and a footpiece. The knee is suspended in a sling with the pull directed upward at a slight angle, as illustrated. Suspension of the thigh may or may not be necessary.

multiple pin method by attaching the pins to an extension bar lying parallel to the extremity (external to the skin), thus obtaining fixation without the use of a cast.

External fixation is ordinarily achieved by bandages, adhesive strips, wood, metal or wire mesh splints, plaster casts, etc. There are three major methods for obtaining external fixation or immobilization of fractured bones. (*a*) *Wooden and flat metal splints* have the advantage of simplicity and ease of application. They may be tightened readily as swelling subsides, thus maintaining efficient fixation. On the other hand, they cannot be used in fractures of major bones where extensive immobilization is necessary. (*b*) *A plaster cast* is perhaps the most widely used method and has a greater range of applicability than others. If reduction can be obtained immediately, fixation is usually so efficient that hospitalization is no longer necessary. However, the subsidence of swelling and atrophy of tissues beneath the cast may be sufficient in many instances to allow displacement to recur. This is particularly true of fractures of the shaft of the femur. (*c*) *Suspension and traction* are particularly useful when complete reduction under anesthesia is not obtained. The constant traction improves the position of the fragments and occasionally results in satisfactory spontaneous reduction. This method has the advantage of permitting inspection and dressings, but has the disadvantage of necessitating prolonged confinement of the patient to bed. The limb is suspended in one of a variety

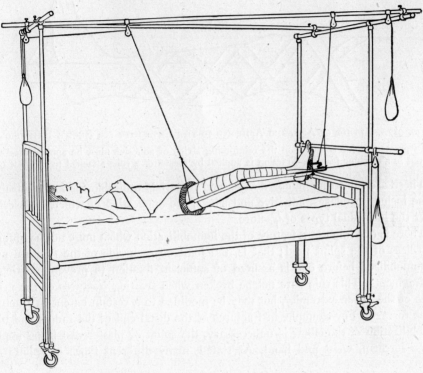

FIG. 216.—SUSPENSION AND TRACTION WITH THE THOMAS SPLINT.

This is perhaps the most commonly used method, and may be employed in the treatment of fractures of the shaft of the femur and fractures involving the upper portion of both bones of the leg, when traction for correction or prevention of overriding is desired. The advantage of traction in a Thomas splint over fixation in a plaster cast lies in the fact that if the fracture is oblique and cannot be locked in position after reduction and fixation in a cast, overriding of fragments is not apt to develop.

of splints (Hodgen, Thomas, Böhler, etc.) and traction is exerted either by skin traction or by skeletal attachments (Kirschner wire, Steinman pin, calipers). *In skin traction* the pull is exerted on the soft tissue of the limb distal to the fracture by means of adhesive strips applied to the skin (Buck's extension[9]); in *skeletal traction,* the metal appliance is first passed through the distal fragment or other bone distal to the fracture, and the pull thus exerted on skeletal tissue. Skeletal is obviously more efficient than skin traction, requiring only slightly more than half as much weight as used in skin traction to obtain a given amount of pull on the bone, but necessitates an aseptic operative procedure. This method of immobilization by continuous traction (during suspension), though commonly requiring bed rest, can be achieved in the ambulatory patient in certain fractures (hanging cast for the humerus, see Figure 240). The method of continuous traction is often used in the early stage of treatment and changed to plaster cast immobilization as soon as sufficient healing to preserve reduction has taken place, thereby allowing the patient to leave the hospital.

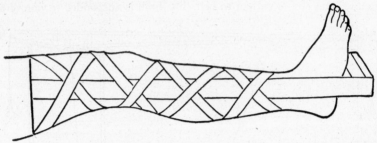

FIG. 217.—METHOD OF APPLYING ADHESIVE TO THE EXTREMITY FOR BUCK'S EXTENSION.

To prevent undue constriction the reinforcing strips of adhesive must be applied diagonally and not in a circular fashion. Traction is applied by means of a rope attached to the foot piece.

There are numerous minor devices and materials utilizable for immobilization. These include bandages, adhesive and slings, the application of which is described under the individual types of fracture.

There is one important feature of the immobilization which must not be ignored, regardless of the splint used; that is, the joint on each side of the fracture must be immobilized before one is assured of sufficient fixation to prevent shifting of the fragments. This rule dare not be broken when treating fractures of the major bones of the lower extremity, but may be modified to a certain extent in fractures of the forearm. For example, in fractures of the distal end of the radius and ulna, immobilization of the elbow is unnecessary, the splint or plaster cast being applied to the forearm, wrist and hand. As stated, many different types of splints and

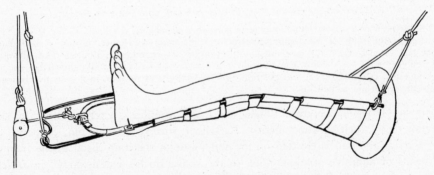

FIG. 218.—SKELETAL TRACTION WITH THE KIRSCHNER WIRE.

Frequently, skeletal traction is the most suitable means of obtaining traction, particularly when much overriding is present or the fracture site is so near a joint that skin traction is not practical. The skeletal traction shown above is attained by inserting the wire through the os calcis; the ends of the wire are attached to a stirrup, to which traction is applied.

appliances have been used and recommended for each of the various types of fracture. It is doubtful if we can truthfully say that one type is better than the other. It is important, however, that as a surgeon becomes trained in the use of one particular type of appliance he should experiment with other types only when there is a definite indication for doing so.

4. *After-Care of Fractures.*—It is essential that all fractures of consequence be under constant observation, particularly when the fracture is in traction, because of the great tendency for ropes, knots, pulleys, adhesive plaster, canvas slings, pads, etc., to become disarranged, thereby allowing fragments to become dislocated. Bony prominences must be free from pressure because of the danger of development of decubital ulcers. Complaints of pain from the patient *must not be ignored,* particularly when the injured part is immobilized by a plaster cast because pain is so commonly indicative of undue pressure over a bony prominence which may result in a decubital ulcer, or perhaps ischemia of an entire limb, which is much worse. If fragments are properly reduced and the immobilization apparatus properly adjusted, pain disappears within a few hours after reduction. Local tenderness over the fracture site may remain for days or weeks but diminishes as healing progresses. The duration of immobilization is determined to a great extent by the size of the bone. A metacarpal bone, for example, should be solidly united after 3 weeks, whereas the shaft or the neck of the femur will require 4 to 6 months. In general, immobilization is a prerequisite for the healing of fractures but there are occasions when weight-bearing (in a walking cast) is indicated in order to accelerate healing, especially in fractures in the distal third of the tibia where delayed healing and nonunion is common.

Early Motion and Physiotherapy are very important in preventing muscle and bone atrophy. The ill effects of prolonged immobilization were emphasized nearly fifty years ago by the French surgeon, Lucas-Championniere, who was the pioneer in the use of massage and movements in the treatment of fractures.[10] Every surgeon now realizes the importance of early active motion which, however, is not often possible for several weeks or more. Physiotherapy, utilizing active and passive movements, local heat, massage, etc., aids in the return to normal function, but requires expert attention and close coöperation of the physiotherapist with the surgeon. In the case of simple fractures, especially those involving joints, such as the elbow and knee, complete immobilization should be maintained no longer than a week or ten days; the ultimate function of the joint will be improved if the cast or splint is removed for a few minutes every day or two and active motion instituted. At no time, however, should the position of the fragments be jeopardized by a zealous desire to institute early mobilization; it should also be emphasized that any motion, active or passive, is apt to be harmful if it provokes pain. In general, active motion is much more effective in preventing atrophy and stiffness of joints than is passive motion.

Compound Fractures.—If the fracture is *compound* the most important feature in the treatment is the prevention of infection (gas gangrene, septicemia, osteomyelitis, etc.). As in open wounds of soft tissue, a delay of many hours (six to twelve) after the accident minimizes the efficiency of preventive treatment, or may contraindicate such radical procedures as débridement (see pp. 195-199). If by such a delay, infection is already present, even reduction of the fracture is unwise, local treatment being limited to immobilization by traction or plaster.

Débridement is in reality more strongly indicated in compound fractures than in soft tissue wounds, because infection is more apt to develop, and when it does is so much more serious than in soft tissue wounds. Naturally, the patient must first be examined for other injuries (*e.g.*, intracranial, thoracic, etc.) which might be even more serious than the compound fracture. The opening through the skin and fascia is enlarged sufficiently to afford good exposure of the most distant crevices. Skin edges must be trimmed and all devitalized tissue along with dirt and other

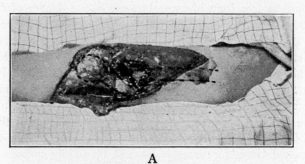

A

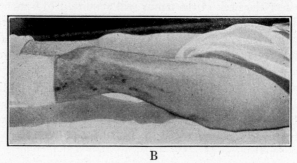

B

FIG. 219.—COMPOUND FRACTURE OF THE FEMUR IN A BOY AGED ELEVEN, SUSTAINED IN AUTO ACCIDENT.

A, appearance of the wound at time of admission to the hospital. The bone ends were visible in the wound, but have been outlined in ink to illustrate more clearly their relative position. A radical débridement was performed and the extremity put in traction in a Thomas splint; *B*, the wound healed without the development of an osteomyelitis. A piece of skin near the knee failed to survive, but in the interval (twelve weeks) between photographs, the defect has closed over.

types of foreign bodies must be removed. All small loose fragments of bone must be removed since they tend to become infected, forming sequestra. All operative manipulation should be performed as gently as possible. Nonabsorbable suture material (particularly cotton) decreases the possible development of infection, and seems preferable, although it is realized that many surgeons fear the danger of persistent sinus formation with such sutures; in reality this is not a very sound argument in favor of catgut since if sufficient infection takes place to cause a persistent sinus, the accompanying osteomyelitis will minimize or obliterate the importance of the type of sutures used. The wound may be irrigated (with physiologic saline) at the conclusion of the débridement, but with care that the flow of fluid is from the depth of the wound toward the surface, so that foreign substances may be washed out rather than in.

Accurate reduction of fragments is a second prerequisite in the treatment of compound fractures, and must be done early. Good reduction minimizes greatly the likelihood of infection presumably because all structures, including particularly blood vessels, nerves and lymphatics, are returned to their normal position, thereby encouraging normal function. Moreover, inaccurate reduction is usually associated with a dead space which is so apt to lead to infection. If reduction cannot be achieved at the time the débridement is performed, manipulation should rarely be done at a later date because of the danger of the inevitable trauma initiating an infection, regardless of the type of fixation or immobilization used. To obtain reduction it may be necessary to insert pins or wires through the bone and obtain traction by some type of apparatus. If a plaster cast is used for immobilization the pins may be incorporated in the cast and removed later when union has taken place.

Although careful débridement and immediate reduction of the fracture are considered necessary in the treatment of compound fractures by all surgeons, two features in therapy, namely, the question of *closure* or *drainage of the wound* and *type of immobilization,* present points of disagreement among certain surgeons, particularly during recent years. According to one group, after débridement compound fractures could and should as a general rule be closed if received up to 6 hours after injury. In 1923 Orr[11] introduced a new principle of packing the wound open with vaseline gauze (after careful débridement and reduction) and applying a plaster cast which is left on for 6 to 8 weeks before changing. Although the practice of open drainage in wounds less than 6 hours old seems contrary to surgical principles, the method has been used by many other surgeons (Heyl,[12] Pfeiffer and Smyth,[13] Trueta[14] and others) and has been found to result in healing with low incidence of infection or death. On the other hand, there is so much criticism of the method, particularly because of the prevalence of a low-grade infection in such open wounds, that it may not be adopted generally in civilian life. The greatest usefulness of the open method would appear to lie in military surgery (where the fractures are so commonly seen late, and where contamination is maximal) particularly since it is so often impossible to furnish the necessary convalescent care incident to treatment with traction. In the recent Spanish revolution, Trueta reported very good results with the open method. With few exceptions the method is being used universally by the Allies in World War II, and with a low incidence of complications. Additional data on the military aspects of compound fractures will be found in Chapter XXXIII.

It appears justifiable to use sulfanilamide or an allied compound orally and locally in the wound (Jensen and associates[26]; Key and Burford[15]) in practically all cases of compound fractures. In 212 consecutive cases treated locally with sulfanilamide Jensen and associates[26] noted that infection was reduced from a previous level of 27 per cent down to 3.3 per cent; the average hospital stay was reduced from 96.3 to 30 days. In their series there was an incidence of gas gangrene of 1 per cent (2 cases) compared to an incidence of 7.3 per cent in the control series not treated with sulfanilamide. In three successive series of about 50 patients each, Jackson[17] found that with débridement, implantation of sulfanilamide and closure of the wound under a plaster, the incidence of infection dropped to 5.6 per cent, with an average period of hospitalization of 6 to 8 days. In the World War II, English surgeons [16] have noted that with its use the percentage of amputations in late cases of infected compound fractures has been reduced from about 75 per cent (in World War I) to a relatively insignificant figure. They have been unable to estimate exactly how much influence the sulfonamide compound had on mortality rate, etc., because in World War II plaster cast fixation (Orr) was being used instead of splints as used predominantly in World War I. After the Pearl Harbor attack (Dec. 7, 1941) compound fractures were treated by placing several grams of sulfanilamide in the wound as soon after injury as possible, followed by débridement, reduction, packing the wound open with vaseline gauze and sulfanilamide, and application of a plaster cast. It is notable that no serious infections (or gas gangrene) were encountered, for at least two weeks following injury.

Complications of Fractures.—It should be emphasized that the surgeon must not be so engrossed in a particular fracture that he is oblivious of other injuries. By other injuries we refer not only to other fractures, but to more serious injuries, such as those involving the internal abdominal organs, thorax and the brain. Not uncommonly the other injuries and the associated shock are of such a serious nature that treatment of the fracture is postponed until the shock is treated or until more serious injuries are taken care of. Ordinarily a fracture of itself is not sufficient to produce surgical shock, except when the larger bones are fractured, and especially when the patient has been transported a considerable distance without proper immobilization. Other injuries also include those to soft tissue, nerves, joints and blood vessels.

1. *Injuries to Soft Tissues.*—By far the most common complication of fractures is injury to the soft tissue. Usually it is of minor significance, consisting merely of contusion of the subcutaneous tissues and muscles with mild hemorrhage. On other occasions the skin will be broken and a *compound fracture* results. The seriousness of this complication and the indication for immediate débridement and reduction have already been discussed. On rare occasions muscles or tendons will be cut by bony fragments. Repair of these structures has been discussed in Chapter X. Infrequently, myositis ossificans, which implies a deposition of calcium and other constituents of bone in a muscle, will develop.

One of the most unfortunate complications from the standpoint of the patient and surgeon is Volkmann's contracture.[18] This is caused by replacement of muscle with fibrous tissue and according to Brooks [19] is due to an obstruction of the venous blood returning from the involved muscles. This lesion is often produced by the application of a bandage or plaster cast too tightly. Usually, however, it is due to arterial hemorrhage beneath unbroken deep fascia which causes subfascial tension and compresses the vessels. Incision of fascia to relieve pressure and evacuate the hematoma may be necessary early. The resultant flexion contracture of the hand, wrist and fingers is hideously deforming and disabling (see page 484). Since the lesion is usually preventable, extreme care must be taken in these injuries.

2. *Injury to Nerves.*—Because of the proximity of nerves to the bone, fractures of the shaft of the humerus and elbow (internal condyle) are apt to be associated with injury of the radial and ulnar nerves respectively. Fractures about the knee and

eg may also involve injury to nerves. In every fracture, *examination for nerve injury should be made carefully before reduction is attempted.* Occasionally the manipulation of bone incident to reduction may compress or tear the nerve. Usually, however, if proper position of fragments is obtained, any compression of the nerve will be released. Only on rare occasions (*e.g.,* immediate complete paralysis, in spite of reduction, and not due to swelling) will it be justifiable to resort to an open operation to release or suture the nerve.

3. *Injury to Joints.*—On many occasions the fracture may extend into the joint. If displacement is present it is imperative that it be corrected in order to prevent disability, which may arise later because of pain or disturbed function. Active motion must be instituted early in order to minimize atrophy of disuse and the possibility of limitation of motion. It may be necessary to aspirate the joint contents (usually blood) in order to prevent undue distention. Frequently, the cartilaginous surface is injured even though the fracture line does not extend into the joint. Such a condition is often referred to as traumatic arthritis which in reality is a low grade inflammatory process involving the joint surface resulting usually from bony irregularities in the joint and characterized by pain, loss of motion and disturbed function of the joint. Increase in the amount of exercise of the joint usually aggravates the symptoms and frequently immobilization must be resorted to before a satisfactory result is obtained (see also page 466).

4. *Injury to Blood Vessels.*—On rare occasions the jagged end of the fractured bone will tear into or sever a major vessel. If the vessel is an artery the swelling created by the hemorrhage may be tremendous. The swollen area may pulsate, and a false (dissecting) aneurysm may be formed. In such an instance the pulsation of the vessel below the fracture is usually absent, the extremity distal to the fracture is cold and pale and the danger of gangrene is imminent. If a vein is injured the resultant hematoma may be large, but will not pulsate. The extremity distal to the fracture is apt to be cyanotic and edematous. Conservative treatment is usually the procedure of choice on account of the tendency for spontaneous restoration of the vascular flow through collateral circulation (see Volkmann's contracture).

5. *Malunion, Delayed Union, Nonunion.*—If a fracture is incorrectly reduced or if the correct position of fragments is lost by inadequate immobilization, the bones may heal in an abnormal position (malunion) and produce a deformity with or without disability. Shortening or disturbance in alignment (angulation) due to malunion is usually not so serious in bones of the upper extremity as it is in the lower extremity.

Delayed union may result from numerous causes, but occasionally a demonstrable factor cannot be found. The same may be said about nonunion. The difference between delayed union and nonunion obviously is one of time. Occasionally, fractures require months for final healing. In such instances a diagnosis of delayed instead of nonunion should be made. Only after the reparative process has come to an end, and at least six months have elapsed without solidification, should a diagnosis of nonunion be made. The distal third of the tibia, the neck of the femur, anatomical neck and shaft of the humerus and carpal bones are the most common sites of delayed union or nonunion.

It has been emphasized by Speed[20] and others that the cause of nonunion is

almost invariably local, *i.e.,* at the site of fracture and not of systemic origin. Ther
are numerous factors, singly or in combination, which are capable of producin
nonunion: (*a*) The factor most commonly associated with ununited fractures i
defective blood supply. When nonunion occurs it usually affects the neck of th
femur, lower third of the tibia, etc., where the blood supply is obviously less tha
elsewhere. (*b*) Unsatisfactory approximation is frequently responsible for nonunio
because of the interposition of muscle and other soft tissue between the fragments
(*c*) Failure of contact at the bone ends is a common cause; lack of adequate reduc

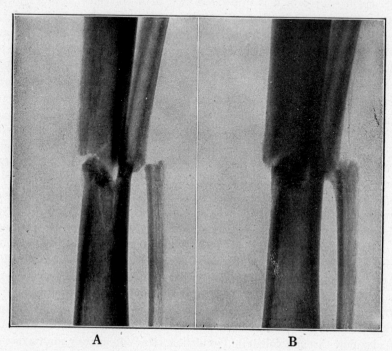

A   B

FIG. 220.—DELAYED UNION FOLLOWING COMPOUND FRACTURE OF THE TIBIA AND FIBULA AT
THE JUNCTION OF THE LOWER AND MIDDLE THIRD.

The bone ends were so dirty that an extensive débridement was necessary; no infection
occurred. *A,* two months after fracture no callus can be seen; *B,* three months after fracture.
Note that even after this long period the only callus visible is a small deposition between the
fractured ends of the fibula. A plaster cast was re-applied to the leg, extending above the knee,
and the patient allowed up on crutches. Weight-bearing after this fashion usually accelerates
union when healing is delayed. In this instance firm union was attained four and one-half months
after fracture.

tion may be the responsible factor. On certain occasions traction may be so intense
as to pull the bone fragments apart. Absorption of bone may take place to such
an extent as to prevent contact of living bone with living bone. (*d*) Lack of immobilization may occasionally be the sole cause of nonunion, especially in untreated
cases. Undue enthusiasm in the early institution of active and passive motion may
likewise result in nonunion. Likewise, numerous manipulations undertaken in an
endeavor to obtain proper position of fragments may be the sole factor producing
nonunion. (*e*) Infection as sustained by a compound fracture is apt to prevent

union. (f) Foreign bodies such as bullets, metal plates, etc., act as a hindrance to the union of bone. (g) Compound fractures sustained in conjunction with serious injury to soft tissue are frequently followed by nonunion, presumably on account of the local escape of blood which prevents the formation of the blood clot between the bone fragments. The importance of the blood clot in the union of bone has already been mentioned. Removal of large fragments of bone in the operative treatment of a compound fracture may be a major factor in the production of nonunion. (h) Constitutional diseases, such as Bright's disease, syphilis, etc., were originally thought to be important factors in the prevention of bony union, but careful clinical analysis suggests that such diseases are rarely true causes of nonunion, but are frequently used as excuses by the surgeon. It is true, however, that in extreme senility and serious debilitating disease, nonunion is more apt to occur than in healthy young people. (i) The incidence of nonunion in spontaneous ("pathological") fractures is high, especially when a malignant growth is responsible for the fracture. The reason for nonunion in such cases is, of course, easy to understand.

The *treatment* of delayed or nonunion is varied. Although too early and too vigorous efforts toward resumption of function may be a direct cause of nonunion there are many occasions (*e.g.,* nonunion of fracture of distal third of tibia) when weight-bearing with proper fixation, *i.e.,* a walking plaster ("skin") cast, may accelerate union. Although the ancient remedy of administration of calcium and phosphorus probably exerts no beneficial effect on the healing, any deficiencies in diet (particularly as related to vitamins) should be corrected. Of the operative procedures perhaps the simplest is drilling holes in the ends of the bone at the fracture site, a method in use for many years and recently described in detail by Griswold.[21] Adequate fixation by operative means is frequently sufficient to obtain union. The older methods of utilizing beef bone, ivory pegs, etc., for fixation have been superseded by the use of autogenous bone grafts. A type of graft commonly used is the so-called inlay graft which is cut with a saw from the tibia and driven into a trough made for it in the two ends of bone. Obviously any soft tissue intervening between the bone ends should be removed; many surgeons prefer also to freshen the bone ends. If the ends of the bone are in good position, the onlay graft (flat graft) as described by Harkins and Phemister[22] may result in union; it is placed over one side of the fracture site and may not need any fixation besides that afforded by pressure of adjacent soft tissue. Treatment is discussed further under the individual fractures.

6. *Infection.*—This is a serious complication, but rarely occurs unless the fracture is compound. The development of infection of the bone (osteomyelitis) in compound fractures is dependent largely upon four factors: (a) the amount of contamination; (b) the length of time intervening between injury and treatment; (c) the amount of traumatized tissue; and (d) the efficacy of treatment. These factors are similar to those influencing the development of infection in open wounds of the soft tissues, but it must be remembered that the soft tissues are more resistant to infection than is bone. Reference has already been made to the necessity of débridement in compound fractures (see page 367). Infection is a serious complication not only because of the delayed healing and loss of bone associated with the osteomyelitis, but also because of the threat made upon life by the systemic invasion of the infection.

The streptococcus and staphylococcus are the organisms most frequently encountered, but infection with a gas bacillus is by no means rare, especially in massive wounds, and is associated with a very high mortality.

7. *Miscellaneous Complications.*—An unfortunate complication of fractures which reflects upon the nursing and medical care given the patient is the development of bed sores or pressure sores. If a plaster cast is improperly padded or ill-fitted, or if the sharp edges are not trimmed away, a necrosis of the skin and subcutaneous tissue at that site may occur. If a patient with a plaster spica is not turned frequently, these *pressure sores* may develop, especially over bony prominences, such as the sacrum and anterior superior spines. This is especially apt to happen in elderly people and without warning, since pain may be absent. A bed sore or decubitus may result merely from the pressure of a part of the body (for example, the heel) on the bed, particularly in aged people.

Fat embolism associated with fractures is no doubt extremely common, but only rarely to the extent that symptoms are produced and still more rarely to the extent that death ensues. Lehman and Moore [23] have emphasized the fact that the amount of fat encountered in the lungs, brain and other organs of the fatal cases is too great to be accounted for by liberation of the fat of the marrow cavity. They have suggested that the physical state of the emulsion of the fat in the blood is altered in some way so that the fine droplets are changed into coarse droplets large enough to plug capillaries. By this latter mechanism fat embolism may produce death, especially when capillaries to vital centers of the brain and medulla are involved. Dark field examination of the blood and search for fat droplets in the urine may be of value in making the diagnosis (Scuderi [24]) (see also p. 171).

Acute traumatic atrophy of the bone, as originally described by Sudeck, fortunately is rare, but when it occurs, manifests itself as an osteoporosis affecting chiefly the bones distal to the fracture, but presumably affects the blood and nerve supply as well. Thus, the extremity may be cold, cyanotic and painful and the motions of the joints included in the atrophy so limited by pain as to frequently create a permanent disability following the fracture. Treatment is usually unsatisfactory, from the standpoint of rapidity of recovery, and consists chiefly of physiotherapy; diathermy, contrast baths and graded activity are advised. A diet rich in vitamins and calcium should be given; cod liver oil may be of value. Paravertebral sympathetic block or lumbar sympathectomy may be helpful (Miller and de Takats [30]).

There are *numerous diseases,* such as pneumonia, etc., which may occasionally result from limitation of activity, especially in aged people. The severity of various diseases, such as nephritis, diabetes, etc., may be accentuated by a fracture of a major bone.

Epiphyseal Separation.—This injury might be classified as midway between a dislocation and a fracture. It occurs, of course, only before puberty, usually during childhood when the epiphyseal line consists of cartilage, thus permitting easy separation of the epiphysis from the shaft. While accurate reduction of the separation is important the danger of nongrowth from injury to the epiphyseal line *must* be avoided meticulously. Unusually careful manipulation must be practiced; open operation is distinctly contraindicated. Moreover, as well emphasized by Aitken,[25] deformity following epiphyseal separation is rapidly and spontaneously corrected.

Except for the danger of nongrowth, Wolff's law seems unusually effective in this type of injury.

DISLOCATIONS

A dislocation of a joint may be defined as a persistent separation of the articular surfaces of the bones constituting the joint. This condition is contrasted to a sprained joint, the articular surfaces of which may be separated at the time of injury, but after the force of impact is over, the articulating surfaces regain their normal position (see page 376). Dislocations may be congenital or traumatic, but only the latter will be considered here. Most of the dislocations occur in the upper extremity, chiefly because the joints in the upper extremity are more mobile and have less supportive structures surrounding them. The most common joints affected are the shoulder, elbow, acromioclavicular joints, joints of the fingers, hand and ankle. Contrary to what might be expected, dislocations of the hip are rarely observed. Dislocations are much less common than fractures, but not infrequently are associated with them.

A variable amount of damage may be inflicted by the dislocation, but there is always a rupture of the capsule of the joint and a stretching or tearing of the ligaments supporting the joint. The muscles and tendons surrounding the joint are frequently traumatized and may be frayed or torn.

The mechanism of production of dislocations is, of course, dependent upon external violence, usually of an indirect character involving leverage. Dislocations of the shoulder are usually sustained by falling in such a way that the hand catches the weight of the body while the arm is sharply abducted. If the arm is more perpendicular to the ground and the elbow is hyperextended as the impact of the body weight is sustained by the hand, a dislocation of the elbow (with or without fracture of the coronoid process) is apt to occur. Joints of the fingers may be dislocated by sudden forceful hyperextension or by impact to a phalanx at right angles to the bone while the proximal phalanx is held rigid.

The complications of dislocations are similar to those accompanying fractures. However, injuries to major vessels are less common in dislocation. Since the articulating surfaces of the joints are reasonably blunt, a compound dislocation is not so apt to occur as a compound fracture. When the healing process in the structures injured by the dislocation has been completed, a rent in the capsule occasionally remains and the ligaments which were torn or irreparably stretched fail to lend support to the bony components of the joint. Under such circumstances recurrent dislocations are not uncommon. A dislocation of the shoulder, for example, may recur subsequently as the result of only mild injury.

Diagnosis.—A dislocation may easily be mistaken for a fracture and *vice versa*. The x-ray, of course, will reveal the true diagnosis and should always be used before resorting to treatment. On many occasions the situation is so complicated from the diagnostic standpoint by the association of a fracture with the dislocation that the x-ray is the only means of arriving at a correct diagnosis. The pain produced by a dislocation is more apt to be constant and of a type associated with nausea. A careful examination should reveal features which are ordinarily distinguishable from those accompanying a fracture. For example, when a posterior dislocation of the elbow exists, the triangular relationship between the olecranon and the condyles of the humerus is lost and the tip of the olecranon is observed to lie posterior to its normal position. In a dislocation of the upper end of the humerus there will be a flattening of the deltoid curve, the head of the humerus cannot be felt in its usual position and there will be inability to adduct the arm across the chest. Crepitus will be absent unless there is an associated fracture. A rather constant muscle spasm and rigidity about the injured part is maintained when a dislocation is present, whereas an abnormal mobility will be demonstrable in a complete fracture. The deformity accompanying a dislocation is, of course, confined to the region of the joint. The tenderness present in a dislocation is apt to be less intense and more diffuse than it is in a fracture.

General Principles of Treatment.—Dislocations should be reduced as soon after injury as possible. The type of manipulation necessary for reduction varies with different joints. Some of the smaller joints, such as interphalangeal joints, may be reduced without anesthesia by simple forceful traction in hyperextension or flexion, depending upon the type of dislocation. On many occasions dislocation of joints as large as the shoulder can likewise be reduced without anesthesia of any kind, except a dose of morphine, if the surgeon can obtain the patient's confidence and perform traction and manipulation carefully and painlessly. Prolonged traction over several minutes may tire the muscles sufficiently to allow the head of the humerus to be pulled out of its new location and be replaced in its socket. Ordinarily, a general anesthesia, preferably ether, will be necessary for reduction of the major joints. With complete relaxation it is rarely difficult to stretch the muscles enough to obtain reduction. It should be emphasized that x-ray films must be taken after, as well as before treatment, in order to verify the success of the reduction. If a delay of a day or two has elapsed since the injury, the subsequent edema and hemorrhage will, of course, make reduction more difficult. If a period of two or more weeks has elapsed since injury, sufficient scar tissue may have been deposited about the head of the bone to greatly interfere with or prevent replacement. Moreover, the rent in the capsule may have healed sufficiently to prevent reduction of the head of the bone through it. In such instances operative reduction may be necessary. Regardless of whether an open or closed reduction has been performed, it is necessary to immobilize the joint for two or three weeks to prevent a recurrence. Until the torn capsule and the ligaments have healed, a dislocation may recur with the slightest trauma. The deposition of scar tissue about the joint after three weeks is usually sufficient to prevent a recurrence.

When a patient suffers from frequent recurrent dislocations it may be necessary to resort to operative procedures to prevent them. Any rents or tears in the capsule should be repaired and the supportive ligaments shortened. If torn completely, they should be approximated by suture if possible. On many occasions these procedures are not sufficient and it becomes necessary to resort to other methods, such as transplantation of bone at a strategic point on the rim of the socket, or to fix the head of the bone in its socket by a strip of fascia.

If a dislocation is compound, the demand for immediate treatment becomes more urgent because of the danger of infection. The head of the bone protruding through the skin should be washed thoroughly and the skin about the wound cleansed and treated with iodine and alcohol or soap and water. Under anesthesia the dislocation is then reduced, taking care that no foreign bodies are left in the joint. The rent in the capsule should be closed by suture and any damaged ligaments repaired. The wound is closed without drainage, but must be watched closely for the development of infection.

SPRAINS

A sprain may be defined as a partial or complete tear of some of the supporting ligaments of the joint produced usually by a temporary dislocation or separation of the articular surfaces. This separation of the articular surfaces is, of course, only momentary so that when the patient is seen the bony portions have regained their normal position. The ankle, which is probably afflicted more often than any other joint, is usually sprained by forcible plantar flexion and inversion of the foot, usually while running or by stepping in a hole. The knee and wrist are likewise commonly sprained, but the hip and shoulder, which normally have a wide range of mobility, are more susceptible to dislocations than to sprains. When there is a tearing of a fragment of bone or a strip of periosteum from the bone at the site of insertion of the ligament the injury is spoken of as a "sprain fracture." Sprains of the knee are frequently associated with injury to the internal semilunar cartilage.

The pain complained of at the time of injury may be so severe as to be indistinguishable from that suffered from a fracture. For this reason it is nearly always advisable to obtain an x-ray film in all sprains, particularly the severe ones, in order to rule out the presence of fracture. The pain associated with sprains is usually located diffusely about the joint, but is more intense at the site of the injured ligaments.

The treatment of sprains is variable, depending upon the severity. If the sprain is seen immediately after injury, the application of cold for an hour or two will minimize the degree of edema and extravasation. In general, the joint should be immobilized with the torn ligament in a relaxed position. This immobilization can usually be obtained by adhesive and bandage. In severe sprains it will be necessary to apply a light plaster cast in order to achieve relief of pain. The application of heat aids in the reparative process. Motion and function are started as soon as subsidence of pain permits.

BIBLIOGRAPHY

1. KEY, J. A., and CONWELL, H. E. *The Management of Fractures, Dislocations and Sprains*, C. V. Mosby Co., St. Louis, 3rd ed., 1942.
2. MAGNUSON, P. B. *Fractures*, J. B. Lippincott Co., Philadelphia, 1942.
3. BÖHLER, Lorenz. *Treatment of Fractures*, 4th ed., Translated by E. W. Hey Groves, Wm. Wood & Co., Baltimore, 1935.
4. SCUDDER, C. L. *The Treatment of Fractures*, 11th ed., W. B. Saunders Co., Philadelphia, 1938.
5. SPEED, Kellogg. *A Textbook of Fractures and Dislocations*, Lea and Febiger, Philadelphia, 4th ed., 1942.
6. HAMM, A. W. A Histological Study of the Early Phases of Bone Repair, *J. Bone & Joint Surg.*, 12:827, 1930.

RHODE, Carl. Does Bone Form from Osteoblasts or from a Metaplasia of the Surrounding Connective Tissue? *Surg., Gynec. & Obst.*, 41:740, 1925.

7. DUPUYTREN, G. *Injuries and Diseases of Bones,* translated and edited by F. LeGros Clark, London, The Sydenham Society, 1847, p. 41.

8. WOLFF, Julius. Das Gesetz der Transformation der Knochen, Berlin, 1892.

9. BUCK, Gurdon. An Improved Method of Treating Fractures of the Thigh, *Bull. New York Acad. Med.*, 1:181, 1860-1862.

10. WILSON, Philip D. *Physical Therapy in the Treatment of Fractures, in Principles and Practice of Physical Therapy,* Vol. 2: Chapter 5. W. F. Prior and Co., Hagerstown, 1932.

11. ORR, H. W. Treatment of Compound Fractures, with Special Reference to Military Surgical Procedures, *Arch. Surg.*, 40:825, 1940.

12. HEYL, G. H. The Treatment of Compound Fractures of the Long Bones, *Ann. Surg.*, 111:470, 1940.

13. PFEIFFER, D. B. and SMYTH, C. M., JR. Treatment of Compound Fractures with Special Reference to the Orr Method, *Ann. Surg.*, 102:1059, 1935.

14. TRUETA, J. *Treatment of War Wounds and Fractures with Special Reference to the Closed Method as Used in the War in Spain,* London, H. Hamilton, 1939.

15. KEY, J. A. and BURFORD, T. H. The Local Implantation of Sulfanilamide in Compound Fractures, *South. M. J.*, 33:449, 1940.

16. FOREIGN LETTERS. The Chemotherapy of War Wounds, *J. Am. M. Ass.*, 115:2194, 1940.

17. JACKSON, Ruth. A Comparative Study of the Treatment of Compound Fractures, *South. M. J.*, 34:319, 1941.

18. VOLKMANN, Richard. Die ischaemischen Muskellähmungen und Kontrakturen, *Zent. F. Chir.*, 8:801, 1881.

19. BROOKS, B. Pathologic Changes in Muscle as a Result of Disturbances of Circulation, *Arch. Surg.*, 5:188, 1922.

20. SPEED, K. Nonunion after Fracture, *Ann. Surg.*, 90:574, 1929.

21. GRISWOLD, R. A. The Treatment of Delayed Union and Nonunion of Fractures by Subcutaneous Drilling, *Ann. Surg.*, 109:135, 1939.

22. HARKINS, H. N. and PHEMISTER, D. B. Onlay Graft for Ununited Fracture, *J. Am. M. Ass.*, 109:1501, 1937.

23. LEHMAN, E. P., and MOORE, R. M. Fat Embolism: Including Experimental Production without Trauma, *Arch. Surg.*, 14:621, 1927.

24. SCUDERI, C. S. Fat Embolism, *Arch. Surg.*, 36:614, 1938.

25. AITKEN, A. P. The End Results of Fractured Distal Tibial Epiphysis, *J. Bone & Joint Surg.*, 18:685; 1036, 1936.

26. JENSEN, N. K., JOHNSRUD, L. W., and NELSON, M. C. The Local Implantation of Sulfanilamide in Compound Fractures, *Surgery,* 6:1, 1939; JENSEN, N. K., and NELSON, M. C. Local Sulfanilamide in Compound Fractures, *Surg., Gynec. & Obst.*, 75:34, 1942.

27. CALDWELL, G. A. *Treatment of Fractures,* Paul Hoeber, Inc., New York, 1943.

28. VENABLE, C. S., and STUCK, W. G. Clinical Uses of Vitallium, *Ann. Surg.*, 117:772, 1943.

29. LEWIS, K. M., BREIDENBACH, L., and STADER, O. The Stader Reduction Splint, *Ann. Surg.*, 116:623, 1942.

30. MILLER, D. S., and DE TAKATS, G. Posttraumatic Dystrophy of the Extremities (Sudecks Atrophy), *Surg., Gynec. & Obst.*, 75:558, 1942.

31. COLE, W. H., and PUESTOW, C. B. *First Aid, Surgical and Medical,* 2nd Edition, 1943, D. Appleton-Century Company, New York.

CHAPTER XVIII

FRACTURES, DISLOCATIONS AND SPRAINS: SPECIFIC TYPES

The Skull
The Facial Bones
The Spine and Ribs
The Shoulder Girdle

The Upper Extremity
The Pelvis
The Lower Extremity

THE SKULL

Although the serious aspects of head injuries are frequently thought of as being produced by fracture of the skull, in reality they are secondary to intracranial injury and increased intracranial pressure. Naturally, fracture of the skull may be accompanied by tenderness along the fracture line, but even this manifestation which is so consistently present in other fractures, may be absent. Therefore, it may not be possible to make an accurate diagnosis without an x-ray, except through manifestations produced by the intracranial injury. Obviously, bone fragments may actually be visible in compound fractures, and deformity demonstrated in depressed fractures. However, since most of the manifestations and serious effects encountered in fractures of the skull are secondary to intracranial injury we have included the entire subject in the chapter dealing with the nervous system.

THE FACIAL BONES

The Nasal Bones.—Fracture of the nasal bones is frequent, particularly in children, football players and boxers. Occasionally the injury consists merely of a separation of the nasal cartilage from the bone. Fracture of the bones usually results in a depression, or lateral deviation of the contour of the nose. If the nose is depressed, the nasal septum usually is buckled and deviated. Bleeding from the nasal cavity occurs commonly and is indicative of a tear of the mucous membrane, produced usually by a broken edge of the bone or cartilaginous septum. Swelling appears early and is usually so pronounced as to obscure mild deformity. Absence of external deformity, therefore, does not justify the physician in excluding the presence of fracture. In such instances, intranasal examination should be made and will frequently reveal deformity indicative of the type of displacement. Lateral deviation can usually be corrected readily by molding the fragments with the fingers. When a depression is present, the bones are best elevated by pressure exerted by a curved, blunt-nosed artery forcep from within the nasal cavity. After reduction of fragments, position can usually be maintained by the insertion of a small rubber tube up each nostril or by packing the cavity loosely with a strip of vaselin or iodoform gauze. In complicated cases it may be advisable to maintain position of the fragments by a splint anchored to the teeth of the upper jaw (Blair[1]). It is occasionally necessary to resect the septum at a later date if the septal deviation obstructs the airway in the nasal cavity.

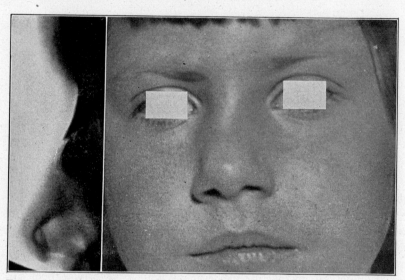

FIG. 221.—FRACTURE OF NASAL BONE SUSTAINED A FEW WEEKS PREVIOUSLY.

Note the deflection of the nose. Insert shows appearance of the fracture in the x-ray. After breaking up the callus, reduction was attained by pressure made by a blunt instrument through the nasal cavity with patient under an anesthetic.

The Zygoma (Malar Bone).—Depression of the zygomatic arch is perhaps the most common type of fracture about the malar bone. In more various injuries the orbital border is detached and an obvious deformity of the orbit, with disturbance in function of the muscles of the eye, is produced. Reduction can usually be made by the insertion of a hook-shaped instrument through the skin, engaging the bone and manipulating the fragment until reduction is attained. Occasionally it will be necessary to wire the fragments in position by operative procedures. A detailed discussion of the various methods of treatment may be found in a recent report by Kanthak.[2]

The Maxilla (Upper Jaw).—Fracture of the upper jaw is not common and occurs only in violent accidents. Fractures of other bones of the skull are apt to be present. Usually, there is very little displacement of fragments. Considerable swelling and ecchymosis of the face about the site of fracture is commonly present. If one side of the maxilla is completely detached from the body of the bone, but is not displaced, fixation by interdental wires may be necessary. The fixation should be achieved by wiring corresponding teeth of the upper and lower jaw on the uninjured side. If the entire body of the bone is detached and is displaced downward, it will be advisable to reduce it, and in some manner maintain reduction, e.g., by a dental-splint held in position by an elastic band anchored over the head (Brown[3]).

The Mandible.—Because of its exposed position and relatively slender shaft, the mandible is a frequent site of injury.

Fracture of the Mandible.—This injury is produced most commonly by a direct blow on the bone, but unfortunately occurs occasionally during extraction of molar teeth. The fracture occurs most commonly near the mental foramen or angle, and not infrequently is bilateral. Most fractures of the mandible are compound chiefly

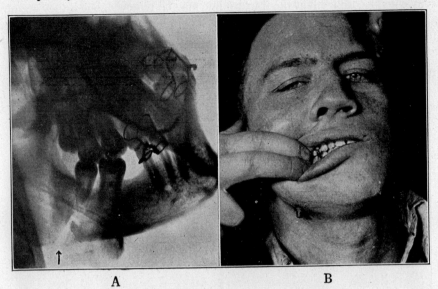

A   B

FIG. 222.—FRACTURE OF THE MANDIBLE.

A, x-ray showing wires in place and fragments reduced. The arrow indicates the site of fracture; *B,* photo of a patient with fracture of the mandible, after wiring of jaw and insertion of a drain alongside the fracture site. The drain is important in the prevention of osteomyelitis and abscesses about the fracture.

because the gum fits so tightly over the alveolar margin that the mucous membrane is torn when even a slight displacement of fragments occurs, and also because the fracture line tends to break into a tooth socket. Inspection of the mouth will reveal asymmetry or deformity in the position of the teeth, with loss of occlusion, if displacement of fragments exists. Bleeding from the gum margin and the presence of a tear in the alveolar mucous membrane are indicative of a compound fracture. Pain and tenderness over the site of fracture are nearly always present. An x-ray should be taken to establish the diagnosis and determine the amount of displacement; more than one view is preferable.

Treatment consists of immobilization of the entire mandible. This is undoubtedly most readily and completely obtained by wiring appropriate teeth of the upper and lower jaw together. This procedure should not be performed while the stomach is full or with the patient under a general anesthesia, because vomiting might result in aspiration of gastric content with perhaps fatal choking. A preliminary sedative and local anesthesia are usually sufficient to allow performance of the procedure with little pain. Experience has shown that since most of these fractures are compound, infection frequently gets into the soft tissues about the broken bones and may lead to development of an abscess at the site of fracture, or to a deep cervical abscess. Osteomyelitis may also be produced. Because of this possibility it is advisable to establish drainage of the tissue at the site of fracture by a small incision along the inferior margin of the jaw, and insertion of a drain upward alongside the bone. This rarely fails to prevent the development of soft tissue abscesses which so commonly accompany compound fracture, and thus minimizes the possibility of osteomyelitis. Loose teeth at the fracture line may be removed, but if they are offering support for the posterior fragment they should be left in place and removed ten to fourteen days later, after fixation is secured by callus. The wires should be left

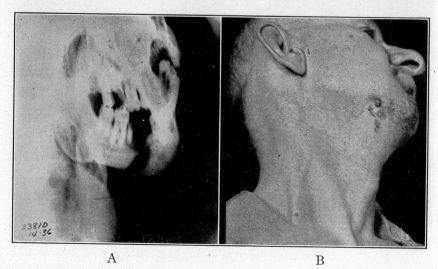

A   B

FIG. 223.—UNTREATED FRACTURE OF MANDIBLE.

A, x-ray at time of admission, five weeks after injury; note separation of fragments. *B,* patient developed an abscess which ruptured spontaneously with the formation of a sinus as noted in the photograph. An osteomyelitis is now present.

in place four to six weeks, depending upon the rapidity of healing. When no teeth are present, immobilization may be accomplished by driving a wire through both fragments (Brown and McDowell [35]), by bandages, or dental splints. On certain occasions it may be advisable to wire the fragments together by an operative procedure. While fixation is being maintained, obviously only liquid food can be ingested. Oral hygiene is important; cleansing mouth washes should be used frequently.

Dislocation of the Jaw.—Dislocation of the jaw is a relatively uncommon injury; the condyles are usually displaced forward, *i.e.,* anteriorly. The mouth is held open. Pain is moderate and talking or chewing difficult, if not impossible. Reduction is effected by placing the thumbs in the mouth on the lower molars and depressing the mandible downward while it is likewise being pushed posteriorly. (The operator must be prepared to remove the thumbs instantly as reduction is accomplished lest they be crushed.) It may be necessary to obtain greater traction by placing a solid object between the upper and lower molars as a fulcrum and pressing upward on the chin. Reduction may be attempted without anesthesia, but anesthesia of some type is usually necessary, preferably ether. The patient should be instructed not to open the mouth very widely for two or three weeks after reduction, since dislocation might easily recur by such a simple mechanism as yawning.

Repeated mild dislocation of the temporomandibular joint is a frequent cause of chronic pain for which many patients seek relief. Often they complain also of an annoying click whenever the jaw is used. Relief may often be obtained by using only the molar teeth for chewing and avoiding the use of the incisors for biting. Although operative therapy has been used for the severe cases, Schultz[4] has described a simple method by which a fibrosis and shortening of the joint capsule is achieved by the intra-articular injection of a solution of sodium psylliate.

THE SPINE AND RIBS

Fractures of the vertebral column may be divided into those of the dorsolumbar and those of the cervical region. The sacrum and coccyx are discussed under the pelvis.

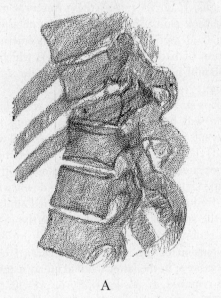 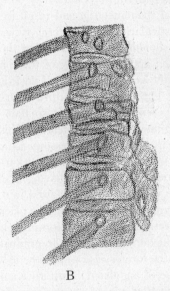

A   B

FIG. 224.—COMPRESSION FRACTURE OF THE BODY OF THE NINTH DORSAL VERTEBRA IN A FIFTY-THREE-YEAR-OLD WOMAN WHO FELL OUT OF A SECOND STORY WINDOW.

The illustrations are drawings made from the lateral x-ray films, A, before and B, after reduction. The patient was hyperextended over a bent Bradford frame for several weeks and a plaster cast then applied. Paralysis and incontinence were complete on admission but slowly disappeared. The Queckenstedt test revealed no spinal block, although the spinal fluid was bloody.

Dorsolumbar Spine.—Of the twelve dorsal and five lumbar vertebrae, the most important ones are those of the lower dorsal and lumbar region, since these are the most movable. The upper dorsal vertebrae are held rigidly by the ribs and are less subject to injury.

Compression Fracture.—The most common site of fracture is the body of the vertebra which is crushed or compressed, hence the frequent use of the term compression fracture. The injury is caused by forced flexion or force applied to the spine while flexed and is often due to a fall with the weight of the body striking the buttocks or feet, or a heavy weight falling on the stooped shoulders. In many cases, however, the degree of force is apparently slight. Dislocation of dorsolumbar vertebrae is rare except in severe injuries. Injury to the spinal cord is also encountered only in the more serious fractures and is discussed in Chapter XXII. Occasionally associated with spine injuries are abdominal symptoms, which simulate general peritonitis (*e.g.*, distention, vomiting and abdominal rigidity). If intra-abdominal injury is excluded these manifestations are due to reflex ileus or to retroperitoneal hemorrhage (see pp. 759 and 749 resp.).

The *clinical manifestations* of a compression fracture may be so slight that the lesion is overlooked. Spine injury should be suspected whenever the patient has fallen so that the body weight has been transmitted to the spine, or when force has been applied which might have flexed the spine acutely, such as overturning in an automobile. Deformity may be absent. Local tenderness at the level of the injury, and pain on movement may be the only signs. If unrecognized, these fractures may heal spontaneously and result in persistent back pain. An x-ray should be obtained, particularly in the lateral view, in order to demonstrate a compression fracture. It should be emphasized that the designation of back sprain (see p. 420), which is often applied to many of these injuries, should not be made unless adequate x-ray study has failed to reveal an injury to bone.

The important feature of *treatment* consists of prolonged immobilization in a hyperextended position so that solid bone will be deposited without altering the alignment of the vertebrae. This will prevent further injury to the cord and will even relieve such pressure as may already be present, by restoring the fracture to more nearly normal position. The hyperextended position is so important that patients suspected of having a spinal injury should be transported face down with the vertebral column bowed into extreme lordosis or, if he is being carried supine, a large blanket roll must be placed under the small of the back to achieve the same effect. If a flexion deformity (kyphosis or dorsal angulation) is already present, reduction by forceful or gradual hyperextension of the spine is first carried out. In the former case an anesthetic will be necessary; in the latter method an adjustable type of angulated Bradford frame will be required. If no deformity is present the patient is placed prone (face down) over a canvas strip and a plaster body cast applied in the hyperextended position. In such a cast the patient may be allowed up within a few days, provided he is comfortable and in no pain. If gradual hyperextension is instituted or if other injuries make bed rest necessary, the cast may be omitted by placing the patient in the supine position over a Bradford frame bent at the site of fracture. Immobilization is continued for two months, and since the new bone is easily softened by weight bearing, a brace which supports the spine is usually advised for a further period of many months. In most cases support of one kind or another will be needed for from 6 to 10 months.

Fractures of other parts of the vertebrae, such as the spinous or transverse processes, lamina and articular facets, are rarer and some of them difficult to demonstrate even in the x-ray. The clinical manifestations consist of local pain and tenderness, rarely deformity. Prolonged immobilization is the proper form of treatment.

Traumatic spondylitis (Kümmell's disease) is a painful lesion of the spine associated with a definite kyphos (gibbus) and occasionally with manifestations of spinal cord compression. It is presumably due to a compression fracture which had been overlooked or inadequately treated. Treatment consists of prolonged immobilization in a hyperextended position.

Cervical Spine.—This part of the vertebral column is more movable and hence more easily dislocated than fractured. The force producing the dislocation may be trivial, such as a sudden twist of the neck, but is usually a severe blow or fall on the head which is transmitted to the spine. The clinical diagnosis of a cervical spine injury is usually easy, because of the pain produced on movement of the neck and the abnormal position in which the head is held. Fracture dislocations are common and unfortunately are more serious even than dislocations.

Dislocation of the Articular Facets.— The most common lesion is an *unilateral dislocation* of the articular facet, usually of the third, fourth or fifth vertebra, which is displaced anteriorly over the one beneath. This is usually evident in the lateral x-ray film because the body of the dislocated vertebra is dislodged forward. The patient's head is turned away from the dislocated side, the chin elevated and the head flexed toward the lesion, producing an attitude similar to that in torticollis. Attempts at rotation of the head toward the dislocated articular facet meets a definite block and produces severe pain. When both facets of the vertebra are dislocated, the head and chin are forward and movement to either side is limited and painful. Much more serious are injuries to the first and second cervical vertebrae (atlas and axis), particularly if the odontoid process is fractured, because of the danger of compression of the medulla which results in immediate death. The disability and pain in fracture or dislocation of the atlas and axis are similar to, but more severe than, injuries to the other cervical vertebrae. Diagnosis depends largely on adequate x-ray films; to show the atlas and axis an anteroposterior view taken through the wide open mouth is essential (see Fig. 227).

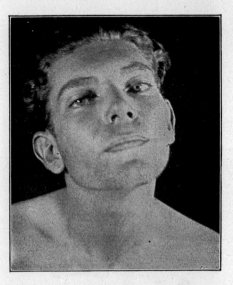

Fig. 225.—CHARACTERISTIC ATTITUDE IN UNILATERAL RIGHT DISLOCATION OF THE ARTICULAR FACETS IN THE CERVICAL SPINE.

This patient, a twenty-one-year-old clerk, gave a history of having his neck manipulated as a therapeutic procedure to relieve a sore throat. X-ray revealed a dislocation of the second on the third cervical vertebra; reduction was easy.

Treatment of dislocations of the lower cervical vertebrae consists of immediate reduction and immobilization in a plaster cast (Brookes [5]). The manipulations which are used (Taylor or Walton) may be carried out with general anesthesia or with only a basal anesthetic (avertin, evipal). Permanent traction in bed with a halter, in place of immediate reduction, is a much less effective method of treatment and should not be used unless the patient's general condition contraindicates the manipulation. The presence of injury to nerves emerging from the spinal cord does not contraindicate reduction; in many instances the manifestations of nerve injury will disappear after a successful anatomical replacement of the injured vertebra. The reduction is usually evident by a bony click and by the complete mobility produced; it should be verified by a lateral x-ray film. Immobilization is achieved by a plaster cuirass which incorporates the head and chest. If primary reduction and plaster fixation is not indicated or is unsuccessful, skeletal traction by tongs inserted into

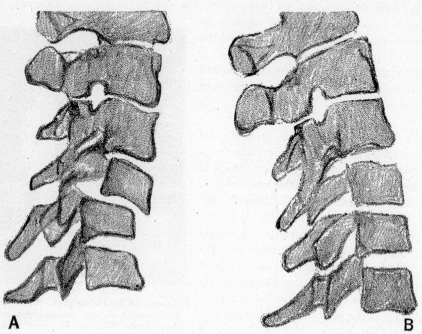

A   B

Fig. 226.—Marked Forward Displacement of Fourth on Fifth Cervical Vertebra due to a Dislocation of the Left Articular Facet.

The patient, a forty-year-old chauffeur, could not turn his head to the left and suffered pain and weakness of the left arm and shoulder which disappeared completely after reduction. *A*, before reduction, and three weeks after an auto collision in which the patient was thrown violently from his car; *B*, after reduction, while patient was in a plaster cuirass, similar to that illustrated in Figure 227 *B*.

the outer table of the skull, as described by Crutchfield,[6] is very effective. The treatment of injury of the atlas and axis consists of immobilization in a plaster cast which protects the base of the skull and immobilizes the spine down to the pelvis. Manipulation is avoided in order to minimize the danger of medullary compression.

Any patient suspected of having a fracture or dislocation of the cervical spine must be transported with great care with the head firmly immobilized; danger of damage to the spinal cord is ever-present until fixation is adequately achieved.

Ribs.—*Fractured ribs* are frequent in any crushing injury and, if the patient is conscious and rational, produces characteristically sharp pain on deep respiration. The acts of sneezing and coughing are particularly painful. A history of difficulty in getting in or out of bed because of pain in the neighborhood of the fractured ribs is almost always obtainable. To protect the injured bones from movement the patient will frequently use only abdominal respirations. Palpation of the individual ribs will nearly always indicate the site of fracture by eliciting the point or points of maximum tenderness. X-ray films may reveal the fracture, but in general are comparatively unreliable, particularly if there is no displacement and the break is in the axillary line (unless a lateral or oblique view is also obtained).

Associated with fractured rib, and of much more serious significance, is injury to the underlying lung. The existence of subcutaneous emphysema (a crepitant

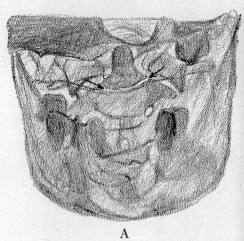

A

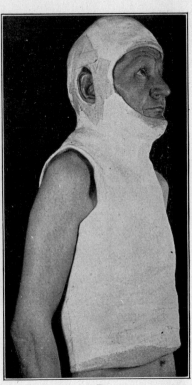

B

FIG. 227.—FRACTURE OF THE ODONTOID PROCESS OF THE AXIS WITHOUT DISPLACEMENT.

The patient, a sixty-year-old laborer, fell and struck his head, following which he had local pain and inability to move his neck. *A*, x-ray taken through the open mouth; the arrows point to the line of fracture. *B*, plaster cuirass for complete immobilization of the cervical spine; this was worn for two months and replaced by a collar brace.

sensation on light palpation) is suggestive of pulmonary lacerations; the presence of air and blood in the pleural space (pneumo- and hemothorax) is more conclusive; occasionally hemoptysis occurs. Physical examination will reveal evidence of pneumo- and hemothorax, but an adequate x-ray is most conclusive of all. The x-ray should be taken in the upright position to show a fluid level, or if that position is inadvisable, an anteroposterior view should be taken with the patient lying on his sound side. The presence of collapsed lung, shifting of the trachea and heart, as well as the demonstration of a fluid level, are of special significance. Clinical manifestations of lung damage may be absent, but evidence of respiratory difficulty, such as a rapid rate and cyanosis, indicates serious impairment of gaseous interchange and makes treatment more urgent.

In simple fracture of the ribs, *treatment* is directed toward immobilization of the thorax, largely to relieve pain. This is best achieved by a firm circular bandage (Fig. 228) which is applied at the time of deep expiration when the chest is collapsed. A chest binder may also be used. Elastic adhesive (elastoplast) applied completely about the chest in expiration is effective and comfortable. Adhesive strips which embrace half the thorax are ineffective. However, adhesive strips placed all the way around, except for about two inches on the side opposite the fracture, will

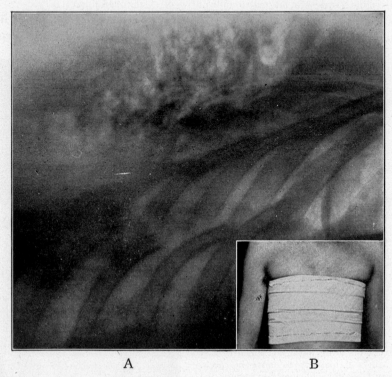

A   B

FIG. 228.—FRACTURED RIBS WITH SUBCUTANEOUS EMPHYSEMA IN AN EIGHTY-YEAR-OLD WOMAN, AFTER BEING STRUCK BY AN AUTO.

A, print from the x-ray film, a lateral view taken while the patient was lying on the sound side. A hemopneumothorax was also present on the injured side. Recovery was uneventful following conservative care, especially immobilization of the chest; *B,* an excellent method of immobilizing ribs; several circular bands of adhesive, or other material are fastened over a layer of soft stockinette during expiration.

be fairly effective in supplying immobilization and relieving symptoms. Relief of pain and easier respirations should follow the application of an adequate support. This treatment is performed even in the face of internal injuries which are insufficient to demand more than rest and conservative care. The operative and other treatment of the injuries to the lung associated with fractured ribs are described in Chapter XXIX.

Sternum.—Fractures of the sternum may be produced by direct blows or crushing injuries, but are comparatively rare. Manifestations consist of tenderness over the line of fracture and pain in this area upon deep breathing, coughing, etc. The patient prefers to allow the head and shoulders to droop forward, since this position relieves the pain. Since the fracture line can rarely be palpated, any patient complaining of significant pain and tenderness in the region of the sternum should be submitted for an x-ray. Usually only the lateral x-ray is of any value. Displacement of fragments should be corrected if possible, but healing with fragments in poor position is rarely accompanied by any permanent difficulty. If pain is considerable, strapping with adhesive may be inadequate and immobilization in bed may be necessary. Contusion of the heart may complicate injuries of the sternum (Beck[7]).

THE SHOULDER GIRDLE

Under this heading will be included fractures and dislocations of the clavicle, scapula and shoulder joint.

Clavicle.—This bone, popularly called the collar bone, is frequently the site of fracture. Occasionally it is dislocated at its acromial attachment; rarely at its sternal end.

Fracture of the Clavicle.—This injury is due to a direct blow or a transmitted force which is directed at the lateral side of the shoulder. Moderate disability, including pain upon movements of the arm and shoulder (particularly active motion) is universally present. The break is usually transverse, but may be slightly oblique

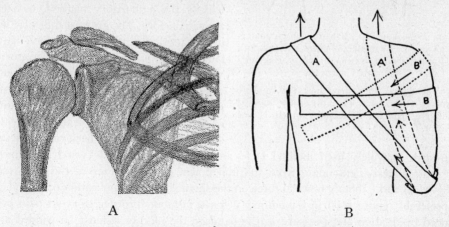

A   B

FIG. 229.—FRACTURE OF THE CLAVICLE AT A COMMON SITE.

A, sketch from an x-ray film, showing the usual displacement; the patient sustained this injury by falling on her shoulder; *B*, rear view of a patient illustrating two common methods by which upward and backward traction (indicated by the arrows) may be exerted by means of strips of adhesive. Note especially the pad under the elbow which prevents pain and pressure irritation at this point. With *A* the upward pull is carried around the opposite shoulder, with *A'* on the same shoulder (but obviously proximal to the fracture line); with *B* the backward pull is exerted on the upper arm, with *B'* it is exerted on the part of the shoulder covered by the deltoid.

and occasionally is comminuted. Owing to the pull of trunk muscles (pectoralis major, serratus, etc.) displacement with overriding is common. The distal fragment is usually displaced downward and medially. Diagnosis is readily made by the relative immobility of the affected arm, the shoulder drop on the affected side and the ease with which deformity and point of tenderness are detected, because the

clavicle is subcutaneous over its entire extent. If there is a displacement of fragments there will be a shortening of the distance on the side of the fracture between
the sternum and acromium, as compared to the uninjured side. X-ray films in the
anteroposterior view reveal the lesion perfectly. On only rare occasions is the
fracture compound; other complications are also uncommon.

Treatment consists of immobilization of the shoulder with force exerted upward
and posteriorly against the shoulder. The functional result following such a simple
procedure is always good and ordinarily that is the chief consideration. In young
women, however, a perfect anatomical reduction of the deformity may be essential
in order to achieve a good cosmetic result as well; immobilization by bandages

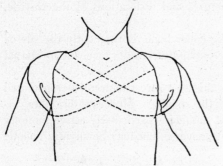

may not always achieve perfect anatomical
reposition. Treatment by bed rest, as described on the following page, is to be preferred if accurate approximation is to be desired; only rarely will it be necessary to
perform an open reduction of the fracture.

There are a great many methods of
maintaining reduction and immobilization
of the fragments in a fracture of the clavicle by the ambulatory method, but few
are satisfactory. The greatest difficulty lies

FIG. 230.—ANOTHER METHOD OF IMMOBILI-
ZATION IN FRACTURE OF THE CLAVICLE, THE
FIGURE EIGHT BANDAGE; IT IS PARTICU-
LARLY USEFUL IN CHILDREN.

in the fact that many methods which maintain the position of fragments satisfactorily
will be uncomfortable for the patient,

The dotted lines show how the bandage
crosses on the back. The arm on the affected
side is supported in a sling which is not
shown.

chiefly because of pain. It should be emphasized that the two important features
of treatment are immobilization with the
shoulder anchored (1) backward and (2)

upward. A widely used method is to anchor the shoulder backward by a piece
of wide adhesive extending from the upper arm posteriorly across the back (see
Fig. 229) and to obtain upward force on the shoulder by the application of a bandage
(preferably gauze roll) in a modified Velpeau fashion. In order to avoid pain produced by fixation and pressure of the bandage the olecranon must be padded and
the elbow fixed at an angle only slightly less than a right angle. Because of irritating
effect no adhesive is placed on the skin except the posterior strip pulling the shoulder
backward, and perhaps another strip holding the proximal fragment of the clavicle
down. To prevent loss of position of the fragments by stretching of the gauze
dressing, wide adhesive strips are placed over the dressing in various places. Another
efficient method which relies more on adhesive than bandages is that described
by Conwell.[8] A figure-of-eight bandage around both shoulders drawing the scapulae
toward each other posteriorly is often sufficient. A felt pad held in place with
adhesive may be placed over the site of the fracture to correct anterior angulation
if present. A clavicular cross is another popular method and consists of a T-shaped
splint which is placed back of the shoulders and spine. After three to four weeks
the bandages may be removed and free motion permitted.

If it is extremely important that a good cosmetic result be obtained, or if the patient is confined to bed because of other injuries, a sand bag or small pillow placed or anchored between the scapulae, will aid in the reduction of fragments and main-tenance of position. In order for this therapy to be most effective, the patient should lie on her back most of the time so that gravity will aid in pulling the shoulder backward. The arm on the affected side should be abducted and should lie in a plane posterior to the body in order to hold the distal fragment upward and outward. In severe cases lateral traction will be advisable according to the method, for example, illustrated in Figure 229.

Dislocations of the Clavicle.—The articulations at each end of the clavicle, though movable, are diarthroses and not true joints. Through injury of various

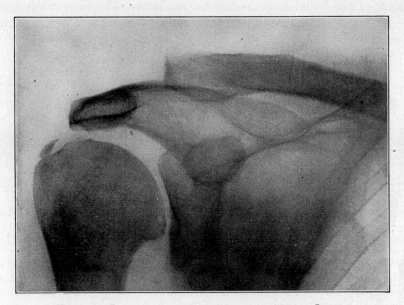

FIG. 231.—DISLOCATION OF THE ACROMIOCLAVICULAR JOINTS.

Reduction was maintained for four weeks but healing was insufficient to prevent recurrence. The patient, a sixty-year-old salesman, suffers no disability and does not therefore require further (operative) treatment. Note that there is also an associated chip fracture of the greater tuberosity of the humerus.

types, the ligaments at either the acromial or sternal end may be torn. *Acromio-clavicular* dislocation, however, is the more common of the two. The articular capsule is readily torn, but rarely does sufficient displacement occur to tear the coracoclavicular ligaments. Examination rarely fails to disclose the true nature of the injury. The distal end of the clavicle is prominent and the acromion is de-pressed to a lower level. Tenderness and pain are present at this site. Abduction of the arm is painful. Treatment is simple. Any type of bandage which presses down on the clavicle and upward on the elbow will be adequate. Most commonly, a felt pad is placed over the distal end of the clavicle and a band of adhesive anchored from the anterior chest over the pad to the back. The shoulder may then be lifted up by a strip of adhesive or modified Velpeau dressing with adequate padding under the olecranon. The outside of the dressing should be reinforced with adhesive in order to prevent stretching of the dressing with consequent loosening. To be effective, this dressing must be tight at all times and be worn for five or six weeks. It should be inspected every four or five days and reinforced or changed lest the shoulder be allowed to droop and tear the early fibrous union at the joint. Firm healing with correction of deformity is not always attained. However, the disability which follows is usually slight. Occasionally, when sufficient disability is present or when the coracoclavicular ligament has been completely torn, operative repair, which will require the use of fascial sutures or wires, may be advisable.

Sternoclavicular dislocation is uncommon; when it occurs the sternal end of the clavicle is usually displaced upward and anteriorly. Tenderness and pain upon movements of the shoulder are present, but not severe. Treatment consists of fixation of the sternal end of the clavicle in its normal position by adhesive for two or three weeks.

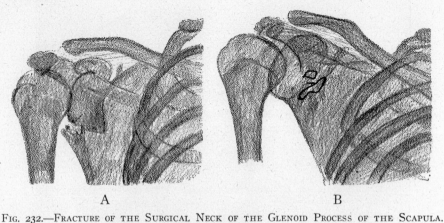

A   B

FIG. 232.—FRACTURE OF THE SURGICAL NECK OF THE GLENOID PROCESS OF THE SCAPULA.

A closed manipulation as well as lateral traction failed to effect a reduction. *A,* before open reduction; *B,* after open operation with wiring of fragments.

Scapula.—This bone is rarely fractured and even then the fragments are not usually displaced. The clinical evidence of fracture may be very meager. If the fracture involves that portion of the bone not covered with much muscle, tenderness will be present and localized. Otherwise, the tenderness and pain will be diffuse, poorly localized and perhaps mild. Immobilization in a sling or modified Velpeau dressing for three weeks is usually adequate treatment. If the surgical neck of the scapula is fractured, more disability will be produced. Motions of the shoulder joint in any direction will be painful. If the fracture is complete and displacement of the glenoid is present, reduction must be carried out. This is usually best accomplished by traction on the arm and manipulation. After reduction it is usually advisable to put the patient to bed with his arm in traction in a Thomas arm splint for two or three weeks. Fixation in abduction for two or three weeks, perhaps with traction may also be indicated in fractures through the glenoid fossa. An open operation is sometimes necessary.

Dislocation of the Shoulder.—This is the most common of all dislocations; it is due to transmitted violence which forces the head of the humerus out of the shallow glenoid depression of the scapula by tearing through the joint capsule.

Anterior or Subcoracoid Dislocation.—This is the most common type and is sustained by the patient falling on the hand or elbow with the arm abducted. The head of the humerus tears through the weakest spot in the capsule, *i.e.,* at the inferior border. However, such a force more commonly results in a fracture of the head of the humerus with which a dislocation is not infrequently confused, and with which it may be associated. Clinical examination, however, usually reveals a characteristic deformity when a dislocation is present. The normal roundness of the

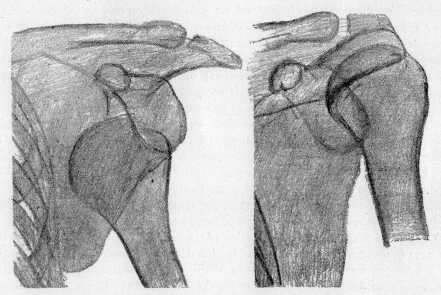

FIG. 233.—ANTERIOR DISLOCATION OF THE SHOULDER IN A FORTY-FIVE-YEAR-OLD LABORER.

Reduction was readily accomplished with the Kocher maneuver but recurrent dislocation finally necessitated an open operation.

shoulder beyond and below the tip of the acromion is lost so that the upper arm forms a straight line at a right angle with the axis of the clavicle (sometimes called deltoid flattening). The acromion is prominent. The axillary fold is depressed to a lower level. The head of the humerus can usually be palpated in its abnormal position beneath the coracoid, particularly if the arm is rotated gently. All the muscles about the joint are held rigidly. The arm is carried in mild abduction and the patient usually prefers to support the forearm with the opposite hand. A characteristic sign is inability to touch the opposite shoulder with the hand of the injured side. There may be numbness of the ulnar side of the hand because of pressure of the head of the humerus on the brachial plexus.

Treatment consists of reduction of the displaced head. If the dislocation has just been sustained and inflammatory swelling has not occurred, reduction can be effected rather easily, but a general anesthetic is usually necessary in order to achieve muscular relaxation. The procedure most often used is called the Kocher maneuver. With the wrist and elbow of the patient in each hand of the operator, the upper arm of the patient is externally rotated. Reduction is then effected by adducting the arm, bringing the elbow forward and across the chest as the upper arm is internally rotated by bringing the hand of the patient over to the opposite shoulder. Another method consists of steady traction of the entire extended arm either in a longitudinal direction or at right angles to the body. After reduction, the arm is immobilized by bandaging it to the chest in a modified Velpeau fashion for from two to three weeks, after which gradually increasing motion may be started. In dislocations up to two weeks' duration the difficulty becomes greater, although reduction may still be effected in some cases up to two months. After this period, or when closed reduction is ineffectual, an open operation may be indicated.

Posterior Dislocation.—This type of injury is rare; it is produced by falling upon the elbow with the arm rotated internally and adducted. The tear in the capsule occurs in the posterior portion and the head comes to rest at the posterior margin of the acromion (subacromial dislocation) or beneath the spine of the scapula (subspinous dislocation). Reduction is accomplished by traction on the arm, and pressure on the head of the humerus in an outward and anterior direction.

Recurrent Dislocation of the Shoulder.—If the tear in the capsule inflicted at the primary injury is large and healing is inadequate, the resultant scar may not offer sufficient support to prevent subsequent dislocation. *Subcoracoid* dislocations are most prone to recurrence; muscular strain on the extremity when the arm is abducted is one of the most frequent mechanisms. Recurrent dislocation can be prevented to a certain extent by binding the arm to the chest, but this entails considerable inconvenience. Operative procedures are usually necessary to correct the condition. Reefing of the inferior portion of the capsule may be tried. Any openings (tears) in the capsule must, of course, be closed. Other procedures, such as insertion of a bone peg into the inferior margin of the glenoid, fixation of the head of the humerus with straps of fascia lata, or transplantation of the biceps tendon through the head (Nicola [9]), are performed in obstinate cases.

THE UPPER EXTREMITY

Fractures and dislocations of this part of the body will be considered under the following headings: humerus, elbow joint, forearm and hand. In contrast to fractures of the lower extremity in which the function of weight-bearing is of primary importance, fractures of the upper extremity are of importance in relation to the finer movements, especially of the hand and wrist. Next in importance to the hand and wrist are the movements of the elbow, including pronation and supination of the forearm, whereas movements in the shoulder are the least essential. Another difference between fractures of the upper and lower extremity, from the therapeutic standpoint, is the importance of alignment; in the leg good alignment is essential to satisfactory weight-bearing but in the arm it is less necessary, although the correct carrying angle of the elbow must be maintained if the patient is to use the arm for this purpose. Fractures of the upper extremity are less subject to muscle pull and the bones, being smaller than those in the lower extremity, heal more rapidly. Hence, immobilization is less prolonged, early motion more necessary and important.

Humerus.—Fractures of the humerus are customarily divided into three groups: the upper end, the shaft and the lower end (supracondylar). Their manner of occurrence is similar, *i.e.*, they are commonly due to indirect trauma transmitted through the outstretched palm, although direct violence is occasionally responsible. Injuries to nerves are not infrequent in fractures of the humerus. Because of its close relation to the bone the radial nerve is most commonly involved. Brachial plexus injury is also seen.

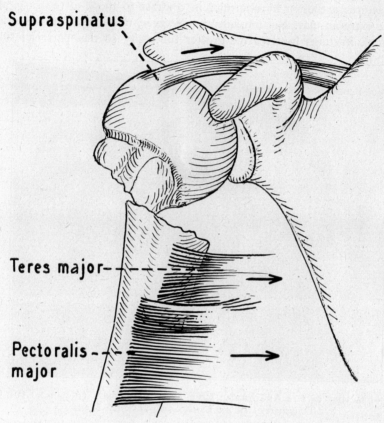

Supraspinatus

Teres major

Pectoralis major

Fig. 234.—Diagram of a Fracture at the Surgical Neck of the Humerus, showing a Few of the Various Muscles which Produce Deformity.

Most important of those pulling the upper fragment into abduction and flexion is the supraspinatus, as indicated. The teres major and pectoralis major adduct the distal fragment. Great variations exist; the position assumed by the fragments depends, in general, upon the relation of the line of fracture to the points of insertion of the various muscles.

Although treatment of fractures of the humerus varies with the site and type of fracture as described in detail below, a simple and ambulatory method applicable to most of them has been described by Griswold, Goldberg and Joplin.[10] The method is often referred to as the "hanging cast" procedure; it has a great many advantages and can be extensively used. Reduction is carried out under local or general anesthesia and the position maintained by the weight of a cast applied to the elbow and forearm which exerts traction in the position of neutral muscle pull.

Fractures at the Upper End of the Humerus.—Various types occur which are difficult to classify. The traditional separation into fractures of the anatomical and surgical neck is maintained here because of the difference in their clinical occurrence in older and young patients respectively. Less frequent types are epiphyseal separation and fractures involving the tuberosity alone. Fractures of the *anatomical neck,* including those of the head, occur nearly always in older individuals and often produce relatively few clinical manifestations of fracture aside from disability. These fractures are often intracapsular in contrast to those of the surgical neck which are extracapsular. Not infrequently, however, the line of separation in anatomical neck fractures involves the greater tuberosity so that part is inside and

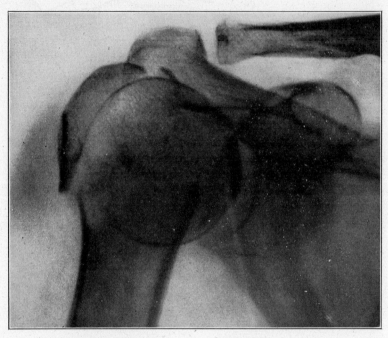

Fig. 235.—Fracture of the Anatomical Neck of the Humerus (including the Greater Tuberosity) in an Eighty-two-year-old Man.

No reduction was attempted; the arm was immobilized in slight abduction in a Velpeau bandage. Moderate permanent disability does not interfere with the patient's work as a watchman.

part outside the joint. Likewise, fractures of the surgical neck may be so close to the head as to extend into the joint. These considerations influence greatly the problem of reduction. Fractures entirely inside the joint capsule are difficult to reduce, particularly because the proximal fragment is loose and cannot be controlled, and is obviously too short for the surgeon to grasp with his hand. In their treatment, therefore, one usually immobilizes the arm with the distal fragment in a position which lines up as well as possible with the short proximal fragment. The x-ray is essential in obtaining this alignment. Although these fractures usually occur in elderly people, a satisfactory result is usually obtained even if the fragments are inaccurately reduced, because a poorly functioning shoulder joint in these patients results in disability which is not often a cause of serious complaint. Fixation, however, in abduction of 45 degrees is in general advisable because this position is comfortable, but more particularly because a greater range of movement will be preserved if the shoulder joint becomes the site of fibrous ankylosis, as it frequently does (see also p. 479); this is due to the motion of the scapula. These patients are best treated in a splint or appliance or light cast, but if aged are kept ambulatory. In younger patients in whom good shoulder movement is important open operation may be advisable.

The *surgical neck* of the humerus is fractured more frequently in early adult life and in children than in elderly people. A displacement, if present, will depend on the site of the fracture and the muscles attached to the proximal fragment. The muscles which pull on the proximal fragment are the subscapularis, the supra- and infra-

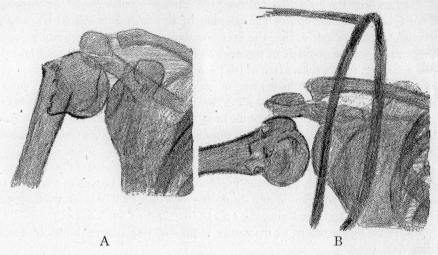

A   B

FIG. 236.—FRACTURE OF THE SURGICAL NECK OF THE HUMERUS IN A TWENTY-SIX-YEAR-OLD LABORER.

Note the abduction of the proximal fragment and the overriding of the distal fragment. *A,* before treatment; *B,* after exerting traction in bed with the arm in full abduction. Note the satisfactory alignment.

spinatus, teres minor; those which pull on the distal fragment (see Fig. 234) are the pectoralis major, teres major and latissimus dorsi. Depending upon the activity of these muscles the proximal fragment may be adducted or abducted in varying degrees or rotated internally or externally. It is often flexed forward as can be shown when lateral x-rays are taken. X-ray is decisive in determining the degree of deformity. The most common deformity is abduction and external rotation of the proximal fragment. The fracture is usually transverse, but may be oblique or comminuted. Disability is immediate and marked; swelling is apt to be masked by the deltoid and other shoulder muscles.

Treatment depends to a large extent on the kind of fracture and on the deformity present. Transverse fractures in which the jagged ends tend to remain intact are best reduced under complete anesthesia and the arm immobilized in a position which maintains alignment. Since the proximal fragment is usually abducted it is necessary to maintain immobilization of the arm in abduction, the degree of which depends on the position of the proximal fragment. If reduction is achieved by manipulation, fixation must be maintained by a supportive splint or plaster cast which includes the entire arm and embraces the body as well. When reduction by manipulation is not indicated (oblique fractures), or has been unsuccessful, suspension and traction is carried out. This implies bed rest, but a Jones humeral splint, or a hanging cast, will permit a certain degree of traction while the patient is ambulatory. If traction in a Thomas arm splint is used, it is best to fix the extremity with the elbow flexed (see Fig. 239) to prevent stiffness and slow recovery of motion in the elbow. When an impacted fracture is present, an aeroplane or abduction splint which carries the arm out at an angle of 90 degrees is occasionally used since no traction is required. On many occasions, however, particularly in young people, it may be preferable to break up the impaction and treat the fracture by plaster cast, or suspension and traction as outlined above. The position of the fragments should be carefully ascertained by the x-ray during the first few days of treatment and any necessary changes made in the position of the arm as indicated. Abduction should be maintained for about four weeks, after which time immobilization for three or four more weeks may be carried out in a sling or similar fixation. Movements of the arm should not be allowed unless x-ray films reveal the deposition of the proper amount of callus. Occasionally reduction cannot be effected because of extreme displacement of the proximal fragment, or because of muscle lodged between the ends of the bone; in such cases open operation may be necessary.

In a few patients the proximal fragment is not abducted or may even be slightly adducted. This simplifies the problem of treatment in that the arm may be immobilized (after reduction of any displacement which may be present) by putting a pad in the axilla and bandaging the arm to the chest in the Velpeau position (see p. 390). If no displacement or deformity is present this type of immobilization is instituted at once.

Epiphyseal separation, while not common, is diagnosed only by the x-ray. It occurs chiefly in children. Treatment requires accurate reduction and complete immobilization. If reduction is obtained and adduction of the arm against the chest wall does not disturb the position of the fragments, immobilization with the arm in a sling or bound against the chest with pads in the axilla is the simplest procedure. This immobilization should be maintained for four weeks or longer. Immobilization in abduction may at times be advisable for the first two or three weeks. Fractures of the *greater tuberosity,* especially if displacement is great, require immobilization in abduction in an aeroplane splint. There is often an associated injury to the supraspinatus tendon which inserts into this part of the humerus, and trauma in the subdeltoid bursa which lies over the tendon. Both injuries heal better with the arm in abduction.

Fractures of the Shaft of the Humerus.—Fractures of the shaft are not uncommon and occur by direct violence or by a transmitted force in falling with the arm outstretched. Transverse, oblique, spiral and comminuted fractures occur, depending upon the degree and direction of the violence. Important is the fact that the radial nerve entwines around the shaft of the humerus at its midportion, thereby accounting for the frequency of radial nerve injury in this type of fracture. The deformity produced by fracture of the shaft varies and is dependent largely upon whether the break is below or above the attachment of the deltoid. If above, the upper fragment is generally pulled inward (adducted) by the pull of the pectoralis major, teres major and latissimus dorsi; if below, the deltoid generally abducts the proximal fragment. Overriding is due to the pull of all muscles acting longitudinally.

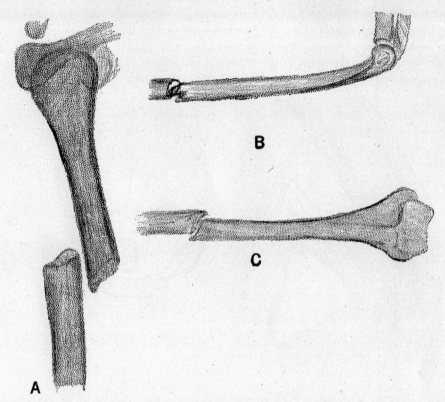

FIG. 237.—FRACTURE OF THE SHAFT OF THE HUMERUS WITH COMPLETE DISPLACEMENT IN A FORTY-TWO-YEAR-OLD HOUSEWIFE, STRUCK BY AN AUTO.

Because of an associated intracranial injury immediate reduction and immobilization under anesthesia was not justified but the patient put to bed and lateral traction exerted as illustrated in Figure 239. Two weeks later the arm was put up in a triangular splint and body cast (see Fig. 238 A) which enabled her to be up and about at home. A, before treatment; B, lateral view and C, anteroposterior view after several days of traction (x-rays taken by a portable machine).

The clinical manifestations of fracture of the shaft are pronounced, the affected arm hanging uselessly, immobile and completely disabled. The site of the fracture can often be detected by gentle palpation, preferably along the lateral aspect of the arm where the muscles are less prominent. Wrist drop, if present, is an indication of radial nerve injury and is associated with anesthesia over the dorsum of the thumb and first finger.

Treatment varies with the type of fracture. If the fragments can be reduced and kept in place, as is usually the case in jagged transverse fractures, an anesthetic is administered and, with the muscles relaxed, traction is used to bring the broken bones end-on in good alignment. Immobilization is then instituted by means of a triangular splint and body support (see Fig. 238) or by a plaster cast embracing the chest, shoulder and arm. Sufficient abduction is used to bring the distal fragment in line with the proximal one and the elbow is flexed at a right angle. If reduction cannot be achieved or maintained it may be necessary to treat the patient in bed by suspension and traction. If possible, traction should be maintained with the elbow flexed. It may be difficult to obtain sufficient skin traction with the elbow flexed in this position, particularly when the fracture is in the distal third. In such a case it may be advisable to exert skeletal traction by a wire passed through the condyles of the humerus, or olecranon. A slight amount of continuous traction, however, need not require bed rest; with the hanging cast this can be achieved satisfactorily in the

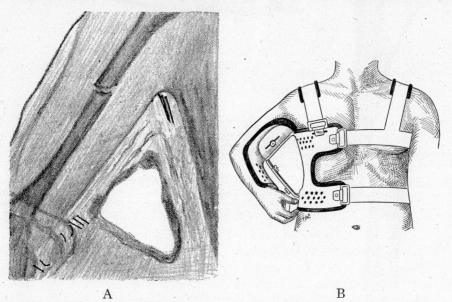

A   B

FIG. 238.—TWO METHODS OF FIXATION FOR THE AMBULATORY TREATMENT OF FRACTURES
OF THE HUMERUS.

A, triangle and body cast; this is from an x-ray film of patient described in Figure 237.
B, Magnuson abduction humerus splint which achieves the same purpose.

ambulatory patient (see Fig. 240). Immobilization for at least four to six weeks is necessary before union takes place. Nonunion, however, cannot be said to exist until at least three months have elapsed with false motion still present. Radial nerve injuries often require open operation with repair of lacerations of the nerve, or freeing of the nerve from infringement between fragments or from callus. Involvement of the radial nerve may, on rare occasions, develop during the course of treatment due to pressure from callus formation. It should be detected early, by frequent examinations so that operative therapy may be instituted before atrophy occurs.

Supracondylar Fractures.—This is a common injury during childhood and comprises fractures of the distal end of the humerus, nearly always transverse with displacement of the distal fragment backward. Lateral displacement also occurs; only occasionally is the distal humerus displaced anteriorly. The force is nearly always transmitted to the elbow by a fall on the outstretched arm (usually with the elbow partially flexed). Examination reveals a deformity of the elbow which is apparent.

The bony landmarks of the elbow are distorted, as may be best demonstrated by comparison with the uninjured side. Both olecranon and condyles are displaced posterior to the shaft of the humerus. At first glance the deformity may appear

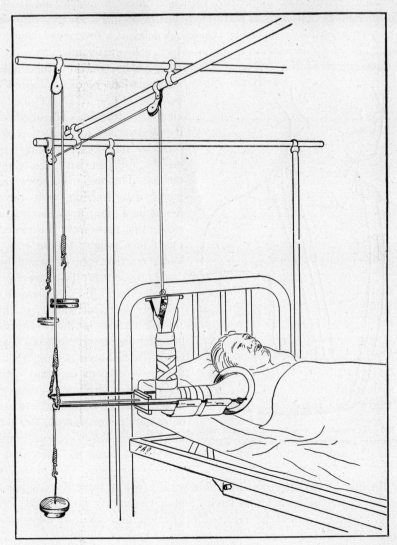

FIG. 239.—SUSPENSION AND TRACTION OF THE UPPER ARM FOR FRACTURE OF THE HUMERUS.

In this case traction is exerted by adhesive strips. When the fracture is close to the elbow, skeletal traction may be necessary; this is achieved by a wire or pin through the olecranon. Note the right angled flexion at the elbow, a position which is advantageous whenever possible because it produces less disability to the joint than that resulting from immobilization in complete extension.

similar to that produced by a posterior dislocation of the humerus, but examination will reveal the fact that the condyles are displaced backward with the olecranon, which does not occur in posterior dislocation. Swelling is rapid and usually intense, however, and tends to hide the type of deformity present. X-ray films in both views should be taken. Supracondylar fractures which involve the joint are discussed under the elbow joint.

Treatment consists of immediate reduction under complete anesthesia with fixation in acute flexion. This is performed even in the presence of severe swelling. Delay of even a few hours should be avoided. A delay of a few days is more serious because it allows the deposition of callus which will greatly interfere with subsequent replacement of the fragments and may make reduction impossible. The manipulations required depend on the position of the fragments but consist chiefly of traction. The method commonly described for reduction of supracondylar fractures is to exert traction on the forearm with the elbow extended. The authors, however, have noted that traction with the elbow flexed at a right angle is just as efficient, and apparently associated with much less trauma to the soft tissue. While traction is being maintained, the distal fragment is pushed anteriorly and molded into position. Reduction is surprisingly easy, particularly in children. Immobilization is then instituted by bringing the forearm in acute flexion. If reduction has been accomplished acute flexion is easy to maintain with very little force. If swelling is great or if the flexed position obliterates the radial pulse the *forearm must be extended until the circulation returns,* even at the expense of losing the reduction. If the patient complains of coldness, numbness or tingling in the fingers at any time within two or three days following reduction, he should be seen immediately, and if circulatory impairment seems to exist, the dressings should be released or flexion decreased to allow adequate circulation. This is important because of the danger of Volkmann's contracture (see p. 484). For this reason nothing should be placed in the fold of the elbow. If closed reduction is impossible, operation may be carried out; a simpler procedure is to insert a Kirschner wire through the olecranon for skeletal traction as recommended for intercondylar fractures (see Fig. 243). Fixation is produced by adhesive straps or bandages which embrace the supinated forearm and upper arm, or by a plaster splint which is molded along the arm posterior to the elbow. A bandage then holds the flexed arm to the side of the chest. Gradually increasing extension is begun in the second or third week. Seldom does any permanent disability result from this type of fracture, providing reduction has been achieved. This is explained

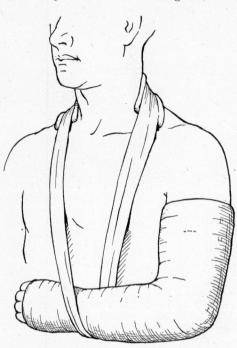

FIG. 240.—HANGING CAST, PARTICULARLY ADAPTABLE FOR THE AMBULATORY TREATMENT OF FRACTURES OF THE SHAFT OF THE HUMERUS.

for the most part by the fact that immobilization is carried out with flexion of the elbow and not extension.

The Elbow Joint.—Injuries to joints are of special significance largely because of the seriousness of damage to the articular cartilage. The nature and extent of the injury to the joint surfaces often determines the ultimate function of the joint, though it is often difficult to demonstrate clinically. The complicated structure

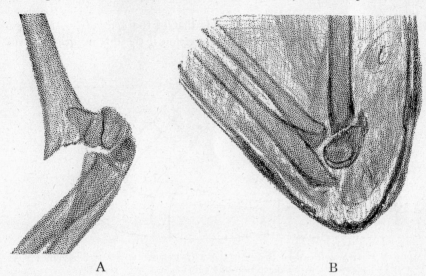

A   B

Fig. 241.—Supracondylar Fracture in an Eight-year-old Boy who Fell on the Outstretched Arm.

A, lateral view before reduction; *B*, after reduction and immobilization in a posterior plaster splint.

of the elbow joint makes it particularly prone to disability because of the possibility of bony blocks due to comminuted fragments which resist replacement. As mentioned elsewhere in regard to the knee, aspiration of blood in elbow joint injuries has great therapeutic value.

Intercondylar Fractures.—Most injuries of the humerus involving the elbow joint are varieties of supracondylar fractures which, in addition to the transverse break across the humerus, also exhibit a longitudinal fracture into the joint, thus producing two or more distal fragments. They are called intercondylar or *Y- or T-fractures* and since they are produced by severe violence are occasionally comminuted. The diagnosis depends on careful x-ray films. Treatment in general is the same as that of supracondylar fractures as already outlined. Immediate reduction, however, is frequently impossible because of the tendency of muscle pull and upward pressure of the olecranon which maintains separation of the fragments. Continuous traction with a wire through the olecranon with the elbow at a right angle is often successful. In a few instances the fragments will have to be approximated and held together by an open operation. In going from one method to the other, too much time must not be lost because of the rapidity with which new bone forms and hinders further procedures. In any event, immobilization in flexion is with few exceptions the position of choice in fractures into the joint, because it tends to maintain proper position of fragments. Perhaps of more importance is the fact that if ankylosis should result, this position of flexion is much less disabling than that of extension. As mentioned in the preceding section it must be remembered that immobilization of the elbow in flexion is apt to produce serious circulatory disturbance distal to the fracture with the consequent development of Volkmann's contracture. The precautions previously mentioned must be heeded vigilantly in any fracture about the elbow.

A second type of elbow joint fracture is that of the *epicondyles*. Diagnosis is made by x-ray. Treatment is simple immobilization if there is no displacement. If

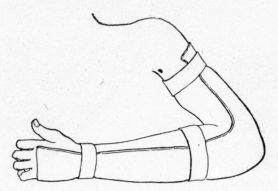

FIG. 242.—A POSTERIOR PLASTER SPLINT WITH THE ELBOW IN ACUTE FLEXION FOR THE TREATMENT OF SUPRACONDYLAR FRACTURES OF THE HUMERUS.

the epicondyle is displaced markedly, open operation may be necessary. This is particularly true of the inner epicondyle which is often forced into the elbow joint. Important is the close relation of the ulnar nerve to the inner epicondyle; during the operation the nerve may have to be transposed in order to avoid involvement in the callus. Fracture of the entire single condyle is similar in nature to the intercondylar fractures already described.

Fracture of the Olecranon Process.—This injury may occur because of a direct blow or because of violent contraction of the powerful triceps muscle. Since the anterior surface of this bone forms part of the elbow joint, just as does the patella in the knee, a complete fracture is associated with manifestations of acute synovitis and the elbow joint becomes filled with fluid and blood. The fragments, if separated, can easily be felt through the skin. Treatment, as in the case of the patella, is best carried out through open operation which enables evacuation of the blood in the joint and accurate approximation of the fragments which are best held in place by silver or stainless steel wire. If the fragments are fixed securely at the time of operation, the joint is best immobilized at a right angle, thereby assuring earlier return of motion in flexion. It is important to begin active motion in two or three weeks in order to prevent delayed restitution of motion in the joint, *i.e.,* limitation of flexion.

Dislocations of the Elbow.—Complete dislocation of the elbow without fracture is produced usually by a fall on the outstretched hand with the elbow extended and in most instances is of the posterior type; the coronoid process of the ulna is displaced backward over the trochlear surface of the humerus so that it (the coronoid process) lies in the olecranon fossa. The radius of necessity is also dislocated. The deformity is striking; the displacement of the olecranon posterior to its usual position is pronounced. The bony landmarks are disturbed, *i.e.,* the ole-

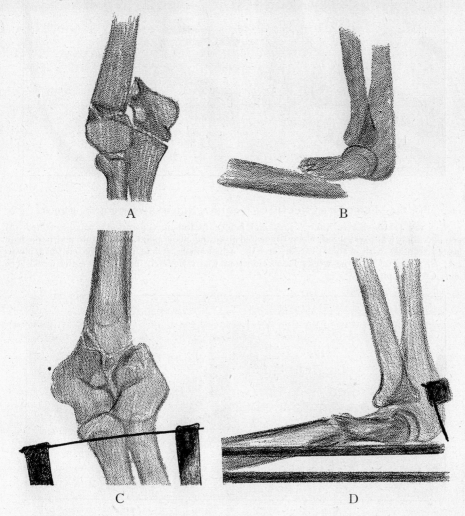

A   B

C   D

FIG. 243.—INTERCONDYLAR FRACTURE IN A THIRTY-FIVE-YEAR-OLD SALESMAN.

Treatment by suspension and traction with a wire through the olecranon. *A,* anteroposterior, and *B,* lateral views on admission showing marked displacement; *C,* anteroposterior, and *D,* lateral view several days after continuous traction reveal satisfactory reduction. Patient allowed up in four weeks, and motion begun two weeks later; function almost complete.

cranon lies far posterior to the epicondyles when compared to the uninjured side. A moderate amount of medial or lateral displacement of the forearm is usually also present. The elbow is held in semiflexion and the slightest motion of the joint produces pain. Reduction should be immediate, under general anesthesia, and aided by supination, hyperextension, traction and gentle lateral manipulations. Immo-

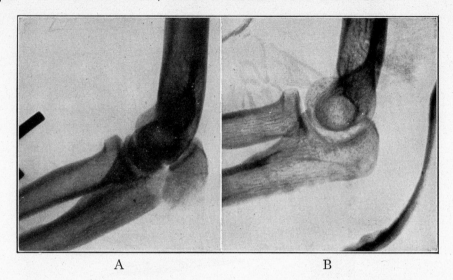

A   B

FIG. 244.—FRACTURE OF THE OLECRANON IN A NINETEEN-YEAR-OLD SCHOOLGIRL.

A, x-ray taken shortly after injury and before treatment (operation) was instituted. An open operation was carried out, blood evacuated from the elbow point, the capsule and periosteum sutured securely with chromic catgut, and the arm immobilized in partial flexion by a plaster cast; *B*, x-ray taken three weeks later. Function was completely normal in eight weeks (St. Louis City Hospital).

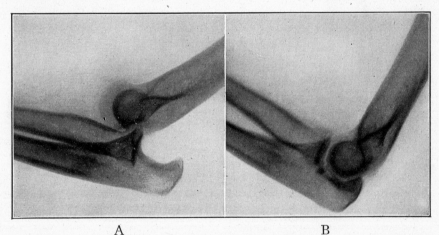

A   B

FIG. 245.—POSTERIOR DISLOCATION OF THE ELBOW.

Note that the word describing the displacement (*i.e.,* posterior) refers to the distal bone. *A*, before and *B*, after reduction.

bilization in moderate flexion in a sling is followed by early motion, but full motion should not be allowed for three or four weeks. *Fracture of the coronoid process* of the ulna is sometimes an associated injury. Its presence requires fixation in more acute flexion.

Dislocation of the Head of the Radius.—This usually occurs anteriorly and is commonly accompanied by a fracture of the upper third of the ulna. However, if the blow is sustained over the posterolateral surface of the forearm, dislocation of the radius may occur without other significant injury. The elbow is held in a semi-flexed position with the hand pronated. The head of the radius can usually be seen and felt anterior to its usual position. Reduction is best achieved under anesthesia by extension of the forearm, traction and pressure in a posterior direction against the head of the radius. The forearm should be immobilized in a sling with the elbow flexed and the forearm supinated for three weeks. Difficulty in reduction is usually caused by portions of the articular ligament being displaced into the depression

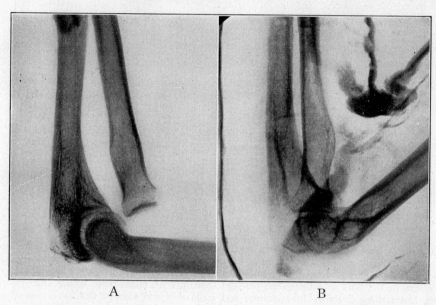

A   B

FIG. 246.—DISLOCATION OF THE HEAD OF THE RADIUS IN A TWENTY-FIVE-YEAR-OLD MAN.

Note also the fracture of the ulna, at the top of the illustration. This patient was first seen six weeks after the injury; an open operation was necessary. *A*, before and *B*, after reduction (courtesy Dr. F. E. Walton).

normally occupied by the head or by an unreduced ulnar angulation. In young children the entire head may be pulled out of its annular ligament by forceful traction of the forearm. In such instances reduction is spontaneous or may be achieved under general anesthesia by manipulation during flexion and supination.

Fracture of the Head of the Radius.—The radial head really forms part of the elbow joint moving against the capitellum of the humerus during flexion of the elbow and during supination and pronation. While rare, fracture at this site is an important injury because of its importance in the motion of pronation and supination. Clinical manifestations include local tenderness, limitation of motion of the joint and pain on performing these movements. An important diagnostic feature is the inability to pronate or supinate the forearm because of pain in the region of the head of the radius. X-ray is essential to determine the degree and type of displacement which varies considerably. Mushrooming of the head with impaction of the shaft into it is a frequent deformity. In the extensive injuries, immediate operative removal of the head is advisable. With moderate displacement, open, or if possible, closed reduction with immobilization in moderate flexion and full supination for 10 to 14 days is adequate therapy. If function remains impaired, removal of the head may be carried out later. When little or no displacement exists, treatment by immobilization without attempt at reduction may be preferable. As already mentioned, aspiration of blood in the joint will greatly hasten the reparative process and shorten disability.

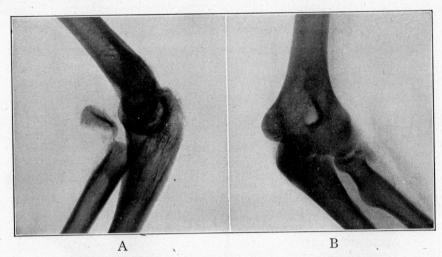

A   B

FIG. 247.—TWO EXAMPLES OF FRACTURE OF THE HEAD OF THE RADIUS.

A, with complete displacement, in a forty-two-year-old woman. There was an associated dislocation of the elbow which was reduced before this film was taken. Patient refused operative removal of the detached bone. Functional result unknown; *B,* fracture with "mushrooming" of one side of the head in a thirty-one-year-old woman. Film taken three weeks after injury; patient had serious disability in pronation and supination and also in flexion of the elbow. Physiotherapy resulted in great improvement of function.

The Forearm.—The forearm, comprising the ulna and radius, is probably the most frequent site of fracture in the upper extremity. Both bones are often involved. Their fractures are arbitrarily divided into fractures of the shafts of ulna and radius alone, of both bones, and Colles' fracture. Of these, the last two are the most frequent.

Fracture of the Shaft of the Ulna Alone.—This is not a frequent fracture and ordinarily presents no great problem in treatment since reduction of any displacement, if present, can readily be achieved by ordinary manipulation. Fixation in the midposition with splints (or plaster slabs) which immobilize the elbow and wrist, but leave the fingers free, is maintained for three to four weeks.

The radial head is occasionally dislocated at the same time that the ulnar shaft is fractured. It is obviously essential that this injury be detected. Reduction of the dislocation is effected first, before the ulna is manipulated.

Fracture of the Shaft of the Radius Alone.—This is a common fracture especially in children. (Those which involve the distal end are especially frequent and are considered separately under the heading of Colles' fracture.) Fractures of the radius are usually transverse and are most often located at the middle third or distal to it. Those in the proximal third are more rare. Displacement, if present, is usually confined to overriding or slight angulation. When the break is above the pronator teres, however, the proximal fragment is flexed and supinated, and hence markedly displaced. The treatment consists of reduction under anesthesia by manipulation and traction followed by fixation as for a fracture of the ulna. Fractures near the elbow will require sufficient flexion and supination at the joint to bring the distal fragment in line with the proximal. Fractures which resist attempts at closed reduction should be promptly operated upon and the fragments approximated under direct vision, fixed with a metal plate and screws and the arm immobilized.

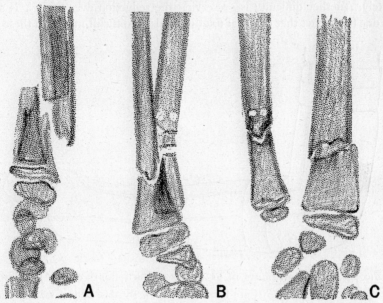

Fig. 248.—Fracture of Both Bones of the Forearm in a Six-year-old Child.

A, lateral view before treatment. Closed reduction of the radius was achieved but the ulna resisted all attempts at manipulation and an operation was performed; B, lateral and C, antero-posterior views after open reduction. Note the drill holes in the ulna which permitted internal fixation with chromic catgut.

Fracture of the Shafts of Both Ulna and Radius.—The shafts of both bones of the forearm are more frequently broken than either alone, particularly in childhood. The force is usually direct or indirect by a fall on the outstretched palm. Considerable variation occurs in the severity of these fractures. Many are simple greenstick fractures of both bones, without displacement, but occasionally exhibiting considerable angulation. Many children sustain a complete and displaced fracture of one bone (usually the radius) with a greenstick of the other. In a considerable number both bones are broken and overriding or angulated, or both. The fracture may be compound.

Treatment consists of immediate reduction of the displacement, if present. The promptness with which reduction is carried out is almost as important in these fractures as it is in supracondylar fractures. If possible, the procedure should be instituted before swelling and muscle spasm have become pronounced, that is to say, within an hour or two after the injury. Greenstick angulations may often be corrected with a local or basal anesthetic. When overriding is present, a deep anesthesia is necessary with complete relaxation. It is particularly important in these fractures that the radius and ulna be kept from coming in contact with each other across the interosseous membrane, lest a bony bridge grow across and seriously interfere with subsequent supination and pronation. This danger is revealed by appropriate x-rays which must show a clear separation between the two bones in at least one view. Reduction of these fractures is not easy and the surgeon must in a few patients resort to open reduction and internal fixation in order to approximate the fragments adequately. Another difficulty is preserving the reduction even after it is achieved. This is due to the fact that external fixation is also a difficult matter in these injuries,

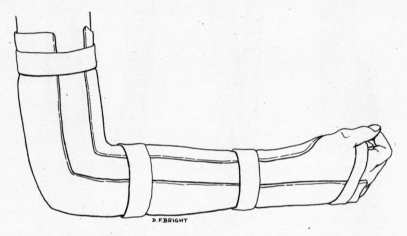

D.F.BRIGHT

FIG. 249.—PLASTER SPLINTS IN FRACTURES OF BOTH BONES OF THE FOREARM.

Note that the elbow and wrist are both immobilized. By this method the fixation may be kept secure by daily tightening of the straps holding the anterior and posterior slabs; this is impossible with a circular cast.

particularly when the fracture is in the distal half of the forearm. The best position for immobilization is with the elbow at right angles and the forearm in supination or in semisupination (the midposition with the palm perpendicular to the ground). The elbow and wrist must both be immobilized. Another feature of importance is the necessity for tightening the fixation during the days after reduction when swelling subsides and permits the fixation to become loose. For this reason board splints are *superior* to a circular cast unless the fracture is put up so early that swelling has not yet occurred. Because reduction is often difficult to maintain, the site of fracture should be checked by x-ray in order to determine the position of the fragments during the first few days. The wrist is usually fixed in straight extension, but in fractures of the distal third it is often necessary to put up the forearm with the wrist in acute flexion in order to maintain the alignment and prevent volar angulation. After fixation in this abnormal position, for a week or ten days, the fore-arm is then replaced in a straight splint for the remainder of the four or five week period. Recurrence of deformity is rare after healing has been in process for a week.

Colles' Fracture.—This is a common fracture of the distal end of the radius, and frequently involves also the styloid process of the ulna. The line of fracture is usually about 1 to 3 centimeters from the articular surface. It is nearly always transverse with displacement and angulation of the distal fragment toward the dorsal surface, thus producing the well-known "silver fork" deformity. However, the fracture is not infrequently impacted and thus may show little or no deformity. In rare instances the distal fragment is displaced toward the palmar side, producing a reverse Colles' (Smith's fracture). Deformity may be obscured if the patient is seen many hours after the injury because of the resulting edema and extravasation of blood. Palpation reveals the site of fracture rather accurately since the radius is so superficial above the wrist; tenderness confined to the fracture site is a constant and important diagnostic sign. Point tenderness over the styloid process may also be detected. The

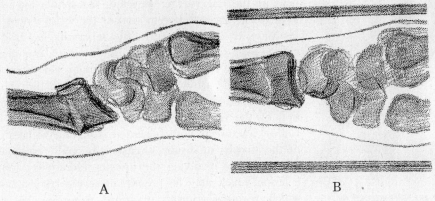

A   B

FIG. 250.—COLLES' FRACTURE IN AN EIGHTY-YEAR-OLD WOMAN WHO FELL ON HER OUTSTRETCHED PALM.

A, before reduction; note the typical silver fork deformity. There is only slight impaction in this case; *B*, after reduction, which was easily effected after the injection of 15 cc. of novocain between the ends of the bone. Immobilization in an anterior and posterior splint; early motion was started on the sixth day.

history, moreover, is usually so characteristic as to lead to almost an immediate diagnosis in most cases. Colles' fractures are particularly common in older individuals, usually women, who fall and allow the weight of their body to be directed against the outstretched palm which is used to break the fall. The force is one of forced extension and compression, transmitted to the distal end of the radius in a dorsal direction which accounts for the usual deformity. If the force is directed more in the axis of the forearm, an impacted fracture occurs. In children the same force usually fractures the bones higher up; occasionally, however, there is an *epiphyseal separation*. The treatment of epiphyseal separation is the same as that of Colles' fracture.

Treatment is mandatory when angulation is demonstrable, even when the fracture is several weeks old. Otherwise the patient will be unable to flex the wrist for proper function and a permanently weak, disabled and painful hand will result. There is considerable dispute as to whether an impacted Colles' fracture without deformity should be broken up before immobilization. Reduction, if performed early, is easy to effect and maintain, because of the absence of muscle pull on the distal fragment. Deep anesthesia for reduction may not be necessary. Injection of novocain into the site of fracture is often adequate. The distal fragment is molded and forced into alignment with the proximal radius, aided by strong flexion and radial abduction. If reduction is adequate the hand will easily fall into 90 degrees flexion at the wrist as the forearm is raised. The wrist is immobilized by a volar splint which allows the fingers and elbow free motion. Most surgeons place the wrist midway between flexion and extension in slight ulnar deviation although full supination is highly recommended by H. F. Graham;[11] some flex the wrist acutely as routine, at least for several days. If the fracture has been reduced soon after the injury and before much swelling has occurred, one must particularly watch for the danger of interference with the circulation by the splints (after edema and extravasation occur). If pain, swelling, coldness of the fingers then develop, the splints must be loosened at once. Active motion of the wrist should be instituted as soon as absence of pain permits, but gradually because of the *danger* of dislocation of fragments before callus forms. This active motion can often be started within a few days by unfastening the splint for short periods every day or so. Disability in the function of the wrist and hand may follow treatment of Colles' fracture if immobilization is prolonged, because of the atrophy of disuse. Occasionally, poor results are due to injury involving the inferior radio-ulnar joint, a lesion which may be present in severe trauma, and which requires accurate fixation. According to the studies of Taylor and Parsons,[12] it is necessary to treat the serious fractures in this region more carefully, and after reduction, the wrist is placed in the Cotton-Loder position, *i.e.,* palmar flexion and extreme pronation, in order to maintain position.

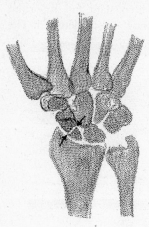

Fig. 251.—Fracture of the Carpal Scaphoid (Indicated by the Arrows) in a Forty-five-year-old Clerk Who Fell and "Sprained" his Wrist.

Fixation of entire hand and wrist in a plaster cast for six weeks; restoration of function almost complete. Nonunion is apt to follow unless complete and prolonged immobilization is instituted at once.

The Hand.—Under this heading will be included fractures and dislocations which involve the carpus, metacarpal bones and phalanges. The wrist joint itself is rarely injured. The classification used will be a purely arbitrary one. It should be emphasized that all injuries of the hand are of special importance since the function of the fingers and wrist are so readily impaired. This is due to the relatively poor blood supply, the paucity of soft tissues and the multiplicity of important structures contained in the hand (see also chapter on infections of the hand).

Fracture of the Carpal Scaphoid.—A fall on the hand or a severe extension at the wrist may produce sudden pain, local tenderness and swelling in the carpus which is often diagnosed as a sprain, but which is actually due to a fracture. Any sprained wrist which has failed to heal within a reasonable length of time should be suspected of having a carpal fracture. Significant, if the scaphoid bone is fractured, is point tenderness over the bone which is best palpated on the dorsal surface in the floor of the triangle formed by the extensor and abductor tendons of the thumb (anatomical snuff box). X-ray, however, is the only certain way of establishing the diagnosis. This is important because adequate treatment of this injury is essential if one is to avoid permanent disability (due to nonunion) which may follow an unrecognized fracture. There is rarely any displacement, merely a crack in the bone which, however, undoubtedly extends into and involves the articular space of the carpal joints. Oblique, as well as anteroposterior, and lateral x-rays may be necessary to make the diagnosis.

Treatment consists of prolonged and complete immobilization of the hand in dorsiflexion with the thumb fixed and the fingers flexed. This is continued for six weeks even at the expense of the atrophy of disuse since otherwise nonunion of the scaphoid bone and subsequent pain will result. If the fragments are displaced preliminary manipulation will be necessary. Although excision is sometimes advisable [13], drilling of both fragments, and insertion of a bone graft into the drill holes, should be tried before excision.

Dislocation of the Semilunar (os lunatum) Bone.—In forced hyperextension (dorsiflexion) the semilunar bone may be squeezed out of place and forced into the palm. The resulting deformity and local pain are usually sufficient to point to the seriousness of the injury and the x-ray easily reveals the nature of the lesion. *Treatment* consists of manual replacement of the bone under complete relaxation (general anesthesia) aided by hyperextension at the wrist and often by the judicious use of a Thomas wrench. Immobilization in the midposition for two weeks is adequate. Neglected dislocations or those impossible to reduce will necessitate open reduction, or excision of the bone. The latter should be avoided, if possible.

Fractures of the Metacarpal Bones.—These injuries are rather frequent, but only a few are seriously displaced, and are therefore rarely difficult to treat. The mode of injury is usually a direct force on the knuckles with the fist clenched. Transverse fractures, if displaced, are often merely angulated, usually toward the dorsal surface. Overriding is rare, but oblique fractures are not uncommon. Fractures accompanied by shortening can be detected by a loss of prominence of the corresponding knuckle. Deformity leads to disability and should be corrected. If angulation alone is present it is usually in a dorsal direction and is best treated by immobilization in a dorsal splint which extends from the tips of the fingers to the mid forearm. With no displacement a ball splint in the palm with the fingers fixed around it is adequate. When significant displacement is present, reduction is required before fixation. If manipulation is ineffective, the hand may be put up in a banjo type of splint with continuous traction or an open operation carried out. In oblique fractures traction in a splint is probably preferable, but in transverse fractures an open operation under local anesthesia is best.

Fracture of the Base of the First Metacarpal Bone (Bennett's Fracture) is a special type of injury which is often overlooked or considered to be a sprained thumb, especially when swelling masks the deformity, and diffuse pain interferes with accurate anatomical palpation. X-ray is, therefore, essential in the diagnosis. Significant displacement demands manipulation; fixation in wide abduction is essential and is best achieved with a plaster spica which embraces the wrist and thumb. The "banjo" splint is often effective when reduction by manipulation fails.

Fractures of the Phalanges.—Fractures without displacement are treated with simple fixation over a padded tongue depressor, or if several fingers are involved, over a ball which fixes the palm and digits in a semiflexed position; this position prevents volar angulation. If significant displacement is present, and attempts at reduction are unsuccessful, continuous traction in a modified banjo splint is used.

Dislocations in the Hand.—In the wrist joint itself the inferior radio-ulnar joint is occasionally displaced and requires immediate reduction and immobilization; radiocarpal dislocations are even more rare and also require immediate reduction and fixation. Carpometacarpal dislocations are rare except that in the thumb the metacarpal bone may suffer a dislocation as well as a fracture. At the metcarpo-phalangeal joints dislocation is more common, at least in the thumb, and is due to forceful hyperextension with tearing of the anterior capsule. Reduction is not always easy and usually demands a general anesthetic; it can only be achieved by *increasing*

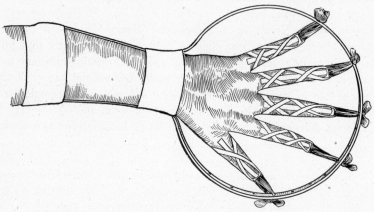

FIG. 252.—THE SO-CALLED "BANJO SPLINT" FOR EXERTING PERMANENT TRACTION IN FRACTURES OF THE PHALANGES AND METACARPAL BONES.

the deformity (hyperextension) and by traction and direct pressure on the dislocated bone. Occasionally interposition of joint capsule or of the flexor pollicis longus tendon of the thumb will prevent closed reduction and open operation must be carried out to remove the interposed tissue. Dislocation of the interphalangeal joints usually presents no great difficulty in either diagnosis or treatment. Reduction is usually easy by manipulation and traction in the line of the finger.

A special but frequent type of injury to the terminal end of the finger is mallet or baseball finger, trauma frequently being sustained by a baseball striking the end of the extended finger. The primary injury consists of rupture of the extensor tendon at or near its insertion, with a consequent subluxation deformity. Occasionally a small chip fracture of the articular surface of the terminal phalanx is sustained. Treatment consists of immobilization in extension with a wooden splint (tongue depressor) but function will be more completely restored by operative repair of the ruptured tendon with subsequent fixation for four to six weeks.

THE PELVIS

Fracture of the Pelvis.—Fracture of the pelvis is usually sustained by direct impact of a crushing type from either the anteroposterior or lateral direction. Fractures through the rami of the pubis and ischium are perhaps most common. Frequently, these fractures are bilateral. Another common injury is fracture through the ramus of the pubis and ischium with a fracture through the region of the sacro-iliac joint on the same or opposite side. Because it is unprotected, fracture through the wing of the ilium frequently occurs. Fracture of the sacrum (usually in a transverse direction) and coccyx, are important because of the tendency for such injuries to be followed by a chronic type of pain and backache, particularly in women. Rarely is there roentgenologic evidence of fracture in patients (usually women) who complain of pain in that region following injury. Pain in the region of the coccyx is fre-

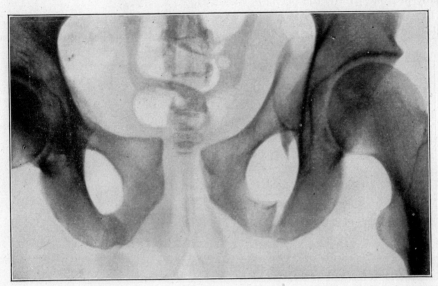

FIG. 253.—FRACTURE OF THE PELVIS SUSTAINED IN AN AUTO ACCIDENT.

Note separation of the symphysis and fracture of the ramus of the pubis and ischium on each side with greatest displacement on the patient's left. While correction of displacement of the degree here present is not absolutely essential, the commonly used method of suspending the patient's pelvis in a canvas sling frequently effects reduction. In this patient the separation of the symphysis was corrected 50 per cent; the functional result was perfect.

quently spoken of as *coccygodynia* and may not be associated with any injury whatsoever. Because of resiliency maintained by the attachment of numerous ligaments and muscles to the pelvic ring, there is a strong tendency for fractured bones of the pelvis, even though displaced considerably at the moment of impact, to shift immediately into correct position. Obviously if the injury is severe this spontaneous immediate reduction does not occur. As with other fractures, injury to neighboring structures is always searched for. Fractures of the pelvis may be accompanied by injury to the urethra, bladder or intra-abdominal injury. These associated injuries are considered separately.

Clinical Manifestations.—The manifestations produced by fractures through the pelvic bones are extremely variable. When a fracture is sustained through the entire portion of the body of the *ilium* or through the region of the *sacro-iliac joint* the patient is rarely able to walk. The pain in such instances is poorly localized and is described as being present over the entire side of the pelvis. If merely the *pubis* or *ischium* is fractured, walking may be possible, but will be painful. When the pubis is involved, pain and tenderness will characteristically be located in the groin. Ecchymosis will likewise appear in this region. Deformity will seldom be demonstrable except when there is a separation at the symphysis pubis, or when there is a fracture through the region of the sacro-iliac joint with displacement. The amount of shock produced by fracture of the pelvis is variable, but may be considerable when the fracture extends through the supporting bones of the pelvis. Pressure on the anterior superior spines, or on the wing of each ilium simultaneously, will usually provoke pain if the pelvis is fractured.

Fracture of the *sacrum* is usually transverse and located in the lower portion. Dislocation of fragments is not frequent. Fracture of the *coccyx* is uncommon and

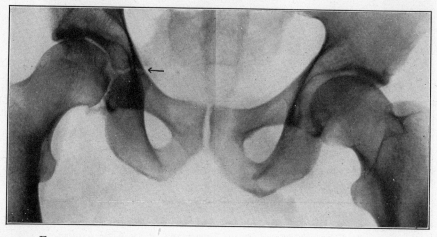

FIG. 254.—FRACTURE OF THE ACETABULUM SUSTAINED BY A FALL FROM A PAINTER'S SCAFFOLD.

Treatment consisted of traction of the extremity in a Thomas splint for five weeks. The ultimate result was good; very little pain or limitation of motion of the hip resulted.

is frequently associated with tearing of the ligaments supporting it. Diagnosis of fracture of the sacrum or coccyx is best made by x-ray, but digital examination through the rectum may be of value in revealing tenderness and extravasation of blood.

Fractures of the *acetabulum* may be one of two types. The most frequent consists of a fracture of the *rim or lip of the acetabulum* with displacement accompanying dislocation of the hip. As the head of the femur is being driven posteriorly and out of the acetabulum the posterior lip of the acetabulum is carried with it. The *floor of the acetabulum* may be fractured and the head driven inward by a direct impact over the trochanter or by a fall with the patient landing on his feet. This type of fracture occurs chiefly in middle-aged people, but is not common; in elderly people the neck of the femur gives way before the floor of the acetabulum. There are few features diagnostic of this type of injury, although the patient is usually unable to walk and complains of pain upon motion of the joint. There is no characteristic change in posture of the foot or other portion of the extremity, although slight shortening may be present.

Treatment.—The type of treatment varies considerably, dependent upon the location of the fracture and the amount of dislocation of fragments. However, in a

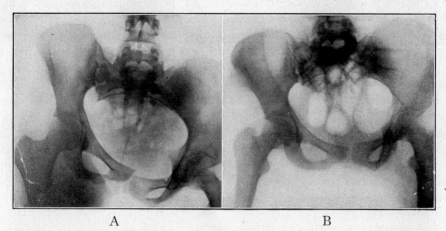

A   B

FIG. 255.—FRACTURE OF THE PELVIS THROUGH THE REGION OF THE SACRO-ILIAC JOINT.

A, before reduction; note marked displacement. Manipulation revealed an impaction of fragment; *B*, the impaction was broken up under anesthesia and reduction attained by application of an Anderson splint (see Fig. 256).

large percentage of patients the fracture is not complicated and no treatment other than bed rest up to six weeks in a firm bed with a fracture board under the mattress,

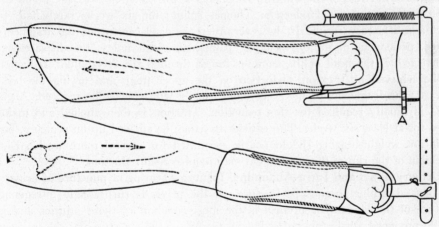

FIG. 256.—THE "WELL LEG" ANDERSON TRACTION (DE PUY TYPE).

A steel pin is inserted through the tibia of the injured extremity and a plaster cast applied up to the knee; the yokes of one side of the splint are incorporated in the plaster. A plaster cast is applied to the uninjured extremity up to the hip, incorporating the yokes of the other side of the splint. By turning a screw pin at *A*, traction on the injured side is obtained by counterbalanced pressure upward on the uninjured side. Except for an occasional severe fracture of the pelvis, the use of this splint is confined chiefly to intertrochanteric fractures.

is all that is required. Attempts need not be made to reduce fractures of the rami of the pubis or ischium, even though considerable displacement of fragments exists.

In addition to bed rest some type of fixation such as a belt, binder, or adhesive strapping around the pelvis, may be applied. If there is a separation at the symphysis or a fracture through the body of the ilium, the pelvis should be suspended in a canvas sling which tends to exert pressure inward from the sides. The extremities can be suspended in Hodgen splints or elevated on pillows so that slight flexion at the knees is obtained. The patient should remain in the canvas sling for four to six weeks, depending upon the severity of the fracture. Only on rare occasions is traction necessary.

If the fracture is located near the sacro-iliac region and associated with much upward displacement of the pelvic fragment, reduction should be attempted. Such fractures are usually impacted so that simple traction will rarely be effective. The patient should be anesthetized and the impaction broken up (usually most effectively by forceful flexion of the thigh and adduction across the opposite hip). Heavy traction on the extremity is necessary to pull the fragments into position. This traction is probably best obtained by the Anderson splint, a type of "well leg" traction (see Fig. 256).

Unfortunately, treatment of fractures of the *sacrum* are rather unsatisfactory unless complete immobilization in bed is resorted to. Adhesive splints and belts obviously do not offer much relief from the pain which may be present for many weeks unless the patient is confined to bed. Fractures of the coccyx, which are rare, are likewise benefited very little unless bed rest is obtained. Occasionally, if pain persists and is severe, removal of the coccyx may be indicated.

The treatment of fractures of the *acetabulum* is usually satisfactory if no displacement of the head of the femur or fragments of the acetabulum exists. Immobilization in traction (in a Hodgen or Thomas splint) for six weeks rarely fails to effect a satisfactory result. If, however, there is displacement of the fragments inward, permanent disability, including pain, may result unless the displacement is corrected. If the head of the femur is forced through the acetabulum, reduction can be achieved by traction, abduction on the upper thigh and prying the head outward; the fragments of the acetabulum usually will likewise be reduced. Anesthesia is usually required for this reduction. Traction is then applied and maintained for at least six weeks. The patient may then be allowed up on crutches, but significant weight-bearing should not be permitted for several more weeks. Displacement of the rim of the acetabulum may require open reduction.

Urinary Tract and Intra-Abdominal Injury.—Tearing or puncture of urinary and intra-abdominal organs in fractures of the pelvis is surprisingly infrequent. Rupture of the bladder or urethra is the most common of these injuries and is usually produced not by puncture, but by tearing of the structures at the moment of impact when displacement may have been considerable. Rupture of either of these two structures will be accompanied by urinary extravasation, intraperitoneal or extraperitoneal—usually the latter. The possibility of rupture of these two organs should be investigated at once. The patient is asked to void, and the urine examined for gross blood. Should the patient be unable to void, a soft rubber catheter is inserted. If a large amount of blood-stained urine is obtained, a rupture of the base of the bladder or urethra near the bladder is suggested, provided trauma to the kidney can be excluded. If only a few drops of bloody fluid is obtained by catheterization, there is a strong probability of a rupture of the bladder into the peritoneal cavity; evidence of intraperitoneal inflammation will of course be present. In this case, laparotomy for repair of the bladder is necessary. If the catheter cannot be inserted all the way through the urethra, and a few drops of bloody fluid are obtained, rupture of the urethra should be suspected; if present, suprapubic drainage of the bladder is usually indicated to prevent serious extravasation about the urethra, scrotum and anterior perineum. If extraperitoneal perforation at the base of the bladder exists, the application of a retention catheter usually is sufficient to prevent serious urinary extravasation. If urinary extravasation develops in spite of treatment, radical incisions may be necessary to prevent fatal infection and toxemia (see also Chapter XXXII).

Obviously any signs of peritoneal irritation in patients with fracture of the pelvis should be viewed with alarm. Besides extravasation of urine from a ruptured bladder, the patient may have perforation of another viscus (particularly the intestine) or may have active severe hemorrhage. Abdominal pain, muscle rigidity, nausea and vomiting are manifestations which should direct attention to the possibilities mentioned above. Laparotomy will obviously be indicated if perforation of the intestine, active severe hemorrhage, or intraperitoneal rupture of the bladder exists. It should be emphasized, however, that signs of peritoneal irritation may be produced by retroperitoneal hemorrhage alone, for which conservative care is indicated (see p. 749). Signs of paralytic ileus (distention and vomiting) may also be of reflex origin (see p. 759).

Sacro-iliac Joint.—Although strong ligaments (sacro-iliac and sacro-sciatic), and rough articulating surfaces allow but little motion in the sacro-iliac joint, it is a true articulation since it is lined with fibrocartilage. The mechanism of production of *sacro-iliac sprains* is not clear. Child-bearing, unusual strains, etc., may be etiologic factors, but frequently there is no discernible etiologic agent. Occasionally the disease is cured by eradication of a focus of infection, suggesting that infection may at times be important in the pathogenesis. There appears to be no doubt that occasionally there is actually a slip in the position of the articulating surfaces so that a definite subluxation exists.

The *manifestations* are varied. The pain is usually unilateral, confined chiefly to the region of the sacro-iliac joint, but may be located in the lumbosacral region or down the course of the sciatic nerve. The patient usually experiences considerable pain when stooping. Attempting to touch the floor with the hands is particularly painful. The disease may develop suddenly with severe pain and complete disability or may appear gradually with only mild symptoms. The duration of the disease is likewise extremely variable. Tenderness over the sacro-iliac joint is usually demonstrable. Muscles about the joint may be spastic.

Treatment is frequently unsatisfactory, but one of the most important factors in the treatment of the acute cases is bed rest. This simple type of therapy, supplanted with the application of local heat is frequently followed by a cure in a week or two. Occasionally the application of adhesive or a belt around the pelvis offers sufficient support to obtain relief. There seems to be a growing belief that at least a mild dislocation of the articulating surfaces exists and for that reason manipulation should be performed, particularly in the stubborn cases. The exact mechanism or maneuver in this manipulation which effects relief is poorly understood, but the fact remains that manipulation is frequently followed by remarkable relief, particularly in those with no "sciatic" pain. In the severe cases, fixation of the pelvis and extremities in a plaster cast for a few weeks may be tried, but does not commonly afford permanent relief.

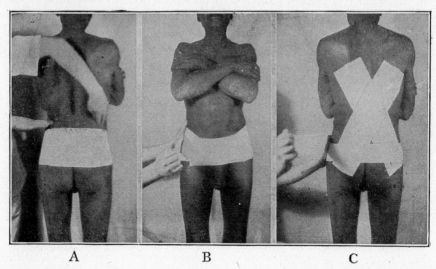

A   B   C

FIG. 257.—METHOD OF STRAPPING THE BACK WITH ADHESIVE, USED IN THE TREATMENT OF ACUTE SACRO-ILIAC STRAINS.

A, seen from the back; note that the strapping is below the brim of the pelvis; *B*, seen from the front, one of the anterior pieces being applied; *C*, one type of adhesive strapping used in the treatment of acute lumbosacral strains. The cross strapping should extend almost up to the axilla. (From Key and Conwell, *Fractures, Dislocations and Sprains*, p. 341, C. V. Mosby Co., 1934.)

Lumbosacral Sprain.—Sprains in the lumbosacral region may likewise be acute or chronic. Usually, the pain comes on suddenly while the patient is performing some simple action such as stooping to the floor and lifting a very light object. People who lead a sedentary life as far as graded, routine exercise is concerned are most apt to be afflicted with the disease. On many occasions faulty posture such as "round shoulders" appears to be an important contributory factor. Faulty posture at times may be so pronounced as to allow such deviation of the lumbar axis so far from the horizontal plane as to actually allow a slipping forward of the last lumbar vertebra on its sacral articulation. Protracted cases may be associated with congenital anomalies, involving, for example, the transverse processes or articular facets.

Pain is located in the lumbosacral region, but radiates outward in all directions but rarely extends down the thigh. Occasionally abdominal pain occupies the center of the stage (see page 556). The patient is unable to stoop over except by flexion at the hips. The spine is usually rigid throughout the entire lumbar region (poker spine). Mild tenderness is present over the lumbosacral region, but proportionally much less than the pain. During the first few days the pain is frequently so severe that the patient is unable to get out of bed.

Treatment during the acute stage of the severe cases consists of rest in a bed fitted with a "fracture board"; in severe cases it may be necessary to apply a plaster cast extending from the midthoracic region down to the femoral trochanters. If recovery is slow the cast may be substituted for a stiff supportive jacket. In mild cases, adhesive splinting of the back may offer sufficient immobilization to effect relief. The daily application of heat, by a bake or otherwise, adds much to comfort and no doubt facilitates healing. Any procedure which encourages relaxation of muscles, even spinal anesthesia, is apt to be helpful. The patient may have to wear a support (*e.g.*, Osgood belt) of some kind for many weeks or even months. He should be instructed not to lift heavy objects until he is completely well. If pain and disability become prolonged, operative procedures, such as spinal fusion, may be indicated. In all of these cases the possibility of a dislocated intervertebral disk (nucleus pulposus) must be kept in mind as a cause of symptoms (see p. 577). Many patients with low back pain are markedly improved or even cured by manipulation (Jostes [14]); the explanation of relief by manipulation is not clear since not all patients relieved have actual dislocation cf bony structure.

THE LOWER EXTREMITY

There are numerous features about fractures of the lower extremity which are peculiar to fractures in this location; these features must be constantly borne in mind if good results are to be obtained. For example, the bones which are associated with weight-bearing must obviously be immobilized longer than other bones. Furthermore, it is particularly important that correct alignment with proper position of fragments be obtained and maintained, because alignment vitally affects the function of weight-bearing; subsequent pain and disability are apt to be severe if position and alignment are not good, chiefly because of disturbances in the line of weight-bearing. In the anteroposterior plane the line of weight-bearing should pass from the anterior superior spine, bisect the patella and approximate the inner border of the navicular (scaphoid) bone. In the lateral plane the weight line should pass from the great trochanter downward through the head of the fibula and external malleolus (see Figure 258).

Neck of the Femur.—Fractures through the neck of the femur are to be considered serious, not only because of their frequency and high initial mortality (up to 25 per cent), but particularly because of the high incidence of nonunion. A high incidence of 30 to 40 per cent nonunion often followed the old closed reduction methods. Nonunion has been considerably reduced by the introduction in recent years of methods of internal fixation, as will be described later. Fractures of the neck of the femur may be either intracapsular or extracapsular, *i.e.*, medial or lateral to the attachment of the capsule of the hip joint. The explanation for the frequency of nonunion in fractures of the hip lies in the fact that the blood supply of the head of the femur is seriously impaired by fracture of the neck, particularly when the break is intracapsular, because the ligamentum teres is then the sole source of nourishment; in many instances the head of the femur receives no blood supply whatever through the ligamentum teres. Because of the more profuse though still meager blood supply furnished by the joint capsule, union is much more apt to occur if the fracture is distal to this point, *i.e.,* extracapsular. The outlook as to union of fragments is much more favorable if impaction is present.

Fractures of the hip are most common after the age of fifty and are particularly prone to occur in women; a variable amount of shock may be produced in these patients. The fracture may be sustained with no more injury than a fall to the ground from a standing position and is presumably produced in most instances by direct impact on the great trochanter. In many instances the fracture is the cause of the fall and not the result, particularly in the aged. Decalcification and other organic changes incident to old age may make the bone so weak and brittle that a sudden twist or strain on the hip may result in fracture at the weak point, namely, the neck of the femur.

Clinical Manifestations.—Invariably the patient is unable to walk, except in the occasional instance when the fragment is solidly impacted. In the absence of impaction a rather typical deformity is usually present. The leg is externally rotated, the thigh slightly abducted, and the knee flexed a few degrees. Comparative measurements of the extremities from the anterior superior spine to the internal malleolus will reveal a shortening of a few centimeters on the injured side. The base of Bryant's triangle will be shortened over that of the normal side and the trochanter will be above Nélaton's line (see Fig. 260). There will, of course, be no shortening in the measurement from the great trochanter to the external malleolus. To avoid error all measurements involving comparison of the two extremities must be made with the uninjured extremity in the same position as the injured. It must be remembered that the results of the measurements just mentioned may be the same in a dislocation of the hip as they

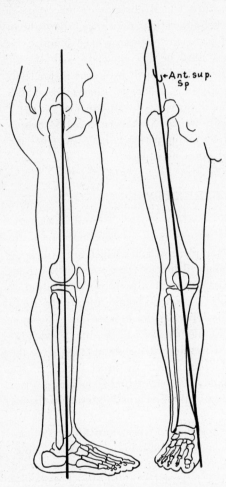

FIG. 258.—LINES DRAWN THROUGH THE BONES OF THE LOWER EXTREMITY SHOWING THE OPTIMUM AXIS OF WEIGHTBEARING.

are in fractures of the neck of the femur. The amount of pain will be variable, but frequently is trivial; it will naturally be increased markedly upon motion. Tenderness is diffuse over the region of the hip. Rotation of the thigh will reveal the fact that the trochanter turns in the palm of the hand instead of rotating in a large arc, as is the case when the neck is intact. Such maneuvers as traction on the extremity, or pressure upward on the heel will reveal changes in the measurement between the anterior and superior spine and internal malleolus. However, these maneuvers usually produce so much pain as to be justifiable only in patients with nonunion. If the fracture is impacted, there may be no deformity or deviation in measurements from the normal side. If examination is painful, it should be omitted and an x-ray taken, thereby enabling one to discern the exact extent of injury. An x-ray is particularly indicated in injuries about the hip, especially in elderly people, since disability and other evidences of fracture may be slight if impaction is present; moreover, the clinical diagnosis may be inaccurate when an impacted fracture is present.

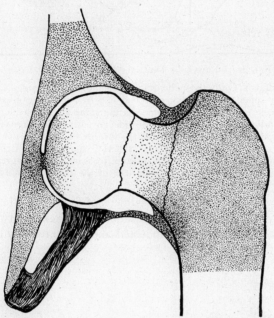

Fig. 259.—The Density of the Shaded Areas Represents the Relative Blood Supply of the Region of the Neck of the Femur.

The two fracture lines illustrated in the drawing are both located in the neck of the femur, but one is intracapsular and the other extracapsular. The latter, since it occurs near the trochanter, is less apt to result in nonunion, because of the greater blood supply at this point, supplied largely through the capsule of the joint. When the break is inside the capsule, the head derives all its meager blood supply from the ligamentum teres; as stated in the text, on many occasions there will be no blood circulation whatsoever through this ligament.

Treatment.—In many instances *emergency treatment* can be instituted before arrival at the hospital. The most important feature in emergency therapy is fixation of the extremity, thereby preventing movement of the fractured ends upon each other which is painful and contributes to shock. One of the best agents available for obtaining fixation in these emergency situations is the Thomas (full ring) or Keller (half ring) splint. If either of these is not available, a Liston board splint extending from beyond the foot to the axilla should be applied. A hypodermic of morphine will be effective in eliminating pain and minimizing the development of shock. The splint should be left on during transportation of the patient to the hospital and even while the initial x-ray film is being taken. If the patient is in shock, treatment of the fracture should be postponed until the shock is relieved.

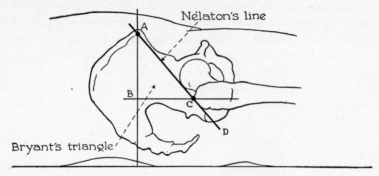

FIG. 260.—BRYANT'S TRIANGLE AND NÉLATON'S LINE.

The triangle is drawn (with the patient lying supine) by dropping a perpendicular from the anterior superior spine, and carrying a second line *BC*, from the greater trochanter, perpendicular to this line. A third line, *AC*, connects the spine and trochanter. If the line *BC* is shortened over such a line drawn on the opposite side, an upward displacement of the trochanter, such as would be produced by a dislocation or fracture of the neck of the femur, is indicated. Nélaton's line *AD* extends from the anterior superior spine to the ischeal tuberosity, and normally should pass through the tip of the greater trochanter. If the greater trochanter lies above this line a dislocation or fracture of the neck of the femur probably exists.

The oldest modern method in the treatment of fracture of the hip is reduction of the fracture by traction and immobilization of the extremity and pelvis in a plaster spica with the thigh widely abducted and the extremity rotated internally (Whitman's position).

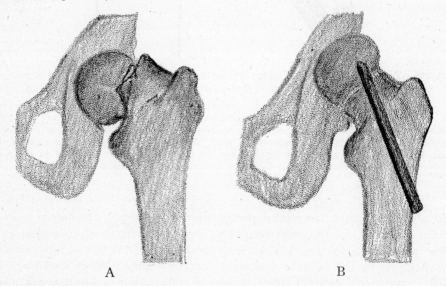

A   B

FIG. 261.—TREATMENT OF FRACTURE OF THE FEMUR BY A SMITH-PETERSEN NAIL.

A, fracture showing moderate upward displacement. *B*, the fracture was reduced and the fragments engaged by the Leadbetter maneuver; fixation and apposition of fragments was attained by driving a Smith-Petersen nail through the trochanter into the head.

The closed method of treatment, as mentioned above, has been supplanted entirely in recent years by operative fixation of fragments by means of some type of nail or pin. This method has the great advantage of requiring no external fixation, shortens the period of bed rest, and allows weight-bearing much earlier. These two factors are very desirable not only from the standpoint of the patient's health and comfort but are also very conducive to healing of the fracture.

Several methods of inserting these pins or nails have been described. Regardless of which method is used reduction must first be obtained. In order to first achieve good reduction, manipulation is carried out, under a local or general anesthetic, by the Leadbetter [15] maneuver which is an excellent method of correcting the displacement (see Fig. 262). This Leadbetter maneuver consists of manipulation with the hip and knee flexed and the pelvis fixed; while the leg is in this position, traction is exerted upward on the thigh which is gently rotated internally to engage the fragments. When the reduction is effected the hip is brought out into extreme abduction with the foot and leg in internal rotation, fixation of the pelvis being maintained by abduction of the other thigh. An efficient reduction is indicated if the heel of the affected leg will remain in the palm of the surgeon in an abducted and internally rotated position (heel-palm test).

One method of internal fixation consists of making an incision one or two inches long over the trochanter, and inserting two or three heavy wires through the trochanter into the head of the femur by means of a drill. A Smith-Petersen [16] nail of proper length is threaded over the wire, which is shown by x-ray to be in the best position, and driven through the trochanter into the head to obtain complete fixation. Some surgeons prefer to drive the nail without the aid of the guide wire, particularly if a protractor of the type devised by Westcott [17] is used to guide the direction of the nail. Regardless of the method of "nailing" used, the x-ray will be of inestimable value in determining whether or not the position is satisfactory. A lateral as well as an anteroposterior film is necessary. These films should be made, developed and read after reduction and before incision has been made. They should be repeated and read after the internal fixation material is in place and before the wound is closed. After closure of the wound the patient is placed in bed with the affected leg suspended with the aid of a few pounds traction for about four weeks, after which time he may be allowed up, using crutches for a period of four to six months, permitting only slight weight-bearing at first. The nail need not be removed unless complications develop.

Instead of using a large nail as a means of internal fixation, more recent procedures have employed four smaller pins (Moore [18]) threaded at the end, which engage the head of the femur. Ordinarily, the x-ray will be of value in determining whether or not union is taking place in so far as decalcification with decrease in density takes place in the head of the femur under normal circumstances of healing.

Another modification of internal fixation, using an originally designed incision and flange as reported by Cubbins, Callahan and Scuderi,[19] promises to be very satisfactory. Even though the incision appears extensive, incising the capsule and allowing full view of the fracture line, they report only one death in 105 patients operated upon; union was obtained in 90 per cent of the fresh fractures. The incision has an important advantage in so far as pieces of periosteal synovial membrane, which might lodge between the bone fragments and encourage nonunion, can be seen and removed. The incision has an added advantage in that the extent of reduction by the Leadbetter maneuver can be observed. A summary of the various methods of internal fixation in use for fracture of the neck of the femur has recently been published by Callahan.[20]

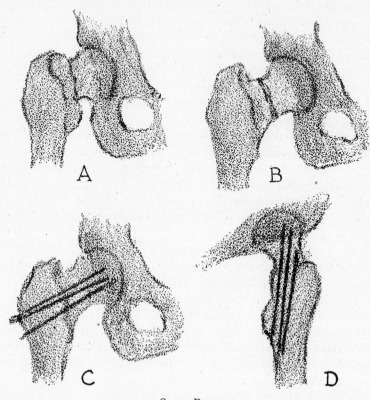

STEEL PINS.

A, fracture showing mild displacement; *B*, reduction has been achieved by the Leadbetter maneuver; *C*, three pins have been introduced fixing the segments in apposition; *D*, lateral view showing proper position of pins through the neck. Four pins are preferable to the three shown.

If the x-ray shows signs of necrosis of the head, or erosion of the neck of the femur, protection by means of the caliper splint will have to be extended and weight-bearing postponed for several months (Speed [21] and Phemister [22]). Phemister has discussed the features of aseptic bone necrosis in detail. X-ray changes consisting of increased density of the head may be the first evidence of necrosis.

As already mentioned, *nonunion* in fractures of the neck of the femur occurs frequently, even when treated in expert hands. However, a positive diagnosis of nonunion cannot be made earlier than six months after the injury, even with the aid of the x-ray. Nonunion is suggested in the x-ray by an absorption of bone at the line of fracture, but particularly by a more dense appearance of the head of the femur, or at the fracture line. This apparently paradoxical condition (*viz.*, increased density of the head of the femur associated with nonunion) is due to the fact that normal bones with adequate blood supply always exhibit decalcification following immobilization. The absence of the absorption of calcium, therefore, is indicative of inadequate or absent blood supply.

Five major types of procedures (all operative) are available in the treatment of nonunion of fracture of the neck of the femur.

1. Internal fixation, using nails or pins as described for the treatment of fresh fractures, may be successful, but obviously in a lower percentage of cases.

2. A bone graft may be inserted through the trochanter into the head, a procedure more difficult than nailing, but perhaps associated with a higher percentage of success.

3. The Brackett operation may be very successful if the head is viable. In a series of 59 operations for ununited fracture of the neck of the femur, Magnuson,[23] utilizing a modified type of Brackett operation, found it appropriate in 41 of the 59 cases. The operation consists of excavating the central portion of the head of the femur and inserting the fashioned end of the shaft. The trochanter must be cut off and transplanted lower down to avoid interference in motion. Weight-bearing is permitted in eight weeks.

4. The Whitman operation, consisting of removal of the head and insertion of the fashioned end of the shaft into the acetabulum with transplantation of the trochanter as in the Brackett operation, may be very adaptable, particularly when any of the other procedures for nonunion have resulted in failure.

5. Osteotomy (cutting through the entire thickness of the shaft), either high or low, as described by McMurray[24] and Schanz[25] respectively, may be performed to eliminate shearing action at the fracture and to bring the line of weight bearing at a right angle to the fracture surfaces. This operation is less extensive and shocking than the reconstruction procedures and may be employed in patients who would not stand more extensive operations. A high percentage of union has been recorded following these procedures.

The choice of the five procedures will depend largely upon the features of the case under consideration. It must be remembered that some of them are quite formidable procedures, and will not be tolerated by patients who are poor risks, particularly the aged. Moreover, the fixation incident to fibrous union not infrequently will eliminate most of the pain and disability of nonunion, and will contraindicate any operative procedures, particularly in the aged.

Dislocation of the Hip.—Dislocations of the hip are relatively uncommon and may be either of two types, namely, posterior or anterior. By far the majority are of the former type. Occasionally they are complicated by fractures of the acetabulum, consisting usually of merely the rim of the acetabulum (see p. 416).

A complication of dislocation of the hip only recently appreciated lies in the possibility of aseptic necrosis of the head of the femur (Phemister[22]), a phenomenon which occurs, however, more commonly in fracture of the neck of the femur.

Posterior Dislocation.—The mechanism producing this type of injury usually consists of an upward thrust on the knee with the thigh flexed, adducted and rotated internally. The head of the femur is forced through the posterior capsule and lies on the ilium posterior to and above the acetabulum. The deformity, consisting of internal rotation and adduction of the extremity with mild flexion of the thigh, is quite characteristic. There is a shortening of the distance between the anterior superior spine and the internal malleolus compared to the uninjured side. The amount of pain produced by the injury is variable, but frequently is surprisingly

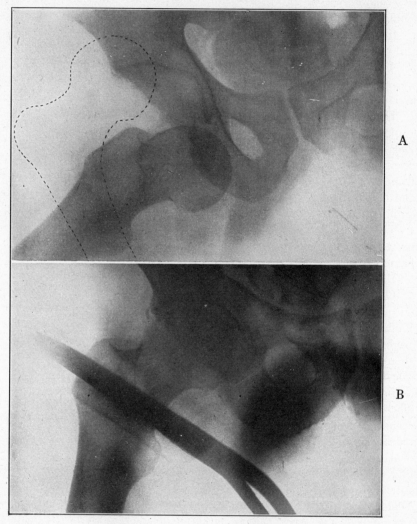

FIG. 263.—DISLOCATION OF THE HIP.

A, roentgenogram shows an anterior dislocation, with the head of the femur lying in the obturator foramen. The dotted line illustrates the usual position of the head in posterior dislocation of the hip which is more frequent than the anterior type; *B,* x-ray film after reduction.

mild. On many occasions, however, the amount of pain, tenderness and local findings is so similar to the manifestations encountered in fracture of the hip that a differential diagnosis cannot be made without the aid of an x-ray.

Reduction may be performed in one of several ways. The Bigelow manipulation as herein described is one of the effective procedures. A general anesthesia should be administered. Usually nitrous oxide produces sufficient relaxation, but if not, ether or spinal anesthesia should be given. The thigh is flexed, adducted, and rotated internally while traction is being made by the operator's arm hooked under the patient's bent knee. This procedure should disengage the head of the femur. The thigh is then abducted, and increased traction made upon the extremity while it is being rotated. Completion of this maneuver usually results in reduction, but if ineffective should be repeated. After reduction the patient should be kept in bed for at least two or three weeks. Walking may then be permitted since there is no tendency for the ordinary motions of walking to produce recurrence through the rent in the capsule, which is located posteriorly. As intimated previously, the greatest danger from the standpoint of complications in convalescent care lies in the possibility of aseptic necrosis of the head of the femur resulting from destruction of the blood supply through the round ligament. Therefore, too early and extensive weight-bearing may give rise to collapse of the head with subsequent permanent lameness (Phemister). The x-ray may be helpful in determining the development of necrosis as noted by increased density, but would rarely be noted under two or three months.

Anterior Dislocation.—Injury of this type with dislocation of the head of the femur through the anterior or lower portion of the capsule so that it rests anteriorly upon the obturator foramen, is usually produced by violent abduction of the hip. The deformity produced is much different than that observed in posterior dislocation. The thigh is abducted and flexed with external rotation. The knee is also flexed. The extremity cannot be extended or adducted while the dislocation exists. Reduction is performed by flexing and abducting the thigh (after administration of an anesthetic) and the use of traction on the extremity. The thigh is then rotated inward and extended. Reduction may be facilitated by having an assistant exert pressure laterally against the proximal part of the thigh.

The Trochanters.—Intertrochanteric fractures are sustained in a manner similar to fractures of the hip, but occur in older people, and are probably associated with more violence and trauma. Although extracapsular fractures rarely lead to nonunion because of the richer blood supply, they are more common and are associated with a slightly higher mortality; according to the report of Rowlette et al.[26] there was a 38 per cent mortality in 214 trochanteric fractures and a mortality of 25.9 per cent in 166 intracapsular fractures over the same period. Most of these patients were treated according to older methods; the mortality has accordingly been reduced sharply during recent years. The fracture line may extend through both trochanters. The amount of displacement is usually small and separation of fragments is not marked. The clinical manifestations are similar to those of fracture of the hip, except that shortening is not as pronounced. Treatment may be carried out by several methods including traction with the Thomas or Hodgen splint, plaster cast, or Anderson's "well leg" traction splint. In some cases internal fixation with the use of Moore nails may be used to facilitate the handling of the patient and thus decrease mortality. Usually, however, the outer fragment is too badly comminuted to give good fixation. A simple "well-leg" plaster splint has recently been devised by Weiner.[27] It enables the patient to be lifted out of bed into a wheel chair almost immediately. Weight-bearing is discouraged until union is quite firm. Ordinarily firm union will take place several weeks earlier than in intracapsular fractures because of the large surface involved and the increased blood supply, each of which factors will result in the formation of more callus. If shortening occurs, and it often does, the disability may be minimized by using a shoe with a built-up heel on the affected side. McKibbin [36] has recently described an ambulatory method of treatment, using four pins for fixation, and a short plaster cast to the thigh for stability.

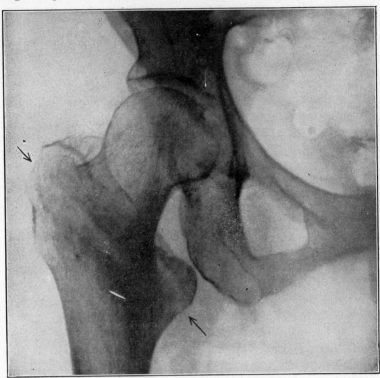

FIG. 264.—INTERTROCHANTERIC FRACTURE.

No reduction is necessary. Plaster cast as illustrated in Figure 265 was applied without an anesthetic.

Shaft of the Femur.—The type of violence producing a fracture of the shaft of the femur may be either direct or indirect. Shock may be produced by this type of injury and may be as pronounced as in fracture of the neck of the femur. Pain is usually severe and complete disability is present. Because of the depth of the tissue overlying the fracture, tenderness is diffuse, and though considerable swelling is present, ecchymosis is delayed or absent. Measurements between the trochanter and external malleolus reveal a shortening on the injured side unless a fracture exists without displacement. Crepitus will be present but no attempt should be made to elicit it because of pain and trauma inflicted. Slight and gentle rotary motion of the knee or leg will reveal a failure of the trochanter to move with the shaft. Because of the pain and shock produced by transportation, immobilization should be effected by some type of metal or wood splint *at the scene of the accident,* and before the patient is transported to the hospital or other suitable place for

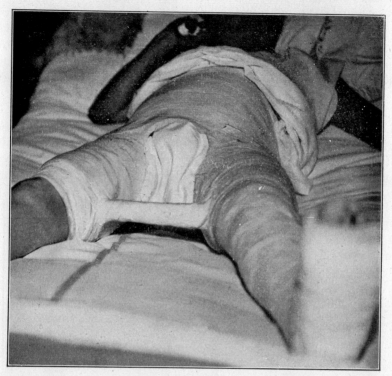

FIG. 265.—PLASTER SPICA.

This cast was applied to a patient with an intratrochanteric fracture as shown in Figure 264. When a plaster spica is used for treatment of a fracture of the neck of the femur, more abduction (to the Whitman's position) is necessary.

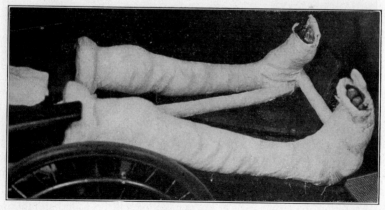

FIG. 266.—WEINER MODIFICATION (UNPUBLISHED) OF THE WELL LEG TRACTION FOR THE TREATMENT OF INTERTROCHANTERIC FRACTURE OF THE FEMUR.

About 20 cc. of 1 per cent novocain is injected into the fracture site, a pin inserted through the tibia under local anesthesia, and a plaster cast applied with supporting crossbars as illustrated.

roentgenograms and treatment. A traction splint, such as the Thomas or Keller, is most effective in preventing and in reducing displacement during transportation. Displacement as well as overriding of fragments is nearly always great, owing to the number and strength of the muscles attached to the femur. The amount and type of displacement depends to a great extent upon the location of the fracture. In fractures of the *upper third* of the shaft, the iliopsoas and glutei muscles tend to abduct and flex the proximal fragment so that it usually lies anterior and lateral to the distal fragment. The deformities of fractures of the *middle third* are apt to be variable, but the proximal fragment usually lies anterior and lateral to the distal fragment as in fractures of the upper third, but with less displacement. The anterior convexity of the thigh is lost. In fractures of the *lower third,* the pull of

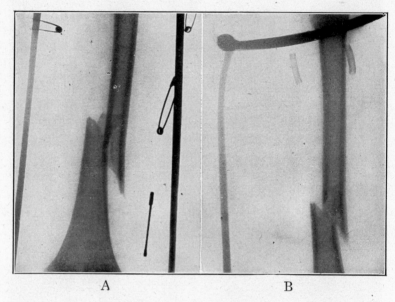

A   B

FIG. 267.—FRACTURE OF THE SHAFT OF THE FEMUR.

A, before treatment; *B,* position of fragments after 5 days traction in a Thomas splint. Ultimate result good with only ½ inch shortening.

the gastrocnemius displaces the distal fragment posteriorly. Fractures in this location are apt to be associated with injury to the popliteal artery or nerves; severance of the artery is serious because of the danger of gangrene.

Treatment.—Simple reduction and immobilization in a plaster cast is not satisfactory, because reduction is difficult to achieve, and even more difficult to maintain. Fractures of the shaft are, therefore, usually best treated by suspension and adhesive or skeletal traction. In either case a Thomas splint will be found suitable to obtain suspension of the limb. Bending the splint to allow a few degrees flexion at the knee, or the use of the Pierson attachment will add to the comfort of the patient and to a slight extent encourage the return of motion in the joint. If adhesive traction is used, either a Hodgen or Thomas splint will be found satisfactory. An important feature of the traction lies in the necessity of placing the extremity in a position with sufficient abduction and flexion of the thigh to bring the distal fragment into alignment with the proximal fragment. Moreover, with the thigh flexed the weight of the body aids in attaining efficient counter traction. If the fracture is oblique, and there is little over-riding, adhesive traction should be adequate to obtain satisfactory results. However, if the fracture is transverse (usually with pronounced over-riding), reduction is much more readily obtained by skeletal traction. Skeletal traction can be carried out by the insertion of a Kirschner wire through the condyles of the femur and application of traction to the stirrup attached to the wire. The application of 30 to 40 pounds usually corrects the overriding in two to three days, at which time spontaneous reduction of fragments frequently occurs, but if not, very little manipulation is necessary to bring the fragments into position. Frequent observations by x-ray may be necessary lest overpull result in separation of the fragments. Attempt need not be made to secure perfect end-to-end approxi-

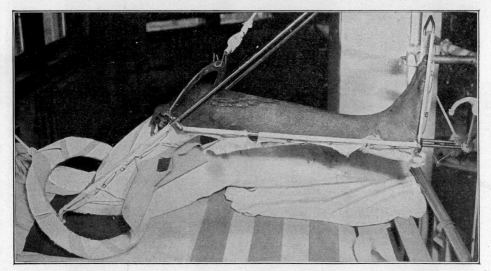

Fig. 268.—Pierson Attachment for Thomas Splint in Skeletal Traction for Treatment of Fracture of Shaft of Femur.

mation; if the two fragments are merely locked at the edge, good results may be expected provided alignment and proper immobilization are maintained. After the fragments are locked end on, the amount of traction should be reduced to 10 to 15 pounds. Regardless of the type of traction used, the splint will have to be suspended in some type of overhead (e.g., Balkan) frame. In many cases suspension and traction may be replaced by a plaster cast after three to four weeks; at this time there is no danger of losing the position of the fragments. If the fracture is located in the *upper third,* traction will have to be maintained in wide abduction with considerable flexion of the thigh so that alignment of fragments may be achieved. Usually some type of skeletal traction as previously mentioned will have to be used. Adhesive traction will not be very useful in fractures in this location but will find its greatest usefulness in the fractures in the *middle third,* care being taken that the posteriorly displaced distal fragment is held forward by the flannel or canvas bands or by a sling attached to the frame in traction. Only slight abduction is indicated in fractures of the middle third.

If the fracture is in the *lower third,* the distal fragment will be so firmly displaced posteriorly by the gastrocnemius muscle that adhesive traction will be inadequate in obtaining proper position of fragments. Skeletal traction is much more

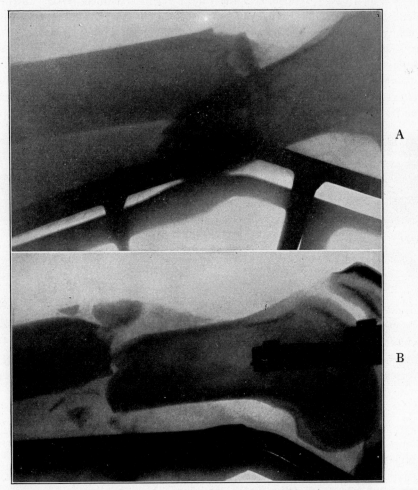

FIG. 269.—FRACTURE OF THE FEMUR AT THE JUNCTION OF THE MIDDLE AND LOWER THIRD.

A, before treatment. Note the marked posterior displacement due to the pull of the gastrocnemius muscle; *B,* reduction achieved by skeletal traction (wire through the condyles). In adults, adhesive (skin) traction is rarely successful in obtaining reduction in a fracture in this location. (Courtesy Dr. J. A. Key.)

efficient, especially because it permits a greater degree of flexion at the knee. It may be obtained by the application of a Kirschner wire through the condyles or through the upper end of the tibia, depending upon the proximity of the fracture to the joint. Occasionally it may be wise to reduce the fracture under an anesthetic and apply a plaster spica with the knee flexed. If so, the position of the fragments must be checked from time to time by x-ray and the circulation of the leg carefully watched.

Griswold [28] has described a method of treating fractures of the shaft of the femur, involving application of metal pins through the fragments, reduction, and the application of a non-padded plaster cast. He very appropriately warns that surgeons should have experience in the application of the non-padded plaster cast in minor cases before attempting to use it in a spica. A great many of the patients treated by this method may be made ambulatory, a procedure which will play a great part in speeding union and in preventing soft tissue atrophy. The Stader [33] method of fixation of the pins (after placement through the fragments) to a bar external and parallel to the skin represents another method of avoiding prolonged hospitalization. Open reduction with internal fixation may be indicated at times, if proper reduction is unobtainable by manipulation alone.

The *after treatment* of fractures of the shaft of the femur is extremely important. Regardless of the type of traction apparatus used (with the exception, perhaps, of the skeletal fixation method just described), it must be watched daily and adjustments made as indicated. Such precautions include application of pressure over fragments to aid in alignment, watching skin for pressure sores, guarding against knots slipping, use of counter or secondary traction, etc. When traction is chosen as the method of treatment it must be maintained for six to eight weeks, after which time a plaster cast may be applied for an additional six weeks or more depending upon the type of fracture and rate of healing. However, it is usually desirable, eight to twelve weeks after the fracture, when union is fairly solid, to allow the patient up in a convalescent caliper splint which takes the weight off the foot. Actual weight-bearing should not be allowed to any significant degree up to six months following fracture. Active and passive motion, as well as massage should be instituted as soon as possible without disturbing the traction and position of fragments.

Compound fractures of the femur are uncommon because of the large amount of muscle surrounding the bone. Usually the amount of bone projecting beyond the skin is so small that extensive débridement may not be necessary. Traction and immobilization may be carried out as outlined above. If skeletal traction is used, the wire or pin must not be inserted through the bone near the fracture line because of the danger of osteomyelitis. See page 367 and Chapter XXXIII for details.

Fractures of the Shaft of the Femur in Children.—Most fractures of the femur sustained by children are located in the shaft. Up to the age of five or six years they are best treated by Bryant's overhead suspension and traction. Adhesive is applied to the extremity which is then suspended upward at right angle to the bed, and sufficient traction applied to just raise the buttocks from the bed. Immobilization in traction for four weeks followed by fixation in a plaster spica for four or five more weeks usually is sufficient immobilization to begin weight-bearing (see Fig. 271).

For children over six years of age the Russel [29] traction consisting of adhesive traction from the knee down, with flexion of the knee created by a sling, will be found very useful. This mechanism can often be used advantageously in adults, particularly when a maximum amount of traction is not needed. Its great advantages are simplicity and freedom of movement by the patient. One disadvantage is that it requires constant care and adjustment (see Fig. 215, page 364).

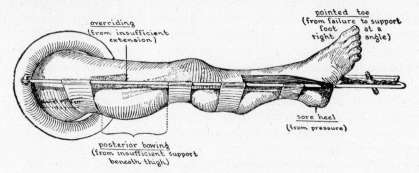

FIG. 270.—COMMON ERRORS IN THE TREATMENT OF FRACTURES OF THE SHAFT OF THE FEMUR
CAUSING PROLONGED AND PERMANENT DISABILITY.

(From Babcock, *Text-Book of Surgery*, p. 313. W. B. Saunders Co., Philadelphia, 1928.)

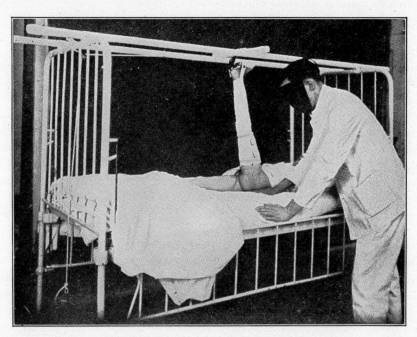

FIG. 271.—BRYANT'S OVERHEAD TRACTION FOR FRACTURE OF THE FEMUR IN CHILDREN;
SUFFICIENT WEIGHT IS USED TO BARELY LIFT THE BUTTOCK OFF THE BED.

(From Cole, *Arch. Surg.*, 5:702, 1922.)

The Knee.—*Fracture through the Femoral Condyles.*—This fracture may be inflicted when violence of unusual degree is sustained by a fall upon the feet or knees. The condyles are usually split in a T fashion so that the fracture extends into the joint; commonly the fragments are displaced posteriorly and spread apart.

Such a fracture is serious because of the difficulty in obtaining adequate reduction and in preventing stiffness or ankylosis of the knee. Skeletal traction, obtained by a Kirschner wire inserted through the tubercle of the tibia, is usually the treatment of choice because in this way sufficient flexion of the knee may be secured to relax the pull of the gastrocnemius. Occasionally, operative reduction with some type of fixation of fragments will be necessary. Frequently, closed reduction by instrumental manipulation will be indicated and successful, although difficulty will usually be experienced in maintaining reduction.

In children *separation of the lower epiphysis of the femur* is encountered as a result of violent trauma such as an automobile accident. The distal fragment is displaced anteriorly. Reduction should be carried out under anesthesia and is usually accomplished with ease. The extremity is immobilized in a plaster cast with the knee flexed. An open reduction should never be done because of the danger of nongrowth.

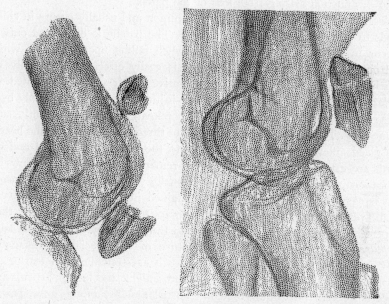

FIG. 272.—FRACTURE OF THE PATELLA WITH WIDE SEPARATION OF THE FRAGMENTS.
A, on admission; *B,* operative reduction, fixation secured by chromic catgut. (From St. Louis City Hospital.)

Fracture of the Patella.—This is a common injury and is usually sustained by a direct blow over the knees. Effusion into the joint is usually profuse and contains a large amount of blood. The patella may be comminuted with or without displacement, but the fracture is usually transverse. When complete, the lateral tendinous attachment of the joint ligaments are usually torn and wide separation of the fragments is produced. In such cases, operative reduction is adopted unless sufficient injury has been inflicted to the skin about the patella to jeopardize asepsis, a complication which commonly occurs. The danger of infection in such a situation may be so great that it will be necessary to delay operation for many days until the skin has healed. Adequate fixation of the fragments by operation allows early motion, thereby tending to prevent stiffness of the knee, which is a frequent complication of fractures of the patella. Fixation is usually accomplished by absorbable sutures such as chromacized catgut. In severe comminution the use of strips of fascia lata may be indicated. Wire sutures through small drill holes in the anterior surface of the patella are occasionally used; the solidity of the repair obtained by metal sutures allows early motion and is, therefore, very advantageous in fractures about the knee in general. To obtain good results the tear in the capsule *must* be closed. A cast is applied in extension, bivalved early and active motion begun in three or four weeks. If no separation of fragments exists, simple fixation of the knee by a thin plaster cast will be the method of choice. Excision of small distal fragments and suture of the patellar tendon to the proximal fragment is widely used (Thompson). Dobbie and Ryerson [37] recommend excision of the fragments in fracture of the patella, as originally advised (1937) by Brooke of England; they noted no dysfunction arising from loss of the patella.

Dislocation of the Patella.—This is uncommon and usually occurs in childhood, but tends to recur with only slight violence. The patella is dislocated outward. It may occur in adults, particularly women, when falling upon the knee with force exerted outward on the patella. Reduction is easily effected and usually without an anesthetic. In recurrent dislocation operative repair may be indicated.

Dislocation of the Knee.—This is a rare injury and is sustained only by severe violence. Injury to the peroneal nerve or popliteal vessels is frequently sustained simultaneously. The dislocation may be one of three types, *i.e.,* with the head of the tibia displacd anterior, posterior or lateral to the femur. The lateral and cruciate ligaments are usually torn, thereby allowing remarkable mobility. The anterior type of dislocation is the most common and is usually produced by hyperextension. Reduction is easy, but fixation must be maintained in a plaster cast for five or six weeks to prevent a relaxed joint which is so apt to follow such injuries; therefore, open operation with repair of the ligaments at time of injury is frequently advisable.

Rupture of Cruciate Ligaments.—Rupture of the cruciate ligaments is fortunately not common, but minor injuries, such as stretching and tearing, are no doubt sustained in many sprains and fractures about the knee, particularly when the knee is overextended and rotated. Unusual mobility of the knee, particularly in the anteroposterior direction, is the most diagnostic sign. If the anterior cruciate ligament is torn, the mobility is apt to be most prominent when the knee is extended. When the posterior cruciate is torn the mobility will be most marked when the knee is flexed. For treatment of torn cruciate ligaments, immobilization of the knee in a plaster cast for several weeks is probably the method of choice. Operative repair of neglected cases is recommended by some surgeons, and may be facilitated by the use of fascial strips (Hey-Groves,[30] and Gallie and Le Mesurier [31]).

Injury to the Semilunar Cartilages of the Knee.—The semilunar cartilages are flat circular structures which are attached by their ends near the center of the joint, and furnish a concavity for articulation of the condyles of the femur. Their lateral attachments to the capsule and lateral ligaments are so insecure that detachment or injury at this point is frequent. The medial cartilage is injured much more frequently than the lateral. The injury may consist of a detachment, tear, or a crush, and is usually sustained by sudden extension of the joint with twisting. Considerable pain is usually experienced at the time of the initial injury. If a piece of cartilage is torn off or displaced there may be "locking" of the joint with inability to completely extend it. Tenderness is usually present along the articular surface of the tibia on the medial side. Commonly, reduction occurs spontaneously, in which case the characteristic "locking" will be absent. Diagnosis may then be difficult and can be made on the basis of recurrent attacks of pain in the knee without x-ray changes. Acute injury of the cartilage is usually associated with an accumulation of clear, straw-colored fluid in the joint.

Treatment should be directed toward reduction of the cartilage (if dislocation is present) with immobilization in a plaster cast for two or three weeks. Commonly, however, conservative treatment is a failure and operative excision of the cartilage will be necessary to obtain relief. Likewise, if reduction is not attained after a few days, operation will be indicated at the time of the initial attack (see p. 468).

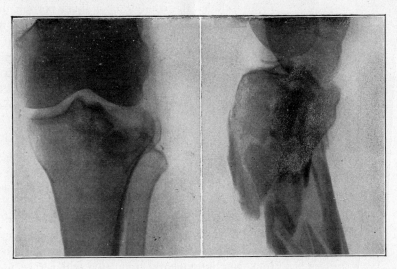

FIG. 273.—TWO TYPES OF FRACTURE OF THE UPPER END OF THE TIBIA; EACH EXTENDS INTO THE JOINT.

Permanent disability with a varying amount of pain and limitation in the knee is apt to result in such fractures because of proximity to the knee joint.

Sprain of the Knee.—Injuries of this type are common and consist primarily of a stretching or tearing of the lateral ligaments which are in reality thickened portions of the capsule of the joint. Fluid commonly accumulates within the joint so that the patella is floating and the normal joint landmarks are obliterated (acute traumatic synovitis). Ecchymosis may be present. Flexion of the joint is painful, but unless the semilunars are likewise injured, extension is free and painless. Lateral mobility of the knee may be increased because of the tearing or stretching of the ligaments. The internal lateral ligament is most often affected. It is particularly important to get an x-ray of the joint if disability is very pronounced because a sprain fracture (*i.e.*, avulsion of a small fragment of bone at the attachment of the ligament) is so often present.

Treatment consists of rest of the affected part for two or three weeks, depending upon the severity of the sprain. In severe cases it may be necessary to resort to immobilization with a plaster cast or similar type of fixation. The joint should be aspirated if fluid is present.

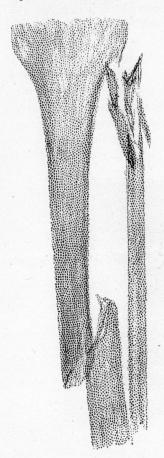

FIG. 274.—FRACTURE OF THE TIBIA AND FIBULA AT DIFFERENT LEVELS FREQUENTLY OCCURS IN INDIRECT VIOLENCE.

Because of this feature, any x-ray film taken for fracture of the tibia should include the entire shaft of the fibula.

The Tibia.—Under this heading will be included fracture of the upper end of the tibia, and fracture of the shaft of the tibia and fibula.

Upper End of the Tibia.—Fractures may be sustained through either or both condyles of the tibia. They are commonly due to direct violence when the patient is struck by the front bumpers of an automobile; hence, they are called "bumper fractures." The fracture line in the "high bumper fractures" almost invariably extends into the joint. If the fragment includes the condyle or a small portion thereof it is usually displaced downward. There is nearly always a concomitant injury to the cartilage, particularly if there is much displacement of fragments. Pain is unusually severe. The joint is filled with fluid, the greater part of which is blood. It is particularly important to obtain as complete reduction as possible, because of the danger of development of a permanently painful joint. Furthermore, if the condyle is not replaced upward into its normal position, genu valgum or genu varum is apt to develop, depending upon which condyle is displaced. Traction will usually be the most adaptable method of treatment. Reduction of fragments by direct manipulation is difficult, but may be facilitated by the application of a clamp over the fracture site to compress the fragments into position. Not infrequently, reduction will not be possible by traction and manipulation, making it necessary to resort to operative reduction. On account of the active blood supply in this region, union takes place rapidly (within six weeks), but weight-bearing should not be allowed for ten or twelve weeks. In recent years "bumper fractures" occur lower down on the leg because the newer cars are made with lower bumpers. Frequently, therefore, they do not involve the joint; treatment is similar to that of fractures of the shaft.

Shaft of the Tibia and Fibula.—Fractures of the shaft of the tibia and fibula may occur at any level, but are most frequent at the junction of the lower and middle thirds where nonunion is also most common. The fractures may be transverse, oblique or spiral, with or without comminution. The lower fragment of the tibia is usually displaced posteriorly. The fractures may be caused either by direct or indirect violence. In the former case, as when the direct blow is sustained, the fracture in the two bones is apt to be at the same level. In indirect violence, the tibia usually breaks near the junction of the middle and lower thirds, and the fibula at a higher level. For that reason it is particularly important that the x-ray include the entire leg from the ankle to the knee. Diagnosis of a fracture of the tibia is usually made without difficulty because the bone is subcutaneous over its entire anterior surface. The patient is unable to walk unless the fracture is impacted or incomplete. Pain and local tenderness point to the location of the fracture. Swelling and ecchymosis develop, after a few hours. When the fracture affects only the upper

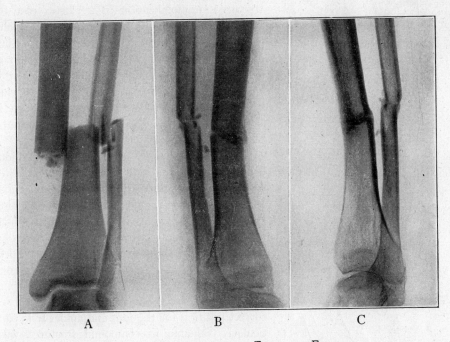

A   B   C

Fig. 275.—Fracture of the Tibia and Fibula.

A, anteroposterior view on admission; *B*, two months after reduction; note that union is taking place but is delayed and associated with a very small amount of callus; *C*, six months after injury healing is more advanced, but still not sufficiently advanced to safely allow normal weight-bearing. Note that the callus is confined to the space between the ends of the bone. Walking in a skin cast as shown in Figure 276 frequently accelerates union.

two-thirds of the fibula the manifestations will be less severe; the patient may be able to walk with only a moderate amount of difficulty, since the fibula has little to do with weight-bearing of the body.

Treatment.—There are several anatomical features which must be borne in mind during the treatment of a fracture of the tibia. For example, the articulation at the ankle and knee must be restored to the normal position; otherwise a painful joint with disability may result. It is essential then that proper alignment be obtained in the anteroposterior, as well as the lateral plane. A mild degree of shortening is tolerated without detriment to the patient as far as function is concerned. However, a posterior bowing (*i.e.*, convexity posteriorly) is particularly disabling to the patient and for that reason it may be wise to overcorrect this deformity at time of reduction by producing a mild anterior angulation. Usually the fragments can be reduced manually without difficulty and molded into position with the patient under proper anesthesia. Flexion of the knee frequently facilitates reduction. If reduction is obtained, it is obviously important to maintain position of the frag-

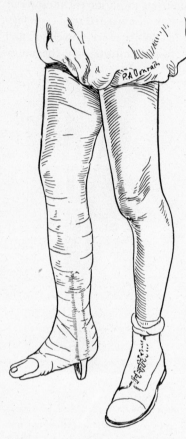

Fig. 276.—Skin (Unpadded) Cast with Metal Foot Piece Incorporated in the Cast.

This is particularly useful in patients with delayed union of the tibia and fibula as shown in Figure 275. The skin cast is often used as a primary form of treatment; its fixation is more secure and it permits ambulatory care.

ments while the cast is being applied. Care must likewise be taken to avoid medial and posterior bowing. The foot is placed at right angles to the leg and in mild inversion. If the fibula alone is fractured, immobilization in a plaster cast for three weeks should be sufficient to obtain solid union. However, if the tibia is fractured, immobilization in a cast must be maintained for at least eight weeks. Following this the patient is allowed to walk with crutches, weight-bearing being permissible and encouraged, particularly if a walking iron has been incorporated into the cast (see Fig. 276).

Occasionally, and particularly when both bones are fractured and complete dislocation of fragments exists, apposition of fragments cannot be obtained or maintained by simple reduction and the application of a plaster cast. In such instances it may be advisable to insert a Kirschner wire through or above the os calcis and secure constant traction to the stirrup connected with the wire. Traction by this means encourages correct alignment and maintains a correct position for the foot and ankle. It is particularly valuable in compound fractures with great destruction of tissue when open drainage and irrigation are indicated. Delayed union or nonunion is fairly common when the fracture of the tibia is located at the junction of the middle and lower thirds, presumably because of the obvious deficiency of blood supply at this point. For this reason, it is particularly important that the reduction of fragments in this area be accurate. If, after six to eight weeks of immobilization, there is no evidence of union, the deposition of callus may frequently be encouraged or hastened by allowing the patient to bear weight on the foot, providing, of course, a close-fitting plaster cast (skin cast) from the toes to the midthigh maintains position and alignment (see Fig. 276). This method may also be used as the primary procedure when displacement is not marked. Griswold [32] has emphasized the value of the ambulatory treatment with a nonpadded cast and walking iron, in fractures of the tibia and fibula, in the prevention of bone atrophy and nonunion. Satisfactory reduction and fixation can likewise be achieved by other types of apparatus as designed by Roger Anderson, Haynes and Stader.

Compound fractures occur more frequently in the tibia than in any other bone, chiefly because the tibia is subcutaneous over such an extensive area. If the break in the skin is small and there is reason to suspect that very little and unimportant contamination has taken place, the fracture may be treated as a simple fracture with reduction and application of a plaster cast or splint as indicated. However, if the bone has protruded, or if the wound is large and obviously seriously contaminated, thorough débridement must be done immediately unless contraindicated by serious injury elsewhere. Extreme care must be taken in the removal of foreign bodies, dead tissue, blood clots and small fragments of bone. After the fragments are reduced, the wound including the skin is closed. Rarely is a drain justified. Immobilization is then obtained by a plaster cast. A window may be cut in it at the site of fracture so that the wound may be inspected, only if fever or undue pain develops. If infection of serious consequence develops, it may be necessary to open the entire wound. If the injury is more than seven or eight hours old, but with no evidence of infection, débridement should still be carried out; the wound is then packed open with vaseline gauze (Orr [33]), and a plaster cast applied. In serious cases continuous traction with metal pins and some type of frame, may be indicated (see also p. 440). As discussed in the preceding chapter, the use of sulfanilamide and sulfathiazole (locally, by mouth, or both) is receiving considerable attention as a means of preventing infection in compound fractures. See also page 367 and Chapter XXXIII.

The Ankle.—Because of the relatively small size of the structures existing in articulations at the ankle and the great weight of the body, injuries in this region are common and usually produced by indirect violence. As will be discussed later in the text, injuries involving the joints (particularly of the tarsal bones) are most serious since permanent dysfunction due to pain is so apt to develop; position of fragments becomes very important in such injuries.

Pott's Fracture.—The term, Pott's fracture, is loosely applied to a variety of fractures of the lower end of the fibula and tibia about the ankle joint. The most common type consists of a fracture of the fibula an inch or two above the ankle and an avulsion of the tip of the internal malleolus. Most commonly the fracture is produced by a fall or impact in which so much strain is put on the foot in *eversion* (*abduction*) as to carry it beyond its normal range of motion. In this way the anterolateral border of the astragalus infringes on the external malleolus, producing a fracture (usually oblique) of the fibula an inch or two above the lowermost tip. If the impact or force is more severe, the strain is exerted on the internal lateral ligament which usually pulls off the tip of the internal malleolus (tibia) before rupturing it. Occasionally the fracture extends through the entire shaft of the tibia as well as fibula a few centimeters above the joint. This usually occurs, however, only when the trauma is quite severe. If the foot is also forcibly extended (*i.e.,* in plantar flexion) during the injury, a posterior fragment of the tibia may break off, including a considerable portion of that bone. Although the ligamentous attachment between the lower portion of the tibia and fibula is quite strong, there is a tendency toward tearing or stretching of this ligament with separation of the two bones and a mild lateral displacement of the astragalus. One type of deformity which is of extreme importance in Pott's fracture is a posterior dislocation of the astragalus, at the

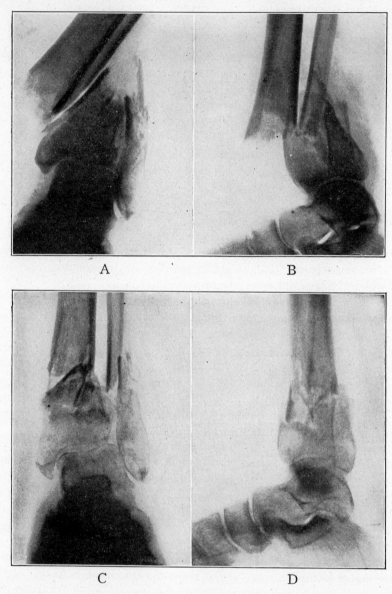

A   B

C   D

FIG. 277.—COMPOUND FRACTURE OF THE TIBIA AND FIBULA.

A and *B*, anteroposterior and lateral view before treatment which consisted of débridement, reduction and application of a plaster cast. *C* and *D*, three months after reduction; union is taking place. Two months later union had advanced sufficiently to allow weight bearing with crutches.

tibial articulation. This is particularly apt to occur if the injury is produced by forcible extension of the foot. Less commonly, a Pott's fracture is sustained by forcible adduction or inversion of the foot. In this case, the external malleolus is pulled away and the internal malleolus is broken by infringement of the astragalus. Occasionally the entire shaft of the tibia is broken.

The clinical manifestations of Pott's fracture are extremely variable. The cardinal signs of fracture (as described on p. 443) may be present, but if the fracture is limited to the fibula and not complete or displaced, the patient may be able to walk with only moderate difficulty. Local tenderness will, of course, be present over the external malleolus and perhaps over the lower border of the internal malleolus. However, there may be no way of differentiating this type of a fracture from a

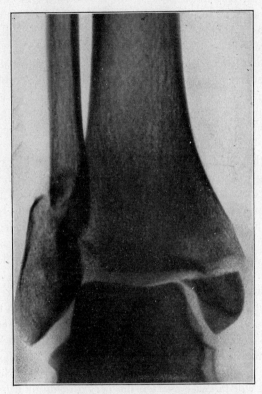

FIG. 278.—TYPICAL POTT'S FRACTURE.

Note the slight medial displacement of the proximal fragment of the fibula. The medial malleolus (of the tibia) is also fractured.

sprain without the aid of an x-ray, which should always be taken in such instances. There may be an obvious eversion or inversion deformity, depending upon the mechanism of fracture. If the fracture includes the shaft of the tibia, the patient will, of course, be unable to bear any weight whatever upon his foot, unless impaction exists. The backward dislocation of the astragalus may not be demonstrable, although the foot is almost always held in a position of extension (*i.e.,* plantar flexion). Part of the swelling about the ankle is accounted for by the bloody effusion into the joint which is no doubt of greater quantity than suspected. The swelling tends to mask deformity and obliterate the bony landmarks.

The *treatment* of Pott's fracture is simple, chiefly because reduction and immobilization are rarely difficult. If the fragments of the fibula buckle inward toward the tibia, or a chip of the internal malleolus is displaced downward, or if fracture of the tibia with displacement exists, reduction under anesthesia will be necessary. Much better results are obtained if reduction is performed as soon as possible after the accident, and not delayed until after the swelling becomes minimal, as was practiced by many surgeons years ago. Proper reduction consists primarily of inversion of the foot, traction upward and flexion of the foot to a right angle with the shaft of the tibia, and the application of a cast as mentioned above. It is important that an x-ray be taken after reduction to be sure that no deformity remains. Attention is directed particularly to posterior displacement of the astragalus because this type of deformity is so frequently overlooked. The simple procedure of placing the foot in a right-angled position tends to correct most of this deformity. Application of a plaster cast from the toes to the knee is the most desirable type of fixation; in fractures with marked displacement, the knee, too, must be immobilized. Anesthesia may be obtained by one of the gases or by injection of several cubic centimeters of 2 per cent procain into the joint and region of the fracture. If dislocation of fragments is slight no anesthesia will be necessary.

The toes must be watched carefully for numbness, tingling, coldness, paralysis, etc., because any great increase in swelling could easily interfere with the blood supply to such an extent as to jeopardize the structures distal to the obstruction. Since immobilization and proper reduction practically always relieve the pain of a fracture within a few hours, pain of more than a slight degree may warrant splitting or bivalving of the cast, thereby allowing room for excessive swelling.

If the fracture involves only the external malleolus (*i.e.*, the fibula), the cast may be removed in three weeks, the ankle strapped and bandaged, and weight-bearing allowed with crutches. If the shaft of the tibia is fractured, the immobilization should be maintained for eight weeks. Weight-bearing with the aid of crutches should be started cautiously. The application of heat by baking, etc., will frequently be efficacious in relieving the stiffness and chronic pain so frequently complained of in fractures about the ankle. Such measures will also tend to shorten the period of disability. The application of a skin cast with a walking attachment, one or two weeks after injury, will likewise shorten the period of disability.

Dislocation of the Ankle.—Posterior dislocation and a mild lateral dislocation may occur in Pott's fracture as already described. On rare occasions complete dislocation, usually posterior or lateral, may occur without fracture. Complete dislocation is usually accompanied by fracture of the external malleolus or tip of the tibia, perhaps both. Reduction of the dislocation is not difficult, but if there is much comminution of the tibia and fibula, considerable difficulty may be experienced in replacing these fragments. Immobilization must be maintained for four weeks, at least. If there has been an accompanying fracture of the entire shaft of the tibia, immobilization for a longer time will be required.

On rare occasions a dislocation of the ankle is *compound*. Treatment is not different from that of a compound fracture. As soon as possible, the wound is subjected to thorough débridement and irrigation, followed by reduction of the dislocation and closure of the wound. Immobilization is best obtained by a plaster cast, but

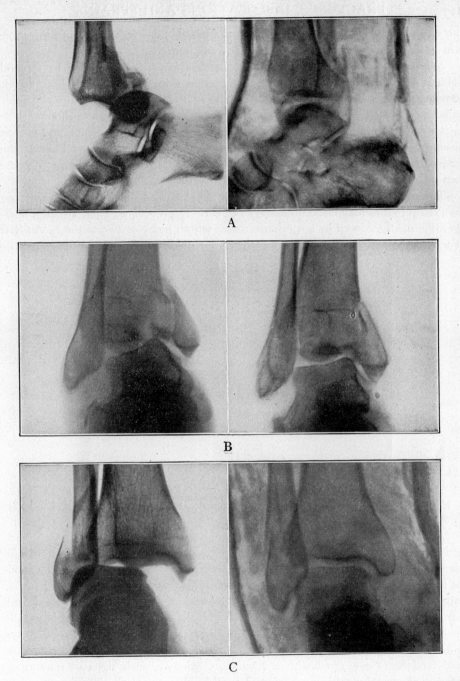

A

B

C

FIG. 279.—THREE TYPES OF DISLOCATION OF THE ANKLE.

Each (as is usually the case) is associated with a fracture. *A,* posterior dislocation, before and after reduction; *B,* slight medial displacement which must necessarily fracture the internal malleolus. In such fractures, it is important that the tilting of the axis of the tibio-astragaloid articulation be corrected. Reduction here is satisfactory, but not perfect; *C,* lateral dislocation, which necessarily must fracture the lower end of the fibula. Reduction is rarely difficult; fixation (in a plaster cast) with the foot inverted is an important feature in the treatment.

the wound must be observed closely for the possible development of an infection, which, if serious, may lead to gangrene and amputation.

Sprain of the Ankle.—This injury is almost invariably sustained by forceful plantar flexion and inversion of the foot beyond normal range of motion, and is commonly inflicted by throwing the weight of the body on the "turned" ankle usually after catching the heel on a stair, or stepping in a hole while running. The injury consists primarily of a tearing of the external lateral ligaments, and is thus produced by a force opposite to that producing a typical Pott's fracture. If the external lateral ligament resists tearing, the tip of the external malleolus may be torn off, constituting what is called a sprain fracture.

The pain inflicted by a severe sprain may be equally as severe as that produced by a fracture and may be so disabling as to entirely prevent walking. Usually, however, the pain produced by a sprain decreases within a day or two to the extent that at least a slight amount of weight-bearing is possible. Forcible pressure against the

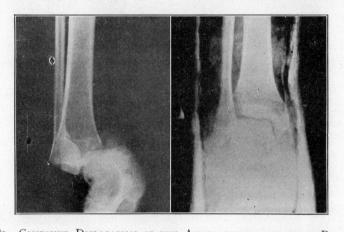

FIG. 280.—COMPOUND DISLOCATION OF THE ANKLE BEFORE AND AFTER REDUCTION.

Healing occurred without infection and the functional result was good. (St. Louis City Hospital.)

heel does not produce appreciable pain when a sprain is present, but is quite painful when there is an associated fracture of consequence. Swelling of the soft parts about the injured ligaments occurs within a few hours and a variable amount of ecchymosis will develop. This ecchymosis is usually less extensive than that associated with a fracture. The joint not infrequently fills with fluid or blood, but this is usually indicative of injury to the joint structures. The *tenderness associated with a sprain is apt to be diffuse* over the injured external lateral ligaments, in contrast to the local tenderness associated with a fracture. Obviously, such signs of fracture as crepitus, abnormal mobility and deformity will be absent. The disability sustained by a sprain is usually not so severe as that associated with a fracture, particularly in regard to weight-bearing, etc. On a few occasions, however, a badly sprained ankle will produce a painful joint for many weeks or months in contrast to the relatively short duration of pain after a fracture confined to a minor bone.

The type of *treatment* is variable, depending upon the severity of the injury. If the patient is seen immediately after injury, the application of cold packs for an hour or two combined with complete rest of the part may lessen the amount of hemorrhage and exudation of serum. The most important feature, however, is immobilization of the joint. Strapping with adhesive in an overlapped fashion until the entire joint and lower third of the leg are encased in an adhesive splint is usually quite efficient. Elastic adhesive (Elastoplast) is comfortable and effective. This immobilization should be carried out with the foot in the position of right angled flexion and eversion so as to afford rest for the external lateral ligament which is usually the ligament torn in a sprained ankle. If the internal ligaments are torn, as happens only occasionally, the foot should be immobilized in inversion. After two or three days' rest the patient may begin to walk about, using a cane or a crutch as indicated. The application of heat for thirty to forty-five minutes, two or three times a day, encourages hyperemia and is efficient in relieving the pain and promoting healing. The patient should not be encouraged to increase the activity of the joint beyond the production of pain, especially during the first ten days when healing is taking place. The adhesive splint usually becomes loose after four or five days and must be reapplied. It should be worn as long as pain is experienced during walking and as long as it affords appreciable relief. When the sprain is severe, immobilization with an adhesive splint will not relieve the pain and it will be obvious within twenty-four hours that more secure fixation is necessary. In this case the application of a light plaster boot for a week or even more will not only decrease the pain, but it will promote healing and allow the patient to walk comfortably with the aid of crutches. After the plaster cast is removed (seven to ten days) the ankle is strapped and the patient allowed to walk more and more each day, depending upon the amount of disability. Obviously the treatment of a sprain should not be undertaken without thoroughly excluding fractures, particularly by x-ray.

The Foot.—*Fractures of Tarsal Bones.*—These injuries consist of those to the tarsal bones, metatarsal bones and phalanges. Fractures of the tarsal bones include chiefly the astragalus, os calcis and scaphoid, and they are usully sustained by a fall in which the foot receives the impact. The type of fracture varies from a single line to a comminution or crushing. The manifestations are so atypical that an accurate diagnosis can rarely be made without an x-ray. Tenderness may be diffuse, as is also ecchymosis and swelling. Walking is very painful, if possible at all. Treatment consists of molding of the fragments into position if possible, and immobilization in a plaster cast for four weeks or more. All fractures of the tarsal bones are serious because of the frequency of permanent disability, due to pain. This is particularly true of fractures of the *astragalus* (*talus*), which are so often followed by persistent pain that many surgeons advise arthrodesis (to promote ankylosis) as the primary treatment immediately after the injury. Occasionally astragalectomy will be necessary when considerable comminution is present and union fails to take place. Fractures of tarsal bones are common in the Navy during wartime, being sustained when a torpedo explodes below decks (see Chapter XXXIII).

Fracture of the *os calcis* is apt to be sustained in such a way that flattening of the arch results. It is a frequent injury most common in roofers and painters who fall from a height, striking on their heels. This is an extremely disabling fracture and should be corrected as completely as possible. The flattening of the foot is due to force transmitted to the calcaneus by the wedge shaped portion of the talus. The calcaneus is crushed and spread laterally, the lateral fragment or fragments coming to rest beneath the lateral malleolus and compressing the structures which pass behind and beneath the malleolus. Marked comminution is a rule, with fracture

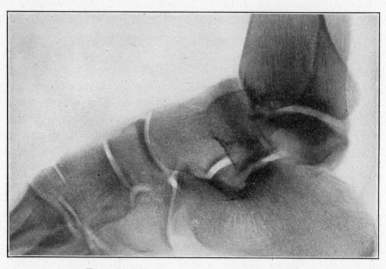

FIG. 281.—FRACTURE OF THE ASTRAGALUS.

Because of the universally poor results associated with comminuted fractures of this bone, astragalectomy was performed in this patient a few days after injury.

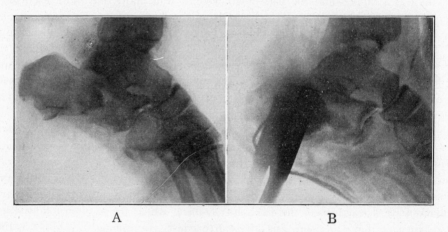

A   B

FIG. 282.—FRACTURE OF THE OS CALCIS.

A, note the usual, but mild, upward displacement of the portion of os calcis to which the Achilles tendon is attached; *B*, correction of deformity by insertion of a wire through the os calcis, and application of traction. (Courtesy Dr. J. E. Stewart.)

lines running into and distorting the astragulocalcaneal joint. The posterior portion of the os calcis is forced upward and held by the tendo Achilles. Böhler [34] has laid great stress upon the tuberosity-joint angle, otherwise known as the salient angle. This is the angle between a line drawn from the upper part of the tuberosity of the calcaneus to the highest point of the bone and another from the anterior angle to the highest point. These two lines normally make an angle open posteriorly of 20 to 40 degrees. Following flattening of the bone in fractures, this angle becomes zero or even negative. Böhler regards restoration of this angle as of primary importance in treatment. Reduction of the fracture requires strong traction by a pin or wire through the upper portion of the os calcis, combined with pressure on both sides to reduce the spreading and the impingement of fragments upon the structures below and behind the lateral malleolus. Traction or skeletal fixation in plaster should be maintained for at least 8 to 10 weeks. Careful weight bearing in a skin tight cast may be permitted after this time. Neglected or unsuccessfully treated fractures may require operative removal of bone from beneath the lateral malleolus and fusion of the astragulocalcaneal joint to reduce the disability from traumatic arthritis.

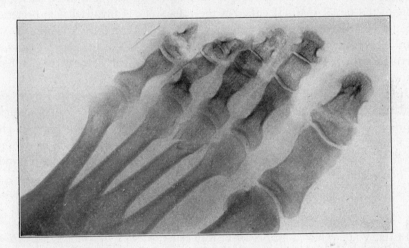

FIG. 283.—FRACTURE OF THE DISTAL END OF THE THIRD METATARSAL BONE, THE TERMINAL PHALANX OF THE GREAT TOE, AND THE PROXIMAL PHALANX OF THE FOURTH TOE.

Dislocation of the tarsal bones may occur, but is uncommon. The astragalus is the bone most often affected. If a severe blow is sustained on the ball of the heel while the foot is plantar flexed, the astragalus may be thrust completely out of position. So much difficulty may be experienced in exerting enough traction on the foot to allow for replacement of the bone that section of the tendo achillis may be necessary.

Fractures of the Metatarsal Bones.—Fractures of these bones are not infrequent, but dislocation is extremely uncommon because the metatarsals articulate with the tarsals at different levels. Any one of the metatarsals (perhaps most commonly the second and fifth) may be fractured at any point in its shaft. The distal end of the bone is apt to be displaced anteriorly. Walking is rarely possible on account of pain. Swelling and ecchymosis may be mild. Displacement of fragments can and should be corrected by manipulation under anesthesia. Immobilization by a plaster cast extending to the upper third of the leg is usually the most logical treatment, although occasionally adhesive strapping and crutches will offer sufficient immobilization.

After three weeks, weight-bearing may be allowed. Nonunion and persistent pain are uncommon. "March" fracture, which involves the metatarsal bones and is sustained so commonly during the strenuous period of military training, is discussed in Chapter XXXIII.

Fractures and Dislocations of the Phalanges.—Fractures of the phalanges of the toes are common. The distal phalanx of the first and fifth toes are the ones most commonly affected. The injury may be of a crushing type, but more often the patient gives a history of having stubbed his toe in the dark. The pain experienced at the time of injury is usually severe. Local tenderness is pronounced; pressure against the end of the toe is invariably extremely painful. Ecchymosis almost always develops after a few hours. The treatment is unsatisfactory, considering the fact that the injury is so trivial. When the fracture involves the first toes, it is best to apply a well-padded thin splint extending from beyond the tip of the toe back past the middle of the tarsal shaft. If either of the other toes is involved it is preferable to strap the injured toe to the one medial to it. In either case, however, it will be painful, if not impossible, to wear a shoe. On such occasions it may be necessary to use crutches for ten or fourteen days. Union is quite firm at three weeks, but pain upon walking may be pronounced for many weeks.

Dislocations of the phalanges are usually confined to the great toe and consist of dorsal dislocation at the metatarsophalangeal joint. They are readily reduced by sharp flexion and simultaneous pressure downward at the base of the first phalanx until it slips over the head of the metatarsal. If the flexor tender has slipped in between the metatarsal head and the phalanx, reduction may be impossible and open reduction required.

BIBLIOGRAPHY

1. BLAIR, V. P. Quoted by Brown in *Key and Conwell's Fractures, Dislocations and Sprains,* C. V. Mosby Co., St. Louis, 1942.
2. KANTHAK, F. P. Fractures of the Zygomatic Bone, *Surgery,* 7:796, 1940.
3. BROWN, J. B. Fractures of the Jaw and Related Bones of the Face, in *Key and Conwell's Fractures, Dislocations and Sprains,* C. V. Mosby Co., St. Louis, 1942.
4. SCHULTZ, L. W. A Treatment for Subluxation of the Temperomandibular Joint, *J. Am. M. Ass.,* 109:1032, 1937.
5. BROOKES, T. P. Dislocations of the Cervical Spine, *Surg., Gynec. & Obst.,* 57:772, 1933; Fractures and Dislocations of the Cervical Spine, *J. Am. M. Ass.,* 109:6, 1937.
6. CRUTCHFIELD, W. G. Fracture Dislocation of the Cervical Spine, *Am. J. Surg.,* 38:592, 1937.
7. BECK, C. S. Contusions of the Heart, *J. Am. M. Ass.,* 104:109, 1935.
8. CONWELL, H. E. Fractures of the Clavicle, *J. Am. M. Ass.,* 90:838, 1928.
9. NICOLA, T. Recurrent Anterior Dislocation of the Shoulder. A New Operation, *J. Bone & Joint Surg.,* 11:128, 1929.
10. GRISWOLD, R. A., GOLDBERG, H., and JOPLIN, R. Fractures of the Humerus, *Am. J. Surg.,* 43:31, 1939.
11. GRAHAM, H. F. An Efficient Method for the Reduction and Immobilization of Colles' Fracture, *Ann. Surg.,* 108:156, 1938.
12. TAYLOR, G. W., and PARSONS, C. G. Fractures of the Lower End of the Radius, *Surg., Gynec. & Obst.,* 69:249, 1938.
13. DAVIDSON, A. J., and HORWITZ, M. T. An Evaluation of Excision in the Treatment

of Ununited Fracture of the Carpal Scaphoid, (Navicular) Bone, *Ann. Surg.*, 108:291, 1938.

14. JOSTES, F. A. Backache: Manipulative Treatment without Anesthesia, *J. Bone and Joint Surg.*, 20:990, 1938.

15. LEADBETTER, G. W. A Treatment for Fracture of the Neck of the Femur, *J. Bone & Joint Surg.*, 15:931, 1933.

16. SMITH-PETERSEN, M. N., CAVE, E. F., and VANGORDER, G. W. Intracapsular Fractures of the Neck of the Femur, *Arch. Surg.*, 23:715, 1931.

17. WESTCOTT, H. H. A Method for the Internal Fixation of Transcervical Fractures of the Femur, *J. Bone & Joint Surg.*, 16:372, 1934.

18. MOORE, A. J. *Internat. S. Digest.*, 19:323, 1935; *Surg., Gynec. & Obst.*, 64:420, 1937.

19. CUBBINS, W. R., CALLAHAN, J. J. and SCUDERI, Carlo. Fractures of the Neck of the Femur. A New Incision and a New Director for the Use of a Simplified Flange, *Surg., Gynec. & Obst.*, 68:87, 1939.

20. CALLAHAN, J. J. Fractures of the Neck of the Femur; Five Year Collective Review, *Surg., Gynec. & Obst.*, 68:411, 1939. (Int. Abst. Surg.)

21. SPEED, Kellogg. Fractures of the Neck of the Femur, *Ann. Surg.*, 96:951, 1932.

22. PHEMISTER, D. B. Fracture of the Neck of the Femur, Dislocations of the Hip, and Obscure Vascular Disturbances Producing Aseptic Necrosis of the Head of the Femur, *Surg., Gynec. & Obst.*, 59:415, 1934; The Pathology of Ununited Fractures of the Neck of the Femur, *J. Bone & Joint Surg.*, 21:681, 1939.

23. MAGNUSON, P. B. Report of Fifty-nine Consecutive Cases of Ununited Fracture of the Neck of the Femur, *Surgery*, 7:763, 1940.

24. McMURRAY, T. P. Fracture of the Neck of the Femur Treated by Oblique Osteotomy, *Brit. M. J.*, 1:330, 1938.

25. SCHANZ, A. Ueber die Nach Schenkelhalsbrüchen Zuruckbleibenden Gehstörungen, *Deutsche med. Wchnschr.*, 51:730, 1925.

26. ROWLETTE, A. P., HASLEM, J. R., SIEGERT, R. B., MORRIS, H. D., and KEY, J. A. Results Obtained by Subcutaneous Pinning of Fractures Through the Neck of the Femur, *J. Am. M. Ass.*, 107:1610, 1936.

27. WEINER, D. O. Unpublished Observations (In Press).

28. GRISWOLD, R. A. A Positive Treatment for Fracture of the Shaft of the Femur, *Surg., Gynec. & Obst.*, 60:848, 1935.

29. RUSSEL, R. H. A System of Traction for the Legs of Children, *Brit. J. Surg.*, 11:491, 1924.

30. HEY-GROVES, E. W. The Crucial Ligaments of the Knee: Function, Rupture and Treatment, *Brit. J. Surg.*, 7:505, 1919.

31. GALLIE, W. E. and LeMESURIER, A. B. Reconstruction of Ruptured Crucial Ligaments of the Knee, *Ann. Surg.*, 85:592, 1927.

32. GRISWOLD, R. A. Fracture of Both Bones of the Leg, *J. Am. M. Ass.*, 104:35, 1935. Double Pin Skeletal Fixation in Fractures of the Leg, *Surg., Gynec. & Obst.*, 68:573, 1939.

33. ORR, H. W. The Treatment of Fractures by Means of Skeletal Devices, *J. Am. M. Ass.*, 98:947, 1932.

34. BÖHLER, Lorenz. *The Treatment of Fractures*, Wm. Wood and Co., Baltimore, 1936.

35. BROWN, J. B., McDOWELL, F. Internal Wire Fixation for Fractures of Jaw, *Surg., Gynec. & Obst.*, 74:227, 1942.

36. McKIBBIN, W. B. An Ambulatory Method of Treatment for Intertrochanteric Fracture, *Surg., Gynec. & Obst.*, 76:343, 1943.

37. DOBBIE, R. P., and RYERSON, S. The Treatment of Fractured Patella by Excision, *Am. J. Surg.*, 55:339, 1942.

38. LEWIS, K. M., BREIDENBACH, L., and STADER, O. The Stader Reducton Splint, *Ann. Surg.*, 116:623, 1942.

CHAPTER XIX

THE ORGANS OF MOVEMENT:
BONE, JOINT, BURSA, TENDON AND MUSCLE

Bones	*Tendons*
Joints	*Muscles*
Bursae	*Miscellaneous Lesions*

Serious disability is commonly due to disease of the organs of movement, not only because they are subject to frequent injury and infection, and are involved in systemic disease, but also because of the dense rigid structure and relatively poor blood supply of some of them, particularly bones and joints; this last factor probably accounts for the slow and often imperfect power they have to overcome the effects of disease. Of special importance too is the tendency for bone, joint and muscle to suffer from serious disability through rest or disuse. Since immobilization is an important aid in treatment, particularly of injuries and infections, it is obvious that such deleterious changes are to be prevented if possible. The term *atrophy of disuse* is used to describe the changes which follow prolonged immobilization. These changes include atrophy of muscles, decalcification of bone, and stiffness and even fibrous ankylosis of joints. They begin very soon, but are apparent only after a few weeks, and become pronounced after months. Care should be taken in each case to utilize only a sufficient period of rest to allow healing without inducing atrophy of tissues. This is often a difficult problem because the healing of bone and joint injuries, and especially infection, frequently requires many weeks and months and sometimes years. Though bones, joints, etc., are not vital structures and are not often the seat of diseases which endanger life, they play an important part in our social-economic structure. Diseases of these organs are frequent causes of loss of time in industry and constitute the main basis for workmen's compensation laws. They, therefore, have a great medicolegal importance.

Many of the diseases discussed in this chapter are to a large extent of orthopedic nature. Detailed descriptions may be found in textbooks on orthopedic surgery, particularly those of Osgood and Allison;[1] Shands and Raney;[2] and Whitman.[3] Of the various lesions which affect the organs to be described in this chapter, pyogenic infection and injury are perhaps the most important.

BONE

Bone is subject to traumatic, neoplastic, infective and constitutional diseases. The traumatic group, *i.e.,* fractures, have been considered in the preceding chapters. Bone tumors are discussed in Chapter XVI.

Pyogenic Osteomyelitis.—This infection of the bone may be considered in three groups, acute (primary), secondary and chronic osteomyelitis.

1. *Acute Osteomyelitis.*—As a primary infection acute osteomyelitis is not uncommon in childhood, but is rare in adult life. It is a hematogenous infection of bone due to the staphylococcus, occasionally the streptococcus which is considered separately. Not infrequently the infection seems to arise from some obvious pre-

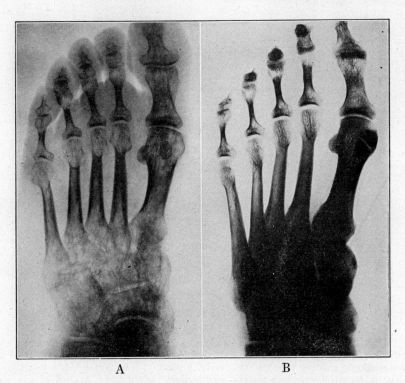

A　　　　　　　　　　　B

FIG. 284.—BONE ATROPHY AND NORMAL FOOT.

A, bone atrophy revealing extreme decalcification in the foot of a forty-eight-year-old man after prolonged immobilization because of an infected compound fracture of the leg; *B,* a normal foot of a man of the same age for comparison.

existing lesion such as a furuncle, septicemia, otitis media, etc., but more commonly through some occult or unknown portal of entry. There is frequently a history of injury at the site of the infection, but its etiological importance is unestablished. The organisms lodge in the marrow cavity of the metaphysis, presumably because the end capillaries at the epiphyseal line turn sharply and slow the blood current sufficiently to allow the bacteria to gain a foothold and multiply. The resulting acute inflammatory reaction being in the closed bony structure develops extreme pressure and causes intense pain and disability. The infection spreads by penetration through the cortex or extends into the medullary cavity. It rarely if ever breaks through the epiphyseal line into the epiphysis, but penetrates the cortex through the Haversian canals, a process which usually takes a number of days. In any case pus finds itself under the periosteum which it strips away from the bone, thus forming a subperiosteal abscess which sooner or later ruptures into the overlying soft tissue and ultimately forms a subcutaneous abscess. Of greatest significance in this process is the actual amount of bone infected and killed by the disease. This is not apparent until later, but it determines the further course of events. In the severe cases when the infection involves the whole medullary cavity, the entire shaft may become necrotic. On the other extreme the infection may break through the cortex so soon

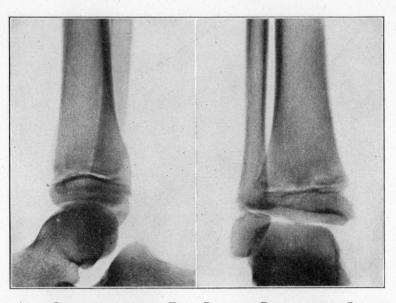

FIG. 285.—ACUTE OSTEOMYELITIS OF THE TIBIA, REVEALING ROENTGENOLOGIC CHANGES WHICH ARE BARELY DETECTABLE.

Lateral and anteroposterior views. The changes in density are slight but can be seen just above the epiphyseal line. The disease started apparently five days previously. It is unusual for roentgenologic changes to occur this early. Operation was performed a few hours after admission. A huge subperiosteal abscess was encountered; a large amount of pus was also present in the medullary cavity. Adequate drainage was instituted and a plaster cast was applied. Extensive destruction of bone had already taken place at the time of operation; this is apparent from the bone involvement which ultimately showed up in the x-ray (see Fig. 288). Staphylococcus was the causative organism.

(or with the aid of the surgeon's drill) that very little bone is killed. Although the infection rarely penetrates the epiphyseal line, it may precipitate a pyogenic arthritis by entering the joint from without after pus has appeared under the periosteum and extended from this point into the joint.

After several weeks, reparative processes are apparent though they really begin much earlier. These steps are first the separation and partial phagocytosis of necrotic bone which becomes demarcated from the viable cortex and is called *sequestrum*. Secondly, nature begins to build new bone to take the place of that destroyed by the infection. Osteogenesis occurs from the lifted up periosteum and probably begins early, although it cannot be seen roentgenologically for two or three weeks. This new bone is called *involucrum;* it eventually becomes dense, hard, rich in calcium, and replaces the necrotic bone. It develops in the presence of the sequestrum and even while the tissue is bathed in pus, regardless of whether treatment has been instituted or not. On rare occasions the infection does not extend or penetrate, but forms a localized lesion in bone and is called *Brodie's abscess* which ordinarily develops insidiously, and is really a manifestation of chronic osteomyelitis. From the primary bone lesion, metastatic foci may develop and it is not uncommon for several bones to become infected one after the other. In a few unfortunate children this succession continues for years so that eventually most of the long bones become the site of osteomyelitis. The bones commonly involved in order of their frequency are, tibia, femur, humerus, radius, ulna, fibula and the metatarsal bones. Abnormal lengthening of the affected bone occurs in many children after many months and is apparently due to the increased blood supply, the hyperemia at the epiphyseal line augmenting local bone growth.

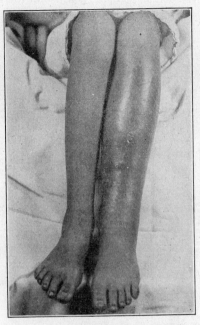

Clinical manifestations are general and local, the former being those of general septicemia with fever, chill, leukocytosis, rapid pulse and prostration. The extreme pain always seems to make the prostration more marked, at least in the first day or two of the disease before the infection has broken through the cortex. In adults the general reaction is apt to be less severe; subacute and chronic forms are more frequently encountered in which the infection develops slowly. The local signs and symptoms in the typical acute case are those of a deep seated infection. The pain is severe and located over the end of the bone close to the joint. While muscle spasm is present to a slight extent, the joint can be moved somewhat without increasing the pain. Acute tenderness over the involved bone on deep palpation is one of the earliest signs. In eliciting this tenderness the bone is carefully

Fig. 286.—Neglected Acute Osteomyelitis in a Twelve-year-old Girl.

The patient was treated as a case of "rheumatism" for four weeks before admission. X-ray showed involvement of the entire shaft of the tibia. As can be seen from the photograph, the leg was literally a "bag of pus"; this was confirmed at operation when a large quantity of staphylococcus pus was evacuated.

palpated, starting at some distance from the lesion which is approached gently and gradually in a manner similar to that used in the detection of point tenderness over a fracture. The overlying tissues may be swollen and edematous, but the skin itself is not red or tender during the early stage of the disease. If the infection has been present for several days there may be evidence of a local abscess, *i.e.,* swelling, redness, local heat and fluctuation.

Streptococcus osteomyelitis differs considerably from osteomyelitis produced by the staphylococcus. The former infection much more commonly occurs as a metastatic invasion of the bone from a primary source such as otitis media, mastoiditis, etc. The manifestations of the streptococcus osteomyelitis are apt to develop more insidiously than the staphylococcus infection. The pain is not so severe; swelling and subcutaneous suppuration develop more slowly and less commonly. There is less destruction of bone; sequestration is therefore less marked. Many such lesions will subside under proper conservative care without gross suppuration. They are particularly prone to occur in infants.

Diagnosis, though more difficult when the patient is seen early, should be made as soon as possible, because of the need for prompt surgical treatment. The diseases

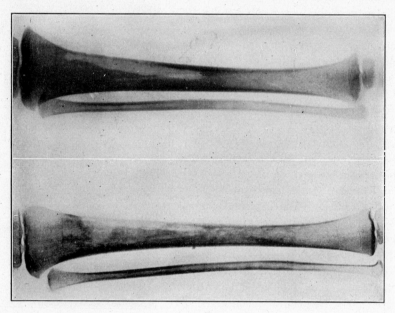

FIG. 287.—ACUTE OSTEOMYELITIS DUE TO THE HEMOLYTIC STREPTOCOCCUS IN A THREE-YEAR-OLD BOY.

There was pain in the leg and fever of twenty-four hours' duration before admission. Because of the atypical nature of the infection, operation was delayed until five days later; the periosteum was edematous and of a dusky pink color and from a hole drilled through the cortex on the diaphyseal side of the epiphyseal line, exuded a dirty gray fluid from which the streptococcus was cultured. More of the cortex was removed releasing more infected fluid. Above, x-ray after operation showing the amount of bone removed. Below, x-ray two months later; note the absence of sequestration. Healing was complete but was complicated by respiratory infections and cervical lymphadenitis (see Fig. 341).

which may be confusing are acute rheumatic fever, acute pyogenic arthritis and acute cellulitis; the first and third do not demand immediate operation and hence must be excluded (see page 471). X-ray is disappointing because the earliest roentgenologic evidence of acute osteomyelitis is absorption of bone which ordinarily is not demonstrable a week or more following the onset. Involucrum formation is seen when calcium becomes deposited under the elevated periosteum and requires at least two weeks. Sequestration may not be demonstrable for an even longer period. The local signs and symptoms are, therefore, of greatest importance and should be carefully noted, and examination repeated at short intervals if necessary.

Treatment in acute osteomyelitis depends on the causative organism which should be identified as early as possible by blood culture, and by the patient's age.

In general, operation is urgent in older children with staphylococcus, and delayed or unnecessary with streptococcus infection especially in infancy; the latter is discussed on page 460. The principles of treatment are first, lowering the mortality, second, minimizing the extent of bone destruction. General measures for septicemia are obviously important and include general rest, immobilization of affected extremity, large fluid intake, sedation, etc. Specific therapy including chemotherapeutic drugs are discussed on page 35. In the case of staphylococcus osteomyelitis in older children operation may be delayed if the systemic manifestations are severe, in order to improve the general condition; otherwise operation should be carried out as soon as the diagnosis is made. Unlike pyogenic infection of soft tissue the surgeon does not wait until pus forms; in this respect the situation is similar to that in acute tenosynovitis, acute pyogenic arthritis and felon. The necessity for early operation depends on the anatomical location of infection within dense unyielding bone; drainage of the pent-up inflammation not only minimizes the amount of bone destroyed, but of more importance it lessens the tendency of extension to other foci. It should be stated, however, that a number of surgeons have become dissatisfied with the operative therapy in acute staphylococcic osteomyelitis and have advised only the nonoperative measures just mentioned, except for incision of subcutaneous abscess. While this conservative therapy may be advisable in infants, older children do much better with a simple osteotomy, particularly when judgment is exercised in regard to (1) operability as just outlined and (2) the extent of the osteotomy as described below.

The operation in acute osteomyelitis is not an extensive procedure, consisting merely of simple decompression of the infected metaphysis. A general anesthetic is necessary and a tourniquet is applied to the extremity if possible. The end of the bone is exposed because the infection is in the metaphysis; drill holes are made, therefore, close to the epiphyseal line which must not be injured because of the danger of producing nongrowth.[4] On the other hand, if the bone is drilled too far from the epiphyseal line the metaphysis may be missed, or, still worse, the open medullary cavity of the diaphysis may be entered with spread of the infection to the entire shaft. At most the bone between such openings may be removed to permit more ready drainage but extensive resection of cortex is unnecessary and may prove deleterious in the very ill children. Pus is ordinarily encountered immediately on incising the periosteum, or mixed with the blood escaping from the drill holes. In early cases the amount of pus may be so slight as to be seen with difficulty; culture of the sanguinous fluid will, however, reveal the staphylococcus. The wound is left wide open by the insertion of vaselin packs and the extremity immobilized. Frequent dressing is to be condemned because it is so painful and deleterious. Orr[5] has popularized the idea of immobilization of the extremity in a plaster cast. The effectiveness of this method has been established by clinical experience and is presumably due to the local and general rest afforded. The application of a cast obviates the need for dressings since the cast is left in place three or four weeks, and is then changed or removed entirely. The draining secretions soak through the cast and soon become the source of an obnoxious odor. An excellent detailed discussion of acute osteomyelitis may be found in a report by Miller.[6]

As suggested already, the treatment in streptococcus osteomyelitis is much more conservative than in the usual staphylococcus infections. Operation is frequently delayed even when a localized destruction of bone is observed in the x-ray. Incision of superficial abscesses which may develop is obviously indicated. Conservatism is particularly indicated in infants regardless of the organism involved; the hazard of an anesthesia and even of a simple osteotomy is often sufficient to create a very high mortality. The basis for this point of view is well presented by Green and Shannon [26]. The conservative treatment consists of local and general rest, a large fluid intake, repeated transfusions of blood containing specific immune bodies, and especially the adequate use of chemotherapy.

2. *Secondary Osteomyelitis.*—This is a type of bone infection occurring as an infection arising not primarily in the bone, but elsewhere, such as that due to compound fractures (see p. 367). Secondary osteomyelitis of the jaw often develops

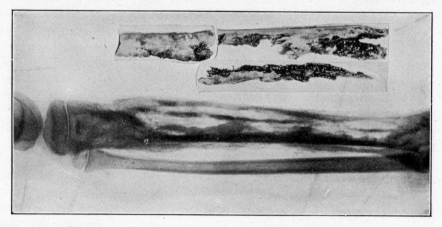

FIG. 288.—CHRONIC OSTEOMYELITIS IN A SIX-YEAR-OLD BOY.

The early stage in this patient is presented in Figure 285. The x-ray film illustrated was taken three months after the first operation and just before sequestrectomy. A photograph of a portion of the sequestra which were removed is also shown. A cast was reapplied; two months later the wound was almost completely healed by granulation.

by extension from a cellulitis about a tooth. If the tooth is pulled at the improper time, osteomyelitis is particularly prone to develop and may lead to a fatal septicemia (see p. 652). The terminal phalanx becomes the site of osteomyelitis following a neglected felon. The other phalanges are frequently infected secondarily from acute suppurative tenosynovitis. Osteomyelitis of the tarsus is sometimes secondary to penetrating infections and may eventually involve the entire foot. Amputation is often necessary as a last resort. The patella and olecranon are sometimes involved by direct extension from an overlying lesion. Osteomyelitis of the skull is secondary to compound fracture or neglected sinusitis. Osteomyelitis is always suspected when an abscess or infected wound located near bone fails to heal, and forms a chronic draining sinus. X-ray may enable one to make a definite diagnosis. During the acute stage treatment is that of the primary lesion. Treatment in the chronic stage is that of chronic osteomyelitis as outlined below. In general, radical surgery is to be avoided. The dead bone or sequestrum is sometimes absorbed or discharged spontaneously, thus allowing healing to occur. However, in many instances it will be necessary to remove the sequestrum by operation.

3. *Chronic Osteomyelitis.*—This lesion is the outcome of acute or secondary osteomyelitis which has resulted in necrosis of bone. Its severity depends on the extent of bone killed by the infection which, as already stated, is influenced to a large extent by the promptness of operation in the acute stage of the primary disease. An extremity which is the site of chronic osteomyelitis shows considerable muscular and bone atrophy and exhibits one or more draining sinuses leading to

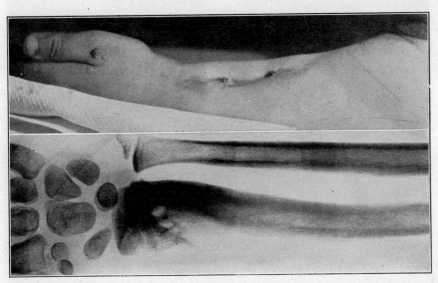

FIG. 289.—CHRONIC OSTEOMYELITIS OF THE RADIUS IN AN EIGHT-YEAR-OLD BOY, AS OBSERVED NINE MONTHS AFTER ONSET.

The operation for the acute infection was performed ten days after onset; x-ray was entirely negative at this time. The wound discharged small sequestra from time to time, and one large one was removed operatively, represented by the bone defect in the x-ray. The photo represents the almost healed incision; the patient is allowed full use of the arm and atrophy has completely disappeared.

diseased bone. X-ray will reveal the extent of the lesion and often will clearly demonstrate the site and size of sequestra.

Treatment of chronic osteomyelitis is to a large extent conservative. When the infection involves a long bone of an extremity, protection of the limb is important to avoid the danger of fracture before a strong involucrum forms. This, indeed, is all that need be done in most patients. Small sequestra are often discharged from time to time or are absorbed. However, as long as dead bone remains, it acts as a foreign body and permanent closure of the sinus will not occur. Operation for removal of sequestra may be carried out as soon as there is roentgenologic evidence that separation between the dead and living bone is well under way and that there is a well developed involucrum. Operation may also be necessary to drain abscesses or cavities which have formed since the initial osteotomy, or as a primary manifestation (Brodie's abscess). Such operations, however, should rarely be extensive except when the dead bone to be removed involves nearly all of the diaphysis. Healthy bone is resected only to remove loose sequestra or to open and drain residual abscesses; saucerization to eliminate dead spaces is, however, justified. Wounds are left wide open, packed with vaselin gauze, and a plaster cast applied. It should also be emphasized that operation is not indicated merely because a chronic sinus is present, since such an operation may be useless and damaging, unless a sequestrum is found and removed, or an abscess drained. Moreover, in adults such sinuses tend to heal, al-

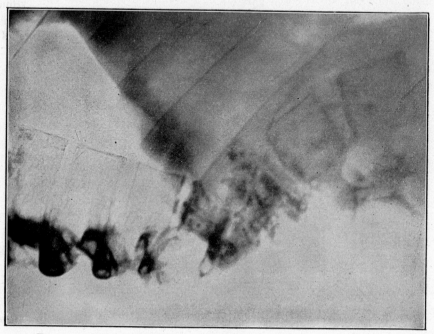

Fig. 290.—Tuberculosis of the Spine; Lateral View of Pott's Disease of the Eleventh and Twelfth Dorsal Vertebrae in a Thirteen-year-old Girl.

Note the destruction of the bodies of the vertebrae and the marked angulation. However, no signs of spinal cord pressure were present. The disease started six years previously with a reputed injury followed by persistent pain in the back. The child's complaints were minimized until an x-ray revealed the true diagnosis six months later. Following the unsuccessful use of more conservative measures spine fusion was performed. This operation is an ankylosing procedure which immobilizes the spine by creating a bony arthrodesis between the articular facets and also between the dorsal spines. (Courtesy Dr. F. A. Jostes.)

though several weeks or months may be required. In children healing takes place less readily (perhaps because of a lesser immunity to the organism during childhood), the sinus occasionally persisting until adult life. However, with proper care and judicious sequestrectomy many of these infections will heal early.

The use of maggots as a therapeutic agent in the treatment of chronic as well as acute osteomyelitis was instituted originally by W. S. Baer,[7] and has been advocated by a number of other surgeons. It has not, however, received general acceptance as a routine method of therapy.

Tuberculosis of Bone.—The distinction between tuberculosis of the bone and of the joint is not always clear since the tubercle bacillus often seems to attack both structures together (see p. 473). In the *spine* (Pott's disease) it starts in the anterior part of the vertebral body, destroying it, producing a deformity (gibbus, kyphosis). Occasionally a cold abscess is formed which, in tuberculosis of the lumbar spine, may burrow along the psoas muscle and present in the groin as a psoas abscess. It does this so silently that the fluctuant inguinal mass may be mistaken for a hernia. The cervical spine is also involved and may be associated with a cold abscess of the neck. Occasionally abscess of the spine produces pressure on the cord, and a spastic paralysis ensues. The head of the *femur* is also frequently involved, especially in children, but the clinical manifestations are so distinctly referable to the joint that it will be included under joint disease. Another favorite site of bone tuberculosis, in Negroes at least, is the sternal end of the *clavicle*.

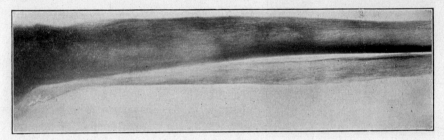

FIG. 291.—SYPHILITIC PERIOSTITIS IN THE TIBIA.

Note the surface irregularity, particularly in the proximal portion of the bone. The patient, a forty-three-year-old woman, had pains in the legs and also had luetic ulcers.

Tuberculosis of bone heals by fibrous replacement or by ankylosis when joints are involved. The disease responds slowly to treatment, which is largely an orthopedic problem and consists of immobilization and general hygiene. It should be emphasized that as a rule healing is best achieved by ankylosis of the adjacent joint surfaces involved. (See also under Tuberculosis of the Joints.)

Syphilis of Bone.—Three types of disease are recognized. (1) Syphilitic periostitis consists merely of a thickening of the periosteum with a roughening of the bone and is commonly seen in the tibia. Local pain and tenderness, especially at night, are complained of in syphilitic periostitis and the x-ray may show characteristic changes. (2) A hyperplastic form occurs commonly in the sternum and the sternal end of the clavicle or the clavicle itself, simulating tuberculosis, particularly in Negroes in whom the two diseases are common. It also occurs in the shafts of long bones as a hypertrophy of the cortex and may simulate Paget's disease. (3) A destructive form (gumma of bone) is seen in the shaft of long bones and in the skull. In the x-ray it may simulate primary bone tumor, metastatic carcinoma or pyogenic osteomyelitis. Diagnosis of bone syphilis is aided by the x-ray and particularly by the finding of a positive Wassermann. Treatment is medical (antiluetic therapy).

Miscellaneous Diseases.—These comprise the following: (1) *Rickets* is less common than formerly and has a surgical interest only in that it causes deformities in the long bones, especially "bow legs" and "knock knees." If the deformities persist in spite of medical treatment, osteotomies may have to be done to correct them.

(2) *Osteochondritis deformans juvenilis* (Legg-Perthes-Calve's disease, coxa plana), is a disease of the upper femur affecting children between five and ten years of age and often confused with tuberculosis. Pain is slight, a limp followed by atrophy occurs and there is seen in the x-ray a progressive flattening of the head of the femur which is characteristic of the disease. Treatment consists of immobilization followed by a walking caliper splint. A similar lesion has been described in the tibial tubercle (Osgood-Schlatter's disease), and in the tarsal scaphoid (Kohler's disease). Diagnosis is made by x-ray. Treatment consists of immobilization when pain is present. (3) *Scurvy,* now a rare disease, is due to vitamin C deficiency and is manifested by bleeding from the gums, tenderness and swelling of the bones about the joints. Subperiosteal hemorrhage is common and in many instances is a source of the pain. The roentgenogram is characteristic. Treatment is dietetic. (4) *Osteomalacia* is probably also due to dietary deficiencies. It is observed mostly in women. The bones become soft, lose much of their content of calcium, are subject to fracture and deformities. Pain and

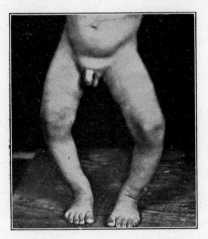

FIG. 292.—BOW LEGS DUE TO RICKETS.

Prevention of this as well as other bony deformities due to rickets is largely a pediatric and orthopedic problem. Osteotomy for correction of deformity as depicted above is carried out only after healing of the active disease has been achieved.

stiffness are noted. Treatment is symptomatic and dietetic (vitamin D). (5) *Paget's disease* (osteitis deformans) is characterized by enlargement and distortion of bones, by pain in the limbs, by a decrease in the height, and by an increase in the size of the head. The condition is uncommon. It has a long course and begins insidiously during middle life; the changes in the skeleton are usually general but they are occasionally confined to a few bones, notably the skull and legs. Roentgenograms are characteristic; areas of softening as well as increased density are noted. The tibiae are much thicker than normal and bowed laterally. The vertebrae are also compressed apparently from the weight of the body. Spontaneous fractures sometimes occur; malignant changes have been observed. The etiology is unknown and the treatment is merely palliative. (6) *Fragilitas ossium* (brittle bones, osteopsathyrosis, osteogenesis imperfecta) is a rare disease of bones manifested by the presence of multiple fractures after slight trauma. It may be present soon after birth, persist into, or be noted first in childhood. Many cases are associated with blue sclerae. The etiology is obscure. There is no treatment except protection of the extremities to avoid trauma. Spontaneous cure often occurs with the advent of adolescence. (7) *Achondroplasia* (dyschondroplasia) is a rare deforming disease of the shafts of bone which softens and shortens them due to the formation of osteoid tissue which has little calcium and contains cartilage. It occurs in childhood and leads to distortions of all kinds and to spontaneous fractures. (8) *Chondroplasia foetalis* is apparent at birth and is a complex disturbance of bone formation which causes dwarfism, deformities and a square, large head. (9) Although the muscle paralysis resulting from *poliomyelitis* constitutes perhaps the most serious complication of the disease (except mortality) *bone shortening* takes place and may be sufficient to prevent restoration of proper function even though muscular deficiencies have been corrected. To combat the disability incident to the shortening,

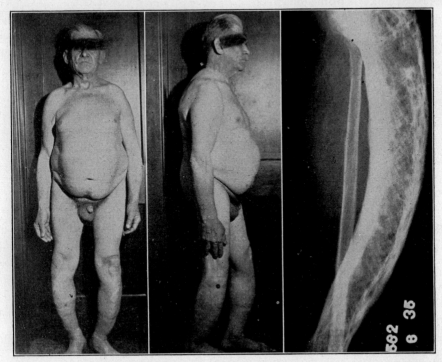

FIG. 293.—PAGET'S DISEASE OF THE BONE; WELL ADVANCED STAGE IN A SEVENTY-YEAR-OLD MAN.

The disease was of slow, almost imperceptible development. In the photographs note how relatively long the arms are; this is due to an actual shortening of the skeleton produced by a collapse of a vertebra and a bowing of the long bones of the lower extremities. The characteristic x-ray appearance of the disease may be observed in the roentgenograms of the lower leg; note the bowing and overgrowth of the cortex, which, however, is composed of soft osteoid tissue and not true bone. (Courtesy Dr. W. B. Gnagi, Jr.)

Abbott [8] has devised a very ingenious method of lengthening the bones of the leg by operative means. Obviously this method could be utilized for bone shortening resulting from various causes (see also Wilson & Thompson, *Ann. Surg.*, 110:992, 1939).

JOINTS

The anatomical structures involved in joint disease consist of the articular (cartilaginous) joint surfaces and the synovial membrane which is a continuation of the cartilaginous layer forming a closed (joint) cavity. The synovial membrane is composed of modified fibrous tissue cells or mesothelium which secrete mucilaginous fluid thereby lubricating the joint surface. It is reinforced on the outside by a supporting layer of dense fibrous tissue called the *joint capsule*. Outside the joint are the ligaments, tendons and muscles which are attached to the bone on either side and which are more important than the capsule in lending stability to the joint. In some joints there are additional structures such as the semilunar cartilages and cruciate ligaments of the knee, and the round ligament of the hip which also help in the proper function of the joint.

Traumatic Joint Disease.—Injury to joints alone, aside from dislocation, is probably rare because the associated structures such as tendons, ligaments, muscles and bone are nearly always involved in trauma of any consequence. Thorough exam-

A   B

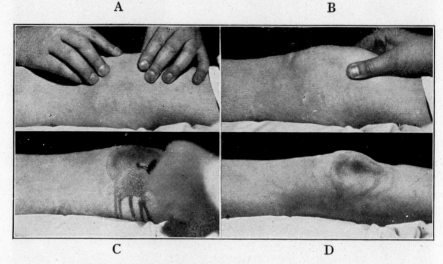

C   D

Fig. 294.—Acute Traumatic Synovitis in a Seventy-year-old Man after Being Struck
by a Motorcycle.

A, the method of demonstrating a patellar click; the index finger of the right hand presses the "floating patella" against the femur. *B*, note the obliteration of the normal bony landmarks of the knee joint by the fluid contained within the joint; the examining fingers detect a definite sense of fluctuation. *C*, aspiration of the joint; nearly 100 cc. of bloody fluid was obtained. The blood pointed to joint damage and an x-ray revealed a tiny but definite fracture into the joint without displacement. *D*, after aspiration; note the normal contour of the knee.

ination is therefore important in order to arrive at a correct anatomical diagnosis. The term acute traumatic arthritis is applied to various injuries which are described separately below.

1. *Acute Traumatic Synovitis.*—This lesion is descriptive of the reaction of the joint itself to injury and consists of the development of *swelling, pain, limitation of motion and muscular spasm.* The same reaction occurs to a lesser extent when normal joints, immobilized for many weeks, are first used, especially if the alignment of an associated fracture has been faulty or other structural defects are still present. The same signs are seen in the early hours of an infection. Fluid in the joint cavity (hydrops, hydroarthrosis) is one of the first signs of synovitis and is manifested clinically in the superficial joints by swelling, obliteration of the normal bony landmarks and by a sense of fluctuation on palpation. In the knee the fluid lifts the patella from its normal contact with the femur (floating patella) which can often be shown by pressing it against the femur producing an audible or palpable click.

In the hip and shoulder these signs may be obscured by the overlying muscle; comparison with the opposite side may be helpful.

Aspiration of the joint is the surest and sometimes the only way of detecting fluid in the synovial cavity and serves the added advantage of revealing the kind of fluid present. If it is blood, proof of hemorrhage is obtained. Investigation of the fluid microscopically and bacteriologically is often useful and important. Blood should be removed from a joint because of the danger of limitation of motion which may result from incomplete absorption of blood clots. Aspiration of fluid may also serve a therapeutic purpose in relieving the pain and swelling when it is severe. Pain, however (in the absence of fracture or sprain) is not apt to be severe. When pain is severe there is usually an associated lesion of bone, ligament, or tendon which is ordinarily detectable by local tenderness. Limitation of motion is usually due to pain and associated muscle spasm, but is also due in part to fluid in the joint. Muscle spasm is a protective reaction which serves to splint the injured part and is prominent in many joint diseases, both acute and chronic. It is sometimes elicited only on movement.

Before *treatment* of joint injury is instituted, injuries to bone and cartilage must be excluded since they may demand special treatment. The key to the spontaneous recovery of simple acute traumatic synovitis is the resorption of the fluid which ordinarily takes but a few days and indicates a subsidence of the inflammatory process. During this time rest and firm bandaging of the joint are advisable. As soon as the pain subsides voluntary motion is started, but weight-bearing is best postponed for at least a week or two. Cold, in general, limits edema due to trauma when applied early (in the first hour or two) though heat, by promoting the circulation, aids in its resorption once swelling develops. Cold or heat may be used for the relief of pain depending to some extent on the preference of the patient.

2. *Laceration of Joint Capsule.*—The treatment of lacerations involving the joint capsule is, in reality, the same as that of any deep wound as already discussed in Chapter X. If the injury is recent, and exploration and débridement is indicated, the wound is treated thoroughly, the joint cavity carefully inspected and irrigated, then the joint capsule *closed without drainage.* If twenty-four hours or more have have elapsed since injury, and infection is already present, conservative measures such as immobilization, cleanliness and perhaps traction are indicated; insertion of drains into joint cavities is as a rule to be condemned.

3. *Rupture of Ligaments (Sprain).*—Sprains are to be suspected in every severe injury about the joint, especially if there is excruciating tenderness over the ligaments and not over the bone. Severe pain which develops on specific motions only, also suggests a sprain if a fracture is not present. Detailed consideration of sprains will be found in Chapters XVII and XVIII.

Sacro-iliac and lumbosacral sprains are special types of sprain and frequently cause back pain and often serious disability. They are discussed in more detail on page 419. Local muscle spasm, tenderness and pain on movement are the most important clinical signs and may develop after a slight or nonapparent trauma or exertion. Indeed, injury to lumbosacral and sacro-iliac joint ligaments is nearly always difficult to demonstrate; in this sense the designation of sprain is perhaps inaccurate. They represent, moreover, an especially difficult group of cases in workmen who have suffered lower trunk injuries because of the variety of lesions produced and the frequency of malingering. Sacro-iliac and lumbosacral sprains are to be distinguished from coccygodynia and various types of synovitis, neuritis, sciatica and bursitis in the region of the back and hip. A detailed discussion of the differential diagnosis may be found in a report by Brahdy.[9] Treatment consists of immobilization which is more readily accomplished in sacro-iliac than in lumbosacral sprains and if effective in relief of pain supports the diagnosis. Immobilization is performed by firm circular adhesive bandage or a specially designed belt which immobilizes the pelvis. Cure is often difficult and recurrences are common. Manipulation sometimes is effective. Many of the chronic types are due to defective posture which may be improved by exercises of various kinds.

4. *Injury to Cartilage.*—At the time of injury it is sometimes impossible to detect evidence of trauma to cartilage which may only become apparent later because chronic joint disability develops. When a fracture extends into a joint, as shown by x-ray, the joint cartilage is obviously injured. In such an instance the fluid in the joint will be bloody and will be demonstrable by aspiration. Severe injuries of this type are best treated by suspension and traction rather than immobilization in a plaster cast, even if there is no displacement of fragments. Aspiration of blood and early motion are also advisable. Treatment of any associated fracture is obviously important.

Injury to the semilunar cartilage of the knee is a special type and may consist of a dislocation or actual rupture or tearing. Injury to the semilunar cartilage frequently follows a severe sprain because of the intimate attachments of this cartilage to the joint capsule and ligaments. The internal semilunar cartilage is most commonly involved, especially following severe twisting and hyperextension of the knee such as catching the foot in a hole while running. The injury may consist of a detachment, tear, or crush. If the cartilage is merely displaced, complete extension may be impossible and the usual local signs of acute injury will develop with severe pain and local tenderness. "Locking" of the knee with inability to extend the joint is a frequent manifestation. Occasionally considerable clear, straw-colored fluid accumulates in the joint. Replacement often occurs spontaneously or may sometimes be achieved by careful flexion and rotation of the tibia, with or without anesthesia, and is evident by the ability to completely extend the leg. The knee is then treated like acute synovitis except that in severe cases immobilization in plaster may be necessary. If, after six weeks of non-operative therapy, symptoms persist, especially pain and instability, the damaged cartilage should be removed although operation should not be postponed over a year after the injury (Cravener and MacElroy [25]). Rupture of the *cruciate ligaments* of the knee sometimes occurs and is to be suspected when abnormal mobility in the anteroposterior direction is elicited. The treatment is prolonged immobilization. Frequently, a stabilized joint can only be obtained by operative repair of the torn ligament, preferably immediately after the accident.

5. *Chronic Joint Lesions.*—Acute injuries to joints and cartilage sometimes give rise to such lesions as chronic synovitis, chronic traumatic arthritis and joint mice. (a) *Chronic synovitis* is an ill-defined term applied to a recurrent and persistent development of pain, swelling and fluid in the joint, particularly after exertion. When chronic synovitis develops after trivial injury, tuberculous disease

of the joint is to be suspected. Often it occurs following trauma with injury to cartilage or because of malunion of an associated fracture. Occasionally an unsuspected joint mouse is responsible. In many cases the cause is to be sought in repeated trauma or perhaps in insidious types of infection. Villous arthritis is a form of chronic synovitis in which the synovia proliferates to form numerous projections or villi into the joint. It may develop spontaneously without previous injury, is most common in older individuals and may be present without symptoms or at most may cause "rheumatic" pains. It is manifested clinically by puffiness about the joint, commonly the knee, and a crepitation on motion and sometimes by fluid in

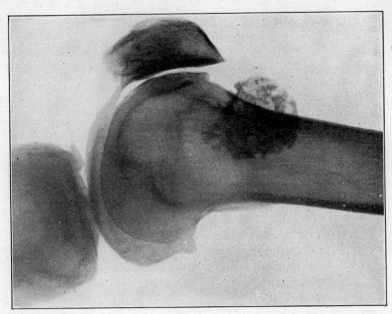

FIG. 295.—JOINT MOUSE OF UNUSUALLY LARGE SIZE IN THE KNEE OF A SIXTY-SEVEN-YEAR-OLD MAN.

Symptoms of mild pain in the knee were not sufficient to justify arthrotomy. There was no history of trauma.

the joint. (b) *Traumatic arthritis* is really a type of synovitis as just discussed except that the symptoms of pain, swelling and disability clearly follow, and are due to a preceding injury (see also p. 466), and are aggravated by use of the part. (c) *Joint mice* are loose bodies in the joint which are composed of fragments of cartilage or bone which becomes covered with cartilage, and which move freely about inside the joint cavity. They may give rise to pain, swelling and disability (often in attacks) by their mechanical interference with joint movements. They are frequently the result of previous joint disease or injury. Loose bodies in the joints are also produced by spontaneous detachment of segments of the articular cartilage and underlying bone (osteochondritis dissecans) or by actual neoplastic growths from the synovial membrane (osteochondromatosis). X-ray usually reveals these loose fragments when they contain bone or calcified areas. Operation for their removal is often indicated when symptoms are sufficiently severe.

Joint Infections.—The effect of pathogenic bacteria on joints are varied and depend on the causative organism. Since all parts of the joint are usually affected, the lesion is really an arthritis.

1. *Acute Pyogenic (Suppurative) Arthritis.*—The joint is not infrequently infected with pyogenic bacteria from without by penetrating wounds, from adjacent osteomyelitis, or most commonly *from the blood stream* as a hematogenous infection. In the latter case evidence of disease elsewhere, such as a pneumonia, endocarditis, otitis media, septicemia, etc., is frequently present. However, the joint involvement

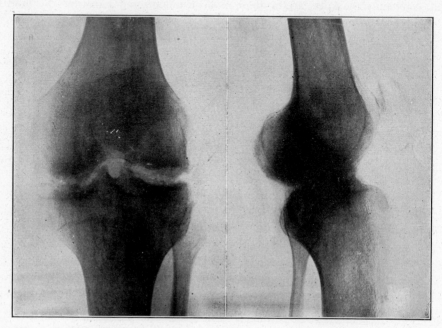

Fig. 296.—Complete Ankylosis of the Knee due to Suppurative Arthritis.

X-rays (anteroposterior and lateral views) taken six months after the onset; the infection has completely subsided. The patient, a healthy eighteen-year-old schoolboy, was treated conservatively in a hospital for several weeks; late in the course of the infection several abscesses were opened above the knee, extensions no doubt of pus breaking through the suprapatellar bursae. Note the complete bony ankylosis; an arthroplasty was done with partial restoration of motion.

may be the first manifestation and occasionally the only site of disease. Like osteomyelitis the disease is most commonly encountered during childhood. The streptococcus, staphylococcus and occasionally the pneumococcus, are the organisms most frequently responsible for the infection. The gonococcus produces a special type of arthritis which is considered separately. The inflammation begins as an acute synovitis, the joint filling with thin, slightly turbid fluid which contains many bacteria and leukocytes of the polymorphonuclear type. As the infection progresses the cellular elements increase so that after a few days frank pus may fill the joint cavity. Of serious importance is the early involvement of the cartilage which is attacked directly and destroyed. On some occasions the loss of cartilage may include most of the articular surface. Pressure of the opposing surfaces aids in destruction of cartilage as pointed out by Phemister.[10] As the inflammation subsides, these denuded areas become filled with granulation tissue, and since this cartilage does not regenerate, the raw areas eventually become united with each other across the more or less obliterated joint space with either fibrous or bony tissue. This end stage of repair leaves the joint in a state of immobility or ankylosis, which if bony, results in absolute immobility, but if fibrous may be only partial.

Clinical manifestations are local and general, the latter being those of septicemia as already described. The degree of fever and prostration may be great and often overshadows the local lesion. Pain is severe and localized to the joint, but is especially excruciating on the slightest attempt to move the joint. Tenderness is also marked and is sometimes so severe that the weight of the bed clothes cannot be borne. Associated with the pain is extreme muscle spasm of the adjoining muscle groups which splint the joint in a fixed position, usually in slight flexion. In hip joint disease flexion is accompanied by abduction and external rotation, a position which corresponds to the greatest relaxation of the joint capsule. Swelling, heat and hyperemia are localized to the region of the joint. In superficial joints the swelling is characteristically confined to the joint cavity which is easily apparent because of the obliteration of the usual bony landmarks. Frequently there is also a prominent superficial swelling due to edema of the subcutaneous tissue overlying the joint. Aspiration is an important procedure, especially in the deeper joints such as the shoulder and hip, in order to establish the existence of joint fluid. Moreover, the examination of such fluid by smear and culture is essential for final diagnosis. Smears may reveal the presence of the organisms; segmented leukocytes also tend to brand the lesion as an acute pyogenic infection. Roentgenologic manifestations occur late, and are due to destruction of cartilage as evinced by obliteration of the normal clear area between the ends of the bone.

Differential diagnosis of suppurative arthritis from acute rheumatic fever, acute osteomyelitis and acute cellulitis is important because of the difference in the type of treatment required. *Acute rheumatic fever* is accompanied by acute joint manifestations for which operative interference is not indicated; the joints are usually involved several at a time in this disease and the general reaction, while marked, is not as severe as in acute pyogenic arthritis; the presence of cardiac signs and symptoms and the more subacute nature of the disease are also helpful. *Acute osteomyelitis* does not cause much joint tenderness or muscle spasm; there is no joint fluid or swelling; limitation of motion is less pronounced; the tenderness, while close to the joint, is located distinctly over the bone. *Acute cellulitis* over the joint may be confusing, and is important to recognize, since treatment of it is conservative and distinctly nonoperative (see p. 48). Usually the superficial location of the redness and swelling accompanying cellulitis is so localized as to be characteristic. Red streaks (acute lymphangitis), when present, point to acute cellulitis since they are absent in the deeper infections. Similarly, regional lymphadenitis, which practically always accompanies acute cellulitis, is absent in infections of the bone or joint, at least in its early stages. The typical joint effusion is absent in acute cellulitis; muscle spasm and limitation of movements are not apt to be present.

Treatment of acute pyogenic arthritis is particularly directed toward avoidance of necrosis to cartilage; this is best accomplished by surgical drainage of the infected fluid *as soon as the diagnosis is made*. Aspiration alone, as a therapeutic procedure, in a large number of cases at least, is an inadequate method of drainage. But if this procedure is chosen it should be repeated frequently. More efficient is *actual incision* into the joint for drainage, which is then maintained by suture of a small rubber drain in place down to the capsule to prevent closure of the wound. The decision to institute drainage depends upon the clinical signs and on finding frank pus; however, even if the pus is thin, the presence of organisms in the stained smear is usually sufficient to warrant operation for drainage. The advantage of irrigating the joint cavity with various solutions has not been established. The application of heat to maintain hyperemia should be continued after operation. Moist warm dressings for a day or two promote drainage. Protection of the joint in a splint is appreciated by the patient to guard against movement which is very painful. Slight traction with Buck's extension also relieves pain considerably and minimizes necrosis of the cartilaginous surface of the bones (Phemister[10]). Harris[11] reports that as a result of arthrostomy with fixation and extension, one-half of his cases in children recovered with normal joint movement. A contrasting view is that of Willems[12] who, as a result of his war experiences, advised early active motion after arthrostomy. However, in suppurative arthritis as encountered in civil life, particularly in children, the lesion is probably different in nature; early active motion is hardly advisable, although it should be urged as soon as subsidence of the pain permits. Inge and Liebolt[13] found the best prognosis followed early arthrostomy and drainage, with institution of mild active and passive motion. The course of the disease is apt to be long and require several months before final healing takes place; great variations in severity, however, are encountered. The use of chemotherapy (see page 35) should precede operation and be continued after operation. When considerable destruction of cartilage has occurred and ankylosis is inevitable, it is important to assure a good position for the fixed joint, *i.e.,* one which gives a maximum usefulness and a minimum of disability (see p. 479). Months after the infection has subsided motion in the ankylosed joint may be restored by various types of arthroplasty.

2. *Gonococcal Arthritis.*—There is usually a history of an acute urethritis or cervicitis preceding the joint lesion by several weeks. It occurs only in adult life and does not follow juvenile vaginitis. While several joints may seem affected at the onset, serious manifestations generally localize in only one. The disease is thus usually mono-articular involving, in order of frequency, the knee, wrist, elbow, shoulder, hip and ankle. The constitutional reaction is confined to fever and leukocytosis, prostration being rare; as in gonorrhea elsewhere toxemia is not prominent. The tenderness and pain over the joint are exquisite so that sometimes even jarring of the bed is feared by the patient. However, great variations in the severity of the infection occur, the lesion varying from a simple serous synovitis to actual suppuration with destruction of cartilage. In the former instance satisfactory restoration of joint function may be expected; in the latter, bony or fibrous ankylosis is the rule. The course of the disease may be prolonged for many weeks before subsidence of the acute manifestations. It may be difficult in the early stages to determine the course of the infection. This inconsistency in the progress of the disease undoubtedly accounts for the wide diversity in method of treatment. In

many cases, especially the milder types, conservative care is adequate. However, in the suppurative type incision and drainage may be indicated. Most forms of treatment used previously have now been displaced by artificial fever therapy and chemotherapy, both of which are as effective in treatment of gonococcal arthritis, as in other forms of gonorrheal infection, including salpingitis, etc. Of great importance in cases ending in bony ankylosis is a useful position of the joint (see p. 479).

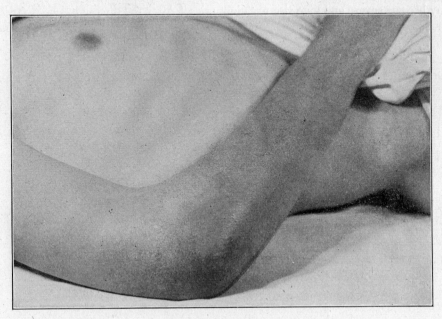

Fig. 297.—Gonococcal Arthritis of the Elbow.

A mild case with spontaneous recovery in a twenty-six-year-old male. Onset two weeks previously; aspiration revealed thin serosanguinous fluid from which the gonococci were grown in pure culture. Patient discharged three weeks later with full function.

3. *Tuberculous Arthritis.*—This lesion is not uncommon in childhood and is a frequent cause of disability and crippling. While constitutional signs and symptoms, such as loss of weight and afternoon fever may be present, the disease not infrequently seems to present only local manifestations in a joint. Whether the bone or joint is the primary point of infection in joint tuberculosis is still a considerably disputed question. A most thorough study of 82 cases of hip joint tuberculosis in children and adults has been made by Hatcher and Phemister.[14] In many of their cases this question could not be answered at all. In 26 the bone bordering on the joint seemed to be the beginning of the infection. In 9 very early cases only the synovia was involved, but the authors mentioned could not be sure that a small bone lesion was not also present. A "cold abscess" occurs late in joint tuberculosis, but an effusion into the synovial cavity is usually present, which is often called "white swelling" because of the absence of acute signs. The hip and knee are commonly affected, but the ankle, shoulder and elbow are also often involved. Years ago before the days of dairy inspection and pasteurization the infections were usually of bovine origin.

The onset is often gradual and insidious. Pain is always present, but may be slight, and is often referred to another joint. Thus the pain associated with tuberculosis of the hip is often referred to the knee. Limping, however, may be the first apparent symptom. In the superficial joints swelling is nearly always apparent. Aspiration will reveal the existence of fluid. There is a gradual atrophy of the adjacent muscles which are tense and spastic. At night when they relax the pain may become severe and give rise to "night cries." After the disease has been present for some time, marked atrophy of bone becomes apparent. Eventually deformity

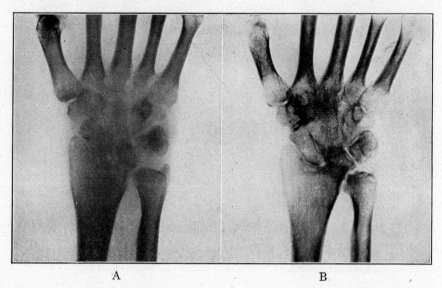

A   B

FIG. 298.—GONOCOCCAL ARTHRITIS OF THE WRIST IN A TWENTY-SEVEN-YEAR-OLD WOMAN.

There was a definite history of genital infection with identification of the organism from the cervix. *A,* x-ray seven weeks after onset of pain and swelling which was severe and disabling. Note the obliteration of joint markings indicating destruction of cartilage. Two periods of artificial fever each of four and one-half hours' duration produced prompt and lasting relief of symptoms; *B,* x-ray four months later; note the bony ankylosis, especially between the radius and lunate bone. The patient, while free from pain and swelling, has a partial limitation of motion. (Courtesy Dr. Peter Heinbecker.)

may develop as a result of the destructive process. If drainage of a cold abscess is established, either spontaneously or by incision, the resultant sinus may drain for months or years. Because of the paucity of clinical manifestations in early cases, diagnosis is often difficult, but is aided by the following procedures: (*a*) tuberculin test, especially in younger children, if positive, is valuable; if negative, tends to exclude tuberculosis at any age. (*b*) X-ray is negative early in the disease, but later shows generalized bone atrophy as compared with the opposite side, and an irregular fuzzy appearance with ill-defined joint outlines. Destructive bone changes are marked only in the more advanced cases. In the spine a lateral view will show erosion of the anterior margin of the vertebral bodies, and destruction of intervertebral discs. Characteristic of bone tuberculosis is the absence of new bone formation in the x-ray; in this respect it differs from pyogenic and luetic infections. (*c*) The joint fluid may be aspirated and produce the disease after injection into a

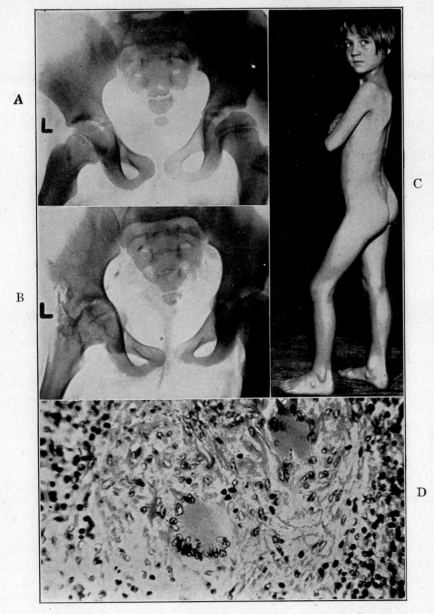

FIG. 299.—TUBERCULOSIS OF THE HIP IN A SEVEN-YEAR-OLD GIRL.

For several months the patient complained of pain and stiffness in the left hip followed by an increasing limp. *A*, the x-ray at this time was negative; nevertheless an operation was performed and a biopsy of the capsule revealed tuberculous tissue on microscopic section. The joint was immobilized in a cast; *B*, x-ray, one year later, shows marked changes and beginning ankylosis; *C*, photograph on admission; note the flexion at the hip and atrophy of the calf on the affected side; *D*, photomicrograph of the biopsy specimen showing typical giant cells.

guinea-pig. It rarely shows bacilli on smear. (d) Arthrotomy with biopsy of the synovia may be the most reliable method of diagnosis. This may be justified in order to start therapy as early as possible.

Treatment includes both operative and nonoperative procedures. The former consists of the production of a bony ankylosis by intracapsular or extra-articular arthrodesis, depending on the age of the patient and the joint involved. Osteotomy for correction of deformity associated with spontaneous ankylosis is also occasionally indicated. Amputation may be indicated when extensive tarsal disease, particularly when secondary osteomyelitis of the tarsus, is present. Radical therapy of this type is especially indicated if rapid economic rehabilitation is necessary. Non-

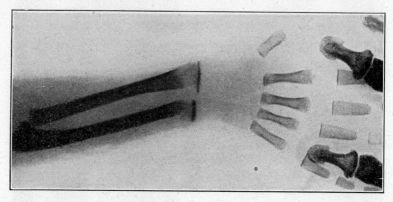

FIG. 300.—SYPHILITIC OSTEOCHONDRITIS IN A THREE-WEEKS-OLD NEGRO INFANT.

Note the increased density along the epiphyseal line. The term "syphilitic epiphysitis" is often applied to the disease. The term "pseudoparalysis" is sometimes used because of the disability produced. The name of Parrott is also associated with this lesion. Although only one wrist is shown in the above photograph the same appearance was noted on the opposite side and in both lower extremities. The mother noted a swelling of the infant's wrists which were painful and tender; a history of a fall was suspected. The Wassermann was strongly positive and after 2 antiluetic treatments the pain and swelling disappeared.

operative treatment consists of immobilization by plaster cast or appliances and general hygienic and dietary measures including heliotherapy. Cold abscesses associated with bone and joint tuberculosis should be treated conservatively; most of them will become absorbed spontaneously following treatment of the primary lesion. Aspiration may be necessary in certain cases, particularly to relieve pressure symptoms or to forestall spontaneous drainage.

4. *Syphilitic Arthritis.*—Two forms are described, one of which is the osteochondritis of infancy which is sometimes the first evidence of congenital syphilis. A history of trauma is not infrequent and the joint is swollen and tender and clinically simulates an acute infection. The x-ray shows characteristic changes in the epiphysis; the Wassermann reaction is positive. It responds to antiluetic treatment though immobilization is necessary for symptomatic relief of pain. The second form of syphilitic arthritis is the painful joint encountered in the secondary stage and is often confused with tuberculosis. The Wassermann reaction is helpful. Treatment is entirely medical (antiluetic therapy). Charcot joints, though of syphilitic origin, are discussed on page 478 under the heading of neurotrophic joints.

Spondylolisthesis.—This lesion consists of a forward displacement of the bodies of one of the lumbar vertebra on the ones beneath; the most common is the fifth which slips forward over the sacrum. The etiology is supposedly due to fracture of the neural arch at birth. Clinical manifestations include pain and weakness in the lower back and inability to bend forward. Examination reveals a striking lordosis; diagnosis is aided by lateral roentgenograms to show the characteristic displacement. Treatment is supportive, manipulative and operative.

Arthritis Deformans.—This designation includes both atrophic and hypertrophic or degenerative arthritis, and comprises a great class of chronic joint disease, always multiple, usually occurring in older individuals, but often attacking

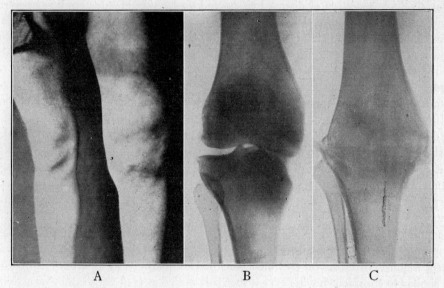

A B C

FIG. 301.—CHARCOT JOINT IN A FIFTY-FIVE-YEAR-OLD TABETIC.

A, note the enlargement of the left knee which was almost a "flail" joint, *i.e.,* movable in all directions without sufficient stability to avoid disability; *B,* anteroposterior x-ray of the joint; *C,* x-ray four months after arthrodesis, showing bony union between tibia and femur.

younger persons and exhibiting a great variety of clinical forms. This indicates that there are either many different diseases grouped under this term or that the disease, if it is a clinical and etiological entity, manifests itself in widely divergent ways, *i.e.,* either acute or chronic and with or without systemic reaction. When the process is acute, and fever and prostration are present, the disease is called infectious arthritis, but *must not be confused,* however, with the acute pyogenic infections already mentioned. Pathologically, the disease exhibits hypertrophic forms in which there is proliferation of the fibrocartilage outside the joint (Heberden's nodes) as well as fibrous tissue and bone; in other cases the joints become atrophic or ankylosed. Although various bacteria have from time to time been isolated from the joints of these cases the cause is still undetermined. One group is called Still's disease and occurs largely in childhood. Further discussion of the various types of the disease and their treatment may be found in medical and orthopedic monographs on the subject.

Neurotrophic Joints.—This term is applied to the so-called Charcot joint which occurs as a manifestation of tertiary syphilis, but may be seen in other diseases of the spinal cord such as syringomyelia. It is a slowly developing, painless, degenerative lesion, although the manifestations may seem to appear acutely. Especially characteristic are the hypertrophic changes which most frequently attack the knee, but also the ankle, foot, hip, spine, shoulder and elbow. The earliest sign may be periarticular edema, but in the late stages the swelling which is due to degenerated collapsing bone and overgrown fibrous tissue and cartilage may be enormous. Pain is absent; instability of the joint is the usual complaint. Treatment may be conservative, *i.e.,* support of the insecure joint by appliances if possible, or operative, *i.e.,* resection of diseased tissue and production of a bony ankylosis.

Constitutional Joint Diseases.—These comprise, according to Allison's classification,[15] gout, hemophilia, hysterical joints and intermittent hydrops. (1) Gout, now a rare disease, is due to the deposition of sodium urate around joints (and also in the cartilage of the ear as tophi). It is most frequent in joints of the great toe and causes episodes of severe pain and disability with relief of symptoms between attacks. Treatment is conservative and dietetic. (2) Hemophilics often have chronic stiffness and enlargement which may resemble a tuberculous joint. The swelling is due to the presence of blood which, on organization, gives rise to fibrous ankylosis. The history is important since the disease is hereditary, transmitted by females, but present only in males. Treatment is largely of a prophylactic nature. Transfusions are useful and endocrine therapy has been recommended. (3) Hysteria is a term of exclusion used in joint disease when thorough examination is negative in a patient with stiffness and limp which, however, are characteristically variable. Contracture may develop from disuse. There may be a history of injury. Diagnosis is important, but often difficult. The finding of a psychogenic factor may help. Treatment requires careful local treatment and psychotherapy. (4) Intermittent hydrops is similar to chronic synovitis except that it is not connected with injury or activity, is not painful and comes and goes without apparent cause. It may be of vasomotor nature (Allison). Treatment is symptomatic.

Congenital Deformities.—These are almost entirely of orthopedic interest. The most important ones are clubfoot and congenital dislocation of the hip. *Clubfoot* is a congenital deformity due to maldevelopment of the bones and joints of the foot. The most common type of deformity is talipes equinovarus or reel foot, though other varieties are seen (talipes varus, valgus, equinus and calcaneovalgus). The disease may be unilateral or bilateral. Treatment in early cases consists of manipulation and application of a plaster cast. Open operation is necessary in some patients. *Congenital dislocation of the hip* is a not infrequent disease and though present at birth usually remains undiagnosed until the child begins to walk when an abnormal gait or limp is observed. The condition is often allowed to progress into later childhood during which the disability becomes more marked, and the anatomical changes more pronounced. Diagnosis is confirmed by roentgenograms which show an abnormally shaped and displaced head of the femur, and a deficient acetabulum. The disease may be unilateral or bilateral. Treatment consists of reduction by manipulation or open operation, and immobilization by plaster cast. The method depends on the age of the patient and the experience of the surgeon.

Of great significance is the fact that the most effective clinical results are obtained when the treatment of clubfoot and congenital dislocation of the hip is started early in life. Unfortunately, there is a tendency, even by physicians, to postpone therapy until the infant grows into childhood. It is important to emphasize, therefore, that *treatment should be begun, whenever possible, as soon as the diagnosis is made.*

Ankylosis of Joints.—Ankylosis is a frequent outcome of previous joint disease. As already mentioned, it occurs after destructive arthritis and tuberculosis. A severe fracture into the joint which involves both articular cartilages may result in bony union across the articular surfaces with complete joint immobility. In the

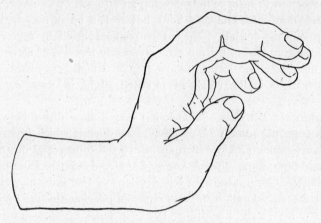

FIG. 302.—DORSIFLEXION.

Slight dorsiflexion is the most favorable position in ankylosis of the wrist; this gives satisfactory function with a useful grasp to all of the fingers and thumb.

operation or arthrodesis such a bony ankylosis is purposely produced. In all such cases the degree of the resulting disability is minimized to a great extent if the joint is fixed in a favorable position and angle. It is important, therefore, that, whenever possible, healing be allowed to take place with the joint fixed in such a position. If the position is poor and ankylosis has not yet taken place, the joint should be manipulated under general anesthesia, followed by immobilization at the proper angle in a plaster cast.

The angle of maximum usefulness is different for each joint as follows: ankle, at right angles with just enough equinus to permit wearing of a shoe with a heel; knee, in slight flexion to clear the ground easily when walking; hip, in moderate (15 degree) flexion and abduction for the same purpose; wrist, in partial dorsiflexion to aid in the grip of the fingers; elbow, in flexion just beyond a right angle with the forearm pronated enabling the hand to be used in most types of work and yet to reach behind the head; shoulder, at about 30 degrees abduction and 15 degrees flexion to enable as extensive motion of the scapula as possible.

BURSAE

Bursae are related to joints in that they are potential cavities lined by modified fibrous tissue or mesothelium which secrete a mucoid lubricant and thus enable tendons or muscles which lie over them to glide smoothly against underlying bone or other structures. In superficial locations the bursa protects underlying structures from trauma inflicted over them. Bursae likewise serve to facilitate skeletal movement. Some of them are present consistently at certain points; others may form in response to special needs when certain movements are repeatedly used. Some bursae, specially about the knee, are continuous with the joint cavity. They are similar to joints in their reaction to injury; they develop an effusion or swelling, may become painful and cause disability. Unlike a joint, however, a bursa may be destroyed or excised without causing disability, but it often replaces itself by regeneration from neighboring connective tissue. Bursae are only rarely the site of an acute pyogenic infection; the most common lesions follow trauma which is sometimes direct and acute, but more often is the result of repeated slight injuries, *e.g.,* prepatellar bursitis.

Acute Traumatic Bursitis.—This lesion may follow direct blows, but more often it results from the same type of forceful movement which gives rise to ruptured tendons or ligaments. After such an injury the differential diagnosis may be quite difficult and often impossible. A knowledge of the exact location of the various bursae is invaluable. Often, acute bursitis develops rather suddenly, manifestations appearing after a relatively slight injury, repeated previous insults or irritations to the bursa. Thus a housemaid may injure her prepatellar bursa each time she scrubs the floor on her hands and knees, but have no acute symptoms until, suddenly, an acute exacerbation follows some slight blow. Symptoms are local pain and swelling, the former aggravated by certain motions and the latter apparent only in the superficial bursae. Disability is usually quite severe on account of the pain, limitation of motion and muscle spasm. Occasionally infection develops in the bursa and progresses to suppuration, thereby demanding drainage by incision. Treatment of traumatic bursitis consists of rest in a comfortable position and local applications of heat until motion is possible without pain. The acute process may last for a week or two and subside without further difficulty. Unfortunately, further attacks are liable to occur. More troublesome is the development of more or less constant or chronic disability and pain.

Chronic Bursitis.—This may follow an acute lesion, but frequently develops insidiously and is often erroneously diagnosed as neuritis, "rheumatism" or chronic arthritis. The pathologic changes in the bursa are similar to those in the joint, in that fluid is present and villous overgrowth of the bursal lining occurs. In addition, however, calcification of the wall of the bursa is not infrequent and can often be seen in a roentgenogram. Symptoms are pain, more or less severe, brought about or aggravated by certain movements which tend to compress or irritate the bursa. Tenderness is often localized to this area. Swelling may develop because of effusion which is always present, and may be demonstrated by aspiration. Treatment is often unsatisfactory, unless the occupation or activities of the patient can be changed in cases due to irritation from certain specific muscular movements. In other patients the decision as to the advisability of motion or rest is not an easy one. The application of penetrating heat is usually helpful. Excision of the bursa is often indicated and is frequently curative, especially when the bursa is calcified and has not responded to conservative treatment.

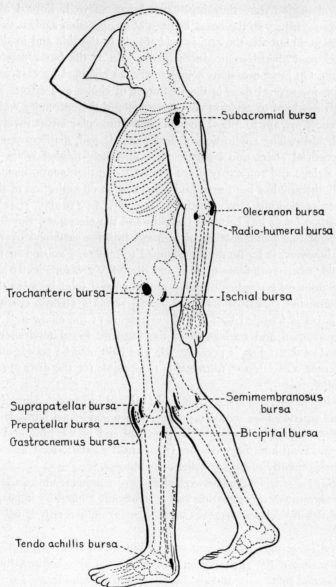

Subacromial bursa

Olecranon bursa

Radio-humeral bursa

Trochanteric bursa

Ischial bursa

Semimembranosus bursa

Suprapatellar bursa

Prepatellar bursa

Bicipital bursa

Gastrocnemius bursa

Tendo achillis bursa

FIG. 303.—THE SITES OF THE MORE COMMON BURSAE.

Specific Types of Bursitis.—Although there are about twenty-six bursae in the human body, only a few are commonly diseased. Discussion will therefore be limited to them. The *subdeltoid (subacromial) bursa* is the most frequent site of bursitis. Its anatomy and clinical importance were emphasized by Codman [16] many years ago. It is located between the deltoid muscle and the humeral tuberosity and aids in the contraction of the deltoid which operates almost at right angles in abducting the arm. It also extends upward and under the acromion lying between it and the insertion of the supraspinatus muscle. Rupture of the supraspinatus tendon from violent abduction may thus injure the bursa as well. Forced abduction in general may cause injury to the bursa because of compression against the acromion. In severe subdeltoid bursitis the arm is held closely to the side and in slight inward rotation. Attempted abduction produces severe pain as the bursa meets the overlying acromion. On most occasions complete rest as obtained by carrying the forearm in a sling for several days is the treatment of choice and effects a cure. The patient is instructed not to perform any movements of the extremity which produce pain. Recurrences are apt to follow sudden severe muscular effort involving abduction of the shoulder. The application of heat (electric pad, diathermy, etc.) appear to have a beneficial effect and analgesics are obviously needed when the pain is severe. The serious and refractory cases often tax the therapeutic ingenuity of the surgeon; radiotherapy has been used and operation on or aspiration of the inflamed bursa has been carried out (see editorial in *J. A. M. A.*, 116:955, 1941).

The *olecranon bursa* lies between the skin and the olecranon. Bursitis (miner's elbow) occurs at this point because of frequent injuries sustained over the bursa. The disease, however, is by no means confined to miners. Excision of the bursa is often indicated, when symptoms of pain and disability are sufficiently severe.

The *radio-humeral bursa* lies over the radio-humeral joint between the extensor carpiradialis and the supinator longus muscles. Bursitis (tennis elbow) develops because the bursa is irritated by forceful movements of the elbow and wrist, associated with pronation and supination of the forearm. Local tenderness over and above the head of the radius is pronounced. The pain may be severe and disabling in some instances. Cessation of movements responsible for the disease often results in prompt relief.

The *prepatellar bursa* is not so commonly injured in present days of mechanical appliances and machines for scrubbing floors. It is a superficial bursa lying between the patella and the skin or between the proximal end of the tibia and skin where irritation occurs from kneeling position (housemaid's knee). Rest and cessation of repeated injuries usually results in relief of symptoms.

The *achilles bursa* which lies between the gastrocnemius tendon and the os calcis is frequently the seat of inflammation and is commonly caused by improperly fitting shoes. Relief usually follows removal of the cause; only rarely is operation indicated.

The *ischial bursa* may be the seat of inflammation (Weaver's bottom) in individuals who maintain the sitting position for long periods because the bursa lies between the ischial tuberosity and the overlying gluteal muscles.

TENDONS

Many tendons move in sheaths which are structurally similar to joints and bursae, but in general are not frequent sites of serious disease. Wounds, tumors and acute infections of tendons have been described in previous chapters.

Traumatic tenosynovitis is a common, but rarely serious injury which produces an inflammation of the sheath with outpouring of an excess amount of the lubricating fluid. Local tenderness is present along the course of the sheath and use of the tendon produces pain. There may be palpable a creaking or crepitation on motion of the tendon. Later, fibrous tissue may replace the fluid and fibrin, thereby resulting in limitation of motion. In general, rest should be maintained as long as acute symptoms are present, but increasing active motion should follow as soon as subsidence of pain permits.

Other lesions depend on special injuries. A *dislocation* of a tendon may occur so that it leaves the groove it normally occupies and finds a new abnormal site. The common ones involved are the long head of the biceps, the peroneal tendons and the posterior tibial tendon. Treatment consists of operative replacement of the tendon, and rest for a week or two until movements without pain are possible. *Stenosing tenovaginitis* (trigger finger, snapping finger) is a rare lesion which produces a temporary impediment of flexion (or extension) of the finger which on further movement suddenly gives way and the finger snaps.

Tuberculous tenosynovitis manifests itself as a thickening of the tendon sheath which becomes filled with thick fluid and caseous material containing "rice bodies." The flexor and extensor tendons of the wrist, hand and forearm are most commonly involved. Treatment may be conservative and hygienic or operative. In the latter case all excessive fibrous and granulation tissue are removed and the wound closed carefully without drainage.

MUSCLE

Unlike bone and joints, muscle is seldom the site of disease or serious injury. However, of all the elements important to movement and locomotion, muscle is the most prone to atrophy, especially of disuse. Paralysis results from denervation; recovery depends on regeneration of the nerve.

Atrophy.—There are several types. Disuse alone, particularly following immobilization or when associated with ankylosis, will produce a rapid and severe muscular atrophy. The presence of infection aggravates the process. However, atrophy of disuse alone is usually relieved rapidly as soon as active motion is restored and leads in most cases to the return of the muscle to its normal state. Frequently the stronger set of muscles contracts and results in a deformity, often called contracture, which is especially apt to follow atrophy due to paralysis of the muscles which follows interference with the nerve supply. Spontaneous subluxation (dislocation) of the joint may thus occur. Atrophy from severance of the nerve supply produces a paralysis as well as atrophy and is much more serious because recovery depends on regeneration of the nerve (see p. 548). Disease of the brain and spinal cord may also produce muscular atrophy, whether the resulting paralysis is flaccid or spastic. *Spastic paralysis* of children (Little's disease) is produced by cortical injury sustained during childbirth, or to prenatal cerebral defects. Mental deficiency frequently accompanies the muscular paralysis. Treatment is a complex neurological and orthopedic problem. *Poliomyelitis* is a serious cause of muscle atrophy which becomes permanent when the infection destroys the anterior horn cells which innervate the muscles. With the onset of paralysis it is very important that the affected muscles should be supported in a plaster cast. The permanent paralysis is frequently accompanied by deformity due to the pull of the uninvolved muscles. The treatment of these deformities is an orthopedic problem, and consists of muscle training, braces of various types, and transplantation of tendons. A rare type of atrophy is *progressive muscular atrophy* which is a slow chronic disease beginning in the intrinsic muscles of the hand. *Birth (Erb's) paralysis* affects the muscles

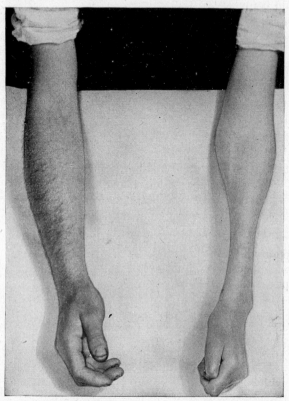

FIG. 304.—PHOTOGRAPH OF BOTH HANDS AND FOREARMS SHOWING A VOLKMANN'S CONTRACTURE ON THE LEFT SIDE, APPROXIMATELY THREE YEARS AFTER ONSET.

(From Hill and Brooks, *Ann. Surg.*, 1936, 103 :448.)

of the upper extremity and is due to injury to the brachial plexus during delivery. The diagnosis should be made as soon after birth as possible. Treatment consists of immobilization and relaxation of the injured structures; operative treatment of the nerves is only occasionally indicated.

Volkmann's contracture (ischemic contracture or paralysis) is a tragic and usually preventable accident which occurs most frequently after immobilization of an elbow fracture in acute flexion. It may also be caused by the application of a cast or splints too tightly about the forearm. Soft tissue injury alone with extensive extravasation of blood about the elbow or forearm may also be the instigating factor. The first symptoms are (*a*) diffuse pain in the forearm and hand, (*b*) cyanosis, especially of the fingers, (c) swelling, (d) inability to move the fingers, and (e) tingling and numbness of the fingers. When the condition complicates fractures about the elbow the damage is presumably done by continued swelling after immobilization of the joint in forced flexion. As a consequence the venous return from the forearm is shut off. The arteries for a time continue to pump blood into the forearm, thus increasing the swelling which ultimately obstructs the arterial supply to some extent. These changes have been studied experimentally by Brooks.[17] It is important to realize that after six or seven hours the damage is done and no form of treatment will bring the muscles back to normal. The end result is the conversion of the contractile cells into fibrous tissue which produces an atrophied forearm and useless "claw" hand (*main en griffe*).

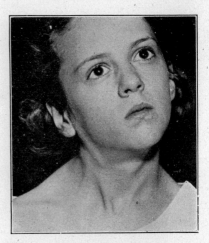

FIG. 305.—CONGENITAL TORTICOLLIS IN A TWELVE-YEAR-OLD GIRL.

Note the attitude and the tense sternomastoid muscle on the patient's right. This muscle was cut across and a cast applied; the result was excellent six months later. X-ray showed only a rotation of the cervical spine (Washington U. Clinics).

Treatment is prophylactic except when the swelling is due to soft tissue injury alone. In this case the only efficient form of treatment is prompt and radical incision of the tense tissues. The greatest danger exists from swelling about joints immobilized with a cast or appliance in a flexed position. This is apt to occur most frequently after fractures about the elbow which are nearly always fixed in flexion. After reduction and immobilization of such fractures the surgeon must palpate the radial pulse since its absence is a sign of serious vascular obstruction. The patient should be either kept under observation for twenty-four hours or emphatically instructed to return at the first indication of severe pain, numbness or paralysis of the parts distal to the lesion. In such an event the constricting dressing or cast must be loosened or removed even at the expense of losing the position of the fracture.

Myositis ossificans is a remarkable posttraumatic condition in which calcium is deposited in muscle which thus takes on the characteristics of bone. It may occur in hematomas of the muscle or may develop in muscles adjacent to a fracture. Tendons are occasionally affected also. Treatment consists of prolonged and complete immobilization; in a good many instances partial or complete absorption of the calcium in the muscle occurs.

Wryneck (*torticollis*) is a disfiguring disease of the cervical muscles (or their motor nerve supply) which by continuous contraction maintain the head in an inclined position to one side or the other. The disease is congenital, though usually only recognized in childhood. An acquired type, often called spasmodic torticollis, occurs in adults and belongs to the group of nervous disorders known as "tics." When prolonged, torticollis produces changes in the cervical spine. Treatment of the congenital type is operative and manipulative and should be instituted as early in life as possible.

MISCELLANEOUS LESIONS

Ingrown toenail, a common lesion, especially in young women, is a frequent cause of suppuration about the large toe as described previously. Although with rest, elevation and local heat, such an acute infection diminishes or subsides, it is apt to recur unless the ingrowing part of the nail finally clears the soft tissue of the toe or is removed and prevented from reforming by an appropriate operation. Tight shoes and too frequent clipping of nails probably do play some role in the

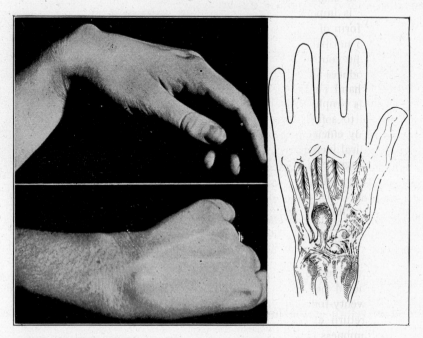

FIG. 306.—GANGLION OF THE WRIST IN AN EIGHTEEN-YEAR-OLD SCHOOLGIRL.

Note in the photograph how the tumor is made more prominent by flexion at the wrist; it was tense but definitely cystic on palpation. The patient complained of constant rheumatic pain in the wrist and arm, aggravated by use. The sketch was based on a drawing made at operation and shows the mass attached to the joint capsule; it contained thick mucoid fluid. Excision of the entire cyst including its pedicle was performed; complete relief ensued.

development of this lesion. More important, however, is the presence of a congenital abnormality in the root of the nail allowing the lateral edge of the nail to grow out obliquely and penetrate the soft tissue. This produces pain and frequently breaks the skin and thus introduces infection which persists because the ingrown nail acts like a foreign body.

Treatment in mild cases consists of shaving off the central portion of the nail from the distal edge back to the cuticle which may encourage growth toward the center to such an extent as to relieve symptoms. Radical treatment consists of removal of a segment of nail including its entire lateral edge and excision of its root so completely that the removed portion will not regenerate. In a detailed study by E. L. Keyes,[18] the results of the various methods of repair have been discussed.

He recommended removal of a wedge of tissue from the hypertrophied portion of the toe adjacent to the edge of the nail, as well as the lateral edge of the nail and its attached root. This procedure, modified after Winograd,[19] not only promotes more rapid healing, but tends to eliminate the possibility of recurrence in case the root has not been removed adequately. Operation is done under local anesthesia with the aid of a rubber tourniquet.

Ganglion is a term applied to a smooth rounded mass (½ to 1½ centimeters in diameter) which commonly appears in the distal portion of the wrist on the dorsal surface, and is made more prominent by flexion of the wrist. It also occurs

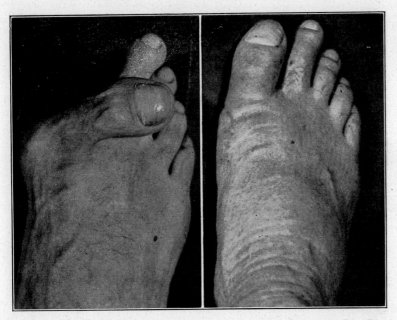

FIG. 307.—HALLUX VALGUS BEFORE AND AFTER RADICAL OPERATION FOR ITS CORRECTION.

A wedge was removed from the medial margin of the joint and the toe immobilized in its normal position (St. Louis City Hospital).

on the ventral surface of the wrist and in some other joints, particularly the knee. It is found in women much more frequently than in men (3:1) and is especially common in young women (Carp and Stout [20]). The tumor, when exposed, is found to lie among the tendons, but nearly always is attached to the joint capsule. It consists of a fibrous sac which contains mucoid material. The lumen of the cyst is commonly a closed cavity, but occasionally it communicates with the wrist joint or a tendon sheath. As to its pathogenesis the most careful studies (Ledderhose [21]), have shown that it originates from the fibrous tissue of the joint capsule as a neoplasm. The cystic nature of the tumor is explained by the presence of secreting mesothelial cells or to mucoid degeneration of the fibrous tissue. Its origin as a herniation of the joint or tendon sheath, a theory which is generally held, lacks definite proof. Clinical manifestations beside the presence of the tumor include pain or "rheumatoid" discomfort which may result in definite disability. Treatment to be curative necessitates complete excision, or recurrence may follow. Breaking the cyst with a well directed blow is sometimes followed by cure. Aspiration and injection of sclerosing solutions has been used, but is obviously dangerous, especially in rare instances in a ganglion whose lumen communicates with the joint cavity.

Corn or clavus is a local hypertrophy of the hornified layer of the skin which develops as a response to chronic pressure or irritation, usually from tight or ill-fitting shoes. The most important clinical manifestation is severe pain which is due to pressure over the lesion and can be relieved by shifting the contact with the shoe from the corn to the surrounding skin by means of a circular pad with a hole in the center, which protects the tumor. This is the principle upon which corn

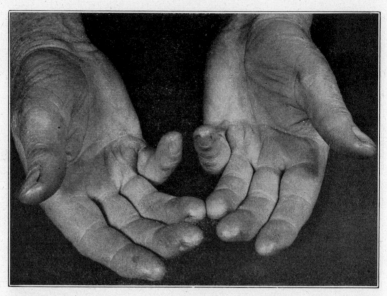

Fig. 308.—Dupuytren's Contracture in a Forty-five-year-old Man.

The photograph indicates the maximum possible extension. Disability was insufficient to justify operation.

plasters are used. Eradication of the lesion may be achieved by elimination of the source of the chronic irritation or by actual excision. Occasionally certain types of corns (particularly those between the toes) can be cured only by removal of part of the base of the phalanx adjacent to the corn. Corns occasionally are the site of infection which is treated by the usual methods.

Hallux valgus is a common deformity of the great toe (outward deflection or abduction) which to a great extent, at least, is caused by wearing ill-fitting, short and pointed shoes. Its importance lies in the frequent formation of a bunion which is often painful and disabling. This knob or bunion consists of an overgrowth of the medial margin of the distal end of the metatarsal bone at the metatarsophalangeal joint and is associated with a true bursal sac which contains fluid and often becomes infected. Relief of pain is often achieved by correcting the normal position of the toe with an appliance, and the wearing of correct shoes. In severe cases operation consists of removal of the bursa and trimming off the excess bone, thus allowing the toe to assume its normal position.

Dupuytren's contracture is a rare, probably hereditary disease and of gradual and insidious onset. This condition is not a contracture of the tendons but of the palmar fascia on the ulnar side of the palm gradually causing a flexion deformity of the 5th and later the 4th finger. The fascia extending into the fingers as well as the overlying skin may also be involved. There is no pain or tenderness, disability being due to inability to extend the fingers. Recurrence is liable to follow any treatment. However, wide but careful and painstaking excision of the sclerotic fascia (and full thickness skin graft in the advanced cases) is the therapy most likely to succeed (Kanavel, Koch and Mason [22]).

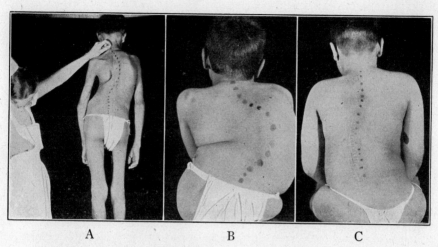

| A | B | C |

FIG. 309.—TWO TYPES OF SCOLIOSIS.

A, idiopathic scoliosis with marked rotation of vertebral bodies. This type of scoliosis is very difficult to treat; *B*, total curvature of the spine without rotation due to infantile paralysis. No rotation of vertebral bodies. This type of curve is easily corrected and held by spine fusion; *C*, same as *B*, after fusion of the spine. (Courtesy Dr. C. H. Crego, Jr., Shriners Hospital for Crippled Children, St. Louis.)

Foot strain is encountered under a variety of circumstances which bring the patient to the surgeon, largely because of foot pain, which may be severe or mild, and may be accompanied by swelling and other anatomical changes. Frequently no definite organic basis can be made out. Foot strain is a common disease, and is often aggravated by the wearing of improperly fitting shoes. It should be emphasized that the form of the arch has nothing to do with the painful symptoms of foot strain. The diagnosis and treatment of foot strain is largely an orthopedic problem; rest of the strained ligaments plays an important part in therapy, especially by the use of a Thomas heel, which gives support to the tarsal scaphoid, which is most frequently the bone involved in the strain (Key [23]). Occasionally adequate support to a low arch will relieve symptoms.

Scoliosis, or lateral curvature of the spine, is a disfiguring and eventually crippling deformity due to gradual deviation and torsion of the spinous processes of several adjacent vertebra. It is a disease of childhood, and in most instances has no known etiology. Treatment is an orthopedic problem, and consists of a variety of manipulative, operative, supportive, and gymnastic methods.

Athlete's foot (epidermophytosis) is really a dermatitis of the skin of the foot, especially in and between the toes, caused by a fungous infection. Symptoms of cellulitis and suppuration may occur whenever secondary pyogenic invasion occurs; treatment is the same as that of infection in general. Eradication of the original ringworm may be achieved by cleanliness, and by the use of a nonirritating fungicide (resorcinol lotion, Whitfields ointment, etc.). Infections about the feet, in general may largely be prevented by ordinary cleanliness, as well as the wearing of properly fitting shoes; this is particularly important in patients suffering from peripheral circulatory disease and diabetes.

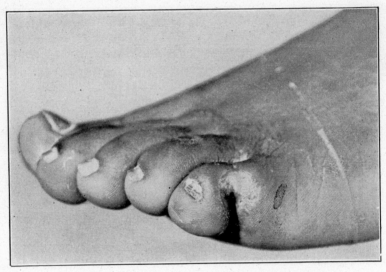

FIG. 310.—AINHUM IN A THIRTY-FIVE-YEAR-OLD NEGRO.

The constriction at the base of the toe was first noted five years previously and has steadily progressed. The patient complained only of mild pain of three weeks' duration, due to a superficial infection which responded to local incision and bed rest. The remnants of the infection can be seen in the scaling of the skin.

Foreign bodies, usually needles, are not infrequently introduced (accidentally) beneath the skin, especially in the hand, and often produce pain and disability, particularly if located over an area which is subject to trauma. Removal of the foreign body is usually indicated. When the needle is deeply seated its removal may be difficult. The x-ray film should be taken just before operation inasmuch as considerable migration of the foreign body may occur even in a day or two. X-ray localization is often aided by placing a lead marker at a convenient point on the skin. Obviously two views are essential. If infection is present the treatment is the same as that of an infected wound, as has already been described.

Metatarsalgia (Morton's disease) consists of severe pain below and between the heads of the metatarsal bones, probably produced by pressure or impingement of the nerves between the heads of the metatarsal bones. Relief is often obtained by rest and support of the anterior arch by a pad or other appliance placed beneath it. *Hammer toe* is an acquired flexion deformity of the toes, most often the middle

ones, due usually to tightly fitting shoes. Severe cases may require a plastic operation (wedge resection of the interphalangeal joint). *Calcaneal spurs* are sometimes
the cause of pain localized to the heel (painful heel, policeman's heel). The pain
may be due to an associated bursitis but is apparently primarily dependent upon
the presence of the spur, which may be unilateral or bilateral. Diagnosis is readily
made by the x-ray. If pain is very severe, and does not respond to conservative
treatment, excision is justifiable.

Ainhum is a rare degenerative disease consisting of a circular constriction at
the base of the toes, usually the little toe; it occurs largely in African countries but
is encountered in this country in Negroes only. The etiology is unknown. The toe
finally drops off; there is no treatment. (See Fig. 310.)

Most of the lesions just described are in the foot; an excellent monograph on
the foot and ankle by Lewin [24] has become available, to which the reader is referred.

BIBLIOGRAPHY

1. Osgood, R. B., and Allison, N. *Fundamentals of Orthopedic Surgery in General Medicine and Surgery*, The Macmillan Company, New York, 1931.
2. Shands, A. A., and Raney, R. B. *Handbook of Orthopedic Surgery*, 2nd ed., C. V. Mosby, St. Louis, 1940.
3. Whitman, R. *Treatise on Orthopedic Surgery*, Lea and Febiger, Philadelphia, 1930.
4. Johnson, R. A. Y. The Effect of Infection on the Epiphyses, *Arch. Surg.*, 32:810, 1936.
5. Orr, H. W. The Treatment of Osteomyelitis and Other Infected Wounds by Drainage and Rest, *Surg., Gynec. & Obst.*, 45:446, 1927.
6. Miller, R. H. Acute Hematogenous Osteomyelitis, *N. Eng. J. M.*, 212:283, 1935.
7. Baer, W. S. The Treatment of Chronic Osteomyelitis with the Maggot (Larva of the Blow Fly), *J. Bone & Joint Surg.*, 13:438, 1931.
8. Abbott, L. C. The Operative Lengthening of the Tibia and Fibula, *J. Bone & Joint Surg.*, 9:128, 1927; Abbott, L. C. and Saunders, J. M. The Operative Lengthening of the Tibia and Fibula, *Ann. Surg.*, 110:961, 1939.
9. Brahdy, L. Mechanics of the Physical Signs in Lower Trunk Injuries, *Surg., Gynec. & Obst.*, 60:802, 1935.
10. Phemister, D. B. The Effect of Pressure on Articular Surfaces in Pyogenic and Tuberculous Arthritides and Its Bearing on Treatment, *Ann. Surg.*, 80:481, 1924.
11. Harris, R. I. Acute Suppurative Arthritis in Children, *J. Bone & Joint Surg.*, 7:849, 1925.
12. Willems, C. Treatment of Purulent Arthritis by Wide Arthrotomy Followed by Immediate Active Mobilization, *Surg., Gynec. & Obst.*, 28:546, 1919.
13. Inge, G. L., and Liebolt, F. L. The Treatment of Acute Suppurative Arthritis, *Surg., Gynec. & Obst.*, 60:86, 1940.
14. Hatcher, C. H., and Phemister, D. B. The Primary Point of Infection in Tuberculosis of the Hip Joint, *Surg., Gynec., & Obst.*, 65:721, 1937.
15. Allison, N. *Surgical Diagnosis*, edited by E. A. Graham, W. B. Saunders, Philadelphia, Vol. I, p. 55, 1930.
16. Codman, E. A. On Stiff and Painful Shoulders: The Anatomy of the Subdeltoid or Subacromial Bursa and Its Clinical Importance. Subdeltoid Bursitis, *Boston M. & S. J.*, 154:613, 1906.
17. Brooks, B. Pathologic Changes in Muscles as a Result of Disturbances of Circulation: An Experimental Study of Volkmann's Ischemic Paralysis, *Arch. Surg.*, 5:188, 1922.

18. KEYES, E. L.   Surgical Treatment of Ingrown Toenails, *J. Am. M. Ass.*, 102:1458, 1934.
19. WINOGRAD, A. M.   A Modification in the Technic of Operation for Ingrown Toenail, *J. Am. M. Ass.*, 92:229, 1929.
20. CARP, L., and STOUT, A. P.   A Study of Ganglion, *Surg., Gynec. & Obst.*, 47:460, 1928.
21. LEDDERHOSE.   Die Aetiologie der Carpalen Ganglien, *Deut. Zeit. f. Chir.*, 37:102, 1893.
22. KANAVEL, A. B., KOCH, S. L., and MASON, M. L.   Dupuytren's Contraction with a Description of the Palmar Fascia, a Review of the Literature, and a Report of Twenty-nine Surgically Treated Cases, *Surg., Gynec. & Obst.*, 48:145, 1929.
23. KEY, J. A.   *The Practitioners Library of Medicine and Surgery*, Vol. IV, p. 937, D. Appleton-Century Co., New York, 1933.
24. LEWIN, Phillip.   *The Foot and Ankle: Their Injuries, Diseases, Deformities, and Disabilities.* Lea & Febiger, Philadelphia. 2nd edition, 1941.
25. CRAVENER, E. K. and MACELROY, D. G.   Injuries of the Internal Semilunar Cartilage, *J. Am. M. Ass.*, 117:1695, 1941.
26. GREEN, W. T., and SHANNON, J. G.   Osteomyelitis of Infants, *Arch. Surg.*, 32:462, 1936.

CHAPTER XX

BLOOD VESSELS

The Arteries
Peripheral vascular disease
The Veins

Probably the first important step in the development of surgery of the blood vessels was the reintroduction of the ligature (first described by Celsus) by the French surgeon, Ambrose Paré. When Koeberlé (another French surgeon) introduced the standard hemostatic forceps in 1865 (Garrison), the entire field of surgery benefited tremendously. The introduction of transfusion of blood in more recent years by Carrel, Crile and others, has been a means of adding greatly to the safety of surgical procedures.

The most recent contribution to the study of the blood vessels is the knowledge of the role of the autonomic nervous system in the control of the caliber of the peripheral arteries and arterioles. These data are of most importance in consideration of vascular diseases of the extremities. Numerous functional tests have been devised in an effort to determine the type of lesion present, particularly with regard to the relative amount of mechanical occlusion and functional spasm present. These tests are discussed on pages 229 and 504.

THE ARTERIES

Anomalies.—Abnormalities of the arteries are extremely common and consist chiefly of *malposition*. Common examples which are of significance in operative surgery consist of abnormalities in position of the hepatic and cystic arteries. When the former vessel is anomalously placed anteriorly, it may be injured or be mistaken for the cystic artery and erroneously ligated during cholecystectomy; this error gives rise to pathological changes resulting in hepatic insufficiency and usually is fatal. Anomalies of the renal artery, particularly aberrant vessels, are not uncommon and tend to give rise to symptoms on account of pressure against the ureter or pelvis of the kidney; this may result in obstruction with consequent infection.

Other anomalies may be considered *structural* in type. Of this group arteriovenous fistulas including cirsoid aneurysms are relatively uncommon but important because of the skill and care necessary in their successful treatment. Because they present individual problems and at times are not congenital, they are considered later in this chapter. Certain *neoplasms,* including various types of hemangiomas are congenital in origin. They are discussed in Chapter XVI.

493

Normally the *ductus arteriosus,* which connects the pulmonary artery and dorsal aorta in fetal life closes shortly after birth. In a study of a large series of infants at post mortem, Christie[1] found the ductus still open in 44 per cent of infants at one month, 12 per cent at two months and 2 per cent at eight months of age. Although many individuals live a comparatively normal life with a patent ductus arteriosus, serious complications including rupture or thrombosis of the ductus, endocarditis or cardiac decompensation may result, and be averted by its ligation. Gross[2] has reported successful ligation of the patent ductus arteriosus in several cases.

Wounds.—When an artery is completely severed the resultant hemorrhage, unless arrested, may prove serious or even fatal, depending upon the size of the vessel and the type of wound. If an artery is torn by avulsion, or cut in a jagged manner, there is a greater tendency for the formation of a clot than if the wound is made by a sharp instrument, largely because the frayed edges tend to obstruct the blood flow, and likewise encourage the development of a clot at that point. Large arteries such as the axillary and the popliteal, when torn across by an avulsion of the extremity, may cease bleeding spontaneously before causing a fatal hemorrhage because of the great tendency for contraction of the open end. However, if the blood pressure is brought back to normal too rapidly by artificial means before the artery is ligated, the clot formed in the lumen of the vessel may be ejected and another hemorrhage will ensue. Incomplete division of an artery, which happens only occasionally, is in reality more serious than complete division because the retraction of the walls of the vessel enlarges the opening, thereby making it more difficult for a clot to be formed and retained. Frequently, an artery is severed by a punctured wound passing through sufficient muscular tissue and fascia to prevent the escape of blood to the exterior. Under such circumstances a hematoma will form under such tension about the injured vessel as to stop further bleeding. Unless the collateral circulation is adequate there will, of course, be danger of production of gangrene. Unfortunately, the extravasation of blood may be so extensive on some occasions as to partially or completely obliterate the collateral circulation. Unless signs of beginning gangrene develop within the first 24 or 48 hours, they are not apt to develop, since with time the collaterals tend to increase in size and efficiency unless the bleeding persists. On certain occasions the pressure in the blood clot surrounding an injured large artery is so great (because of dense fibrous and muscle planes) that bleeding ceases, although an actual communication between the artery and center of the blood clot still exists. When this happens, the periphery of the clot becomes organized forming a fibrous capsule, thus leading to the formation of a false aneurysm. The swelling may pulsate and present all the other signs of aneurysm.

Treatment.—As described in Chapter X, any wound which bleeds vigorously longer than two or three minutes demands immediate attention to stop the hemorrhage. Simple procedures such as pressure, packing, application of a tourniquet or elevation of the limb (when the wound is on an extremity) will usually suffice. If bleeding still persists an attempt should be made to grasp the injured vessel with a hemostat. If this is successful, operative treatment then consists of ligation of the vessel and debridement with closure of the wound as discussed on page 193.

Occasionally the bleeding point cannot be found even in the operating-room because of depth of the wound and extravasation of blood. In this case it may be preferable to expose the injured artery proximal to the bleeding point and ligate it. Occasionally, when large vessels are severed, the ends may be sutured together, using fine silk and approximating intima to intima. Technics for bridging arterial defects utilizing metal (vitallium) tubes lined with vein wall, have been described (Blakemore and associates [22]).

If no external wound is present, or is so small that there is no external loss of blood, it may be difficult to decide whether or not an operation for ligation of the vessel is indicated, particularly if distal arterial pulsation is absent. Under such circumstances conservatism is permissible, particularly if the hematoma is relatively small and is not increasing in size, but the limb must be watched for signs of serious ischemia. This conservative attitude may be wise since some blood may be coursing past the injured point, but not in sufficient quantity to create a palpable pulsation; ligation of the vessel at this time would interrupt circulation entirely and might result in gangrene. However, when the hematoma is increasing in size operation may be indicated in order to forestall gangrene which will follow if the collateral vessels are obliterated by the hematoma; at operation the patency of the collaterals is restored by ligation of the injured vessel and evaculation of the clot.

It was observed during the Boer War by Makins, and later proved experimentally by Brooks and associates,[3] that if the corresponding vein were ligated at the same time the injured artery was ligated, the incidence of gangrene was decreased. It is usually advisable, therefore, to ligate the vein simultaneously with the artery.

Embolism and Thrombosis (Arterial).—An embolus may originate from a thrombus located in any major vein or in the heart itself. When it lodges in a major trunk of an extremity the blood supply to the distal part of the extremity may be interrupted with threatening gangrene. Severe pain, pallor, and muscular weakness along with other manifestations as described in detail on page 131 may develop. Immediate operation with removal of the clot (embolectomy) is usually indicated.

Pulmonary embolism occurs when a thrombus becomes detached from a vein outside the lung and is carried through the right side of the heart into the pulmonary artery. This is a serious postoperative complication and frequently results in death. The clot may originate from various sources including any large vein following operation, particularly if infection exists. Occasionally it arises from one of the heart chambers especially in the presence of cardiac disease such as endocarditis. The symptoms will, of course, vary depending upon the size of the clot and amount of the arterial tree occluded. Chest pain of variable intensity is usually the first symptom. The patient becomes dyspneic, cyanotic and complains of "smothering" and a feeling of weakness. The heart rate is rapid and sounds are feeble. Death may be instantaneous and dramatic, the patient sitting up in bed, suddenly crying out as if in severe pain and falling over dead. More commonly symptoms as mentioned previously, develop; death may take place in a few hours or a few days. Recovery may, of course, be spontaneous. Treatment consists of the immediate administration of ½ grain of papaverine (de Takats [4]) to overcome the vascular spasm. Oxygen therapy is usually strongly indicated. Supportive measures such as intravenous glucose or even ephedrine, may be resorted to, but the latter with caution. The clot may be removed by operation, which, however, if extensively employed, will probably result in more deaths than lives saved (see discussion on page 853). Prophylactic reduction of the incidence of pulmonary embolism will probably follow routine breathing and leg exercises, as emphasized by Potts [5] and others. Increasing the clotting time with intravenous heparin will probably also lessen the likelihood of pulmonary embolism, although the oral use of dicoumarin (Link and associates [42]) is probably preferable. The aim is to keep the prothrombin time between 35 and 60 seconds (Allen and associates [43]) with a dose of about 200 mg. of dicoumarin per day. The incidence of fatal pulmonary embolism will also be lowered by ligation of the thrombosed femoral vein (see page 516).

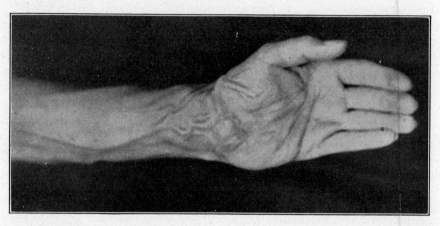

FIG. 311.—CONGENITAL ARTERIOVENOUS FISTULA (CIRSOID ANEURYSM) INVOLVING THE ULNAR ARTERY AND VEIN IN A YOUNG WOMAN AGED TWENTY.

The dilated veins and swelling of the hand and wrist had been present since early childhood and without any preceding history of trauma. Operation is rarely successful in such instances unless all the communicating vessels are ligated or the entire vascular mass can be excised with ligation of the arteries entering the mass. The danger of onset of gangrene of the extremity distal to the excised mass is obviously significant. Frequently the affected extremity is larger than the normal one.

Arteriovenous Fistula.—An abnormal communication between artery and vein may be traumatic or congenital. The *traumatic* type is caused by injury to the wall of the artery and vein by a foreign body (usually a bullet or stiletto) in such a way that blood from the artery finds its way into the vein, either at the time of injury or by erosion of the wall at a later date (usually the latter). The vein then becomes enlarged and tortuous due to the arterial pressure. This entrance of arterial blood into the venous system may cause serious embarrassment of the right heart and cardiac hypertrophy (Holman [7]).

When the communication is *congenital* there is apt to be an enormous number of vessels involved in the mass. In either type a swelling may be present; a thrill can be felt and a systolic and diastolic bruit heard. The temperature of the skin over the involved area is elevated because of the increased blood supply. When vessels of an extremity are involved, actual lengthening of the limb may take place, likewise because of vascularity beyond normal. Blood withdrawn from a surface vein may show increased oxygenation, a fact which in itself may serve to make the correct diagnosis. Common locations for these fistulas are between the common carotid artery and jugular vein, the internal carotid artery and the cavernous sinus, the femoral artery and vein, and between the axillary artery and vein. A *cirsoid aneurysm* is a term which in reality should be applied to any type of congenital arteriovenous aneurysm, but unfortunately is frequently discussed separately, but without any definite differentiating features. The term is commonly applied to congenital arteriovenous aneurysm of the scalp.

The *treatment* is concerned with surgical obliteration of the fistula, or excision of the entire vascular mass. Only on rare occasions indeed will it be possible to ligate the communication between the artery and vein. Congenital arteriovenous fistulas, however, are amenable to treatment in this way. Usually it is necessary to ligate the artery and vein proximal and distal to the mass, and excise all the intervening vascular communications. Although ligation of a normal artery in locations occupied by these fistulas would ordinarily result in gangrene of part of the extremity, it rarely occurs in the presence of a fistula because the condition has usually been present long enough for the development of an adequate collateral circulation. Recurrence following operative treatment may occur.

Aneurysms.—From the standpoint of etiology most aneurysms are syphilitic, but some are traumatic. The mechanical factor responsible for the formation of practically all aneurysms is a weakening or destruction of the media which is the supporting layer of the artery. An aneurysm is considered *fusiform* when the entire circumference is weakened, thereby allowing a more or less symmetrical dilatation. A *sacculated aneurysm* projects from the artery as a globular mass because of a weakness in the media at one point. A *false aneurysm* results usually from puncture of a large artery when the resistance of the soft tissue to the outflowing blood results in encapsulation, with communication still existing between the center of the clot and the lumen of the artery. Obviously the aneurysmal space is not surrounded by an arterial coat, but after a time a fibrous lining forms on the periphery of the blood-filled space.

There is a slight tendency for clots to form within the lumen of aneurysms. When this occurs progressive enlargement is delayed. On rare occasions the aneurysm may be cured by a clot filling the entire sac and becoming organized. Calcification in the wall of the sac sometimes occurs.

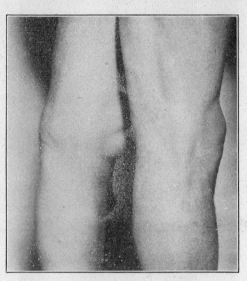

FIG. 312.—SYPHILITIC ANEURYSM OF THE LEFT POPLITEAL ARTERY.

The patient is a Negro, aged forty, who contracted syphilis at the age of seventeen. The mass, accompanied by pain in the thigh and popliteal region, was noted only during the past six months.

The thoracic aorta is the most frequent site of aneurysms. Such aneurysms are practically always syphilitic in origin. The diagnosis is largely a medical problem. Such signs as thrills, bruit, erosion of bone, tracheal tug, palpable pulsation, etc., should be looked for. Fluoroscopic examination is helpful in determining the presence or absence of pulsation. A difference in the volume of the radial pulse on the two sides is of diagnostic significance.

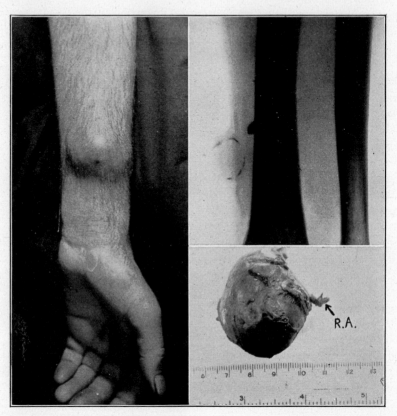

FIG. 313.—TRAUMATIC ANEURYSM SECONDARY TO AN INJURY SIX YEARS PREVIOUSLY.

A small fragment of steel penetrated the forearm, but healing was rapid without any special treatment. A small mass developed shortly after injury; a few weeks before entry it began to enlarge rapidly, aided perhaps by the development of an essential hypertension. The photograph was taken just before operation. The x-ray on the right shows the foreign body lying adjacent to the radius, and calcification in the wall of the aneurysm. Below is a photograph of the aneurysmal sac after removal. The proximal end of the radial artery (R.A.), is indicated.

When the aneurysm is located in an extremity it is frequently *traumatic,* a history of a penetrating injury which has healed is usually obtained. The patient's first intimation of disease is usually swelling or pulsation; the mass may increase in size slowly or rapidly. Soon a weakness or stiffness of the limb is complained of. At times, pain at the site of the aneurysm or along the course of the nerve is experienced because of pressure by the mass. The pain is more severe if bone is being eroded. The extremity may become cold and pale, and on rare occasions gangrene may develop. Rupture of the vascular mass with serious or fatal hemorrhage may occur.

One of the most diagnostic features of aneurysm is the presence of expansile pulsation as detected by careful palpation or by fluoroscopy. This must not be confused with transmitted pulsation which is noted frequently when solid tumors lie against large arteries.

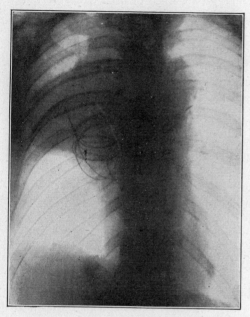

FIG. 314.—X-RAY SHOWING AN ANEURYSM OF
THE AORTA.

The roentgenogram was taken shortly after the aneurysm had been "wired," following which the patient's pain was entirely relieved. This method for the relief of pain is being supplanted almost entirely by paravertebral injection of the upper dorsal sympathetics which is discussed on page 588.

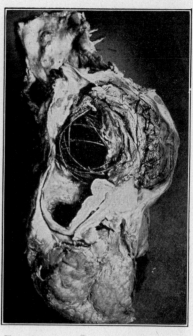

FIG. 315.—AUTOPSY SPECIMEN OF AN
AORTIC ANEURYSM.

The patient died 48 hours after the aneurysm was wired. Note the coils of wire (about 8 feet) within the sac and absence of clot formation which occurs only occasionally.

Treatment.—Paravertebral injections of alcohol into the upper dorsal sympathetics has recently proved to be an effective method for the relief of pain (see page 588); removal of the upper thoracic ganglia by operative means may be advisable in certain cases (White [38]). In sacculated thoracic or abdominal aneurysms the passage of a galvanic current through a coil of silver or steel wire, which is inserted into the sac through an insulated needle, is likewise effective in relieving pain. If a clot forms, as it occasionally does, progression of the aneurysm is arrested temporarily. Aneurysms of the terminal portion of the abdominal aorta can occasionally be treated successfully by ligation without subsequent development of gangrene of the extremities (Brooks, *J. A. M. A.,* 87:722, 1926). If the aneurysm is located in an extremity, ligation of the artery proximal and distal to the aneurysm with excision of the sac is usually curative. The classic monograph of W. S. Halsted [s] on ligation of the subclavian artery describes many interesting cases. Gangrene of an extremity following this type of ligation rarely occurs because of the preformed collateral circulation; ligation of the artery in aneurysms of the popliteal artery is much more apt to result in gangrene, since there is a paucity of anastomotic vessels at this point. Aneurysmorrhaphy as described by Matas may be resorted to if gangrene following ligation is feared. This method consists of opening the sac, folding and suturing the walls of the aneurysm together to such a degree that a lumen of more or less normal size is produced.

PERIPHERAL VASCULAR DISEASES

Under this heading may be considered a group of disorders which interfere with the distribution of blood through peripheral areas. They may be classified as:

I. Diseases resulting from abnormal functional response of the arteries to various stimuli, including the autonomic nervous system which may or may not be at fault: angiospasm; Raynaud's disease; erythromelalgia; acrocyanosis

II. Diseases due to structural changes in vessels: thrombo-angiitis obliterans (Buerger's disease); arteriosclerosis

III. Diseases of the veins: varicose veins; thrombophlebitis.

Angiospasm.—Spasmodic contraction of the smooth muscle in the wall of an artery or in one segment of a vessel may come about in a number of circumstances as a result of vasoconstrictor impulses reaching the muscle through autonomic nerves. There is frequently a large element of vasospasm in organic disorders such as thrombo-angiitis obliterans and even arteriosclerosis. Thrombophlebitis, injury of a nonpenetrating type, or rough handling of an artery at operation may give rise to reflex spasm.

The best known clinical entity of this type is a vasomotor disturbance giving rise to bilateral symmetrical attacks of arterial spasm called *Raynaud's* syndrome. This was described in 1862 as a disease process which frequently resulted in bilateral symmetrical gangrene. Occasionally, long standing cases are seen today in which fibrosis of the arterial wall produces a permanent narrowing of the lumen and atrophic changes in the peripheral part, or even gangrene. The disorder most commonly occurs in women, with its onset in youth or early middle life and usually affects the hands, only occasionally being encountered in the feet. The first attack is often precipitated by some disturbing emotional experience and subsequent attacks may be preceded by some psychic upset; however, the history after the initial spasm is generally that cold produces a painful, persistent blanching of both hands with a later slow return of circulation, sometimes with an abnormal degree of redness, numbness, or paresthesia and pain. Gangrene may develop, but is always superficial and confined to the tips of the fingers. More often an atrophy of the pulp of the tips of the fingers develops, with a dry scaly skin. The nails may be distorted. The attacks may be minimized by preventing exposure to extreme cold, wearing warm gloves, or immersing the exposed hands in warm water. When such measures are of no avail, operation designed to interrupt the constrictor fibers should be done. Sectioning the autonomic nerves as they course along the outer arterial coat (Leriche) or in the postganglionic distribution is unsatisfactory (Smithwick [9]). In many cases there will result an increased sensitivity to adrenalin (Wright, Mulholland, CoTui, and McCloskey [10]), and spasm produced by cold or any other mechanism will be prolonged and extremely painful (Gask [11]). Smithwick [9] has described the operation for section of the preganglionic fibers supplying the upper extremity which will prevent rapid regeneration so common in these

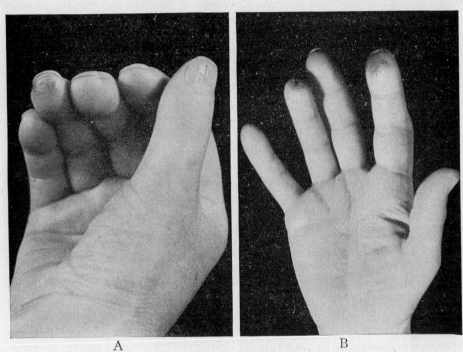

A   B

FIG. 316.—LESIONS ENCOUNTERED IN RAYNAUD'S DISEASE.

A, note slight scaling and atrophy on tip of third or ring finger; *B*, note superficial gangrene of tip of index and ring finger. Lesions of this extent are less common than the lesion noted in *A*.

nerves. The presence of the ganglion seems to complete a nervous arc which will permit vasodilatation after cold or some other stimulus to the periphery has produced normal constriction. Smoking is forbidden.

Arteriolar disease is a term applied by us to a condition showing evidence of arterial deficiency of the spastic type affecting particularly the lower extremities (occasionally the upper). Lack of knowledge regarding the pathogenesis of the disease prevents the application of an accurate name for the syndrome which we refer to here as arteriolar disease, because the disease is apparently primarily confined to the arterioles, at least at the onset. It is much more common than Raynaud's disease and is identified most readily in young or middle-aged people. It is possible that the disease is likewise common in old people, but up to the present time we have been reluctant to make this diagnosis in the aged because of possible confusion with arteriosclerosis. It is slightly more common in men than in women. Occasionally no pulsation will be palpable in the dorsalis pedis or posterior tibial artery, but rarely if ever are both pulsations absent. This feature of the disease suggests that an actual obliteration exists. On the other hand, the fact that the pulsation is occasionally regained following such factors as spinal anesthesia, heat therapy, etc., suggests that angiospasm is an important etiologic element. The first evidence of disease noted by the patient is that his feet are abnormally cold, and in winter require more protection from the weather than the feet of the average person. The patient frequently complains of profuse sweating of the feet and that they readily become tired. Severe pain, however, is rarely present. Injury to the skin of the feet, such as lacerations, heal slowly and are very apt to be accompanied by unusually severe infection and chronic ulcers on the feet or legs. The disease frequently occurs concomitantly with varicose veins and is a frequent cause of failure of ulcers to heal following obliteration of varicose veins. The disease differs markedly from Raynaud's disease in so far as it occurs as often in men as women, is not associated with typical spasmodic attacks of cyanosis or gangrene of any type. It is likewise sharply different from Buerger's disease because of the absence of severe pain. Moreover, absence of pulsation in both dorsalis pedis and posterior tibial artery, which is so characteristic of Buerger's disease, has not been noted in arteriolar disease. The disease probably resembles acrocyanosis more closely than any other disease. Examination reveals a dusky cyanotic blush of the lower extremity which fades to pallor when the feet are elevated. Sweating may be profuse. The feet are cold unless warmed by exercise or heat. Occasionally, chronic ulcers are present on the distal part of the leg, on the toes or plantar surface of the feet. *Treament* is not very important because most patients complain so little that therapy is not strongly indicated except from a prophylactic standpoint. Since open wounds of the lower extremities of patients with this disease are so apt to be followed by severe infection or chronic ulcers, the patients must be instructed to keep the feet clean, avoid injury, limit exercise, etc., to prevent serious complications. Usually the disease is discovered by the physician during the course of a routine examination, particularly where effort is being made to determine the causative factor in the chronicity of an ulcer of the foot or leg which fails to heal. In the severe cases smoking should be prohibited.

There are other disorders of the periphery probably due to some autonomic nervous system dysfunction which are not clearly understood. *Scleroderma,* a sharply localized thickening of areas of the skin, is relieved by preganglionic section of these nerves (see p. 587).

Erythromelalgia (*Weir Mitchell's Disease*).—This disease, as originally described by Mitchell [12] is rare, but its manifestations are dramatic because of its contrast to the manifestations of many other circulatory disturbances. The patient complains of constant frequent attacks of pain in the feet, particularly when they are held in the dependent position. Examination reveals swelling, *redness* and hyperesthesia of the skin which is unusually *warm,* presumably because of a vasodilation. The disease is perhaps slightly more common among men than women. There is no known satisfactory treatment.

Acrocyanosis.—The characteristic feature of this disease is a bluish red discoloration of the extremities (usually the hands and including the fingers particularly). The cyanotic color is aggravated by cold but is usually lost when the extremity is warmed or elevated. The skin of the extremity is cool and moist. In a great many respects this disease is similar to arteriolar disease as just described. In fact, Lewis and Landis[13] are of the opinion that the disease is primarily caused by a local spasm of the arterioles, but in a recent study, C. S. Stone[14] and associates have come to the conclusion that "the primary vascular fault in acrocyanosis is a dilatation and refractoriness to stimuli of the capillaries and venules of the skin." There is no efficacious method of treatment.

Thrombo-Angiitis Obliterans (Buerger's Disease).[15]—This disease is a progressive process involving whole arteries or segments of arteries of medium or

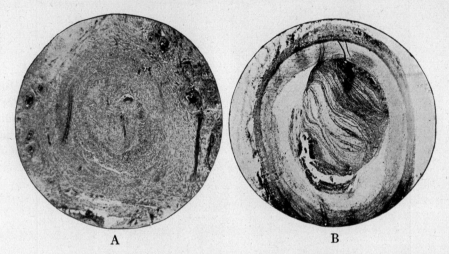

A   B

FIG. 317.—PHOTOMICROGRAPH OF ARTERIES IN BUERGER'S DISEASE; SPECIMENS OBTAINED FROM AN AMPUTATED LEG.

A, the entire artery has been obliterated by a thrombus which is fairly well organized. Note the marked inflammatory reaction, with dense fibrous tissue, surrounding the wall of the artery; *B,* this artery is likewise occluded by a thrombus, but recanalization is taking place. An unusually large amount of proliferation of the intima is present in this specimen.

small caliber characterized by thickening of the intima, thrombosis, periarterial inflammation which may involve the accompanying vein and nerve. The initial pathologic changes and the etiology are little known.

It occurs in men, in most series 100 per cent of cases being males. Tobacco smoking is considered by some writers to be a constant factor in the etiology although some cases have been reported in nonsmokers. Of the Mayo Clinic cases, more than 50 per cent were Jewish (Brown, Allen and Mahorner[16]) The onset is most often between the ages of twenty-five and forty-five.

Clinical Manifestations.—The disease may be ushered in in a number of ways. With sudden thrombotic occlusion of a hitherto patent, but narrowed artery, the onset may be sudden, painful, and with all the manifestations of an acute circulatory deficiency including gangrene. Most often, however, the symptoms like the pathologic process, develop gradually. In many cases the first sign will be a peculiar localized phlebitis of the superficial veins of the leg in areas which subside after a few days—to recur in some other vein or other area of the same vein. This condition is called *migrating phlebitis* and should lead one to an investigation of the state of the arteries. Gradually, developing arterial occlusion may produce the first symptoms of pain on exertion. This pain is situated in the calf muscles and subsides after a short rest. It is called *intermittent claudication*. The slowly developing cir-

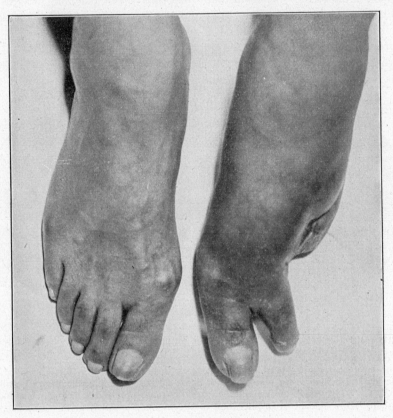

FIG. 318.—BUERGER'S DISEASE.

Onset one year ago with tingling and pain in the toes. Pain increased and became very severe. Six months after onset, the lateral three toes became gangrenous at the tip and were amputated. The incision healed, but later broke down, resulting in the ulcer as noted in the photograph. Note the cyanosis of the skin over the distal part of the foot. Pain is still present and now located in the remaining toes and distal part of the foot.

culatory deficiency promotes the development of a collateral circulation in the vessels of the skin. In patients whose demands are not greater than the collaterals can satisfy, the skin retains its warmth and well-nourished appearance, and retains a remarkable ability to heal small wounds and resist infection. Most patients in this stage who are untreated tax the collaterals beyond their capacity and the peripheral structures suffer from lack of blood. In these patients the skin of the foot may become blue or dusky red in color, shiny and stiff. Changes in the position of the foot result in marked color changes. In later stages of the neglected case, or in the treated case with insufficient collateral circulation the foot will appear swollen from edema; nutritional deficiencies in the skin, indolent ulcers and eventually gangrene of the toes may develop.

The periarterial inflammatory process which involves the vein and nerve gives rise to the most characteristic and distressing symptoms. The foot becomes deep red or blue, the pain becomes intense, and the skin hyperesthetic to a degree which

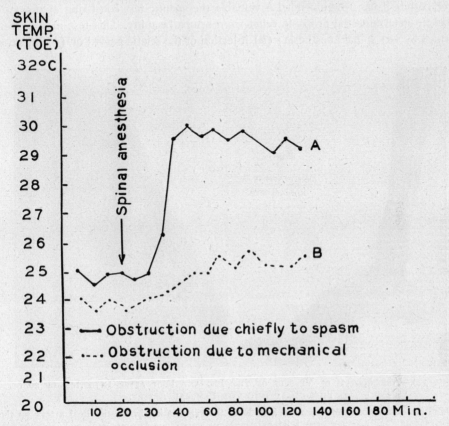

FIG. 319.—GRAPHIC CHART TO ILLUSTRATE METHOD OF DIFFERENTIATING ARTERIAL SPASM FROM ACTUAL MECHANICAL OCCLUSION BY THE RESPONSE OF SKIN (TOE) TEMPERATURE TO PARALYSIS OF VASOCONSTRICTOR FIBERS (VASODILATATION) BY SPINAL ANESTHESIA.

Curve A shows a rise of 5° to 6° C. above normal, indicating that most, but not all, of the obstruction was due to spasm. Patients with normal arteries or obstruction due entirely to spasm would exhibit a rise of 7° to 9° C., depending on the type of vasodilating method used. Curve B illustrates a rise of only 2° or less, indicative of actual mechanical occlusion, which in this instance was due to arteriosclerosis.

will not permit the bed clothes to rest on it. For some reason most relief is obtained with the foot hanging over the side of the bed, the hands grasping the ankle and encircling it. Fortunately, the inflammatory process recedes spontaneously in many patients; but in some, when it persists, it is the reason the patient will beg for amputation. There almost always is a vasospastic element in the circulatory deficiency.

Diagnostic Tests in Circulatory Disease.—It is important to determine the presence of vasomotor spasm which is frequently associated with the anatomical changes in thrombo-angiitis obliterans as well as in other types of circulatory disease. This is of particular value therapeutically since section of the sympathetic nerve supply to the vessels of the extremity affected with considerable vasomotor spasm might lead to beneficial results because of the vasodilatation produced by this procedure (see Chapter XXII). Before any operative procedures are instituted, however, White [17] has recommended a valuable therapeutic test consisting of novocain block to determine the probable relief from sympathectomy. This test may be performed by (a) spinal anesthesia; (b) injection of the sciatic nerve; or (c) injection

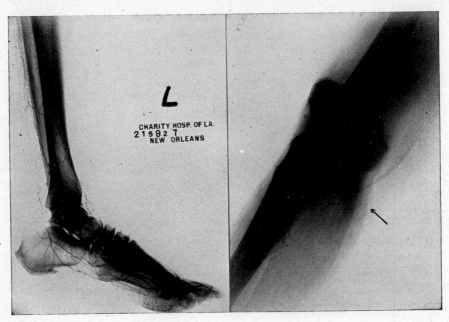

Fig. 320.—Arteriogram of Vessels of the Leg and Foot after Injection of 20 cc. Thorotrast into the Femoral Artery.

The major arterial trunks are blocked. Note the calcification in the popliteal artery on the right. Amputation was performed later because of gangrene. (From Veal and McFetridge, *Ann. Surg.,* 101:770, Fig. 3, 1935.)

of the lumbar sympathetic chain. An appreciable rise in surface temperature (5 to 7° C.) indicates that vasodilatation is still possible and sympathectomy will be followed by beneficial results. Scott and Morton [18] have devised a simpler method of differentiating spasm from organic occlusion by injecting the posterior tibial nerve at the internal malleolus with novocain. If there is a normal response after the anesthesia, *i.e.,* a rise in temperature of the great toe of 7 to 10° C. up to a level of about 30.5° C., the presence of organic occlusion is ruled out. If a moderate rise in temperature is obtained, the deficiency is caused by a mixture of spasm and organic occlusion. If no increase in temperature is noted it is assumed that the walls of the arteries are so badly diseased that dilatation is impossible. Coller and Maddock [19] resort to a still more simple method of determining the amount of vascular occlusion present. They expose the patient's bare body to room temperature for an hour, record the temperature of the skin of the feet, etc., wrap the patient in three woolen blankets for one hour and again record the skin temperature. In normal people and patients with angiospasm uncomplicated by organic obstruction, the temperature of the feet rises to the vasodilatation level, *i.e.*, 33° C. In patients with organic obstruction of their arteries such as that produced by Buerger's disease and arteriosclerosis, the temperature of the feet will rise little or none at all. It is perhaps more accurate to expose the patients to a constant temperature (*e.g.*, 68° F., 20° C.) before wrapping them in blankets, thereby standardizing the method more completely.

There are various types of oscillometers which determine the amount of pulsation in a large artery to an extremity. By injecting the sympathetics to the extremity

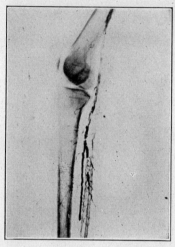

FIG. 321.—ARTERIOGRAM MADE BY INJECTION OF A SUSPENSION OF BARIUM SULPHATE INTO THE FEMORAL ARTERY OF A LEG AMPUTATED FOR ARTERIOSCLEROTIC GANGRENE OF THE FOOT.

Note the filling defect in the artery and the block in the lumen at the juncture of the lower and middle third of the leg.

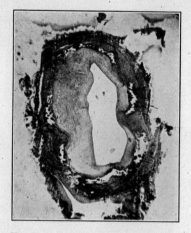

FIG 322.—MICROSCOPICAL TRANSVERSE SECTION (LOW POWER) OF AN ARTERY SHOWING CHANGES DUE TO ARTERIOSCLEROSIS.

Note that the hypertrophy of the intima partially obliterates the lumen. There is an extensive deposition of fat in the thickened intima, which can be seen better in sections specially stained to show fat (*e.g.*, Sudan stain).

with novocain, an increase in skin temperature will be detected if spasm has been present in addition to organic obstruction in the artery. This procedure will be found very helpful in arterial obstruction such as Buerger's disease, since on a few occasions there will be sufficient spasm accompanying the obliterative endarteritis to justify sympathectomy. Temperature changes illustrating the amount of spasm may also be obtained before and after immersing an extremity in warm water or after giving a vasodilating drug such as sodium nitrite (Beck and de Takats [20]).

Arteries as well as veins may be visualized by taking an x-ray picture 1 to 3 seconds after injection of an impervious solution; of the various solutions used, diodrast is the most satisfactory. It may even be used to outline the chambers of the heart (Robb and Steinberg [21]). Details of many of the tests for determining vascular disease may be found in the excellent monograph by White.[23] Other tests including the histamine tests, etc., which are more applicable to determination of the level of amputation, are described elsewhere in the text.

Treatment of Buerger's Disease.—The treatment is essentially the encouragement of a collateral circulation sufficient to meet the needs of the patient, or the adjustment of the needs of the patient to the blood supply available. If the occlusion is progressing at a greater rate than skin vessels are developing, the patient must obviously be put at complete rest. Many cases are known to have enlarged their

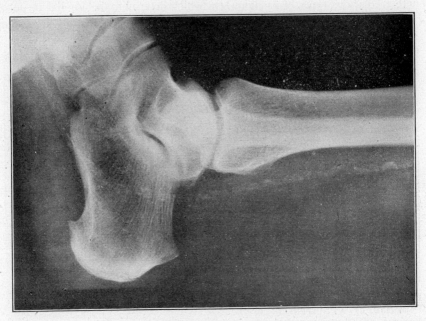

FIG. 323.—X-RAY OF FOOT OF A MAN AGED SEVENTY WITH MODERATE GENERALIZED ARTERIOSCLEROSIS.

The patient did not have gangrene; the only symptom complained of was slight coldness of the feet. Note the calcified posterior tibial artery. The degree of circulatory impairment cannot be determined without an arteriogram because of the variable amount of collateral circulation.

smaller vessels to a degree which compensates for the loss of all major arteries thus restoring them to normal functional activity. Any vasoconstricting factor, such as smoking, should be strictly forbidden [24, 25, 26] and vasodilating measures, such as small doses of alcoholic drinks or the caffeine group of drugs should be encouraged. Buerger's exercises, the alternate elevation and lowering of the legs to empty and fill the collaterals are very helpful. Measures designed to stimulate the dilatation of smaller vessels by alternate suction and pressure (Pavaex machine [27]) or better still by intermittent venous occlusion with a pressure cuff should be tried. It is probably advisable in many cases to section the autonomic pressor nerves, not only because of a spastic element in the occlusion but also because the collaterals develop faster in the denervated extremity. Artificial fever with its accompanying vaso-dilatation may be used.

The pain of intermittent claudication is relieved by rest; the pain of migrating phlebitis is not too severe; the rest pain—due to involvement of the peripheral nerve, is a difficult problem. Smithwick and White [28] first suggested that the peripheral nerves be injected with alcohol, and Laskey and Silbert [29] later suggested cutting the nerves and resuturing them. The latter seems to be the most effective measure and should be used in painful ulcers, or the "rest pain." If morphine is given for pain, care must be taken lest an addiction be developed. Rarely is amputation necessary for pain alone. In gangrene when it is indicated, conservatism in selecting the site is the keynote of modern treatment.

Arteriosclerosis.—This is one of the most common diseases of the arteries, but is chiefly of medical significance. However, arteriosclerotic occlusion of the vessels of the lower extremities producing symptoms of circulatory impairment occurs frequently in the aged and often may lead to gangrene (see Chapter VII). Frequently, arteriosclerosis is the cause of the rupture of an artery within the brain (apoplexy). The coronary artery in the heart may become occluded (angina pectoris), thereby leading to serious myocardial damage.

THE VEINS

In a consideration of diseases of the veins, it is important to remember that in the lower extremity there is a superficial (saphenous) and deep (femoral) venous system which are separated by deep fascia, through which the communicating veins

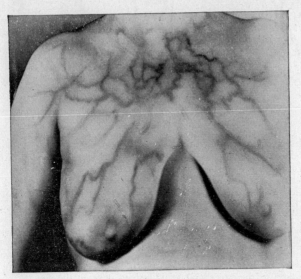

FIG. 324.—PHOTOGRAPH TAKEN WITH AN INFRA-RED PLATE SHOWING THE VEINS OF THE CHEST DILATED AS A RESULT OF VENOUS OBSTRUCTION FROM A SUBSTERNAL GOITER.

(From Pemberton and Haines, in Christopher, *Textbook of Surgery*, W. B. Saunders Co.)

penetrate. The saphenous vein ultimately joins the femoral vein in the upper part of the thigh at the saphenous opening.

Varicose Veins.—The term varix or varicose vein is usually applied to the varicosities affecting the superficial veins of the leg, although esophageal varices, varicoceles and hemorrhoids should perhaps be classified as varicose veins. The deep veins are never the site of varicosities because of the support supplied by the surrounding muscles.

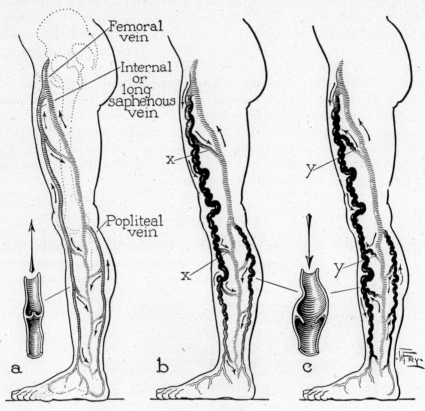

Fig. 325.

a, Diagrammatic drawing showing the relative relationship of the deep to the superficial veins of the lower extremities. As shown by the arrows, the direction of blood flow in the superficial and deep veins is upward, whereas the direction of blood flow in the communicating veins is from the superficial to the deep veins. This is possible because of competent valves in the deep, superficial and communicating veins. *b,* Diagrammatic drawing showing varicosities of the superficial veins with incompetency of the valves in these veins. There is a reversal of blood flow in the superficial veins, *i.e.,* from above downward. Because, however, the valves in the communicating veins (*X*) are still competent, the direction of blood flow is normal, *i.e.,* from the superficial to the deep veins. *c,* Diagrammatic drawing showing varicosities of the superficial and communicating veins with reversal of blood flow in both sets of veins. Because of incompetency of the valves in the communicating veins, as shown in *Y,* the direction of the blood flow is from the deep to the superficial veins instead of from the superficial to the deep as normally occurs.

(From Ochsner, in Lewis-Walters, *Practice of Surgery,* W. F. Prior Co.)

Of the several *etiologic factors* associated with the condition, perhaps the most important is an inherent weakness of the wall of the vein, presumably of congenital origin. Inadequacy or incompetency of the valves, while perhaps also of congenital origin, is more likely a secondary result of the dilatation of the vein. Venous stasis produced by wearing apparel (tight circular garters, etc.) and long hours of standing, are important secondary factors. Venous obstruction associated with tumors and numerous pregnancies also aid in the production of varicose veins. The pressure exerted by the long column of blood is of course an important mechanical factor in the etiology. Women are affected more commonly than men.

Clinical Manifestations.—Important in the pathogenesis of symptoms is the circulatory impairment resulting from the varicosities, since the return flow of blood

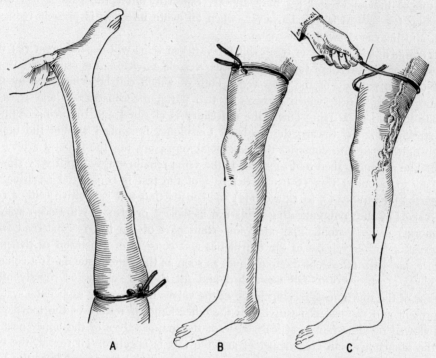

A   B   C

Fig. 326.—Principles in the Performance of the Trendelenburg Test.

A, with the patient lying supine and the extremity elevated, the blood is forced out of the veins by stroking the leg from above downward; a tourniquet is then applied, but only tight enough to constrict the superficial veins and not the femoral. It is easier to determine the correct amount of pressure by holding the ends of the tourniquet in the hands. *B,* negative *constriction test:* the patient was asked to stand and the rapidity of filling of the saphenous system noted. In this case these veins did not fill during thirty seconds observation: the test is therefore negative. *C,* positive *release test;* the tourniquet is released and the fall of the blood column in the saphenous vein observed. In this case the column fell immediately; the test is therefore positive. If the saphenous system is already filled before the tourniquet is released, it must be emptied by again placing the patient on the table. For interpretation of results see text.

is seriously interfered with, thereby leading to local venous stasis. Varicosities usually appear first on the medial side of the leg or thigh, although they may be present on any portion of the lower extremity. As the walls of the vein dilate and stretch, the vessel becomes tortuous. On many occasions the patients present no complaints except from a cosmetic standpoint. The most frequent symptom is a tired sensation which is made more prominent by prolonged inactivity in a standing or sitting position. Itching and tingling of the skin of the leg is not uncommon. Pain is seldom complained of, although occasionally it may be present and cramp like in character. Pigmentation or eczema of the skin of the leg is apt to appear when the varicosities have been present over a long period of time. One of the most important manifestations is the chronic ulcer which may result from the slightest trauma, or appear spontaneously. These ulcers are usually located on the inner side of the lower third of the leg and are rarely painful (see p. 514). Diffuse scarring of the skin may be present as the result of the healing of these ulcers. Edema of the ankle and leg may appear, especially after the patient has been standing for several hours. However, when an acute infection is present redness, pain and increased swelling develop.

Treatment.—The type of treatment for varicose veins will depend upon (*a*) the efficiency of the valves of the communicating vessels as well as the saphenous vein; and (*b*) the patency of the deep veins, both of which can be determined by the Trendelenburg [30] test, which consists of two parts, the constriction and release. While the patient is lying down, the extremity is elevated and the veins emptied by stroking the leg toward the thigh. A tourniquet is applied around the upper thigh tight enough to constrict the superficial veins, but not the femoral artery or vein. The patient is then told to stand. If the veins remain empty or fill very slowly (20 to 30 seconds) this (constrictive) part of the test is considered negative. If the veins fill rapidly (5 to 15 seconds) the constriction test is positive; either (*a*) the valves of the communicating veins are inefficient or else (*b*) the deep system (femoral) is not patent. The other important part of the test is concerned with observations after release of the tourniquet and consists of repetition of the procedure, but with release of the tourniquet as soon as the patient stands. If a column of blood is observed to fall downward and fill the varicose veins rapidly after release of the tourniquet, incompetency of the valves in the upper saphenous system is present and the test is positive. On the other hand, if release of the tourniquet is followed by slow filling, at least some of the major valves of the upper portion of the saphenous vein are competent and the test is negative. To repeat, the two parts of the Trendelenburg test as mentioned above may be referred to as the constriction and release test. If the veins fill rapidly after application of a tourniquet as described above, indicating insufficiency of the valves of the communicating veins, the test may be designated as a *positive constriction test* (*commonly known also as Trendelenburg double positive*). If a column of blood is seen to fall downward and fill the saphenous vein upon release of the tourniquet the test is designated as a *positive release test* (*commonly known also as Trendelenburg positive*), and indicates that the valves of the saphenous trunk are inadequate. As has been emphasized by Sarma,[31] incompetency of the valves of the communicating veins is usually complicated by incompetency of the valves of the saphenous vein which may make it difficult to obtain a clear cut release test. Regardless of whether or not the valves of the saphenous or communicating veins are efficient, injection of a sclerosing agent such as sodium morrhuate as described later, is indicated if symptoms are present. However, if the test reveals an inefficiency of either set of valves mentioned above, recurrence is more apt to occur, and more injections than usual will be necessary to effect a cure. On the other hand, the prognosis is very good if only the valves of the saphenous trunk are incompetent, because ligation of the vein as discussed later, followed by obliteration by injection is usually not followed by recurrence. In the presence of an obliterated deep circulation (*i.e.*, thrombosis of the femoral vein), injection, though rarely disastrous, might be harmful and be followed by recurrence or an increase in the edema.

A simple and practical method for determining the advisability of obliteration of the varicose veins is to instruct the patient to wear an elastic bandage around the leg for a few days while walking. This is, in effect, a therapeutic test. If the bandage causes amelioration of symptoms, relief may be expected from obliteration of the varicose veins. If the bandage has been worn correctly and discomfort is increased, obliteration of the veins may not yield favorable results because of impairment (usually thrombosis) of the deep circulation. If injections are not done an elastic bandage and adjustment of the patient's activities afford much relief.

The *Perthes* test will be found useful in estimating the patency of the deep circulation. A tourniquet is placed around the thigh above the varicosities just tight enough to prevent reflux of blood down the saphenous trunk. The patient is then instructed to walk vigorously for a minute or two. If the communicating and deep veins are patent and functioning normally, the saphenous varicosity will become emptied because exercise has forced the blood into the deep system and into the general circulation. Mahorner and Ochsner [32] have modified the Perthes test into a *comparative tourniquet test* which determines particularly the competency of the communicating veins between the deep and superficial system. By numerous trials, having the patient walk with the tourniquet applied at different levels the level of incompetent valves in the communicating veins can be determined. For example, they remark that "when the tourniquet is below the lowest communicating vein of the thigh in which the valves are competent, the veins of the calf become less prominent. In this instance high ligation alone is not sufficient, and low ligation also must be performed to prevent retrograde flow through communicating veins."

Obliteration by injection of sclerosing substances has during recent years supplanted operative removal of varicose veins. Injection of chemicals such as sodium salicylate, sodium morrhuate, quinine and urethane, etc., are very effective in producing a phlebitis (and usually thrombosis), which obliterates the lumen of the vein. Occasionally recanalization of the obliterated veins may take place. Ochsner and Garside [33] have conducted numerous experiments in an effort to determine the most advantageous sclerosing agent. They concluded that a 5 per cent solution of sodium morrhuate is the most desirable of the solutions now in use. Injection produces no pain; the usual dose is 2 cc. but slightly smaller doses may be injected at two or three different places. It has likewise been our experience that sodium morrhuate * is the most efficient substance in effecting obliteration of the veins; sodium salicylate (5 cc. of 40 per cent solution) produces obliteration with perhaps the least amount of local reaction, although the pain produced by its injection is so intense as to preclude its use in many patients. Care must be taken lest a portion of the fluid escape outside the vein, since most solutions used (especially sodium salicylate) will produce a slough when injected outside the vein. The injections may be given every four or five days as long as no complications are encountered. The sclerosing substance is injected through a fine hypodermic needle with the

---

* Sodium morrhuate is a mixture of the salts of the unsaturated fatty acids of cod liver oil; it is available as a 5 per cent solution with added benzyl alcohol.

patient lying down, sitting, or standing. The application of pressure or a tourniquet several inches above the site of injection may increase the efficiency of the chemical agent. A bandage should be applied after injection to prevent leakage at the site of the needle puncture, as well as to encourage obliteration of the vein by adhesion of its walls rather than by thrombosis. It is preferable that the patient be ambulatory except for bed rest of perhaps one-half hour following each injection. If the thrombosis produced by the injection is complicated by infection, as shown by redness, tenderness, swelling and pain along the site of the vein, injections must not be resumed for several weeks and only after all clinical evidence of the infection has disappeared.

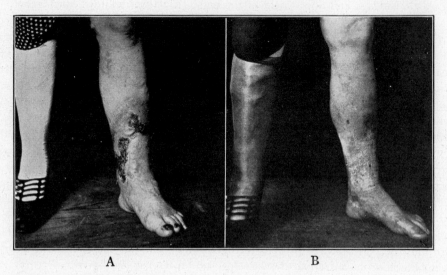

A   B

FIG. 327.—VARICOSE ULCERS OF THE LEG.

A, ulcers due to varicosity are usually single, not multiple. *B,* appearance of leg several months later, after obliteration of the veins by injection of a sclerosing agent (in this instance sodium salicylate). Note that the ulcer has healed and that the varicosities are obliterated. (Washington University Clinic.)

As intimated previously, sodium morrhuate is perhaps associated with less reaction than any of the sclerosing agents. However, anaphylactoid reactions may occur; Dobson[34] reports two serious reactions in 4,000 injections. Reactions are most apt to occur when a second series is begun after a rest period. The initial dose should always be small (0.5 cc.) following rest periods. If a reaction takes place, it is not safe to give additional injections because the reactions will be increasingly severe and perhaps fatal. Sensitivity to the drug may also be determined by doing a patch test.

Ligation of the saphenous vein is an advantageous supplement to injection of the veins, when the valves in the saphenous trunk are incompetent (as noted by the Trendelenburg and other tests). It should be carefully performed, at the saphenofemoral junction with division of the main trunks; all the tributaries of the saphenous at that point should be cut and ligated, even if they are not dilated. When the valves of the saphenous are incompetent, injection alone without ligation is usually followed by recurrence. The details of ligation and its indication have been discussed by Faxon,[35] de Takats,[36] Sarma,[31] and others.

Complications of Varicose Veins.—On rare occasions a varicosity will rupture through the skin with the consequent loss of considerable blood. Elevation of the extremity and application of a pressure bandage will control the bleeding.

After the varicosities have been present for a sufficient length of time to produce malnutrition of the skin, ulcers are apt to appear. Ligation of the saphenous vein in the presence of an ulcer is somewhat unsafe, because of the danger of infection or emboli, but some surgeons do it without undue reaction. If much infection is present about the ulcer it should be treated with bed rest, elastic bandage, elevation and heat before even injections are begun. The clinical appearance of these ulcers and the treatment (other than injection therapy) are discussed in Chapter VII. Lymphatic obstruction due to chronic infection and fibrosis is frequently a salient factor in the chronicity of the ulcer, as is discussed in the next chapter. An associated arteriolar disease of the type described on page 501 is present in a remarkably large number of patients with varicose veins of long standing, particularly those associated with ulcers. Lymphangiectasis is also encountered occasionally (p. 531). Because of the frequency with which more than one lesion is present in patients with circulatory diseases of the extremities, diagnosis is often difficult. See chart, page 517, for differential points.

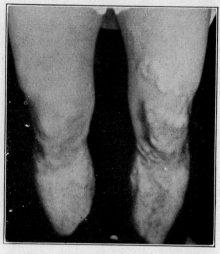

FIG. 328.—MARKEDLY TORTUOUS VARICOSITIES OF THE LEGS, PARTICULARLY THE LEFT.

The constriction as well as the release test was positive on the left. The veins are usually difficult to obliterate by injection alone in such instances, and recurrence is common; a preliminary ligation of the saphenous vein is therefore indicated.

Thrombophlebitis of varicose veins may occur spontaneously at any point in the veins, but usually starts in a sacculated varicosity. Thrombosis, of course, is induced following injection and is, therefore, of therapeutic value. The thrombosis rarely progresses beyond the saphenous system, and practically never gives rise to pulmonary embolism. The thrombosed vessel is usually felt as an isolated cord-like structure free from signs of inflammation. Only rarely is the thrombosis accompanied by redness and tenderness, or other evidence of infection. Treatment of the average thrombosed varix is simple and conservative. After the acute process has subsided it will be safe and advisable to proceed with the treatment by ligation and injection as already described. Bed rest and elevation of the extremity is advisable. On rare occasions when the process appears to be progressing upward or has given rise to a pulmonary embolus, high ligation of the saphenous may be indicated.

Thrombophlebitis of Deep Veins not Varicose.—The most common type occurs in the femoral vein, *i.e.,* thrombophlebitis femoris (milk leg, phlegmasia alba dolens) and is usually secondary to pelvic inflammation accompanying childbirth, pneumonia and operations for suppurative lesions, especially of the pelvis and abdomen. There is no doubt that confinement in bed made necessary by the above conditions is important in the development of the thrombophlebitis because of the slowing of the peripheral circulation, and stasis of the venous return. The extent of the edema cannot be explained on the basis of obstruction of the femoral vein alone. From experience we know that ligation of the vein will not produce it, probably because of the extensive venous collateral system. However, the edema might be explained on the basis of a widespread thrombosis involving the tributaries (de Takats [37]) being secondary to mechanical and inflammatory factors. Obstruction of major lymphatic trunks (Homans [39]) is also an important factor particularly in the production of edema. A variable amount of vascular spasm, involving the arterioles, appears to be present.

Pain is present in the medial part of the thigh; the entire extremity is swollen, pale, somewhat edematous, and colder than normal. A moderate amount of local tenderness along the course of the deep femoral vessels is present. Fever accompanies the onset of the process if not already present. The course of the disease is usually two to three weeks and may be followed by a permanent dilatation of the superficial veins, which then act as the collateral venous circulation and may be mistaken for varicose veins. Permanent symptoms of pain, ulceration and other evidence of circulatory impairment occasionally occur. In most cases of femoral thrombophlebitis the edema and other manifestations disappear in two or three weeks with very few if any residual difficulties. Undoubtedly, the extent of the process upward and the number of tributaries involved are important factors in the duration of symptoms. The thrombosis usually extends past the femoral into the external iliac; frequently, it extends into the common iliac, and less commonly into the vena cava. Thrombosis may involve the *deep veins of the leg* as a result of infection or injuries. Pain is present, and is aggravated by walking up stairs. Swelling may be trivial and is always limited to the leg, but may involve the thigh later, if the thrombosis extends up into the femoral vein as it is apt to do. Dorsiflexion of the ankle produces pain in the calf or back of the knee. Tenderness over the posterior part of the leg is almost always present. Thromboses of the deep veins of the leg are of much importance because of the tendency to give rise to pulmonary emboli, a complication which probably occurs more commonly in postoperative patients.

The *treatment* of thrombophlebitis femoris is conservative, *i.e.,* elevation of the extremity under a cradle, and rest in bed. The patient must not be permitted to sit up or hold the extremity in a dependent position, because circulatory stasis would be increased about the proximal end of the clot, thereby encouraging extension upward. Movement of the leg for two or three weeks following the thrombosis is also avoided in order to insure against embolism, which appears to be more common when the phlebitis involves the veins of the leg. To prevent pulmonary embolism, ligation of the femoral vein is indicated in a large proportion of the cases, as discussed by Allen [44], Fine and associates [45], and others. Division as well as ligation is usually indicated because of the likelihood that complete severance of the vein may interrupt some of the impulses responsible for vasospastic reflexes.

TABLE 6

DIFFERENTIATION OF CIRCULATORY DISEASES OF THE EXTREMITIES

	Buerger's Disease	Raynaud's Disease	Arteriolar Disease	Arteriosclerosis	Varicose Veins	Femoral Thrombophlebitis
Age Sex Frequency	25 to 40 Mostly male Fairly common	25 to 40 Mostly female Rare	Any age Either sex Frequent	Above 50 Either sex Frequent	Above 20 Either sex Most frequent	Any age More often female Frequent
Pathogenesis	Obliterating thrombo-angiitis; vasospasm sometimes present; migrating phlebitis	Vasospasm; sensitivity to adrenalin(?); organic occlusion sometimes present	Probable onset vasospasm; later develops organic occlusion	Organic arterial obstruction by lipoid deposition and calcification	Congenital weakness of wall and defect of valves; occupation, pregnancy, etc.	Secondary to childbirth, appendicitis, and pelvic operations
Site of Disease	Usually feet, rarely hands	Usually hands, rarely feet	Usually feet, also hands at times	Chiefly legs but disease is systemic	Legs and thighs	May spread proximally to iliac veins and vena cava
Clinical Manifestations Pain	Very severe, sometimes intermittent claudication	Severe during attacks	Slight if any	Intermittent claudication	Dull aches and tired feeling relieved by walking	Dull and moderate in degree
Color	Cyanosis	Pallor with cyanosis during attacks	Cyanotic blush on dependency	Pallor with occasional cyanosis	Normal, or brown pigmentation	Pale or normal
Swelling	None	None	None	None	Yes	Most marked
Local Temperature	Markedly reduced	Reduced especially during attacks	Always low	Always low	Normal	Normal or low
Pulse	Absent	Present except during attacks	Present (absent occasionally)	Absent	Present	Present unless obliterated by edema
Ulceration (when present)	Particularly of the toes	Particularly of the finger tips	Foot and ankle (but not frequent)	Only when due to gangrene	Lower leg	Lower leg but uncommon
Gangrene (when present)	Superficial	Superficial	None	Massive	None	None
Treatment	Prophylactic; no smoking; amputation especially for pain, pavaex	Prophylactic; no smoking; sympathectomy(?)	Prophylactic; no smoking	Prophylactic: amputation for gangrene	Elastic bandage; injection of veins; ligation of saphenous vein	Rest in bed; elevation of leg

The preferred site is just below the profunda, thereby allowing collateral blood flow through the profunda and internal saphenous. If the clot has reached this point, ligation is performed higher, or the clot extracted from the incised vein (Allen [44]).

The chief value of bed rest lies in the fact that the inflammatory process subsides more rapidly under immobilization, and the edema is decreased by elevation of the extremity. It is extremely important that the edema by eradicated as soon as possible since the longer it is present, the more permanent it is apt to be. Restriction of fluids and salt are important; the use of salyrgan or calcium gluconate may tend to decrease the edema (de Takats, *Illinois, M. J.,* 79:25, 1941).

Mention has already been made (p. 496) of the use of dicoumarin (orally) and heparin (intravenously) in order to minimize extension of the clot, and decrease the possibility of pulmonary embolism. Dicoumarin has the advantage of being effective when given orally, but an interval of 24 to 48 hours after the first dose is required before the desired prothrombin level is attained.

On the basis that venospasm and arteriospasm are important factors in the production and maintenance of edema in thrombophlebitis, Leriche and Kunlin,[40] Ochsner and DeBakey [41] and others recommend novocain block of the sympathetic trunks every day or two for a few injections, beginning *early* in the course of the disease. Walking in the early stage of the disease aggravates the swelling tremendously because the collateral veins and lymphatics have apparently not thoroughly developed. It is therefore essential that when the patient is allowed out of bed, an elastic bandage be applied to the affected extremity.

When the edema and pain are persistent and disabling, considerable relief may be obtained by the Kondoleon operation (see p. 531) which relieves the obstruction of the deep lymphatics by permitting an anastomosis to develop with the superficial system.

Other types of thrombophlebitis include pylephlebitis, or thrombophlebitis of the portal vein which is not uncommon, and is usually secondary to acute suppurative appendicitis or acute cholecystitis. In addition, thrombosis of the portal vein of a more chronic nature may appear during the course of cirrhosis of the liver, but is perhaps not accompanied by infection, and is rarely fatal of itself. Canalization usually occurs if the patient lives for several weeks following the occlusion. On the other hand, thrombophlebitis of the portal vein of the suppurative type, is often fatal within a short time of its onset, because of the infection and the added effect of the primary disease producing the pylephlebitis. Thrombophlebitis of the *sinuses of the brain* (*e.g.,* cavernous) is a serious condition (usually fatal), and is ordinarily secondary to infection of the upper part of the face (furuncle of the upper lip, etc.) or acute mastoiditis associated with cellulitis. A less common location for thrombophlebitis is the *mesenteric veins* within the abdomen; this lesion is discussed in detail on page 779. Phlebitis of the *axillary vein* is a rather uncommon condition but may occur as a complication of trauma in that region. Moderate swelling of the arm will be present. It does not tend to give rise to pulmonary embolism and gradually subsides. Perhaps more common is thrombosis of the *deep veins of the leg,* likewise associated with trauma and thus different from the thrombophlebitis femoris already described. It occurs also as a complication of local infections in that area and under such conditions is apt to result in pulmonary embolism. Diagnosis may be difficult on account of the slight amount of swelling which of course will not be present above the knee unless the thrombus extends into the femoral vein, not an unusual complication. Tenderness is usually present over the calf; walking produces pain in this area. Treatment is conservative; if extension develops, ligation of the femoral vein may be indicated. Thrombosis of the veins of the *forearm and antecubital fossa* following intravenous injection of glucose and other fluids is extremely common. The use of hypertonic solutions and of repeated vein puncture increases the incidence of this lesion. Tenderness and a variable amount of redness, swelling and pain will be present. Treatment consists of immobilization and application of hot packs. Pulmonary embolism rarely complicates the condition. Obviously, no attempt should be made to use the vein again for intravenous injection until all inflammatory signs are gone; the vein will usually be obliterated.

Postphlebitic Induration and Edema.—On many occasions chronic edema of the extremity, incident to thrombophlebitis of the femoral vein is followed by an induration of the skin and subcutaneous tissues, especially of the leg. As time goes on, pigmentation develops and the skin ultimately turns to a brownish color. This indurated tissue does not pit on pressure. Pain is variable, but at times is extremely annoying. Unless the patient takes considerable care by resting and elevation of the leg, ulcers are apt to appear. An important etiologic factor in the development of this condition appears to be a blockage of the lymphatics by the infection. Perhaps of more importance is the fact that extravasation of serum, high in protein concentration, as occurs in massive thrombosis of veins (de Takats [37]) results in the deposition of considerable amount of scar tisue. This in turn would lead to a variable degree of lymphatic and venous blockage. The scar tissue, however, is probably the chief factor in development of the induration. Treatment consists of restricting activity; the dependent position of the extremity should be avoided as much as possible. If ulcers are present, bed rest and hot wet dressings will be indicated particularly if much infection is present. Wearing an elastic bandage will be of some help. Occasionally, thorough examination by palpation for soft areas will reveal the presence of large varicosities. These should be obliterated by injection, although if ulcers are present, infection must first be cleared. The Kondoleon operation is sometimes of value.

BIBLIOGRAPHY

1. Christie, A. A Normal Closing Time of the Foramen Ovale and the Ductus Arteriosus, *Am. J. Dis. Child.*, 40,323, 1930.
2. Gross, R. E. Surgical Management of the Patent Ductus Arteriosus, *Ann. Surg.*, 110.321, 1939.
3. Brooks, B., Johnson, G. S., and Kirtley, J. A., Jr. Simultaneous Vein Ligation: An Experimental Study of the Effect of Ligation of Concomitant Vein on the Incidence of Gangrene Following Arterial Obstruction, *Surg., Gynec. & Obst.*, 59:496, 1934.
4. de Takats, G. Vascular Accidents of Extremities, *J. Am. M. Ass.*, 110:1075, 1938.
5. Potts, W. J. Pulmonary Embolism, *Ann Surg.*, 111:554, 1940.
6. Murray, Gordon. Heparin in Surgical Treatment of Blood Vessels, *Arch. Surg.*, 40:307, 1940; Murray, D. W. G., Jazues, L. B., Perrett, T. S., and Best, C. H. Heparin and Thrombosis of Veins Following Injury, *Surgery*, 2:163, 1937.

7. HOLMAN, E. Arteriovenous Aneurysm, *Ann. Surg.*, 80:801, 1924.

8. HALSTED, W. S. Ligations of the Left Subclavian Artery in Its First Portion, *J. H. H. R.*, 21:1, 1920.

9. SMITHWICK, R. H. The Problem of Producing Complete and Lasting Sympathetic Denervation of the Upper Extremity by Preganglionic Section, *Ann. Surg.*, 112:1085, 1940.

10. WRIGHT, A. M., MULHOLLAND, J. H., CoTUI, F. W., and McCLOSKEY, K. L. Local Adrenalin Effect After Sympathectomy, *J. Lab. and Clin. Med.*, 20:947, 1935.

11. GASK, G. E. Surgery of Sympathetic Nervous System; Bradshaw Lecture, *Brit. J. Surg.*, 21:113, 1933.

12. MITCHELL, Weir. Rare Vaso-motor Neurosis of the Extremities, *Am. J. M. Sc.*, 76:17, 1878.

13. LEWIS, Sir Thomas, and LANDIS, E. M. Observations Upon the Vascular Mechanism in Acrocyanosis, *Heart*, 15:229, 1930.

14. ELLIOT, A. H., EVANS, R. D., and STONE, C. S. Acrocyanosis: A Study of the Circulatory Fault, *Am. Heart J.*, 11:431, 1936.

15. BUERGER, Leo. *The Circulatory Disturbances of the Extremities*, W. B. Saunders Co., Philadelphia, 1924.

16. BROWN, G. E., and ALLEN, E. V. Thrombo-angiitis Obliterans: Clinical Physiologic and Pathologic Studies. Collaborating in Pathology, with H. R. Mahorner, *Mayo Clinic Monographs*, W. B. Saunders and Co., 1928.

17. WHITE, J. C. Diagnostic Novocaine Block of the Sensory and Sympathetic Nerves, *Am. J. Surg.*, 9:264, 1930; *J. Am. M. Ass.*, 94:1382, 1930.

18. SCOTT, W. J., and MORTON, J. J. Differentiation of Peripheral Arterial Spasm and Occlusion in Ambulatory Patients, *J. Am. M. Ass.*, 97:1212, 1931; *N. Eng. J. M.*, 204:955, 1931.

19. COLLER, F. A., and MADDOCK, W. G. Differentiation of Spastic from Organic Peripheral Vascular Occlusion by Skin-temperature Response to High Environmental Temperature, *Ann. Surg.*, 96:719, 1932.

20. BECK, W. C., and DE TAKATS, G. The Use of Sodium Nitrite for Testing the Flexibility of the Peripheral Vascular Bed, *Am. Heart J.*, 15:158, 1938.

21. ROBB, G. P., and STEINBERG, I. Visualization of the Chambers of the Heart, *J. Am. M. Ass.*, 114:474, 1940.

22. BLAKEMORE, A. H., LORD, J. W. Jr., and STEFKO, P. L. Restoration of Blood Flow in Damaged Arteries, *Ann. Surg.*, 117:481, 1943.

23. WHITE, J. C. The Autonomic Nervous System, Macmillan Co., New York, 1935.

24. MADDOCK, W. G., and COLLER, F. A. Peripheral Vasoconstriction by Tobacco and Its Relation to Thrombo-angiitis Obliterans, *Ann. Surg.*, 98:70, 1933.

25. WRIGHT, I. S., and MOFFAT, D. Effects of Tobacco on Peripheral Vascular System, *J. Am. M. Ass.*, 103:318, 1934.

26. LAMPSON, R. S. Quantitative Study of Vasoconstriction Induced by Smoking, *J. Am. M. Ass.*, 104:1963, 1935.

27. HERRMANN, L. G., and REID, M. R. The Conservative Treatment of Arteriosclerotic Peripheral Vascular Diseases, *Ann. Surg.*, 100:750, 1934.

28. SMITHWICK, R. H., and WHITE, J. C. Elimination of Pain in Obliterative Vascular Disease of Lower Extremities; Technique for Alcohol Injection of Sensory Nerves of Lower Leg, *Surg., Gynec. & Obst.*, 51:394, 1930.
———— Peripheral Nerve Block in Obliterative Disease of the Lower Extremity, *Surg., Gynec. & Obst.*, 60:1106, 1935.

29. LASKEY, N. F., and SILBERT, S. Thrombo-angiitis Obliterans; Relief of Pain by Peripheral Nerve Section, *Ann. Surg.*, 98:55, 1933.

30. TRENDELENBURG, F. Ueber die Unterbindung der Vena Saphena Magna bei Unterschenkelvaricen, *Beit. z. Klin. Chir.*, 7:195, 1890.

31. SARMA, P. J. Saphenous Vein Ligations, *Surg. Cl. N. A.*, 18:129, 1938.

32. MAHORNER, H. R., and OCHSNER, A. A New Test for Evaluating Circulation in

the Venous System of the Lower Extremity Affected by Varicosities, *Arch. Surg.*, 33:479, 1936.

33. OCHSNER, Alton, and GARSIDE, E. Intravenous Injections of Sclerosing Substances, *Ann. Surg.*, 96:691, 1932. OCHSNER, A., and MAHORNER, H. R. Comparative Value of Intravenous Sclerosing Substances, *Arch. Surg.*, 29:397, 1934.

34. DOBSON, L. Sodium Morrhuate Reactions, *Ann. Surg.*, 111:645, 1940.

35. FAXON, H. H. Treatment of Varicosities; Preliminary High Ligation of Internal Saphenous Vein with Injection of Sclerosing Substances, *Arch. Surg.*, 29:794, 1934.

36. DE TAKATS, Geza. Causes of Failure in the Treatment of Varicose Veins, *J. Am. M. Ass.*, 96:1111, 1931.

37. DE TAKATS, G. Management of Acute Thrombophlebitic Edema, *J. Am. M. Ass.*, 100:34, 1933; ZIMMERMAN, L. M., and DE TAKATS, G. The Mechanism of Thrombophlebitic Edema, *Arch. Surg.*, 23:937, 1931.

38. WHITE, J. C. Angina Pectoris; Treatment by Paravertebral Alcohol Injection or Operation Based on Newer Concepts of Cardiac Innervation, *Am. J. Surg.*, 9:98, 1930; Technic of Paravertebral Alcohol Injection, *Surg., Gynec. & Obst.*, 71:334, 1940.

39. HOMANS, J. Phlegmasia Alba Dolens and Relation of Lymphatics to Thrombophlebitis, *Am. Heart J.*, 7:415, 1932.

40. LERICHE, R., and KUNLIN, J. Traitement immediat des phlebites post-operatoires par l'infiltration novocainique du sympathique lombaire, *Press med.*, 42:1481, 1934.

41. OCHSNER, A., and DeBAKEY, M. Therapy of Phlebothrombosis and Thrombophlebitis, *Arch. Surg.*, 40:208, 1940.

42. STAHMANN, M. A., HUEBNER, C. F., and LINK, K. P. Studies on the Hemorrhagic Sweet Clover Disease: V. Identification and Synthesis of the Hemorrhagic Agent, *J. Biol. Chem.*, 138:513 (April), 1941.

43. ALLEN, E. V., BARKER, N. W., and WAUGH, J. M. A Preparation from Spoiled Sweet Clover which Prolongs Coagulation and Prothrombin Time of the Blood, *J. Am. Med. Ass.*, 120:1009, 1942.

44. ALLEN, A. W. Peripheral Circulation in Relation to Trauma, *Am. J. Surg.*, 59:177, 1943.

45. FINE, J. F., FRANK, H. A., and STARR, A. Recent Experiences with Thrombophlebitis of the Lower Extremity and Pulmonary Embolism, *Ann. Surg.*, 116:574, 1942.

CHAPTER XXI

THE LYMPHATIC SYSTEM

The Lymphatic Vessels
The Lymph Nodes
Differential Diagnosis of Tumefaction of the Neck

The lymphatic system is composed of vessels or channels which collect fluid (lymph) from the tissue spaces, and the lymph nodes through which these channels must pass before they finally empty into the veins of the neck. This system is really a part of the circulation of the blood since it carries away fluid brought to the tissues by the blood and brings it back again. Analysis of tissue lymph reveals only one essential difference from blood plasma, *i.e.,* normal lymph contains much less pro-

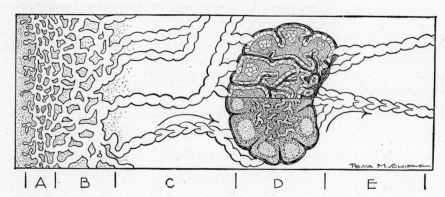

| A | B | C | D | E |

FIG. 329.—THE STRUCTURAL BASIS OF THE LYMPHATIC SYSTEM (SEMIDIAGRAMMATIC).

A, the irregular, blindly ending lymph capillaries. *B,* the reticular network. *C,* the afferent tubular lymphatics containing valves. *D,* the lymph node, presenting (above) the lymph sinuses and (below) the histologic picture. *E,* the efferent lymph vessels, showing above the arrow numerous valves. (From Curtis, in Christopher, *Textbook of Surgery,* 1936, W. B. Saunders Co., p. 188.)

tein; although it contains fibrinogen and coagulates, it does so much more slowly than blood. However, in the presence of infection, lymph contains more protein and usually coagulates more rapidly than plasma. Chyle is a milky mixture of emulsified fats and lymph which is found in the vessels draining the small intestines. Small lacteals in the villi of the intestine collect the emulsified fats and conduct them to larger trunks in the mesentery. Obviously, this lymph will contain but little emulsified fat during starvation. Chyle is of surgical importance in injuries to the thoracic duct or its tributaries.

Lymphatics have been known for 300 years, but our knowledge of the growth and development of these channels has been advanced during recent decades particularly by the work of Florence Sabin.[1] It is now known that lymphatic channels are present everywhere in the body (except the brain) and that they form a number of definite networks, each of which drains into regional lymph nodes. These nodes are composed of lymphocytic cells arranged along a labyrinth of channels, through which the lymph flows on its way centralward in gradually enlarging vessels, finally entering the thoracic duct which empties at the junction of the left jugular and left subclavian vein in the neck. A second smaller duct drains into the right side and carries lymph only from the right upper extremity and right side of the neck. The lymph vessels are thin endothelial lined channels equipped like the veins with valves.

This auxiliary circulation of body fluids has important functions in the interchange of fluid in the tissue spaces, much of which is even now under intensive investigation. Especially significant in surgery is the role the lymph vessels play in draining fluid from areas of acute inflammation. They also serve as a carrier of bacteria and of cancer cells, thus playing an important part in the extension of infection and of cancer. But the lymph nodes are means of protection; they halt, for a time at least, further invasion. In the case of cancer they act merely as a sieve, holding back the malignant cells for a while. With infection, however, their function is more useful; the cells lining the lymph spaces actively fight the invaders, and indeed in most cases succeed in killing them, thus protecting the rest of the body. In the process the nodes always enlarge and sometimes soften and suppurate. The lymph vessels, although usually passive agents, are not infrequently involved in surgical lesions, i.e., lymphangitis, lymphedema and elephantiasis. The neoplastic diseases of lymphatic vessels and nodes are described in Chapter XVI; the following discussion will therefore be largely confined to the inflammatory lesions.

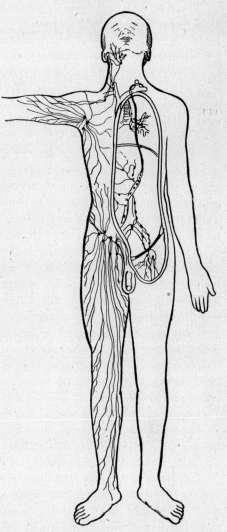

Fig. 330.—DIAGRAMMATIC SKETCH OF THE LYMPHATICS TO SHOW BOTH DEEP AND SUPERFICIAL SYSTEMS AS WELL AS THE MAIN REGIONAL GROUPS OF LYMPH NODES.

Note that the superficial lymphatics of the leg converge and enter the saphenous opening to join the deep lymphatics which then ascend along the iliac vessels to the thoracic duct.

THE LYMPHATIC VESSELS

The flow of lymph from tissue spaces is always active even in the resting limb. Under conditions of inflammation it is often tremendous. Experimental studies by Field, Drinker and White [2] have cast much light on lymph flow after such simple inflammation as occurs on immersion of the extremity in very hot water. Not only is the lymph pressure increased, but the protein content, normally about 1 per cent, rises to a value four times greater. The inability of the lymphatics to drain all of this exudate rapidly enough is probably responsible for the swelling in such areas and even outside the actual field of inflammation (*i.e.,* lymphedema) as discussed in more detail on page 526.

In the lower extremity at least, the lymphatics, like the veins, are composed of a deep and superficial group, separated by the deep fascia. Unlike the veins there are no communicating channels through this barrier, although they do converge and join at the saphenous opening below the inguinal ligament.

Trauma to Lymph Vessels.—Such injury is probably frequent, but is usually nonevident, for even if a large channel is cut the lymph clots at once or the flow is so slow as to escape detection, especially if much bleeding is present. Detailed experimental studies by McMaster and Hudack,[3] however, indicate that the tiny lymphatics severed by incisions remain open for as long as forty-eight hours, and may absorb infectious material for this length of time. Later, however, they proliferate extensively into the inflammatory area (as described in a previous chapter) and play an important role in healing and repair. On rare occasions clear fluid pours out of a wound profusely and for many days or weeks. Such an event is called lymphorrhea or lymphorrhagia. It is apt to be especially severe if the *thoracic duct* itself is torn as it enters the subclavian vein in injuries or operations in the left lower part of the neck. However, the flow of lymph usually stops spontaneously. Packing or closure of the wound controls the leakage.

Reëstablishment of lymph flow after complete division of lymphatics to a limb has been studied by Reichert.[4] He found that it occurs through regeneration of new channels, which is a rapid process, taking but a week in absence of infection.

Infection of Lymph Vessels.—Even in severe infections the larger lymphatics usually play but a passive role in carrying exudate and occasionally bacteria from the inflammatory area. On some occasions bacteria may gain access through a slight wound and be carried to the lymph node without provoking any significant reaction in either the skin or lymphatic channels. In such a case the first defense takes place in the node.

Acute Lymphangitis.—Acute inflammation of the major lymphatics does, however, frequently occur, and to distinguish it from the diffuse lymphangitis of the smaller channels is called *acute tubular lymphangitis*. It is evident clinically as red streaks which extend up the arm or leg from the local portal of entry. It may be seen following relatively mild infections, but usually means a serious invasion and is frequently accompanied by the signs of systemic infection, *i.e.,* chills, fever and prostration. In such a case the visible lymphatic vessels are intensely red, swollen and often surrounded by an area of edema. Tenderness is slight. Except in the severe or fatal cases, the process usually subsides in two to five days. However, the regional lymphadenitis which so frequently develops following the lymphangitis, usually subsides more slowly; in fact suppuration occasionally takes place in the involved lymph nodes. Treatment of the lymphangitis is strictly one of *noli me tangere*, except that application of hot moist packs along the involved extremity will be helpful. Immobilization of the extremity, however, is extremely important and

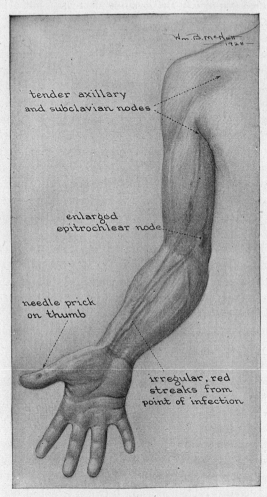

FIG. 331.—ACUTE TUBULAR LYMPHANGITIS.

Streptococcus lymphangitis and lymphadenitis in a physician following a needle prick during an operation for appendiceal peritonitis. (From Babcock, *Textbook of Surgery*, W. B. Saunders Co., 1935, p. 387.)

should be as complete as possible. Incision is used *only* if a local abscess forms along the course of the lymphatic; this *rarely* occurs. Treatment of the primary infection has already been described (p. 47). Since the organism causing lymphangitis is usually the streptococcus, sulfanilamide will be an important factor in therapy.

Acute diffuse (or reticular) lymphangitis is a term applied to a variety of lesions. Its most specific and characteristic, though perhaps least common form, is a type of infection involving the entire subcutaneous system of an extremity, which may occur in patients with lymphatic obstruction (lymphedema). Matas[5] has been influential in describing and emphasizing the importance of this type of lymphatic infection. It is ushered in by chills, fever, prostration and a tender red swelling of the entire limb. A streptococcus has been found in many cases. After the infection has subsided completely the swelling decreases, but a permanent enlargement persists due to the deposition of fibrous tissue. Repeated attacks eventually lead to elephantiasis.

The second and most common type of reticular lymphangitis is that produced by a spreading infection which involves the smaller local lymphatic channels. Clinically, the redness, swelling, induration, etc., is differentiated with difficulty from acute cellulitis. Indeed, there undoubtedly is always a certain degree of diffuse reticular lymphangitis present in acute cellulitis. Another entirely different type of reticular lymphangitis is erysipelas (see Chapter VI). Erysipeloid, however, is a mild type of reticular lymphangitis which occurs most commonly following injury to the skin of individuals who work with oysters or other types of sea food. Treatment is simple inasmuch as the infection usually subsides spontaneously.

Another form of acute lymphangitis, still different, is the inflammation noted by Homans[6] around the iliac and femoral vessels in a patient with thrombophlebitis femoris as already discussed (see p. 516).

Chronic Lymphangitis.—This lesion is of importance in certain patients with indolent, long standing ulcers of the lower leg which refuse to heal. The subcutaneous tissue is the site of edema and permanent swelling in the form of fibrous overgrowth which is believed to be due to chronic infection of the lymphatics through the open lesion (see p. 120).

Chronic lymphangitis is also important in patients, without obvious portals of entry for infection, who have localized chronic swelling or enlargement, usually of the leg, which is often called lymphedema. Similiarly chronic lymphangitis is also found in patients with more pronounced swelling called elephantiasis. Histologically, chronic lymphangitis exhibits primarily an extensive round cell infiltration of the finer subcutaneous lymphatic channels (Fig. 332). In addition there may also be edema and fibrosis; the former feature, strictly speaking, is marked only in lymphedema, the latter only in elephantiasis. Unfortunately microscopic study of the subcutaneous tissue in these cases is not often possible; it is usually only when the Kondoleon operation is performed that tissue is excised for examination. As indicated below, there is considerable confusion between lymphedema and elephantiasis, and as might therefore be expected the relation between chronic lymphangitis and its clinical manifestations are similarly difficult to establish.

Lymphedema.—Lymphedema is a term used to describe a localized though diffuse collection of lymph in the vessels and tissue spaces, especially of an extremity; the condition is manifested clinically by an edematous swelling which pits on pressure. It differs in etiology and extent from the *symmetrical edema* due to cardiorenal disease. Lymphedema is due in most cases to regional lymphatic obstruction, to increased lymph formation secondary to the venous stasis in varicose veins, to an increased permeability of the channels, or to an accumulation of lymph faster than the existing vessels can remove it; the latter is commonly due to an

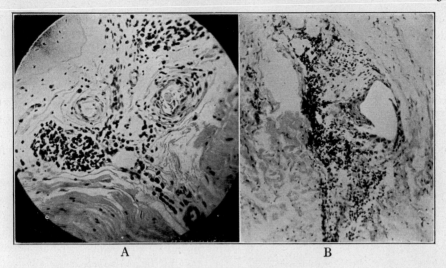

A   B

FIG. 332.—CHRONIC LYMPHANGITIS.

Photomicrographs from two cases of unilateral swelling of the leg in which the Kondoleon operation was done. *A,* note the round cell infiltration; only moderate fibrosis is present. The inflammation present in this case was not due to infection entering through ulcers of the leg for this patient had none. The onset of the swelling was insidious but there was a definite history of several attacks of acute infection (subcutaneous cellulitis) involving the entire affected leg; these attacks are characteristic of elephantiasis (see p. 530). *B,* note the dilated lymphatic vessel and extensive round cell infiltration; only moderate fibrosis was present. The inflammation in this case is probably similar in nature to that in *A;* there was a history of episodes suggesting acute infection of the subcutaneous tissues of the entire leg. The photograph of the leg is shown in Figure 336.

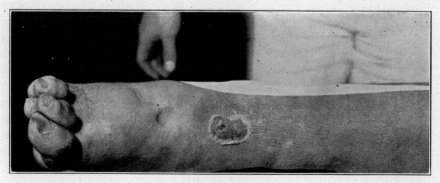

FIG. 333.—TRANSIENT ACUTE LYMPHEDEMA SECONDARY TO A TRAUMATIC INFECTED ULCER IN A THIRTY-SEVEN-YEAR-OLD MAN.

Note the pitting edema. This swelling subsided promptly after several days of rest and elevation, and the ulcer healed (St. Louis City Hospital).

acute inflammation in the neighboring tissues. One type is represented by the painless edema of the dorsum of the hand which so constantly accompanies palmar infection. Such lymphedema is *transient* and disappears as the primary site of infection sudsides. The edema of the leg following thrombophlebitis femoris as already described (p. 516) is due in part to obstruction of the lymphatics by inflammation associated with the phlebitis, and in part to venous obstruction incident to widespread thrombosis of collateral veins (de Takats) as well as the femoral (see p. 516).

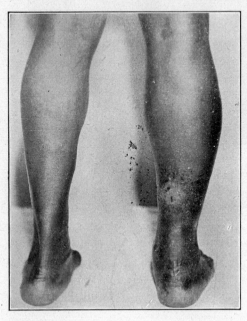

FIG. 334.—LYMPHEDEMA IN A FIFTY-NINE-YEAR-OLD NEGRO OF GRADUAL ONSET ONE AND ONE-HALF YEARS PREVIOUSLY FOLLOWING A HISTORY SUGGESTIVE OF A VENOUS THROMBOSIS.

Many months afterward the ulcers appeared, which are evident in the photograph although now almost healed following conservative care and elastic bandaging. The swelling pitted on pressure and decreased markedly on rest and elevation.

There is another more mysterious type of lymphedema which seems to occur spontaneously or after some apparently trivial injury. In certain patients there seems to be an hereditary factor as the sole cause (Milroy's disease). This group of cases has been excellently summarized by Allen.[7] The swelling, usually confined to one leg or one arm, may subside completely on rest and elevation, the limb returning to its normal size. On ordinary use, however, the swelling recurs. Such an extremity is subject to infection of the lymphatics (reticular lymphangitis) which may lead to elephantiasis.

It should be mentioned, however, that the group of chronic or persistent lymphedema shades off, as the disease becomes more severe, into elephantiasis. Indeed, there is considerable confusion in the use of the two terms. The term lymphedema should be confined to swellings which pit deeply on pressure and subside completely on rest and elevation. Chronic swelling particularly when sufficiently advanced to be called elephantiasis is probably due to chronic lymphangitis, as already indicated; diagnosis of this lesion depends, obviously, on microscopic section, particularly in patients with no history of infection and no ulcers or other obvious portals of entry for infection.

Treatment of lymphedema is often unnecessary since the swelling subsides on removal of the cause. In the absence of a known etiology effective therapy is difficult to institute, although considerable relief of symptoms and edema may often be achieved with a tightly fitting elastic stocking or bandage. However, if an acute inflammatory process is present such therapy is contraindicated; the extremity should be immobilized by bed rest. In a few patients the Kondoleon operation has been successful, although its results are much more effective in true elephantiasis (see p. 531).

Elephantiasis.—Although often classified under lymphedema, elephantiasis is really a different disease since the swelling is only partly due to lymphedema, most of it consisting of actual hypertrophy of the skin and subcutaneous tissue because of

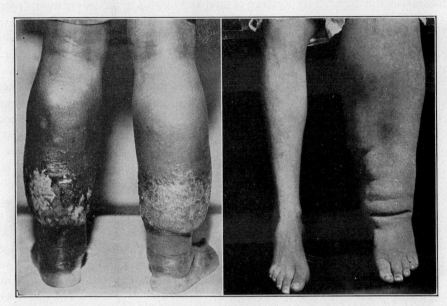

Fig. 335.   Fig. 336.

Fig. 335.—Elephantiasis Affecting Both Legs in a Fifty-year-old Negro.

The swelling was insidious, without cause, beginning two years previously. It would diminish on rest and elevation, due presumably to a simple lymphedema of unknown etiology. The superficial ulceration noted in the photograph is of one year's duration and has been getting worse. The swelling now is brawny and hard, pits only slightly on pressure. After several weeks in bed the edema subsided to a moderate extent and the infection abated considerably.

Fig. 336.—Elephantiasis Affecting the Left Leg in a Fourteen-year-old Girl.

The swelling was of insidious onset at the age of eight and became progressively worse, especially following mild attacks of a few days' duration, consisting of fever and redness, tenderness and pain in the leg. On admission the leg felt bulky on palpation and scarcely pitted on pressure. A Kondoleon operation was performed; a chronic lymphangitis was present in the excised tissue (see Fig. 332B). Although the patient was discharged with both limbs the same size, the swelling recurred in the left leg and persisted (except for mild subsidence during prolonged rest in bed). This case illustrates the difficulty in differentiating lymphedema from elephantiasis since it presents features characteristic of both.

fibrous tissue overgrowth. As its name implies, elephantiasis is a remarkable swelling or enlargement which may affect an entire extremity, usually the leg, or in rare cases the scrotum or vulva. Though more common in the tropics, it is seen everywhere, especially in mild forms.

The clinical variations are great. The remarkable cases are usually seen only in the tropics. Though slight pitting edema is present, it disappears on rest and elevation, leaving a limb only slightly smaller than before, but indurated, somewhat pale and larger than its fellow. Occasionally both legs are involved. Ulcers are present in some cases and as already mentioned (Chapter VII) their indolence and lack of healing is no doubt due to the disturbance in lymph flow. Elephantiasis of the arm may follow radical breast amputation whenever the interruption of the lymphatics is associated with an infection; it has been designated by Halsted [8] as elephantiasis chirurgica. The presence of fluid and fibrosis in the subcutaneous tissue can sometimes be differentiated by the study of soft tissue roentgenograms of the limb as pointed out by Reichert.[9]

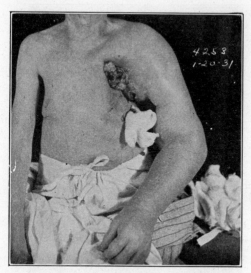

FIG. 337.—ELEPHANTIASIS CHIRURGICA FOLLOW-ING REMOVAL OF A FUNGATING CARCINOMA OF THE BREAST SIX MONTHS PREVIOUSLY.

Note the tremendous swelling of the arm and hand. Usually, edema of the arm following radical excision of the breast is due to infection involving lymphatic vessels and veins. However, in this instance the condition is complicated by the enormous mass of recurrent carcinomatous tissue in the axilla. (Courtesy Dr. J. W. Gale.)

Lymphatic obstruction plays a great role in the pathogenesis of elephantiasis, but obstruction alone cannot explain the presence of the fibrous tissue overgrowth which is responsible for the greatest part of the enlargement. This is due, as pointed out by Matas [10] and also Halsted, to a type of superimposed infection which is responsible for the deposition of fibrous tissue. In some patients such infection (reticular lymphangitis) occurs in acute attacks with chills, fever and prostration, the red swollen part finally subsiding and leaving an aftermath of diffuse fibrosis. It is after a history of many such episodes that the limb finally attains a huge size. In other instances the infection is more chronic, due, as already mentioned, to the presence of an indolent ulcer which acts as a permanent portal of entry. That lymphatic stasis by itself cannot cause elephantiasis is shown by the study of tropical elephantiasis in which filarial obstruction of the lymphatics has been erroneously assumed to be the sole causative factor. As pointed out by Matas, many patients infected with filaria do not have elephantiasis; conversely, in many patients with elephantiasis, no organisms can be found. Moreover, in those having elephantiasis with demonstrable filaria a history can often be obtained of recurrent acute attacks of the above mentioned reticular lymphangitis from which a streptococcus has been isolated. Thus, it is clear that even in filarial elephantiasis it is necessary that both infection as well as obstruction to the lymphatics occur before the disease is produced. Each alone will not lead to the disease.

The dual significance of lymphatic infection and obstruction lies in the fact that the fibrosis which follows infection in itself obstructs a free lymphatic drainage. A vicious circle is thus doubtlessly established. Lymphedema is the primary event; secondary infection leads to fibrosis which interferes with lymph flow. This in turn leads to lymphedema which most likely renders the part less able to resist further infection. Such a conception of the dual role of lymphatic infection and obstruction is confirmed by the striking experiments of Drinker, Field and Homans [11] who have produced lymphedema and elephantiasis in dogs by inducing lymphatic obstruction of the extremity which in the successful experiments was accompanied or induced by infection, streptococcal in nature. Typical fibrous tissue overgrowth was noted.

Treatment.—Therapy is based on the dual pathogenesis mentioned above and is often quite efficient. Infection is first guarded against by avoiding injuries of any kind. Infection which may be already present, *i.e.,* ulcers and indolent wounds, are treated by elevation, rest, hyperemia and skin graft. The progress of the disease may sometimes be halted in this way by closing the portals of entry for chronic infection in spite of the existence of a certain amount of lymph stasis. In many cases the ulcers will not heal unless lymphatic obstruction is relieved by operation. Trout,[12] for example, has described many patients with chronic ulcers which healed following the Kondoleon operation, a procedure consisting of removal of the fascial barrier between deep and superficial lymphatics, thus relieving the obstruction in the latter system. The operation as described by Homans [13] is often done in stages and consists of (1) the excision of as much skin as necessary and all the scarred, hypertrophied, edematous, subcutaneous tissue. (2) the removal of a large area of the deep fascia. The second procedure denudes muscle which because of its good blood supply offers an excellent bed for the overlying skin. Although muscle has no lymphatics, lymphatic drainage from the skin probably occurs through numerous intramuscular septa. Operation is always preceded by a period of several weeks during which the limb is elevated and kept at rest to diminish infection and lymph stasis as much as possible.

Lymphangiectasis.—Although often used synonymously with lymphangioma, lymphangiectasis is distinctly different because it is in reality not a true neoplasm. Lymphangiectasis consists primarily of dilatation of the lymph vessels, and is commonly a sequela of lymph stasis. A differentiating clinical feature lies in the fact that lymphangiectasis is compressible whereas lymphangioma is not. Small localized areas are frequently encountered in the intestinal mesentery in association with carcinomatous metastases, but extensive lesions are perhaps most common in association with varicose veins of the legs. Transition from lymphangiectasis to a true neoplasm (lymphangioma) does occur, however, thereby accounting for considerable clinical and pathological confusion between the two lesions.

Treatment consists of excision of the involved tissue.

Neoplasms of the Lymph Vessels.—Neoplasms confined to the lymph vessels are not common; they have been described in Chapter XVI. Lymphangioma is a true tumor of the lymphatic vessels. It consists primarily of an actual dilatation and proliferation of the vessels. On rare occasions, considerable endothelial proliferation is present, giving rise to the term endotheliomatous lymphangioma. Commonly, lymphangioma is found in areas where a network of lymphatic vessels exists, but it may occur almost any place in the body. When the dilatation of the vessels is pronounced, the tumor is spoken of as a *cavernous lymphangioma.* Such tumors occur in the tongue (macroglossia) and in the lip (macrocheilia or macrolabia) as congenital tumors. Such neoplastic growths are soft and painless, and are not compressible. They may grow to a large size, resulting in serious deformity, particularly those occurring in the tongue. *Cystic hygroma* of the neck is another type of cavernous lymphangioma. The tumor contains large cyst-like cavities (usually multilocular) and is seen only in infants. Aspiration may yield fluid with characteristics

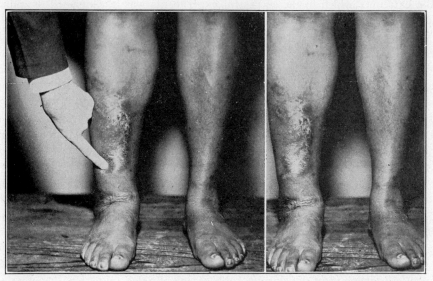

FIG. 338.—LYMPHANGIECTASIS.

The photographs were taken a few seconds apart. Note the compressibility of the swelling which is not due to a pitting edema; release of pressure as shown on the right results in an immediate return of the compressed point to normal. A portion of tissue which was removed showed dilated lymph channels as well as areas resembling hemangioma.

similar to lymph. Such tumors tend to infiltrate the structures of the neck. Treatment is surgical but in large tumors excision may be associated with a high mortality due to the extensive nature of the operation and perhaps injury to adjacent structures. Radium and x-ray therapy may be helpful; in the tumors of the tongue and lip they are particularly effective.

LYMPH NODES

Anatomical knowledge of the various regions of the body draining into each of the many groups of lymph nodes is of great clinical importance; such knowledge helps considerably in finding the source of many apparently spontaneous lymph node enlargements which are seen by the physician. The superficial nodes are located in the subcutaneous tissue of the following areas and go by these names: cervical, occipital, axillary, epitrochlear, inguinal, femoral (subinguinal) and popliteal. The deep nodes include, among others, the iliac, mesenteric (abdominal) and thoracic (mediastinal) groups. In general the two groups are separated by the deep fascia; they join, however, before they empty into the main lymph channels which enter the venous system by way of the thoracic duct.

Of the inflammatory diseases affecting these nodes the following will be considered: acute lymphadenitis, chronic pyogenic lymphadenitis, tuberculous and syphilitic lymphadenitis. Obviously only localized lymphadenitis will be considered because generalized lymph node enlargement is usually a manifestation of systemic disease which is nearly always of medical rather than surgical interest.

Acute Lymphadenitis.—Acute infection of the lymph nodes is always regional and secondary, therefore, to inflammation in the area drained by the node or nodes; it may, however, follow the entrance of bacteria through a portal of entry which, for some reason, exhibits no inflammatory signs. Thus, the local lesion may be prominent and severe, or it may be hardly noticeable. In either case the node serves as a

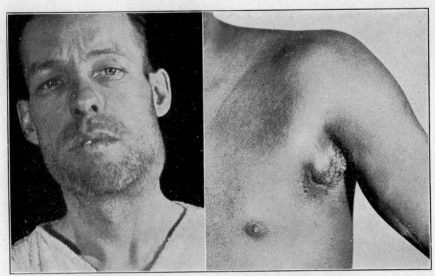

FIG. 339.   FIG. 340.

FIG. 339.—ACUTE CERVICAL LYMPHADENITIS WHICH SUPPURATED AND WAS INCISED AFTER TWO WEEKS OF CONSERVATIVE CARE.

On culture a streptococcus and staphylococcus were recovered; healing was uneventful but delayed. No portal of entry for the infection was found in spite of careful search of the oral and pharyngeal cavity.

FIG. 340.—ACUTE AXILLARY LYMPHADENITIS WHICH SUPPURATED AND WAS INCISED TWO WEEKS AFTER ONSET.

A hemolytic streptococcus and staphylococcus were also isolated in this case. Ten days before the node began to swell, the patient injured the index finger with subsequent transient superficial infection.

sieve to prevent further invasion of the body. The effectiveness of the lymph nodes in removing bacteria entering them, has been shown in perfusion experiments reported by Drinker, Field and Ward.[14] They found that no organisms were able to pass through the lymph node at least during the early stages of inflammation. Recent evidence has also shown that specific antibodies may be produced in lymph nodes and that they, therefore, also play a role in resistance against the invasion of infection in an immunological manner. During the process of acute reaction the node enlarges not only because of edema and exudation, but also because of the multiplication and infiltration of phagocytes and other leukocytes.

The organisms most commonly responsible for the development of acute lymphadenitis are those of the pyogenic group, such as the staphylococcus and streptococcus, but in certain locations Ducrey's bacillus, the Bacillus tularense, and the virus of venereal lymphogranuloma (see Chapter VI) are the etiologic factors. The lymph nodes most commonly invaded are the cervical and axillary group and those in the groin, *i.e.*, the inguinal and femoral nodes. The cervical nodes are perhaps the most frequently infected; in most instances they follow acute infections of the oral cavity, including upper respiratory infections such as pharyngitis and tonsillitis, and also dental abscesses. In the latter case, however, it may be the deeper tissue of the neck rather than the superficial lymph nodes which become infected and swollen.

Clinical Manifestations.—The manifestations of acute lymphadenitis may develop as early as twelve to twenty-four hours following the entrance of bacteria at the

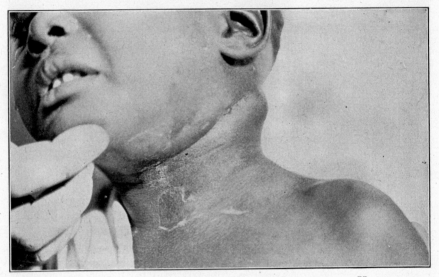

Fig. 341.—Acute Cervical Lymphadenitis due to the Streptococcus Hemolyticus in a Three-year-old Child.

During the course of over two months five of such abscesses formed and were incised for drainage, each time yielding the same organism in pure culture. The child had otitis media, pharyngitis and a streptococcus osteomyelitis. Recovery was finally complete. This type of cervical lymphadenitis (produced by the hemolytic streptococcus) which occurs so frequently in children following otitis media, etc., is particularly prone to persist for many weeks before subsiding. Chemotherapy, however, often hastens final healing.

portal of entry. As stated already, however, there may be no evidence of inflammation at the primary site, or in the channels which transmit the offending organism. Enlargement of the affected node, accompanied by local heat and tenderness, is one of the earliest manifestations. As the enlargement progresses pain develops; disability of variable extent likewise occurs early and becomes progressively more marked. For example, a severe *cervical lymphadenitis* provokes so much pain and discomfort that the patient may be unable to turn his head from side to side. In severe cases fever will be noted early; its degree will depend, of course, on the severity of the infection. Accompanying the fever may be other symptoms such as general malaise, weakness, anorexia, prostration, etc. After a day or two the tissue about the lymph node will become swollen and edematous (periadenitis). As the infection proceeds neighboring nodes are apt to become involved. These nodes are at first discrete, but later become confluent. In a few days redness of the skin over the involved nodes begins to appear; this usually indicates the development of suppuration and is frequently produced by the escape of pus into the subcutaneous tissues through rupture of the capsule of the infected nodes. It should be pointed out, however, that in a majority of instances acute lymphadenitis is a transient process and subsides rapidly without suppuration as soon as the primary infection is overcome. It usually takes several days, however, before the node recedes to its normal size. In adults this is the usual outcome; in children, however, suppuration is more frequently encountered.

If suppuration occurs, the pain persists and usually increases. Fluctuation will be demonstrable in most instances except when the node is deeply seated. In such a circumstances, suppuration will be suggested by the continued fever and local pain. Occasionally deep suppuration is accompanied by a variable degree of cellulitis because the undrained abscess breaks through the capsule of the node into the surrounding tissues; there is, however, a distinct tendency for the pus to remain localized and point outward toward the skin.

Manifestations of septicemia may occur when the infection breaks through the line of defense within and around the lymph node, and enters the general circulation. This is particularly apt to occur when the causative organism is a hemolytic streptococcus arising from an upper respiratory infection. In such instances a more serious outcome may occur as has already been discussed under septicemia.

When the *inguinal nodes* are involved, the local manifestations may be confused with other diseases, particularly strangulated inguinal hernia. The disability and local pain produced by both conditions are the same. However, an important differential feature lies in the fact that the development of the local manifestations produced by lymphadenitis is gradual, whereas those associated with a strangulated hernia appear suddenly. If there is any doubt as to the nature of the swelling, a careful search should be made of the area drained by the nodes, *i.e.*, the perineum and especially the anus (*e.g.*, infected fissures) and the genitalia. The primary lesion may be no more conspicuous than a small scratch or infection about a hair follicle, or a tiny ulcer under the foreskin.

When a *retroperitoneal or deep inguinal* (*iliac*) *lymph node* is involved, the manifestations may simulate those of a local peritonitis; if the infected node is on the right side acute appendicitis will be simulated. This diagnostic confuson will be particularly apt to occur in the early stage of the lymphadenitis, before the node is sufficiently enlarged to be palpable. Fever is more apt to be present in lymphadenitis; vomiting, however, is less apt to occur. Children are much more commonly infected than adults. When a mass is palpable it is felt under Poupart's ligament or in the abdomen just above the ligament. In case the nodes do enlarge so that they become readily palpable, suppuration usually develops sooner or later and demands incision and drainage. It is frequently impossible to demonstrate the portal of entry for these infections. A series of 18 of such cases have been well described by Irwin.[15]

In other parts of the body acute lymphadenitis may produce local effects which may or may not be characteristic. *Mesenteric lymphadenitis* is not uncommon in children, and produces manifestations which simulate general peritonitis as discussed in Chapter XXV. *Mediastinal lymphadenitis* is described in the chapter on the thorax.

The duration of acute lymphadenitis varies from one to two weeks, except that if suppuration demands incision, the sinus may require longer to heal. However, there is a type of acute cervical lymphadenitis in children secondary usually to pharyngitis, otitis media, and mastoiditis, which may persist for many months and require incision at intervals because of successive involvement and suppuration of various nodes. This type of infection in encountered chiefly in winter and sometimes in an epidemic form. Systemic manifestations, such as fever, malaise, weakness, anorexia, tachycardia, etc., are particularly apt to be present. The elevation in temperature may persist every day for weeks, or may recur intermittently, apparently as new lymph nodes become involved and suppurate. The offending organism in these cases is usually the hemolytic streptococcus; on rare occasions it may be the hemolytic staphylococcus.

Treatment.—To a great extent the treatment of acute lymphadenitis is the same as that of acute infection in general, as already discussed in previous chapters. One of the most important features is the immobilization and rest of the involved part. For example, a patient with axillary adenitis should carry the arm in a sling in order to prevent massage of the infected nodes by motion of the arm; if the infection is severe, bed rest may be advisable. Cervical and inguinal adenitis are best treated by bed rest, particularly if fever is present. The primary site of infection producing the lymphadenitis should receive early attention; immobilization, application of hot wet packs and incision of abscesses when they form, are indicated. Tonsils and teeth are prone to cause cervical adenitis, particularly in repeated attacks; if such a history is obtained the tonsils and offending tooth or teeth should be removed, *but only after all the evidence of acute infection has subsided.*

The nodes should be examined daily for the development of fluctuation; when found, incision and drainage is indicated without delay. When doubt exists as to the presence of pus, aspiration may be utilized as a method of diagnosis, but not if the nodes are deeply situated and lie adjacent to the large vessels of the neck; the danger lies more in the production of an infected thrombus by puncture of a vein, than in producing hemorrhage. Occasionally, when fever persists for days, and local tenderness is marked, exploration of the deep nodes will be justified; in such instances the surgeon is usually rewarded by finding pus in one of the nodes (see also section on deep cervical infections in Chapter XXIV). The acute manifestations of infection, both local and general, usually subside rapidly after incision of the suppurating node. It is not uncommon for more than one node to suppurate, as already mentioned above. An interval of several days usually occurs before the second infection is manifested by a recurrence of fever, local tenderness, swelling, etc. The necessity of repeated incisions is best illustrated by the persistent type of cervical lymphadenitis in children, as described on page 534. The sulfonamide drugs are extremely useful in acute lymphadenitis, especially when the streptococcus is the offending organism. Its early use will undoubtedly lower the incidence of suppuration. Once pus has formed the drug is useful only in conjuction with incision and drainage or in the prevention of further spread.

Chronic Pyogenic Lymphadenitis.—Slight enlargement of lymph nodes occurs frequently as a result of chronic or recurrent mild pyogenic infections of low grade virulence in the field drained by the nodes. Such infections are commonly seen in active boys who frequently injure their extremities, so that the resulting mild infections produce a moderate painless enlargement of the femoral and axillary nodes. The cervical region is also a common site because of the frequency of mild repeated or chronic respiratory infections. Chronic pyogenic lymphadenitis of this type has little clinical importance except for the fact that it is often mistaken

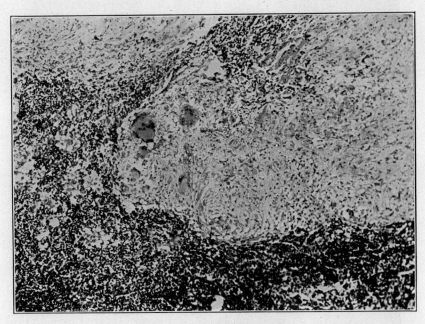

FIG. 342.—PHOTOMICROGRAPH OF A LYMPH NODE REMOVED FROM A YOUNG WOMAN WHO COMPLAINED ONLY OF A SMALL MASS IN THE SIDE OF HER NECK OF SIX MONTHS' DURATION.

There was a history of transient pleurisy some years previously, which may have been tuberculous. Note the tuberculous tissue in the midst of normal lymphoid cells. Giant cells are obvious and there is considerable necrosis although caseation is not as pronounced as it often is (see Fig. 43). No other evidence of tuberculosis was found in this patient, who remained perfectly well.

for tuberculosis or some type of malignant disease. Removal of one of the nodes for microscopic examination is usually necessary in such instances to solve the diagnostic difficulty. When possible, of course, the primary infection responsible for this type of adenitis should be investigated and eliminated.

On rare occasions, the sinus produced by the drainage of an acute lymphadenitis persists; the associated lymph nodes also remain enlarged and palpable. In such instances a total excision of the sinus and involved nodes may be indicated; such an operation rarely results in any spread of infection and is almost always curative. In many instances the question of whether the infection is tuberculous or not is impossible to answer on clinical evidence alone; microscopic examination of the excised tissue will nearly always result in a positive diagnosis.

Tuberculous Lymphadenitis.—The cervical and mediastinal lymph nodes are most commonly involved by tuberculous infection, but none is exempt. Though tuberculosis of the cervical nodes probably follows some portal of entry in the oral or pharyngeal cavities, such a lesion is practically always indetectable. It is rarely encountered as a manifestation of a systemic (pulmonary) infection. The lesion

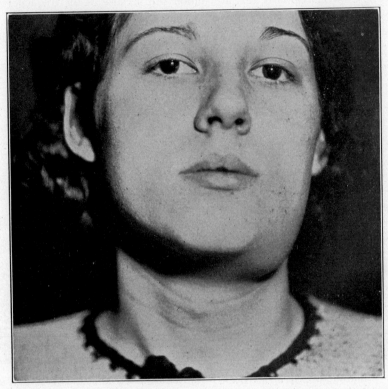

FIG. 343.—CHRONIC CERVICAL LYMPHADENITIS, PROBABLY TUBERCULOUS, OF TWO
MONTHS' DURATION.

This mass grew slowly in size, was not tender or painful but finally became fluctuant. A small amount of thick pus was aspirated which showed only lymphocytes and no bacteria on smear, yielded no growth on culture and did not produce tuberculosis after injection into a guinea-pig. Oral cavity, nose and throat revealed no source for the infection. The swelling disappeared following radiotherapy, and the patient has remained well.

is common in infancy and childhood and at any age among Negroes, who are particularly susceptible to all forms of tuberculosis. It is probably due to the bovine form of bacillus. In the United States, at least, massive and extreme enlargement of tuberculous nodes is not seen as commonly as formerly. This is apparently due to a diminished consumption of tuberculous milk because of the more rigid inspection of cows for the presence of tuberculosis and because of the rather general use of pasteurized milk in the cities.

Pathologically, the disease first causes infiltration of endothelial and giant cells or actual tubercle formation, which brings about a simple hypertrophy of the node. Softening or caseation may occur by the gradual breaking down and digestion of tissue by the organism or its products. Tuberculosis is also prone to lead to a deposition of calcium in the node, especially when caseation occurs. Spontaneous drainage of such softened lesions is not infrequent. The calcareous deposit in such instances acts as a foreign body and may lead to the formation of a permanent sinus until the calcified node is removed surgically.

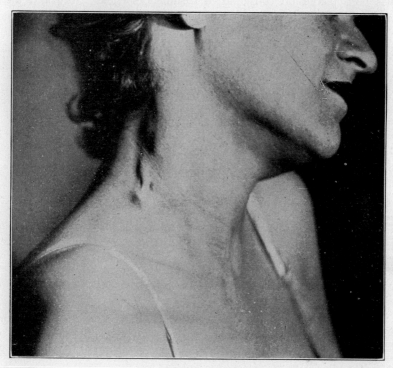

FIG. 344.—HEALED TUBERCULOUS LYMPHADENITIS OF THE NECK IN A TWENTY-SIX-YEAR-OLD WOMAN.

For five years at intervals small nodes would appear, enlarge and suppurate without pain or tenderness (cold abscess). Tubercle bacilli were demonstrated on smear of this pus. With the aid of radiotherapy healing has always occurred. The patient has evidence of a quiescent pulmonary lesion. A few nodes 1 to 2 centimeters in diameter are still present, and may be seen above the scars of the healed sinuses.

Clinically, the nodes in the early stages are moderately enlarged, firm, elastic and not tender. When several are involved they are discrete, though as they enlarge they may coalesce. They may remain in a chronic stage of enlargement indefinitely and gradually subside or soften. The occasional softening of tuberculous nodes is due to the formation of pus; the fluctuant mass is called a *cold abscess,* because it is without acute inflammatory signs. These may open spontaneously or by incision, following which thick creamy pus escapes (occasionally thin, watery pus containing much caseous material is seen). The resulting wound frequently fails to heal and becomes a chronic draining sinus or indolent ulcer. Often the overlying skin adheres to the fibrosed skeleton of the node. A positive tuberculin test will be obtained in these patients but is of diagnostic value only in young children.

Treatment.—Local treatment depends upon the presence or absence of fluctuation and a chronic draining sinus. (1) When no fluctuation is present treatment may be merely symptomatic and hygienic. Excision has the advantage of actually removing the tuberculous focus; excision also has the advantage of insuring a definite diagnosis by microscopic study of the tissue. Recently, however, much reliance has been placed on conservative treatment such as x-ray and ultraviolet radiation (particularly the former) which often results in a subsidence and even

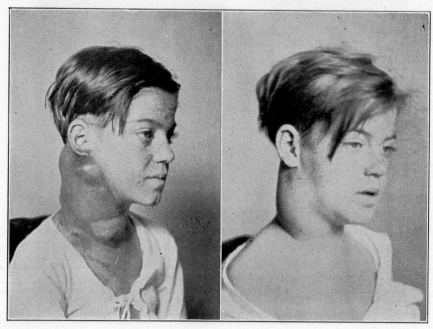

FIG. 345.—HODGKIN'S DISEASE IN AN ELEVEN-YEAR-OLD BOY, BEFORE AND AFTER RADIOTHERAPY.

The diagnosis was based on biopsy at the site shown in the left photograph. The patient also had a palpably enlarged spleen, irregular fever, slight anemia and a leukocytosis of 19 to 23,000. The photograph on the right was taken three weeks after the one on the left, following a course of radiotherapy; the mass disappeared entirely shortly afterward as did the enlargement of the spleen. Recurrent tumors of the neck and axilla occurred three years later, which likewise responded to radiotherapy. The patient was asymptomatic for eight years when he became anemic because of persistent melena due apparently to bleeding from the stomach which seems to be the site of a recurrent infiltration.

disappearance of the swelling. In any case removal of one of the more superficial nodes is advisable to establish the diagnosis before beginning treatment. (2) When the node is fluctuant, repeated aspirations may forestall its opening spontaneously, but may occasionally lead to the development of a chronic draining sinus. In any case the usual conservative measures are also used. However, if spontaneous drainage is imminent it is better to incise the abscess in order to hasten the reparative process. The danger of a chronic draining sinus resulting from such an incision, for reasons mentioned above, is not as great as it was two or three decades ago. Excision of all of the diseased tissue will, however, result in the most rapid healing and is often justified. (3) When chronic draining sinuses do occur, healing will frequently be hastened by x-ray radiation. However, a careful excision of the sinus and its attached node, which is frequently calcified, will usually save months of care, and lead to rapid healing, even in the face of an open secondarily infected wound.

Syphilitic Lymphadenitis.—Enlargement of the lymph nodes is constantly associated with the primary and secondary stages of this disease. Within a few days or weeks after appearance of the primary lesion, the nodes draining the area become discretely enlarged and firm, but do not suppurate unless secondary infection develops. When the secondary lesions of the disease appear, there is apt to be a gen-

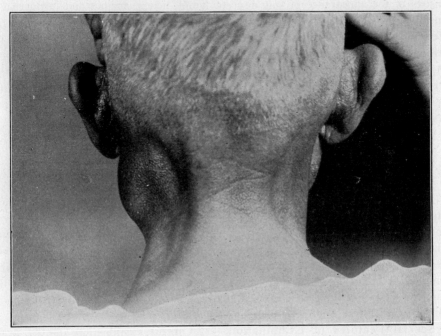

FIG. 346.—METASTATIC CARCINOMA OF THE CERVICAL LYMPH NODES.

This patient, a fifty-nine-year-old farmer, first noted a painless swelling in the left side of the neck. Later salivation developed. An extensive ulcerating carcinoma of the left tonsil was seen on inspection of the oral cavity. This patient is a suitable case for radiotherapy, preferably with the fractionated Coutard technic.

eralized lymphadenopathy. This is more pronounced in the negro race than in the white. Differentiation from tuberculous lymphadenitis is rarely difficult because syphilitic nodes are apt to be generalized at some time in the disease and do not suppurate; the Wassermann reaction is of value after the primary stage.

Neoplasms of the Lymph Nodes.—The inflammatory lesions as just described constitute most common causes of enlargement of lymph nodes. The neoplasms affecting the lymph nodes will be considered only briefly here since most of them are discussed in detail in Chapter XVI. Almost all of them are malignant. *Hodgkin's disease* is characterized by a progressive enlargement of the lymph nodes, anemia, loss of weight, and cachexia, finally terminating in death, except perhaps in rare cases. *Lymphosarcoma* is a malignant tumor so similar to Hodgkin's disease that differentiation can often be made only by microscopic section. One type of lymphosarcoma is sometimes called *reticular cell sarcoma*. *Carcinoma* readily metastasizes to lymph nodes and produces manifestations characteristic of the disease as described elsewhere. *Lymphatic leukemia* may or may not be considered as a true neoplasm; it is characterized by a generalized invasion of the lymph nodes which enlarge; there is an associated lymphocytosis of the blood. The nodes remain discrete and do not adhere to the skin or ulcerate. Microscopically, the node is composed of a finely reticulated tissue, which is densely infiltrated with small lymphocytes. An acute form is commonly encountered in children and is rapidly fatal; the illness consists of the appearance of soft discrete lymph nodes, anemia and hemorrhages beneath the skin and from the mucous membranes; it may terminate in death within a few days. The chronic form occurs chiefly in adults and is characterized by remissions of anemia, weakness, enlargement of the lymph nodes and lymphocytosis. An aleukemic form, characterized by an absence of leukocytosis but a relative increase in the lymphocytes of the blood is also encountered. The leukemias, including the myelogenous type are primarily medical diseases, and are of interest surgically only from the diagnostic standpoint.

DIFFERENTIAL DIAGNOSIS OF TUMEFACTION OF THE NECK

No region of the body is so frequently the site of tumefaction as the neck. Whether small or large these swellings always present a difficult diagnostic problem. Most of them are lymph node enlargements; many are due to acute or chronic inflammation. There are many other lesions, neoplastic and congenital, which occur often enough to add to the diagnostic possibilities. The history and complete physical examination are of primary importance. A detailed chart containing a list of the commonest types of tumefaction, whether of the neck or of other parts of the body, will be found on the following page.

Special Features in Examination.—1. Careful examination of the areas drained by the cervical lymph nodes should include the scalp and the oral and pharyngeal cavities. In the latter case special laryngeal mirrors are necessary to inspect all the possible sites for ulcer, tumor, chronic infection, etc. Sinusitis and infections about the teeth are also noted.

2. The Wassermann or Kahn reaction is of value in the diagnosis or elimination of secondary and tertiary syphilis.

3. The tuberculin test if positive is of value only in children, chiefly in the very young. A negative test is of value at any age; however the test is so frequently positive in older children and adults that it is not even used on them.

4. Aspiration of fluctuant tumors will give valuable information provided the lumen of the needle is large enough to convey the contents, which sometimes are viscid and thick. Pus should be smeared, stained and also cultured. If tuberculosis is suspected, some of the pus should be injected into a guinea-pig. If nothing can be aspirated the fluid is either too thick, *i.e.,* contains sebaceous or fibrinous material, or the mass is a solid tumor, *i.e.,* a nonsuppurating lymph node, lipoma, lymphangioma, etc. Aspiration should not be used deeply below the surface because of the danger of entering the large vessels of the neck.

TABLE 7

COMMON TYPES OF TUMEFACTION

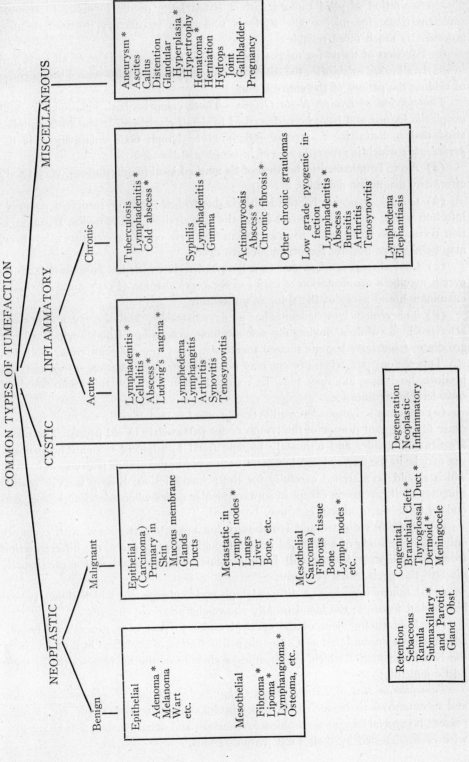

* Lesions likely to occur in the neck.

5. Aspiration of solid tumors with a sharp large needle in order to remove sufficient tissue for microscopic study is sometimes satisfactory. Surgical biopsy, however, is much more reliable.

6. Excision of tissue for microscopic study is the most decisive of all tests and in nearly all cases establishes the diagnosis. In many cases it also serves the purpose of ridding the patient of the entire lesion.

Tumefaction of Lymph Node Origin.—These comprise both inflammatory and neoplastic lesions and have been described in detail elsewhere. It should be emphasized that a distinctive feature of inflammatory lymph node enlargement is the *periadenitis* which is generally absent in neoplastic diseases.

(*a*) Acute lymphadenitis, because of its marked local manifestations, very rarely offers any diagnostic difficulty.

(*b*) Chronic pyogenic lymphadenitis is due to low grade or recurrent pyogenic infection whose source is searched for in the area drained by the nodes. If suppuration occurs, the pus usually shows pyogenic bacteria on smear; cultures, however, may be negative because the organisms are dead.

(*c*) Cold abscess is often due to a lymphadenitis which has suppurated. However it may be a manifestation of caries of the cervical spine (Pott's disease). Local examination and x-ray of the spine is important.

(*d*) Tuberculous lymphadenitis has no demonstrable portal of entry, and is characterized by a painless, moderately soft swelling, consisting of nodes which at first are discrete but later become matted together. Biopsy reveals giant cells, tubercles, etc. Tuberculous pus, when present may not show the organisms on smear, but will produce the disease in guinea-pigs. In young children a positive tuberculin test is of considerable significance.

(*e*) Metastatic lymphadenopathy (carcinoma) is undoubtedly the most frequent cause of malignant disease of the lymph nodes particularly in old people. The nodes are firm, nontender and ultimately become fixed to adjacent tissue. The primary site may be in the face or head, but more commonly in the oral or pharyngeal cavities which should be searched carefully for the primary lesion. Biopsy usually reveals squamous-cell carcinoma except in supraclavicular nodes when adenocarcinoma, secondary to breast, stomach, etc., may be found.

(*f*) Hodgkin's disease and lymphosarcoma are often diagnosed with certainty only after the study of an excised node although in a few cases, the differentiation from nonmalignant lesions will be impossible. The enlarged nodes are usually discrete and periadenitis is absent.

(*g*) Leukemia produces a diffuse lymph node enlargement which shows typical histological features; the blood usually shows characteristic changes.

(*h*) Mild enlargement of the cervical nodes as part of a generalized lymphadenopathy is encountered as a systemic manifestation of syphilis. On rare occasions the lymphadenopathy which accompanies a chancre of the lip is a source of diagnostic difficulty.

Tumefaction Not of Lymph Node Origin.—(*a*) Benign neoplasms of the skin and subcutaneous tissue such as lipoma, fibroma, lymphangioma, nevus, etc., usually present no special diagnostic problem. Aneurysm and arteriovenous fistula are likewise easily detected by their local manifestations.

(*b*) Congenital cysts are rare; they may be of branchial cleft origin if on the lateral side, or of thyroglossal duct origin if in the midline. The cyst may be a part of a lymphangioma (hygroma). The fluid is clear (colorless or straw colored) unless infection is present.

(*c*) Sebaceous cysts are not common in the neck, but present no diagnostic difficulty.

(*d*) Dermoid cysts are likewise uncommon and are often confused with branchial cleft cysts.

(*e*) Carotid body tumor is rare, may be associated with circulatory episodes (fainting, etc.), but is usually diagnosed only after excision.

(*f*) Tumors of thyroid origin (adenoma, hyperplasia) are characteristically in the normal position of the gland, but aberrant thyroid tissue though somewhat rare may be present in the lateral cervical region, and less commonly at the base of the tongue.

(*g*) Actinomycosis and mixed tumor of the parotid are often considered in the differential diagnosis of cervical tumefaction but they really involve the lower portion of the face and jaw and thus are strictly speaking not of cervical origin. Swelling of the submaxillary gland is rare but is most often due to obstruction of the duct by a stone. Acute tumefactions such as Ludwig's angina and deep cervical abscess have such striking manifestions as to rarely cause any diagnostic difficulty.

BIBLIOGRAPHY

1. SABIN, F. R.   Method of Growth of the Lymphatic System, *Science*, 44:145, 1916.
2. FIELD, M. E., DRINKER, C. K., and WHITE, J. C.   Lymph Pressures in Sterile Inflammation, *J. Exper. M.*, 56:363, 1932. *See also* DRINKER, C. K.   The Lymphatic System, *Lane Medical Lectures,* Stanford U. Press, 1942.
3. McMASTER, P. D., and HUDACK, S. S.   Participation of Skin Lymphatics in Repair of Lesions Due to Incisions and Burns, *J. Exper. M.*, 60:479, 1934.
4. REICHERT, F. L.   Regeneration of Lymphatics, *Arch. Surg.*, 13:871, 1926.
5. MATAS, R.   The Surgical Treatment of Elephantiasis and Elephantoid States Dependent upon Chronic Obstruction of the Lymphatic and Venous Channels, *Am. J. Trop. Dis.*, 1:60, 1913.
6. HOMANS, J.   Phlegmasia Alba Dolens and Relation of Lymphatics to Thrombophlebitis, *Am. Heart J.*, 7:415, 1932.
7. ALLEN, E. V.   Lymphedema of Extremities, *Arch. Int. M.*, 54:606, 1934.
8. HALSTED, W. S.   Swelling of Arm after Operations for Cancer of Breast—Elephantiasis Chirurgica—Its Cause and Prevention, *J. H. H. R.*, 32:309, 1921.
9. REICHERT, F. L.   Recognition of Elephantiasis and of Elephantoid Conditions by Soft Tissue Roentgenograms, with Report on Experimental Lymphedema, *Arch. Surg.*, 20:543, 1930.
10. MATAS, R.   *Loc. cit.*
11. DRINKER, C. K., FIELD, M. E., and HOMANS, J.   Experimental Production of Edema and Elephantiasis as a Result of Lymphatic Obstruction, *Am. J. Physiol.*, 108:509, 1934.
12. TROUT, H. H.   Ulcers Due to Varicose Veins and Lymphatic Blockage; New Principle in Treatment, *Arch. Surg.*, 18:2281, 1929.
13. HOMANS, J.   Treatment of Elephantiasis of Legs; Preliminary Report, *New England J. Med.*, 215:1099, 1936.
14. DRINKER, C. K., FIELD, M. E., and WARD, H. K.   Filtering Capacity of Lymph Nodes, *J. Exper. M.*, 59:393, 1934.
15. IRWIN, F. G.   Acute Iliac Adenitis; Report of 18 Cases, *Arch. Surg.*, 36:561. 1938.

CHAPTER XXII

THE NERVOUS SYSTEM

Peripheral Nerves   *Spinal Cord*
The Brain   *The Autonomic Nervous System*

So complex and detailed is our knowledge of the nervous system that both medical and surgical specialties, *i.e.*, neuropsychiatry and neurosurgery, are devoted to its study. Nevertheless its functions concern the general surgeon and practitioner at almost every turn and some of its diseases are of importance to all students of medicine. For descriptive purposes the nervous system will be classified into (1) the peripheral and cranial (somatic) nerves, (2) the brain and spinal cord, and (3) the autonomic (sympathetic) nervous system.

PERIPHERAL NERVES

Anatomically the nerve is composed of nerve fibers, the number of which decreases by branching as the terminal end is approached. Each fiber is in reality the axon of a nerve cell. The cells of the motor nerves are located in the brain and cord, whereas the cells of the sensory nerves are in the spinal ganglia.

Injury.—When the continuity of a nerve (motor or sensory) is destroyed, all nerve function distal to this point is lost. Following an anatomic division a peripheral *degeneration* of the nerve occurs. This process, named Wallerian degeneration after its discoverer, consists of fragmentation and absorption of the myelin and the axis cylinder, leaving the sheath of Schwann sufficiently viable and patent to receive a new fiber regenerating from the central stump. Degeneration does not progress proximally from the point of injury. *Regeneration* of the nerve takes place from the central stump and if there is no obstructive barrier the axis cylinders find their way into the distal stump. Growth is slow, averaging perhaps less than 2 millimeters per day and thus taking months before growth is completed. A physiologic connection of the end of the nerve and its end organ requires an additional amount of time. The time required for regeneration and return of function even under favorable conditions varies considerably as mentioned below.

The types of injury vary, but the most common lesion responsible for complete loss of function is severance of the nerve by an incised, or lacerated wound, or by avulsion. Other injuries are those produced by stretching or pressure; these may be followed by total, though perhaps temporary loss of function. It is even possible to stretch the brachial plexus or avulse the spinal nerve roots by suddenly and forcibly jerking a child from the ground by its hand. In fractures, nerves may also become pinched by fragments of bone or be compressed by callus. Injury to the radial nerve by a fracture of the humerus is the most frequent example of this type. Another type of paralysis is the so-called "tourniquet paralysis"; it occurs in extremities and results from the application of a tourniquet too tightly, or over too long an interval. Such paralyses are usually of a temporary nature but on rare occasions recovery takes place only after regeneration of the nerves.

Complete severance of sensory fibers is followed by immediate anesthesia of the skin over the area supplied by the nerve, except for the margin of the area of anatomical distribution where overlapping of adjacent nerves will maintain partial function. This overlapping will be manifested by retention of some sensation (*i.e,* sensibility to pin prick) in this zone, although the sensibility to light touch (epicritic sense) is lost. Deep sensibility and the sensation of position of joints and digits (protopathic) may be retained over the entire anesthetic area, because this function is usually ascribed to a different set of fibers which are present to a large extent at least in motor nerves. The area of sensory loss of pain and temperature is greater in the early stages after section of the nerve than it is later. A decrease in the area of anesthesia appears long before regeneration has occurred; this results from the assumption of function by the neighboring nerves in the region of overlap and must not be confused with recovery of the injured nerve.

The skin over the area of anesthesia is apt to be dry, due to interruption of the sweat fibers, and the nails become brittle and frequently deformed. Tapering of the fingers and atrophy of their pulp also occur. Important is the likelihood of unconscious infliction of trauma such as burns, etc., because of the anesthesia; the patient therefore must be cautioned about this danger.

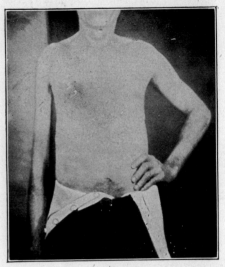

FIG. 347.—FLACCID PARALYSIS OF THE ENTIRE RIGHT UPPER EXTREMITY DUE TO INJURY OF THE NERVE TRUNKS COMPOSING THE BRACHIAL PLEXUS, A SHORT DISTANCE AFTER THEIR EXIT FROM THE INTERVERTEBRAL FORAMINA.

Note the extreme atrophy of the muscles of the arm.

An incompletely severed sensory nerve is followed by less definite disturbances of function. Sensation may be merely diminished (hypesthesia). There is usually considerable tingling and burning (paresthesia) over the area which may likewise be extremely sensitive to touch (hyperesthesia) or painful hypesthesia. Causalgia, as described by Weir Mitchell, is characterized by intense, constant, burning pain and affects most commonly the median and medial popliteal nerves. Wet applications are helpful. Blocking of the sympathetics gives relief (see page 555).

Complete severance of motor fibers is followed by immediate loss of the power of voluntary contraction in the muscle innervated. Contraction to faradic current stimulation is possible, but after a few days even this is lost. Contraction to galvanic current takes place, but gradually diminishes. This diminution in the excitability of muscle is known as the *reaction of degeneration.* As soon as galvanic stimulation fails to produce any contraction whatsoever, recovery of muscle function is said to be impossible. The paralysis of muscles may be recognized in various ways. First, by inspection and palpation of superficial muscles when appropriate movement is attempted, *e.g.*, the deltoids, the biceps, or the adductor of the thumb. Second, by the performance of a movement for which the questionable muscle is solely responsible, *e.g.*, flexion of the terminal phalanges of the fingers by the flexor profundus digitorum. Third, by palpation of the tendon of a muscle when an appropriate effort is made by the patient to use it, *e.g.*, tightening of the tendon of the flexor carpi ulnaris as it attaches to the pisiform bone when wrist flexion is attempted. Fourth, diagnosis by exclusion, *e.g.*, judgment of the flexor sublimis digitorum after ruling out paralysis of the flexor profundus and the intrinsic hand muscles.

Recovery of Function.—Numerous factors affect the range, degree, and character of recovery following division and suture of nerves. The principal nerves of

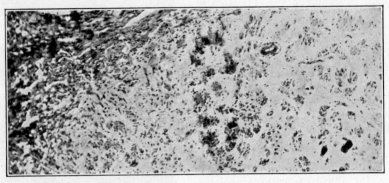

FIG. 348.—PHOTOMICROGRAPH OF AN AMPUTATION NEUROMA.

The patient had an amputation for a crushed leg; four weeks after the wound healed, an extremely tender area developed in the amputation stump. At operation the stump of the posterior tibial nerve was found enlarged and terminated in a bulbous tip 1 centimeter in diameter, which was excised. Note the intermingling of the curled fibrous strands and nerve fibers.

the extremities are mixed—motor and sensory. The accuracy of replacement and suture of the divided nerve ends, and the amount of scar tissue that forms between them, will affect the result as will the distance to be traversed by the regenerating axones in reaching their ultimate destination. In the regeneration of sensory nerves, the sensibility to pin prick is first regained, while that to light touch is the last to recover.

The time of return of motor function, likewise, depends upon the distance from the point of suture to the motor end plate in the muscle. The length of time that paralysis has persisted has much to do with the degree of improvement that follows suture. When it has existed for a long time, the muscle atrophy, degeneration, and fibrosis have become pronounced and some of these changes are permanent. Since overstretched muscles lose their elasticity and contractility, they must be supported during the paralysis and pending recovery. Such factors affect the ultimate result as well as does regeneration of the nerves themselves. It is unlikely that any mixed nerve ever shows complete recovery. Regenerating axons branch, sensory axones may grow along motor routes, and motor fibers find strange muscles, so that function is incompletely restored. Such nerves as the radial, noted for favorable results after suture, have a relatively small number of sensory fibers in proportion to the motor, so fewer of them go astray. In addition, this nerve supplies muscles not highly specialized in function. The manner of action of a muscle has much to do with the apparent functional recovery. For example, a muscle which has regained only slight contractility may, by reason of an advantageous fulcrum, produce a wide though possibly weak movement. For example, slight contraction of the extensor

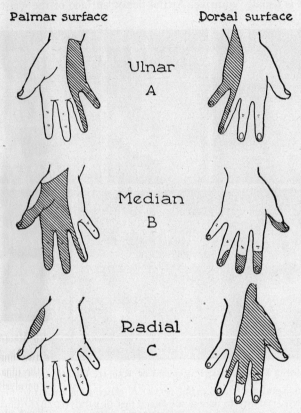

FIG. 349.—AREAS OF ANESTHESIA IN PARALYSIS OF NERVES TO THE HAND.
A, ulnar; *B,* median; *C,* radial.

carpi radialis may produce complete wrist extension. In contrast, a proportionate contraction of muscle fibers in the adductor of the thumb produces a movement with only a slight range and effectiveness.

Treatment.—Operative repair of the severed nerves has already been discussed on page 200. Emphasis should be placed on the importance of postoperative care such as support of the paralyzed muscle, movement of paralyzed joints and physiotherapy during the period of regeneration. Such support or splinting too often takes the form of rigid appliances and immobilization. For lesions of the peripheral nerves, splinting does not mean immobilization which is harmful. Stiff, useless joints often are the result. Elastic and spring supports, though more cumbersome, are less likely to be injurious. When rigid splints are used, they should be removed twice daily or oftener and the joints manipulated through their full range of motion. If the axis cylinders are prevented from reaching the distal stumps because of the presence of a fibrous tissue barrier or for other reasons, the proximal stump may grow in a coiled fashion with the ultimate formation of a tumor known as a *neuroma*. If the resulting pain and paresthesia are sufficiently severe, the neuroma may be resected and the freshly cut ends sutured. Such tumors are also likely to form in amputation stumps and may be the cause of severe pain and local tenderness. Operative removal of the neuroma is usually curative. At the flexor surface of the wrist large sensitive

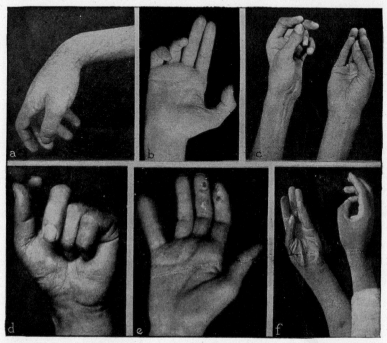

Fig. 350.—Motor Findings in Paralysis of Radial, Ulnar and Median Nerves.

a, wrist drop in paralysis of the radial nerve; *b*, clawing of inner two fingers in paralysis of the ulnar nerve; *c*, inability to oppose all finger tips in paralysis of the ulnar nerve, the left compared with the normal right hand; *d*, inability to make a fist in paralysis of the median nerve; *e*, trophic ulcers in paralysis of the median nerve; *f*, inability to oppose the thumb to the little finger in paralysis of the median nerve. (From Christopher, *Textbook of Surgery*, W. B. Saunders Company, 1936, p. 317.)

neuromas are likely to follow suture and to recur if removed. A mechanical protection is sometimes needed.

Injury to Special Nerves.—Lack of space prohibits discussion of the clinical findings accompanying the various nerves which may be injured, but there are a few (ulnar, radial and median) which are injured so frequently as to justify individual discussion. The ulnar and median are readily severed or injured by lacerations of the forearm which are so commonly sustained in both industrial and automobile accidents. Obviously, the findings will vary somewhat, depending upon the level at which the nerve is injured.

The *ulnar nerve* is injured most commonly by incised wounds of the forearm and wrist, penetrating wounds of the palm, and by fractures which involve the medial condyle of the humerus. The area of sensory impairment in complete division of the ulnar nerve includes the fifth finger, the neighboring half of the ring finger and the corresponding portions of the palmar and dorsal surfaces of the hand to the wrist. The only area, however, from which *all* forms of sensation are lost is the terminal joint of the little finger. Complete sensory loss of the terminal phalanx is proof of complete sensory interruption. Several types of motor disability are also produced by injury to this nerve depending on the level of injury. Since the ulnar nerve supplies most of the intrinsic muscles of the hand (excepting the two lateral

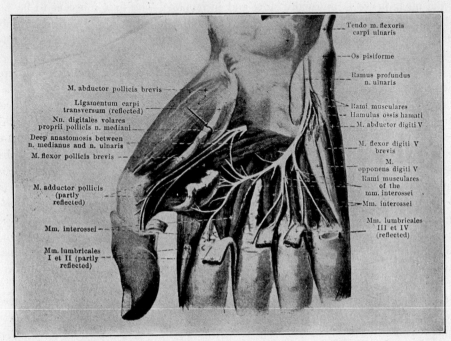

FIG. 351.—DISSECTION TO SHOW THE DEEP BRANCHES OF THE ULNAR NERVE AS THEY ARE DIS-
TRIBUTED TO THE FINGERS AND MUSCLES OF THE HAND.

(From Spalteholz, *Hand Atlas of the Human Body,* 5th ed., Vol. III, Philadelphia, J. B. Lippincott Company.)

lumbricales) division of this nerve results in considerable motor disability for finger movement of the hand (see Fig. 350). On account of paralysis of the interossei muscles, there is a weakness of the power of flexion at the metacarpal phalangeal joints, especially of the ulnar side of the hand. Abduction and adduction of the fingers are impossible because of paralysis of the dorsal and palmar interossei, although other muscles can perform this function to a slight degree. Paralysis of the interossei also prevents extension of the tips of the fingers, particularly when the metacarpophalangeal joints are bent at a right angle. Paralysis of the adductor pollicis muscle prevents the patient from bringing his thumb against and in front of the base of the index finger. If the nerve is injured at the elbow as frequently occurs at the groove of the internal condyle of the humerus, there will also be a weakness of the flexors of the fourth and fifth fingers.

As time elapses and the intrinsic muscles atrophy, a flexion deformity of the fingers (most marked on the fourth and fifth fingers) known as the "claw hand" (main en griffe), is produced. This deformity is produced chiefly because of paralysis of the interossei muscles. Since the power of flexion of the fingers at the metacarpophalangeal joints, and extension of the second and third phalanx, is controlled by the interossei, their paralysis will allow the opposing muscles to draw the fingers into flexion with extension at the metacarpophalangeal joint. This deformity is similar to but actually quite different from that observed in Volkmann's contracture and other lesions (p. 484). Restoration of function following suture of the ulnar nerve is unusually slow and incomplete. The first function to be regained is sensibility to pin prick. Function of the intrinsic muscles returns only after a year or two (depending somewhat upon the level of injury), but is rarely complete. After two years further restoration is unlikely.

The *median nerve* is often severed by deep lacerations above the wrist. It supplies the abductor and opponens pollicis, two outer lumbricales and the deep head of the flexor brevis pollicis muscle of the hand. Paralysis of the opponens pollicis muscle, which is one of the most diagnostic features of injury to the median nerve, prevents rocking of the thumb, so that apposition of the tip of the thumb to the base of the little finger is impossible. Abduction of the thumb, which is performed by the abductor pollicis, is inefficient if the median nerve is severed. If the nerve is injured at or above the elbow, flexion of the distal phalanx of the thumb and of the index finger is impossible because of paralysis of the flexor muscles to those digits. The sensory disturbance accompanying injury to the median nerve is the same regardless of the level of injury above the wrist; *i.e.,* the radial side of the palm and tips of the index, middle and ring finger (see Fig. 349). The terminal phalanx of the index finger is the only part that is totally anesthetic in complete median lesions. Recovery of sensation is of the greatest importance in the median nerve supply. Permanent loss of sensation in the index finger and thumb involves great disability. Sensory restoration in this nerve is more important than motor improvement.

The *radial (musculospiral) nerve* lies in direct contact with the humerus, winding around just below the insertion of the deltoid. It is, therefore, frequently injured, especially by fracture or by compression in the callus accompanying the healing of fractures of the middle third of this bone. Pressure paralyses are occasionally encountered in the operating room by carelessly allowing the arm to hang over the side of the operating table during an operation. If such pressure exists for a short time only, the paralysis is usually transient. The motor disturbance created by injury to the radial nerve is confined chiefly to the extensors of the wrist, fingers and thumb, and produces the disability commonly known as "wrist drop." If the nerve is injured high in the arm paralysis of the triceps may also occur, resulting in inability to extend the forearm. The sensory areas involved are located on the medial side of the dorsum of the hand and the medial side of the wrist (see Fig. 349).

Regeneration of the radial nerve after operative repair of the injury is generally satisfactory and a favorable prognosis as to restoration of the power of extension of the wrist and fingers can usually be offered. It is important that wrist drop be prevented by supporting the hand in a dorsiflexed position. This is achieved if the hand is kept in a "cock-up splint" during the several months that regeneration is taking place.

Neuritis.—This term is greatly abused, not only by the laity, but also by the medical profession. In reality it should be confined to a lesion of the axons, which at times may progress to actual degeneration. Such a lesion may present either sensory or motor manifestations, or both, and may be produced in one of two ways. First, the degeneration may be produced by a toxin or chemical poison affecting also other parts of the body, *e.g.,* lead, alcohol, and arsenic poisoning. The symptoms produced by this type of neuritis, which is frequently designated as *polyneuritis,* consists of paresthesia and various motor nerve paralyses, especially wrist drop. It has been shown that a great majority of these patients are suffering from vitamin deficiencies incident usually to a poorly balanced dietary intake or deficient absorption. Vitamin B_1 is the one most commonly deficient. Administration of this vitamin along with a well balanced diet is helpful and even curative. Important surgically is the use of splints and appliances to prevent contractures. In diphtheria the nerves involved in respiration may be affected, producing respiratory paralysis. Trauma itself represents the second mechanism in the production of neuritis; the injury is obviously partial, since complete destruction would result in paralysis.

Traumatic Neuritis.—The most frequent of this type of neuritis is produced by pressure or irritation of a nerve, and manifests itself by pain, paresthesia, tingling, numbness, hyperasthesia, paralysis, etc., in the region of the nerve and its distribution. Stretching of the peroneal and ulnar nerves during manipulation for the correction of deformities and pressure on the brachial plexus by spinal injury are examples of this type of neuritis. Other examples are injury to the peroneal nerve just below the head of the fibula by a plaster cast, injury to the ulnar nerve accompanying fixation of a fractured elbow put up in flexion, and paralysis of the median nerve from kinking at the annular ligament when a swollen wrist and hand is put up in flexion. The pathologic changes in and about the nerve are variable, depending upon the type of injury but consist chiefly of hemorrhage with crushing of a small amount of tissue, followed by deposition of scar tissue in and adjacent to the nerve. Brown[1] has emphasized the necessity of early operation in injuries of this type because of the muscle atrophy, stiffness of joints and nerve degeneration which might result from delayed therapy. He advises operation within a month following injury if no improvement is noted by that time, or if partial involvement progresses. Operative treatment consists of removal of constricting bands of scar tissue about the nerve, neurolysis (*i.e.,* excision of the thickened sheath), and transfer of the nerve to a new position out of its bed of scar tissue if possible. On some occasions removal of the cause may be followed by rapid amelioration of symptoms. On other occasions contusion of the nerve may be so severe as to produce paralysis (sensory or motor) until regeneration takes place. Since the nerve itself is usually not severed, regeneration takes place readily after removal of the cause, unless sufficient scar has been deposited to actually interfere with the growth of the axon down the sheath. If motor paralysis remains after removal of the cause, protective measures, such as splinting of the part to prevent contracture due to an overpull by the antagonistic muscles, must be instituted.

Cervical ribs have a surgical interest only because they may produce a type of traumatic neuritis. This congenital anomaly is almost always confined to the seventh cervical vertebra; the ribs vary considerably as to their stage of development. Very few are sufficiently developed as to be attached to the manubrium. More commonly the rib is short; it may or may not terminate in a fibrous band which is attached to the first rib near the scalene tubercle. Most cervical ribs are found accidentally in x-ray films, and do not produce symptoms. When symptoms are produced the

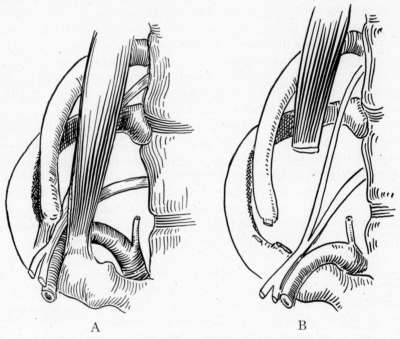

A   B

Fig. 353.—Diagram Illustrating How Cervical Ribs may Produce Disorders of Nerves and Blood Vessels on Side Affected.

Cervical ribs may compress the nerve trunks constituting the brachial plexus and produce a type of traumatic neuritis. They may likewise create a diminution in the volume of the radial pulse, with decreased blood pressure on the side or sides affected. *A*, the end of the cervical rib or its fibrous attachment (when present) to the first rib may compress the subclavian artery and nerve trunks against the scalenus anticus muscle; *B*, section of the scalenus anticus near its attachment to the rib allows the artery and nerve trunks to slide medially and downward, thereby eliminating the pressure on them.

most common manifestation is numbness and tingling of the hand in the distribution of the ulnar nerve. The fibers of this nerve are contained in the lower cord of the plexus, and are therefore most susceptible to pressure by the cervical rib. However, other fibers may be involved. Actual weakness of muscles of the hand or flexors of the wrist may be present. Less often there may be evidence of compression or spasm of the subclavian artery as exhibited by coldness and cyanosis of the fingers and decrease in volume of the radial pulse, particularly when the arm is held in a dependent position with the shoulder relaxed. On rare occasions superficial areas of gangrene will develop on the fingers.

The *treatment* of cervical ribs which produce symptoms is satisfactory and consists of release of the pressure upon the artery and nerve trunks. Although this may best be accomplished by removal of the rib in the more rare instances of completely formed ribs, it will not be necessary when the rib is very short or terminates in a fibrous cord. Adson and Coffey (*Ann. Surg.*, 85 :839, 1927) noted that in most instances, the artery and nerve trunks were compressed against the scalenus anticus muscle by the cervical rib or its fibrous attachment. They noted that section of this muscle at its insertion would allow the artery and nerve trunk to slide forward with subsidence of symptoms. Under such conditions removal of the cervical rib is, therefore, not necessary.

Brachial plexus neuritis, described by Murphy [2] and Naffziger [4] produces symptoms similar to those produced by cervical rib, but occurs in absence of a cervical rib. The term *scalenus anticus syndrome* (Ochsner and associates [3]) seems to classify it about as effectively as any designation, because section of the scalenus anticus muscle is almost universally curative. The pressure on the nerve fibers of the plexus is probably brought about by an abnormally high position of the first rib, or by drooping of the shoulder to an unusual extent. The condition is most commonly observed in women. Symptoms may be varied. Probably the most significant and reliable diagnostic sign is marked sensitiveness to pressure over the scalenus anticus at its attachment to the first rib. One of the most common symptoms complained of is a heavy dragging sensation in the shoulder (Naffziger [4]). Pain and paresthesia indicative of a neuritis as in the disease accompanying cervical ribs may be encountered. Motor weakness including the muscles of the hand and the flexors of the wrist may be observed. Certain exercises which lower the shoulder and stretch the nerves aggravate the symptoms. *Treatment* consists of section of the scalenus anticus muscle (scaleniotomy). This procedure allows the plexus and subclavian artery to slide forward, but, of perhaps more importance, it allows the first rib to drop.

Causalgia is a form of traumatic neuritis, characterized by severe burning pain, occurring at varying intervals following injury. Weir Mitchell, who originally described the condition, noted it was observed most commonly following war wounds. The pain occurs in attacks and is commonly revived by a touch or slight jar to the affected extremity; at times the discomfort is severe, demanding specific therapy. However, treatment is unsatisfactory. Of the radical procedures available sympathectomy should offer the best chance of relief.

Hiccup (*Singultus*).—This common complaint, produced by a sudden spasm of the diaphragm associated with the closure of the glottis, has been classified as a type of neuritis, but seemingly incorrectly. The abnormal impulse is transmitted by the phrenic nerve. In its most frequent form it is apparently of reflex origin from disorders of the stomach or intestine. It is commonly encountered as a complication of abdominal operations; in other instances it is instigated perhaps by irritation or inflammation of the diaphragm as produced by peritonitis, mild or severe. Occasionally the condition is caused by intracranial tumors but in such instances, is not severe. Various methods of treatment have been suggested (see p. 170). They have been summarized in detail by Mayo.[5] Sedation (morphine, etc.), gastric lavage, inhalation of carbon dioxide, rebreathing into a paper bag, and many other remedies have proven effective. When the above conservative measures fail and the condition is proving to be an exhaustive complication, the phrenic nerve may be isolated by operative procedures and the impulses broken by various means (Weeks[6]).

Neuralgia.—Unlike neuritis, neuralgia is caused primarily by an organic disturbance of the terminal ends of the nerve or of the ganglion cells. The pain may be of severe stabbing character and radiate over a wide area. Common examples are trigeminal neuralgia (see below), and toothache, in which the pain may be referred over the entire jaw and side of the face. Of special interest to surgeons is chronic neuralgia of the lower thoracic nerves due to various vertebral lesions, producing pain and tenderness *in the abdominal wall* and thus often mistaken for referred pain of visceral origin such as appendicitis which leads to an unnecessary operation (see Carnett, J. B., *J. Am. M. Ass.,* 102 :345, 1934). The pain is often of the sacro-iliac or lumbosacral type.

Trigeminal Neuralgia (Tic Doloureaux).—This is a serious malady producing severe excruciating pain distributed along one or more of the divisions of the nerve (usually the second and third). The onset is usually abrupt with severe pain radiating to the upper or lower jaw. If the second division is involved the pain will be confined chiefly to the cheek and upper lip. Although the disease usually affects one division at first, there is a tendency in time for all three to become affected. Although there are no objective sensory changes in the skin over the area of the face affected, it has a peculiar reflex sensitivity in so far as a slight touch may at times set off a paroxysm of pain which characteristically is located in the upper jaw but may extend to the mandible and nose. In character it is sharp, lightning-like, stabbing or electric in quality. One shock may succeed another over a few seconds. In the intervals there may be no pain whatever, though at times there is a more or less persistent discomfort. Remissions of weeks or months characterize the disease. The average age of the sufferers is between fifty and sixty. In the very young there may be an association with other nervous diseases such as disseminated sclerosis. The pain is apt to occur in paroxysms and is extremely severe, requiring sedation, although narcotics such as morphine should be avoided because of the danger of drug addiction. The only permanent cure is by section of the sensory root of the fifth nerve, either in whole or in part. The motor division can be spared. The anesthesia is permanent. If the pain does not involve the first division, that portion of the root should not be sacrificed, as permanent anesthesia of the cornea involves obvious dangers.

It may be wise first to inject the nerve with alcohol. This is usually effective in relieving the pain for several months or years. It may be repeated, or avulsion of the root be performed by operation. Alcohol injection may be a useful therapeutic test for what may be accomplished permanently by operation. Trethylene inhalations, 25 drops three times per day, is effective in controlling the attacks in a minority of cases.

Herpes Zoster (Shingles).—This condition is caused by a lesion, often of infective origin, located presumably in the spinal ganglia in which, on some occasions, actual pathologic lesions have been demonstrated. The ganglia associated with the intercostal nerves are most commonly affected, and severe pain which is usually of a constant debilitating character radiates along the course of these nerves. The skin over the area supplied by the nerves becomes red and edematous and vesicles soon appear. Such vesicles may become infected secondarily. In the severe cases the pain is so intense as to demand constant narcosis which of course must be used with care, because of the consequent danger of addiction. The disease occurs, however, in all variations of severity, and frequently is so mild or of such short duration as not to demand special treatment. Since pain precedes the herpes, which in some cases may be absent, the disease may be mistaken for other lesions.

Treatment may be unnecessary in the mild cases; in the severe cases unfortunately it is often unsatisfactory. However, the intravenous administration of heavy doses of sodium iodide (as much as 5 grams in forty-eight hours) is frequently specific in eradicating the disease. In the early stages, many workers have found arsenic (endoarsen 1 cc. every day for five doses) to be most effective. It seems to prevent most of the postherpetic pain. It should be emphasized that to be effective the sodium iodide must be given in large doses as mentioned for postherpetic pain. X-ray therapy to the spine, injection of the nerve roots with alcohol, sensory root sections and various other palliative procedures have been recommended, but none has proved very successful. If conservative measures fail, section of the spino-thalamic tract may be tried as a last resort in the severe cases. Local treatment of the skin lesions are obviously necessary, especially in order to insure against secondary infection.

The Cranial Nerves.—The *first* or *olfactory* nerve carries impulses responsible for the sense of smell, and by this means likewise contributes to a great extent to the sense of taste. Its chief surgical significance lies in the fact that loss of the sense of smell aids in the localization of brain tumors and site of brain damage in head injuries, particularly those accompanying fracture of the skull.

The *second* or *optic* nerve, transmitting stimuli which give rise to the sense of sight, is one of the most important of the cranial nerves. Although injuries or diseases of the retina may create blindness or disturbances in vision, lesions affecting the optic nerves or visual pathways are more important surgically, because defects in the visual fields created in this way may be due to the presence of an intracranial tumor. *Choked disk* (papilledema), which is in reality an edema of the nerve trunk ending in the retina, is secondary usually to an increased intracranial pressure of subacute or chronic nature. This condition may be brought about by a number of causes including brain tumor, brain abscess, intracranial injury, etc. If the intracranial pressure is allowed to persist, the choked disk passes into the stage of "secondary atrophy" with serious impairment of vision or permanent blindness.

The *third* (*oculomotor*), *fourth* (*trochlear*) and *sixth* (*abducens*) nerves innervate the external muscles of the eye. Inflammatory or neoplastic lesions of the brain or fractures of the base of the skull may create a disturbance in the normal movements of the eyeball by injury to these nerves. A carotid aneurysm, however, is a frequent cause of oculomotor paralysis, and is to be particularly suspected if the onset of the paralysis is sudden. Careful examination of the movements of the eye is obviously important.

The *fifth* (*trigeminal*) nerve is rarely injured, but is frequently the seat of a neuralgia which is known as *tic douloureux* (see preceding page).

The *seventh* (*facial*) nerve, which is a motor nerve supplying the muscles of the face is occasionally injured by operative procedures, fractures of the base of the skull or disease processes such as infection about the middle ear and mastoid. Paralysis of the facial nerve results in a disfiguring deformity on account of the unilateral loss of facial expression, and shifting of the mouth toward the unaffected side. Since the nerve divides into its branches in the outer surface of the parotid gland, operations in this area for parotid tumors, cervical lymphadenitis, etc., may result in injury to the nerve. Spontaneous, though often transient facial paralysis also occurs as the result of various infections, toxins, etc. (*Bell's palsy*). These types of seventh nerve paralysis are of the peripheral type which is characterized by

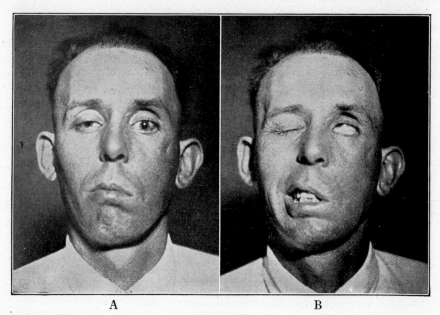

A   B

Fig. 354.—Paralysis of the Seventh Nerve Produced by a Gunshot Wound of the Face.

A, with the facial muscles at rest the only evidence of paralysis (in this instance) is a slight deviation of the mouth toward the unaffected (right) side, and a lack of wrinkles on the paralyzed (left) side; *B,* when the patient is instructed to close his eyes and "show his teeth," a marked distortion results because of the paralysis of muscles on the left side.

inability to close the eyes or wrinkle the forehead. In contrast to this are the lesions which are of central or cortical origin in which only the lower facial muscles are affected. Thus the patient retains the ability to close the eye and wrinkle the forehead. In permanent facial paralysis of the peripheral type, the facial deformity may often be corrected by plastic operation, which includes the transplantation of fascial strips. In peripheral facial palsy where there is some possibility of recovery, the facial muscles should be supported and kept relaxed to prevent overstretching. Adhesive straps attached to a band about the head may be used.

The *eighth* (*acoustic*) nerve is occasionally injured in fractures of the skull, but more commonly the equilibratory sensation is impaired by cerebellar lesions (tumor). The nerve itself may be the seat of neoplastic growths, *e.g.,* acoustic neurinoma, von Recklinghausen's disease, etc. Ménière's disease has been successfully treated by the intracranial section of the eight nerve or of its vestibular portion.

The *ninth* (*glossopharyngeal*) nerve is of little surgical significance except for *glassopharyngeal neuralgia,* which is similar to trigeminal neuralgia except that it is more rare and is confined to the anatomical distribution of this nerve. Treatment consists of the intracranial section of the ninth nerve. Occasionally cerebral lesions (tumors, etc.) compress the fibers constituting this nerve and produce an impairment in taste and deglutition.

The *tenth* (*vagus*) nerve is of special significance since section or destruction of both nerves in the cervical region is fatal to man. It contains fibers which carry autonomic impulses of the parasympathetic type to and from the abdominal and thoracic organs. Occasionally tumors compress the vagus in such a manner as to create an irregularity in the cardiac rhythm. Because of its position in the posterior portion of the carotid sheath it has no doubt been mistaken for the phrenic nerve or sympathetic trunk and occasionally removed.

The *eleventh* (*spinal accessory*) nerve supplies the sternomastoid and trapezius muscles and may readily be injured or severed during operations upon the lower part of the neck, such as dissection for carcinoma. The degree of disability and discomfort following such paralysis is variable; at times it is extreme.

The *twelfth* (*hypoglossal*) nerve which supplies the muscles of the tongue should be avoided in block dissection beneath the jaw for carcinoma. Severance of one hypoglossal nerve results in unilateral atrophy of the tongue with deviation to the side of the injury. Disturbances in deglutition and articulation are not marked, so that this nerve is often severed and crossed with the facial nerve in instances of permanent facial palsy.

THE BRAIN

Craniocerebral Injuries.—The term *head injury* is often used to include three groups of trauma, which occur so frequently together that they are described here in the section on brain: (1) injury to the scalp; (2) fracture of the skull; and, (3) intracranial injury. This classification will be used in the following discussion, except that most of the space will be devoted to varieties of intracranial injuries which, it should be emphasized, represent the most important of the three groups, being responsible for the serious and often fatal results.

1. *Injury to the Scalp.*—In any patient with such an injury it is obviously important to know whether or not a skull fracture and intracranial injury are present. Examination of the head may reveal contusions, hematomas, or ecchymotic patches anywhere about the scalp. The presence of a laceration of the scalp is of extreme importance because of the possibility of detecting an underlying fracture which may demand repair as will be discussed later. Local tenderness may be elicited even if the patient is only partially conscious. Pitting of the scalp extends along linear fractures. Presence of pitting and tenderness may permit the diagnosis of linear fissures. A hematoma with a soft crater may sometimes simulate a depression in the skull though continued pressure on its margins may alter it and indicate its character; frequently differential diagnosis between it and a depressed fracture may be possible only by x-ray. Aside from the opportunity to estimate damage to the underlying bone and brain, a simple scalp injury presents no other feature of

importance. The treatment of this uncomplicated lesion has been described under Wounds; such injuries heal readily, on account of the profuse blood supply. Antitetanic serum or tetanus toxoid (if war wound) should be given as discussed elsewhere.

2. *Skull Fracture.*—Fracture of the skull rarely occurs alone; injury to the underlying brain is often associated, and injury to the overlying scalp is frequently present. The serious and often fatal effects of skull fracture are *due to injury of the brain or a blood vessel, and not to the fracture itself,* except in basal fractures when meningitis may develop, regardless of the presence or absence of brain injury. When the compressing force acts from pole to pole the fracture is apt to be linear. If the head is struck a direct blow with a small object, a stellate fracture, with lines radiating outward from a central point, is apt to be produced. Such a blow, if severe enough, will result in a depressed fracture. An important example of the indirect localized depressed type is a fracture of the base of the skull sustained when the patient falls to the ground from a height, and lands on his feet or buttocks so that the impact of the heavy head strikes against the vertebral column and literally caves in the base of the skull. Such injuries, of course, are very serious and usually fatal, because of the damage to the adjacent vital medullary centers. Because of the thinness of the bone in certain parts of the base of the skull, fractures in this region are particularly common.

Bullet wounds produce a variable amount of shattering, depending on the speed and softness of the bullet. Fractures of the skull may be classified in many different ways but the classifications themselves are not sufficiently important to deserve much discussion. If considered from the standpoint of the mechanism of production they may be bursting, indented or expansile. If classified according to the character of the fracture itself they may be linear, stellate, comminuted, depressed or penetrating.

On a few occasions a fracture of the skull may be diagnosed by simple clinical observations. The fracture may sometimes be palpated when depression and comminution is present; it may be seen and felt occasionally through a laceration; local tenderness is usually present over the fracture. Bleeding from the nose or ear is indicative of skull fracture if the soft tissue can be excluded as the source of the hemorrhage. Escape of cerebrospinal fluid is nearly always pathognomonic of cranial fracture.

The diagnosis of skull fracture, however, on most occasions cannot be made clinically, but requires x-ray films taken in several views and often stereoscopically. From the therapeutic standpoint, x-ray is necessary in so far as it may reveal a depressed fracture which might otherwise be undemonstrable and which may require operative correction. Views taken with the ray tangential to the depression are necessary to show its depth. On the other hand, it may not be permissible to subject severely shocked patients to the strain of roentgenologic examinations. From the medicolegal standpoint, x-ray films showing a skull fracture are extremely valuable because of the importance of demonstrating the fracture itself during court proceedings.

Treatment of skull fractures is to a large extent that of the associated intracranial and scalp injuries, unless a depressed or compound fracture is present. Even in the absence of demonstrable intracranial injury, the patient is kept at rest in bed for at least ten days, since it is probable that brain damage is present although it is not evident clinically. When the fracture is depressed or compound, operation is indicated. (See also under types of intracranial injury.)

Depressed fractures are important because they are frequently associated with brain injury which may be of the local type or may be diffuse, and associated with so much edema that any of the manifestations described on page 564 may be produced. However, Naffziger and Glaser [8] have shown that the "changes in the brain are caused by the force producing the injury rather than the depression of the bone." Persisting depressions do not cause adhesions or localized softening. The problem with depressed fractures depends upon the management to avoid infection

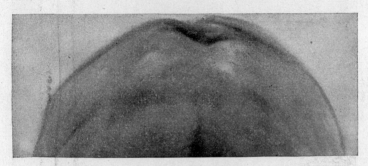

FIG. 355.—DEPRESSED FRACTURE OF VERTEX OF SKULL.

Patient was unconscious for two hours after the accident. Several hours later craniotomy was performed and the depressed fracture elevated. (Courtesy Dr. Ernest Sachs.)

and removal of devitalized material to minimize gliosis, scar contraction, and later sequelae such as convulsions.

The skin may or may not be broken over the site of injury. Not infrequently, the depressed fragment may be detected by palpation. An x-ray should always be taken, however, since the conformity of a blood clot in the scalp may frequently simulate a depressed fracture. A careful neurologic examination is particularly important, especially the search for pathologic reflexes. If the injury occurs in a "silent" area (*e.g.,* frontal lobes) there will be a paucity and perhaps even an absence of neurologic manifestations. If the injury is located in the motor area, weakness or paralysis of motor function may be noted. If the lesion is posterior to the fissure of Rolando, cortical types of sensory disturbance, and frequently astereognosis (inability to recognize shape of objects by touch) may be demonstrable. Obviously, the operative treatment of depressed fractures consists of craniotomy with elevation of the depressed fragment; if the underlying dura and cortex have been torn, débridement of the damaged tissue is also performed, but closure of the dura is essential.

Compound fracture is frequently associated with laceration of brain tissue; at times considerable brain tissue may actually be lost. The neurologic manifestations may include any of those described later under Varieties of Intracranial Injury.

A compound fracture is obviously a serious injury, but by no means necessarily fatal. The treatment consists of immediate operation.

Excision of the wound of entrance, enlargement of it by a tripod incision, removal of a block of bone if the wound of entrance is small (*e.g.*, made by bullet), is to be done by separate perforator and burr openings so that a rectangle of bone, perhaps 3 cm. square, can be lifted out. With larger and extensively comminuted depressed or in-driven fractures, portions of bone can be moved directly.

In the conscious patient, who by straining or blowing can raise intracranial pressure, a large amount of the completely disintegrated and devitalized material will extrude from the opening in the dura. Irrigation, suction and removal of re-

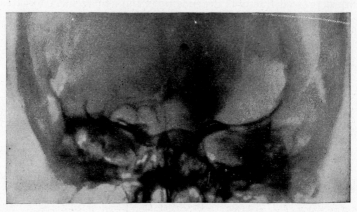

FIG. 356—COMPOUND FRACTURE OF THE SKULL IN A THIRTY-FIVE-YEAR-OLD POLICEMAN.

The trauma was so extensive that a fragment of bone shown by the defect on the x-ray has been lost. Laceration of the brain was extensive, and at time of admission considerable macerated brain tissue was visible about the scalp wound. Operative treatment in this case was entirely successful and an excellent functional result was obtained. Such injuries are not necessarily fatal, providing proper débridement can be done immediately, and the trauma to the brain is sustained in a "silent" area such as the frontal lobe. (Courtesy Dr. Ernest Sachs.)

tained foreign bodies with forceps are used. Portions of metal far removed from the wound of entrance, should not be sought. This involves added damage to surrounding tissues. These are less apt to carry infections than are other foreign bodies. Small vessels of the brain are controlled either by electrocoagulation or the use of silver clips. The wound is then liberally irrigated and closed (with cotton or silk), after 2 to 5 grams of sulfanilamide are sprinkled into it. Sulfathiazole should not be used. Wounds penetrating the ventricles are associated with a very high mortality rate. Other details of the treatment of compound fractures, particularly those related to war injuries, may be found in Chapter XXXIII.

3. *Intracranial Injury.*—In any trauma to the skull it is obviously important to know whether or not damage to the brain tissue has occurred; still more important is the estimation of the degree and type of injury. The varieties of intracranial injuries are described at some length under a separate heading. It should be emphasized that the existence of scalp injury, and even skull fracture, does not necessarily mean brain damage; on the other hand, the brain is occasionally injured, sometimes severely, with no other associated lesion either in the skull or scalp.

At times, patients may sustain a head injury which produces trauma to the brain without exhibiting any clinical manifestations. This is particularly true if the damage is sustained in the frontal lobe. Because of this fact many surgeons advise lumbar puncture to determine the presence or absence of bloody spinal fluid in order to establish or rule out the existence of intracranial hemorrhage. Obviously, of course, bloody spinal fluid indicates (in absence of trauma due to the needle itself) bleeding into the ventricles or subarachnoid space; however, not all injuries result in such hemorrhage. Nevertheless, when bloody fluid is found, a diagnosis of some type of intracranial injury is obvious, and routine treatment must be carried out even in the absence of positive neurologic signs or x-ray evidence of fracture. The danger associated with lumbar puncture in patients with severe intracranial injury does not apply to the border-line cases just mentioned; the precautions mentioned on page 566 should nevertheless be observed.

The simplest manifestation of intracranial injury is transient unconsciousness sustained immediately after the accident, followed later perhaps by dizziness, headache, or visual disturbances which clear up within a few hours without producing any permanent effect. This type of manifestation is often called *concussion,* a physiopathologic state assumed to be due to microscopic or perhaps only functional trauma to the brain cells. Of considerable interest is the fact that repeated episodes of this type may lead to permanent brain damage which is observed in boxers who are said to be "punch drunk." Organic injury, consisting chiefly of minute hemorrhages particularly in the pons, is responsible for this condition. In the severe cases the mental disturbances may develop into almost complete imbecility.

More obvious manifestations of intracranial injury consist of a great variety of specific signs and symptoms. Many of them have already been discussed to a certain extent in Chapter XV. These manifestations include disturbances in the peripheral circulation, *e.g.,* surgical shock, abnormalities in respiration, manifestations of increased intracranial pressure, and various types of sensorial changes from coma to hyperactivity; other evidences comprise those more local in character, such as cranial nerve paralyses, papilledema and leakage of cerebrospinal fluid from wounds, ear or nose. So important are these various types that they are discussed in some detail. Treatment is also described under each variety of injury; it is naturally unsatisfactory when the damage (*e.g.,* laceration) is sustained in vital centers.

There are *several varieties of intracranial injury* consisting of contusion and laceration of brain tissue, of hemorrhage, edema and compression, and of actual destruction or loss of brain tissue. The hemorrhage may be massive and local, or diffuse and petechial in type; it may be within the brain, subdural or extradural. The contusion or laceration of brain tissue may be diffuse or localized; cerebrospinal fluid may escape subdurally (extra arachnoid) where it is absorbed slowly, thus increasing intracranial pressure, or it may leak externally when a compound fracture exists. Most of these various lesions may be differentiated clinically. Often a combination of two or more will be present, thus complicating differential diagnosis. Nevertheless, the therapy may be so different in each type that the surgeon should seriously attempt to diagnose the type and severity of the injury and particularly its development by frequent observation. In the following classification *four types of injury* are discussed: (1) diffuse injury with edema, (2) local brain damage, (3) extradural hemorrhage and (4) subdural hemorrhage. The treatment indicated will be described in each type.

1. DIFFUSE INJURY WITH EDEMA.—This group represents the most serious type of injury and is frequently fatal. Contusions and lacerations may be extensive throughout the brain. A variable amount of tiny and massive hemorrhages within the brain or along the meningeal surfaces is associated with the injury. The contusions and lacerations are responsible for the development of edema which, along with hemorrhage, may readily give rise to sufficient compression to produce serious manifestations purely from the mechanism of the increased pressure alone.

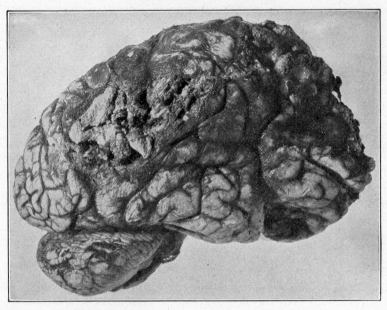

FIG. 357.—FATAL BRAIN INJURY IN COMPOUND FRACTURE.
Note the laceration and diffuse subarachnoid hemorrhage. (Courtesy Dr. S. A. Levinson.)

A variable degree and duration of *unconsciousness* will be present, dependent upon the severity of the injury. In many instances vertigo and headache will be fairly constant complaints. Nausea and vomiting may be present. The skin is usually pale and the extremities are cold and moist. When complete unconsciousness is produced and maintained over a period of several hours, the objective manifestations just mentioned may be more prominent. Urinary and fecal incontinence, particularly the former, may be noted. Variable changes may be found in the reflexes, including hyperactivity or absence. Abnormal reflexes, *i.e.,* Babinski, Oppenheim, Gordon or ankle clonus may be present. Pathologic "eye signs," such as inequality of pupils and lack of reaction to accommodation or to light, are not uncommon. If the patient is conscious a paralysis of extraocular muscles may be revealed. Paralysis of various muscle groups of the extremities may also be noted.

Manifestations of *increased intracranial pressure* (produced by edema and hemorrhage may be noted within a few hours; if active hemorrhage is the cause of the compression (see p. 567) these manifestations may be noted sooner. As a rule, the blood pressure rises and the pulse rate decreases (down to 40 to 60 per minute). A sudden decrease in blood pressure, particularly if it drops below normal, is usually serious and may be a sign of impending death. The same may be said of an increase in pulse rate, particularly if it rises to above 120 or 130 per minute. The optic disks rarely show swelling. The respirations become abnormal and are commonly slow and deep, but may be stertorous or of the Cheyne-Stokes variety.

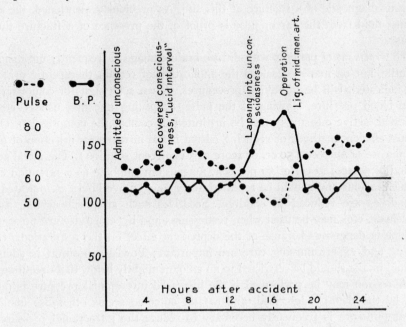

CHART 6.—EXTRADURAL HEMORRHAGE FROM THE MIDDLE MENINGEAL ARTERY.

Note that as the patient recovered consciousness (lucid interval) the pulse and blood pressure remained unchanged. The rise in blood pressure and drop in pulse rate at about the fourteenth hour was caused by the pressure effect of the bleeding from the torn artery. While this type of chart is almost pathognomonic of middle meningeal hemorrhage, it should be emphasized that this is not always present in such lesions.

Signs of compression of the brain may be produced by the simple accident of rupture of the arachnoid, thus allowing fluid to escape into the subdural space. However, the manifestations of this injury are more apt to simulate those of middle meningeal hemorrhage, except that the rise in blood pressure may not be so great.

In those injuries which are so severe as to be fatal, the blood pressure falls and the pulse rate rises as death approaches. Other manifestations of shock, including pallor, cold extremities, etc., become more pronounced. The breathing becomes more abnormal, particularly slower and more irregular. A terminal rise in temperature is commonly noted in patients who have survived longer than a few hours.

Fractures of the base of the skull are usually associated with diffuse damage to the brain, but it is occasionally true that the damage is purely local and may be of trivial consequence. They are usually serious (because of the proximity of the vital centers) even though the damage is local. The patient is usually uncon-scious. Any or all of the eye signs previously mentioned may be present. Involve-ment of the facial nerve and nerves supplying the eye are the most valuable from a diagnostic standpoint. If the fracture passes through the petrous portion of the temporal bone, bleeding from the ear may be noted. In fact bleeding from the ear, not arising from the external ear or canal, is usually indicative of a basal fracture. Bleeding from the nose and mouth may be produced by a basal fracture, but is by no means diagnostic of a fracture at this site. As previously mentioned, the escape of spinal fluid from the ear or nose is proof of the presence of a fracture through the base.

The *treatment* of patients with diffuse brain damage is frequently unsatisfactory and futile, but on many occasions the application of certain therapeutic principles, when indicated, will be lifesaving procedures. When such signs of compression as rise in blood pressure, slowing of the pulse, deepening unconsciousness, etc., are manifested, active measures must be instituted to combat the compression. One of the most efficient methods of reducing edema is the intravenous injection of hyper-tonic glucose or sucrose (50 cc. or more of 50 per cent solution). The rectal admin-istration of 90 to 120 cc. of 50 per cent magnesium sulphate as a retention enema is also efficacious and should be repeated every four or five hours as indicated. The above doses are reduced in children. Sedatives such as phenobarbital, aspirin, paraldehyde, etc., may be used when restlessness and hyperactivity are present, but morphine is dangerous because of the depressant effect on the respirations. Gentle handling and expert nursing care are important; Fowler's position is advisable. The fluid intake should be restricted to an amount slightly below daily requirements. Decompression may be performed if the increased intracranial pressure is not re-lieved by the therapy described, and a fatal outcome seems otherwise imminent. Lumbar puncture is frequently necessary to reduce the intracranial pressure, but only when other means fail. Lumbar puncture may be dangerous because on rare occasions it results in death by sudden compression of the medulla against the foramen magnum. Because of this danger not all surgeons recommend its use in intracranial injury. However, this danger can be eliminated by using an appropriate manometer during the puncture and by removing cerebrospinal fluid slowly and in sufficient amount to reduce the pressure to the desired level. In any case, lumbar puncture must be considered as a serious procedure and utilized only on sufficient indication. It is repeated only when indicated; the routine use of lumbar puncture in intracranial injury is to be condemned. Complete bed rest is absolutely essential inasmuch as activity of the patient during the first day or two is apt to incite serious hemorrhage. Of equal importance is the fact that bed rest for ten to twenty days tends to prevent chronic headaches, vertigo, etc., which are so apt to follow any brain injury associated with fractures of the skull.

2. LOCAL BRAIN DAMAGE.—A fracture may or may not accompany this type of injury. When a fracture is present, as is commonly the case, it is usually of the depressed type. In this instance there may be laceration of brain tissue near the fracture site. Various types of hemorrhage, including subcortical, extradural or sub-dural, may be produced. Occasionally there is a superficial contusion and laceration of brain tissue at one point with hemorrhage of variable degree from the surface

vessels. When this type of injury is encountered on the side opposite to that of the fracture it is spoken of as a *contrecoup injury*. Patients with local injury may be unconscious because of the associated edema and compression, or may be merely drowsy. Local manifestations, such as weakness of muscles of the face or an extremity on the side opposite the brain damage, may be encountered. Various signs, including visual defects, may be demonstrable. On rare occasions convulsions of the Jacksonian type may develop. Pathologic reflexes may be elicited. Occasionally the patient may be aphasic. Treatment consists of the general measures already mentioned and of operative repair of depressed or compound fractures which has already been discussed.

3. EXTRADURAL HEMORRHAGE.—In most instances, extradural hemorrhage arises from the middle meningeal artery which is torn by a fracture. On rare occasions a fracture is not present. There is usually a history of at least a short period of unconsciousness followed by a lucid interval of variable duration (two to eighteen hours). The patient then becomes stuporous and sinks into total unconsciousness. The blood pressure usually rises sharply, and when it occurs, is perhaps the most valuable diagnostic sign of middle meningeal hemorrhage, with the exception of the periods of unconsciousness just described. The slowing of the pulse rate is a more constant finding. The respirations may become stertorous. Swelling of the optic disks may develop. Localizing symptoms are not commonly observed except in late cases indicating that the clot has progressed upward over the motor area; weakness of one side of the face or an extremity (usually the arm) opposite the side on which the hemorrhage is located, constitutes the chief local sign. Convulsions occasionally are noted. It will be noted that most of the manifestations accompanying middle meningeal hemorrhage are in reality those of a gradually increasing intracranial pressure. Death may follow in a few hours; for that reason it is important that the condition be recognized at once and immediate operative procedure undertaken. At operation, a subtemporal decompression is performed, the blood clot evacuated and the artery ligated. The dura is not opened.

4. SUBDURAL HEMORRHAGE.—Hemorrhage of this type usually arises from rupture of veins on the surface of the brain in the subdural space between the dura and arachnoid. The amount of bleeding is extremely variable and the symptoms may arise shortly after the injury, or their appearance may be delayed for weeks or even months. It is in the chronic cases that a history of injury is often lacking; in such instances the organized clot is termed chronic subdural hematoma (see Furlow[9]). The term pachymeningitis hemorrhagica was first applied to this type of lesion, regardless of its cause, by Virchow. If the hemorrhage is profuse, acute manifestations are likely to occur and detection will be readily possible, but it will naturally be difficult to determine whether the lesion consists primarily of hemorrhage or laceration. The two stages of unconsciousness and the fall in pulse rate, so characteristic of hemorrhage in the extradural space, will not be elicited because the hemorrhage, being venous in type, is rarely severe enough or localized sufficiently to cause acute compression of the brain. The blood may be clotted or liquefied. Occasionally rather clear fluid is found; this is either cerebrospinal fluid or fluid formed by transudation. If the bleeding occurs so slowly that a chronic subdural hematoma is produced, it may be weeks or months after the accident before mani-

festations are noted. The most common symptoms are those seen in increased intracranial pressure such as headache, vomiting, irritability, change in personality, sometimes mental deterioriation including inattentiveness, forgetfulness and even stupor
or unconsciousness. Weakness of an extremity and exaggerated reflexes on the side
of the body opposite the hemorrhage may be demonstrable. Choked disks are usually
present. The diagnosis is usually difficult, particularly in the chronic cases, because
the trauma producing the injury may be so slight as to have been forgotten. Moreover, symptoms and signs may be few in number and atypical. It is extremely important, however, that this lesion be recognized inasmuch as conservative treatment is
so unsatisfactory, whereas operation is usually curative. Treatment consists of
removal of the blood clot and fluid through a posttemporal trephine opening, by
means of irrigation through a small catheter. Rarely will it be necessary to turn
down a flap. The sac surrounding the clot need not be removed. Occasionally,
localization is difficult; it is not uncommon to find the clot on the side opposite to the
site originally suspected, or to find a clot on each side, thereby illustrating the
necessity of making a bilateral trephine opening. If a clot is not found, ventriculograms may be made. Details may be found in an article by Groff and Grant [60].

Summary of Therapy in Head Injuries.—Lacerations of the scalp are treated
like similar wounds elsewhere, provided the other injuries present have been
diagnosed and treated adequately. Fractures of the skull in themselves require only
rest in bed unless a depressed or compound fracture is present which requires
operative repair. In general, depressed fractures, compound fractures, certain types
of active bleeding (*e.g.,* middle meningeal) and blood clots demand operation;
decompression may rarely be indicated after conservative measures have failed to
halt an increasing intracranial pressure.

Conservative measures for the treatment of intracranial injuries imply absolute
bed rest and sufficient sedation in patients exhibiting hyperactivity. Most important
is the reduction of increased intracranial pressure, when present, by the use of
dehydration, *i.e.,* limitation of fluid intake, intravenous injection of hypertonic
solutions and retention enemas of concentrated magnesium sulphate solution as described. Lumbar puncture as a means of reducing intracranial pressure is also used
but only when indicated and when properly carried out, never as a routine procedure.

Repeated and careful clinical observation is essential to estimate changes in the
degree or type of injury. The surgeon should be prepared to change the type of
therapy, dependent upon changes in the clinical manifestations exhibited by the
patient. This is particularly important during the first twenty-four hours after the
accident, but also for several days afterward.

The after-effects of severe intracranial injury are important and often serious.
They belong to the domain of neurology.

Nontraumatic Intracranial Lesions (Tumor and Abscess).—A few decades
ago surgical diseases of the brain, especially tumors, were thought to be uncommon
lesions. During the past twenty-five years the fallacy of this idea has become
apparent; there are only four or five organs which are more often the seat of tumors
than the brain. For this reason it becomes necessary for graduates in medicine to
familiarize themselves with the manifestations produced by such lesions. It must
be remembered, too, that the brain is the site of metastatic carcinoma (primary

most commonly in the bronchus) which may produce the same clinical picture as that presented by a primary tumor. It should also be emphasized that there are numerous diseases, including meningitis, encephalitis, syphilis (gumma, tabes, paresis), tuberculosis (tuberculoma and meningitis), etc., which may produce symptoms and signs similar to those produced by tumor. Detailed descriptions of brain tumors with classification, treatment, etc., may be found in the publications of Sachs,[10] Bailey,[11] Penfield,[12] Davis [13] and others.

Tumors of the brain are perhaps of greater variety than those occurring in any other organ of the body. In the brain tissue itself the glioma, a primary tumor, is most common; there are several types of gliomas, some of which are very malignant whereas others are comparatively benign. Of the gliomas, astrocytomas, which are composed largely of well differentiated glia cells, are perhaps more common than the other varieties. They are relatively slowly growing tumors; many are cystic. Medulloblastomas which are considerably less common, are on the other hand quite malignant. They are composed of a primitive type of cell of the round cell variety. They are usually encountered in the cerebellum of young people, particularly children. Glioblastomas are likewise comparatively malignant but occur chiefly in adults and in the cerebrum. They are made up of glia cells. Oligodendrogliomas are relatively uncommon and are comparatively benign. They are usually found in the cerebrum and are frequently readily diagnosed by a plain x-ray film because of deposition of calcium in the tumor. Metastatic growths are extremely common and offer the neurosurgeon a great deal of trouble from the diagnostic standpoint, particularly when the initial tumor is located internally and is insidious. Carcinoma of the bronchus and breast are particularly prone to metastasize to the brain. Tuberculomas and syphilomas likewise simulate primary brain tumors but are, of course, primarily infectious in origin. There are several varieties of primary tumors arising in accessory tissue of the brain, *e.g.,* meningiomas in the meninges, hypophysial duct cysts, adenomas of the pituitary and tumors of the cranial nerves. The *treatment* of brain tumors is confined to operative removal and x-ray therapy. Obviously, if practical the tumor should be removed. Electrical cutting and coagulating instruments are of great assistance in removal of brain tumors. Even if the tumor cannot be totally removed, it is commonly good practice to remove as much as possible because this procedure will relieve the devastating effects of intracranial pressure, of which impending blindness is one of the most important. Moreover, when the tumor is comparatively benign the patient may be relieved of symptoms for years and live a comfortable, useful life. Obviously, cysts should be evacuated, or removed if possible; if they cannot be removed a nodule of neoplastic tissue on the wall should be looked for and removed if possible, or coagulated by the diathermy.

Brain abscess is a serious condition, frequently difficult to diagnose, but since proper surgical treatment is commonly curative, diagnosis should be made as soon as possible. Abscess of the brain is usually secondary to neighboring infectious lesions such as suppurative mastoiditis and frontal sinusitis, but may be metastatic particularly from various infections of the lung and pleural cavities. Foreign bodies imbedded in the brain as a result of trauma may result in the development of an abscess. Largely because of the lack of lymphatics in the brain, it fails to produce the ordinary manifestations of an infection unless it ruptures into a ventricle. Symptoms may, therefore, be similar to a brain tumor, presenting pressure symptoms such as headache, dizziness and choked disk. If located in the cerebellum, ataxia and nystagmus will be produced; if in the temporal lobe, perhaps an homonymous hemianopsia. The treatment of brain abscess is surgical, usually consisting of drainage. Ordinarily it is best to make a small opening in the dura and evacuate the pus (even though this procedure must be repeated) because drainage through a large opening in the dura is apt to result in a brain fungus, which ultimately usually results in death. During recent years there is a tendency to attempt to enucleate the entire abscess if at all possible. Obviously if the abscess is enucleated without rupture, the complicating features of persistent drainage with danger of spread of the infection are avoided. Enucleation will be more feasible in small superficial abscesses with a thick wall. A summary of the various features of brain abscess may be found in the collective review by Grant (*Surg., Gynec. and Obst.,* 72:118, 1941, *Internat. Abst. Surg.*)

The clinical manifestations of brain tumors may conveniently be classified into general and focal. In the following brief description we have taken the liberty of consulting freely the monograph by Sachs.

General Manifestations of Intracranial Lesions.—Sooner or later in their development and growth, tumors and abscesses (especially the former) will produce an increase in intracranial pressure.* Until that time there may be no means of discovering their presence unless, as occasionally happens, focal signs develop. The general manifestations may be listed as follows:

1. *Headache.*—This is no doubt the most common of the symptoms of intracranial disease and may be the first to appear. As the tumor increases in size the headache increases in intensity, although there may be days when it is practically absent. It may be confined to any or all parts of the head, but the location is of no significance in the localization of the tumor. Neither is the type of headache different from that encountered in the numerous other diseases producing them.

2. *Vomiting.*—After the increase in the intracranial pressure become significant, vomiting becomes a prominent symptom. The vomiting may be projectile, but more characteristic is the fact that it may occur with little or no nausea.

3. *Choked Disk (Papilledema).*—Only on rare occasions does a brain tumor fail to produce a choked disk, especially if the increased intracranial pressure has been present for some time. The "choking" of the disk (papilla) is presumably due to obstruction of the veins of the disk, created by the increased intracranial pressure. Hemorrhage and exudate in the retina is also present and is more important in determining the age of the process than is the amount (number of diopters) of swelling.

4. *Convulsions (General).*—Although the cause of generalized convulsions (clonic, without aura) is not clear, they are frequently observed and are presumably of irritative origin. They appear to arise in the cortex and are especially common when the tumor involves the cerebral cortex.

---

* The relation of trauma to the symptoms and signs of increased intracranial pressure has already been discussed. Ordinarily, however, trauma produces increased pressure so much more rapidly that the clinical manifestations are quite different.

5. *Mental Dullness.*—As the intracranial pressure increases there is a tendency for the patient to become mentally dull. Cerebration is slow, and at times the patient may become so stuporous as to be aroused with difficulty. It is not uncommon, however, for a normal sensorium to be retained even in the presence of marked increase in intracranial pressure. Lesions in the temporal lobe are more apt to be associated with mental dullness than lesions in other areas. It is usually possible to differentiate the type of mental dullness caused by diffuse pressure, from that

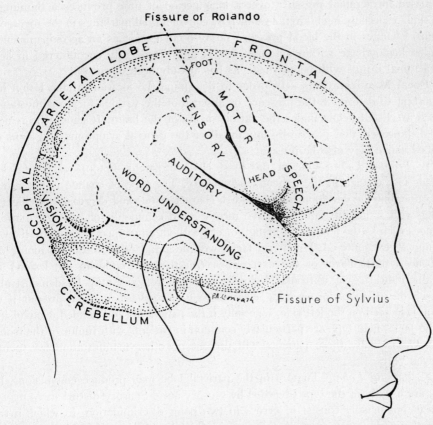

Fissure of Rolando

Fig. 358.—Diagram of the Brain to Show its Anatomical Divisions and a Gross Localization of Some of the Important Centers.

produced by a focal lesion, by noting changes induced after the administration of hypertonic fluids, since in the latter instance the dullness is usually not relieved.

6. *Slow Pulse.*—Slowing of the pulse rate (presumably of medullary origin) is frequently observed, but is much more common in brain abscess than tumor. The rate may be as slow as 45 beats per minute.

7. *Unconsciousness.*—A pronounced increase in intracranial pressure may lead to unconsciousness and may progress to deep coma. If it appears suddenly the possibility of hemorrhage (into the tumor) should be considered; however this is of infrequent occurrence. More commonly ventricular obstruction is the cause of the unconscious state.

8. *Miscellaneous Manifestations.*—Vertigo and dizziness are frequently produced by an increased intracranial pressure, but on many occasions are focal signs, *i.e.,* produced by lesions involving the eighth nerve, which supplies the semicircular canals. Yawning and sighing respirations are evidences of medullary compression and therefore are usually serious symptoms. Respiratory difficulty of various types may be observed (including cessation) and is usually caused by pressure of the cerebellar tonsils against the medulla in the foramen magnum. The presence of increased intracranial pressure over a long period of time produces a thinning of the skull, especially in children as shown by convolutional markings in the roentgenograms. Changes in the blood pressure rarely occur except as an accompaniment of sudden hemorrhage within a tumor, but is more frequently encountered in acute intracranial injury with hemorrhage, as has already been discussed.

Focal Manifestations.—In order to determine the location of the lesion it is important to determine the presence or absence of the various focal manifestations which are listed below under the various areas of the brain. It should be remembered, however, that practically any or all of the general symptoms and signs described above may also be present.

1. *Frontal Lobe.*—One of the most characteristic symptoms of frontal lobe lesions is a change in the patient's personality. The type of change is not always the same, but the development of childish characteristics and decreased intelligence, along with irritability and defective memory are commonly observed. Emotional changes such as the tendency to laugh or cry without ample provocation are likewise commonly encountered. Unilateral facial weakness and other muscular motor disturbances, particularly of the extremities (on the side opposite the lesion) are usually indicative of a frontal lesion. Pathologic reflexes may be demonstrable. Speech disturbances, progressing even to complete aphasia may be present if the lesion is located on the left side, especially if the patient is right handed. Convulsions of the Jacksonian type are particularly common in patients with tumor of the frontal lobe. Occasionally these patients will present no other manifestation for months or even years.

2. *Parietal Lobe.*—Tumors in the parietal lobe may produce convulsions, but they are usually of the type preceded by sensory aura. Sensory disturbances may be present but usually consist of errors in two point discrimination, in which a true hypesthesia does not exist. Astereognosis (inability to identify objects placed in the hand) is occasionally demonstrable. Pathologic reflexes as well as motor and sensory disturbances may be present. Occasionally, aphasia of varied types will be present, but usually only when the tumor is located low down near the fissure of Sylvius.

3. *Temporal Lobe.*—Lesions in the temporal lobe commonly produce a characteristic defect in the visual field, consisting of varying degrees of homonymous hemianopsia. For example a patient with a left sided temporal lobe tumor would have blindness on the left side of each retina; this is called a right homonymous hemianopsia because the patient is unable to see objects on his right. Disturbances in smell such as inability to detect odors, and the presence of the sensation of a disagreeable odor, are commonly found. A characteristic symptom is the "dreamy state" which has been described in detail by Kennedy.[14]

4. *Occipital Lobe.*—Lesions in the occipital lobe commonly produce homonymous hemianopsia which usually does not extend to the center of vision. Visual aura (usually color) are not uncommon and are frequently followed by focal convulsions. Frequently the symptoms and signs produced by occipital lesions simulate those located in the cerebellum.

5. *Cerebellum.*—Ataxia is one of the most characteristic features of cerebellar lesions. When the patient walks there is usually a tendency to fall toward the side of the lesion. Adiadokocinesis (inability to rapidly pronate and supinate the hand) is likewise usually present. Nystagmus is commonly observed. Occasionally the attitude of the head may be characteristic, *i.e.,* flexed toward the side of the lesion with slight rotation so that the chin is pointed to the opposite side. The general symptoms and signs of increased intracranial pressure are usually present to a marked degree when cerebellar lesions are present, because of the obstructive hydrocephalus which is produced.

Diagnostic Tests.—These may be extremely helpful in making a diagnosis of various lesions affecting the brain or spinal cord. Of the various procedures *spinal puncture* is perhaps most often used. This is performed by having the patient lie in a right recumbent position, and inserting a needle into the spinal canal usually through the third and fourth interspace. Not more than 10 or 15 cc. should be taken for study. It may be used therapeutically for a few lesions as described but must be employed with caution. If a pressure reading is desired, a needle with a two-way stopcock attached to a manometer must be used. The normal pressure is 60 to 180 millimeters of water.

An effective method of detecting a block in the subarachnoid space is the *Queckenstedt test,* which consists of observations of the pressure while the cervical veins are compressed. If no obstruction is present the pressure should rise to 150 to 300 millimeters (of water) and return shortly to normal after release. A combined cistern and lumbar puncture will be more effective in discovering a partial block. The cistern puncture is performed by inserting the needle cautiously through the skin about 2 centimeters above the spine of the axis with the neck moderately flexed. The needle should take a direction toward the glabella. Any difference in pressure between the fluid in the lumbar region and cisterna, when the patient is horizontal, is suggestive of a subarachnoidal obstruction. Spinal fluid may be examined in numerous ways, cell count, test for protein, determination of color and sugar content, Kahn test, etc. The x-ray may be of extreme value in determining the presence of lesions in the vertebrae.

Injection of lipiodol into the subarachnoid space and observation by the x-ray, of its movement, looking for filling defects, may be helpful in detecting tumors, etc., but the lipiodol results in so much irritation locally that many neurosurgeons are reluctant to use it without clear indications. However, the procedure will detect spinal cord tumors and dislocated intervertebral disks quite accurately.

Encephalograms are performed by injecting a gas (*e.g.,* air, oxygen or ethylene) through a lumbar puncture needle with the patient in a sitting position. In this way the subarachnoid space is filled with air, and obstructions may be noted by the x-ray. The ventricles may not be well filled. It is a dangerous procedure to employ when increased intracranial pressure with choked disks is present.

Ventriculograms, made by injecting air or oxygen (preferably the latter) into the ventricles, through trephine openings, gives a much more accurate outline of the ventricles by means of the x-ray than that obtained by an encephalogram. It is therefore a very valuable aid in the localization of intracranial tumors. However, the procedure is not without danger (fatalities being sustained in the best of hands) and therefore must not be used indiscriminately.

SPINAL CORD

Trauma to the spinal cord is of the greatest importance surgically. Next come the neoplasms, and lastly are the infections which are largely of medical interest. Congenital lesions such as spina bifida have already been mentioned (see page

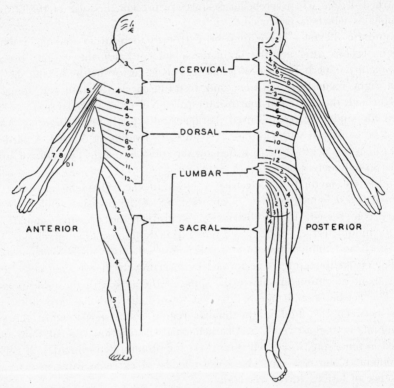

Fig. 359.—The Anterior and Posterior Segmental Sensory Distribution of the Cervical, Dorsal (Thoracic), Lumbar and Sacral Nerves.

Note that the sacral nerves supply chiefly the posterior perineum and the medial and posterior surface of the thigh; this distribution of paralysis constitutes what is called "saddle anesthesia."

346). Detailed discussion of these diseases may be found in publications by Elsberg [15] and Frazier and Allen.[16]

1. *Injury to the spinal cord* may be caused by penetrating wounds, or by fracture or dislocation of the vertebrae. Evidence of serious cord injury in such cases is based on the presence of flaccid paralysis and anesthesia. Complete severance

is rare; total paralysis is therefore usually produced by a crushing injury of serious type which may be hopeless as far as recovery of function is concerned. Partial paralysis is usually associated with considerable hemorrhage or edema. By review-

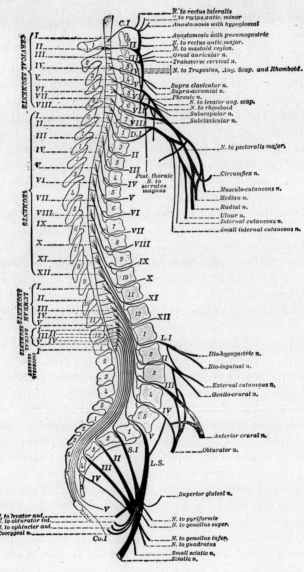

FIG. 360.—RELATION OF THE SEGMENTS OF THE SPINAL CORD AND THEIR NERVE ROOTS TO THE BODIES OF THE VERTEBRAE. (After Frazier and Allen.)

ing the history of the accident and mechanism of trauma, it may be possible to obtain valuable data as to the actual type of damage inflicted upon the cord. For example, a fracture of a cervical vertebra sustained by striking the head on the bottom of a swimming pool while diving is apt to result in serious damage to the cord. Whereas a crushing of a thoracic vertebra sustained by falling upon the buttock is not apt to result in much damage to the cord. Since the spinal nerves are distributed segmentally it is possible, by carefully mapping out the level of anesthesia, to locate accurately the level of the injury (see Fig. 360). Motor paralysis, if confined to the lower extremity, indicates a lesion below the first thoracic segment; if the arms are involved the cervical cord is damaged; if the injury is at the third cervical vertebra or above, respiratory movements will be affected and respiratory paralysis may occur. Injuries of the cord also frequently produce retention of urine or a dribbling incontinence. Injury at the 7th cervical with motor paralysis is often associated with priapism and involuntary ejaculation. In rare cases there may be a unilateral motor paralysis combined with anesthesia of the opposite side. This is called Brown-Séquard paralysis, and is due to an injury of one-half of the cord.

Less serious injuries of all degrees may occur and produce variable sensory and motor changes. After industrial accidents, when large compensation claims are at stake, serious signs and symptoms of cord injury may be apparent in the absence of an actual lesion (malingering).

The outcome of the injury also varies and depends, of course, on the seriousness of the damage to the cord. Complete severance results in immediate paralysis which is permanent because of the inability of the cord to regenerate. Hemorrhage into the spinal cord or canal may also cause immediate and complete paralysis, yet recovery is apt to occur as the blood is absorbed, though some disability usually remains. Edema, on the other hand, produces symptoms more slowly, and allows the best prognosis since it usually results in complete recovery when the inflammation subsides.

Evidence of recovery can be detected by repeated sensory and motor examinations, even as early as the first or second week. Further progress varies and may be very slow, requiring months or years to reach its maximum. Recovery may be aided by appropriate muscle stimulation and muscle reëducation. If the injury is due to complete severance and no recovery is possible, the situation may be distressing indeed. A few such patients may still lead useful lives in spite of complete paralysis. Many become helpless invalids, but succumb later to intercurrent disease. Transportation and other details of war injuries are discussed in Chapter XXXIII.

Treatment may be conservative or operative. It is imperative, however, that the patient be handled with utmost care, particularly during transportation to the hospital, because of the danger of increasing the cord damage. The decision as to operation (laminectomy) is determined to some extent by the time elapsing since injury. For example, in the acute cases operation is indicated if the symptoms of spinal cord compression are progressive, or if the symptoms are stationary and the Queckenstedt test shows a complete block. If considerable period of time has elapsed since injury the operative indications are less definite. Operative procedures are concerned with the removal of a hematoma, a foreign body, or spicule of bone pressing on the cord. Dislocations, particularly in the cervical region, must obviously be reduced and immobilized (see p. 385). In those cases in which conservative therapy is indicated nursing care is particularly important, especially because of the loss of sphincter control and the danger of skin injury and decubitus. The use of an air mattress is often of value. Opinions differ somewhat as to the care of the bladder which cannot be emptied by the patient. There is a growing tendency, however, not to let it empty by overflowing but to insert a retention catheter and empty the bladder every four or five hours, hoping to encourage automatic control. A better procedure is to set up apparatus for tidal irrigation by using 1 to 3000 potassium permanganate somewhat after the principle advised by Munro,[17] hoping to keep down infection while automatic bladder control is being established. Further discussion of the problems presented by such a "neurogenic bladder" will be found on page 1007. When the bodies of the lumbar or thoracic vertebrae are fractured, fixation in an hyperextended position is advisable either by placing the patient on a Bradford frame or in a body cast. The efficacy of spinal puncture in relieving pressure from edema or hemorrhage may be sufficient in some cases to warrant its use. Constant care of paralyzed muscles by traction and support will minimize the tendency to contracture. Other features of the care of the vertebral fracture will be found in Chapter XVIII.

2. *Tumors of the spinal cord* may be of numerous varieties including gliomas, neurofibromas, meningiomas, lipomas, dermoids, etc., the latter four of which are relatively slow growing. Gliomas, which are intramedullary tumors, are malignant but may grow slowly and are sufficiently encapsulated to be removed surgically. Most of these tumors will, in time, produce clear cut evidence of compression, and be easily detected by carefully mapping out the level of motor and sensory paralysis. Such cases offer little diagnostic difficulty when they develop rapidly. More commonly the growth is so slow that the early symptoms (particularly pain) are apt to be misleading, and the patient may be treated for various kinds of neuritis, arthritis or neuralgia, or even be considered as a neurotic. Careful examination, however, will reveal sensory changes. Motor changes which manifest themselves along with sensory changes may not produce manifestations more significant than slight lameness or stiffness, indicative of a mild spastic paralysis. Occasionally crossed paralysis of the Brown-Séquard type (frequently atypical and indefinite) may be demonstrable. Exaggerated knee jerks or ankle clonus are usually present early. Loss of sphincter control comes late. Important in the diagnosis, is lumbar puncture which may reveal yellow fluid (xanthochromia) or a pressure reading which does not increase on jugular compression, thus indicating a block in the spinal subarachnoid (Queckenstedt test). X-ray following air or lipiodal injection may be diagnostic, although the latter is considered irritating by some. Confusing, however, are certain inflammatory lesions (arachnoiditis, etc.) which may simulate tumor.

Treatment is entirely surgical, *i.e.,* laminectomy to expose and remove the tumor.

3. *Protrusion of an Intervertebral Disk* (*Nucleus Pulposus*) has been shown during recent years to be responsible in many instances for pain in the lumbar region, and pain extending down along the course of the sciatic nerve (sciatica). Protrusion of the disk into the spinal canal with consequent pressure of the nerve trunks is the mechanism most responsible for the symptoms. Naffziger and associates[18] have emphasized the fact that localizing thickening of the ligamentum flavum may likewise produce pressure with consequent symptoms. The disks in the lumbar region (particularly the one between the third and fourth lumbar vertebrae) are the most commonly involved, largely because they are thicker in this region. The anterior convexity of the vertebrae at this point likewise would be important

in the production of the dislocation of the disk at this point. Trauma commonly is an initial cause (see also Chapter XXXIII for dislocation in military life); Naffziger and associates emphasize that lifting imposes comparatively a greatly increased amount of pressure upon the intervertebral disks because of the leverage action, thereby encouraging damage and protrusion. Other points in mechanism of the production of the lesion are discussed in detail by them. As stated, the pain is apt to be located over the distribution of the site of the sciatic nerve, being mild at first and becoming more intense as time passes. It may be located in the lumbosacral region, and even in the hip joint. Pain is apt to occur in attacks, but is not completely absent in the intervals. A spinal nerve may be compressed by either the ligamentum flavum or the intervertebral disk or both. The degree of protrusion may be significantly influenced by flexion and hyperextension of the spine. It may be difficult to differentiate the condition from a tumor of the spinal cord. Lumbar puncture together with the Queckenstedt test will be of assistance in differentiating. Cell count, and other spinal fluid findings which are relatively normal in nucleus pulposus will eliminate the chronic forms of meningitis. The spinal fluid in the presence of a protruding disk frequently has an excessive amount of protein in it. It must be stated, however, that this disease is not the only cause of sciatic pain. The injection of air or lipiodol for diagnostic purposes should be avoided, if possible; the latter is irritating to the nerve roots. The clinical picture is so well understood that such procedures are practically never necessary (Dandy [61]).

The treatment of protrusion of a disk is chiefly surgical. Very little relief of a permanent nature can be obtained without removal of the disk, which occasionally lies fairly loose in the spinal canal. Dandy calls attention to the danger of overlooking a "concealed" disk which does not protrude. If an injured disk cannot be found, thickened areas of ligamentum flavum should be removed if present. The operation itself is not disabling since neurosurgeons are now finding it necessary to remove only a small portion of one lamina (occasionally no bone) to obtain exposure.

4. *Infections of the spinal cord and meninges* are largely of medical interest, *i.e.*, spinal meningitis and the various types of myelitis. Multiple sclerosis of various kinds present problems only when they simulate tumor. Infection following penetrating wounds presents the usual signs of meningitis; fever, leukocytosis, muscular rigidity, hyperactive reflexes, etc. Frequent or continuous drainage of spinal fluid by laminectomy or lumbar puncture may reduce somewhat the high mortality in types of pyogenic meningitis not responding to serum therapy. Drainage by spinal puncture cannot be used in pneumococcus meningitis because of the thickness of the pus. Sulfonamide compounds should be utilized early in the disease and in large doses; sera will be indicated in the presence of such organisms as the meningococcus and pneumococcus. Tuberculosis of the spine (Pott's disease), whether in the lumbar, thoracic or cervical region, occasionally forms a cold abscess which may compress the cord and produces characteristic neurological manifestations.

5. *Operative Procedures for the Relief of Pain.*—Severe intractable pain, particularly in the lower extremities, as produced by malignant tumors, etc., may be eliminated by operative procedures. Spiller and Martin [19] initiated chordotomy, *i.e.*, cutting the spinothalamic tracts. The operation is usually performed in the upper thoracic region but may be done at a higher level. Another procedure for the relief

of pain, namely, section or crushing of the posterior roots, is available but not very satisfactory. Intraspinal injection of 5 to 8 minims of absolute alcohol is of recent years more popular but has not been found to be very satisfactory. Injection of more than 14 to 16 minims may lead to motor paralysis. Details of the method are obtainable in a publication by Adson.[20]

THE AUTONOMIC NERVOUS SYSTEM

The nerve cells and fibers comprising the autonomic nervous system are concerned in general with the control and regulation of the so-called involuntary or automatic functions of the body such as the heart activity, intestinal movements, respiration, glandular secretion, vasomotor caliber, sweating, etc. It should be emphasized, however, that many of these involuntary functions (particularly digestive and endocrine) are also influenced by hormones of various types. Of great importance is the fact that in its control of important and vital visceral functions, the autonomic system is greatly influenced through the emotional states and through the stresses and strains to which the individual is exposed in his work and play (Cannon [21]). This influence is not only able to produce abnormal function with its resultant symptoms, but is probably able to initiate definite organic visceral and peripheral disease which are of great surgical interest and importance. Of great clinical importance, too, is the fact that the autonomic nerves carry impulses of visceral pain, which is discussed later in this chapter, and can frequently be abolished by severing the appropriate fibers. Though the autonomic system is a complex ramification of nerve cells and fibers, there are certain general anatomic features which are simple. One may identify three elements in the autonomic system aside from their central sources in the brain and cord; (1) fibers (preganglionic) which connect these centers with (2) ganglion cells outside the central nervous system (see Fig. 361) and (3) fibers (postganglionic) which connect these ganglion cells with the end organs. The arrangements and pathways of these three elements or components are complicated and have been under especially intensive investigation during recent years. The autonomic system is usually divided into two groups: (a) the sympathetic or abdomino-thoracic-cervical chain, and (b) the parasympathetic or craniosacral group. These two divisions have a different segmental origin and have antagonistic functions as will be mentioned below. (It should be noted that the word sympathetic is often loosely used as an all-inclusive term synonymous with autonomic. It is used in this chapter to designate only one part of the system as opposed to its complementary part, the parasympathetic.)

Because of the antagonistic character of the functions of the two systems (sympathetic and parasympathetic) it is obvious that a clear conception of the disease processes associated with these systems is dependent upon an accurate anatomic discrimination between the two. The fibers of the two systems may be identified separately at the points of origin, but distal to the prevertebral ganglia (celiac, pulmonic, etc.) this is impossible.

The *sympathetic chain* is so-called because its ganglion cells are arranged in a chain on each side of the vertebral bodies in the form of tiny ganglia which are called paravertebral ganglia. In general, the fibers entering the ganglia are called preganglionic or white rami communicantes, and those leaving are called post-ganglionic or gray rami. In the neck there are three pairs of ganglia: the superior, middle, and inferior cervical, and in the thorax, twelve, one for each segment.

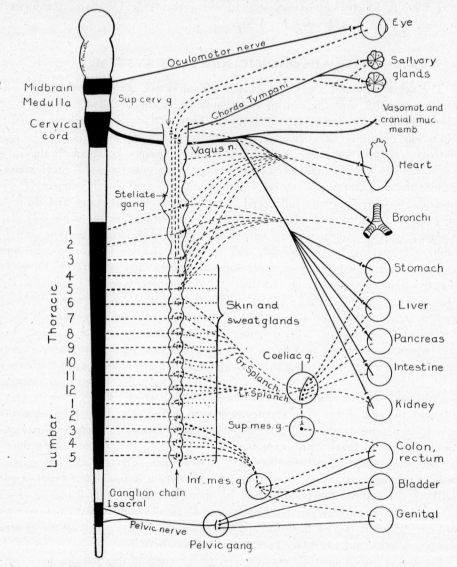

FIG. 361.—SCHEMATIC DRAWING ILLUSTRATING THE COMPONENTS OF THE AUTONOMIC NERVOUS SYSTEM.

The solid black lines indicate the craniosacral or parasympathetic nerves, whereas the broken lines indicate the thoracolumbar or sympathetic nerves. (Modified from Kuntz, *Autonomic Nervous System,* Lea and Febiger, 1929, p. 24.)

Occasionally the inferior cervical and the first thoracic ganglia are united into one, which is known as the stellate ganglion. In the lumbar region the number of ganglia on each side is variable, but usually four.

The sympathetic fibers supply the various viscera *via* special nerves and plexuses. The innervation of the heart (sensory as well as motor) is derived from the cardiac plexus which receives the superior, middle and inferior cardiac nerves (from the superior, middle and inferior cervical ganglia respectively) and also thoracic cardiac nerves from the first to the fifth thoracic ganglia. In addition to these fibers the cardiac plexus receives branches from both vagi (parasympathetic). The celiac (solar) plexus, which surrounds the celiac artery and overlies the aorta at this point, is the most extensive of the prevertebral plexuses. It is supplied primarily by the greater splanchnic nerve which is formed by the union of fibers from the fifth to the ninth or tenth thoracic ganglia. However, the celiac ganglion also receives parasympathetic fibers (from the vagus). There are a series of small plexuses including the aortic, ureteral, hypogastric, iliac, etc., which are for the most part extensions of the celiac plexus lying in approximation with the aorta. The abdominal organs are innervated by this series of plexuses, but also receive parasympathetic fibers from the vagi, some of which enter the plexuses and some of which do not.

The sympathetic fibers going to the periphery (skin, muscle, blood vessels, sweat glands, etc.) are distributed largely through somatic nerves, *i.e.,* the peripheral (spinal or cranial) nerves which carry voluntary motor and ordinary sensory impulses as well. The sweat glands (supplied only by the sympathetics) comprise one of the few organs which definitely do not appear to have also a parasympathetic innervation.

The *parasympathetic* system, which consists primarily of the craniosacral portion of the autonomic system, innervates, by means of the vagus and pelvic nerves, practically all the thoracic and abdominal organs which likewise have a sympathetic innervation. As mentioned in the preceding paragraph, the thoracic and upper abdominal organs receive their parasympathetic innervation by the vagus nerve which supplies fibers either directly, or by traversing the prevertebral ganglia. Shortly after piercing the diaphragm the vagus nerves divide into three main divisions: left, middle and right. The left and middle branches of the left vagus innervate the fundus and pyloric region of the stomach, respectively, and the right branch passes to the liver. The left and middle branches of the right vagus go to the stomach, but the right enters the celiac ganglion (Kuntz [22]). Within the wall of the digestive tube are two systems of plexuses (the submucous or Meissner's and the myenteric or Auerbach's) which are associated with peristalsis and glandular secretion. The nerves supplying these plexuses are preganglionic, arising from the vagus and sacral nerves. The pulmonary plexus which distributes fibers to the lungs (particularly the bronchi) is really continuous with the cardiac plexus, but consists primarily of vagus fibers. The pelvic nerve arising from the sacral nerves is distributed to the distal part of the colon, the bladder, and perhaps to parts of the genital system.

Functions of the Autonomic System.—These are manifold and for the most part motor (efferent), but also include sensory (afferent) impulses which are important in initiating reflex activity and the sensation of visceral pain which, as mentioned previously, is frequently referred to skin areas. Motor function is of two kinds, excitatory and inhibitory. A functional or physiological balance between these two activities is maintained by the opposing innervation of the sympathetic and parasympathetic systems, with one or two exceptions (*e.g.*, the sweat glands).

TABLE 8

The Balanced Motor Function of the Autonomic System

Organ	Sympathetic	Parasympathetic
Heart (rate)	Acceleration	Slowing
Intestines { peristalsis / secretion	Inhibits	Stimulates
Anal Sphincter	Contracts	Relaxes
Urinary bladder { wall / sphincter	Relaxes / Contracts	Contracts / Relaxes
Eye { pupil / lid slit	Dilates / Widens	Constricts / Narrows
Arteries	Constricts	Dilates (?)
Sweat glands	Stimulates	———
Bronchi	Dilates	Constricts

Motor Functions.—The motor functions of the *sympathetic system* as contrasted to the parasympathetic system comprise acceleration of the heart rate, arterial constriction, inhibition of intestinal peristalsis and secretion, contraction of the bladder and anal sphincters, etc. (see Table 8). There is considerable evidence that sympa-

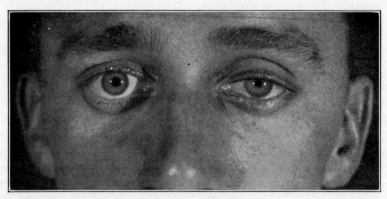

Fig. 362.—Horner's Syndrome (Left Eye) Produced by Gunshot Wound Injuring the Left Cervical Sympathetic Chain.

The two important signs of Horner's syndrome, namely, constricted pupil and drooping of the upper eyelid, were present in this patient. Narrowing of the lid slit in Horner's Syndrome leads to the false impression that an enophthalmos is present.

thetic stimulation through excitation of the adrenals causes contraction of the spleen with consequent outpouring of blood. It is likewise responsible for the outpouring of adrenalin which occurs during excitement. Adrenalin has in general an action similar to that of the sympathetic nerves, *i.e.*, it is responsible for liberation of glucose from the liver, for increases in the heart rate, and inhibition of digestive secretion. The sympathetic system is important in the maintenance of vital processes of the cells of skeletal as well as smooth muscle, and has a definite effect on muscle metabolism (Kuntz [22]). Cannon [21] has emphasized the fact that the bodily functions which are stimulated by the sympathetics are those necessary for the efficient mobilization of forces and energy, which are required in times of stress (mental as well as muscular, but especially the latter). Important also in this way are the emotional states, such as fear, rage, etc.

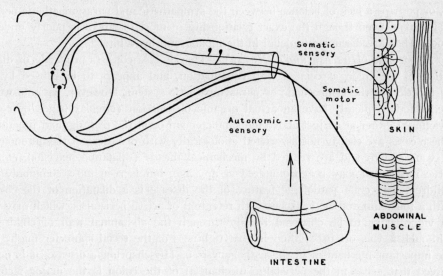

FIG. 363.—THE NERVE PATHWAYS PRODUCING REFERRED PAIN AND INVOLUTIONARY MUSCLE SPASM.

The impulse originates in the intestine or other viscus and travels along the autonomic sensory fibers (indicated by the arrow) to the central nervous system. Here it reaches ganglion cells which normally are excited by impulses reaching them over somatic pathways entering the central nervous system at the same level. The pain is experienced as coming from the region supplied by these somatic fibers. The activation of these central sensory cells provokes reflex muscular contraction by way of the somatic motor nerves; this reaction is called involuntary muscle spasm.

The motor functions of the *parasympathetic system* include such activities as slowing of the heart rate, excitation of the digestive glands, intestinal peristalsis, contraction of the bladder and rectum along with relaxation of their sphincters, etc. (see Table 8).

Sensory Function.—Although of less physiologic significance than the motor, the sensory function of the autonomic nervous system is nevertheless important. For example, the integrity of many reflex arcs is dependent upon sensory stimulation. Moreover, visceral pain, especially that of cardiac origin, is obviously dependent upon afferent autonomic fibers for transmission and may be eradicated by severance of these fibers. Visceral pain as transmitted by autonomic fibers, may be intense but is poorly localized; because of this fact it is often referred to parts of the body other than its site of origin (see Fig. 363). In addition to visceral pain, the sensory autonomic fibers may carry impulses which reach consciousness and are perceived as discomfort, or fullness, etc.: in many hypersensitive individuals impulses due to normal peristalsis are perceived. The various types of visceral sensation are important in the diagnosis of abdominal disorders, particularly those of non-organic or functional nature.

Additional data on the anatomy and physiology of the autonomic system may be found in the books by Larsell,[23] Kuntz [22] and Ransom.[24]

Disorders of the Autonomic Nervous System.—There are a number of diseases whose pathogenesis is associated, at least to a great extent, with dysfunction of, or perhaps a lack of balance between the sympathetic and parasympathetic nervous system, even though the exact relationship in most instances is poorly understood. They are discussed in detail in the monograph by White.[25]

Megacolon (Hirschsprung's Disease).—This disease consists primarily of dilatation of the colon associated with constipation, and appears to be caused by a dysfunction of the sympathetic or parasympathetic system. However, patients with megacolon frequently have an actual organic obstruction (circular bands or constrictions) either at or just above the sphincter ani or at the rectosigmoid junction. These cases are clearly not associated etiologically with disorders of the autonomic nervous system and are treated by mechanical means (dilatation, excision, etc.). True megacolon may be encountered at any age, but is seen most commonly in children. The chief pathologic feature of the disease is a dilatation of the colon with a thickening of the wall, but with retention of active peristalsis, which may be so vigorous as to be observed readily through the abdominal wall of children. Although it was originally thought that tightness of the rectal sphincter might be the important mechanism in the pathogenesis of Hirschsprung's disease, it is now agreed that error in the peristaltic mechanism of the colon is the major factor. Learmonth and Markowitz [26] have shown that sympathetic nerves relax the musculature of the rectum and lower portion of the colon, and that the parasympathetics increase the tonus and peristaltic mechanism. This appears to prove the supposition that the disease is caused by an error in the peristaltic mechanism, particularly in view of the fact that Adamson and Aird [27] were able to produce the disease in cats by excision of the parasympathetic sacral rami. Whether the disease is produced purely by relaxation of the wall of the rectum and lower colon alone, or whether there is an additional error in type of peristalsis, cannot yet be definitely proved. The fact that dilatation of the sphincter improves the condition markedly in some cases does not disprove the points mentioned above, particularly since the beneficial effect is probably reflex in origin. Histologically, Cameron [28] has reported replacement of the ganglion cells of Auerbach's plexus by inflammatory cells at the pelvirectal flexure in two fatal cases of Hirschsprung's disease.

The patient may have few symptoms in spite of the fact that the dilatation may be enormous and affect the entire colon. Constipation is, of course, universally present except that occasionally there are periods when bowel movements are relatively normal in frequency. Very little pain is experienced in spite of the fact that peristalsis may be very vigorous indeed. The amount of abdominal distention varies with the dilatation and distention of the colon. Symptoms including headache, nausea and vomiting occur occasionally, but are rare.

Therapy has undergone drastic changes in this disease during recent years. One or two decades ago colectomy was performed frequently. In 1927 Wade and

Royle [29] recommended lumbar sympathectomy for megacolon. Morton and Scott [30] introduced the use of the spinal anesthetic as a therapeutic test in determining the probable effect of sympathectomy. If a copious bowel movement with decrease in the size of the colon is obtained within a few minutes following the spinal anesthetic, they expect favorable results from a sympathectomy on that patient.

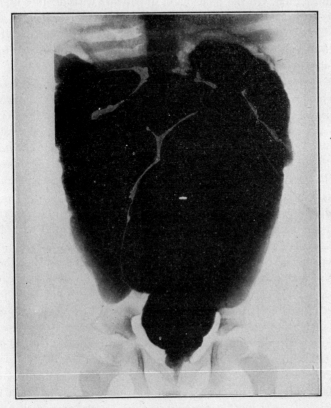

FIG. 364.—HIRSCHSPRUNG'S DISEASE.

The redundant, extremely dilated colon is clearly shown by the roentgenogram which was taken after a barium enema.

Operation is fairly effective and should consist of removal of the inferior mesenteric and presacral (superior hypogastric) plexuses (Rankin and Learmonth).[31] In male patients it is preferable to utilize resection of the lumbar chain, since resection of the presacral plexus results in a loss ejaculation (White [25]). Dilatation of the anal sphincter may be very helpful, especially in mild cases; dilatation must be more than momentary and is best performed under a general anesthesia. Hurst [32] has made the suggestion, and a logical one, of inserting a conical bougie into the rectum every day and retaining it in position for one-half hour. This procedure may prove to be important because of its simplicity.

Vascular Disease of the Extremities.—These diseases have already been discussed in Chapter XX. In Raynaud's disease particularly, it is assumed that vasoconstriction of the smaller vessels produced presumably by overstimulation of the sympathetic system, is an important factor in the pathogenesis of the disease. It is thought by some that the fault is a local one in the vessels themselves (Lewis [33]) in that patients suffering from Raynaud's disease have been found to be unusually sensitive to adrenalin (Heinbecker and Bishop [34] and others). It should be emphasized, however, that in many instances organic obstruction of the vessels also exists as a late manifestation. On the other hand in patients with definite organic changes in the vessels such as Buerger's disease vascular spasm often plays an important role. In so far as vasoconstriction is present in some patients with obliterative vascular disease, a disorder of the autonomic system is assumed also to be present. The various diagnostic methods have been discussed in Chapter XX.

Carotid Sinus (Body) Syndrome.—The carotid sinus which exerts a regulatory effect on the blood pressure and heart rate, has nervous connections with the vagus nerve and cervical sympathetic; it may become hypersensitive and give rise to symptoms (Heymans and associates [35]). Manifestations consisting of weakness, dizziness, fall in blood pressure, and unconsciousness with or without convulsions, occur in attacks. Pressure over the bifurcation of the carotid may reproduce an attack. Excision of the periarterial tissue at the carotid bifurcation may be curative. Details of the syndrome are described by Weiss and associates.[36]

Tumors of the carotid body are comparatively rare, but are important because most of them are malignant or potentially so, yet are associated with a good prognosis when completely removed. Most of them produce no symptoms other than gradual growth of the tumor; fainting is rare. Complete removal of the tumor will require ligation and excision of the carotid artery in about half the cases. Since ligation of the common carotid is associated with hemiplegia and death in the majority of patients (particularly in the older group), it will be necessary to compress the vessel for an increasing length of time every day preoperatively for a period of time so as to encourage the development of collaterals in the brain. Details of the condition may be found in an article by Harrington and associates [62].

Neurocirculatory Asthenia.—The etiology of this condition cannot definitely be ascribed to the sympathetic nervous system, but the symptoms support the relationship. The disease is seen most commonly in thin, poorly nourished women except that a similar condition (effort syndrome) is encountered in soldiers. The complaints consist of weakness, nervousness, irritability, palpitation, diffuse pains, and even syncope. Excessive sweating, particularly in the palms of the hands, is almost constant. The hands are cold and blotchy blue. The heart rate is fast and accelerates rapidly with exercise, but decreases to its original level quite slowly. The basal metabolic rate may be slightly elevated. Considerable difficulty is encountered in differentiating the disease from hyperthyroidism, pulmonary tuberculosis, etc.

Miscellaneous Disorders.—It is possible that many of the disorders of intestinal peristalsis, including especially *spastic colon,* as discussed in Chapter XXIV, are due to an imbalance of the sympathetic and parasympathetic innervation, resulting, perhaps, in a defective peristaltic mechanism.

There is a strong probability that derangements of the sympathetic nervous system are frequently responsible for the pain in many of the cases of so-called *chronic appendicitis.* The reports referable to this possibility are presumably based on the histologic studies of Masson [37] who described staining methods revealing microscopic changes in the sympathetic fibers of the appendix, lesions which are visible but not clearly delineated in ordinary sections. Thus Hosoi [38] reported 195 instances of appendicular neuromas in 344 consecutive appendices removed at operation showing no gross or microscopic acute inflammation. All except 3 or 4·per cent had at least a moderate amount of abdominal pain.

Scleroderma, a rare disease, is assumed by many to be due to a derangement of the sympathetic nerve supply to the skin. Manifestations consist of the deposition of a dense fibrous layer beneath the skin, associated with a sclerosis of the smaller arteries. The skin may become pigmented, the extremities cyanotic and the face mask-like. Edema is usually present, but is not of the pitting type. The outcome is frequently fatal, but sympathetic neurectomy has been advised for certain types of the disease.

Operative Procedures Upon the Autonomic System.—Perhaps the earliest significant operation upon the autonomic nervous system was performed by Jaboulay [39] who resected the cervical sympathetic chain and ganglia for exophthalmic goiter. This procedure has, of course, been supplanted by partial operative removal of the thyroid gland and medical treatment. Several years later Royle [40] introduced the operative procedure of lumbar sympathectomy in spastic paralyses of the lower extremities. The efficacy of this procedure is doubtful. A short time later Wade and Royle [29] applied this operative procedure to *Hirschsprung's disease.* Additional reports indicate successful results in a large percentage of cases. It should be remembered, however, that in this disease the presacral nerve or plexus should also be removed. Leriche [41] has recommended various types of sympathectomy for *scleroderma,* asthma and a type of polyarthritis with vascular deficiency to the extremities. Sufficient reports are not available to determine the efficacy of the operation in these diseases. Lumbar sympathectomy combined with excision of the presacral plexus has been used successfully by Learmonth [42] in the treatment of various types of *pelvic pain,* especially those of uterine, tubal and ovarian origin. Section of the appropriate sympathetic nerves has been successfully performed for *localized hyperhidrosis.* Sympathectomy is fairly efficient in relieving the shortening, atrophy and cold skin of a limb paralyzed by *poliomyelitis.* Presacral neurectomy is sometimes performed for *spasm of the neck of the bladder* in "cord bladders" (Learmonth [42]).

Periarterial sympathectomy was popularized by Leriche in the treatment of spastic vascular disease of the extremities, but cannot be considered logical since the nerves supplying the vessels enter at numerous points and do not traverse the entire length of the artery. On the other hand sympathectomy (*i.e.,* removal of ganglion or preganglionic fibers) is becoming popular. The better results which are being obtained are produced by a more accurate choice of patient for operation and improvements in operative principles. Naturally, since sympathectomy results primarily in vascular dilatation with elimination of vascular spasm, one of the diseases most readily amenable should be Raynaud's disease. Results support this prediction; many cases of Buerger's disease in which diagnostic tests (see p. 505) reveal a strong element of spasm along with the organic obstruction, are also improved markedly by sympathectomy. In the upper extremity, the modifications as recommended by Telford [43] (cutting the whole rami from the second and third thoracic nerves) and Smithwick [44] (removing proximal segments of the second and third thoracic nerves), are equally effective, as long as the sympathetic trunk below the third thoracic ganglion is sectioned. These modifications which do not include removal of the ganglia, avoid Horner's syndrome. White [45] and de Takats [46] have corroborated the successful results obtained by this type of operation, *i.e.*, preganglionic section instead of ganglionectomy. In the lower extremity it is now agreed that removal of the sympathetic trunk with the lumbar ganglia as performed with very little modification for the past several years, is an effective procedure.

Cervical sympathectomy for the treatment of pain of *angina pectoris* was first performed by Jonnesco,[47] but has been supplanted by the more simple method of paravertebral injection of the upper thoracic nerves (as they give off their sympathetic rami) with alcohol (Mandl [48] and Swetlow [49]). The same effect may be attained, at least to a certain extent, by total thyroidectomy, as shown a few years ago by Blumgart [50] and associates. Paravertebral injection of thoracic nerves has been used extensively by White [51] who has extended its use to the treatment of the *pain caused by aneurysms and aortitis*. The mechanism of relief of thoracic pain, particularly cardiac, obtained by paravertebral injections and other methods has been discussed in detail by White,[51] Heinbecker [52] and Davis and Pollock.[53] Learmonth [54] has discussed the operative procedures available for the relief of the various types of visceral and peripheral pain.

The use of spinal anesthesia in the determination of the probability of relief from operation (sympathectomy) in Hirschsprung's disease and spastic vascular disease of the extremities, as recommended by White, and by Morton and Scott has already been discussed.

In the surgical treatment of *essential hypertension* numerous technics have been adopted (Peet [55] and others), but the method recommended by Smithwick [56] appears to be superior to others. This operation combines sympathectomy above and below the diaphragm and concentrates on removal of as many preganglionic fibers as possible. Utilizing this procedure, most of the patients will obtain relief from symptoms if the patients are well chosen for operation (de Takats and associates [57]), and a large percentage of them will have a permanent decrease in blood pressure. In selected cases of unilateral renal disease, complicated by hypertension, nephrectomy will be effective in lowering the blood pressure. An extensive review of this subject has been made by Abeshouse [63]. However, in view of the recent report of Page and associates [58] showing a decrease in hypertension following administration of kidney extracts, it is possible that the surgical treatment of hypertension will ultimately be displaced by medical therapy.

It must be apparent from the great diversity of operative procedures noted above, that much remains unknown of the anatomy and physiology of the autonomic system. Predictable results following severance of specific fibers must depend on specific knowledge of the impulses they carry. This type of investigation will undoubtedly contribute greatly to the surgery of the sympathetics in the years to come, and extend the field of many other types of disease. The indications for operations on the autonomic nervous system have been discussed by Adson.[59]

BIBLIOGRAPHY

1. BROWN, H. A. Contused Injuries of Peripheral Nerves. The Value of Early Treatment. *California and West Med.*, 41:166, 1934.
2. MURPHY, T. Brachial Neuritis Caused by Pressure of First Rib, *Australian M. J.*, 15:582, 1910.
3. OCHSNER, A., GAGE, MIMS, and DeBAKEY, MICHAEL. Scalenus Anticus (Naffziger) Syndrome, *Am. J. Surg.*, 28:669, 1935.
4. NAFFZIGER, H. C. The Scalene Syndrome, *Surg., Gynec. & Obst.*, 64:119, 1937; NAFFZIGER, H. S., and GRANT, W. T. Neuritis of the Brachial Plexus Mechanical in Origin, *Surg., Gynec. & Obst.*, 67:722, 1938.
5. MAYO, CHARLES. Hiccup, *Surg., Gynec. & Obst.*, 55:700, 1932.
6. WEEKS, CARNES. Surgery of Phrenic Nerve in Treatment of Intractable Hiccup, *Ann. Surg.*, 93:811, 1931.
7. DANDY, W. E. Ménières Disease: its Diagnosis and Method of Treatment, *Arch. Surg.*, 16:1127, 1928.
8. NAFFZIGER, H. C., and GLASER, M. A. An Experimental Study of the Effects of Depressed Fractures of the skull, *Surg., Gynec. & Obst.*, 51:17, 1930.
9. FURLOW, L. T. Chronic Subdural Hematoma, *Arch. Surg.*, 32;688, 1936.
10. SACHS, ERNEST. *Diagnosis and Treatment of Brain Tumors,* C. V. Mosby Co., St. Louis, 1931.
11. BAILEY, P. *Intracranial Tumors,* C. Thomas Co., Springfield, Illinois.
12. PENFIELD, W. *Cytology and Cellular Pathology of the Nervous System,* Paul Hoeber, Inc., New York, 1932.
13. DAVIS. L. *The Principles of Neurological Surgery,* Lea and Febiger, Philadelphia, 2nd Ed., 1942.
14. KENNEDY, FOSTER. The Symptomatology of Tempero-sphenoidal Tumors, *Arch. Int. Med.*, 8:317, 1911.
15. ELSBERG, C. A. *Surgical Diseases of the Spinal Cord,* Paul B. Hoeber, 1941.
16. FRAZIER, C. H., and ALLEN, A. R. *Surgery of the Spine and Spinal Cord,* D. Appleton & Co., New York, 1918.
17. MUNRO, D. The Urinary Bladder in Injuries of the Spinal Cord, *Am. J. Surg.*, 38:120, 1937.
18. NAFFZIGER, H. C., INMAN, V., and SAUNDERS, J. Lesions of the Intervertebral Disk and Ligamenta Flava, *Surg., Gynec. & Obst.*, 66:288, 1938.
19. SPILLER, W. G., and MARTIN, E. The Treatment of Persistent Pain of Organic Origin in the Lower Part of the Body by Division of the Anterolateral Column of the Spinal Cord, *J. Am. M. Ass.*, 58:1489, 1912.
20. ADSON, ALFRED. The Value of, and Indications for, Intraspinal Injections of Alcohol in the Relief of Pain, *Minnesota Med.*, 20:135, 1937.
21. CANNON, W. B. *Bodily Changes in Pain, Hunger, Fear and Rage,* D. Appleton & Co., New York, 1929.
22. KUNTZ, A. *The Autonomic Nervous System,* Lea and Febiger, Philadelphia, 1934; *A Textbook of Neuro-Anatomy,* Lea and Febiger, Philadelphia, 3rd Ed., 1943.
23. LARSELL, O. *Anatomy of the Nervous System,* D. Appleton-Century Co., New York, 1942.
24. RANSON, S. W. *The Anatomy of the Nervous System,* W. B. Saunders Co., Philadelphia, 1943.
25. WHITE, J. C., and SMITHWICK, R. H. *The Autonomic Nervous System,* Macmillan, New York, 1941.
26. LEARMONTH, J. R., and MARKOWITZ, J. Studies on the Function of the Lumbar Sympathetic Outflow: I, The Relation of the Lumbar Sympathetic Outflow to the Sphincter Ani Internus, *Am. J. Physiol.*, 89:686, 1929; Studies on the Innervation of the Large Bowel: II, The Influence of the Lumbar Colonic Nerves on the Distal Part of the Colon, *Am. J. Physiol.*, 94:501, 1930.

27. ADAMSON, W. A., and AIRD, I. Megacolon: Evidence in Favor of Neurogenic Origin, *Brit. J. Surg.*, 20:220, 1932.

28. CAMERON, J. A. M. On Etiology of Hirschsprung's Disease, *Arch. Dis. Child.*, 3:210, 1928.

29. WADE, R. B., and ROYLE, N. D. Operative Treatment of Hirschsprung's Disease, *Med. J. Australia,* 1:137, 1927.

30. MORTON, J. J., and SCOTT, W. J. Studies on Activity of Lumbar Sympathetic Nervous System, *Ann. Surg.*, 92:919, 1930.

31. RANKIN, F. W., and LEARMONTH, J. R. Sympathetic Resection for Megacolon, *Ann. Surg.*, 92:710, 1930.

32. HURST, A. F. Anal Achalasia and Megacolon, *Guy's Hospital Reports,* 84:317, 1934.

33. LEWIS, T. Raynaud's Disease, *N. Eng. M. J.*, 206:1192, 1932.

34. HEINBECKER, P., and BISHOP, G. H. On Mechanism of Spastic Vascular Disease, *Proc. Soc. Exper. Biol. & M.*, 32:152, 1934.

35. HEYMANS, C., BOUCHAERT, J. J., and REGNIERS, P. *Le Sinus Carotidien et la Zone Homologue Cardio-Aortique,* Paris, G. Doin et Cie, 1933.

36. WEISS, S., CAPPS, R. B., FERRIS, E. B., and MUNRO, D. Syncope and Convulsions due to a Hyperactive Carotid Sinus Reflex, *Arch. Int. Med.*, 58:407, 1936.

37. MASSON, P. Sympathetic Neuromas of Appendicitis, *Lyon. Chir.*, 18:281, 1921. Section XXV, W. PENFIELD. *Cytology and Cellular Pathology of the Nervous System,* Paul Hoeber, New York, 1932.

38. HOSOI, KIYOSHI. Neurogenic Appendicitis, *Am. J. Surg.*, 22:428, 1933.

39. JABOULAY, M. Chirurgie du Grand Sympathetique et du Corps Thyroide: ed. by Dr. Etionne Martin, Lyon and Paris, 1900.

40. ROYLE, N. D. Treatment of Spastic Paralysis by Sympathetic Ramisection, *Surg., Gynec. & Obst.*, 39:701, 1924.

41. LERICHE, R. Surgery of Sympathetic System; Indications and Results, *Tr. Am. Surg. Ass.*, 46:150, 1928. *Ann. Surg.*, 88:449, 1928.

42. LEARMONTH, J. R. Operations on the Nerves of the Bladder, *Proc. Staff Meetings Mayo Clin.*, 5:234, 1930.

43. TELFORD, E. The Technique of Sympathectomy, *Brit. J. Surg.*, 23:445, 1935.

44. SMITHWICK, R. The Value of Sympathectomy in the Treatment of Vascular Disease, *New Eng. J. Med.*, 216:141, 1937; Surgical Intervention of the Sympathetic Nervous System for Peripheral Vascular Disease, *Arch. Surg.*, 40:286, 1940.

45. WHITE, J. Recent Developments in the Surgery of the Sympathetic Nervous System, *New England J. Med.*, 216:91, 1937.

46. DE TAKATS, GEZA. The Effect of Sympathectomy on Peripheral Vascular Disease, *Surgery,* 2:46, 1937.

47. JONNESCO, T. Angine de poitrine guerie par la résection du sympathique cervico-thoracique, *Bull. Acad. de Med.*, Paris, 84:93, 1930.

48. MANDL, F. Paravertebral Injection of an Anesthetic in Treatment of Angina Pectoris, *Arch. f. klin. Chir.*, 136:495, 1925.

49. SWETLOW, G. Paravertebral Alcohol Block in Cardiac Pain, *Am. Heart J.*, 1:393, 1926.

50. BLUMGART, H. L., LEVINE, S. A., and BERLIN, D. D. Congestive Heart Failure and Angina Pectoris, *Arch. Int. Med.*, 51:866, 1933.

51. WHITE, J. C. Painful Aneurysms of Aortic Arch; Relief by Paravertebral Injections of Procaine and Alcohol, *J. Am. M. Ass.*, 99:10, 1932; Experimental and Clinical Studies in the Surgical Treatment of Angina Pectoris, *Ann. Int. Med.*, 7:229, 1933.

—— Angina Pectoris; Treatment by Paravertebral Alcohol Injection or Operation Based on Newer Concepts of Cardiac Innervation, *Am. J. Surg.*, 9:98, 1930; Technic of Paravertebral Alcohol Injection, *Surg., Gynec. & Obst.*, 71:334, 1940.

52. HEINBECKER, P. Anatomic and Physiologic Criteria for Surgical Relief of Cardiac Pain, *J. Thor. Surg.*, 2:517, 1933.

53. DAVIS, LOYAL, and POLLOCK, L. J. The Rôle of the Autonomic Nervous System in the Production of Pain, *J. Am. M. Ass.*, 106:350, 1936.

54. LEARMONTH, J. R. Surgeon and Pain, *Brit. M. J.*, 1:47, 1935.

55. PEET, M. M. Splanchnic Section for Hypertension: Preliminary Report, *Univ. Hosp. Bull.*, Ann Arbor, 1:17, 1935; The Surgical Treatment of Hypertension, *Proc. California Acad. Med.*, 1935-36.

56. SMITHWICK, R. H. A Technique for Splanchnic Section for Hypertension, *Surgery*, 7:1, 1940.

57. DE TAKATS, G., HEYER, H. H., and KEETON, R. W. Surgical Approach to Hypertension, *J. Am. M. Ass.*, 118:501, 1942.

58. PAGE, I. H., HELMER, O. M., KOHLSTAEDT, K. G., FOUTS, P. J., and KEMPF, G. F. Reduction of Arterial Blood Pressure of Hypertensive Patients and Animals with Extracts of Kidneys, *J. Exper. Med.*, 73:7, 1941.

59. ADSON, A. W. Indications for Operation on the Sympathetic Nervous System, *J. Am. M. Ass.*, 106:360, 1936; Indications for and Value of Various Types of Sympathectomy, *The Military Surgeon*, 83:275, 1938.

60. GROFF, R. A., and GRANT, F. C. Chronic Subdural Hematoma, *Surg., Gynec. & Obst.*, Internat. Abst. Surgery, 74:9, 1942.

61. DANDY, W. E. Recent Advances in the Diagnosis and Treatment of Ruptured Intervertebral Disks, *Ann. Surg.*, 115:514, 1942.

62. HARRINGTON, S., CLAGETT, O. T., and DOCKERTY, M. B. Tumors of the Carotid Body, *Ann. Surg.*, 114:820, 1941.

63. ABESHOUSE, B. S. Hypertension and Unilateral Renal Disease, *Surgery*, 9:942, 1941; *ibid.*, 10:147, 1941.

CHAPTER XXIII

LIVER, GALLBLADDER, PANCREAS AND SPLEEN

Liver	*Pancreas*
Gallbladder	*The Spleen*
The Bile Ducts	

LIVER

Only during recent years have we appreciated the number of functions performed by the liver, and the vital importance of a great many of these physiologic processes to life. The fact that it is the largest organ in the body should offer proof of this importance. Complete removal is incompatible with life. It is quite true, however, that the liver probably has a wider margin of safety from the standpoint of the amount of tissue necessary for the performance of its functions than other organs, but this wide margin of safety is obviously necessary in times of stress, such as illness and excessive exertion. It is one of the few organs which has the power to regenerate rapidly after injury. For example, Mann and associates [1] and others have proved that after removal of 70 per cent of an animal's liver, regeneration takes place so rapidly that the normal size is regained within a few weeks following removal.

The various *functions* of the liver are summarized herewith; details may be found in a report by Mann [2]: (1) *Carbohydrate storage and metabolism,* including conversion of monosaccharides (glucose) to glycogen and *vice versa,* as demonstrated by Claude Bernard in 1857, are among the most important functions of the liver. (2) The secretion of *bile* is well known and its significance can be readily appreciated. The role of bile constituents in the splitting of fat is undisputed. (3) From the standpoint of systemic protection from toxic substances the liver is no doubt one of the most important organs because of its remarkable ability to *detoxify* various deleterious substances, particularly those of enteric origin. Bacteria which gain access to the portal system are also eradicated by the liver. (4) The role of the liver in the metabolism of *proteins and amino-acids* is complex and very inadequately understood. Notable contributions on the catabolic role of the liver, especially as the site of formation of urea, have been made by Mann and his associates.[1] On the anabolic side the liver is undoubtedly the site of formation of at least some of the plasma proteins, certainly fibrinogen, prothrombin and perhaps albumin. A brief but excellent discussion of the relation of liver to plasma protein is that of Luck.[3] (5) *Bilirubin* is made in many organs besides the liver, but it is excreted only by the liver. (6) Many inert as well as *toxic substances* coming to the liver from the intestinal tract or through the blood stream are *excreted* into the bile and thus eventually eliminated. (7) The importance of the liver in *hematopoiesis* is clearly demonstrated by the effect of liver extract on pernicious anemia. (8) There are many *miscellaneous hepatic functions,* including the formation of blood-clotting elements, such as fibrinogen and prothrombin (Andrus and associates [4]), and perhaps innumerable enzymes and hormones, most of which are as yet undiscovered. Among the other important functions may be mentioned storage of blood proteins, vitamins, and fat, the first of which is important in hemorrhage and other functional stresses; the latter two are important in nutrition.

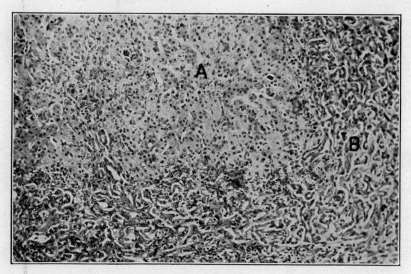

FIG. 365.—Photomicrograph (Biopsy from Operation) to Illustrate the Remarkable Regenerative Power Possessed by the Liver.

The patient had been jaundiced for several weeks because of an acute hepatitis of unknown etiology. Represented at *A* are recently regenerated cells; the portion of the section marked *B* represents a compressed mass of bile ducts and remains of necrotic hepatic cells. In the process of hepatic necrosis, the bile ducts are the last to be destroyed; the deeper staining tubular structures probably represent newly regenerated bile capillaries. It is probable that considerable fibrous tissue will be deposited in this area, *B,* and in time, the liver will present a picture like that of cirrhosis.

Because of the vital importance of the liver in the maintenance of health, numerous attempts have been made to devise tests which would reveal disease processes and identify the type of disease. Up to the present time no single completely satisfactory test has been found. This is no doubt explained for the most part by the fact that there are so many different functions performed by the liver. A few of the innumerable liver function tests devised are of definite clinical value; their diagnostic application is discussed under Jaundice.

Injury.—The liver may be injured by a crushing blow over the upper abdomen or by a penetrating wound such as a bullet, knife, etc. The lesion in the liver is usually a laceration or penetration but may at times be entirely subcapsular. Hepatic insufficiency (see p. 598) may be produced if the injury to the liver has been massive, but in most cases the symptoms are due to the escape of blood or of bile or of both. Signs of peritoneal irritation will obviously be present, *i.e.,* local tenderness, muscle spasm, nausea and vomiting. Pain may be present over the liver or may be referred to the shoulder. If there has been extensive hemorrhage there may be clinical evidence of fluid in the peritoneal cavity. More important are the manifestations of surgical shock which are seen in liver injury even when the hemorrhage has not been severe. The manifestations of intra-abdominal hemorrhage (regardless of origin) are described in more detail on page 749. Of even greater seriousness in liver injury is the possibility of a bile peritonitis which may follow if the injury has involved a large bile radical permitting bile to escape into the peritoneal cavity.

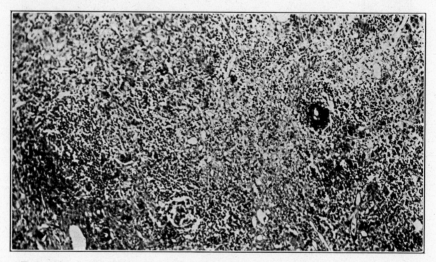

Fig. 366.—Acute Hepatitis with Necrosis, of the Inflammatory Type.

Note the extensive destruction of the hepatic cells, and the marked lymphocytic infiltration throughout the entire section; polynucleated leukocytes are also occasionally found. This type of hepatitis (*i.e.,* inflammatory) like chemical hepatitis, is serious and commonly fatal. The patient had had a cholecystogastrostomy one year previously to the present operation for jaundice of four weeks' duration due to an inflammatory tumor of the pancreas. At the second operation marked hepatitis was noted, particularly about the gallbladder. The infection in the gallbladder produced by the anastomosis presumably gave rise to the hepatitis.

Treatment demands laparotomy if there is evidence of a severe injury which is producing a continuous hemorrhage or if the various manifestations do not respond rapidly to shock therapy, especially if the physical signs do not decrease in severity. The development of shifting dullness is an important operative indication not only because it suggests continuous bleeding but also because of the possibility of bile leakage. This last possibility usually adds to the necessity for operation. Laparotomy is also indicated because of the possibility of other injuries, especially of penetrating wounds which usually produce multiple injuries, with perforation of hollow viscera. At operation hemorrhage from the liver may be controlled by suture of the laceration (aided by the use of muscle grafts) or by gauze packs which are left in place as drains and brought out through the abdominal incision.

Before operation it will usually be necessary to give the patient supportive therapy such as subcutaneous saline, intravenous glucose, transfusion, etc. In a study of 60 cases of hepatic injury, Krieg [5] noted that hemorrhage and shock were the cause of death in 73 per cent of the fatal cases. Peritonitis, due to micro-organisms or bile, may also be important factors in the lethal outcome.

Hepatitis.—The term hepatitis is an inclusive one and comprises various types of inflammations of the liver, which may be classified roughly into those produced by chemicals and by various types of infection. In many instances, however, the etiology of hepatitis, particularly the noninfectious type, is unknown.

Whether inflicted by chemicals or bacteria, the injury may be difficult to detect microscopically. Frequently, nothing more than a cloudy swelling is noted, but there is no doubt that considerable damage to the function of the cell may be sustained without revealing microscopic change. On the other hand, the damage may be so severe as to cause necrosis of the cells without producing very serious clinical mani-

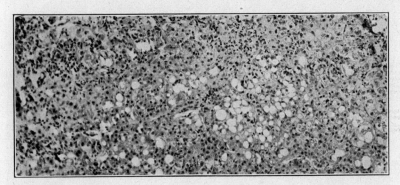

FIG. 367.—ACUTE HEPATITIS WITH NECROSIS, PROBABLY OF CHEMICAL ORIGIN.

Note the diffuse destruction of hepatic cells with mild infiltration of lymphocytes and fat. The liver was small and yellow, and of the type described as "acute yellow atrophy." The patient, a forty-year-old woman, complained of slight abdominal pain and jaundice of three weeks' duration, and had been taking a drug almost daily for many months, for arthritis. Among other ingredients the drug contained cinchophen, a chemical noted for its toxic action on the liver.

festations. This, no doubt, happens frequently, but the remarkable power of cellular regeneration in the liver replaces the damaged cells very rapidly.

Types of Hepatitis.—As already mentioned two general groups of hepatitis are recognized: (a) chemical or toxic and (b) bacterial (infectious). In a few cases however both mechanisms may play a role. It is possible also that other types of etiologic agents may be responsible in obscure cases.

(a) *Chemicals* responsible for the cellular necrosis may be of intrinsic origin. Various toxins formed in the intestinal tract during the process of digestion and absorption may reach the liver by way of the portal vein and exert direct damage on the parenchymal cells so that actual necrosis occurs. The so-called "acute yellow atrophy" may be an example of this type of cellular damage which is encountered frequently surgically because of its confusion with lesions obstructing the bile ducts. Cellular destruction of this type may also be produced by such drugs as arsenic, chloroform, atophan (cinchophen), etc.

(b) *Hepatitis due to infection* may be divided into those produced by (1) pylephlebitis (*via* portal vein), (2) cholangitis (*via* bile ducts) and (3) pericholangitis (*via* lymphatics).

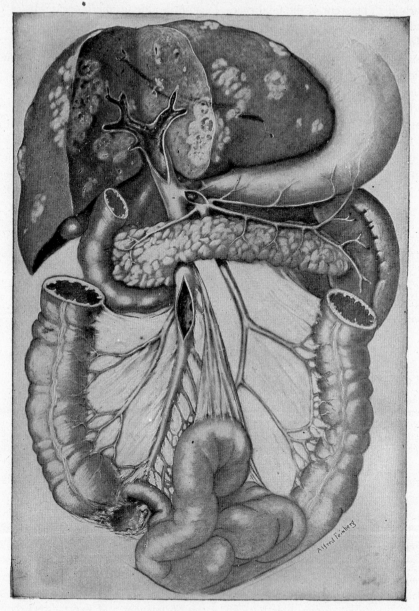

FIG. 368.—SUPPURATIVE PYLEPHLEBITIS ARISING FROM APPENDIX ABSCESS.

Numerous abscesses in the liver. (From MacCallum, *Text-book of Pathology,* 5th ed., 1932. Courtesy of W. B. Saunders Co., Philadelphia.)

1. *Pylephlebitis* or inflammation of the portal vein may arise in the vein itself or in its tributaries. Complete thrombosis of the large trunk may or may not be produced. Extension into the portal tributaries within the liver takes place readily

and produces serious symptoms of surgical significance. Such a condition appears usually as a complication of suppurative appendicitis, but may occasionally accompany cholecystitis. The symptoms of pylephlebitis involving a large portion of the portal system are difficult to differentiate from such complications as intra-abdominal suppuration of various kinds. As stated previously, if thrombosis occurs during convalescence of a patient operated on for suppurative appendicitis, the temperature which might have been receding to normal will gradually ascend along with various symptoms such as prostration, tachycardia, malaise, anorexia and occasional vomiting. Jaundice may or may not be present. Chills are common. The patient is obviously very ill and usually symptoms progress until death intervenes. There is a tendency for production of multiple small abscesses throughout the liver. These abscesses along with obstruction of the portal vein and the suppurative process

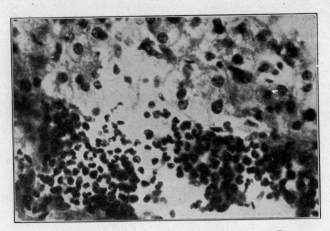

FIG. 369.—ACUTE CHOLANGITIS FROM BIOPSY TAKEN AT LAPAROTOMY.

Note the infiltration of polymorphonuclear cells: this is in the periportal area, and in reality, constitutes a miliary abscess. The patient's illness was of four weeks' duration and was manifested by high fever, jaundice and large liver with elevated diaphragm. A liver abscess was suspected and the patient operated on, but no abscess was found. For some unexplainable reason sharp improvement took place beginning a day or two following operation; the temperature dropped to normal and all symptoms subsided within a few more days.

about the original focus are, of course, ample cause for the fatal termination. Occasionally when the obstruction of the portal vein is complete there may be numerous intestinal hemorrhages secondary to the portal obstruction. The production of such symptoms is readily understandable after consideration of the effects of portal ligation in animals (Elman and Cole [6]).

2. *Cholangitis* is primarily an inflammation of the bile ducts and may be acute or chronic. The acute suppurative type of infection is usually secondary to acute infectious processes in the gallbladder, especially when there is obstruction of the common duct by stone. The infection may extend upward into the tributaries of the biliary ducts and involve the entire liver. Microscopically it may be difficult to differentiate this type of infection from pylephlebitis; multiple abscesses may likewise be formed. Edema occluding the walls of the ducts is frequently sufficient to produce biliary obstruction, thereby leading to jaundice. Acute catarrhal icterus is

pathologically a type of acute cholangitis; its etiology and pathogenesis, however, remain obscure.

3. *Pericholangitis* is an infection which in most instances is of lymphatic origin. This infection is in reality a type of hepatitis (Graham) which, as already mentioned, arises primarily from cholecystitis, but also from other infectious processes within the abdominal cavity. The liver in such instances is slightly swollen and the edges rounded. The polynuclear and lymphocytic infiltration extends throughout the portal spaces. A variable amount of necrosis of adjacent hepatic cells may be present. Such processes may be secondary to acute infections not only in the gallbladder, but also in the appendix, pancreas and other organs and are associated occasionally with jaundice, fever, etc.

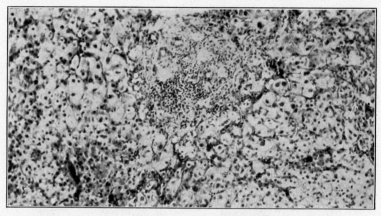

FIG. 370.—PERICHOLANGITIS PRODUCED BY CHRONIC CHOLECYSTITIS, FROM A BIOPSY OF THE LIVER OBTAINED AT TIME OF CHOLECYSTECTOMY.

The patient had several attacks of pain in the right upper quadrant during the past several months, but no jaundice. Note the lymphocytic infiltration with beginning scar formation in the periportal area, surrounding three or four small bile ducts.

Clinical Manifestations of Hepatitis.—The manifestations of hepatitis depend of course on the existence of associated lesions, particularly in the infectious group. In themselves the signs and symptoms produced by the hepatic lesion may be very meager indeed, consisting of nothing more than mild dyspepsia and occasionally slight jaundice. Mild tenderness in the right upper quadrant over the edge of the liver may be present. When significant infection is present more definite and local manifestations occur, which are discussed under types of hepatitis as just described. However, if the damage to the liver is great enough *hepatic insufficiency* may be produced, a condition producing manifestations which may be few in number, but serious in so far as death may ensue. Hepatic insufficiency occasionally develops following operations upon the biliary tract in which severe hepatitis is already present. Weakness and lassitude are usually the first symptoms complained of and become noticeable on the second or third postoperative day. The pulse rate and temperature usually remain near normal until shortly before death, but the pulse itself is soft and poorly sustained. A fall of blood pressure may accompany a collapse which simulates that due to a severe hemorrhage. Anorexia and nausea are prominent, but vomiting is unusual. Difficulty in "getting his breath" may be complained of by the patient, but there is no change in the rate or depth of respirations. Drowsiness often develops but in the severe cases pronounced restlessness and hyperactivity may occur. Although the patient may complain of severe abdominal distress examination of the abdomen rarely reveals anything abnormal. Jaundice may or may not be present. Edema of the ankles is not uncommon, and after several days the urinary output decreases alarmingly. Urobilin is found in the urine in large quantities. Helwig[7] and his associates have called attention to an associated renal damage. The patient continues to grow weaker and more drowsy until eighteen or

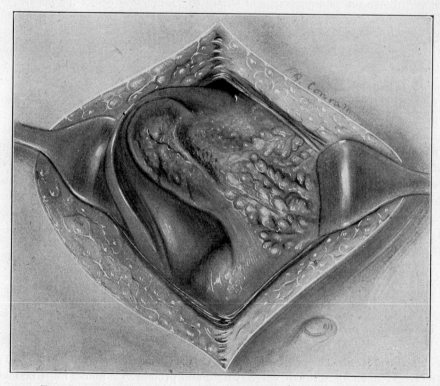

FIG. 371.—THE ROUNDED EDGE OF THE LIVER (DUE PRESUMABLY TO SUBACUTE HEPATITIS) WHICH CAN BE DEMONSTRATED GROSSLY AT THE TIME OF OPERATION.

This finding is not uncommon as a complication of acute and subacute cholecystitis.

twenty-four hours before death when he is apt to become irrational. Death which occurs near the eighth or tenth day is preceded by coma. The term "hepatic asthenia" would appear to be appropriate when referring to patients suffering from this disease because of the debility and weakness associated with the malady.

From the above discussion it will be noted that hepatic insufficiency may be of great importance surgically, particularly because it is so frequently unrecognized. Although such a clear cut clinical picture as described above is uncommon, there are no doubt many instances when this disease, in a more insidious form, is a major factor contributing toward a fatal outcome. Years ago, Graham[8] and associates called attention to the danger of operating on patients with hepatic insufficiency. Symptoms of hepatic insufficiency may develop in toxic hepatitis (acute yellow atrophy, etc.) as well as in infective hepatitis.

Differential Diagnosis of Hepatitis due to Chemical or Toxic Substances.—As is mentioned elsewhere, symptoms of hepatitis are so insidious that the damage may progress to the point that considerable hepatic insufficiency exists before the lesion is recognized. By the time the condition is recognized, jaundice which is produced in this instance by inability of the damaged liver to excrete bilirubin at the required rate, is usually present. However, certain tests including the flocculation test of Hanger,[9] the serum phosphatase, and others will frequently detect the hepatic disease before jaundice develops. Such tests will be of still more value in differentiation of the different types of jaundice as discussed on page 609.

It is extremely important that the cause of the hepatitis be determined if possible because the factor causing the damage may at times be controllable, and thereby eliminated. Hanger and Gutman [9, 13, 25] have emphasized the importance of an elevated serum phosphatase as pointing to extra hepatic obstruction as the cause of jaundice, whereas the positive cephalin flocculation test indicates an intrahepatic damage to the liver cells preventing bile excretion, the result of a toxic or chemical factor. These two tests are a most valuable aid in the differential diagnosis of the etiology of jaundice. If the etiology of the hepatitis is unknown, it is usually advisable to stop all drug medication, since certain people are at times sensitive to drugs which are ordinarily harmless in the usual doses utilized. The age of the patient may be helpful since acute catarrhal jaundice (a so-called toxic or infective type of hepatitis) is not common in late adult life. Chemical hepatitis due to drugs could of course be present at any age.

Treatment of Hepatitis.—Treatment of the infectious types of hepatitis differs only slightly from that described below for hepatic insufficiency. However, there is perhaps a stronger indication to find and correct, if possible, any local infectious processes which may be a factor in the production or maintenance of the hepatitis. In the chemical group the agent responsible should be eliminated if possible.

The treatment of hepatic insufficiency in most instances is chiefly of a medical nature. The most obvious prerequisite is the maintenance of fluid intake to 3,000 cc. or more per day. An adequate carbohydrate and protein [10, 11] intake must be maintained. If the patient is not able to take this by mouth it will be necessary to administer glucose (5 or 10 per cent solution) intravenously once or twice a day in amounts up to 3,000 cc. per day, depending upon the amount of fluid taken by mouth. The observations of Maddock and associates [78] conclusively prove the beneficial effect of glucose on maintenance of liver glycogen. They noted an average level of 5.03 per cent liver glycogen in patients given supplementary glucose feedings for 12 hours previous to operation, contrasted to an average of 3.96 per cent found in normal control patients. Inasmuch as hypoalbuminemia is frequent in liver disease, repeated and large plasma or whole blood transfusions may be necessary. Intravenous amino acids may also be of value (see p. 152). Since bile salts are known to be good cholagogues, their oral administration may be tried in an endeavor to stimulate hepatic secretion. Obviously an effort should be made to determine the cause of the hepatic insufficiency. Any drugs which could possibly have been a factor in

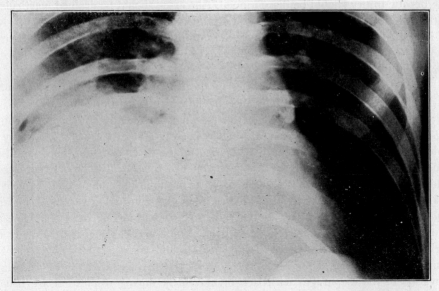

FIG. 372.—PYOGENIC ABSCESS OF THE LIVER; ROENTGENOGRAM SHOWING MARKED ELEVATION OF THE RIGHT DIAPHRAGM, WHICH WAS ALSO IMMOBILE.

Operation was performed for drainage by resection of the ninth rib in the posterior axillary line; about 300 cc. of foul smelling pus was evacuated. Recovery was uneventful (see Chart 7).

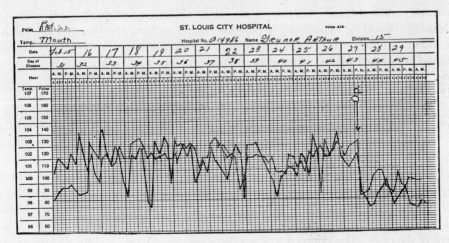

CHART 7.—TEMPERATURE CHART OF PYOGENIC ABSCESS OF LIVER SHOWN IN FIGURE 372.

The patient, aged thirty-seven, was first operated on one month previously for drainage of a large intra-abdominal abscess, presumably of appendiceal origin. The abdominal and general condition gradually improved and the temperature returned to normal. Four weeks after admission, the fever recurred (as noted above on the second day of the chart) and assumed a swinging septic form. Twelve days later, as indicated on the chart, operation was performed. Following drainage of the hepatic abscess the temperature returned to normal. Recovery was uneventful.

the hepatic injury should be discontinued. Abscesses should be drained, particularly if they are intra-abdominal. Bed rest is necessary. Sufficient narcotics must be given to insure adequate sleep. If the hepatitis is of infective origin, sulfonamide therapy should be tried. It has been found effective in pylephlebitis even in the presence of small multiple abscesses.

Abscess of the Liver.—Abscesses of the liver may be of two types, namely, pyogenic which is usually multiple, and amebic which is usually solitary.

Pyogenic Abscess.—Abscesses of this type most frequently accompany suppurative processes in the abdomen (appendicitis, etc.) and are usually secondary to pylephlebitis. Occasionally they may be secondary to cholangitis. The organisms most frequently responsible for the infection are the *Bacillus coli,* streptococcus and staphylococcus. The abscesses are apt to be multiple unless they happen to coalesce and form one or two large cavities. Symptoms, including weakness, malaise, anorexia, chills and mild pain in the right upper quadrant or right shoulder, are similar to the severe manifestations of pylephlebitis and cholangitis as already described. Ochsner and associates[12] noted nausea and vomiting, loss of weight and jaundice in one-third of the series reported by them. Intermittent fever and slight elevation of the diaphragm with lack of movement during respiration are usually the most objective diagnostic signs. Differentiation from subphrenic abscess may be difficult or impossible when a large single abscess is present. Leukocytosis is pronounced and usually higher than that noted in amebic abscesses. The *treatment* of these abscesses may be operative, but they are not so amenable to drainage, chiefly because of the fact that they are usually multiple. The mortality is therefore high; however, when there are but one or two large abscesses treatment is more hopeful. Drainage should be established if possible, but in such a way that the pleural and peritoneal cavities are not contaminated; the retroperitoneal approach (Ochsner) should be utilized whenever possible. Sulfonamide therapy in large doses has in the past three years proved curative in a few cases of liver abscess following pylephlebitis with appendicitis.

Amebic Abscess.—Years ago amebic abscess of the liver was thought to be a tropical disease but it is well known now that it is common in the temperate as well as tropical climate. As the name implies the causative organism is the Endameba histolytica. The lesion is much more common in males than females. The relationship of the development of the abscess to the initial intestinal infection is extremely variable. Furthermore, a history of diarrhea may be absent. In a series of 741 collected cases (including their own) Ochsner and DeBakey[14] noted a history of diarrhea in only 58 per cent of cases and diarrhea at time of entry in only 21 per cent of the cases. The symptoms of amebic abscess are fever, weakness, malaise and mild pain in the epigastrium, right upper quadrant or right shoulder. Fever is apt to be of the remitting type, accompanied by sweating and exhaustion; loss of weight is common. Examination may reveal nothing more specific than a mild degree of tenderness over the liver. However, as the abscess increases in size the area of hepatic dullness likewise increases. The diaphragm may be elevated, and upon fluoroscopic examination is usually found to be immobile. Perforation of the diaphragm may occur with the production of an empyema. More rarely the pus breaks through the lung into a bronchus, producing a bronchial fistula. The pus found in an abscess of the liver is characteristically of a brick red color. The amebae may be found in the pus, but with more certainty from the wall of the cavity.

The treatment is largely medical. Rogers [15] was perhaps the first to demonstrate the truth of this statement; he noted a decrease in mortality from 56 per cent after open drainage, to 14 per cent after conservative treatment including closed drainage (aspiration) and medicinal therapy. Rogers attributed the high mortality following open drainage to secondary infection of an abscess cavity which was initially sterile. Occasionally spontaneous secondary infection develops; if micro-organisms are found in the pus, open drainage is usually indicated. The drug most commonly used is emetine, given intravenously in daily doses of 1 grain. Because of the toxic effects of the drug on the heart it is not safe to continue it longer than 10 consecutive days.

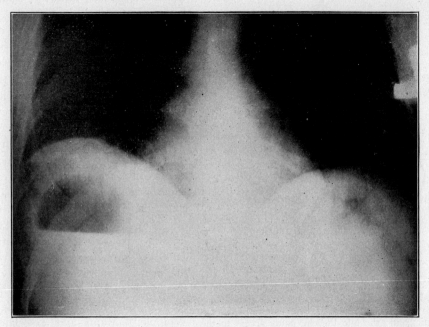

FIG. 373.—AMEBIC ABSCESS OF THE LIVER.

The patient, a forty-five-year-old male, complained of loss of weight and strength; examination revealed an intermittent fever and a palpably enlarged liver. The roentgenogram was taken in the upright position after part of the aspirated pus had been replaced by air; note the fluid level. Emetine was injected into the cavity; it was also given by mouth. Recovery was uneventful without operation (St. Louis City Hospital).

This "course" may be repeated later or other amebicides tried, as indicated. If feasible, the cavity may be irrigated with 1 to 2500 emetine solution. When the abscess perforates through the diaphragm, the resulting empyema may have to be treated by rib resection, inasmuch as the pus in such a case is usually secondarily infected. If the abscess perforates into a bronchus without producing an extensive empyema, as it occasionally does, cure is usually spontaneous.

Jaundice.—To understand the mechanism of production, and the significance of jaundice, it is necessary that the chief factors in the metabolism of bile pigments be understood. Bilirubin is present in the blood normally in quantities equal to 1 to 2 milligram per 1000 cc. of serum (quantitative Van den Bergh). When the content is raised to 20 or 25 milligrams per 1000 cc. of serum, macroscopic or tissue jaundice results. Thus, it is obvious that a hyperbilirubinemia may exist without visible discoloration of the tissues; this is often spoken of as latent jaundice. Bilirubin is made by the reticulo-endothelial system, *e.g.*, the bone marrow, lymph nodes, spleen, Kupffer cells of the liver, etc., but is normally excreted only by the liver. Bilirubin is formed from hemoglobin probably through the intermediary product hematin. When bilirubin is excreted with the bile into the intestine, the action of the bacteria converts it into urobilin which is absorbed and reconverted in part at least into bilirubin, chiefly in the liver. Urobilin is found normally in human bile and in traces in the urine. The stools, however, contain large amounts. Urobilin may be found in the urine in certain diseases. It is assumed that in such instances a slight degree of hepatic insufficiency exists to the extent that the urobilin cannot be converted into bilirubin, and is therefore excreted by the kidney. In other instances, urobilinuria occurs when the liver, though normal, is unable to remove the urobilin from the blood stream when produced in excess by such conditions as hemolysis. On the other hand, when no bile reaches the intestine, as in complete obstructive jaundice, urobilin disappears from the urine. The basis for the above remarks about bile pigment metabolism may be found in the work of Whipple,[16] Mann and associates,[1] Elman and McMaster[17] and others.

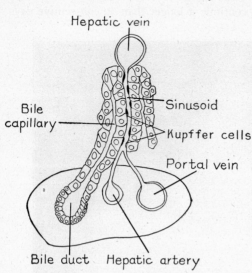

FIG. 374.—DIAGRAM TO ILLUSTRATE THE MECHANISM OF OBSTRUCTIVE JAUNDICE.

If the bile duct becomes obstructed, the bile obviously is blocked from its normal exit and "spills" over into the sinusoid, which empties into the hepatic vein; the bile thereby gains access to the general circulation. The manner in which the capillaries of the portal vein and hepatic artery unite to form the sinusoid is not clearly understood and is illustrated in a diagrammatic fashion. (Modified from McNee, *Quart. J. M.*, 16:390, 1923).

Jaundice first appears in the sclerae and conjunctivae and gradually becomes noticeable over the skin and mucous membranes throughout the rest of the body. When severe jaundice has been present for a long time the skin turns to a dark greenish bronze color because of the transformation of bilirubin to biliverdin.

For obvious reasons it may frequently be of considerable advantage, from the surgical as well as medical standpoint, to determine the intensity of jaundice and to follow its course with reference to a decrease or increase.

As stated previously, jaundice is dependent upon the amount of bilirubin in the blood. There are several methods of estimating the bilirubin content of the blood; the quantitative Van den Bergh and icterus index are the two most commonly used tests. Normal readings for the quantitative Van den Bergh are given on page 603. The normal icterus index is about 5 (which represents a purely arbitrary figure). Gross jaundice is evident if the reading is above 15. In patients with intense jaundice the index may be as high as 150 or above.

Types of Jaundice.—Aside from hemolytic jaundice which is really a disease of the spleen and hemopoietic system, and not of the biliary apparatus, jaundice is due to the failure of bile to reach the intestine. Because bile is constantly formed this failure obviously results in the accumulation of bile in all of the tissues of the body and in the blood, as already mentioned. There are a variety of diseases which result in a failure of bile to reach the duodenum; these can be conveniently divided into two general groups, *hepatogenous* and *extrahepatic,* each of which is described in more detail later on. In hepatogenous jaundice the liver parenchyma itself is diseased so that it cannot excrete bile; such lesions include acute and subacute yellow atrophy, toxic hepatitis, primary hepatitis, cirrhosis, etc. In extrahepatic jaundice the disease is in the biliary ducts which become obstructed by one lesion or another, usually either stone or tumor; this type of jaundice is therefore called obstructive. Hepatogenous jaundice is in general a medical disease; surgery has little to offer aside from the value of laparotomy in making the diagnosis. Obstructive jaundice, on the other hand, is a surgical disease because operation often permits relief of the obstruction or even cure of the lesion producing it. The importance of both types of jaundice to the surgeon is that the clinical differentiation is sometimes difficult or impossible to make, thus justifying an operation for such a purpose.

Regardless of the cause of the jaundice it is important to recognize the existence of any damage to the liver parenchyma for reasons to be discussed later. For this purpose the patient's symptoms may be of value but *tests of hepatic function* are often more informative. Of the many tests which have been devised, the hippuric acid test (Quick[18]), galactose tolerance tests, dye excretion tests (bromsulphalein and phenoltetraiodophthalein), serum phosphatase, Hanger's flocculation test, and a fall in albumin (and rise in globulin) of the plasma proteins (Keeton and associates[19]) are the most important. On the basis of the results of these tests it is frequently possible to differentiate extrahepatic types of jaundice from hepatogenous jaundice as will be discussed later. Regardless of the absence or presence of infection, the retention of bile salts alone if continued long enough will eventually produce hepatic damage and actual necrosis of many of the cells. The liver then will become enlarged and a mild edema as well as a lymphocytic infiltration will take place. Ultimately, scar tissue will be deposited and an actual microscopic biliary cirrhosis will be produced.

In all types of jaundice bile pigment is found promptly in the urine but does not appear in the tissues until the serum attains a certain concentration, *i.e.,* 2.0 to 2.5 mgm. per cent; only when values above this level are reached is clinical jaundice evident. Because of this latent period in the clinical appearance of jaundice the determination of the amount of bilirubin in the blood may be a valuable method of identifying occult or latent jaundice and also in following the variations in the degree of jaundice, as discussed on page 604.

Postoperative hemorrhage in jaundice is a more serious and not infrequent complication; it may occur at any time during the first ten postoperative days but perhaps most commonly between the fourth and sixth day. Hemorrhage occurs because blood clotting is defective due to a deficiency in the prothrombin content of the blood (Dam,[20] Almquist and Stokstad,[21] and Quick[22]). Although the bleeding and clotting time is usually normal the clot is defective or fragile because of a diminution in the conversion of fibrinogen to fibrin. This is an indirect result of the prothrombin deficiency (hypoprothrombinemia) which in turn is due to a lack of vitamin K. This vitamin is fat-soluble and therefore requires the presence of bile salts in the intestines for its assimilation; a deficiency follows complete jaundice and also complete external biliary fistula because of the absence of bile in the intestinal tract thereby preventing absorption of the vitamin from the food. An excellent discussion of the mechanism of jaundice is that of McNee;[23] various aspects of obstructive jaundice may be found in the excellent survey of Boyce and McFetridge.[24]

1. Hepatogenous Jaundice.—In this group the disease is primary in the liver producing so much cellular damage that bile is not being excreted into the ducts which are, indeed, normal grossly and microscopically; at times edema or fibrous tissue about the bile ducts may be sufficient to exert an additional intrahepatic obstructive mechanism. Hepatogenous jaundice comprises a great variety of conditions; some of them are called infective or toxic jaundice but the cause in many cases is really unknown. The simplest type is the so-called "acute catarrhal jaundice," which runs its course in a few weeks, leaves little or no trace and does not recur. It presents little diagnostic difficulty unless the jaundice persists for many weeks; in such an event it may shade off imperceptibly into the most serious types sometimes called chronic yellow atrophy or chronic hepatitis. Other examples are sepsis of various types (including pneumonia), spirochetal icterus (Weil's disease) and various types of poisoning (chloroform, atophan, carbon tetrachloride, etc.). Acute yellow atrophy represents still another type which is more serious and nearly always fatal. The cause of the injury or damage to the liver cell in these cases is still unknown; however, they present clinical manifestations quite similar to the so-called toxic hepatitis which is known to follow the ingestion of poisons, or use of drugs such as arsphenamine, sulfanilamide, etc., to which certain persons may be sensitive. Fever and leukocytosis are variable. Anorexia is usually present but vomiting is not common; pruritus is usually absent. The stools are not acholic. Urobilin will be found in the urine but only a small amount of bile pigment will be present. Allied to these examples of primary liver disease are patients with various types of cirrhosis. Cirrhosis, when it produces jaundice, must be considered in this group, even though the large amount of scar present in the liver may produce a variable degree of duct obstruction. In many instances ascites may also be present which helps considerably in the differential diagnosis because ascites, though occasionally present in other types of hepatogenous jaundice, is extremely rare in obstructive jaundice unless there are peritoneal metastases from carcinoma.

The surgical problem in hepatogenous jaundice is largely a diagnostic one, i.e., that of differentiation from extrahepatic jaundice for which surgery has much to offer. Actually, in many patients such a differentiation is impossible to make without operation. It is the possibility that the patient has a stone or a carcinoma for which surgery offers the only hope of relief or cure that often tips the balance in favor of laparotomy. At operation on a patient with hepatogenous jaundice the

liver is somewhat swollen or cirrhotic or nodular but is not usually enlarged. The
gallbladder is normal in size and appearance; the common duct appears normal and
the pancreas is not enlarged. Palpable lymph nodes may be felt in the hilus of the
liver. Biopsy of the liver reveals a microscopic picture which varies from mild
leukocytic infiltration to extensive, necrotic or fibrotic changes, cystoplasmic vacuo-
lization and deposition of fat. (See discussion on hepatitis, p. 595.)

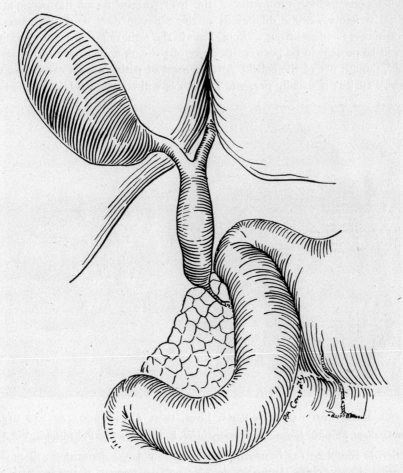

Fig. 375.—Diagram to Illustrate One of the Types of Obstructive Jaundice.

The duodenum has been rolled back to expose the pancreas. In this instance the common
duct is distended because of compression of the terminal end of the common duct by the pancreas.
The pathologic process in the pancreas capable of producing this compression may be either
carcinoma or pancreatitis. In obstruction of this type (absence of infection in the biliary system)
the gallbladder is distended, fulfilling part of the requisites of Courvoisier's law (see text).

2. Obstructive Jaundice.—Obstructive or extrahepatic jaundice really comprises two entirely different types. In one the obstruction is outside the ducts which
therefore remain uninfected; the usual lesion responsible is a carcinoma at the head
of the pancreas (see Fig. 375). Clinical manifestations are apt to develop insidiously
and thus simulate some types of hepatogenous jaundice. The second type is due to

an obstruction within the common or hepatic ducts, usually to stone (see Fig. 386, page 623) ; infection is inevitable, often severe, and usually spreads upward and produces a cholangitis. The clinical manifestations produced by these two types of obstruction will be readily distinguishable if stones in the common duct are associated with enough cholangitis to produce fever, chills, etc., since such inflammatory symptoms are absent in carcinoma of the pancreas. Other noninflammatory or aseptic obstructive lesions include carcinoma of the liver, carcinoma of the common duct, congenital strictures, cystic dilatations of the common duct, and other neoplasms which compress the ducts from without. Pain in the right upper quadrant and epigastrium will be present in 80 per cent or more of patients with stones in the common duct and, though not of the colicky sort, in most of patients with carcinoma of the pancreas. Pruritus is usually present. The stools will contain no bile pigment if the

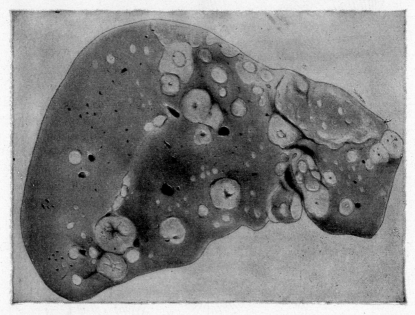

Fig. 376.—Metastatic Adenocarcinoma, Liver, from a Carcinoma of the Breast. (From Graham, *Surgical Diagnosis*. Courtesy of W. B. Saunders Co., Philadelphia, Vol. III.)

obstruction is complete (as is usually the case), but large quantities will be found in the urine. Fever, chills, leukocytosis, etc., will be present if the lesion is associated with hepatitis. It should be stated, however, that of the many lesions mentioned in the obstructive group, stones in the common duct represent about the only group associated with hepatitis of the infectious type.

Contrary to general opinion, jaundice due to obstruction alone, may exist for some time without producing significant damage to the liver. This is particularly true in the slowly developing jaundice which follows an obstruction by carcinoma at the head of the pancreas. However, if there is an accompanying infection, as for example, in the presence of stones in the common duct, there is very obvious and often severe damage inflicted upon the hepatic parenchyma as will be demonstrable by liver biopsy.

As mentioned already, jaundice of the hemolytic type has much more relation to the spleen than the liver. Splenomegalia is fairly consistent. Splenectomy in selected cases is curative. The role of the liver in this disease is limited for the most part to the fact that the amount of bilirubin converted from the hemoglobin (due to excessive destruction of erythrocytes) is so great that the liver is unable to excrete it in a normal fashion. The bilirubin accumulates in the blood stream resulting in jaundice. The condition is therefore discussed under diseases of the spleen.

Differential Diagnosis in Jaundice.—It is extremely important to differentiate hepatogenous from extrahepatic obstructive jaundice because in general, the therapy in the former is conservative whereas in the latter it is surgical. Unfortunately the presence or absence of pain which used to be considered of great diagnostic aid is now known to be of relatively little value. For example, "painless jaundice" was supposed to point to carcinoma of the pancreas which actually is accompanied by abdominal pain in a great many cases, whereas pain may be absent in about 10 per cent of patients with stones in the common duct. It is true, however, that the most severe pain of all the groups is encountered in patients with stones in the common duct. The presence of chills may be helpful since they are rarely present except in patients with common duct stones or with septicemia accompanying serious sepsis such as pneumonia, septicemia, etc. Fever which may be present in hepatogenous jaundice or stones in the common duct, in itself will be of little value except that its presence would exclude carcinoma of the pancreas.

The age of the patient will frequently be very helpful, since acute catarrhal icterus, which is one of the common types of hepatogenous jaundice, is usually encountered in young adults whereas stones in the common duct, and carcinoma are usually encountered in later adult life. Sex will be of no value in differentiation.

The onset of the disease is apt to be more acute in acute catarrhal jaundice and in patients with stones in the common duct. In the former disease the patient may appear quite ill, whereas in carcinoma of the pancreas the onset is frequently insidious. The course of the disease frequently establishes the diagnosis with certainty, that is, allows the surgeon to arrive at the correct decision as to whether or not operation is indicated. For example, if the patient's history reveals a rather sudden onset of relatively painless jaundice, and during two or three weeks' observation shows decrease in symptoms including a lowered bilirubinemia and more pigment in the stool, the decision to refrain from operative interference will rarely be erroneous. In many types of hepatogenous jaundice the spleen will be enlarged, whereas in obstructive jaundice it rarely will be. The size of the liver will not be of much diagnostic assistance, since it will be moderately enlarged in both types of jaundice. However, marked enlargement of the liver is practically never seen in obstructive jaundice due to stone unless a liver abscess is present.

There is slight difference of opinion as to the value of intensity of jaundice, but Hanger [9] reports an average icterus index of 144 in hepatogenous jaundice (normal is 5 to 10) and 61 in patients with stones in the common duct. In hepatogenous jaundice as well as in jaundice due to stones in the common duct there will be intermittent attacks of acholic stools with pigment slightly more common in the former disease. In carcinoma of the pancreas bile rarely is found in the stool once it is noted to be absent. *Stool examinations* may therefore be of great value in making a differential diagnosis. Urobilin will be present in the urine of patients with hepatogenous jaundice but rarely in patients with obstructive jaundice. Pruritus is much more common in obstructive jaundice than in hepatogenous jaundice.

Tests of hepatic function may be extremely helpful. For example, the galactose test, hippuric acid test and dye tests will usually reveal an hepatic insufficiency in hepatogenous jaundice, but normal readings in obstructive jaundice except when an accompanying hepatitis is present. Determinations of serum proteins may be of much diagnostic value since a tendency toward reversal of the albumin-globulin ratio is noted in hepatogenous jaundice (Keeton and associates). In severe hepatic damage, vitamin K is apt not to restore the prothrombin time to normal as it will in jaundice with little hepatic damage. The serum phosphatase test, which is dependent upon the amount of phosphatase (produced in the liver or bones or both) in the blood, may be of great diagnostic assistance. In a detailed clinical study, Gutman [25] found that the level of serum phosphatase with few exceptions was over 10 units in obstructive jaundice and under 10 in hepatogenous jaundice (normal of 4). The flocculation test of Hanger [9] will also be of great value in differentiation between the two types of jaundice. Flocculation is negative or 1 + in extrahepatic jaundice and 4 + in intrahepatic jaundice; like other tests, it will be positive in those cases of extrahepatic jaundice in which significant liver damage is also present.

Treatment of Jaundice.—Obviously the first requirement in the treatment of jaundice is to determine the cause. This may require extensive study including a large amount of laboratory data. Frequently it is extremely difficult to determine the exact cause of the jaundice. On such occasions exploratory laparotomy may be indicated on the assumption that a lesion will be found which can be effectively treated surgically. If the jaundice is produced by mechanical obstruction, particularly if extrahepatic (*e.g.,* stone), operation is obviously indicated for its correction. On the other hand, if the jaundice is due to a diffuse damage or infection of the liver alone (acute yellow atrophy, catarrhal jaundice, etc.) operation will be therapeutically useless. Nevertheless, there are times when an exploratory laparotomy for diagnostic purposes will be indicated and justified.

Medical treatment includes a high carbohydrate intake, supplemented by intravenous glucose (Schreiber,[26] Ravdin,[27] and others), if the oral intake is insufficient. The necessity of maintaining a high glycogen content of the liver is due to the fact that a liver rich in glycogen is able to withstand the effects of injurious agents much more effectively (Graham [28]); an adequate protein intake is also important (Ravdin [10]). Postoperative hemorrhage can be averted to a great extent by intravenous glucose and transfusion, but more effectively by vitamin K and bile salts (Snell and associates [29] and others). Klotogen which was initially used to combat prothrombin deficiency, is gradually being replaced by synthetic products (such as 2-methyl 1, 4 naphthoquinone, and 4 amino 2 methyl naphthol) with vitamin K activity. Each of these two drugs is given in doses of 3 mg. per day or less. The latter is soluble in water and may be given subcutaneously or intravenously. In severe hepatic disease these compounds will not relieve hypoprothrombinemia; repeated transfusions should then be given. See treatment of Hepatitis, page 600.

Neoplasms.—The liver is frequently the site of tumors, especially of a malignant type, secondary to a primary focus elsewhere. Carcinoma of the stomach, intestine and other intra-abdominal organs tend to metastasize first to the liver. Fortunately for the patient such metastases rarely produce many symptoms other than mild discomfort and tenderness, although the liver on some occasions becomes greatly enlarged. If the metastatic nodules are sufficiently numerous, jaundice may be produced. Increasing dyspepsia, weakness, loss of weight, and other systemic manifestations of malignant disease will develop as the disease progresses.

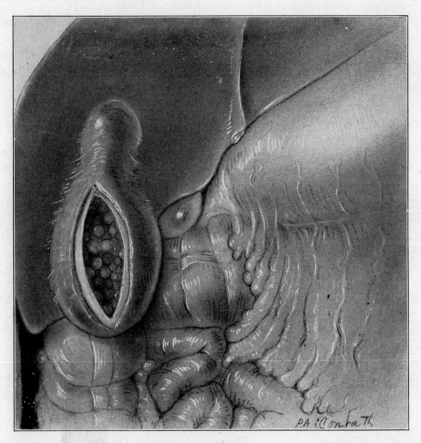

FIG. 377.—DRAWING OF ECHINOCOCCUS CYST OF THE LIVER FROM SKETCH MADE AT THE TIME OF OPERATION.

The gallbladder was normal; its dome may be identified to right of the cyst. The symptoms consist of mild pain in the right upper quadrant of three years' duration and simulated cholecystitis. The cyst was evacuated at the time of operation and drained; the fluid contained hundreds of daughter cysts of variable size. The wound healed after several weeks. Patient was alive and well when last seen, seven years after operation.

On rare occasions carcinoma may be primary in the liver, arising in most instances in the bile ducts. It sometimes occurs also in association with or as a complication of atrophic cirrhosis. The clinical manifestations are no different from those encountered in metastatic carcinoma in the liver. Attempts should be made to arrive at a diagnosis as early as possible because on rare occasions local excision of the tumor in the liver may be possible.

Miscellaneous Diseases of the Liver.—The liver may be afflicted with various types of *cirrhosis,* the most important of which surgically is the atrophic (Laënnec) type. When cirrhosis has progressed to the point where the portal circulation has been obstructed sufficiently to produce an ascites, surgical relief may be offered. Such procedures as implantation of the omentum in the abdominal wall (omentopexy) with scarification of the liver, diaphragm and spleen, may partially relieve portal obstruction and ascites by establishing collateral vessels.

Echinococcus cysts, although rare in this country, occur more frequently in the liver than in other organs. They are apt to develop insidiously with only a moderate amount of discomfort and pain in the upper abdomen. Examination usually reveals a large liver because of the development of the cyst. Evacuation of the cyst by operative procedures is successful in eradicating the disease (see p. 104).

GALLBLADDER

The gallbladder is of extreme importance clinically because of the frequency of its diseases, especially cholecystitis. Unlike the appendix, however, the gallbladder does have definite functions and should not be removed unless the disease process demands it. The normal gallbladder acts largely as a storehouse for bile which accumulates within its lumen because of the resistance of the sphincter of Oddi and the relaxation of the gallbladder which occurs between meals. Large amounts of bile are thus stored in spite of the small size of the viscus because the normal gallbladder mucosa absorbs water and thereby concentrates the constituents of the bile (Rous and McMaster [30]). At mealtime and during the process of digestion the musculature of the gallbladder, aided perhaps by breathing, intra-abdominal pressure, etc., causes expulsion of bile through the relaxed sphincter. Removal of the gallbladder causes dilatation of the extrahepatic ducts (Judd and Mann [31]) and a slight dilatation of the intrahepatic ducts (Counseller and McIndoe [32]).

Infection is known to be important in the *pathogenesis* of cholecystitis but the inflammation may frequently be nonbacterial. Andrews [33] has called attention to the importance of an increase of bile salts in the bile, in the development of chemical cholecystitis (corroborated by Womack and Bricker [35]). Likewise Wolfer [34] has shown that reflux of pancreatic juice into the gallbladder by way of the common duct may instigate cholecystitis. Chronic obstruction of the cystic duct may initiate this inflammation because of resultant overconcentration of bile, etc. (Cole and Associates [35]); in their experiments infection was superimposed in 30 per cent of cases, representing about the same incidence of positive culture noted in human cholecystitis. The ability to find bacteria in only a portion of diseased gallbladders has also led observers to doubt that the inflammation is always bacterial in origin. It is possible however that the bacteria may have been eradicated by the time the gallbladder was removed. Bacteria commonly isolated from diseased gallbladders are *streptococcus, Bacillus coli,* the *Bacillus typhosus* and the *Staphylococcus.* The role of the *Bacillus typhosus* in the production and maintenance of cholecystitis is of particular importance since typhoid "carriers" are usually those patients afflicted with a chronic cholecystitis of typhoid origin. Cholecystectomy, usually, but not always, eliminates the organisms from the stool, thereby eliminating the contagious factor. In 100 cases Illingworth [36] noted that of 62 positive cultures obtained from the wall of the gallbladder, 34 were *Streptococci* and 17 were *Bacillus coli*. On the other hand, of the 40 instances of positive culture from the bile in the 100 cases, 16 were *Streptococci* and 20 were *Bacillus coli*.

There are four chief ways in which bacteria may reach the gallbladder: (1) hematogenous, (2) lymphogenous, (3) spreading infection from a contiguous organ and (4) hepatogenous by way of the bile. Of these 4 methods of development of cholecystitis, the lymphogenous route would appear to be the most important. Graham [37] and associates have called attention to this mechanism of transmission of infection. Due to the rich anastomosis of the lymphatic vessels between the gallbladder and liver, spread of infection from one organ to the other, and *vice versa*, is no doubt a common occurrence. On some occasions the infection perhaps breaks through the mucosal barrier of the intestine, and is carried to the liver by the lymphatics or blood stream, particularly the latter. It is apparent that a vicious circle may be established by an infection between the gallbladder and liver, because of the rich lymphatic anastomosis mentioned above. It may therefore require removal of the gallbladder to break up the vicious circle. Infection of the gallbladder may be acute or chronic.

Acute Cholecytitis.—Acute inflammation of the gallbladder is not so common as chronic cholecystitis, but it is of importance surgically because of the acute abdominal symptoms produced. It is usually associated with cholelithiasis. Indeed, in many cases a stone impacted in the neck of the gallbladder, with the consequent production of obstruction of the cystic duct, is frequently an important factor in pathogenesis. When the organ is the seat of an acute infection the wall becomes thickened and edematous, with a reddened serosal surface upon which fibrin may be deposited. This external reaction is probably a precursor of the formation of numerous adhesions to other organs. The cystic duct may be obstructed by a stone or by edema and adhesions created by inflammation. When this occurs in the presence of an acute infection the contents of the gallbladder are apt to become purulent, thereby producing a condition known as *empyema of the gallbladder*. The secretion of mucus, the pouring out of exudate and the production of pus, increase the distention and the size of the gallbladder. Within a few days after the production of the obstruction, the greenish color of the contents fades to a gray or grayish brown, due presumably to bacterial action on the bile pigment. Empyema of the gallbladder is usually associated with cholelithiasis; it requires operative correction (usually cholecystostomy). The inflammation at the onset of acute cholecystitis may be infectious in origin, but probably is more frequently chemical in origin, infection being superimposed later. The rarity of peritonitis following early operation for acute cholecystitis is almost proof of this point.

In most instances acute cholecystitis subsides spontaneously, but occasionally gangrenous or necrotic areas may form in the wall of the gallbladder, thereby leading to perforation of the organ. The process is slow, however, and the omentum or contiguous organs are usually plastered against the gallbladder in such a way that perforation does not occur into the peritoneal cavity, but rather forms a pericholecystic abscess. On rare occasions perforation may occur into the liver, the duodenum, colon or through the anterior abdominal wall.

Clinical Manifestations.—The onset of symptoms in acute cholecystitis is usually sudden, consisting primarily of pain in the right upper quadrant, nausea and vomiting. Fever usually accompanies the disease, as do other systemic manifestations of severe inflammatory processes, such as tachycardia, malaise, weakness, etc. Not infrequently there is a history of a chill at the onset. Frequently the pain, which is usually severe, radiates backward to the tip of the scapula. Deep respiration may be painful. Palpation will reveal tenderness and muscle spasm localized over the right upper quadrant, persisting for several days, depending upon the intensity of

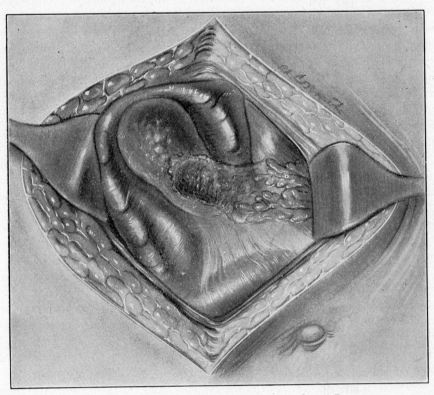

FIG. 378.—ACUTE CHOLECYSTITIS OF ONLY A FEW DAYS' DURATION.

Note the dilated vessels and the attachment of adjacent organs (omentum) to the gallbladder by exudate and fibrin. The gallbladder is slightly distended, but the walls are not greatly thickened as yet.

the attack. The gallbladder will frequently be palpable as a tender mass even in the face of muscle spasm over it. Jaundice induced either by a coincidental obstruction of the common duct or by hepatitis associated with the cholecystitis (Graham), may be present. The leukocyte count is sharply elevated, frequently reaching 25,000 or higher. The acute symptoms, including nausea, vomiting and severe pain are apt to diminish sharply after the first twenty-four hours, whereas local muscle spasm and tenderness are more likely to persist. If perforation of the gallbladder occurs, a local abscess is usually formed and the local findings, including tenderness, pain and muscle spasm, will be much more pronounced.

The disease is perhaps encountered more frequently in a mild form with pain of less intensity and duration (two or three days) and accompanied by only slight fever. Such attacks commonly masquerade as acute dyspepsia or indigestion. It is difficult to decide whether such attacks should be classified as acute cholecystitis or exacerbations of chronic cholecystitis.

Differential Diagnosis.—The location of the pain in the right upper quadrant combined with the characteristics of the pain which is usually severe and sometimes cramplike in nature, will usually point to the correct diagnosis. Occasionally it may be confused with acute appendicitis when the appendix is retrocecal and high, but rarely does the tenderness of appendicitis localize itself so definitely in the right upper quadrant. Acute appendicitis is usually a disease of young people, whereas cholecystitis usually occurs in later adult life. Acute cholecystitis may be confused with perforated peptic ulcer, but the onset of the pain, etc., in the latter condition is apt to be more sudden, and associated with prostration and more generalized abdominal rigidity. Moreover, in perforated ulcer there may be a history of dyspepsia relieved temporarily by food or alkali. X-ray of the abdomen with the patient in a sitting position will rarely fail to reveal air under the diaphragm if perforation of an ulcer is present. Frequently the pain produced by acute pancreatitis is indistinguishable from that of acute cholecystitis, but is usually confined to the midline in the epigastrium or to the left upper quadrant (see p. 633). Patients with acute cholecystitis are apt to have a history of previous attacks of a similar character. The pain of acute cholecystitis is similar to renal colic except that the pain in the latter instance is apt to radiate downward even into the thigh or genital organs. Tenderness associated with renal colic is more apt to be acute posteriorly; examination of the urine rarely fails to reveal erythrocytes or pus cells; fever and leukocytosis are usually absent in nephrolithiasis. Occasionally the pain encountered

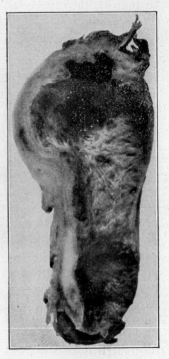

Fig. 379.—Subacute Cholecystitis.

Note the enormously thickened wall and the beginning perforation in the fundus. A large stone was present in the neck of the gallbladder.

in gastric crises associated with tabes dorsalis may be similar to that produced by acute cholecystitis. Muscle spasm and abdominal tenderness, however, are usually much less prominent. Moreover, fever and leukocytosis are absent in the gastric crises. Neurologic examination should reveal signs of tabes. Pain of cardiac origin occasionally simulates that of cholecystitis, but rarely indeed will a careful consideration of the manifestations fail to establish differentiation between these two diseases.

Treatment.—Previous to the past few years an attitude of conservatism had been adopted by practically all surgeons when dealing with acute cholecystitis.

Since acute peritonitis is rarely produced by perforation, conservatism is rarely detrimental in this respect. By waiting a few days the fever practically always disappears and the clinical signs diminish. After ten to fourteen days the inflammation about the gallbladder has usually subsided sufficiently to permit operative interference if that is indicated. However, if the symptoms do not subside in 24 to 48 hours, and particularly if there is an increase in such manifestations as pain, muscle spasm and fever, along with a rising leukocyte count, operation will be indicated on the assumption that a serious complication, such as gangrene or perforation, may be present, thereby demanding surgical relief. At operation cholecystostomy or cholecystectomy may be performed, depending upon the age of the patient and the condition of the gallbladder. If the gallbladder is so badly diseased and densely

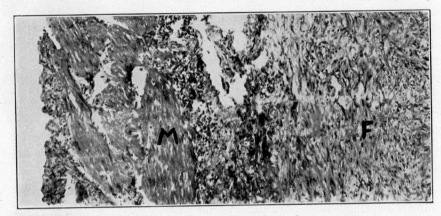

FIG. 380.—PHOTOMICROGRAPH OF SUBACUTE CHOLECYSTITIS.

Note that the mucosa has been eroded away and the submucosa is covered with exudate. The muscularis (M) is comparatively normal. Most of the thickness of the wall consists of fibrous tissue (F), only a part of which is shown.

adherent that removal will jeopardize the patient's life, it may be advisable to perform cholecystostomy. Frequently, operative interference will not be indicated, especially if the attack is the first one and is mild in character. Operation likewise may not be indicated in elderly patients who are poor operative risks. On account of the acute illness of the patient and associated hepatitis, it is usually necessary to institute preoperative restorative procedures such as intravenous administration of glucose, subcutaneous administration of physiologic saline, etc.

For the past several years some surgeons (H. F. Graham,[38] Zinninger[39] and others) have advocated immediate cholecystectomy in acute cholecystitis. There is now fairly complete agreement that if cholecystectomy is performed in the first twenty-four to thirty-six hours after the onset of the attack, removal of the organ will be simple, and postoperative reaction, including mortality, will not be serious. Moreover, immediate operation eliminates much discomfort during resolution of the acute attack, and shortens the period of disability.

Chronic Cholecystitis.—This is an extremely frequent condition, but on many occasions offers marked difficulty in diagnosis. There is sufficient difference in the manifestations, treatment and prognosis of patients with cholecystitis with or without stones that the two conditions are considered separately. Cholelithiasis is discussed later in this chapter.

Pathology.—Chronic cholecystitis may develop as a sequel to acute cholecystitis, but more frequently develops insidiously. The gallbladder wall, because of bacterial invasion or a chemical inflammation becomes thickened, largely because of the deposition of scar tissue. Adhesions in varying degree are found externally (pericholecystitis) and may involve the contiguous organs. If the cystic duct becomes obstructed because of adhesions or a stone in the cystic duct, a condition

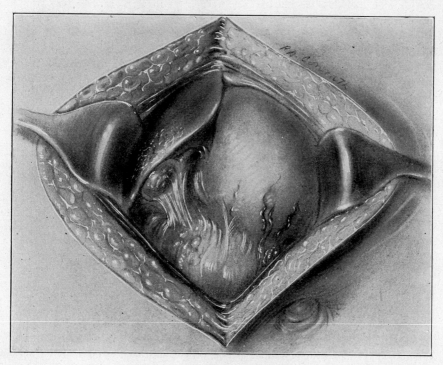

FIG. 381.—CHRONIC CHOLECYSTITIS.

Numerous adhesions to contiguous organs, particularly the omentum, may be noted. There is also a localized area of hepatitis on the superior surface of the liver, adjacent to the gallbladder.

known as *hydrops* may develop. The brownish green color fades because of destruction or absorption of bile pigment and the contents become colorless. The gallbladder becomes distended because of the secretion of mucus by the mucosa and may attain an enormous size, often becoming palpable as a smooth, only mildly tender mass in the upper abdomen. The contents of the gallbladder in such an instance is sterile and is known as *white bile* since the most important constituent is mucus excreted by the gallbladder, and because bile pigments are absent. If the contents become infected an empyma, as discussed previously, will result.

The function of the chronically inflamed gallbladder as determined by cholecystography may or may not be seriously impaired. It is quite probable that during the acute attack, the gallbladder function is lost, but when healing takes place, is to a great extent regained. Microscopically the wall is thickened by fibrous tissue and infiltrated by lymphocytes. Granulation tissue and plasma cells are abundant. The muscle and elastic tissue may be destroyed and replaced by fibrous tissue and fat cells. On rare occasions the wall of the gallbladder becomes calcified to such an extent that it may be demonstrable by x-ray.

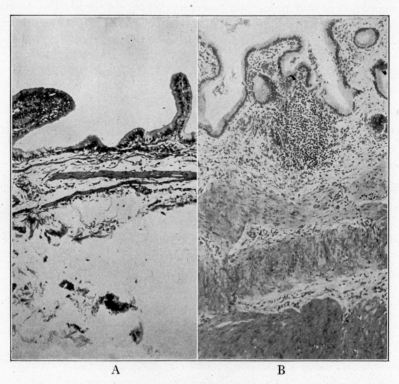

A   B

FIG. 382.—PHOTOMICROGRAPHS SHOWING CHRONIC CHOLECYSTITIS.

A, diffuse mild lymphocytic infiltration and only slight thickening of the wall; the mucosa is intact. *B*, the wall of this gallbladder is greatly thickened because of numerous attacks of subacute inflammation. Lymphocytic infiltration is more extensive than in *A*.

Frequently the gallbladder mucosa is the seat of polypoid enlargement of the villi. These villi contain yellowish deposits of cholesterol or cholesterol esters which are visible to the naked eye. The term *strawberry gallbladder* has been applied by MacCarty[40] to this condition, although it was probably first recognized by Moynihan.[41] The pathogenesis of this type of disease has been discussed by Elman and Graham,[42] and others. Years ago this lesion was considered a type of cholecystitis for which cholecystectomy was thought to be indicated. During recent years, however, there has been a growing tendency to consider the lesion of slight importance, for which cholecystectomy is not indicated unless stones are present.

Clinical Manifestations.—The presence or absence of stones influences the clinical picture as discussed later. One of the most common symptoms complained of in chronic cholecystitis is *dyspepsia,* which may include such symptoms as epigastric distress, flatulence, anorexia, belching, mild pain, etc. It must be emphasized, however, that innumerable diseases may produce dyspepsia; the presence of this group of symptoms alone is, therefore, only suggestive evidence of the presence of gall-bladder disease. Pain is of much more value in establishing the diagnosis. The pain usually varies in extent, occurring in mild cramp-like attacks which in reality may be due to transient acute inflammation and are localized in the right upper quadrant, but frequently radiate toward the tip of the scapula. Nausea is encountered frequently, but vomiting is uncommon except during severe attacks. Rarely is there any relation of the pain and discomfort to meals, except that fatty food is poorly

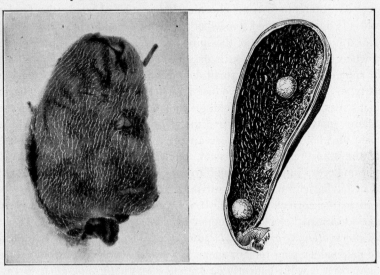

A   B

FIG. 383.—CHOLESTEROSIS OF THE GALLBLADDER.

A, without stones. *B,* with stones.

tolerated. Constipation is a frequent complaint. Fever and leukocytosis are rarely present. Jaundice, if present, is usually associated with a stone in the common duct except that mild jaundice is occasionally produced by an associated hepatitis. Occasionally, patients with chronic cholecystitis have dyspepsia of more or less constant severity without attacks of severe pain. Such a clinical picture, however, offers great diagnostic difficulty since it is produced by so many other diseases.

Examination of the abdomen reveals tenderness over the right upper quadrant, the intensity of which varies with the severity of the disease. Frequently the infection subsides to such an extent that the patient will be free from symptoms or signs for months at a time only to have them recur. Tenderness under the right costal margin (over the liver edge) may be present and is a manifestation of the associated hepatitis (Graham).

Evidence has been presented (Alvarez, Necheles and associates [43]) to suggest that allergy may affect the gallbladder. Whether or not it is a true allergy cannot be determined, but it is definitely known that certain foods such as chocolate, bananas, etc., may initiate attacks of severe right upper quadrant pain.

Differential Diagnosis.—It may be extremely difficult to differentiate chronic cholecystitis from peptic ulcer but symptoms of the former disease are rarely related to meals, whereas in peptic ulcer there is usually a history that discomfort occurs two or three hours after meals and is relieved by eating or ingestion of alkali. The most reliable method of distinguishing peptic ulcer from cholecystitis is by x-ray, especially cholecystography and the barium meal. The two diseases frequently occur together. Recurring attacks of mild acute appendicitis may simulate chronic cholecystitis if the appendix is adherent high in the abdominal cavity. However, appendicitis is rarely associated with dyspepsia; pain and tenderness are the chief manifestations. Spastic colitis associated with constipation is perhaps the most difficult disease to differentiate from chronic cholecystitis. Usually the tenderness in spastic colitis is diffuse, limited somewhat to the colon, and not localized to the right upper quadrant. Osteo-arthritis of the spine is commonly confused with cholecystitis, and even when the latter condition is present the most annoying symptoms may be due to the spinal lesion. At times, small diaphragmatic hernias (particularly those of the hiatus type, see p. 800) will produce a variety of digestive symptoms including epigastric distress, bloating and belching so commonly observed in cholecystitis. Intestinal allergy may likewise simulate the manifestations of chronic cholecystitis, but the pain and tenderness are more apt to be diffuse. On rare occasions tuberculosis of the spine may produce pain, tenderness, etc., in the upper quadrant. This condition occurs just often enough to demand inspection of the spine in patients suspected of having chronic cholecystitis. In all these conditions, cholecystography should lead to the correct diagnosis. It should be emphasized, however, that the demonstration of a pathologic gallbladder by cholecystography *does not necessarily mean that the symptoms are of cholecystic origin,* inasmuch as it is known that a pathologic gallbladder may remain silent for years. Moreover, chronic cholecystitis is so common that it will frequently *be present along with some other disease which may be producing the symptoms,* and be of much more importance than the gallbladder disease. Duodenal drainage, with study of the centrifuged sediment, is of real diagnostic value. The finding of cholesterol crystals, calcium bilirubin, bile pigment particles, and pus cells is positive evidence of gallstones and bladder pathology, and by some surgeons is considered more valuable than cholecystography.

Treatment.—There is little to offer the patient with chronic cholecystitis other than surgical procedures (cholecystectomy and, rarely, cholecystostomy), except that occasionally changes in the diet, such as elimination of fatty food, will be helpful. It should be emphasized, however, that operation should not be recommended unless the diagnosis is definite and symptoms, especially pain, are sufficient for the patient to demand relief. It has been emphasized recently (Graham and Mackey [44]) that relief frequently does not follow cholecystectomy in the absence of stones and other gross pathologic lesions, particularly when symptoms are not typical of those commonly found in chronic cholecystitis.

Cholecystectomy is much to be preferred over cholecystostomy because of the great tendency for the latter to be followed by recurrence of symptoms at a later date. The *operation* for removal of the gallbladder is associated with certain technical pitfalls which, if not avoided, will lead to deleterious sequelae. During the procedure of cholecystectomy, extreme care must be exercised in the identification of the cystic and common duct lest the latter structure be injured. Such a tragedy is avoided by careful dissection at the neck of the gallbladder which will facilitate identification of the ducts and thereby minimize the possibility of inflicting injury upon them. The carefully isolated cystic duct is clamped, cut, and the stump ligated. Identification of the cystic artery will also enable its ligation so that removal of the gallbladder from below upward may then be performed with little or no bleeding. Most surgeons insert a rubber dam drain down to the stump of the cystic duct, if drainage is slight; it is usually removed in forty-eight hours. Cholecystectomy is apt to produce more postoperative discomfort (gas pains, etc.) than most other types of abdominal operations. For this reason adequate amounts of morphine or similar hypnotic should be given during the first two or three days. If nausea or

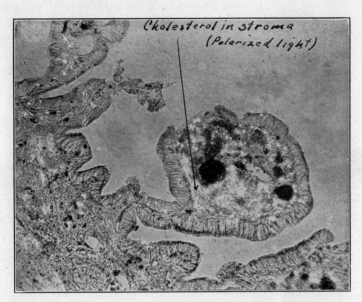

Fig. 384.—Photomicrograph of Gallbladder with Cholesterosis to Illustrate One of the Possible Mechanisms in the Formation of Gallstones.

The section was made from unfixed frozen tissue and is unstained, but is viewed under polarized light for determination of the presence of cholesterol; the white material in the enlarged villus is cholesterol. It seems logical to assume that the large cholesterol containing villus might be detached by rupture of the stalk, and become the nucleus of a gallstone.

vomiting is present to a significant degree, gastric lavage is indicated and will be effective in relieving distress and preventing gastric dilatation. In biliary operations on aged individuals, particularly if jaundice is present, transfusions minimize the danger of shock and other circulatory accidents. The use of vitamin K in operations for obstructive jaundice is discussed on page 610.

Poor results following cholecystectomy may be attributed to such factors as error in diagnosis, overlooked stones in the common duct, pancreatitis, technical errors at operation, biliary dyskinesia,[45] etc. By the latter term is meant spasm of the common duct sphincter (Westphal, Walters et al); the term postcholecystectomy syndrome is often used.[62]

Cholelithiasis.—Gallstones nearly always contain cholesterol; many also contain calcium and bile pigments. They may be solitary or multiple. They vary in shape from the round single stone to the faceted multiple stones. Occasionally the surface is nodular (mulberry stones). Numerous factors, as recently summarized by Phemister and associates,[46] including (1) obstruction, (2) infection, (3) reflux of pancreatic or duodenal secretions, (4) altered cholesterol metabolism, (5) increased bile pigment (in hemolytic icterus), (6) over-concentration of bile acids with resultant injury to the gallbladder wall, and (7) reduction in the ratio of cholesterol to fatty acids or bile acids by absorption of bile salts through a damaged gallbladder wall with partial obstruction of the cystic duct (Andrews [47]) are important in the formation of gallstones. Attention should be directed to the importance of formation of cholesterol stones by altered cholesterol metabolism, as indicated by the high incidence of cholesterol stones in the absence of gallbladder disease. On the contrary, calcium carbonate stones are almost always found in gallbladders with a diseased wall and associated with a complete or high grade obstruction of the cystic duct (Phemister and associates [48]).

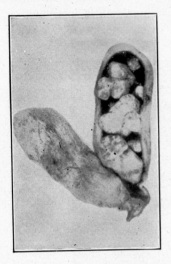

FIG. 385.—CHOLELITHIASIS.

The stones in this instance completely filled the gallbladder.

About 50 per cent of the gallbladders removed surgically throughout the country contain stones. Autopsy statistics, including deaths from all causes, show an incidence as high as 25 per cent in persons past the age of 45. They occur in women about three times as often as in men. Multiple pregnancies and obesity are strongly predisposing factors. Cholecystitis caused by the typhoid bacillus may be encountered with or without stones.

The *clinical manifestations* produced by biliary calculi vary tremendously. On many occasions the patient may carry gallstones in his gallbladder the greater part of his life without experiencing any symptoms whatever. On the other hand, symptoms may develop as soon as the stones are formed and provoke a wide variety of clinical manifestations.

The clinical picture produced by gallstones *depends on their location*. When in the *gallbladder,* stones frequently are silent or cause only mild symptoms of dyspepsia. As a rule, however, the pain associated with stones in the gallbladder is more severe and more apt to occur in attacks than it is in chronic cholecystitis without stones. When a stone becomes lodged in the *cystic duct* the pain is usually severe; the clinical picture produced by this condition is frequently spoken of as biliary colic. The origin of the pain is uncertain but may be associated with such factors as spasm or contraction of the gallbladder, by distention of the duct, or by the inflammation associated with the stone. The pain is apt to occur in paroxysms with tenderness and pain remaining in the intermissions. These attacks are apt to last for several days, but unlike stone in the common duct are not associated with jaundice, except when a coexisting hepatitis is present. If the obstruction to the cystic duct does not subside, the gallbladder distends and its contents become colorless (white bile) because of the disappearance of the bile pigment (hydrops of the gallbladder). If the contents of a hydrops become infected, empyema of the gall-bladder results.

When the stones are located in the *common duct* a different clinical picture manifests itself, although stones may occasionally be present and produce very few manifestations. Usually, however, the common duct at the sphincter of Oddi becomes occluded by the stone; more severe manifestations then develop. An intermittent colicky pain in the epigastrium or right upper quadrant is usually present. At the onset of obstruction, nausea and vomiting may occur. Within thirty-six to forty-eight hours gross jaundice will appear. The skin and mucous membranes become yellow, and bile pigment appears in the urine. The stools will be

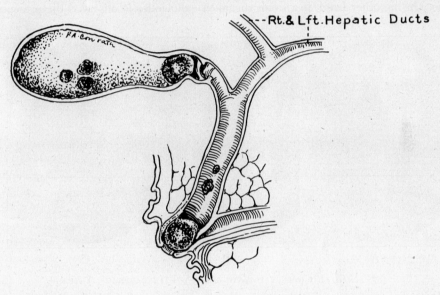

FIG. 386.—DRAWING TO ILLUSTRATE THE COMMON LOCATIONS OF GALLSTONES IN THE BILIARY SYSTEM.

Impaction in the cystic and common duct as depicted in the illustration is quite common.

clay-colored because of their lack of bile pigment. The amount of fever is dependent largely upon the amount of associated infection in the common duct, gallbladder and liver, and will be accompanied by the usual febrile manifestations. Occasionally the fever is of the intermittent type (Charcot's hepatic fever) produced supposedly by the ball valve action of the stone on the sphincter of Oddi. If the stone becomes dislodged or the associated infection and edema subside, jaundice diminishes or disappears. On rare occasions the stone may be passed. Dilatation of the common duct may be sufficient to allow reëstablishment of the flow of bile into the intestine around the stone. If the infection spreads by traveling up the bile ducts (cholangitis) chills may be encountered. Occasionally the infection leads to the accumulation of pus in the common duct above the stone. If the obstruction is complete (without infection) and of sufficient duration the bile pigments disappear, and mucus (white bile) secreted by the wall of the duct accumulates within its lumen. This is indicative of at least a partial suppression of bile formation and is usually considered a serious sign as far as prognosis is concerned. In spite of the fact that obstruction by stone in the common duct causes a retention of bile in the biliary tree, the gall-bladder is rarely dilated. This is due in part at least to the fact that the infection in the wall of the gallbladder has resulted in the deposit of so much fibrous tissue that distention is impossible. With obstruction of other kinds, however, including carcinoma of the pancreas, etc., distention of the gallbladder usually occurs. This phenomenon is known as *Courvoisier's law.* The practical value of this law lies in the diagnostic aid it affords during the course of a laparotomy performed on a jaundiced patient. If the surgeon observes a large dilated gallbladder, a diagnosis of extrahepatic biliary obstruction (*e.g.,* carcinoma of the head of the pancreas) is made. On the other hand, if a small shrunken gallbladder is observed the presence

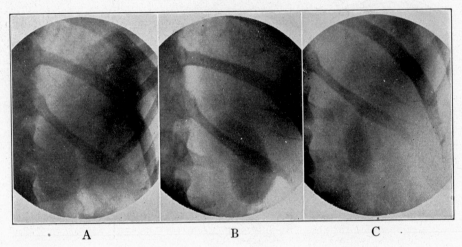

A   B   C

FIG. 387.—NORMAL CHOLECYSTOGRAM AFTER THE INTRAVENOUS TECHNIC.

A, four hours after administration of the dye; *B,* eight hours after injection. Note that the shadow is denser; *C,* twenty-four hours after injection, the shadow is fainter and much smaller, indicating contraction and emptying of the gallbladder. The shadow of a normal gallbladder may or may not persist through twenty-four hours.

of a primary gallbladder disease, with or without stones, is indicated. In the absence of jaundice, a dilated gallbladder indicates obstruction of the cystic duct, and as discussed on page 617, is spoken of as hydrops of the gallbladder.

Treatment of cholelithiasis does not differ from cholecystitis except when stones are present in the common duct. The presence of stones in the common duct will usually be manifested by the presence or at least a history of jaundice, and by finding dilatation of the common duct at operation; such circumstances will demand additional operative work. Incision must be made in the choledochus, the interior explored, the stones removed and a T-tube sewed in the common duct for drainage of bile (choledochostomy). Thus a biliary fistula is produced (see below). In these patients it is usually necessary to institute special preoperative preparations such as bed rest, high carbohydrate and fluid intake, etc. (as on page 610). Extreme precaution must be taken against hemorrhage during and after operative procedures in the presence of jaundice since such patients frequently have a delayed coagulation time of the blood. Administration of vitamin K with bile salts, intravenous glucose and transfusions are effective in treatment. (See also p. 610.)

Cholecystectomy in patients with gallstones is also indicated as a means of preventing carcinoma of the gallbladder (Graham [49]).

Biliary Fistula.—As mentioned above, a biliary fistula is purposely produced after the common duct is opened for exploration and the removal of stones. Ordinarily such a fistula is of short duration, the T-tube being removed in two or three weeks. Drainage of bile through the resulting sinus tract may continue for a few days, after which time it closes spontaneously; closure is accompanied by a gradually increasing amount of pigment in the stool which changes from an acholic to a pigmented character.

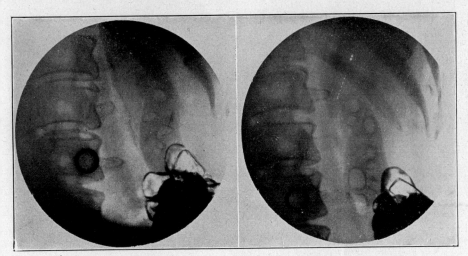

Fig. 388.—Cholecystograms Fourteen and Eighteen Hours after Oral Administration of the Dye, Showing Negative Filling Defects of Cholesterol ("Soft") Stones.

The film taken before cholecystography revealed no evidence of the stones. Note that the density of the shadow in the films is only slightly impaired, indicating that the concentrating function of the gallbladder is practically normal, although the stones were responsible for numerous attacks of gallbladder colic. The dense shadow in lower right hand corner of the films is the hepatic flexure of the colon, filled with barium and gas.

Persistent drainage of bile for more than several weeks is usually indicative of an obstruction in the common duct distal to the opening made at operation. Injection of radiopaque substances such as hippuran or lipiodol into the tract will allow visualization of the larger bile ducts by x-ray. The obstruction can readily be demonstrated by this procedure (cholangiogram); if produced by a stone left in the common duct, the stone can usually be visualized. Regardless of the cause of the persistent obstruction, a secondary operation will usually be indicated.

Persistent loss of bile is poorly tolerated by all patients, particularly in males of advanced age. An important symptom is a severe degree of anorexia which may be so marked as to create a positive loathing for food. Rapid loss of weight occurs. There is often a tendency toward spontaneous bleeding due to vitamin K deficiency; the mechanism is the same as in jaundice (see p. 606). Treatment is difficult but the symptoms rapidly improve as soon as bile flow into the intestine becomes reëstablished. Bile by mouth may be effective; but it induces a further loss of bile since it is a cholagogue. If the fistula does not close in a few weeks operation will be indicated to relieve the obstruction. Preoperative preparation including administration of vitamin K, etc., as previously described will be necessary.

A spontaneous biliary fistula is rare but may occur if the gallbladder becomes adherent to the abdominal wall and ruptures to the outside. Rare, also, is rupture of the gallbladder or a large bile duct (usually by abscess formation) through the

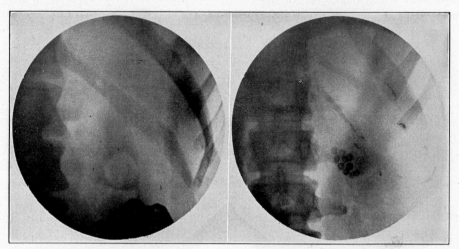

FIG. 389.   FIG. 390.

FIG. 389.—X-ray Showing Gallbladder with Faint Shadow following Oral Cholecystography, and Revealing a Huge Single Negative Filling Defect, Indicating the Presence of a Large Cholesterol Stone.

The stone was not visible in the film taken before ingestion of the dye.

FIG. 390.—X-ray Showing Gallbladder with Faint Shadow following Oral Cholecystography, and Revealing Several Small "Positive" Shadows.

These stones, which contain a large amount of calcium, were visible in the "plain" film taken before the cholecystogram.

diaphragm into the lung and bronchus, thereby producing a bronchobiliary fistula, which is characterized by the expectoration of bile-stained sputum.

Cholecystography.—Cholecystography refers to the visualization of the gallbladder in an x-ray film following the administration to the patient of a radiopaque substance which is carried in the bile to the lumen of the gallbladder, and is concentrated there in sufficient amount to cast a shadow on the x-ray film. This diagnostic procedure was discovered in 1924 by Graham and Cole.[50] A substance capable of fulfilling such requirements must have two prerequisites, namely, be excreted primarily by the liver and contain elements of sufficient atomic weight (*e.g.,* iodine) to be impervious to the x-ray. In individuals with a normal gallbladder, a shadow of the organ is obtained within a few hours after oral or intravenous administration of the contrast medium. Before the advent of cholecystography there was no direct clinical method of gaining objective information as to the presence of abnormal changes in the gallbladder; only rarely did a flat x-ray film reveal diseased conditions (calcified gallbladder, calcified stones); the drainage of gallbladder bile through a duodenal catheter (Lyon's test) yields but indirect evidence of disease and often gives equivocal findings.

Production of a dense shadow of the gallbladder (which usually reveals a change in size on successive films) is indicative of a normal gallbladder. Absence of shadow and evidence of stones within the gallbladder shadow (as produced by the dye) are extremely reliable indications of a pathologic gallbladder. It is de-

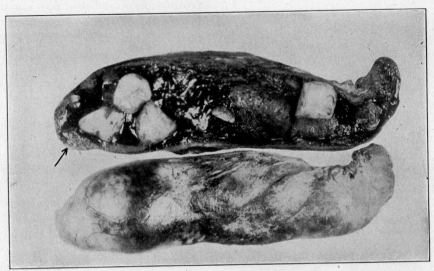

Fig. 391.—Carcinoma of the Gallbladder.

The organ contained stones, and, as is likewise common in carcinoma of the gallbladder, considerable inspissated bile and mucus. The patient had symptoms typical of chronic cholecystitis. Although longitudinal section of the gallbladder revealed an unusual thickening at the fundus, as indicated by the arrow, the presence of the carcinoma was not evident until the microscopic section was obtained. In spite of the performance of a cholecystectomy in this early stage, the patient returned eighteen months later with a metastasis in the liver, thereby illustrating the extremely invasive character of carcinoma of the gallbladder.

sirable, however, to obtain a preliminary open film of the gallbladder region, because putty-like material or calcium deposited in the wall may cast a shadow which resembles a normal gallbladder but is not due to administration of dye. One of the most serious pitfalls in cholecystography occurs because asymptomatic cholecystitis is frequent and that clinicians, on finding cholecystographic evidence of a diseased gallbladder, may cease searching for other diseases such as carcinoma of the colon, etc., and thus overlook the lesion which may in reality be producing symptoms.

Nonvisualization of the gallbladder after cholecystography may mean that the concentrating power of the gallbladder has been lost or that an obstruction at the cystic duct is present. If a shadow of the gallbladder is obtained, stones will show up as "negative" or "positive" defects in the films, i.e., cholesterol stones displace dye and produce negative shadows, whereas hard calcium stones show up as areas of increased density, which are spoken of as "positive" shadows. A distortion of the gallbladder shadow, which is consistent in more than one film is indicative of adhesions (pericholecystitis). It should be emphasized, however, that the dye must be excreted by the liver before it can enter the gallbladder; the presence of jaundice interferes markedly with the production of a gallbladder shadow, because of numerous factors such as inability of the liver to excrete the dye, edema of the gallbladder wall, etc.

At the present time tetraiodophenolphthalein and its isomer phenoltetraiodophthalein are used in the performance of this test. If a simultaneous estimation of liver function is to be made the latter substance must be used (intravenously) since

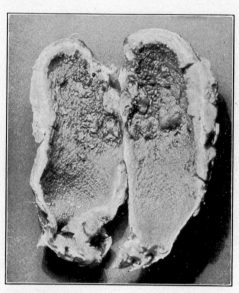

FIG. 392.—ADENOMA OF THE GALLBLADDER IN THE PRESENCE OF CHRONIC CHOLECYSTITIS.

This tumor is flat and large, in contrast to the pedunculated type of tumor which is much smaller, and in reality only hypertrophied villi.

tetraiodophenolphthalein does not stain blood serum. Either of these substances may be given orally or intravenously except that if estimation of hepatic function is desired the intravenous method must be employed. The oral dose of tetraiodophenolphthalein is 4 to 5 grams and the intravenous dose 3 to 3.5 grams. Because of its apparent rapidity of excretion the dose of the isomeric compound phenoltetraiodophthalein may be reduced 30 per cent from that of tetraiodophenolphthalein. In doubtful cases a "double" dose (several hours apart orally) may increase the accuracy of the test.

For purposes of cholecystography x-ray pictures are taken on two or three occasions following the administration of the dye (four, eight and twenty-four hours after intravenous and twelve, eighteen and twenty-two hours after oral administration). The oral method is used more extensively now than the intravenous and is about as accurate as long as certain pitfalls such as vomiting, lack of absorption, etc., are kept in mind. Diagnosis is based upon intensity of the shadow, its shape, mottling, etc., as mentioned above. Many roentgenologists utilize the "fat meal" as suggested by the experimental work of Boyden[51] and Whitaker[52] for the diagnostic aid afforded by its effect on the gallbladder shadow. The normal gallbladder empties almost completely within two or three hours following a meal consisting particularly of egg yolks, cream and butter. When a gallbladder shadow is obtained the meal may be given to determine the distensibility and rate of emptying of the gallbladder.

Tumors of the Gallbladder.—*Primary carcinoma* of the gallbladder is the most common of these tumors and constitutes about 5 or 6 per cent of all cases of carcinoma. Carcinoma of the gallbladder rarely occurs without the presence of stones in the organ. The relative frequency of carcinoma compared to cholelithiasis varies in different clinics, but on the average 2 to 6 per cent of all patients proved to have stones in the gallbladder by operation or autopsy have associated carcinoma of that organ. Unfortunately, carcinoma of the gallbladder may develop insidiously. The symptoms may occur late and be insignificant; they resemble those discussed under chronic cholecystitis. In the early stages of the disease pain is usually slight, but may be very troublesome later on. The diagnosis is rarely made before operation. If the disease is found to be local at the time of operation the gallbladder obviously should be removed (see Fig. 391). The tumor is so invasive that even though it is early and small, cholecystectomy is rarely curative.

Small *benign papillomas* which consist in reality of hyperplasia of the villi are rather common. Papillomatous structures due to deposition of cholesterol have already been mentioned. Other tumors such as adenoma and sarcoma do occur, but only on rare occasions. True adenomas have very little clinical importance.

THE BILE DUCTS

Inflammation of the intrahepatic bile ducts (cholangitis) is common and has already been discussed. Infection of this type may also affect the extrahepatic bile ducts, especially when a stone is impacted in the common duct. On such occasions white bile and even pus may be found in the choledochus at operation. *Strictures* are not uncommon and may occur either in the ductus choledochus or the common hepatic duct, usually the former. They may be infectious or traumatic in origin. Probably the most common etiologic factor is accidental injury during operative procedures upon the biliary tract. The stasis of bile created by the obstruction encourages infection and symptoms are apt to occur in attacks consisting of chills, fever, jaundice, pain, malaise, etc. The only hope for relief lies in surgical therapy. Such procedures as resection of the stricture with anastomosis around a Vitallium tube (Pearse [79]), or implantation of the end of the duct just proximal to the stricture into the stomach or duodenum, are satisfactory methods of repair. Not infrequently no remnants of the common duct can be found. In such instances it will be necessary to anastomose the stump of the hepatic duct at the hilus of the liver to a loop of jejunum around a Vitallium tube. Results with this type of repair have been brought to a fairly satisfactory level by the use of the Vitallium tube. Rubber tubes previously used were usually passed, and a stricture with renewal of symptoms such as pain, chills, and fever (caused by cholangitis) would develop a few months later.

On rare occasions such tumors as *carcinoma,* adenoma, polyp, etc., may be primary in the ducts. Of this group, carcinoma of the ampulla of Vater is perhaps the most common. The symptoms produced by such tumors are similar to those observed in carcinoma of the pancreas (as described later). Cysts of the common duct are extremely rare and usually are congenital in origin.

PANCREAS

The pancreas is one of the smallest and most deeply placed of the abdominal viscera. Lying transversely in the epigastrium, it extends from the curve of the first part of the duodenum to which it is firmly attached and through whose wall its two ducts penetrate, to the hilus of the spleen; it crosses the bodies of the twelfth thoracic and first lumbar vertebrae. It is entirely retroperitoneal, the anterior surface forming part of the posterior wall of the lesser peritoneal sac. Topographically its axis is represented by an oblique horizontal line halfway between the xiphoid and umbilicus. Most of the organ is located to the left of the midline, but its thickest part, the head, lies to the right. Important is its relation to the common bile duct which, on passing through pancreatic parenchyma to the duodenum, can be easily compressed through edema or neoplasm of the head of the pancreas. Another clinically important anatomical feature is the fact that the common bile duct and the main pancreatic duct terminate in the duodenum through a common ampulla at the sphincter of Oddi in a certain proportion of cases. In about one-half of normal

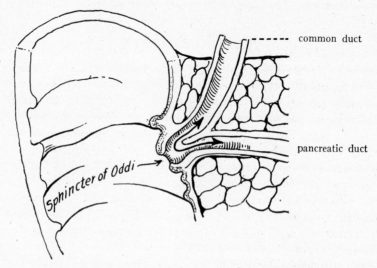

common duct

pancreatic duct

Sphincter of Oddi →

FIG. 393.—DIAGRAM OF THE RELATIONSHIP BETWEEN THE COMMON BILE DUCT AND PANCREATIC DUCT, FOUND NORMALLY IN ONE-HALF OF ADULT HUMANS.

Note the free communication between the two lumina. Note also the lower end of the common duct which is completely surrounded by pancreatic parenchyma, thus permitting a biliary obstruction by inflammation or neoplasm in the pancreas at this point.

individuals the common sphincter can, when it is closed, convert the bile and pancreatic ducts into a common channel so that bile can flow into the pancreatic duct or pancreatic juice into the common duct. However, the chance of such an intercommunication between the two ducts being produced by a stone impacted in the ampulla is much more remote because the septum between the termination of the two ducts will prevent it, even with a tiny stone, except in 3 to 5 per cent of normal individuals (Mann and Giordano[53]). The significance of this anatomic relationship concerns the possibility of regurgitation of bile into the pancreatic duct which has a possible bearing on the pathogenesis of acute pancreatitis as is discussed later.

Physiologically the pancreas plays a double role, endocrine and secretory; these functions are concerned with carbohydrate metabolism and digestion, respectively. Its endocrine function is concerned with the production of insulin which is formed n the islets of Langerhans. Besides its surgical considerations in diabetes, the islets have become of recent importance to the surgeon because of the occurrence of umor (*adenoma of the pancreas*), which produces manifestations of hypoglycemia (see Chapter XXX). The external secretion is produced by the acinar tissue and is a clear alkaline fluid which neutralizes gastric acidity and contains three ferments, ipase, amylase and trypsin. The latter is in an inactive form (trypsinogen) but is activated normally as the secretion pours into the duodenum by enterokinase, a substance present in and produced by the duodenal mucosa. Being a proteolytic ferment trypsin plays a large role in the pathogensis of acute pancreatic necrosis (see p. 633). Of the two functions of the pancreas the endocrine one is essential for life. There is evidence to show that a substitute for the pancreatic juice may, if necessary, be manufactured by other digestive glands (succus entericus) in the duodenum, especially by Brünner's glands. Thus the suppression of pancreatic juice may result only in temporary digestive difficulty. The development of frequent fatty, bulky, grayish stools is supposed to be due to interference with normal secretion and is called pancreatogenous diarrhea. Of surgical importance are the inflammatory lesions, carcinoma, and cyst of the pancreas. The reader is referred to the excellent monograph of Brunschwig [54] and to a series of yearly reviews [80].

Pancreatic Function Tests.—Attempts have been made for decades to measure the external secretory function of the pancreas, largely as an aid in the diagnosis of diseases affecting the acinar tissue. A detailed description of these various tests, most of them now largely of historical interest only, will be found in another publication [55]. Although a fairly extensive study of pancreatic ferments in the duodenal contents, urine and feces has been made, there is perhaps more advantage in studying the blood itself. Thus, blood is always available, is sterile, of a more or less constant reaction and composition; blood moreover reflects changes in pancreatic secretion almost at once, unlike the urine and feces which require hours and days respectively. Of the three enzymes in the pancreatic juice, lipase and amylase have been studied most; of these the latter has received the greatest attention.

Serum amylase may be measured quantitatively by one of three methods. The oldest one is based on the starch-iodine reaction and is usually associated with the name of Wohlgemuth. The second method depends upon the amount of sugar produced during a given period of time when a starch suspension is acted upon by the amylase present in a specimen of the patient's serum. Obviously the more amylase present, the more sugar will be created from the starch. This method (as modified by Somogyi *) is perhaps the simplest to perform as a routine in most laboratories.

---

* A colloidal suspension of 1½ per cent washed (C.P.) corn starch is prepared as a starch solution which if sterile keeps fairly well; the formation of molds makes it unsuitable. To 5 c.c. of this suspension, 1 c.c. of the patient's plasma or serum and 2 c.c. of 1 per cent sodium chloride is added, and the mixture incubated for thirty minutes at 40° C. Then 1 c.c. of 5 per cent $CuSO_4$ is added immediately, the mixture is shaken and 1 c.c. of 7 per cent sodium tungstate is added; the mixture is again shaken and filtered. Sugar determination is made on 5 c.c. of the filtrate. From the total amount of sugar formed by the hydrolysis of the starch, is subtracted the amount of sugar present in 1 c.c. of the patient's serum. The result is expressed in milligrams of sugar per 100 c.c. of blood. Normally 70 to 200 milligrams of sugar will be produced by 100 c.c. of blood serum in this way. At the height of an acute pancreatic obstruction or inflammation this value may reach a figure as high as 3000 milligrams (*i.e.*, milligrams per 100 c.c. of blood).

A third method utilizes the measurement of the viscosity of a colloidal starch solution; as the starch is acted upon by the amylase-containing serum the viscosity falls progressively. For the determination of high amylase values any of these three methods are adaptable.

The value of blood amylase determinations in the diagnosis of acute pancreatic disease has been indicated in a number of studies by various observers. Thus in pancreatic cyst, in acute pancreatic necrosis, and in acute pancreatitis without necrosis it has been found to be many times the normal value. It should be emphasized, however, that the level of blood amylase depends to a great extent on the stage of the pancreatic disease. When transient inflammation (or obstruction to the duct) occurs, the blood amylase will be high only at the height of the attack,

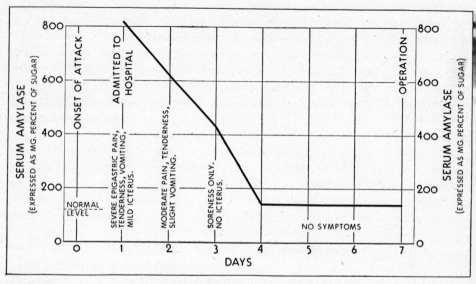

Fig. 394.—Acute Interstitial Pancreatitis: Curve Showing the Fall of Blood Amylase from the High Level as Attack Subsides.

The patient, an obese 50-year-old housewife, had had previous attacks similar in nature to the present one which had been diagnosed as biliary colic. At operation the gallbladder was full of stones and was removed; the pancreas was swollen, indurated, and exhibited a few areas of fat necrosis, which is seen, but not as commonly in this type as it is in pancreatic necrosis. A biopsy showed the inflammatory changes shown in Fig. 396, page 636. Recovery was uneventful.

and rapidly subsides with the resolution of the acute process. Thus, a determination of blood amylase at a time when the patient is suffering no acute symptoms will probably reveal a normal value and give no indication of the true nature of the disease.

Ordinarily the rise in blood amylase is caused by primary inflammation of the pancreas, but on certain occasions passage of gallstones through the sphincter of Oddi may compress the pancreatic duct (see Fig 393) and give rise to retention (vascular as well as parenchymal) of amylase through obstruction primarily.

As a negative test, the measurement of serum amylase may also be of value, particularly when acute pancreatic necrosis is suspected, a condition which demands operative treatment. This is particularly important if the acute upper abdominal pain is actually due to coronary disease. In such a case, a normal blood amylase, obtained while the patient is having acute symptoms, will rule out the possibility of pancreatic disease; this will obviously greatly simplify the problem of therapy and thus avoid the likelihood of an ill-advised operation which, of course, is apt to be fatal.

Acute Pancreatic Necrosis (Acute Hemorrhagic Pancreatitis).—The general term "acute pancreatitis" is often loosely used to indicate acute necrosis of the pancreas. In reality, there are two different types of acute inflammation, one of which is accompanied by necrosis and hemorrhage, whereas the other is designated as acute interstitial pancreatitis (see p. 635). While the two types may represent merely different degrees of severity of the same disease, the pathologic changes and treatment are quite different; there is considerable practical clinical importance in considering them separately, particularly because the manifestations of the hemorrhagic type are more fulminating than the interstitial type.

Acute pancreatic necrosis is really a rare disease, for, though often fatal, it comprises but 0.2 per cent of the deaths in a large series of routine autopsies (Moench [56]). It is a most remarkable lesion since it represents an autodigestion of living tissue by its own secretions. This is apparent from the degeneration and gangrene which involves the pancreas in these cases; hemorrhage into the gland is diffuse and often profuse. Blood-tinged fluid accumulates in the peritoneal cavity. Suppuration may be found later and if the disease lasts long enough sloughing of the organ may occur. Microscopically, a diffuse necrosis of cells with a widespread infiltration of polymorphonuclear cells is found. The disease can be produced experimentally by injecting a variety of substances into the pancreatic duct under pressure. Infection is assumed to play a role; obstruction to the outflow of the secretion would seem to be obviously necessary. The flow of bile into the pancreas from the common duct due to an impacted stone in the ampulla of Vater (Opie [57]) or to a spasm of the common sphincter (Archibald [58]) is a popular etiologic theory. While bile may undoubtedly provoke inflammation of the pancreas, there is no evidence that it can activate the harmless trypsinogen, a change which is essential before digestion of the tissue can occur. The mechanism of this activation within the gland is not clearly understood. Once trypsin is set free the other pathologic changes are relatively easy to explain. The digestion of the tissue leads to necrosis and eventually to suppuration; the digestion of blood vessels leads to hemorrhage and the digestion of fat leads to another feature of the disease, *i.e.,* multiple fat necrosis which is manifested as tiny white lentiform areas, throughout the great omentum and elsewhere, but especially marked in the neighborhood of the pancreas. It is, however, of some significance to note that fat necrosis is often seen when no sign of digestion of the pancreas is present; indeed fat necrosis may be produced experimentally by obstruction of the pancreatic ducts (Opie). It has been shown by Neal and Ellis [59] that lipase alone is able to produce this lesion. Not only is the reason for the activation of the trypsinogen unexplained, but also the ability of the activated juice to digest living tissue within the pancreas when it never does so in the duodenum or elsewhere. An important feature of the pathology of this disease is the frequent association of gallbladder disease. What significance this has in the pathogenesis is still a matter of speculation and theory.

Besides these local tissue changes which may extend beyond the neighborhood of the pancreas, are the systemic results which follow absorption of the split protein products or of the trypsin itself. The development of circulatory shock is supposedly due to this absorption (peptone shock).

The *clinical manifestations* of a typical case of acute pancreatic necrosis are dramatic. Suddenly, often after a full meal, the patient, previously well, is seized

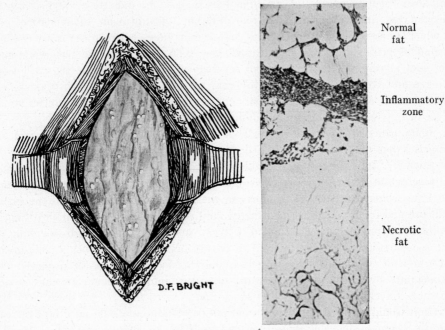

Normal fat

Inflammatory zone

Necrotic fat

D.F. BRIGHT

FIG. 395.—FAT NECROSIS DUE TO ACUTE HEMORRHAGIC PANCREATITIS.

In this disease the characteristic whitish areas are usually widespread and are often found, as indicated in the sketch, in the omentum, thus revealing their presence as soon as the abdomen is opened. Similar areas of fat necrosis are sometimes found in acute interstitial pancreatitis but in this disease the lesion is confined to the pancreas and is noted only if the organ is exposed to inspection. The photomicrograph is from an area of fat necrosis removed at operation; note the zone of inflammatory cells between the normal and necrotic fat.

with most excruciating pain in the epigastrium which radiates to the back, often to the left side and sometimes to the space between the shoulder blades. This is usually followed by vomiting. Severe prostration occurs and evidence of circulatory collapse develops rapidly; the extremities of the patient are cold, there is evident sweating, the color is a peculiar gray cyanosis, the pulse is rapid and weak, blood pressure low and temperature subnormal. Death may occur in twenty-four hours in spite of any form of treatment. In less severe cases the progress may be less rapid and remissions may occur. Jaundice is not often evident clinically, but an elevated icteric index of the blood is found (hyperbilirubinemia). The abdomen is moderately and diffusely distended and tender everywhere, but especially over the epigastrium in the region of the pancreas. There may be a zone of hyperesthesia over the left upper abdomen. Leukocytosis is present in most cases and may be high though not infrequently absent. Examination of the blood for amylase will in nearly all cases yield a high value which is of considerable diagnostic value, as already discussed.

Important in the *differential diagnosis* are lesions which do not require emergency operation. Prominent among these are biliary colic and acute interstitial pancreatitis as discussed presently. Important is coronary occlusion, the pain of which is not infrequently referred to the epigastrium; operation during an acute attack of coronary disease is apt to be fatal. A cardiac lesion is to be suspected when dyspnea, orthopnea, and frank cyanosis are present. The blood amylase as already discussed (p. 631) is normal in this and other acute abdominal diseases not involving the pancreas. If intestinal obstruction, perforated ulcer or acute appendicitis is suspected the error is not so serious, since operation in these diseases is also indicated. However it is obviously important that the surgeon recognize the lesion at laparotomy.

Supportive *treatment* for shock is urgent in the severe cases. If the patient's general condition permits, and the diagnosis is so uncertain that lesions such as perforated peptic ulcers cannot be ruled out, laparotomy must be performed. Frequently it is only after the peritoneum is opened that the existence of acute pancreatic necrosis is first realized. The presence of fat necrosis is diagnostic provided tuberculous peritonitis and metastatic carcinoma can be excluded, since similar white areas are seen in these two diseases. However, fat necrosis may be present when the pancreatitis is of the interstitial type (see below). Blood-tinged peritoneal fluid is also diagnostic provided other sources can be excluded. Exposure of the pancreas will reveal a softened necrotic hemorrhagic organ to which drains are inserted. This allows necrotic tissue to slough off to the exterior and activated secretion to escape, thus minimizing digestion of more tissue. It has been found, too, that biliary drainage (cholecystostomy) is beneficial regardless of whether or not disease of the gallbladder is present.

However, if a diagnosis of acute hemorrhagic pancreatitis can be made with a reasonable degree of certainty conservative (nonoperative) therapy is advisable because of the high mortality which follows operation in these cases. There is some difference of opinion as to the length of time such nonoperative therapy should be pursued, *i.e.*, whether operation (drainage of the lesser peritoneal sac, usually with cholecystostomy) should be carried out as soon as the patient's general condition has improved sufficiently, or whether to await the possible formation of localizing signs indicative of a walled off abscess in which case simple drainage is carried out.

Acute Interstitial (Edematous) Pancreatitis.—This is a lesion, which is not infrequent, and produces manifestations which are commonly mistaken for those provoked by biliary colic, intestinal obstruction and perforated ulcer. A detailed discussion of its pathogenesis and symptomatology will be found in a report by one of us.[61]

Pathologically, acute interstitial pancreatitis is distinguished from acute pancreatic necrosis by the absence of hemorrhage (bloody fluid), necrosis and suppuration of the gland. Fat necrosis, however, may occur but is localized to the pancreas. Fibrosis, edema and acute interstitial inflammation (interlobular polymorphonuclear infiltration) are the only microscopic changes noted. Grossly the organ is swollen, firm, edematous and may be surrounded by tiny areas of fat necrosis, provided, however, that the organ is observed during the period of acute inflammation.

Clinically, there is seldom difficulty in differentiating the disease from pancreatic necrosis in that there is no prostration or evidence of circulatory collapse. Important is the fact that spontaneous subsidence is the rule, thus removing it from the group of cases demanding immediate operation. Blood amylase is high at the height of the attack, but diminishes progressively to normal as the symptoms disappear (see Fig. 394). Jaundice, though not evident clinically except by a slight icteric tint to the sclerae in some cases, can be detected by measuring the degree of bilirubinemia, which is elevated at the height of the attack, but decreases as the symptoms

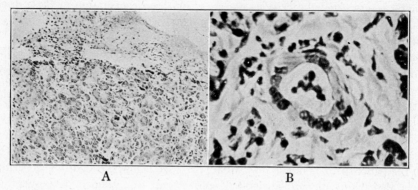

| A | B |

FIG. 396.—ACUTE INTERSTITIAL PANCREATITIS.

Photomicrographs from a biopsy of the pancreas removed at operation. *A*, low power, showing the edge of a lobule with polymorphonuclear cells in the interstitial tissue of the acini as well as the lobule; *B*, high power, showing a tiny duct with similar cells within its lumen and marked edema of the tissue outside.

subside. The jaundice is probably due to a transient compression of the terminal part of the common duct as it passes through the swollen edematous head of the pancreas. Dilatation of the gallbladder in fact has been observed at operation in some cases. On the other hand, it is possible that the jaundice may be due to an associated hepatitis. The relationship of this acute process to chronic pancreatitis is suggested by many observations which point to the fact that repeated attacks of acute interstitial inflammation lead eventually to the development of chronic pancreatitis.

Treatment in patients with acute interstitial pancreatitis is ordinarily that of the associated gallbladder lesion which is nearly always present. Emergency operation is not indicated, provided the correct diagnosis is made. The absence of circulatory collapse is usually sufficient to exclude pancreatic necrosis. If the patient is seen soon enough the attack itself may often be aborted by the prompt use of nitroglycerine, 1/100 grain placed under the tongue and repeated in 5 to 10 minutes. This drug is usually ineffective if used after the attack has lasted for an hour or more. Morphine is disappointing.

In most cases removal of the gallbladder is accompanied by a cessation of the attacks of acute pancreatitis; in many instances, however, cholecystectomy is followed by a recurrence of the pain, which, however, eventually disappears. Occasionally, the recurrent symptoms will be so severe and frequent that a second operation will be indicated with the idea perhaps that a stone is present in the common duct. If this is not the case, drainage of bile through a catheter inserted into the common duct is generally advisable. If prolonged drainage is desired a T-tube is used. There is some evidence to indicate that dilatation of the common sphincter of the common and pancreatic ducts by means of bougies inserted through the open choledochus is of value in these patients; however, many surgeons consider this detrimental and even dangerous. It is probable that some cases of so-called postcholecystectomy syndrome [62] are in reality due to acute interstitial pancreatitis.

Chronic Pancreatitis.—A hard indurated pancreas has frequently been observed by many surgeons in the course of operation for chronic gallbladder disease. This finding has been described as being due to chronic pancreatitis. In absence of actual biopsy, however, such a designation is uncertain. Pathologically, extensive fibrous tissue ingrowth both between the acini, as well as between the larger lobules, is the main manifestation. In some patients these changes may be due to previous attacks of acute interstitial pancreatitis. The clinical manifestations, if any, are overshadowed by the associated gallbladder lesion. In many patients the lesion has been found to accompany other diseases (nephritis, myocarditis, etc.). Its relationship to diabetes has not been established, although in diabetics with chronic cholecystitis, the existence of chronic pancreatitis seems to aggravate the severity of the disease. Removal of the gallbladder in such cases may result in amelioration of the diabetes. Rarely fibrosis at the head of the pancreas becomes marked enough to obstruct the lower end of the common duct. In such a case, symptoms of increasing jaundice will develop which are indistinguishable from those due to a carcinoma at the head of the pancreas.

Treatment of chronic pancreatitis is surgical only if gallbladder disease is present, or if the pancreatic fibrosis is sufficient to have produced jaundice; in the latter case an anastomosis between the gallbladder and stomach, duodenum, or jejunum will be indicated.

Carcinoma of the Pancreas.—The malignant tumors of the pancreas are nearly always adenocarcinomas originating from either the acinar tissue or ducts, chiefly the latter. Any part of the organ may harbor the tumor, but the head is most commonly involved. Certainly it is the site which most often produces symptoms because of its proximity to the common duct which it compresses, and thus leads to the development of jaundice which is the most important diagnostic manifestation. The jaundice develops insidiously and is accompanied by moderate or slight pain. Before the onset of the icterus or coincident with it, other symptoms occur, *i.e.*, anorexia, vague epigastric distress, diarrhea, extreme weakness and rapid loss of weight. Diagnosis in absence of icterus, however, is difficult if not impossible without operation. Of interest is the preponderant incidence of the disease in males.

Aside from the jaundice, the bed-side examination of a patient with carcinoma of the head of the pancreas is apt to be negative. Abdominal examination will only rarely reveal a palpable gallbladder, though an enlarged liver can nearly always be detected after the jaundice has been present for some time. The diagnosis, in general, resolves itself into the differentiation from other causes of extrahepatic jaundice (*e.g.,* stone in the common duct) and from hepatogenous jaundice (*e.g.,* primary hepatitis, cirrhosis, etc.). Because of this diagnostic difficulty, operation is frequently indicated. In a few cases the clinical impression of carcinoma will prove erroneous and a stone in the common duct will be found unexpectedly and removed. In this case the gallbladder will be shrunken. If the gallbladder is dilated and tense (including the cystic and common ducts) a diagnosis of stone may be excluded and one of carcinoma of the head of the pancreas or of the ampulla of Vater made (Courvoisier's Law). In the latter case a successful anastomosis between the gallbladder and stomach, duodenum, or jejunum, will relieve the jaundice. Special preparations for laparotomy are necessary because of the jaundice (p. 610). The course of carcinoma of the pancreas is rapid, most patients dying within a year. Radiotherapy has not received adequate trial, but is not satisfactory. Biopsy of the tumor should be done if possible to verify the clinical diagnosis. Excision of the tumor has been performed, and should be done more frequently in the attempt to cure an otherwise hopeless disease. The work of Whipple and associates [63] has been most important in the development of the surgical treatment of carcinoma of the ampulla of Vater and head of the pancreas. They do a cholecystenterostomy at the first stage, and at the second remove the head of the pancreas and duodenum, reestablishing intestinal continuity by a gastro-enterostomy; one stage resections are also done. Details of various types of operations on the pancreas may be found in the splendid monograph by Brunschwig [54].

Carcinoma of the body and tail of the pancreas is much less common than in the head (1:6). Because of the absence of jaundice in patients with tumors of the body and tail, diagnosis is difficult indeed; the more important clinical manifestations, as reported in a study by Levy and Lichtman [64] are rapid, unexplained loss of weight, anorexia and persistent pain of a noncolicky type frequently radiating posteriorly (Keeton, Med. Cl. N. A., March, 1935).

Cyst of the Pancreas.—Though many different types of pancreatic cysts have been described, only one is of sufficient frequency to merit discussion. This is a remarkable tumor which fills the lesser peritoneal cavity behind the stomach and transverse colon, is attached to and originates from the pancreas and is filled with clear or slightly brownish or straw-colored fluid containing at least one of the three pancreatic ferments, usually amylase. The wall of the cyst is composed of a thin or thick layer of fibrous tissue and has no epithelial lining and is hence often called pseudocyst. The connection with the pancreas when it can be demonstrated consists of a communication with the lumen of one of the finer ducts. The pathogenesis is apparently dependent on a rupture of one of the ducts, usually by direct trauma (or inflammation) allowing pancreatic juice to leak out into the lesser peritoneal cavity. The fibrous tissue reaction around it forms a limiting membrane which increases in size as more secretion pours into it. Finally the cyst becomes large and produces a bulging, smooth epigastric swelling. X-ray observations, utilizing the barium meal and barium enema simultaneously will be very helpful in differential diagnosis. In pancreatic cysts involving the body and tail, these studies almost always will reveal the stomach to be displaced upward and to the right with the transverse colon and splenic flexure displaced downward and to the left.

Treatment is surgical. The cyst is exposed and incised, and the contents evacuated slowly. Occasionally bits of necrotic pancreas can be seen floating in the fluid, which is evidence of previous disease even though no history is obtained thereof. The incised edges of the cyst are then sutured to one end of the wound (marsupialization) in order to permit continuous drainage. The cystic cavity gradually decreases in size, sooner or later the walls adhere, and obliteration occurs. However,

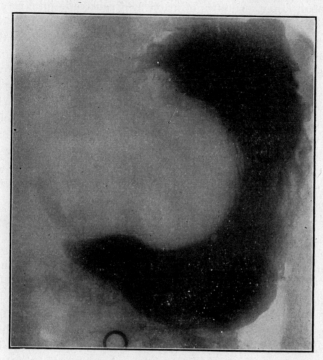

FIG. 397.—PANCREATIC CYST.

Roentgenogram of stomach, after ingestion of a barium meal, showing characteristic displacement due to the presence of a tumor presenting above the lesser curvature. The patient, aged forty-six, had noted a gradually increasing upper abdominal swelling associated with epigastric pain and occasional vomiting of two years' duration. The blood amylase was elevated. At operation a large amount of slightly turbid fluid was evacuated; the fluid contained a high concentration of pancreatic ferments. Recovery was uneventful.

recurrence may develop, thereby necessitating reoperation. An excellent clinical summary of many collected cases may be found in a report by McWhorter.[65]

Other Lesions of the Pancreas.—*Pancreatic asthenia* is a syndrome consisting of extreme weakness, fast pulse, anemia, ptyalism, anorexia and vomiting which is sometimes seen following pancreatic operations (Whipple[66]). Treatment is conservative. *Fistula of the pancreas* sometimes occurs following drainage of a pancreatic cyst and as an accident after various gastric and duodenal operations. Serious is the occasional presence of active trypsin in the discharge from the fistula because excoriation and digestion of the skin surrounding the opening will then occur. This is also true of duodenal fistula for the same reason. If unchecked, the results are disastrous because of loss of electrolytes and fluid, and because of digestion of the wound edges which is associated with excruciating pain. Various substances (HCl, oil and protein paste, aluminum powder, etc.) are used to protect the skin from the secretion, or to neutralize the trypsin. However, a much more effective way of preventing digestion is to resort to continuous aspiration of the secretions as they pour out into the wound. *Injury to the pancreas* produces no serious immediate effect unless hemorrhage is considerable or if the leaking secretion becomes activated. Large quantities of inactivated pancreatic juice may escape into the peritoneal cavity because of injury to a large duct without deleterious results, except that a pancreatic cyst occasionally develops following trauma to the pancreas, as already mentioned.

Pancreaticohepatic Syndrome.—During recent years fatty infiltration of the liver has been increasingly noted in association with clinical pancreatic lithiasis and pancreatic atrophy. These findings are similar to the older observations by physiologists that pancreatic insufficiency is followed by hepatic deposition of fat. It has long been known that raw pancreas as well as choline will prevent or cure such a fatty liver. Dragstedt [67] and his associates have produced a pancreatic extract (lipocaic) which has the same therapeutic effect, and is considered by them to be a lipotropic hormone. The extract has been used clinically with beneficial results (Snell and Comfort,[68] Rosenberg [69]).

THE SPLEEN

The spleen is a major component of the reticulo-endothelial system, but is not indispensable to life. One of its chief functions is the formation of lymphocytes. The phagocytic endothelial cells are instrumental in the destruction and disposal of erythrocytes and blood platelets, and are likewise phagocytic for other foreign bodies such as parasites, etc. The organ also acts as a reservoir for blood, and by contraction in times of stress may liberate a large quantity of blood. There is evidence, but very little proof, that the spleen is an important link in the mechanism of production of immunity. Conforming to the function of the reticulo-endothelial system elsewhere, the splenic parenchyma is a site for the formation of bilirubin from the hemoglobin of the broken down erythrocytes. Removal of the organ has few if any detrimental effects.

Rupture.—In spite of the fact that the spleen is well protected by the ribs and spine, it is not uncommonly the seat of lacerations which often are the source of so much hemorrhage that operative treatment is necessary. Such lacerations are produced usually by blows sustained over that area and, in a large percentage of the cases, are not associated with any other significant intra-abdominal injury. Loss of blood may be sufficient to produce a tachycardia, drop in blood pressure and other manifestations of shock as described in Chapter XIII. Evidence of peritoneal irritation, including tenderness and muscle spasm, are present to a varying degree, but vomiting is apt to be absent. *Pain is often referred to the left shoulder.* If the signs of shock do not respond to conservative treatment, it is safe to assume that bleeding has not ceased, and laparotomy is indicated. Transfusions are usually necessary, preoperatively, to combat shock before operation is safe. In emergencies, the blood in the peritoneal cavity may be mixed with sodium citrate and given to the patient (autotransfusion), unless it is contaminated by intestinal contents. The laceration may rarely be repaired by suture; usually it is more advisable to remove the entire organ. On rare occasions spontaneous rupture occurs, particularly in patients with splenomegalia, especially if the enlargement is of recent origin.

Splenomegalia.—There are many diseases which may produce splenic enlargement, but only a few are of surgical significance. For example, enlargement is encountered in such diseases as malaria, syphilis, and chronic sepsis of various types, but treatment of the splenomegalia is surgical only on rare occasions when splenectomy may be indicated. Enlargement of the spleen is also encountered in lymphatic and myelogenous leukemia, especially the latter, but splenectomy is rarely beneficial. On many occasions the enlargement of the spleen is due entirely to mechanical factors such as portal obstruction associated with hepatic cirrhosis, tumors, etc.

The diseases associated with splenomegalia, which are particularly of surgical significance are hemolytic jaundice, so-called Banti's disease, thrombocytopenic purpura and Gaucher's disease. In these conditions splenectomy is frequently indicated. The large variety of splenic diseases which are commonly or constantly associated with splenomegalia are thoroughly discussed in the excellent report of Whipple.[70]

TABLE 9

ANALYSIS OF CASES OBSERVED IN PRESBYTERIAN HOSPITAL, NEW YORK CITY
(A. O. WHIPPLE) UP TO OCT. 15, 1940.

Type of Case	No. Cases	With Splenectomy	Postop. Deaths	Without Splenectomy
Typical Hemolytic Icterus	57	42	3	15
Atypical Hemolytic Icterus	15	7	2	8
Idiopathic Thrombocytopenic Purpura	54	31	0	23
Atypical Thrombocytopenic Purpura	62	12	2	50 *
Splenomegaly—Obstructive Factor Undetermined..	31	24	1	7
Splenectomy with Cirrhosis	117	27	6	90
Schistosomiasis	13	12	0	1
Thrombosis of Splenic Vein	4	3	0	1
Cavernous Transformation of Portal Vein	2	2	1	0
Stenosis of Portal Vein	3	3	0	0
Miscellaneous Splenectomies	27	27	1	0
Splenomegaly of Undetermined Origin	59	8	1	51
Normal Splenectomy	23	23	0	0
Traumatic Splenectomy	7	7	2	0

Total Cases 474
Total Splenectomies 228
Number of Operative Deaths 19
Percentage of Mortality 8%

Hemolytic Jaundice.—Up until recently the hemolytic anemias were divided into congenital (familial) and acquired types, largely because in the former group hereditary tendencies could be discovered, whereas in the latter group they were not. Careful study reveals the fact that the pathologic manifestations of the two

* Of the 50 without splenectomy, 22 were secondary and 28 symptomatic thrombocytopenic purpura.

types are identical. The only notable difference lies in the observation that patients who present acute hemolytic crises uncommonly reveal hereditary tendencies. In reality there is no longer any justification for the division of the group into the two types except to signify whether or not the family history reveals other members of the family with the disease. Occasionally the disease is associated with infections of various types, which at times may appear to have some etiologic relationship to the disease process. On other occasions the etiology can be traced to a poisonous drug such as benzol, toluol, etc.; such types are frequently spoken of as secondary hemolytic anemia.

The mechanism of production of the jaundice is dependent upon an increased destruction of red blood cells and not upon hepatic insufficiency. In other words, the large amounts of bilirubin resulting from the breakdown of so much hemolyzed blood is more than the normal liver can excrete, and it therefore appears in the blood.

The typical case of hemolytic jaundice or anemia is diagnosed without difficulty. Cardinal manifestations are jaundice (of variable intensity), splenomegalia, and anemia of the spherocytic, reticulocytic type. Immature forms of erythrocytes, particularly reticulocytes are found in the blood in large numbers. Still more characteristic cells in the blood are spherical microcytes, which may constitute as many as 10 to 20 per cent of the total number of erythrocytes. The actual level of bilirubinemia is lower than that encountered in the average case of obstructive jaundice. A characteristic finding in this disease is urobilin in the urine in large quantities, erroneously thought by many to be indicative of hepatic insufficiency in this disease. The urobilinuria is presumably due to the fact that the excess amount of bilirubin excreted by the liver into the intestine results in the transformation and absorption of an excess amount of urobilin which cannot be handled by the liver, since this organ is already overwhelmed by the excretion of the excess bilirubin resulting from the increased hemolysis. The increased production of urobilin is due to the conversion in the intestinal tract of the excess amount of bilirubin excreted by the liver. A large amount of both bilirubin and urobilin will be found in the stool (producing stools of normal color or even darker than normal), but there is relatively little bilirubin in the urine in contrast to its high concentration in obstructive jaundice. This latter feature is an important diagnostic sign.

Increased fragility of the red cells is fairly constant. In normal individuals, hemolysis of the erythrocytes *in vitro* begins in 0.45 per cent salt solution and is complete in 0.35 per cent solution. In hemolytic icterus, hemolysis may begin in a concentration as high as 0.65 per cent and be complete at 0.45 or 0.50 per cent. The various hepatic function tests reveal no significant indications of hepatic insufficiency. Small pigmented gallstones (calcium bilirubinate) are often present in the gallbladder, but only rarely produce manifestations of biliary disease.

Splenectomy is specific in relieving the jaundice in the typical cases, since it results in a cessation of the excessive blood destruction. Removal of the spleen, however, does not change the fragility of the erythrocytes. If possible splenectomy should be avoided during acute crises, because of the high mortality contrasted with a mortality of only 2 to 5 per cent when operation is performed during a remission. At times the acute crises will be so severe and prolonged that splenectomy will be indicated. Post-splenectomy thrombosis, a not rare danger, may be controlled by x-ray radiation to the heart, or better by injections of heparin (Ladd and Gross [77]).

Banti's Disease (Splenic Anemia).—In 1894 Guido Banti wrote a paper entitled "Splenomegaly with cirrhosis of the Liver." The condition which goes by his name at the present time applies to a disease or a group of diseases of unknown and perhaps variable etiology, characterized primarily by splenomegalia, anemia and mild leukopenia. The relationship of obstruction of the portal vein to the pathogenesis of at least a major portion of the patients classified in this group is suggested by the report of Dock and Warthin,[71] years ago. More recently Rousselot [72] has shown that the obstruction may be either in the portal or splenic vein and concludes that the obstruction is the major etiologic factor; to this condition McMichael (*Jour. Physiol.,* 75:241, 1932) has applied the term "portal hypertension."

The disease affects children as well as adults. The patient commonly notices a gradually increasing weakness, anorexia and abdominal discomfort. Pallor is noted and examination of the blood reveals an anemia, but the resistance of the erythrocytes is apt to be increased. Frequently the liver is enlarged, but only in the late stage; as the disease progresses the liver becomes cirrhotic and finally ascites manifests itself. However, many of these patients do not develop hepatic cirrhosis at all (Rousselot). The course of the disease is not uniform since exacerbations are common. During the acute attacks fever of unknown origin may be present and the anemia becomes more pronounced. In the later stages the abdominal symptoms increase and attacks of vomiting are frequent. Hemorrhage from the stomach is not uncommon (esophageal and gastric varices). Urobilin is found in the urine. The spleen usually gradually increases in size. Jaundice is apt to occur before death. Considerable difficulty may be encountered in differentiating splenic anemia from Laënnec's cirrhosis of the liver. In general there is more fibrosis of the spleen and less fibrosis of the liver in splenic anemia than in cirrhosis of the liver. The spleen is usually smaller in the latter disease.

On many occasions splenectomy will result in great improvement, and in some patients, particularly in children, will result in cure; in adults, splenectomy is rarely curative. In the group of patients having hypertension, splenectomy will result in cure if the obstruction is in the splenic vein. However, if the obstruction is in the portal vein, splenectomy will offer only slight improvement and will exert little or no effect on hemorrhage from esophageal varices which usually results in the patient's death sooner or later (Rousselot). If hepatic cirrhosis with ascites is encountered at the operation, an omentopexy may be helpful. This operation consists of implanting omentum into the subcutaneous tissue through the abdominal incision. Thus, portal blood may, through anastomosis reach the general circulation, thereby relieving the portal obstruction. Operative procedures should not be carried out during an acute stage. In any event the patient should be adequately prepared by transfusion, etc., because occasionally splenectomy is difficult due to the presence of adhesions. The mortality rate for splenectomy in Banti's disease will be high if done in the late stages because of hepatic insufficiency and postoperative hemorrhage. Symptomatic results will also be poor in the advanced cases, however, splenectomy is fairly effective in eliminating ascites (Barg and Dulin [73]). Hemorrhage from esophageal varices is always of serious prognostic importance. Ligation of the left gastric and left gastro-epiploic arteries in addition to splenectomy may be advisable. Injection of the varicosities with sclerosing agents may be tried (Walters and associates [74]).

Thrombocytopenic Purpura (Purpura Haemorrhagica).—This is perhaps not accurately classified as a disease of the spleen, but slight to moderate enlargement of the spleen is quite constantly present. It is a relatively rare disease, but is most common in young women and children. The first manifestations to appear are usually ecchymotic patches under the skin and mucous membranes and a tendency to bleed from insignificant wounds. Frequently spontaneous bleeding from the gums or nasal cavity is manifested and may be of a serious nature. Petechiae are common. As the disease progresses the hemorrhages become more severe and the anemia more pronounced. A diagnostic feature is the appearance of petechiae on the skin of an extremity when its venous blood supply is obstructed (tourniquet test) by a tourniquet or blood pressure cuff.

A low platelet count (100,000 per c.mm. or lower) is one of the most diagnostic features of the disease. The bleeding time is prolonged for hours, although the clotting time may be unaltered. When the blood is allowed to clot in a test tube, the clot does not retract. The degree of anemia varies, depending upon the amount of blood lost, but may be severe and associated with nucleated erythrocytes even when hemorrhage is insignificant. These findings must be distinguished from those encountered in hemophilia, a disease in which the thrombocyte count and bleeding time are normal, but the clotting time prolonged. As in hemorrhage from other causes, bone marrow studies show a myeloid, erythroid and megakaryocytic hyperplasia. The platelets are reduced equally in the bone marrow and blood (Limarzi and Schleicher [75]), suggesting that the disease is one of faulty maturation of platelets and not their destruction. If megakaryocytes are absent or markedly diminished in the bone marrow, splenectomy is apt to be ineffective. The platelet count in the blood usually approaches normal after operation, although occasionally this rise is not sustained. The diagnosis of idiopathic thrombocytopenic purpura should always be questioned in the presence of a leukopenia. In such cases an atypical leukemia or aplastic anemia is the more probable diagnosis for which splenectomy is not indicated.

Splenectomy is remarkably effective in stopping the hemorrhage in the properly selected cases. On numerous occasions, hemorrhage has been observed to cease immediately as soon as the splenic vessels were ligated. Years ago it was thought that splenectomy should not be performed in the acute phase of the disease. It is now generally agreed that more patients in the acute stage will be saved by splenectomy than by medical therapy, *providing proper preoperative, operative and postoperative care* is utilized. The most important adjunct to surgical therapy is probably transfusion of an adequate amount of blood. Patients in an extreme state of exsanguination need three or four transfusions before operation (continued throughout the operation) and as many after operation. Utilizing such precautions the mortality rate will not be more than 5 or 10 per cent. However, bleeding into the central nervous system, though rare, may lead to a fatal outcome.

Gaucher's Disease.—This is a rare disease occurring most commonly in young girls and characterized by a marked enlargement of the spleen in the absence of many debilitating symptoms. The skin, especially over the face and neck, becomes pigmented. After the disease has been present for years the patient may become anemic and the liver enlarged. A characteristic pathologic feature of the disease is the presence of large lipoid-containing cells in the reticulo-endothelial organs, especially the spleen, bone marrow and lymph nodes. Splenectomy is usually very beneficial unless the reticulo-endothelial system elsewhere (especially the bone marrow) is diseased.

Miscellaneous Types of Splenomegalia.—There are many other types of splenomegalia, including those due to malaria, syphilis, etc., but perhaps the most important surgically is a relatively rare disease (observed chiefly in children) consisting of splenomegalia and on many occasions, hemorrhage from dilated esophageal varices. Smith and Farber [76] have recently made a study of the disease with a report of 15 cases. It is very significant that anemia is not present except when produced by hemorrhage, and that there is no tendency toward the ultimate development of cirrhosis and ascites, thus differentiating it from so-called Banti's disease. It appears that in many instances the chief etiologic factor is obstruction of the portal vein produced by congenital malformation or by thrombosis representing a group of cases already discussed in the group designated as so-called Banti's disease. Treatment may be conservative, but if hemorrhage occurs, splenectomy with ligation of the left gastric artery or occasionally the coronary vein may be indicated. Laënnec's atrophic cirrhosis is usually associated with a mild degree of splenomegalia. Splenectomy is occasionally performed in mild, well-chosen cases, but in general is followed by poor results. Moreover, the operative mortality will be high (near 20 per cent) because of the severe impairment of liver function in addition to postoperative hemorrhage from the operative site and esophageal varices.

BIBLIOGRAPHY

1. MANN, F. C., and BOLLMAN, J. L. Liver Function Tests, *Arch. Pathol.*, 1:681, 1926; MANN, F. C. Rôle of the Liver as the Commissariat of the Body, *Am. J. Digest Dis.*, 4:355, 1937-38; Physiology and Pathological Reactions of the Liver. *South. M. J.*, 31:425, 1938.
2. MANN, F. C. The Liver and Medical Progress, *J. Am. M. Ass.*, 117:1577, 1941.
3. LUCK, J. M. The Liver Proteins, in Weedham, J., and Green, D. E., *Perspectives in Biochemistry*, Cambridge, University Press, 1937.
4. ANDRUS, W. DEW. and LORD, J. W. Clinical Investigations of Some Factors Causing Prothrombin Deficiencies: Significance of the Liver in their Production and Correction, *Arch. Surg.*, 41:596, 1940.
5. KRIEG, E. C. Hepatic Trauma; Analysis of Sixty Cases, *Arch. Surg.*, 32:907, 1936.
6. ELMAN, R. and COLE, W. H. Hemorrhage and Shock as Causes of Death Following Acute Portal Obstruction, *Arch. Surg.*, 28:1166, 1934.
7. HELWIG, F. C., and ORR, T. G. Traumatic Necrosis of Liver with Extensive Retention of Creatinine and High Grade Nephrosis, *Arch. Surg.*, 24:136, 1932; SCHUTZ, C. B., HELWIG, F. C., and KUHN, H. P. A Contribution to the Study of So-called Liver Death, *J. Am. M. Ass.*, 99:633, 1932.
8. GRAHAM, E. A., COLE, W. H., COPHER, G. H., and MOORE, SHERWOOD. *Diseases of the Gall Bladder and Bile Ducts,* Lea and Febiger, Philadelphia, 1928.

9. HANGER, F. M. Serological Differentiation of Obstructive from Hepatogenous Jaundice by Flocculation of Cephalin-Cholesterol Emulsion, *J. Clin. Investigation,* 18:261, 1939; The Differential Diagnosis of Jaundice, *Virginia M. Monthly,* 67:1, 1940; GUTMAN, A. B., and HANGER, F. M. Differential Diagnosis of Jaundice by Combined Serum Phosphatase Determination and Cephalin Flocculation Test, *M. Clin. North America,* 25:837, 1941.

10. RAVDIN, I. S. Recent Advances in Surgical Therapeusis, *Ann. Surg.,* 109:321, 1939; ELMAN, R., and WEINER, D. O. Intravenous Alimentation, with Special Reference to Protein (amino acid) Metabolism, *J. Am. M. Ass.,* 112:796, 1939.

11. ELMAN, R., and HEIFETZ, C. J. Experimental Hypoalbuminemia, *J. Exp. Med.,* 73:417, 1941.

12. OCHSNER, A., DeBAKEY, M. and MURRAY, S. Pyogenic Abscess of the Liver, *Am. J. Surg.,* 40:292, 1938.

13. HANGER, F. M., and GUTMAN, A. B. Postarsphenamine Jaundice Apparently due to Obstruction of Intrahepatic Biliary Tract, *J. Am. M. Ass.,* 115:263, 1940.

14. OCHSNER, A. and DeBAKEY, M. Diagnosis and Treatment of Amebic Abscess of the Liver, *Am. J. Digest. Dis.,* 2:47, 1935; Amebic Hepatitis and Hepatic Abscess, *Surgery,* 13:460, 1943.

15. ROGERS, L. Amebic Liver Abscess, *Lancet,* 1:463, 569 and 677, 1922.

16. WHIPPLE, G. H. Origin and Significance of Constituents of Bile, *Physiol. Rev.,* 2:440, 1922.

17. ELMAN, R., and McMASTER, P. D. Urobilin Physiology and Pathology, *J. Exper. M.,* 41:503, 1925; 41:513, 1925; 41:719, 1925.

18. QUICK, A. J. Clinical Value of Test for Hippuric Acid in Cases of Disease of Liver, *Arch. Int. Med.,* 57:544, 1936.

19. FOLEY, E. F., KEETON, R. W., KENDRICK, A. B., and DARLING, D. Alterations in Serum Protein as an Index of Hepatic Failure, *Arch. Int. Med.,* 60:64, 1937.

20. DAM, H. Antihemorrhagic Vitamins of the Chick, *Biochem. J.,* 29:1273, 1935.

21. ALMQUIST, H. J., and STOKSTAD, E. L. R. Hemorrhagic Chick Disease of Dietary Origin, *J. Biol. Chem.,* 111:105, 1935; ALMQUIST, H. J. Vitamin K, *Physiol. Rev.,* 21:194, 1941.

22. QUICK, A. J. The Nature of Bleeding in Jaundice, *J. Am. M. Ass.,* 110:1658, 1938.

23. McNEE, J. W. Jaundice: A Review of Recent Work, *Quart. J. M.,* 16:390, 1923.

24. BOYCE, F. F., and McFETRIDGE, E. M. Obstructive Jaundice, *Surgery,* 4:280, 1938.

25. GUTMAN, A. B., OLSON, K. B., GUTMAN, E. B., and FLOOD, C. A. The Effect of Disease of the Liver and Biliary Tract upon the Phosphatase Activity of the Serum, *J. Clin. Investigation,* 19:129, 1940.

26. SCHREIBER, E. Uber Stillung innerer Blutungen durch intravenose Traubenzucker-Injektionen, *Zentralbl. f. Chir.,* 40:1200, 1913.

27. RAVDIN, I. S. Some Aspects of Carbohydrate Metabolism in Hepatic Disease, *J. Am. M. Ass.,* 93:1193, 1929.

28. GRAHAM, E. A. The Resistance of Pups to Late Chloroform Poisoning in its Relation to Liver Glycogen, *J. Exper. M.,* 21:185, 1915.

29. SNELL, A. M., BUTT, H. R., and OSTERBERG, A. E. Treatment of the Hemorrhagic Tendency in Jaundice; with Special Reference to Vitamin K. *Amer. Jour. Digest Dis.,* 5:590, 1938.

30. ROUS, P., and McMASTER, P. D. Concentrating Activity of Gall Bladder, *J. Exper. M.,* 34:47, 1921.

31. JUDD, E. S., and MANN, F. C. The Effect of Removal of the Gall Bladder, an Experimental Study, *Surg., Gynec. & Obst.,* 24:437, 1917.

32. COUNSELLOR, V., and McINDOE, M. B. Dilatation of Bile Ducts (Hydrohepatosis), *Surg., Gynec. & Obst.,* 43:729, 1926.

33. ANDREWS, E. Pathologic Changes of Diseased Gallbladders, *Arch. Surg.,* 31:767, 1935.

34. WOLFER, J. A. The Rôle of Pancreatic Juice in the Production of Gallbladder Disease, *Surg., Gynec. & Obst.,* 53:435, 1931.

35. WOMACK, N. A., and BRICKER, E. M. Pathologic Changes in the Gallbladder Wall Due to Action of Bile, *Proc. Soc. Exp. Biol. & Med.*, 45:710, 1940; COLE, W. H., NOVAK, M. V., and HUGHES, E. O. Experimental Production of Chronic Cholecystitis by Obstructive Lesions of the Cystic Duct, *Ann. Surg.*, 114:682, 1941.

36. ILLINGWORTH, C. F. W. Types of Gall-bladder Infection, *Brit. J. Surg.*, 15:221, 1928.

37. GRAHAM, E. A. Hepatitis, a Constant Accompaniment of Cholecystitis, *Surg., Gynec. & Obst.*, 26:521, 1918. GRAHAM, E. A., and PETERMAN, M. G. Further Observations on Lymphatic Origin of Cholecystitis, Choledochitis and Associated Pancreatitis, *Arch. Surg.*, 4:23, 1922.

38. GRAHAM, H. F. Value of Early Operation for Acute Cholecystitis, *Ann. Surg.*, 93:1152, 1931.

39. ZINNINGER, M. M. Surgical Treatment of Acute Cholecystitis, *Ann. Surg.*, 96:406, 1932.

40. MacCARTY, W. C. The Pathology of the Gall-bladder and Some Associated Lesions, *Ann. Surg.*, 51:651, 1910.

41. MOYNIHAN, B. G. A. A Disease of the Gall-bladder Requiring Cholecystectomy, *Ann. Surg.*, 50:1265, 1909.

42. ELMAN, R., and GRAHAM, E. A. Pathogenesis of "Strawberry" Gall Bladder (Cholesterosis of Gall Bladder), *Arch. Surg.*, 24:14, 1932.

43. ALVAREZ, W. C. "Pseudocholecystitis" Apparently Caused by Food Sensitiveness, *Proc. Staff Meet. Mayo Clin.*, 9:680, 1934; NICHELES, H., RAPPEPORT, B. Z., GREEN, R., MARCUS, P., and MESOROW, S. Allergy of the Gallbladder, *Am. J. Digest Dis.*, 7:238, 1940.

44. GRAHAM, E. A., and MACKEY, W. A. Consideration of Stoneless Gall Bladder, *J. Am. M. Ass.*, 103:1497, 1934; MACKEY, W. A. Cholecystitis without Stone, *Brit. J. Surg.*, 22:274, 1934.

45. WESTPHAL, K. Muskelfunction, Nervensystem und Pathologie der Gallemege, *Ztschr. f. klin. Med.*, 96:22, 1923; McGOWAN, J. M., BUTSCH, W. L., and WALTERS, W. The Use of Glyceryl Trinitrate for the Control of Pain Following Cholecystectomy, *Ann. Surg.*, 104:1013, 1936.

46. PHEMISTER, D. B., ARONSOHN, H. G., and PEPINSKY, R. Variation in the Cholesterol Bile Pigment and Calcium Salts Contents of Gall Stones Found in Gall-bladder and in Bile Ducts with the Degree of Associated Obstruction, *Ann. Surg.*, 109:161, 1939.

47. ANDREWS, E., DOSTAL, L. E., GOFF, M., and HRDINA, L. The Mechanism of Cholesterol Gall Stone Formation, *Ann. Surg.*, 96:615, 1932.

48 PHEMISTER, D. B., REWBRIDGE, A. G., and RUDISILL, H. Calcium Carbonate Gall Stones and Calcification of the Gallbladder Following Cystic Duct Obstruction, *Ann. Surg.*, 94:493, 1931.

49. GRAHAM, E. A. Prevention of Carcinoma of Gall Bladder, *Ann. Surg.*, 93:317, 1931.

50. GRAHAM, E. A., and COLE, W. H. Roentgenologic Examination of the Gall Bladder, a New Method Utilizing Intravenous Injection of Tetrabromophenolphthalein, *J. Am. M. Ass.*, 82:613, 1924.

51. BOYDEN, E. A. The Effect of Natural Foods on the Distention of the Gall Bladder with a Note on the Change in the Pattern of the Mucosa As It Passes from Distention to Collapse, *Ant. Rec.*, 30:333, 1925.

52. WHITAKER, L. R. Mechanism of the Gall Bladder, *Am. J. Physiol.*, 78:411, 1926.

53. MANN, F. C., and GIORDANO, A. S. Bile Factor in Pancreatitis, *Arch. Surg.*, 6:1, 1923.

54. BRUNSCHWIG, A. *The Surgery of Pancreatic Tumors*, C. V. Mosby Co., St. Louis, 1942.

55. ELMAN, R. In Graham's *Surgical Diagnosis*, Vol. II, p. 550, W. B. Saunders, Philadelphia, 1930.

56. MOENCH, G. J. Acute Pancreatitis with Erosion of the Splenic Artery and Fatal Hemorrhage, *J. Am. M. Ass.*, 82:360, 1924.
57. OPIE, E. L. *Diseases of the Pancreas*, Philadelphia, 1910.
58. ARCHIBALD, E. Acute Edema of Pancreas, *Ann. Surg.*, 90:803, 1929.
59. NEAL, M. P., and ELLIS, M. M. Etiological Factor of Fat Necrosis, *South M. J.*, 23:313, 1930.
60. CASBERG, M. A. Acute Pancreatic Necrosis and Acute Interstitial Pancreatitis; Treatment without Operation: Clinical Study of Ten Cases, *Arch. Surg.*, 39:247, 1939.
61. ELMAN, R. Surgical Aspects of Acute Pancreatitis, *J. Am. M. Ass.*, 112:1265, 1942.
62. ――― The Post-Cholecystectomy Syndrome, *Surg. Cl. N. A.*, 20:1247, 1940.
63. WHIPPLE, A. O., PARSONS, W. B., MULLINS, C. R. Treatment of Carcinoma of Ampulla of Vater, *Ann. Surg.*, 102:763, 1935; WHIPPLE, A. O. Surgical Treatment of Carcinoma of the Ampullary Region and Head of the Pancreas, *Am. J. Surg.*, 40:260, 1938.
64. LEVY, H., and LICHTMAN, S. S. Clinical Character of Primary Carcinoma of the Body and Tail of the Pancreas, *Arch. Int. Med.*, 65:607, 1940.
65. McWHORTER, G. L. Cysts of Pancreas, *Arch. Surg.*, 11:619, 1925.
66. WHIPPLE, A. O. Pancreatic Asthenia as Postoperative Complication in Patients with Lesions of the Pancreas, *Ann. Surg.*, 87:176, 1923.
67. DRAGSTEDT, L. R. The Present Status of Lipocaic, *J. Am. M. Ass.*, 114:29, 1940.
68. SNELL, A. M., and COMFORT, M. W. Hepatic Lesions Presumably Secondary to Pancreatic Lithiasis with Atrophy, *Am. J. Digest Dis.*, 4:215, 1937.
69. ROSENBERG, D. H. A Proved Case of Recovery from Fatty Metamorphosis of the Liver After Treatment with Lipocaic, *Am. J. Digest. Dis.*, 5:607, 1938.
70. WHIPPLE, A. O. The Combined Spleen Clinic: Results with Medical and Surgical Therapy in Splenopathies, *Surg., Gynec. & Obst.*, 64:296, 1937.
71. DOCK, G., and WARTHIN, A. S. A Clinical and Pathological Study of Two Cases of Splenic Anemia, with Early and Late Stages of Cirrhosis, *Am. J. M. Sc.*, 127:24, 1904.
72. ROUSSELOT, L. M. Rôle of Congestion (Portal Hypertension in So-called Banti's Syndrome): Clinical and Pathologic Study of Thirty-One Cases with Late Results Following Splenectomy, *J. Am. M. Ass.*, 107:1788, 1936; The Late Phase of Congestive Splenomegaly (Banti's Syndrome) with Hematemesis but without Cirrhosis of the Liver, *Surgery*, 8:34, 1940.
73. BARG, E. H., and DULIN, J. W. Splenectomy in the Treatment of Banti's Syndrome, *Arch. Surg.*, 41:91, 1940.
74. WALTERS, W., MOERSCH, H. J., and McKINNON, D. A. Bleeding Esophageal Varices: Evaluation of Methods Directed Toward their Control, Especially by Direct Injection of Sclerosing Solution, *Arch. Surg.*, 41:1101, 1940.
75. LIMARZI, L. R., and SCHLEICHER, E. M. The Reaction of Peripheral Blood and Bone Marrow in Chronic Hemorrhage and in Essential Thrombopenic Purpura, *J. Am. M. Ass.*, 114:12, 1940.
76. SMITH, R. M., and FARBER, SIDNEY. Splenomegaly in Children with Early Hematemesis, *J. Pediat.*, 7:585, 1935.
77. LADD, W. E. and GROSS, R. E. P. 244. *Abdominal Surgery of Infancy and Childhood*, W. B. Saunders, Philadelphia, 1941.
78. MacINTYRE, D. S., PEDERSON, S., and MADDOCK, W. The Glycogen Content of the Human Liver, *Surgery*, 10:716, 1941.
79. PEARSE, H. E. Vitallium Tubes in Surgery, *Ann. Surg.*, 115:1031, 1942.
80. ELMAN, R. Contributions Made to Knowledge in Regard to the Pancreas, *Am. J. Dig. Diseases*, 6:233, 1939; 7:227, 1940; 8:105, 1941; 9:303, 1942.

CHAPTER XXIV

THE ALIMENTARY TRACT

Oral Cavity
Stomach and Duodenum
Small Intestine
The Appendix

The Cecum and Colon
Rectum and Anus
The Umbilicus

Knowledge of the alimentary tract, especially of the stomach and intestines has advanced much in recent years and leans importantly on roentgenologic study with barium sulphate as a contrast medium for diagnosis. Also important in diagnosis is the use of the esophagoscope and gastroscope for the visualization of the upper gastro-intestinal tract, and the proctoscope and sigmoidoscope for direct vision of the distal colon and rectum. The peritoneum may also be inspected with an instrument similar to a cystoscope called peritoneoscope. Of primary surgical significance are the emergency lesions which, as will be indicated (Chapter XXV), are frequent causes of peritonitis, *e.g.,* perforated peptic ulcer and ruptured appendicitis. Primarily surgical, too, are the malignant diseases, notably carcinoma of the stomach, colon and rectum. Consideration of peptic ulcer, aside from its complications (perforation, hemorrhage, pyloric obstruction) belongs primarily to internal medicine, although it frequently requires operative treatment.

ORAL CAVITY

Many of the diseases which occur in the upper end of the alimentary tract do not properly belong to the domain of general surgery. Although often primary in the mouth or its contents, the lesions are frequently but local manifestations of disease elsewhere. The teeth contribute greatly to the diseases of the oral cavity. Much of the material in the following discussion has been based on the text of Blair and Ivy.[1]

The Mouth.—*Congenital Clefts.*—These defects are a result of embryonic maldevelopment; various types occur, though one of the most frequent of congenital anomalies, cleft lip and palate, occurred only twenty-four times in a series of 28,000 births (Davis[2]). A cleft which involves the upper lip may be single or double and is often called a harelip but a better term is *cleft lip*. Extending backward, the alveolus and the palate may also be cleft. The *cleft palate* may involve only the soft palate, but frequently includes the hard palate as well, so that the floor of one or both nasal cavities is exposed. Because of difficulty in nursing, the infant may suffer from malnutrition; respiratory infections are more likely to occur because of the defect. The diagnosis is obvious on inspection. Treatment is entirely surgical. Operative closure of the cleft lip may be performed soon after birth. Forceful closure or wiring of the alveolus is usually omitted at this early date in order to avoid later deformity of the dental arch. The cleft palate is best repaired in early childhood; because of its interference with speech, the operation is usually done about the second year. The best results are obviously obtained by those specially trained in plastic surgery.

Infections.—Inflammation of the mucous membrane of the mouth is generally described as *stomatitis,* of which there are several types. Most of them are secondary

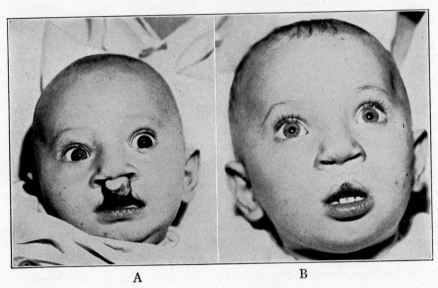

A   B

FIG. 398.—DOUBLE HARELIP BEFORE AND AFTER OPERATIVE REPAIR.

A, at four months of age just before repair of the lip. *B,* at one year of age; a cleft palate was repaired at this time (St. Louis Children's Hospital).

to specific causes such as infected teeth, chemical or physical irritants, or known bacterial invaders. Many are secondary to digestive disturbances of various types and are in general associated with poor hygiene and undernutrition, being frequent in neglected children. Mercury, bismuth and lead poisoning produce stomatitis. Bacterial infections of the Vincent's angina type have been described in Chapter VI. The clinical manifestations of stomatitis depend on the severity of the inflammation and consist of local pain and tenderness, foul breath and evidences of generalized infection. The nature of the lesion is noted on inspection and may be characterized by a catarrhal inflammation, by the appearance of grayish-white spots with a reddened border (aphthous stomatitis), or by actual ulceration. In severe cases a gangrenous stomatitis may occur with necrosis and destruction of tissue; this type of lesion is called *noma* and is described in the following paragraph. *Treatment* consists of removal of the cause, if known. Simple cleanliness and an alkaline mouth wash combined with general hygienic care are usually effective. The ulcers may be touched with 10 per cent silver nitrate or chromic acid. However, a warning should be issued against the use of strong escharotics such as the silver nitrate stick; severe destruction of tissue may follow its use in these patients. In the gangrenous type a fatal outcome is not uncommon (see Fig. 52). *Thrush* is a superficial infection of the anterior part of the tongue, gums and cheeks of infants who are fed starchy foods and live in unhygienic and unclean surroundings. It is due to a fungus, *Oidium albicans*. The disease is characterized by the appearance of white patches with an uneven surface. Removal of the crust or membrane reveals

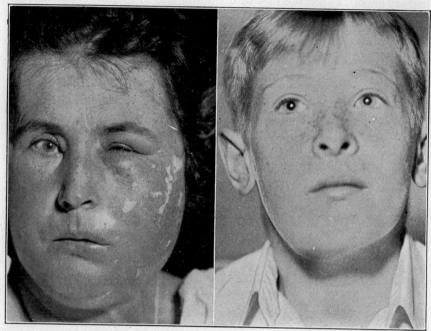

FIG. 399.   FIG. 400.

FIG. 399.—ACUTE DENTO-ALVEOLAR ABSCESS OF THE UPPER JAW IN A FORTY-YEAR-OLD HOUSEWIFE.

The swelling began nine days previously, forty-eight hours after the extraction of a left upper molar which had been painful for two weeks. The abscess opened into the mouth spontaneously shortly after the above picture was taken; a large amount of greenish, foul-smelling pus escaped (Barnes Hospital).

FIG. 400.—ACUTE DENTO-ALVEOLAR ABSCESS OF THE LOWER JAW OF ONE WEEK'S DURATION.

Incision and drainage of the abscess was followed by rapid healing with no evidence of osteomyelitis.

a red, soft, bleeding mucous membrane. Treatment consists of cleanliness, proper diet and local applications of gentian violet in aqueous solution.

Noma (Cancrum Oris).—This infection is in reality a progressive gangrene of the mouth, starting in a tiny portal of entry, usually about the lip or gum, in debilitated children weakened by some other disease, usually measles or pertussis. The disease also occurs in adults but is similarly a secondary manifestation of some general disease such as severe anemia, leukemia, etc. A variety of organisms have been held responsible for the disease, including the bacillus and spirochete found in Vincent's angina. Evidence of general infection is present. Spontaneous healing may occur but usually only in children; treatment, however, should be promptly instituted, particularly by measures designed to relieve the systemic effects of the infection, *e.g.,* transfusion, chemotherapy, etc. In order to halt the local destructive process, the cautery may be used to destroy diseased tissue. Plastic repair is usually necessary later to correct deformities (see also p. 92).

The Jaw.—Although infections of the teeth properly belong to dentistry many of them are important because they so frequently lead to surgical complications.

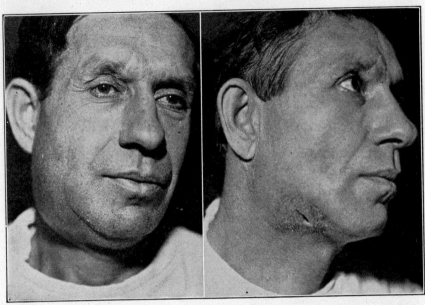

Fig. 401.—Acute Dento-alveolar Abscess followed by Chronic Osteomyelitis.
Three lower molars had been extracted several weeks previously. The two photographs are taken four days apart before and after incision and drainage. Foul-smelling pus was evacuated containing many types of mouth organisms (Barnes Hospital).

Acute Dento-alveolar Abscess.—If such an abscess (also called root abscess) is seen early, it should be drained just as an abscess elsewhere. In neglected cases the pus may burrow through the gum and present outside and rupture through the cheek, producing a draining sinus and disfiguring scar; in other instances the abscess may rupture on the lingual aspect of the mandible and enter the tissue spaces of the floor of the mouth and upper part of the neck, thereby producing a deep cervical infection. Involvement of bone of variable severity nearly always occurs, leading to osteomyelitis of the jaw, which is discussed below. Drainage of root abscesses should be instituted by a properly placed incision as soon as pus forms. The extraction of a tooth not worth saving is justified as a means of instituting drainage, but judgment should be exercised in *choosing the time for extraction.* In the early stages of the infection, at a time when the pain is severe, the temptation is great to relieve the patient by extraction. Yet such a procedure is often as prone to aggravate the infection as an early incision into an area of cellulitis (see p. 48). The danger lies in the conversion of a case of simple toothache into a serious and often fatal case of general septicemia.

Osteomyelitis of the Jaw.—Infection of the bone may develop as a sequel to acute dento-alveolar abscess; in reality every acute root abscess is a localized osteomyelitis, which, when slight, has little clinical significance. On the other hand, when healing of the abscess does not take place promptly, a spreading infection in the bone, or at times a block necrosis of the jaw, is to be suspected. However, x-ray is often necessary for its detection but will not show block necrosis under three weeks. Treatment should always be conservative; however, simple external dependent drainage is necessary in the severe cases. Loose fragments generally are discharged or are absorbed spontaneously. Fortunately, the osteomyelitis following most root abscesses remains local, does not involve the whole mandible, and therefore requires no special treatment.

Dental caries and pyorrhea alveolaris have an important medical significance as a source of focal infection.

Tumors of the jaw have been described on page 338.

The Tongue.—Among the congenital deformities, *tongue-tie* is the only one of importance. It is due to an abnormally short frenum which prevents the tip of the tongue from being extruded. The deformity may interfere with nursing and perhaps with speech later. The treatment in the mild cases is simple and consists of snipping the taut part of the frenum with the tongue elevated. However, in the severe cases, in which the tongue is bound down firmly to the floor of the mouth, a plastic operation will be necessary. *Simple ulcers* of the tongue are frequent and may be due to trauma or irritation from a sharp tooth or may follow a herpetic blister. If the lesion is chronic and in an older individual, a suspicion of cancer should be aroused, and biopsy performed if necessary. Microscopic examination of the whole lesion or part of it should be carried out, particularly if it persists for one month after ordinary therapy. *Tuberculous ulcers* of the tongue occur but rarely and may be associated with lupus of the face, starting as a nodule, as a traumatic ulcer, or spontaneously. It is indolent with a pale, uneven base. The ulcers are painful in late stages. Treatment depends on the extent of the lesion and the presence of disease elsewhere. Local excision is advisable when possible. *Syphilitic ulcers* may be due to primary, secondary, or tertiary disease. The chancre and mucous patch have the usual characteristics. Fissures occur along the border of the tongue due to irritation of the teeth. *Glossitis,* or inflammation of the tongue, has characteristics similar to those of stomatitis. Chronic glossitis assumes a variety of forms, such as keratosis and leukoplakia, which are important as precursors of carcinoma (see p. 302) and lesions suggesting sprue and other medical diseases.

Lingual thyroid is the designation of one type of aberrant thyroid tissue, which, however, is itself a rare anomaly. The tumor is located at the foramen cecum at the base of the tongue. If symptoms are produced by its presence excision may be indicated but must not be performed unless a normal thyroid is present, else myxedema will occur.

Tumors of the tongue include most of the benign neoplasms and squamous cell carcinoma; adenocarcinoma also occurs rarely. Cavernous hemangioma is not uncommon. Enlargement of the tongue (macroglossia) is often due to lymphangioma affecting nearly all of the tongue. Treatment has been discussed under neoplasms (Chapter XVI).

The Tonsils.—Of importance to the surgeon is the presence of *peritonsillar abscess* which may require incision and drainage. The history of tonsillar infection precedes the development of the abscess. There is local pain, inability to swallow or open the jaw widely, and salivation. Inspection will reveal a bulging of the anterior pillar with deviation of the uvula. Treatment consists of incision (always under local anesthesia and with the head dependent to avoid aspiration of pus) and drainage as soon as pus is present; suppuration is evident by the local appearance of the tonsillar region or by retropharyngeal swelling. *Retropharyngeal abscess* is not uncommon in young children, and produces interference with breathing and swallowing; respirations may be of a snoring type. The mouth is usually held open as it is when the child has enlarged adenoids. Diagnosis is made by palpation and inspection of the throat. Incision and drainage should be done with precautions against aspiration of pus, but only when the diagnosis is certain.

The Salivary Glands.—Though important in the mastication and digestion of food, the salivary glands are not often the seat of disease. Tumors and cysts have been considered previously (Chapter XVI). Infection and obstruction will be discussed here. Acute infection occurs practically only in the parotid gland.

Acute Parotitis.—This designation is most frequently applied to the swelling which occurs as an acute infectious disease (mumps) chiefly in childhood; the swelling, usually in both parotids is painful but transient in character.

Acute parotitis, which is not due to mumps, is nearly always unilateral at the onset but usually involves the other side sooner or later. The infection occurs most often as a postoperative complication, often in weak, debilitated patients. The disease is ushered in with pain and tenderness over the gland, fever and other manifestations of a generalized infection. In the severe cases there is a pronounced induration of adjacent tissue which accounts for the "lockjaw" so frequently present. If the excretory (Stensen's) duct is visualized by retracting the lips so as to expose the inner side of the cheek, the orifice is swollen and reddened, and often exudes pus, particularly when the duct is stroked toward the orifice. It is probable that the infection is an ascending one through the duct, rather than a blood-borne invasion. It is probable, therefore, that prophylactic measures such as oral hygiene will prevent a great many of these infections; this is particularly important in patients with severe gastro-intestinal lesions in whom "nothing by mouth" is necessary as a postoperative order. The dry infected oral mucous membrane should receive adequate local care in such cases.

Treatment, aside from the prophylactic measures just mentioned, consists of the insertion of a tiny probe into the duct, a procedure which may augment drainage and thus aid in the subsidence of the infection. In many instances spontaneous resolution of the disease occurs either with or without such a procedure. In other patients the course is steadily downward with all the manifestations of acute septicemia. There is a growing tendency toward conservatism in the treatment of this type of acute parotitis, and delay of incision until fluctuation is demonstrable. Fluctuation is often difficult to elicit through the tough aponeurotic capsule; an area of softening, however, can usually be made out at some point on the surface of the gland. The incision should be adequate in order to drain all the pockets. Incision and drainage may at times be indicated in the absence of demonstrable suppuration, particularly when significant fever and toxemia is present, and life seems to be threatened. Radiotherapy to the side of the gland has also been recommended.

Obstruction to the Salivary Ducts.—While obstruction may occur in the parotid, it is much more common in the submaxillary gland. The sublingual gland presents a different problem because it really consists of many tiny glands, each with its own

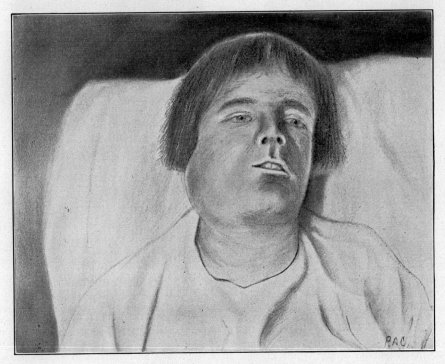

FIG. 402.—ACUTE PAROTITIS.

The patient is a thirty-five-year-old woman upon whom a rectal operation had been performed ten days previously under general anesthesia. The swelling began on the seventh postoperative day;. five days later the opposite parotid became similarly involved. The patient was treated conservatively and several days later small abscesses were incised; recovery was eventually complete.

excretory duct. When one of them becomes obstructed a ranula may develop (see Fig. 195). The most common cause of obstruction to the parotid or submaxillary gland is sialolithiasis, *i.e.,* the presence in the duct of a stone which is usually composed of calcium salts, thus making it radiopaque. The obstruction may be associated with a certain degree of chronic infection which accounts for the variations in the degree of occlusion. There may be no symptoms during periods when saliva is able to flow around the calculus, but with the onset of edema and complete occlusion, localized pain occurs and swelling of the gland develops. An almost diagnostic feature is the exaggeration of the swelling and often of pain during mastication of food; such an effect is probably due to a distention of the intraglandular ducts with saliva. The stone can sometimes be palpated with the finger and often can be seen in the roentgenogram. Removal of the calculus is usually a simple procedure if it is in the distal part of the duct, but if it is embedded in the gland and extensive disease of the secreting parenchyma is present, total excision of the organ may be indicated.

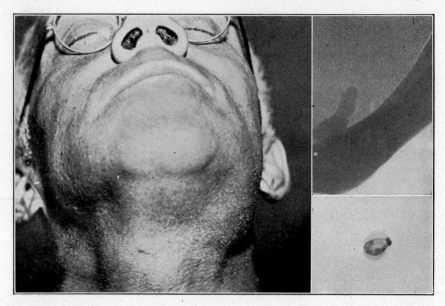

FIG. 403.—OBSTRUCTION OF THE SUBMAXILLARY DUCT DUE TO STONE (SIALOLITHIASIS).

The patient, aged sixty, had been aware of a mass, more or less tender, under the left jaw for many years. It enlarged during and following meals; occasionally it disappeared entirely. A lump under the left side of the tongue was also noted; the symptoms have become more pronounced the past few months. Note the swelling under the angle of the left side of the mandible. The photograph shows the enlarged submaxillary gland, and the x-ray reveals the stone. A photograph of part of the calculus after removal is also included in the lower right hand corner of the illustration.

Mikulicz's disease is a rare condition causing a bilateral enlargement of the salivary and lachrymal glands; few manifestations are produced aside from the swelling. Excision may be indicated; radiotherapy has been recommended.

Deep Cellulitis and Abscess of the Neck.—The portion of the neck which lies beneath the deep fascia, and including also the floor of the mouth, is not infrequently involved secondarily to the infections of the oral cavity which have already been described. Often however, the nature of the primary portal of entry is difficult to demonstrate although careful search should always be made. In most instances the deep cervical infection will be preceded by some type of stomatitis, an alveolar abscess, acute lymphadenitis, or tonsillitis; occasionally it may be produced by direct contamination through a deep wound, or from an inadequately treated or neglected fracture of the mandible (p. 382). It may be a manifestation of agranulocytosis (agranulocytic angina) or of leukemia. Most of these cervical infections are located so deeply that there is no difficulty in distinguishing them from the superficial infections of the neck which are so commonly due to skin lesions or subcutaneous lymphadenitis (p. 534). Acute diffuse cellulitis of the tissue in the sub-maxillary triangle, involving also the floor of the mouth, is generally classified as Ludwig's angina which has already been described on page 92.

The typical cases of deep cervical infections are much different from Ludwig's angina in that they assume a less diffuse form and exhibit localized redness, indura-tion and often a brawny edema, confined first to one side of the neck, but not in-frequently spreading across the midline. They are often due to a deep cervical lymphadenitis (see p. 536). The systemic manifestations of septicemia which accom-pany such an infection are severe; pressure symptoms may produce sufficient respiratory obstruction to demand tracheotomy.

Treatment of any acute deep cervical infection is operative but should in all cases be preceded by a period of rest in bed, general care, chemotherapy, and an attempt to localize the process as much as possible by the application of heat and immobilization. However, incision and drainage are frequently indicated, even if suppuration is not definitely demonstrable. The site and extent of the incision de-pends on the location of the swelling and on the path of the infection as demon-strated after opening the lesion at one point. X-ray treatment may be of great benefit in some cases, but in general merely accelerates the normal inflammatory processes.

ESOPHAGUS

The esophagus or gullet is a muscular tube concerned with swallowing or deglutition; the upper portion is under voluntary control whereas the lower and larger portion is involuntary and is composed of smooth muscle fibers. As might be expected, therefore, diseases of the esophagus produce clinical manifestations by interfering with normal deglutition. Difficulty in swallowing is called dysphagia, which varies greatly in severity, from a transient impediment to the ingestion of solid foods, to a complete inability to swallow even liquids. Regurgitation must always be distinguished from true vomiting. Usually the patient will know when gastric contents are ejected because of the sour taste. The material regurgitated in esophageal disease may merely be swallowed saliva; it may consist of fluids taken just a few minutes before; it may be composed of food eaten many hours previ-ously in patients harboring a large diverticulum or dilated esophagus of sufficient size to retain such food.

Dysphagia may develop as an acute symptom or be of gradual evolution. Sudden dysphagia is usually due to the immediate effects of swallowing corrosive materials, to a foreign body, or acute lesions in the neck or mediastinum such as abscess, thyroiditis, and lymphadenitis which involve the esophagus by contiguity. Chronic dysphagia may be produced by strictures and tumors within the gullet, or by aneurysms, vertebral disease, mediastinal tumors, or other masses pressing on it from without. Occasionally, paralysis of the ninth and twelfth cranial nerves is responsible for dysphagia. *Gradually increasing dysphagia in an otherwise healthy elderly person, particularly in a male, is nearly always due to carcinoma.*

For purposes of diagnosis, special examinations are essential. These special methods include (1) fluoroscopic and x-ray study during and after ingestion of a barium meal, and (2) direct inspection of the interior of the esophagus by a special instrument, the esophagoscope, which is similar to a bronchoscope. Both types of examination will yield valuable information when carried out by those expert in their use. It should be emphasized, however, that the passage of a bougie or tube into the esophagus of a patient with dysphagia is apt to be a dangerous procedure if an aneurysm or acute ulceration is present, and should not be performed unless such lesions are definitely ruled out.

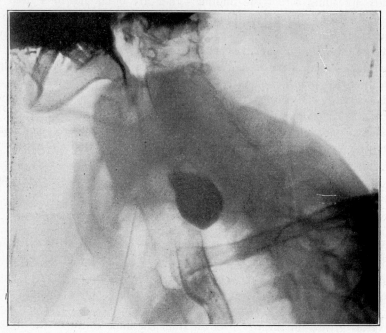

FIG. 404.—PHARYNGEAL (ESOPHAGEAL) DIVERTICULUM.

The roentgenogram is an oblique view after the ingestion of barium and shows the pouch well outlined. The patient, a sixty-three-year-old male, first noted regurgitation of food following meals, especially when lying down; often a gurgling sound preceded the vomiting. Excision was performed in one stage with uneventful recovery. (Courtesy of Dr. V. P. Blair.)

Diverticulum of the Esophagus.—This lesion (also called pulsion diverticulum) is really located in the *pharynx* and is a sac which forms as a herniation through the posterior pharyngeal wall, presumably because of a congenital defect. Traction diverticulum represents another type, but is small in size and has no clinical significance, being noted usually only at autopsy. They are asymptomatic, usually located in the midportion, and are the result of traction by a scar produced by an inflammatory process (*e.g.,* suppurating lymph node). Pulsion diverticulum develops at the weakest point in the muscular wall of the posterior pharynx, just above the cricoid cartilage where the constrictor fibers merge with the circular fibers to form the cricopharyngeus muscle. Although the neck of the sac is thus in the midline, it presents to either one side or the other, nearly always to the left, as it increases in size, but rarely becomes large enough to be visible as a definite mass. Symptoms of slight difficulty in swallowing may date back to childhood. Pronounced manifestations, however, are not produced unless the sac attains a fairly large size and contains food which may be retained for variable periods of time. The patient may be conscious of peculiar sounds, or slight discomfort associated with the deglutition. There may be regurgitation of soured or foul food retained in the diverticulum. The sac may become large enough to produce a definite mechanical obstruction. In the severe cases malnutrition may develop. The diagnosis will usually be obvious by x-ray visualization of the sac (lateral view especially) after ingestion of a barium meal. *Treatment* consists of surgical excision, which is performed ordinarily by dividing the procedure in two stages. Because of the danger of a fatal mediastinitis, it is preferable to mobilize the diverticulum at the first stage, thus allowing adhesions to form about the sac so that it may be excised at the second stage without the possibility of any of the foul contents of the sac contaminating the easily invaded tissue of the deep structures of the neck which communicate directly with the mediastinum. However, there is a growing tendency to excise the sac completely, with careful closure of the esophagus at one stage. Shallow,[3] for example, has reported a series of 76 cases in which a one-stage operation was performed without a single instance of mediastinal infection.

Cardiospasm.—When slight, cardiospasm produces only transient difficulty in swallowing, being thus related to the functional esophageal spasm, known popularly as "globus hystericus," but which is common only in the upper part of the gullet. Cardiospasm, however, when it is severe and of long standing, produces a marked *fusiform dilatation* of the esophagus. After a time the gullet may become so large that it retains considerable amounts of ingested food and liquids. The patient may seem to eat and drink normally but when regurgitation occurs, it may be so profuse as to be mistaken for vomiting. In spite of the marked retention, sufficient food may pass through the obstruction to maintain the patient's normal weight. This is in contrast to other types of obstruction (stricture, carcinoma) which lead to severe emaciation. Cardiospasm may also be distinguished from carcinoma and stricture by x-ray and fluoroscopic study, which is often of decisive importance.

Treatment may be instituted from above by means of procedures designed to dilate the cardia through various manipulative devices. In severe cases the obstruction becomes organic; the term achalasia of the esophagus is often used. For such a lesion an abdominal operation may be necessary in order to relieve the obstruction; the procedure is often called an esophagoplasty (Womack[4]).

Stricture of the Esophagus.—Stricture is due to the contraction of fibrous tissue deposited in the esophageal wall. Such fibrous tissue is always formed in response to a previous ulceration, which is usually produced by the accidental ingestion of corrosive chemicals. The most common example is the swallowing of lye by young children. When fatal poisoning or perforation does not occur, the cicatricial contraction of the resulting scar will gradually result in difficulty in swallowing followed by regurgitation. Stricture formation or stenosis also occurs after other ulcerative lesions, particularly carcinoma, which, however, ordinarily has an entirely different history (see p. 661). X-ray and fluoroscopic study also enables an accurate diagnosis to be made. Many patients may suffer only mild disability because of the stricture, but in most cases the dysphagia becomes severe as the stenosis becomes complete.

Treatment in the severe cases consists of a preliminary gastrostomy (see p. 663) followed by gradual dilatation of the stricture. Many methods of dilatation are available; one procedure (retrograde bouginage) consists of having the patient swallow a thread which is fished out of the stomach through the gastrostomy opening, and to which beads of increasing caliber are attached and pulled gently through the stricture by traction from above. According to another method the solid beads are attached to the thread on the oral side and pulled through the stricture by traction exerted through the abdominal wound. Both methods may also be used alternately.

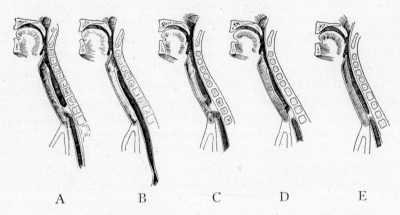

A   B   C   D   E

Fig. 405.—Types of Congenital Malformation of the Esophagus.

A, the type in which the proximal portion ends blindly, the distal portion communicating with the trachea; this type is found in from 80 to 90 per cent of the anomalies; *B*, constriction without atresia, usually occurring at the distal end of the esophagus; *C*, communication between the trachea and each segment of the esophagus; *D*, communication between the trachea and the proximal segment (rare), and *E*, atresia of the esophagus without a tracheal fistula. (From W. H. Cole, *Arch. Surg.*, 23:820, 1931.)

Coöperation between the surgeon and esophagoscopist achieves the best results. In most instances a functioning gullet will result, especially if dilatation is repeated at intervals, and particular attention is paid to the diet and to thorough mastication, in order to avoid swallowing large particles. Eventually the gastrostomy wound may be closed; during the periods of active treatment it is used to administer liquid feedings. In most instances the narrowing of the lumen is not sufficient to prevent swallowing of food, particularly liquids, by the time the patient is seen by the physician. On these occasions, the dilatation may often be carried out by the esophagoscope through the mouth and upper esophagus, without the necessity of gastrostomy.

Congenital stricture and other anomalies of the esophagus are rare but are apparent immediately after birth (see Fig. 405). In addition to various degrees of occlusion or absence of the esophagus, abnormal communications between the distal or proximal gullet and the trachea occur, thereby making the problem of surgical relief difficult or impossible.

Foreign Bodies in the Esophagus.—This condition is of common occurrence in children. The history of the accidental swallowing of a foreign body such as a plaything is usually obtained, but in many instances the first intimation of difficulty may be pain and inability to swallow, followed by regurgitation. If cough and respiratory difficulty occurs, the foreign body is probably in the trachea. If the patient is seen immediately after the accident, a sedative (morphine) is given as soon as possible to allay apprehension and muscular spasm. After relaxation the object is frequently swallowed and reaches the stomach where its presence is of much less concern (see p. 677). Sometimes the object is regurgitated spontaneously. If neither occurs, the child should be brought to a hospital where an x-ray is taken in order to reveal objects which are radiopaque. If the object is sharp, its removal is urgent, in order to prevent esophageal perforation, inasmuch as perforation

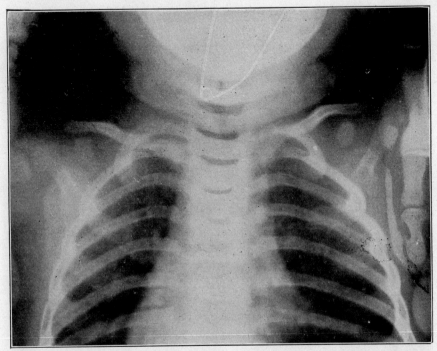

FIG. 406.—ROENTGENOGRAM TAKEN IMMEDIATELY AFTER ADMISSION SHOWING OPEN SAFETY PIN, WHICH THE PATIENT, A TWO-YEAR-OLD CHILD, HAD SWALLOWED A FEW HOURS PREVIOUSLY.

A few minutes after this x-ray was taken the child swallowed several times and the pin passed into the stomach (see Fig. 416).

may lead to a mediastinal infection which is nearly always fatal. On the other hand, the manipulations incident to its removal may produce such a perforation unless performed by an expert. The use of solid food to aid in enabling the esophagus to force the object into the stomach may be used in some instances but only when there is no danger that a sharp point may thereby be made to puncture the wall of the gullet.

Carcinoma of the Esophagus.—This neoplasm is usually of the squamous-cell type arising from the mucous membrane; a few arise from the submucous glands and are therefore adenocarcinomas. It is not a common cancer, comprising about 5 per cent of all malignant disease. The growth rapidly ulcerates the mucosa, and later, by its growth or by fibrous tissue contraction, leads to obstruction of the lumen. The disease occurs in males far more frequently than in females, and in individuals of more advanced years. The disease may occur at any level of the gullet but is more common in the distal portion. Perforation may occur; metastases unfortunately may be widespread when the patient is first seen.

The *clinical manifestations* are due to a gradually increasing difficulty in swallowing, first of solid food and later even of liquids. Regurgitation of food and drink soon develops after stenosis becomes severe. Loss of weight is progressive and is due largely to starvation. Pain is entirely absent. Diagnosis is made by

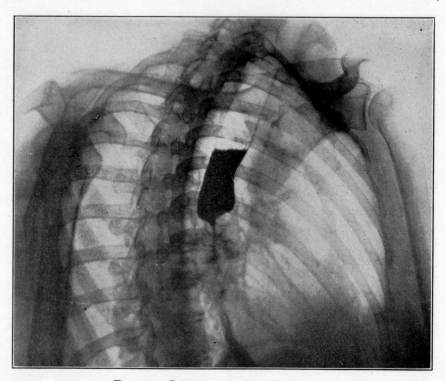

FIG. 407.—CARCINOMA OF THE ESOPHAGUS.

Roentgenogram after ingestion of barium (oblique view) in a patient aged sixty-one, with symptoms of but three months' duration. There was an increasing difficulty in swallowing, first of solid food, and a weight loss of 22 pounds. The obstruction in this case is higher than the most common site which is in the lower portion of the esophagus.

noting the deformity produced in the x-ray film after the ingestion of a barium meal. Of considerable aid is the direct vision of the lesion through the esophagoscope; examination of a biopsy specimen removed in this manner will often enable the diagnosis to be made with certainty.

Treatment is usually surgical. If deglutition has become so impaired that even liquid food cannot be ingested, a gastrostomy will have to be performed to permit feeding. Too often this procedure is performed at such a late date that it proves ineffective in halting or combating the emaciation. If the tumor can be excised before metastasis occurs, cure may be expected and indeed has been achieved. With the increasing interest in thoracic surgery many more patients may be offered the possibility of complete excision of their tumors. The literature on the transpleural approach has been reviewed by Carter, Stevenson and Abbott[5] who have described two successful excisions of their own in which the tumor was at the lower end of the esophagus. Carter[6] has also described two successful excisions higher in the esophagus by the Torek technic, by which an extrapleural esophagus is made outside the thoracic cage. Conservative treatment consists of the use of x-ray therapy and radium therapy. Although the results following their use have been disappointing, they may lead to palliation in some cases by keeping the lumen open for a considerable period of time, aided perhaps by dilatation, so that the patient may swallow and thus obviate the necessity of a gastrostomy. If excision of the lesion is contemplated a gastrostomy must first be carried out.

Gastrostomy.—This procedure is often necessary in esophageal obstruction, whether benign or malignant, whenever the amount of food passing through is insufficient to maintain the patient's general nutrition. Gastrostomy is also indicated preliminary to other operative procedures as already mentioned. If the lesion is one to be dilated (*e.g.,* stricture) the opening is made as near the cardiac orifice as possible through a high left rectus incision, so as to facilitate bouginage from the stomach side. On the other hand, if the surgeon plans a resection of a low-lying carcinoma with primary anastomosis according to the procedure mentioned previously (Carter, Stevenson and Abbott), such a gastrostomy would prove a handicap. In such a case the opening is made into a more distal part of the stomach or into the jejunum (jejunostomy).

Many types of gastrostomies have been described; they fall into two general groups depending upon whether the opening is to be permanent or temporary. In the latter case a large catheter is inserted into the stomach through a small incision and the wall infolded with concentric purse-string sutures around the tube which is brought out through the abdominal incision. The Witzel technic is similar except that the infolded stomach wall extends laterally rather than concentrically. In either case the tube is surrounded by connective tissue so that when it is removed the fistula rapidly closes. If a permanent gastrostomy is desired an operation of the Janeway type must be performed. In this procedure a flap of gastric wall is fashioned into a mucous-membrane-lined tube which is sutured around a catheter and the opening in the stomach closed. The external end of the flap is sewed to a part of the abdominal incision, mucosa to skin. There is thus created a short tunnel leading from the gastric lumen to the outside, lined by mucosa and easily entered with the catheter. As long as the mucocutaneous border is intact the fistula will not close. Leakage is prevented by a modification described by Spivack (The Surgical Technic of Abdominal Operations, S. B. Debour, Chicago, 1936), who makes a valve by folding the mucosa at the gastric end of the tube flap.

STOMACH AND DUODENUM

Gastric Ulcer.—Peptic ulcer, while not infrequent in the stomach, is located most commonly in the duodenum. Indeed, even when in the stomach this remarkable lesion is nearly always located in the pyloric region or along the lesser curvature. Its pathogenesis, though apparently similar to that of duodenal ulcer which is considered next, is less clearly understood. Gastric ulcer is of special importance because it is potential cancer, whereas duodenal ulcer never has been observed to undergo malignant change. The transition from gastric ulcer to carcinoma has been proved in many cases, although many ulcers exist for years without undergoing malignant change. Nevertheless, this possibility influences treatment to a considerable extent in that excision of the lesion is more definitely indicated.

Clinical Manifestations.—Peptic ulcer in general should be considered essentially as a chronic disease with long or short periods of remission or exacerbation. Gastric ulcer, though similar to a duodenal ulcer, has a less definite symptomatology.

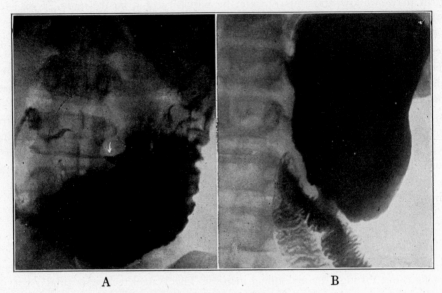

A   B

FIG. 408.—GASTRIC ULCER.

Roentgenograms of the stomach, visualized by the ingestion of a "barium meal," which consists of a suspension of barium sulphate in water or buttermilk. *A,* before operation; note the "niche," indicated by the arrow, characteristic of a peptic ulcer. A gastric resection was performed; the gross and microscopic specimens are represented in Figure 409; *B,* after operation, showing the new stoma between the stomach and jejunum.

Epigastric distress or pain, while periodic and definitely related to food intake, is more apt to be variable, even though often severe. Relief of pain by ingestion of food or alkali is often experienced. Though the pain may be deep (*i.e ,* splanchnic pain, localized to the lesion itself) it is frequently referred to superficial skin areas which are also the site of localized tenderness and sometimes of hyperesthesia. Bolton[7] has studied many patients with peptic ulcers and has found that this superficial pain and tenderness is nearly always referred to the midline of the epigastrium, occasionally, however, to the left and the right. Such areas should be carefully looked for in patients suspected of having pain of gastric or duodenal origin whether functional or organic. Such symptoms as dyspepsia (sour eructations, gas, heartburn) are not infrequent. Vomiting is not uncommon. Diagnosis is readily made by the x-ray after a barium meal by the demonstration of a characteristic niche in the outline of the stomach and by other manifestations which enable the expert radiologist to distinguish the lesions from carcinoma in most cases. Gastroscopic examination is also of value. Although acute perforation of gastric ulcer is less frequent than in duodenal ulcer, chronic gastric lesions which become indurated because

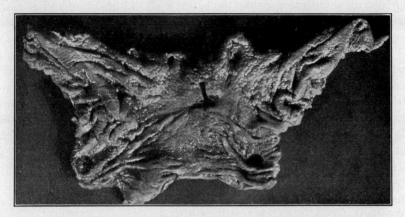

A

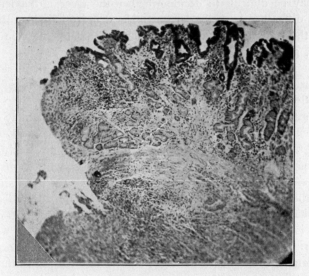

B

FIG. 409.—GASTRIC ULCER IN A TWENTY-NINE-YEAR-OLD WOMAN.

The patient had a long history of epigastric pain unrelieved by medical care. For several days the patient had vomited "coffee ground" material. The x-ray had shown the presence of an ulcer (see Fig. 408); definite organic obstruction was also present. Complete relief of symptoms followed operation. *A,* gross specimen of resected stomach opened along the greater curvature. The block removed for microscopic section is seen as a dark, rectangular area. *B,* photomicrograph of the edge of the ulcer; there is no evidence of malignancy.

of fibrous tissue ingrowth are more common; gradual perforation into adjacent organs, especially the pancreas, are not infrequent and produce severe symptoms. Gastric ulcer is frequently associated with definite gallbladder and appendiceal disease and may, indeed, be overlooked in their presence, not only clinically, but also at operation. Unlike duodenal ulcer it is as common in women as men. Hemorrhage and obstruction will be considered under Complications (see p. 670).

Treatment.—Though uncomplicated gastric ulcer may be started on medical therapy like duodenal ulcer, unlike the latter, it should be considered as essentially a surgical lesion because it may harbor cancer or unsuspectingly develop malignant changes (see Allen and Welch, *Ann. Surg.,* 114:498, 1941). The likelihood of cancer places a grave responsibility on conservative therapy which should not persist beyond a month unless objective evidence of healing is demonstrable. If operation is carried out, resection of the ulcer, including more or less of the adjacent stomach (gastric resection), is the procedure of choice. Removal of the lesion is preferable to gastroenterostomy, not only because it is more effective in relieving symptoms, but also because gastric ulcer is a possible site of malignant degeneration, which often cannot be detected except after microscopic study. The complications of gastric ulcer, *i.e.,* perforation and hemorrhage, are similar to those of duodenal ulcer and will be considered under that heading.

Duodenal Ulcer.—Peptic ulceration occurs far more frequently in the duodenum than in the stomach (5:1). However, it frequently occurs so close to the pyloric ring that it may be difficult to decide whether the ulcer is duodenal or gastric. Ordinarily the difference is easily demonstrable at operation since the pylorus can be located by the transverse pyloric vein; ulcers distal to this vein are duodenal, proximal to it, gastric.

Pathology.—Duodenal ulcers are located nearly always in the first portion of the duodenum, just beyond the pyloric ring at the site where gastric contents first strike the duodenal mucosa. This fact, as will be mentioned later, probably has some significance in the pathogenesis. The lesions vary considerably in their gross anatomy and may be multiple. In the simplest ones the mucosa alone is denuded, but in most instances the necrosis or digestion extends more deeply so that more of the wall becomes involved. If, in the process, a blood vessel is eroded, *hemorrhage* follows; *perforation* of the entire duodenal wall occurs when the lesion reaches the serosa. When the ulcer is on the posterior wall, perforation encounters the head of the pancreas which becomes the site of a fibrous induration. More commonly, however, the ulcer is in the anterior duodenal wall so that perforation, when it occurs, reaches the peritoneal cavity resulting in a general peritonitis unless operation is promptly performed. Rarely does the right lobe of the liver, omentum or the gall-bladder become adherent to such a perforation and seal the leak.

Important also in the pathology of peptic ulcer is the fact that there is a definite healing process which explains the clinical behavior of many of these patients. Undoubtedly, many tiny erosions or even ulcers frequently form in the stomach and duodenum from the mechanical effects of hard or coarse food, or from other factors. Most of them probably heal without being noticed. Even when definite symptoms are present, the frequent spontaneous remissions enjoyed by these patients indicate intermittent healing. Such a healing process has been noted by roentgenologists. Surgeons have frequently seen a scar shining through the serosa of the first part of the duodenum in patients who present an "ulcer history" months or years previously but not at the time of operation. Of special surgical interest is the fact that the scar resulting from the healing of an extensive ulcer may be sufficient to produce an *obstruction* which may lead to serious symptoms as discussed under complications.

The *pathogenesis of peptic ulcer* is incompletely understood, but a few of the salient details will be described. Peptic ulceration is so called because pepsin, the proteolytic ferment in the gastric juice, plays an essential role in its formation; it is true at least that a peptic ulcer does not form in the absence of gastric juice. Thus gastric mucosa is always adjacent to or a few centimeters proximal to the site of the gastric or duodenal ulcer and also of marginal ulcer which, as described later, is chiefly on the jejunal side of the gastro-enterostomy stoma. Ulcers found in a Meckel's diverticulum, a rare lesion which is described under small intestines (p. 679), are always associated with the presence of aberrant gastric mucosa in the pouch (Mason and Graham[8]). Experimental peptic ulcers, likewise, occur just beyond secreting gastric mucosa. It appears, therefore, that not only is the proximity of gastric mucosa necessary for the formation of peptic ulcers, but that they form very close to the point where its secretion first comes in contact with the affected tissue.

The role of a high gastric acidity in the formation of peptic ulcer has long been realized because of the frequency of the abnormally high acid titration found in the gastric contents of patients suffering from ulcer. Indeed, it has been repeatedly noted that peptic ulcer does not develop in the absence of free hydrochloric acid, a fact of practical significance because anacidity is found in about 12 per cent of normal individuals. The beneficial effect of alkali therapy in these patients also suggests the deleterious action of high gastric acidity, not only in producing symptoms, but also in preventing ulcers from healing. It seems logical, therefore, to suppose that not only is the healing process interfered with by a high level of gastric acidity, but that digestion or necrosis continues with its aid. Indeed, it has been shown by Dragstedt[9] that *in vitro* digestion of living tissue by gastric juice occurs only when the acid concentration is above 0.15 per cent (46 degrees or 0.46N) which is about the upper level of normal gastric contents. Thus it seems obvious then that hydrochloric acid is of much more importance in the pathogenesis of peptic ulcer than is pepsin.

Repeatedly in the experimental production of peptic ulcer it has been shown that diversion of alkaline duodenal secretions will be followed by the spontaneous appearance of peptic ulceration, whereas healing occurs when the alkaline secretions are restored. Much of this evidence has been summarized in detail by Matthews and Dragstedt.[10] The assumption seems justified at any rate that a faulty regulation of gastric acidity plays an important part in the pathogenesis of peptic ulcer.

An abnormal motor function of the stomach and duodenum doubtless is another element in the pathogenesis of ulcer. In many patients with ulcer there is an increased gastric motor activity which enables highly acid contents to be forcefully ejected against the duodenal mucosa. Spasm of the pylorus occurs in many instances and may in itself interfere with adequate control of gastric acidity by interfering with regurgitation of alkaline duodenal contents, a theory which rests on a number of clinical and experimental observations. Spasm has also been shown to be a factor in the etiology of peptic ulcers produced experimentally by Steinberg and Starr.[11]

Since both secretory and muscular activities are thus involved, it is obvious that the autonomic nervous system which controls these functions probably has a good deal to do with the pathogenesis. It has long been known that worry, fatigue, and overwork greatly aggravate the clinical severity of peptic ulcer, undoubtedly because of their influence on gastroduodenal secretion and motility via the autonomic nerves, notably the vagus. This conception of autonomic derangement has been advanced within recent years through the well-known observations of W. B. Cannon.[12]

Other etiologic factors are also important, but less easily explainable. Thus, recurrence of symptoms are apt to be worse during the spring and fall seasons. Respiratory and oral infections, especially about the teeth, are also prone to aggravate the severity of the disease.

Clinical Manifestations.—Duodenal ulcer, aside from the complications mentioned below, produces a characteristic type of upper abdominal pain varying from a sense of hunger and distress to a dull gnawing, burning pain; severe disabling pain is relatively uncommon. The pain is not due to the presence of the ulcer *per se*, but to the spasm and cramping which it invokes. The pain is not only variable, but is essentially chronic, yet intermittent, and may disappear for months or years; as stated above, it is apt to be worse in the spring and fall, in times of great mental stress, and following infections, usually respiratory.

The pain is often described as hunger pain, for it occurs characteristically when the stomach is empty, *i.e.*, two to three hours (more or less) after meals. Moreover, it is usually relieved by eating. Patients soon learn this and carry food with them or keep it at the bedside because of the relief it affords. Relief is also achieved by taking alkalis, but it is not as lasting. Other symptoms, such as heartburn, belching, etc., are not characteristic since they are present in so many other conditions. Vomiting is frequent in severe cases, especially when pylorospasm is persistent or actual pyloric obstruction has developed.

On examination there may be deep tenderness in the epigastrium, presumably over the lesion. More superficial tenderness or hyperesthesia is due to the same mechanism which produces referred pain as noted under gastric ulcer. Other physical evidences of ulcer as elicited by the expert radiologist will lead to an accurate diagnosis in most instances. Examination of gastric contents is of value in that it usually reveals a high acid titer, particularly in patients who also show evidence of hypersecretion. However, high acidity may be found in patients without anatomical x-ray or operative evidence of ulcer. Nevertheless, such patients suffer from the same type of pain as described above; pylorospasm may be the explanation in such instances.

More serious manifestations of duodenal ulcer are due usually to the complications as described later. An excellent statistical analysis of the clinical behavior and treatment of peptic ulcer has been reported by Emery and Monroe.[13]

Treatment.—Uncomplicated duodenal ulcer is treated largely by medical means, particularly by modifications of the regimen popularized by Sippy.[14] Rest in bed with exclusion of all disturbing outside influences frequently results in the healing of peptic ulcer. Elimination of the causes for worry is extremely important, since on many occasions exacerbations can be traced to emotional strain.

Surgical treatment in peptic ulcer is ordinarily reserved for the complications of this disease, which are described below. An operation on the stomach and duodenum is necessary in uncomplicated peptic ulcer only rarely, *i.e.*, when symptoms persist in spite of adequate medical treatment. It has been found that the success of operation in the circumstances just noted, depends largely on the effectiveness with which gastric acidity is kept low. In general, two procedures are used in this group of cases: gastro-enterostomy and gastric resection. Gastro-enterostomy has the advantage of being simpler technically, and thus carries a lower mortality. On the other hand, it has a great disadvantage in that it fails to produce a high percentage of permanent cures. While 90 per cent of patients enjoy immediate relief of symptoms following gastro-enterostomy, the percentage rapidly drops with the passage of time so that within five years after operation more than half will be found to be suffering from their old symptoms. In many instances the recurrence of pain is due to the formation of a new ulcer in the jejunum just beyond the operative stoma (jejunal or marginal ulcer). For these reasons gastro-enterostomy is no longer advocated for the routine treatment of uncomplicated duodenal ulcer. Pyloroplasty of the Finney type is occasionally employed, with

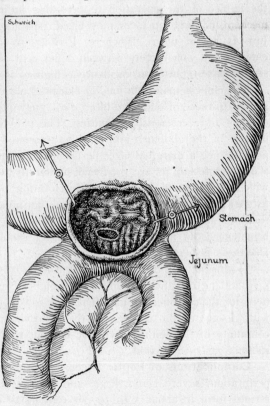

FIG. 410.—JEJUNAL ULCER FOLLOWING GASTRO-ENTEROSTOMY.

Ulcer is not marginal but is actually distal to the stoma and in the jejunum.

or without excision of the ulcer. More commonly used is partial gastrectomy, a procedure which has long been known to result in a more persistent lowering of gastric acidity than is the case following gastro-enterostomy. The reasons for this more effective lowering of acidity are not clear, although it is not due entirely to the resection of the stomach *per se* but also to the altered motor function induced by the anastomosis. Partial gastric resection, because of its effect on lowering gastric acidity, yields a much higher percentage of permanent cures and is followed by a much smaller incidence of marginal ulcers than is the case following gastro-enterostomy. The high mortality which followed gastric resection in the past has been steadily reduced within the past decade, due largely to more adequate pre-operative preparation and postoperative care. Nutritional deficiencies are frequent in these patients as in others with chronic gastro-intestinal disease. Correction of deficiencies, particularly hypoproteinemia, dehydration, lack of vitamin C and B_1, has been found to lower mortality tremendously (see p. 150).

Gastrojejunal (Marginal) Ulcer.—This is a distressing postoperative complication, usually following a gastro-enterostomy. It is a true peptic ulcer whose formation, no doubt, is due to the persistence of a high gastric acidity because of the failure of the operation to favorably influence the secretory or neutralizing mechanism. Such an ulcer may bleed, perforate, or lead to cicatricial contracture just as peptic ulcer elsewhere. Estimations of its incidence following gastro-enterostomy vary widely between 2 per cent and 10 per cent, although some observers have reported an incidence as high as 25 per cent.

The clinical manifestations of marginal ulcer are generally quite severe and are similar to those of duodenal ulcer, *i.e.,* "gnawing" pain, anorexia, nausea, epigastric distress and occasionally vomiting. The pain is often located to the left of the midline of the abdomen and may be associated with local tenderness at the same point. When a marginal ulcer perforates into the free peritoneal cavity sudden and acute manifestations are produced similar to those of a perforated duodenal ulcer which is discussed later. When perforation occurs into the colon (gastro-colic fistula) the manifestations are less acute but none the less severe; great wasting and fecal vomiting are usually produced. Bleeding may also occur and be severe; hematemesis is not as common as tarry stools but anemia may be prominent. Diagnosis is best made roentgenologically.

Treatment of a dietetic nature is usually tried but operation is generally necessary and nearly always requires a prolonged and difficult procedure. The operations for the treatment of marginal ulcer consist chiefly of (1) excision of the stoma with closure of the opening in the stomach and reëstablishment of the original continuity of the jejunum with or without the creation of a new stoma, and (2) subtotal gastric resection.

Complications of Peptic Ulcer.—The three most important complications are perforation, severe hemorrhage, and pyloric obstruction; together they occur in serious form in about 5 to 10 per cent of all cases. Hour-glass contracture also occurs, but is rare; it produces symptoms of obstruction and is associated only with gastric ulcer.

These complications apply both to gastric as well as duodenal ulcer, though the differentiation is nearly always clear. Carcinoma is a fourth complication of peptic ulcer, but applies only to gastric lesions. Duodenal ulcers practically never become malignant. The treatment of carcinoma is discussed separately.

PERFORATION.—A few ulcers may perforate slowly or into a solid viscus (liver, pancreas) and thus be manifested by rather indefinite, though severe pain and local tenderness. More commonly the perforation of a duodenal ulcer is of dramatic suddenness. It occurs practically only in males (95 per cent). The patient may have had previous digestive disturbances, but frequently the perforation is his first intimation of disease. It rarely occurs in treated cases; in untreated patients, 20 per cent perforated (Emery and Monroe). The pain is of excruciating severity and precipitates immediate prostration or collapse due apparently to the severity of the pain itself. The patient lies on his side with his knees drawn up and will not move for fear of aggravating the pain. He may break out into a sweat and his brow and extremities may be cold; there is, however, no other evidence of surgical shock, for the pulse and blood pressure are usually normal. Vomiting is nearly always present. On examination the abdomen presents the most pronounced rigidity and is aptly called "board-like." The slightest pressure elicits exquisite pain and the resistance of the spastic muscles cannot be overcome. It is most evident over the right rectus, however, particularly in the epigastrium. The patient's face is anxious, but only because of pain. Laboratory examination is negative except for a leuko-

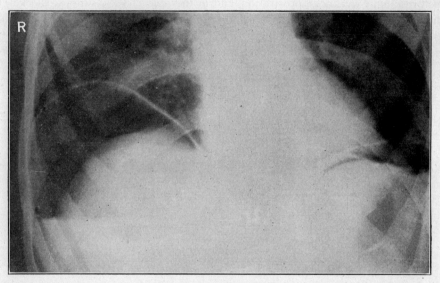

Fig. 411.—Pneumoperitoneum due to a Perforated Duodenal Ulcer in a Twenty-nine-year-old Male.

The roentgenogram was taken in the upright (sitting) position and shows air between the diaphragm and both the liver and stomach. The amount of air above the liver is unusually large; ordinarily only a narrow band can be made out. The patient was seized with severe pain and prostration 6 hours before admission. At operation a tiny round opening was found in the anterior surface of the duodenum just distal to the pyloric vein. The perforation was closed and recovery was uneventful; no further gastric symptoms developed subsequently (St. Louis City Hospital).

cytosis characteristic of peritoneal irritation. After a few hours a roentgenogram taken in the upright position will, in nearly all cases reveal air under the diaphragm (pneumoperitoneum). Differential diagnosis is discussed elsewhere (see Chap. XXV).

Treatment is entirely surgical and when the perforation is free into the peritoneal cavity represents an acute emergency. The mortality increases in direct proportion to the period elapsing between perforation and operation. If performed under six hours the mortality is very low, under twelve hours it is slight, between twelve and eighteen hours it is considerable, whereas after twenty-four hours the prognosis is grave indeed. The minimum requirement at operation is, of course, closure of the perforation. Additional procedures, such as gastro-enterostomy, pyloroplasty or resection are rarely indicated except in patients with a long ulcer history who are operated upon in excellent general condition within a few hours after the perforation.

HEMORRHAGE.—This is the most frequent of the complications occurring in significant degree in over 25 per cent of all cases; only a few are serious, however. Duodenal and gastric ulcers are equally liable to bleed. Wide variations in severity occur; only 5 per cent prove fatal (Emery and Monroe). A duodenal or gastric ulcer may bleed slowly, but persistently, and produce the clinical picture of secondary anemia. Of more importance surgically is the sudden severe hemorrhage which results in weakness, prostration, and in the severe cases, surgical shock. The patient will be pale, sweating, have cold extremities, a low blood pressure, and may die if the bleeding is severe enough. If the blood passes on into the intestine, the cause of the symptoms may be obscure unless the tarry character of the stool is noted

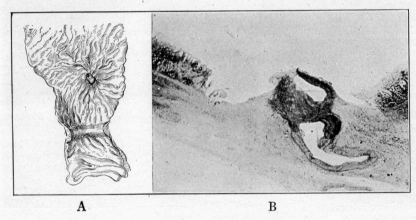

A   B

FIG. 412.—GASTRIC ULCER LEADING TO A FATAL HEMORRHAGE IN A TWENTY-SIX-YEAR-OLD MALE.

A, the gross appearance of the specimen of stomach opened along the greater curvature. Note the "pipe-stem" artery projecting into the base of the small ulcer; B, photomicrograph showing cross-section of the artery which was responsible for the hemorrhage. Operation in this patient would have been the only way of controlling the bleeding from such a vessel.

later. Ordinarily, however, the blood or part of it is soon vomited (hematemesis). However, even this does not necessarily establish the diagnosis of hemorrhage from a peptic ulcer. Unless such a lesion has been demonstrated before, or the history points to it, the bleeding may be due to other causes among which are esophageal varices. Pain is absent.

Treatment is in most cases essentially conservative. The treatment for shock mentioned on page 258 is carried out. Sedation is essential. Although "nothing by mouth" is generally ordered in these patients in order to keep the stomach at rest, the case against starvation therapy and in favor of liberal feeding is well reviewed by LaDue.[15] As long ago as 1906, Lenhartz treated 146 bleeding patients by feeding liberal amounts of egg and milk. Andresen in 1916 adopted a similar regime; Meulengracht popularized this form of therapy in 1935. The advantage of this principle of conservative therapy over unqualified starvation seems well established. Parenteral fluids are nevertheless often essential in the severe cases, especially the use of transfusions. Transfusion should be given when a great deal of blood has been lost, particularly, of course, when shock is present or seems imminent. The danger of precipitating further hemorrhage because of the resultant rise in blood pressure should be borne in mind; because of this, blood should be given slowly, guarding against sudden or pronounced increases in pressure.

Operation for bleeding peptic ulcer is rarely indicated because conservative therapy is so often followed by cessation of the bleeding. Occasionally this does not occur and operation may be necessary to control the hemorrhage. Acute massive

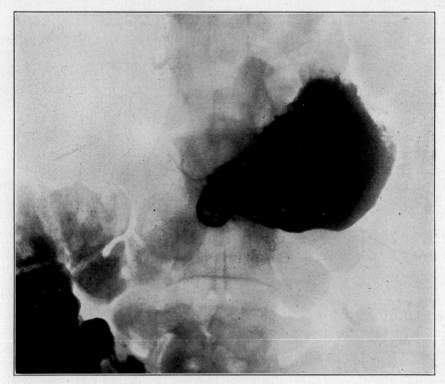

Fig. 413.—Pyloric Obstruction in a Thirty-six-year-old Male with a History of Many Years of Epigastric Pain Relieved by Alkali and Food.

Vomiting had been present for the past six months; in the vomitus could be recognized the food eaten the day previously. The print represented above is from an x-ray taken twenty-four hours after the ingestion of the barium meal; note that while much of the barium has passed, a large part is still within the stomach. At operation a stenosis of the pylorus due to an ulcer was noted; the patient remained asymptomatic following gastroenterostomy but required further surgery 10 years later due to the formation of a bleeding and painful jejunal ulcer.

and repeated hemorrhage is usually due to the presence of a rigid "pipe-stem" artery at the base of a calloused ulcer (see Fig. 412) which explains the failure of conservative therapy. It is, of course, impossible to tell at the bedside which patients harbor such a lesion. In general, however, it should be suspected when severe repeated bleeding continues for 24 or 48 hours. Operation is advisable under such circumstances, especially in the better risk patients. An excellent clinical study of this problem has been made by Allen.[16] If operation is carried out the bleeding point must be found and controlled. This often requires a direct approach to the posterior wall of the duodenum when the ulcer is at this site or a simple excision when the ulcer is in the stomach. It is sometimes also wise to operate in the face of continuous small hemorrhages as well as after several repeated massive ones. It should be emphasized, however, that if operation is performed for massive hemorrhage, it must, as pointed out by Allen, Finsterer and others, be done early; operations carried out more than forty-eight hours after the first of several severe bleedings is associated with a very high mortality, particularly in the older age group.

OBSTRUCTION.—Obstruction due to peptic ulcer is nearly always at the pylorus because both gastric and duodenal ulcers are frequently located near the pylorus. Such ulcers are indeed often spoken of collectively as pyloric ulcers and the obstruction resulting therefrom as pyloric obstruction. Gastric ulcer may rarely lead to an obstruction higher up, producing what is known as an hour-glass obstruction or contracture. Obstruction represents the late stage of a peptic ulcer which has healed partly or completely and in healing has led to cicatricial contraction, *i.e.,* stricture formation. The symptoms of vomiting and dehydration are essentially those of high intestinal obstruction (see pp. 757, 758). Pyloric obstruction is always suspected when the patient vomits material which he can recognize as food he has eaten 24 hours or more before. If a barium meal is swallowed the amount remaining in the stomach, as shown by x-ray, at 6 and 24 hours, yields accurate information as to the degree of completeness of the obstruction. In complete occlusion no barium will be found to leave the stomach even after 24 hours. A simpler bedside method is to empty the stomach by tube, measure the intake for 24 hours, empty the stomach again and calculate by difference the amount which has passed the pylorus. Such measurements are often useful in estimating the type of therapy to be followed. The progression of symptoms from those of ulcer to those of obstruction can usually be noted in the history. As long as no obstruction exists there will be a distinct tendency for the patient to be relieved of symptoms after meals or alkali. As obstruction develops, vomiting becomes more prominent, and less or no relief is obtained from eating or taking alkalis; indeed, eating usually aggravates the distress after obstruction becomes significant. Treatment consists of gastric lavage and parenteral fluids (to relieve dehydration if present) followed by operation for the relief of the obstruction through some type of anastomosis such as pyloroplasty or gastro-enterostomy. It may be difficult to tell even by x-ray, how much of the obstruction is due to pylorospasm and how much is due to stricture formation. A period of conservative care (small frequent feedings, alkali and antispasmodic drugs and daily gastric lavage) may be tried in such cases, as a therapeutic test. Progressive decreases in the amount of 24-hour retention indicate a favorable response to conservative treatment and that part of the obstruction was due to edema or spasm or both.

Gastric Cancer.—Carcinoma of the stomach is important not only because of its frequency but also because it is one of the so-called "silent" neoplasms, producing relatively few symptoms in its early stage, a stage during which surgical excision is a hopeful procedure. Unfortunately, in a large percentage of these patients the tumor has progressed beyond the stage of excision at the time operation is performed. As with cancer elsewhere, the symptomatology and the rapidity of growth vary greatly. Thus, a tumor at the pyloric end will produce symptoms early because of obstruction and be more easily detected. In the fundus, on the other hand (which is fortunately an uncommon site) the neoplasm may reach a large size before its presence is manifested. Except for the fact that a benign peptic ulcer may occasionally precede the cancer, no warning of the neoplasm occurs. The tumor usually takes the form of a surface growth which ulcerates and bleeds. Some are more fungating in type, others develop scirrhous characteristics. The tumor soon penetrates the stomach wall or metastasizes to the adjacent lymph nodes and the liver.

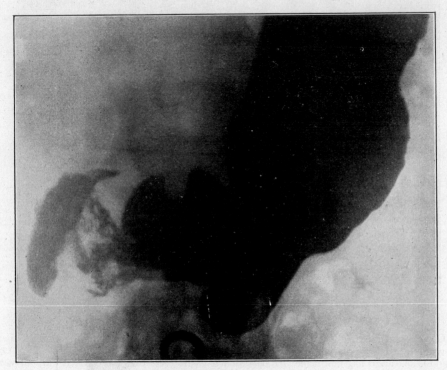

FIG. 414.—ROENTGENOGRAM OF THE STOMACH VISUALIZED BY THE INGESTION OF A "BARIUM MEAL."

Note the irregularity and filling defect in the prepyloric portion of the stomach; a diagnosis of carcinoma was made. The patient, aged fifty-eight, suffered from weakness, anemia, loss of weight and a dull pain in the abdomen relieved by food, dating back only eight months. At operation the growth was inoperable and death occurred shortly after. A biopsy showed on section, adenocarcinoma.

The possibility of cancer of the stomach should be considered in any individual in middle age or older who develops digestive symptoms without cause or precedent. These may be ever so slight, perhaps only an epigastric discomfort and anorexia. If such symptoms persist, the patient should consult his physician and if the symptoms are not readily explainable, x-ray study of the stomach after a barium meal should be made. This examination will be of greatest value when carried out by one expert in its use; it really constitutes our chief objective method of early diagnosis. A filling defect due to the presence of the neoplasm is the significant roentgenologic sign. Gastroscopic examination is useful in some of the more doubtful cases. Less important is the examination of gastric contents which may show blood, lactic acid, anacidity, sarcinae, etc. Anacidity, formerly considered of diagnostic value, is not always found in patients with gastric carcinoma; normal indi-

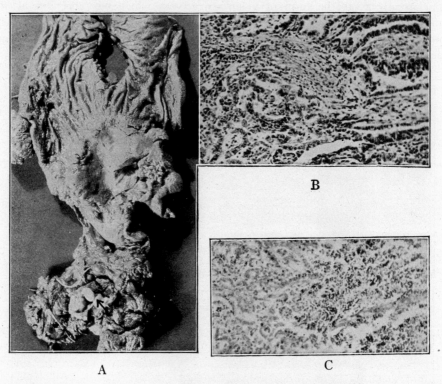

A   C

FIG. 415.—CARCINOMA OF THE STOMACH IN A FIFTY-NINE-YEAR-OLD WOMAN.

Onset was one year previously with epigastric pain and nausea, later vomiting of food eaten twenty-four to thirty-six hours previously. There was 65 pounds loss of weight. An x-ray diagnosis of carcinoma was made. At operation a gastric resection was carried out followed by an anastomosis of the stump of the stomach to the jejunum (modified Polya operation). A, the resected stomach opened along the greater curvature, with attached mesentery. One of the regional lymph nodes (indicated by the arrow) was cut across and shows metastatic carcinoma in the gross. The block removed from the edge of the crater for microscopic section is clearly seen; B, photomicrograph of the tissue in the block removed from the stomach; it shows the character of the growth which assumes a typical gland-like form and is hence called adenocarcinoma; C, appearance of a regional lymph node which contains malignant cells replacing the normal structure.

viduals, moreover, may have no acid in their gastric contents. Vomiting of food taken several hours previously is generally indicative of obstruction regardless of the cause; the presence of "coffee-ground" material in the vomitus is evidence of extensive ulceration and bleeding associated with gastric retention. Abdominal palpation may occasionally reveal the tumor but only when it has reached a considerable size. Anemia and loss of weight are usually late manifestations. Gastric carcinoma is nearly always associated with a variable amount of bleeding which may be detected by noting occult blood in the stools. A clinical summary of many cases has been published by Gaither.[17]

Treatment of gastric cancer is entirely surgical and consists of gastric resection well beyond the growth, particularly on the proximal side followed by some type of gastro-intestinal anastomosis. The mortality following gastric resection can be lowered considerably by preoperative correction of nutritional deficiencies (see p. 150) and by continuous gastric lavage to relieve the edema of the gastric wall induced by the long periods of gastric retention previous to operation. Obviously the presence of metastases to the liver precludes the chance of cure. In many cases all that can be achieved is relief of obstructive symptoms through gastrojejunostomy. Life may thus be prolonged for months—rarely for years. Excision of the lesion, even if metastases are evident, is frequently justifiable because of the marked symptomatic relief which follows the successful eradication of the infected bleeding ulcer. Radiotherapy has been disappointing. *Linitis plastica* is a special type of gastric carcinoma producing a diffuse scarring of the entire stomach which assumes the appearance of a tough wood-like pouch, hence its name. It represents a rare type of growth which contains a preponderance of fibrous tissue. Total gastrectomy must be performed in order to eliminate all of the diseased tissue and permit a successful anastomosis; this is carried out between the lower end of the esophagus and a loop of jejunum. In the duodenum cancer occurs so rarely as a primary lesion that it does not merit clinical consideration here.

Other Gastroduodenal Lesions.—*Foreign bodies in the stomach* are rare, but occasionally require operative removal. On most occasions such an operation is not necessary because the foreign body is usually passed spontaneously. Even open safety pins are disposed of in this way without perforating the intestinal wall. Progress may be determined by periodic x-ray examinations; if the object is sharp and becomes lodged for several days at some point laparotomy for its removal is indicated. Professional débris-swallowers are sometimes operated on for the removal of glass, nails, chains, etc. Food balls represent another type of foreign body which most often develop around the tough vegetable fiber present in ingested persimmons. They are in general called *bezoars*—if of vegetable origin, phytobezoars, and if of animal origin (hair, etc.) trichobezoars. Bezoars are generally discernible in x-ray examination after ingestion of barium, and produce a variety of symptoms, which are usually so significant as to demand operative removal of the foreign body by gastrotomy.

Polyps of the stomach occur and frequently are multiple. Diagnosis is made by x-ray or gastroscope in most cases. Excision by operation should probably always be carried out even if the symptoms are not severe because of the danger of malignant degeneration.

Occasionally *syphilis* produces a thickening of the wall and mucosal ulceration with symptoms and x-ray findings identical with cancer or peptic ulcer. The differentiation is particularly difficult because ulcer or cancer of the stomach may be present in a patient with a positive Wassermann (see p. 72).

Gastritis, as a pathological and clinical entity is now based largely on observations of the gastric mucosa with the flexible gastroscope. Gastritis is also said to be significant in peptic ulcer; many European observers have maintained that gastritis precedes, and is an etiologic factor in ulcer. *Phlegmonous gastritis,* a rare disease is due to extensive and severe infection of the stomach with systemic manifestations and a rapid fatal course. Treatment is palliative.

Acute dilatation of the stomach has been discussed elsewhere (p. 167). It occurs practically always as a postoperative or posttraumatic complication, especially when peritonitis is also present. The entire stomach gradually becomes more and more dilated with liquid and gas, and produces more or less obvious upper abdominal

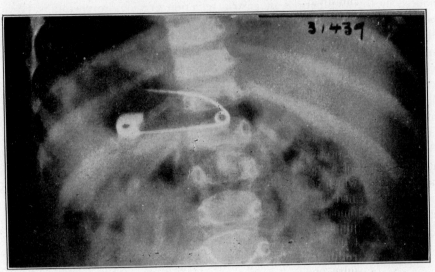

Fig. 416.—Foreign Body (Safety Pin) in the Stomach of a Two-year-old Child.

This roentgenogram was taken six days after the ingestion of the pin which first lodged in the esophagus (see Figure 406). The pin remained at the same point during the six days, although the child suffered no symptoms. Laparotomy was performed and the pin removed through a gastrotomy opening; recovery was uneventful.

distention and serious embarrassment (by pressure) to the heart and lungs. The patient is usually free from pain but vomits continuously, though in small amounts. Diagnosis is generally easy if the condition is suspected; treatment is simple and effective. The passage of a stomach tube will yield one or more liters of stomach contents, and produces an immediate and marked improvement in the patient's local and general condition. It is usually necessary to leave the tube in place for a day or two or until drainage from the stomach becomes insignificant. Indeed, the use of continuous gastric suction for 24 hours or more after operations will prevent the development of acute dilatation of the stomach.

Diverticulum of the duodenum is probably a congenital defect and is not infrequently noted by roentgenologists during an x-ray examination following the ingestion of barium sulphate. Its clinical significance is not great because it rarely produces symptoms and does not lead to serious disease. *Duodenitis* is a poorly understood lesion which is sometimes diagnosed only by the radiologist.

Duodenal fistula is a rare, but distressing postoperative complication following surgical procedures about the duodenum, stomach and pancreas. The destructive action of the discharge from the opening on the tissues is due to the presence of active trypsin. High intestinal fistulas of any type will also produce severe excoriation for the same reason. Treatment has been described on page 139. *Hypertrophic pyloric* stenosis is discussed under high intestinal obstruction in Chapter XXVI.

SMALL INTESTINE

Surprisingly few lesions are located in the small intestine. Polyps, adhesive bands, congenital anomalies (see Fig. 453), intussusception, and postoperative adhesions, which frequently cause intestinal obstruction, are described in Chapter XXVI. Cancer of the small intestine is very rare. Acute infection (enteritis) may result from ingestion of contaminated food and is of interest surgically because it may be confused with acute appendicitis and lead to an ill-advised operation.

Regional Ileitis.—This is a rather remarkable granulomatous lesion of the terminal ileum which has been described in detail by Crohn, Ginzberg and Oppenheimer [18] and others. The disease process is of unknown etiology but is characterized by subacute or chronic inflammation which leads to ulceration of the mucosa, edema and connective tissue proliferation of the remaining portion of the wall. At operation, performed usually for appendicitis, the involved ileum is thicker and more boggy than normal; edema and hyperemic or cyanotic areas are noted in the serosa. The mesentery of the involved ileum is thickened and contains enlarged lymph nodes. The disease occurs in young adults and runs a rather characteristic course, producing symptoms for several months or longer before coming under observation. Clinical manifestations consist of fever, diarrhea, continuous loss of weight and a progressive anemia, thus resembling ulcerative colitis. Stenosis of the bowel producing cramping pain and other symptoms of partial obstruction is common, particularly in the later stages of the disease. In a few patients perforation of the ulcerations leads to persistent fecal fistulas. A mass is present in the right lower quadrant in such cases. Diagnosis may often be made roentgenologically by excluding disease of the colon by the barium enema; the barium meal may give characteristic findings at the site of the diseased ileum. Carcinoma, tuberculosis and actinomycosis of the cecum, being close to the terminal ileum, may produce similar manifestations and must be considered in the differential diagnosis.

Treatment consists of excision of the diseased ileum and ileocecal valve followed by an appropriate ileocolic anastomosis. When a mass is present, particularly with fistulas, a short-circuiting anastomosis is first carried out by dividing the ileum at a point well above the disease, closing both ends and joining the proximal ileum to the ascending colon. Although excision can be done at a later date, symptoms are frequently well controlled by the simpler procedure. However, knowledge of the disease is too recent to make final judgment especially regarding possible extension of the lesion.

Meckel's Diverticulum.—This congenital anomaly is an outpouching of the ileum about one to three feet from the ileocecal valve and in reality is a remnant of the obliterated vitelline duct of embryonic life (see p. 720). It is found in 2 per cent of individuals and usually produces no symptoms. It may become inflamed and produce manifestations similar to acute appendicitis or cause acute intestinal obstruction because of associated adhesions. It sometimes contains aberrant gastric mucosa which commonly produces a peptic ulcer in the adjacent ileum. Such an ulmer may bleed or perforate as peptic ulcer elsewhere. A series of 19 cases of Meckel's diverticulum in which operation was performed was reported by Womack and Siegert (*Ann. Surg.*, 108:221, 1938). The fact that Meckel's diverticulum produces symptoms largely in childhood is shown by the fact that the majority of their cases occurred in children. Only 2 of them were over 21 and 5 of them were under 1 year of age. Most of the patients presented clinical manifestations of intestinal obstruction or perforation. Perforation produces acute abdominal symptoms such as severe pain, nausea, vomiting and manifestations which are not unlike those of peritonitis produced by other causes. In such instances

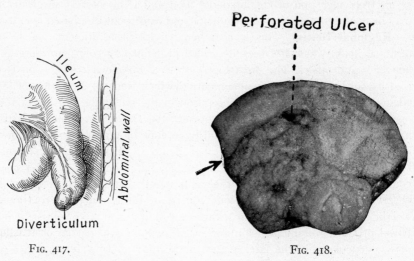

Fig. 417.

Fig. 418.

FIG. 417.—THE USUAL FORM OF MECKEL'S DIVERTICULUM.

Drawing of an intact specimen. Note that the proximal portion of the original vitelline duct persists, but having become closed at its end and detached from the umbilical region, it appears as a pouch hanging free from the convex border of the ileum. The omphalomesenteric vessels run up to its tip. (Redrawn from Kelly, *The Vermiform Appendix*, courtesy of J. B. Lippincott Co., Philadelphia.)

FIG. 418.—MECKEL'S DIVERTICULUM SHOWING A PERFORATED PEPTIC ULCER.

Photograph showing the inside of the specimen which has been opened and laid flat. The patient was a 6-year-old girl and was operated on for manifestations thought to be a general peritonitis of appendiceal origin. However, at operation the appendix was normal but there was a perforation in a Meckel's diverticulum, which was resected, the child making an uneventful recovery. The arrow points to the line of division between the ileal (above) and gastric mucosa (below), each verified by microscopic section. Note that the perforated ulcer is at the juncture of the two types of tissue. Another tiny ulcer can be seen in the middle of the aberrant gastric mucosa (St. Louis City Hospital).

the correct diagnosis will only rarely be made, but the acute manifestations will demand laparotomy during which the true nature of the lesion will be revealed. Blood in the stools in children is sometimes due to an ulcer in a Meckel's diverticulum. The ulcer may be accompanied by abdominal pain of variable severity located in the right lower quadrant or about the umbilicus; a diagnosis of chronic appendicitis is generally made. When symptoms are absent or are of a chronic nature, the x-ray may be the only means of making the diagnosis; however, the lesion frequently cannot be detected roentgenologically. During operations for unexplained abdominal pain the surgeon should always look for a Meckel's diverticulum.

Treatment is urgent only in the acute cases; the presence of abdominal pain, particularly if accompanied by persistent bleeding, will also justify operation in the patient with chronic manifestations. Excision of the sac with inversion of the base is performed.

Intestinal Fistula.—Abdominal wounds or abscesses which fail to heal should always be suspected of being intestinal fistulas. The diagnosis is, of course, obvious if fecal material can be recognized escaping from the wound. If necessary, a colored substance, *e.g.,* carmine, can be given by mouth; it will appear in the wound if a fistula is present. The higher the fistula, the sooner the color will appear, and the more irritated the skin about the wound will become. Most intestinal fistulas have a natural tendency to heal spontaneously. When closure does not occur within a few weeks or months a specific cause must be looked for, and eliminated if possible. These causes are generally one or more of the following: (1) An obstruction is present distal to the fistula. (2) The mucosa of the intestine is continuous with the skin. (3) A granulomatous infection is present, such as tuberculosis, actinomycosis or regional ileitis. Indeed, these lesions (to which must be included colloid carcinoma of the cecum) may lead to spontaneous fecal fistulas.

Acute Mesenteric Lymphadenitis.—The etiology of this condition is obscure; it occurs chiefly in children and is of surgical interest only since it may simulate acute appendicitis (see p. 686) because of the presence of abdominal pain, tenderness, nausea and vomiting. There is usually more fever than is expected with early appendicitis, and the abdominal findings are diffuse. The disease may follow or accompany various types of epidemic infections or of acute upper respiratory infection. If the patient is operated upon, the appendix will be found to be normal or only slightly injected; the mesenteric lymph nodes are enlarged, often to a size 2 to 3 centimeters in diameter. Microscopic section of these nodes reveals only a diffuse hyperplasia. Treatment is conservative; the abdominal manifestations usually subside spontaneously in a few days.

Typhoid fever sometimes causes perforation of the Peyer's patches in the small bowel, which of course represents an acute surgical emergency (p. 733). *Chronic mesenteric lymphadenitis* is usually tuberculous and is described under tuberculous peritonitis (p. 745).

THE APPENDIX

Acute Appendicitis.—This is one of the most frequent and serious of surgical diseases and respects no age, although it is more prone to occur in young adults. In children it is especially serious because of its more rapid, though often atypical course, and its tendency for early perforation. It accounts for nearly 20,000 fatalities a year in the United States alone. This high toll of life is preventable and would be lowered considerably if a prompt diagnosis were made and appendectomy could be carried out in every case. Undoubtedly the widespread use of cathartics, stimulated in recent years by national radio advertising, is an important factor in the maintenance of this high mortality (see p. 687).

The *pathogenesis* of the disease undoubtedly depends on the peculiar anatomy of the appendix. It is a long blind diverticulum with a narrow lumen which is easily occluded by a bit of food or inspissated feces (fecalith), a plug of mucus, or inflammatory edema, particularly at its base where it empties into the cecum. Since the lumen contains innumerable bacteria, such an obstruction allows them to multiply in a closed space and to invade the mucosa and set up an acute inflammation. Interference with the blood supply is no doubt an important factor

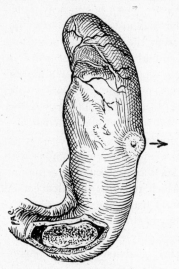

FIG. 419.—GROSS SPECIMEN OF AN ACUTELY INFLAMED, PERFORATED APPENDIX, REMOVED EIGHTEEN HOURS AFTER THE ONSET OF ACUTE ABDOMINAL PAIN.

Note the fecalith impacted at the base of the rather short appendix, producing an acute obstruction to the lumen, and the tense swollen part distal to it in the middle of which is the point of rupture indicated by the arrow.

in this process since the appendicular artery is a terminal vessel without anastomotic connections. Acute appendicular obstruction is a term which Wilkie[19] and Wangensteen[20] have emphasized as an important factor in the pathogenesis of the disease. An actual infection of the appendix then occurs which is serious because of the tendency for involvement of the entire appendiceal wall with subsequent perforation into surrounding tissue, especially into the peritoneal cavity. This perforation may occur rapidly, sometimes within a few hours after onset of the obstruction. Spontaneous healing, however, does frequently occur without perforation, either because of the mildness of the infection or because the obstructing fecalith becomes loose and allows drainage into the cecum. This usually takes several days, however. Indeed, many patients have a history of a succession of such episodes. Whether such repeated inflammation produces scar and fibrous adhesions sufficient to cause symptoms is not definitely known (see Chronic Appendicitis). There are, no doubt, many other factors besides obstruction, which are important in the pathogenesis. For example, it has long been known that lymphoid hyperplasia is associated in many instances with appendicitis.

Subsidence of acute appendicitis, unfortunately, cannot be predicted with certainty at the bedside. Moreover, when acute appendicitis does not subside spontaneously, perforation is usually inevitable and a variety of more or less serious complications may develop provided, of course, that appendectomy is not performed in the meantime. These complications deal most with the development of various degrees of localized or generalized peritonitis, a subject which is discussed in detail in Chapter 25. As applied to appendicitis, these complications present many peculiar features and are therefore also discussed on page 688 of this chapter. Such complications follow in most cases an actual perforation of the inflamed appendix (see Fig. 417), although the same effects follow in certain cases in which the entire appendix is more or less gangrenous without any gross perforation.

Clinical Manifestations.—Abdominal pain, vomiting and tenderness in the right lower quadrant are the three chief abdominal manifestations which should lead the patient or doctor to suspect acute appendicitis. The *pain* is often characteristic, being located in the epigastrium or generalized at first, but soon shifting to the right lower quadrant, *i.e.,* McBurney's point, which in adults is two inches from the anterior superior spine of the ilium on a line drawn from this process to the umbilicus. The pain is only moderately severe but disabling, often inducing the patient

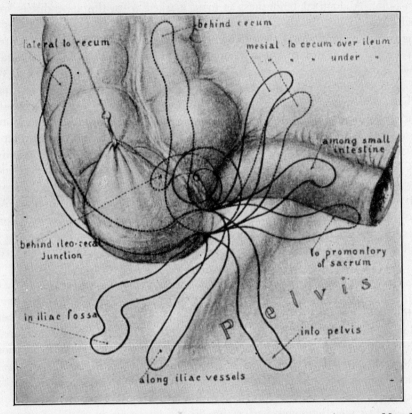

FIG. 420.—DIAGRAM SHOWING THE VARIOUS DIRECTIONS IN WHICH AN APPENDIX MAY POINT.

(From Kelly, *The Vermiform Appendix,* 1909, courtesy of J. B. Lippincott Co., Philadelphia.)

to seek bed rest. Great variations occur, depending on the location of the appendix which may be retrocecal, extend over the brim of the pelvis or upward toward the umbilicus. Indeed, in gangrenous appendicitis, pain may be slight or absent. On the other hand, if the appendix lies along the ureter or near the base of the urinary bladder the pain will radiate into the testicle or thigh or it may produce pain on urination, respectively. Such variations, though exceptional, will influence the severity, nature and location of the pain. *Vomiting* is an important symptom and characteristically is *preceded by pain* and nausea. It may occur but once or twice. On other occasions it is absent, particularly in the early stage of the disease, though nausea is usually present. The importance of pain, spontaneous and provoked, as a minimum syndrome of acute appendicitis has been emphasized by Ivanissevich [21] and others. Provoked pain, *i.e.,* tenderness localized to the acutely inflamed organ, is undoubtedly the most valuable single sign of acute appendicitis because it is the most frequent and least variable.

Abdominal tenderness, though often first noted by the physician, is frequently observed by the patient because of the pressure exerted by his clothes. He frequently prefers to lie with his thighs and knees flexed because of relief of pain afforded by this position. Abdominal tenderness is most marked when the appendix is free in the peritoneal cavity. In such a case there will be a local area of tenderness over the right lower quadrant. Palpation will also elicit muscle spasm, the degree of which varies roughly with the severity of the infection; it becomes generalized only when the appendix has perforated and general peritonitis has developed. When the appendix is retrocecal, tenderness may be slight or elicited only on deep palpation, but tenderness posteriorly may be significant. On many occasions rectal examination will reveal definite tenderness when the appendix lies along the posterior wall, or over the edge of the pelvis. At times localized right lower quadrant tenderness will be elicited only with the patient in the prone position, the examiner's hands being placed underneath the abdomen. Rebound tenderness, *i.e.,* on sudden release of palpation, should be noted when present.

Shortly after the onset a leukocytosis usually appears and is often progressive (12,000 to 18,000 per c.mm.); even when the count is normal, a differential count will usually show an abnormally high percentage of polymorphonuclear forms. Although the pulse rate and temperature rise after the inflammation has progressed sufficiently, the physician *should not have to wait for fever* before he makes a diagnosis of acute appendicitis. Constipation is usually present. Diarrhea is *not* a part of acute appendicitis unless purgation has resulted from the ingestion of cathartics. Diarrhea does accompany appendicitis occasionally, but only when the appendix lies along the anterior rectal wall. In such a case localized acute tenderness may be felt on careful rectal examination. Acute appendicitis may be an expression of acute enteritis which on rare instances becomes an instigating factor in the production of acute appendiceal inflammation.

Acute appendicitis during pregnancy deserves special mention because of the high mortality which follows perforation of the appendix in a pregnant woman. An excellent clinical study of 61 acute surgical emergencies of the abdomen in pregnancy has been made by Smith and Bartlett.[22] They emphasize the importance in acute appendicitis of localized tenderness. They also note that drainage in unruptured appendicitis is associated with a high incidence of miscarriage.

Later manifestations are due to the complications already mentioned, *i.e.,* local or general peritonitis (see Chap. XXV). The pain usually diminishes after rupture of the tense appendix and if it recurs is usually milder and does not manifest itself until several hours later. Vomiting, however, recurs and persists as more peritoneal surface becomes involved, and local tenderness spreads. *Fever* is a delayed manifestation of infection, being significant only at the time of or following perforation; it is therefore *not* necessary in the establishment of an early diagnosis. It is unfortunately true that many practitioners wait for fever to develop before making a definite diagnosis of appendicitis and therefore do not get these patients to the operating table before a local or general peritonitis is present. The manifestations of peritonitis along with other complications, such as pylephlebitis, subdiaphragmatic abscess, intestinal obstruction, etc., are discussed in Chapter XXV.

Differential Diagnosis.—In striving for early diagnosis in order to avoid the high mortality in late cases, one must realize that there are many diseases which simulate acute appendicitis. In many of these, operation is contraindicated and if performed may lead to a fatal outcome. Thus, one is often confronted by a Scylla and Charybdis, a dilemma which in some cases may tax the most experienced and careful observer. The type of pain is important in establishing a diagnosis of acute appendicitis; elimination of this disease, diagnostically, is often made difficult by exaggeration or inaccuracy in the patient's description of the pain. Vomiting is likewise important, especially because in appendicitis it rarely occurs *except when preceded by pain*. Local tenderness usually associated with muscle spasm is undoubtedly the most valuable manifestation, particularly when elicited by careful and expert abdominal palpation, the importance of which cannot be overemphasized.

Of the various specific diseases which simulate acute appendicitis, one may to some extent dismiss perforated ulcer, intestinal obstruction, twisted ovarian cyst, perforation of a viscus, as well as many other conditions, since laparotomy is indicated in these diseases and an erroneous diagnosis will not matter unless the actual lesion is not recognized at operation (see p. 733).

More important are the diseases in which *operations are contraindicated* because of the likelihood of a fatal termination due to the operation itself. In this group are lobar pneumonia, acute nephritis, idiopathic (primary) peritonitis, coronary disease and amebic dysentery. In *lobar pneumonia* the pain may be referred to the abdomen when the diaphragmatic pleura is involved. However, the abdominal signs are absent or confined to the upper abdomen; the patient has a rapid respiratory rate, there is dilatation of the nasal alae and a slight cyanosis. Chest examination in early pneumonia may reveal few signs, and roentgenograms may prove negative. With care, differentiation should not be difficult. In *acute nephritis* there may be vomiting and abdominal tenderness with rigidity of a diffuse character. The presence of abnormal urinary findings (albumin, casts, blood), and evidence of renal insufficiency (high blood urea and nonprotein nitrogen) is characteristic. *Idiopathic peritonitis* produces diffuse abdominal signs and is described on page 743. However, the pre- and postoperative use of the sulfonamides makes operation in this disease much less hazardous. *Coronary thrombosis and occlusion* not infrequently produce abdominal pain which, however, is located in the epigastrium and ordinarily is confused only with perforated ulcer or gallbladder and acute pancreatitis. The presence of dyspnea, orthopnea and cyanosis indicates cardiac, rather than abdominal disease. *Amebic dysentery* produces acute, diffuse, cramplike pain with mucus, pus and blood in the stool and diarrhea. Amebae can usually be found in the stool. Gatewood warns that atypical cases simulate appendicitis and, if erroneously operated upon, are associated with a high mortality (*Ill. M. J.* 71:41, 1937; see also McCoy & Hardy *J. A. M. A.*, 107:1357, 1936).

In another group, operation, while not indicated, is less apt to lead to deleterious results. They comprise the following: fecal stasis (constipation), spastic colitis, acute enteritis, gastric crises (tabes dorsalis), rupture of a Graafian follicle, acute pyelitis, acute right-sided salpingitis, intestinal allergy, acute epididymitis, ureteral stone (renal colic), abdominal wall pain (see page 556), etc. In this group thorough physical and laboratory examination is usually all that is needed to make the diagnosis. Thus it will exclude *pyelitis* (pus cells and bacteria in the urine) and *gastric crises* (absent knee kicks, Argyll-Robertson pupils, etc.). In *fecal stasis* the pain is slight, there are no signs of peritoneal inflammation; rectal examination may reveal sphincter spasm and fecal impaction. An effectual enema usually affords relief. In *spastic colitis* there may be a history of mucus in the stool associated with constipation, perhaps with occasional attacks of diarrhea. A spastic cecum may be palpated. In *acute enteritis* the history of eating spoiled food or of a dietary indiscretion may or may not be obtained; diarrhea is always present and the pain is diffuse and cramp-like in character and does not tend to localize. In *acute mesenteric lymphadenitis* the abdominal signs are marked but not localized. There may be rigidity and severe tenderness almost as great as that found in perforated ulcers, but the signs are diffuse and are usually equal on the two sides. The disease is present only in children and is usually associated with a red inflamed throat, fever, leukocytosis, prostration and vomiting (see also p. 681). In *rupture of a Graafian follicle* the pain, while severe, is momentary and there is only transient local tenderness; its occurrence during ovulation is suggestive. Patients with *salpingitis* due to the gonococcus usually give a history of vaginal discharge and urethritis (frequency and pain on urination). The facial appearance of these patients, even when the pulse is high and temperature is elevated, is characteristic, because it lacks the pained, anxious expression, and they do not appear so ill as do patients with acute appendicitis. The local signs are lower in the abdomen and pelvic examination usually reveals the nature of the lesion. The pain accompanying *intestinal allergy* may be severe, but local signs in the right lower quadrant are usually not present; the differential blood count may shown an eosinophilia. *Acute epididymitis* may simulate the local signs of acute appendicitis when the inflammation extends up into the vas and seminal vesicle, and pain referred up into the abdomen; examination of the testicle, however, is all that is necessary to detect the origin of the symptoms. In *renal colic* the pain ordinarily radiates along the ureter and down one thigh or into the perineum. Blood may be found in the urine and an x-ray may reveal a stone. When the appendix lies along the right ureter, however, it may, when inflamed, produce the same pain as a stone and even lead to hematuria. The local signs and leukocytosis serve to differentiate it from stone. There are many other diseases which on rare occasions offer difficulty, in differential diagnosis, such as Meckel's diverticulitis (see p. 679), tuberculosis of the cecum (see p. 695), regional ileitis (see p. 679), carcinoma of the colon (see p. 696), cholecystitis (see p. 615) and acute interstitial pancreatitis (see p. 635).

In the differential diagnosis of acute appendicitis, the surgeon must recognize the possibility and consequences of a mistaken diagnosis. Two kinds of mistakes may be made, *i.e.,* the surgeon may operate and find no surgical lesion or he may fail to operate and find that the patient has developed a peritonitis from perforation of an acutely inflamed appendix which he has failed to diagnose. In weighing the relative seriousness of these two mistakes he thinks of the following considerations. First, there is the mistake of operating when no surgical lesion is present. Such an

error is disastrous only if the patient is actually suffering from one of the diseases mentioned in the first group just discussed, *i.e.,* pneumonia, coronary disease, nephritis, amebic dysentery, etc. If they can be excluded the mistake is less serious because recovery practically always occurs. It is probable that even the most careful surgeons make such a mistake occasionally, though not more often than in 10 per cent of appendectomies performed for suspected acute appendicitis. On the other hand, to fail to operate on a patient with acute appendicitis is clearly a serious mistake for reasons already mentioned. It is largely because of the danger of peritonitis, that most surgeons, when confronted by a difficult problem in differential diagnosis will obviously prefer to make the lesser of the mistakes discussed above.

Treatment.—It should be emphasized that errors in treatment of acute appendicitis may be dangerous and even fatal. Unfortunately, errors are common. Catharsis, by stirring up an inflamed appendix, aggravates the process, prevents rest and natural healing, and thus promotes perforation and peritonitis. In many cases such dangerous treatment is self-inflicted; sad to relate, physicians are sometimes guilty. Often a cathartic is prescribed over the telephone. A drug clerk frequently advises it in order to sell some medicine. It is fortunate, however, that nature remedies the error in many cases by inducing immediate vomiting with consequent ejection of the cathartic. Nevertheless, the mortality records of acute ruptured appendicitis are filled with instances of unnecessary sacrifices to the great American practice of purgation. Many observers have recorded such evidence; Keyes,[23] for example, found that the mortality of acute appendicitis in patients receiving cathartics was eight times greater than in those not receiving such medication. The rule should be emphasized that *laxative drugs are contraindicated in the presence of abdominal pain.* If a bowel movement is desired, an enema or a glycerin suppository will achieve a result with little or no danger even if acute appendicitis is present.

A second dangerous form of treatment is the indiscriminate use of morphia to allay abdominal pain. This is unfortunately practiced by many careless physicians who make no diagnosis, and who do not perform an adequate abdominal examination. The changes leading to perforation and peritonitis go on while the patient is blissfully sleeping with the aid of the magic hypodermic. But on awakening he may no longer have acute appendicitis—he may have a severe general peritonitis. Such a rapid progress is especially apt to occur in children.

The *safest treatment* for acute appendicitis is, therefore, an immediate and properly performed appendectomy (see p. 690). The mortality following operation before perforation is practically nil. This has been emphasized by Keyes,[23] who noted that the mortality before perforation was 0.75 per cent, whereas after perforation of

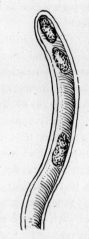

Fig. 421.—Gross Specimen of an Appendix, Bisected, Showing Numerous Fecaliths, Which Produced Appendiceal Colic.

The patient, a sixteen-year-old girl, had had many attacks of right lower quadrant pain, short in duration but severe and becoming so frequent as to produce serious disability. Complete relief followed appendectomy.

the appendix it was 9 per cent; similar observations have been made by many others. Spontaneous subsidence, as already mentioned, frequently occurs, but this is practically impossible to predict, unless the patient is seen at a time when he is obviously recovering from the acute attack and is clearly improving as shown by the history and examination. Appendectomy in such cases may still be indicated, but only as a prophylactic measure, especially if there have been previous attacks. The diagnosis in such a case is *recurrent appendicitis* and the operation is called an interval appendectomy.

Complications of Acute Appendicitis.—Whatever mortality occurs in acute appendicitis, as already mentioned above, is due to the complications of this disease which in nearly every instance follows a *perforation of the appendix*. Thus these complications are practically absent providing the appendix is removed before perforation or shortly thereafter.

The complications of acute appendicitis may be evident clinically when the patient is first seen by the surgeon. This unfortunate situation will probably be improved with increasing education in regard to the significance of abdominal pain. Early in the development of complications manifestations may be rather slight and a bedside diagnosis may be difficult, whereas if the infection extends, the patient becomes extremely ill, prostrated, toxic, dehydrated and distended. In the presence of such severe manifestations the question of operative therapy has been answered in one of two ways. Nearly all surgeons would, of course, combat as many of the symptoms as possible by gastric decompression and parenteral fluids. Many surgeons, however, would operate promptly after such conservative measures had been carried out. Others would pursue a non-operative regime as a definite policy, hoping that localization or even subsidence of the infection might occur.

In spite of this difference in opinion, the practice of prompt appendectomy in acute appendicitis must be emphasized before all other considerations, inasmuch as the treatment of most infections of the peritoneal cavity is based upon the principle of removing perforated lesions as soon after the perforation as possible (see page 737). The justification for this principle lies in the well-known ability of the peritoneal cavity to resist rather severe invasion provided the source of the contamination is removed. If the source is not removed, the repeated contamination may be more than the peritoneum can resist. While it is true that localization around a perforated or gangrenous appendix frequently occurs, it is difficult to be sure that such an event is actually taking place. The proponents of continued non-operative therapy argue that such localization may be interfered with and perhaps prevented by the trauma involved in the operation. On the other hand, such trauma may be perfectly justified if thereby the perforating lesion is eliminated and further contamination of the peritoneal cavity stopped. Moreover, the danger of spreading the infection by operation has been diminished tremendously since the advent of sulfonamide therapy (see pages 693 and 739). Indeed, its local use following operation has proved so effective that many surgeons formerly inclined toward delayed operation in perforative appendicitis are now operating more promptly in such cases. Chemotherapy has influenced this change for another reason, *i.e.*, the hazard of an operation is lowered inasmuch as the systemic effects of the invading organisms are so dramatically reduced by the use of these drugs. Prompt operation even in the presence of the complications of acute disease should be emphasized for another reason which has been suggested already. At the bedside it is frequently difficult to be sure that a complication is present. Many patients, particularly children, may present many manifestations of a perforated appendicitis and yet at operation there is revealed a severely inflamed, but as yet unperforated appendix. It is obvious that delay in operation in such cases might easily result in a perforation. In spite of prompt operation and removal of the perforated or gangrenous appendix, complications are still likely to occur although they are less serious and recovery is the rule.

Thus far complications of acute appendicitis have not been mentioned in detail. In reality they are, of course, variations in the degree and type of peritoneal infection which follows perforation of the appendix or gangrenous appendicitis. Peritonitis is discussed in detail in Chapter XXV, but it has so many special features as a complication of acute appendicitis that they are discussed further under the following headings.

General peritonitis often follows a neglected or mistreated case of acute appendicitis which has perforated or is gangrenous. However, general peritonitis may develop within a few hours after perforation, especially in children. When the infection is well developed the diagnosis is easy (see page 729), whereas its presence may be difficult or impossible to be sure of early in the clinical development of the disease. Indeed, the surgeon at operation in an early case may find it difficult to distinguish between a local, a general or a spreading peritonitis. After the removal of a perforated or gangrenous appendix, general peritonitis is extremely rare.

Appendiceal abscess as a complication of acute appendicitis is suspected in patients with a history and physical findings of acute appendicitis in whom at the time of admission a definite mass is present, indicating that perforation has occurred, but that the infection has remained localized. In a few instances the history may date back for many weeks or months, the mass having been present for this length of time. Under such circumstances, there may be difficulty in the differential diagnosis between an appendiceal abscess and a neoplasm in the iliac fossa. In most cases, however, the history is shorter and there is often no difficulty in deciding that the mass is actually of appendiceal origin. In a few cases, however, such a mass at operation may prove to be indurated omentum firmly adherent to the acutely swollen but still unperforated appendix.

Treatment in a definitely demonstrable appendiceal abscess should still be based upon fundamental principles of prompt appendectomy as already mentioned, although the urgency is not nearly as great and delay for several days may be justified. On the other hand, non-operative treatment for many weeks with an interval appendectomy later often involves a much longer period of convalescence than relatively prompt operation.

Residual abscesses occur not infrequently following operation for perforated or gangrenous appendicitis and are suspected in patients in whom the fever fails to subside in a few days, or recurs after it has returned to normal, usually within the first week or ten days. The various sites of such residual abscesses are illustrated in Fig. 443, page 730. However, in the case of appendiceal infections, the most frequent location is the pelvis. Clinical detection of pelvic abscesses as a complication of perforated acute appendicitis is relatively easy if the surgeon will remember to do frequent rectal examinations. The bulging culdesac into the anterior wall of the rectum as well as localized tenderness and induration are pathognomonic. Treatment of pelvic abscesses is usually conservative inasmuch as practically all of them rupture spontaneously into the rectum with complete relief of manifestations. If such an event does not occur and the general condition of the patient is suffering from the presence of this abscess, it may be necessary to drain the abscess. In such an event, the abscess may be drained directly by an incision through the anterior wall of the rectum; however, some surgeons prefer an abdominal approach.

Wound infections are perhaps the most common complication, particularly if the abdominal wall has been closed without drainage, although its incidence is lessened by the local use of the sulfonamides. Diagnosis and treatment are the same as other postoperative wound infections, as discussed on page 212. *Subdiaphragmatic abscess* sometimes occurs but is usually a late complication; it should be suspected whenever the patient's temperature has returned to normal but recurs in the second week. The detection and diagnosis of subdiaphragmatic abscess is discussed in detail on page 740. *Fecal fistulas* are not infrequent as a complication following operations for perforated acute appendicitis. In most instances such a lesion should be no cause for alarm as healing occurs eventually, particularly if the patient is having normal bowel movements. *Failure of the wound to heal (sinus formation)* is encountered occasionally and is generally indicative of the presence of a fecalith in the depths of the wound, a sponge inadvertently left at operation, or the presence of an unsuspected lesion such as actinomycosis, regional ileitis, colloid carcinoma of the cecum or tuberculosis. These latter conditions should also be suspected in the presence of a fecal fistula which fails to close after a reasonable interval of several weeks. *Pylephlebitis* is a rare but serious complication of acute appendicitis and may develop soon after perforation, even before operation, although in most cases it develops as a postoperative complication. It is to be suspected when the patient develops a chill and high fever (see pages 596 and 741). *Intestinal obstruction* discussed in detail in Chapter XXVI occurs not infrequently as a postoperative complication, usually many weeks, months or years afterwards. *Paralytic ileus,* which occurs so commonly following operation for perforated appendicitis, presents symptoms quite similar to those of mechanical intestinal obstruction; at times it may be difficult to distinguish these two conditions (see page 759).

Appendiceal Colic.—Acute transient attacks of characteristic pain located in the right lower quadrant often occur because of the mere presence of fecaliths, which occlude the lumen with a resultant distention distally, and which perhaps induce hyperperistalsis in the appendix. The pain is usually severe, but transient, and is rarely accompanied by vomiting and only occasionally by nausea. Repeated attacks lasting from a few minutes to a few hours, which leave as rapidly as they come, may occur. There is no leukocytosis, and local tenderness is slight or absent. Attacks may, if frequent, cause disability and offer the danger at any time of leading to a total obstruction and resultant inflammation. Fecaliths, however, may be present without producing symptoms. X-ray study after a barium meal or enema may so visualize the appendix as to produce evidence of their existence. Appendectomy is curative provided the diagnosis is correct, but is not urgent unless evidence of acute appendicular obstruction or inflammation is present.

Chronic Appendicitis.—After one excludes recurrent appendicitis and appendiceal colic there still remains a large group of patients who complain of pain of variable and inconstant or indefinite nature in the right lower quadrant and upon whom a diagnosis of chronic appendicitis is frequently made. This designation has in the past been a common one, often made on insufficient clinical evidence and based, after appendectomy, on little or no pathologic change in the organ. Unfortunately, in many of these patients, operation is followed by no relief and often by an exaggeration of symptoms.

The *pathology* of chronic appendicitis, indeed, has been the subject of much controversy and little general agreement. The presence of inflammatory scar, usually called adhesions, as well as focal obliteration of the lumen, from previous infection, is often definite and may in a few cases be responsible for symptoms. On the other hand, it is not uncommon to find an appendix showing no gross pathologic change

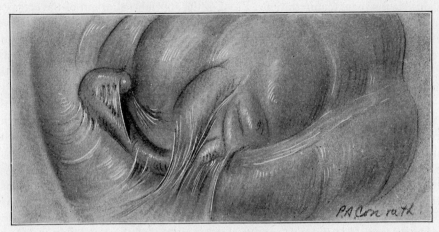

FIG. 422.—CHRONIC APPENDICITIS.

Note the bands of adhesions and the kink in the appendix, produced by inflammatory scar. These fibrous bands are not to be confused with congenital bands which are due to anomalies in the development of the appendix and cecum. In many instances the past history is the only method of differentiation. In this case there was a history of several severe attacks due definitely to acute appendicitis which subsided.

in a patient who is operated on after having recovered from an undoubted attack of acute appendicitis (interval appendectomy). We must assume in such instances that the acute infection has subsided without leaving even a microscopic trace and this conforms with what is known of inflammation in which no necrosis has occurred (see Chap. II). The occurrence of sympathetic neuroma (Hosoi) in patients with chronic pain in the right lower quadrant has been mentioned previously (p. 586). Occasionally a mucocele of the appendix is found; a carcinoid tumor may be encountered. Pinworms (*Oxyuris vermicularis*) are sometimes found in the appendiceal lumen and may be responsible for symptoms. In rare instances small foreign bodies are found. Such evidence of disease as round cell infiltration cannot be accepted as being of clinical importance. The development of atrophy of the appendix in older individuals, the so-called obliterative appendicitis, is a normal change due to senility and probably accounts for the relative rarity of acute disease in the later decades of life. This obliteration of the lumen is not to be confused with the obliteration due to previous acute inflammation as already mentioned.

Clinical Manifestations.—Pain of a mild degree, or perhaps merely a discomfort of a persistent sort located in the right lower quadrant is the main clinical manifestation produced by this disease. The pain is chronic in character and may vary in degree with a variety of circumstances. The surgeon should if possible examine the patient during an exacerbation of pain in the hope of eliciting local tenderness which will be of aid in localizing the source of the pain to the appendiceal area. Otherwise, in most instances abdominal examination will be relatively negative.

Not infrequently, these patients will present manifestations similar to those produced by duodenal ulcer, *i.e.,* epigastric distress with tenderness, sour eructations, etc. X-ray reveals no evidence of duodenal ulcer; pylorospasm is perhaps the factor responsible for these manifestations. Proof of the appendiceal origin of the epigastric complaints lies in the fact that they are completely relieved by appendectomy. Nevertheless, it must be emphasized that most instances of abdominal pain are not due to chronic appendicitis; indiscriminate appendectomy is therefore to be avoided.

Treatment.—A study of clinical results in this group of cases has shown that relief of symptoms is frequently *not* achieved by appendectomy. Indeed, in many of these patients the pain is magnified after the patient leaves the hospital. It is this fact which has led to much doubt as to the existence of true chronic appendicitis, except for the instances already mentioned. Many surgeons believe that such a diagnosis is rarely, if ever, justified. What, then, are the causes of chronic pain in the right lower quadrant? It is of importance to note that most of these patients are young women and girls, many of whom suffer from irregular bowel habits (constipation). Other causes of such pain include many diverse conditions, *i.e.,* spastic colitis, pelvic disease, lumbosacral or sacro-iliac disease (see page 556), and various psychoneuroses. It is through careful clinical study that these possible factors are investigated and eliminated. Only after this is done can appendectomy be advised with reasonable certainty of achieving a cure. The relief of pain following operation under such circumstances is a frequent clinical experience and justifies the diagnosis of so-called chronic appendicitis. In certain patients appendectomy may be justified as a prophylactic procedure, even when the symptoms are obscure, in order to eliminate the appendix as the cause of future manifestations. The operation should be carried out through a rectus incision, particularly if the patient is a female, so that an adequate abdominal exploration can be done at the same time to detect other possible lesions which may be of clinical significance.

Operations for Appendicitis.—Up until fifty years ago surgeons operated upon patients with acute appendicitis only in order to incise and drain an abscess which had formed by rupture of the inflamed organ. Indeed, the role of the appendix was for a long time generally unknown; the clinical diagnosis was usually "phlegmon of the abdominal wall," "right iliac abscess," etc. Because many physicians thought that the suppuration originated in the cecum, a frequent diagnosis was typhilitis or perityphilitis. In many instances, of course, general peritonitis occurred and the attending physician would note no localizing process in the right lower quadrant; the death certificates of such patients usually carried the diagnosis of "acute indigestion." Needless to say, the mortality was exceedingly high, even when an abscess was opened and drained.

Reginald Fitz [24] of Boston, in 1886, published a paper entitled "Perforating Inflammation of the Vermiform Appendix with Special Reference to Its Early Diagnosis and Treatment," which played an important part in the development of the modern operation of appendectomy in acute appendicitis. Although many previous observers, notably Addison and Bright as early as 1838, suggested the relation between appendicular infection and the formation of "iliac abscess" and general peritonitis, the observations and teachings of Fitz, who was primarily a pathologist and not a surgeon, had a tremendous influence in clarifying the subject, in this country at least, and in pointing to the importance of early appendectomy. Surgeons were quick to recognize the importance of Fitz's observations and before the end of the

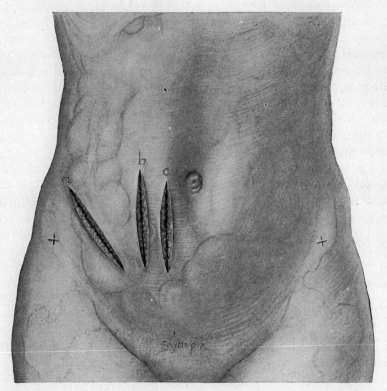

FIG. 423.—THREE TYPES OF INCISIONS COMMONLY USED IN OPERATIONS FOR APPENDICITIS.

A, the McBurney, or gridiron (muscle splitting) incision. *B,* pararectus incision; the rectus muscle is split longitudinally instead of being retracted. *C,* paramedian incision, retracting the muscle laterally; this is used particularly when the diagnosis is uncertain, since it affords better exposure than a McBurney incision. (Schweich, after Brödel.)

century many patients' lives were saved by adequate operative treatment. Among others the names of Charles McBurney, Albert J. Ochsner, and J. B. Murphy should be especially mentioned. As already mentioned above, the most flagrant cause of the high mortality at the present time is the use of cathartics in patients with acute abdominal pain.

There are two types of incision generally used in entering the abdomen for operations on appendicitis. The McBurney incision is located over the McBurney point (see p. 683), is small and utilizes only the separation of the oblique and transversalis muscles in the approach to the peritoneal cavity. Because the fibers of these muscle layers cross each other this approach is often called the gridiron incision. It has the advantages that it requires less dissection, is easier to do, and that there is a minimum of trauma to the abdominal wall. On the other hand, it permits only a limited exposure of, or access to the peritoneal cavity. Its greatest use is in the removal of the acutely inflamed appendix which is known to lie in its normal position in the right lower quadrant; it may also be used in simple drainage of an appendiceal abscess.

More extensively used, especially when the diagnosis is uncertain, is the low right rectus (paramedian) incision in which the right rectus muscle is separated from its sheath medially and retracted laterally. This incision may be made as long as necessary and because it permits adequate exposure results in a minimum of intraperitoneal trauma during exploration and appendectomy, especially of an abnormally placed appendix. In chronic appendicitis this incision is particularly indicated since it permits inspection and palpation of the other abdominal viscera. Exploration should be an essential part of the operation in this type of patient, particularly if there is even the slightest doubt as to the appendiceal origin of the patient's pain. It is practically impossible to gain any information of pelvic and upper abdominal structures through a McBurney incision.

When a perforated appendix is present less contamination of the peritoneal cavity will be produced by the McBurney incision. This is likewise true if an abscess is present, because direct drainage of the cavity is thereby more easily achieved. In a few instances the abscess will be found to lie in an extremely lateral or posterior position; in such an event a counter incision for more dependent drainage may then be made. It is important that the perforated appendix be located and eliminated so as to remove necrotic tissue and prevent further contamination of the peritoneal cavity; on a few occasions, however, the amount of trauma necessary to do so may be too great to justify further search. Careful exploration is also necessary to locate and remove fecaliths, which if overlooked are a frequent cause of failure in healing of the abdominal wound. In no domain of surgery is gentleness and care more necessary than in the operative therapy of perforated appendicitis. In walling off the infected area abdominal packs should be used with great care and gentleness because they traumatize intestinal loops, and tend to spread infection, besides encroaching on the abdominal opening. Contamination is also minimized by removing pus as soon as encountered, with a suction apparatus if possible. Postoperative complications, particularly intestinal obstruction, may in general be minimized or completely avoided by an adequate incision and gentle handling of the peritoneum and intra-abdominal viscera.

The question of drainage in operations for acute appendicitis must be decided at the time of operation. The principles upon which drainage is based have been described by Yates (see p. 737). A drain is used in general because the surgeon wishes to create and maintain an open wound so that any excessive infection or source of contamination may reach the outside rather than become enclosed in the depths of the wound and thus lead to the danger of a local abscess or of a spreading peritonitis. In general, a drain is not needed when the appendix is not ruptured except when an excessive amount of peritoneal reaction is evident. If a local peritonitis is present most surgeons feel safer with the area exteriorized with a single drain. When an abscess is present, drains are inserted into the cavity. Drains consisting of rolled rubber dam are preferable, and should be removed in four to seven days. In severe cases drainage may persist for two to three weeks. Occasionally a fecal fistula follows operation for perforated appendicitis; in such instances the fistula usually closes spontaneously unless an associated obstruction is present distal to the opening in the intestine.

The sulfonamide drugs though discussed elsewhere under the treatment of peritoneal infections, are mentioned here also because of their great value during and after operations for acute appendicitis with perforation. For example, the local use, in the peritoneal cavity, of 4 to 8 grams of the sulfanilamide powder, in early perforations at least, has already lowered considerably the number of cases requiring drainage. Moreover, the intensive use for several days after operation of sulfanilamide subcutaneously or sodium sulfathiazole or sulfadiazine intravenously has greatly reduced the high mortality in this group of acute appendicitis.

Tumors of the Appendix.—These lesions are rare and noted usually only at operation. *Carcinoid tumors,* consisting of glandular or other elements of embryonal origin, have been described. They are usually encountered accidentally, inasmuch as they do not produce any specific clinical manifestations. Often the diagnosis has been chronic appendicitis, or the appendix is removed during the course of an operation performed primarily for another purpose. Grossly the carcinoid tumors of the appendix produce slight to moderate enlargement of the organ which is firm in consistency. *Mucocele* is not infrequent and may be a rare cause of chronic appendiceal pain (see p. 689). Sympathetic *neuroma* in the appendix has been described on page 586. True *carcinoma* of the appendix, likewise, is infrequent and may or may not produce specific clinical manifestations, dependent on its rapidity of growth and involvement of the cecum.

THE CECUM AND COLON

The cecum and colon comprising the large bowel are the site of a number of surgical diseases the most serious of which is carcinoma. There are also a number of medical conditions which so simulate the diseases requiring surgical treatment that the diagnosis is often difficult. Although abdominal pain is a frequent manifestation of disease of the colon it is often not sufficiently characteristic to be of much differential value. More frequent clinical manifestations are symptoms concerned with alterations in the character and nature of the stool. For this reason a careful history of the bowel activities of the patient as well as a knowledge of the character of the stool is an important part of the diagnostic data. Too often in obtaining a routine history this information is inaccurately or incompletely elicited or carelessly overlooked entirely.

Definite delay in colonic motility is of surgical importance when an occlusion of the intestinal lumen is present. A sudden change in bowel habits from normal to constipation may be indicative of obstruction. If the obstruction is incomplete (frequently called chronic intestinal obstruction) few acute manifestations such as pain, nausea and vomiting may be present. In complete occlusion (acute intestinal obstruction) more significant manifestations are produced, but they will still be less than those encountered in obstruction of the small intestine. The pathology, clinical manifestations and treatment of obstructive diseases of the colon in general is described in the section devoted to intestinal obstruction (Chap. XXVI).

Ordinarily the patient becomes aware of a change in the bowel function because of a less serious change in the motility of the colon. Actually, however, he describes the change in terms of *frequency* of bowel movements, *i.e.,* he suffers from a delayed motility which is called constipation, or he complains of an increased motility which is called diarrhea. These terms are, however, inexact; an accurate measure of colonic motility may be made by special methods including the use of the x-ray.

Important also is the character of the stool itself, entirely apart from its frequency. Many patients are entirely unaware of such changes because they do not or cannot inspect the stool after defecation. In such cases negative statements are obviously valueless. Alterations in color, consistency and shape may in many instances prove of great diagnostic value. Tarry stools as an indication of bleeding high up in the alimentary tract, and acholic stools as evidence of obstructive jaundice, are obviously due to lesions outside the colon. Hard, marble-like feces, however, are usually associated with spastic constipation; soft pencil- or ribbon-shaped stools may be due to hypermotility as well as spasm of the terminal colon, provided organic lesions are ruled out; frequent liquid stools may be due to extracolic lesions but are often a sign of inflammatory, neoplastic or functional disease in the colon itself.

Abnormal elements in the stool are frequently of great importance. Fresh blood obviously indicates an ulcerative lesion, benign or malignant, in the distal portion of the colon or rectum. Mucus and pus are found in many kinds of ulceration, inflammatory as well as neoplastic. Mucus alone may be present in purely functional conditions, notably spastic colitis, which is discussed under Constipation. Parasites of various types may be noted grossly, but microscopic search of the stool for their larvae will be a more accurate method for determination of their presence. Because of the prevalence of amebiasis, proper facilities for the warm stage microscopic examination of the stool should be available to all physicians. This may be of particular significance to the surgeon because of the similiarity of manifestations produced by acute amebiasis and many lesions producing peritonitis (see p. 96).

Abdominal pain as a manifestation of disease of the colon is often of limited value, as already mentioned, because of its nonspecific character. This is also mentioned in the differential diagnosis of various types of acute abdominal disease because of the frequency with which the pain produced by colitis and other medical conditions is mistaken for acute surgical diseases. The colon is indeed well supplied with autonomic nerve fibers carrying impulses of pain, which are poorly localized. The abundance of autonomic innervation may also explain the frequency of functional diseases in the colon which often masquerade as organic lesions, and make the problem of diagnosis and treatment especially difficult.

Ordinary physical examination of the abdomen is always carried out but is often of limited value in the recognition of disease of the colon. Cancer of the transverse colon is palpable rather frequently; so are those in the right colon (see p. 696). In the descending colon and sigmoid this is not true. Tenderness over the sigmoid and cecum which are the most accessible to palpation may be indicative of acute inflammatory disease; more commonly, tenderness over the sigmoid is indicative of spastic colitis, but less common lesions such as inflamed diverticula, etc., must be considered.

Because of the obvious deficiencies in the history and physical examination as thus outlined, special examinations are usually essential in the diagnosis of disease of the cecum and colon. The use of the sigmoidoscope which enables direct vision of the distal part of the colon is described later in this Chapter. More important is the fluoroscopic and x-ray study of the cecum and colon after they have been visualized by a barium meal ingested some hours before, or better by a barium enema. By these methods an accurate measure of motility is obtained. Moreover the outline of the large bowel, its haustrations, filling defects, etc., are observed, thereby enabling the expert to make an accurate diagnosis in most instances.

Chronic Constipation (Colonic or Fecal Stasis).—Of interest to the surgeon is the fact that fecal stasis is not infrequently associated with abdominal pain, which, though slight, may be mistaken for the pain of mild appendicitis and other diseases. Relief of pain after bowel movements, either spontaneous or induced by enema, always suggests that constipation rather than appendicitis is the cause of the symptoms. Manifestations such as headaches, lassitude, anorexia, weakness and fatigue may accompany constipation but are of medical rather than surgical interest. Fecal impaction as a sign of fecal stasis has already been discussed (p. 172). Fecal stasis in general is a more descriptive term than constipation and should be based on other evidence than the frequency of the bowel movements. Spasm of the colon in its distal portion is often an etiologic factor in fecal stasis. In other patients the colon, instead of being spastic, is relaxed and atonic. Under these conditions delayed motility is produced by the opposite mechanism, *i.e.,* the muscular force is insufficient to propel the fecal contents normally. The terms spastic and atonic constipation are often used to describe these two types.

Of the two groups of fecal stasis the spastic type is of greatest surgical significance, because, as already suggested, it tends to produce abdominal pain which may be confused with surgical diseases. The term *spastic colitis* has been used to describe the type of constipation associated with spasm of the colon. Other terms such as mucous colitis and "irritable colon" have been applied. It is a medical disease but should be recognized by the surgeon lest he mistake it for other abdominal diseases which require a laparotomy, and thus lead him to perform an unnecessary and perhaps damaging operation.

Tuberculosis.—Tuberculous ulceration of the cecum comprises one-half of all intestinal tuberculosis; over one-third of all patients with pulmonary tuberculosis also have demonstrable lesions in the alimentary tract (Granet). Most patients with tuberculosis of the colon also have an active lesion in the lung. Of greatest importance surgically is the ulceration of the cecum; the lesion is accompanied by a fibrous thickening of the wall, producing symptoms and signs which may be at first indistinguishable from those provoked by carcinoma. Abdominal pain, diarrhea and blood in the stool are the chief manifestations in such instances. In the early cases pain is the only symptom, which may simulate mild appendicitis, and lead to an operation for appendectomy. In other cases a stenosis will ensue, which may be sufficient to produce a partial obstruction.

Diagnosis is readily made roentgenologically with the aid of a barium meal and enema. The deformity noted by x-ray may be identical with that produced by carcinoma, but the extreme irritability of the cecum which refuses to allow the barium to remain within its lumen, will usually lead to the correct diagnosis. Pulmonary tuberculosis should always be looked for. Operation for removal of the lesion may be indicated if severe symptoms are present, but there is a growing tendency to treat the disease conservatively, by hygienic and dietary measures, particularly when the pulmonary lesion is active.

Ulcerative Colitis.—This disease is a definite pathological and clinical entity of unknown etiology; it rarely assumes surgical significance. It may produce abdominal pain which may simulate acute appendicitis, but the history of chronicity, the presence of diarrhea, blood and mucus in the stool should eliminate any difficulty in the differentiation. On the other hand, it may be confused with the manifestations of carcinoma. Very important in the differentiation is the expert use of the x-ray following the barium meal and especially the barium enema. Treatment is a medical problem. Surgical procedures, such as colectomy or ileostomy are occasionally helpful (Stone[25]).

Polyps.—These pedunculated tumors, really adenomas, are either single or multiple (polyposis) and occur most frequently in the sigmoid and rectum; they may give rise to bleeding, diarrhea and abdominal pain. Diagnosis may be made by x-ray (barium enema); if situated in the rectum or lower sigmoid they may be directly visualized with a proctoscope or sigmoidoscope. Important is their tendency to malignant degeneration and hence the necessity for excision. When they are multiple, resection of the involved bowel may be indicated (see p. 711).

Carcinoma of the Colon.—Cancer of the colon accounts (with the rectum) for over one-tenth of all deaths due to malignant disease. The neoplasm is usually an adenocarcinoma and may be a bulky, fungating growth filling the lumen of the bowel or a scirrhous or annular type encircling the wall in the form of a stricture. Colloid carcinoma, though rare, also occurs, particularly in the cecum, and is apt to lead to perforation of the wall and abscess formation. Metastases occur by way of the lymphatics to the mesenteric lymph nodes and by way of the portal vein to the liver. The tumor grows at any point in the colon, but increases in frequency as one proceeds from the cecum, being most common in the sigmoid portion of the colon and the rectosigmoid.

Clinical manifestations depend on the location of the tumor and the rapidity of its growth. When the tumor is on the right side of the colon, bleeding is more common, leading to anemia. Weight loss is also common in carcinoma of the right colon and a mass is noted in a large part of the cases. Pain is present and is sometimes mistaken for acute appendicitis, for which appendectomy is occasionally performed (Ransom[26]). When the left side is involved, obstruction of the lumen is more likely to occur; this obstruction may be sudden with few antecedent manifestations.

Regardless of its location, symptoms are not very prominent early in the disease. Usually, evidences of ulceration or obstruction are the first manifestations of disease and should always arouse a suspicion of cancer when present in an individual of middle or old age. Early evidence of ulceration is the appearance of blood and mucus in the stool or the development of frequent liquid stools; early evidence of obstruction consists of increasing difficulty in regular defecation and attacks of cramping, abdominal pain. Frequently, periods of obstructive and irritative symptoms alternate. Such symptoms, unless explainable in some other way, should lead to an *investigation of the colon* by means of the x-ray with the use of the barium enema. Diagnosis in this way may frequently be achieved early in the disease. In

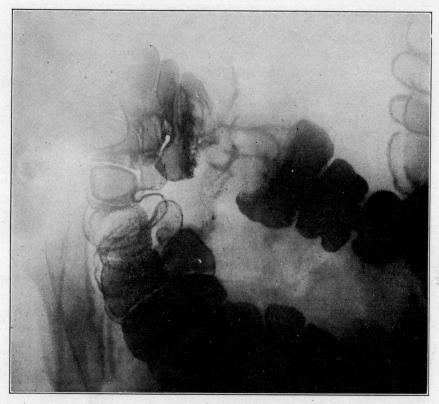

FIG. 424.—CARCINOMA OF THE COLON; AFTER A BARIUM ENEMA.

Note the characteristic filling defect adjacent to the hepatic flexure. The x-ray was particularly helpful in this case inasmuch as the history of abdominal symptoms was vague, consisting merely of anorexia, moderate loss of weight and slight upper abdominal tenderness. At operation the tumor was found and a resection of the colon performed (see Fig. 425) in two stages according to the Mikulicz technic. Seven years have elapsed since operation and the patient, now sixty-four years old, is well, asymptomatic and carries out her duties as housewife.

tumors of the distal colon and rectum direct visualization with a sigmoidoscope may be possible and a biopsy obtained for histologic verification.

Such manifestations as loss of weight, acute intestinal obstruction and severe anemia usually mean an advanced lesion and unfortunately are occasionally the first clinical intimation of disease. Usually, however, a period of weeks or months of lesser symptoms precede them and it is during this earlier period that diagnosis should be made in order to institute hopeful treatment. It should be emphasized that any abdominal symptoms consisting of diffuse pain, distention, anorexia, etc., or change in the defecatory habits of an individual in the cancer age should in most instances raise the question of the presence of early carcinoma of the colon and lead to a thorough examination which will indicate or exclude its presence.

Treatment is entirely surgical, *i.e.,* excision of the tumor after adequate preparation. Numerous types of operations have been described. The tumor may be excised and an anastomosis performed in a one-stage operation, but a high mortality

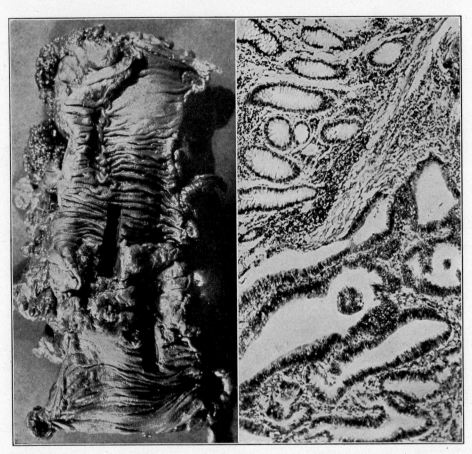

FIG. 425.—CARCINOMA OF THE COLON.

Gross and microscopic appearance of resected specimen in the case described in Figure 424. The rectangular areas at the edge of the ulcer represent blocks of tissue which were removed for microscopic section; note how they include normal as well as diseased tissue. The photomicrograph shows clearly the difference between the normal epithelium of the colon (at the top) and the malignant tissue, *i.e.,* adenocarcinoma (below).

is associated with this procedure, particularly if there has been any signs of obstruction. It is safer to perform a preliminary colostomy (if the position of the tumor permits) and to perform the resection and anastomosis ten or twelve days later. Another type of two-stage operation is an anastomosis between loops proximal and distal to the tumor, followed in twelve to sixteen days by resection of the diseased colon. The Mikulicz procedure which is associated with a still lower mortality, consists of exteriorization of the tumor at the first operation. excision with the cautery several days later, and reëstablishment of the fecal stream by cutting the spur between the two loops of bowel with a special clamp. Similar to the Mikulicz procedure is the Rankin obstructive technic in which more mesentery is removed and the tumor excised with the cautery at the completion of the operation. Primary resection with end-to-end anastomosis utilizing special clamps has been described by Stone.[27] The type of operation to be performed is determined for the most part by the characteristics of the individual case in question. The treatment of the tumor when it occurs in the distal colon is somewhat different and is described under therapy of carcinoma of the rectum. Sulfanilamide, postoperatively and immediately preoperatively, will decrease the incidence of postoperative peritonitis; local implantation at the time of operation has also considerable prophylactic value.

Diverticulitis.—Diverticula are not particularly uncommon in the colon, but rarely produce symptoms unless they become inflamed. In such cases the symptoms may be acute just as in acute appendicitis. Indeed, the clinical picture of acute diverticulitis is that of acute appendicitis located in the left instead of right lower quadrant; this is due to the fact that the diverticula are nearly always located in the sigmoid colon. The inflamed diverticula may perforate into the peritoneal cavity and produce a local peritonitis or abscess. Treatment consists of laparotomy to drain the resultant abscess or the local peritonitis with the idea of preventing a general dissemination; if there appears to be an actual communication with the lumen of the bowel, the opening should obviously be closed.

Occasionally the sigmoid will contain a number of diverticula which become inflamed over a considerable length of the colon; under these conditions the involved bowel becomes the site of an enlarged edematous mass which produces manifestations of a more or less acute intestinal obstruction. In such a case the differentiation from carcinoma will be particularly important because of the obvious difference in therapy. The use of the x-ray following a barium enema will usually lead to a correct diagnosis; even if the obstruction is more or less complete this procedure is often useful but not without some danger. In general the treatment of acute diverticulitis is medical. However, if an acute obstruction exists a laparotomy for its surgical relief will be necessary. In such a case the characteristics of the mass as noted at operation will often enable a true diagnosis to be made. Although occasionally resection may be advisable, it is probable that, in most instances, a colostomy proximal to the occlusion will be the procedure of choice. Diverticulitis may also perforate into adjacent organs and lead to a fistula into the bladder or the cervix or vagina. In such cases surgical therapy will also be required.

The lesser and more chronic types of diverticulitis may produce pain and diarrhea, in occasional cases, bleeding, and are detected only after careful study by roentgenography and sigmoidoscopy; they usually respond to medical care. When there is no evidence of inflammatory changes the designation diverticulosis is usually applied. Such a lesion is often noted accidentally during a routine x-ray study.

Miscellaneous Diseases of the Colon.—Ptosis of the colon is part of a general condition which affects all the abdominal viscera (visceroptosis). The designation refers to an abnormal mobility due to the existence of a long mesentery. When the patient stands, his viscera tend to drop toward the pelvis. As a cause of symptoms its significance is doubtful, although the redundant and mobile sigmoid may tend to encourage the development of a volvulus. Operations for the correction of ptosis are no longer performed. Visceroptosis is probably normal for certain (hyposthenic) types of habitus.

Actinomycosis of the colon, more especially of the cecum, appears to be increasing in frequency and will produce symptoms similar to any of the ulcerative lesions already mentioned, except that actinomycosis is usually associated with the ultimate development of a mass and multiple fistulous openings. Treatment is un-

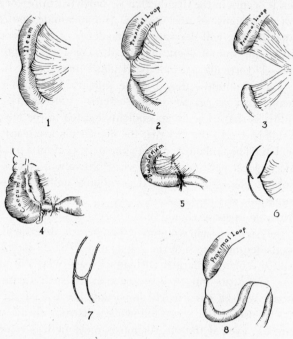

FIG. 426.—CONGENITAL MALFORMATIONS OCCURRING IN THE SMALL INTESTINE.

1, stenosis with partial obstruction; *2,* occlusion with blind loop; *3,* blind loop with a gap in the mesentery; *4,* obstruction by a fibrous band (found usually in the third part of the duodenum or the terminal ileum) ; *5,* obstruction at the ligament of Treitz; occasionally an anomalous superior mesenteric artery is the chief factor in producing the obstruction at this particular site; *6,* cross-section of intestine showing perforated diaphragm; this occurs usually in the duodenum or the terminal ileum; *7,* cross-section of imperforate diaphragm, and *8,* multiple occlusion of the ileum or jejunum; this constitutes about 15 per cent of the atresias of the intestine. Clinically, the dilatation of the proximal loop with collapse of the distal loop, is usually even more pronounced than shown in the illustrations. (From W. H. Cole, *Arch. Surg.,* 1931, 23:820.)

satisfactory in the late stages but if an early diagnosis is made, great improvement and perhaps cure may be achieved by radiotherapy, potassium iodide, and incision and drainage of abscesses (see p. 99) ; a short-circuiting operation (ileocolostomy) is sometimes advisable.

Foreign bodies sometimes become lodged in the colon after their ingestion but with few exceptions all foreign bodies which can be swallowed will be passed in the stool. When their passage becomes arrested (as occurs perhaps most frequently at the hepatic or splenic flexure), symptoms of mild obstruction may develop; if the object is sharp, a slow perforation may occur with the production of local peritonitis, followed usually by abscess formation. Occasionally, abscesses adjacent to and attached to the colon are encountered, when no primary source can be found; the preoperative diagnosis is usually appendiceal abscess or abscess due to diverticulitis. At operation, the nature of the infection is noted for the first time; if the abscess is opened and explored the foreign body may be located and removed. If the infection is merely drained, a chronic draining sinus may follow. If the object is radiopaque it may be identified by the x-ray. A history of swallowing a foreign body (*e.g.*, toothpick or sharp bone) may be obtained, but frequently the patient is unaware of such an occurrence.

Megacolon has been discussed on page 584.

Congenital anomalies are extremely rare and consist of stenosis or atresia. They are usually associated with similar lesions in the small intestine. These lesions, including malrotation, are discussed in Chapter XXVI.

RECTUM AND ANUS

The most serious disease of the terminal large bowel is carcinoma; the most frequent one is hemorrhoids. Inflammatory lesions, such as proctitis, cryptitis, ischiorectal abscess and fistula comprise a frequent and important group of surgical diseases. They are often grouped together as a separate specialty (proctology).

The incidence of anorectal diseases is high. It occurs in all walks of life and respects no single group. Considerable time is lost in the office, the shop and in the home due to common rectal conditions. The study and care of anorectal diseases has only recently received due attention in the general development of medical teaching. In no other branch of medicine has the charlatan exploited the public so severely as in the treatment of anorectal diseases. The medical profession is partially to blame for this condition since little time has been given by medical schools to a careful study of these maladies. Since some of the serious diseases of the rectum, including carcinoma particularly, do not produce marked symptoms until late after onset, it becomes exceedingly important to perform a thorough examination, even in the face of only mild symptoms. Since many patients suffering from rectal diseases visit the pharmacist for the relief of their symptoms, the delay in making a proper diagnosis is often prolonged past the period where successful treatment can be given.

Methods of Examination and Diagnosis.*—Every patient complaining of rectal symptoms, such as bleeding, pain, tenesmus, constipation, etc., should be carefully examined. A diagnosis can frequently be made following a complete history. The important points to be emphasized in questioning the patient are: (1) Is there, or has there been a change in the bowel habit; is there increasing constipation or a tendency to diarrhea? (2) Has there been any passage of blood or blood-tinged mucus from the rectum? (3) Has the patient experienced persistent pain in the perineum at the anal margin and the perianal regions, and if so, is this pain associated with the act of defecation? (4) Is there a discharge of pus? (5) Is there an external swelling?

In acutely painful lesions gentle spreading of the buttocks will frequently reveal

---

* The authors are indebted to Dr. W. R. Rainey for contributing this portion of the chapter.

a fissure; no further examination should be carried out until the patient is an-esthetized. This is likewise true in acutely thrombosed and painful hemorrhoids; in these cases a digital examination is too painful to be considered. With the exception of these two conditions, a digital examination should be made on every patient who complains of any rectal discomfort or other symptoms. Hemorrhoids cannot

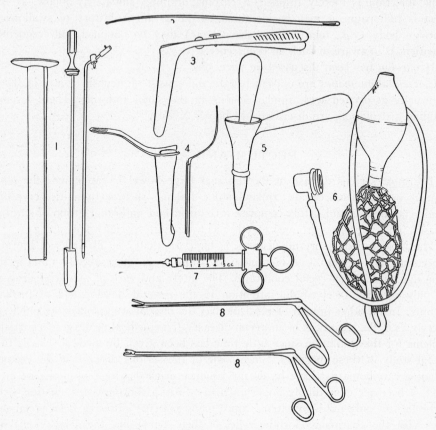

FIG. 427.—INSTRUMENTS ORDINARILY USED IN PERFORMING A COMPLETE ANOSCOPIC AND
PROCTOSCOPIC EXAMINATION.

1, proctoscope. *2*, flexible probe. *3*, bivalve dilating speculum. *4*, speculum (Brinkerhoff). *5*, anoscope. *6*, air dilator and eyepiece for proctoscope; this apparatus is important in the introduction of the proctoscope (see text); *7*, syringe and needle for injection of internal hemorrhoids; the needle should be of small caliber. *8*, biopsy forceps for removal of tissue through the proctoscope.

be diagnosed, however, by a digital examination alone. For the proper protection of the physician, examination should be made with a rubber glove, well lubricated with a jelly or vaselin. The finger cot does not offer adequate protection to the physician in patients with syphilitic anorectal diseases. The author on a number of occasions has been able to find spirochetes in the dark field examination of secretions taken from the anal margin in cases of secondary syphilis. Cases are on record in which venereal lymphogranuloma also has been transmitted to the examining finger.

Examination can best be carried out with the patient lying on the left side or in the knee-chest position under the illumination of a spot light. The well-lubricated, gloved, index finger of the right hand is gently pressed against the anal opening. Slight pressure at regular intervals around the periphery of the anus will determine any painful point. The posterior commissure is the most frequent site of painful lesions. The patient should be assured that the examination will be gentle and that on the slightest indication of pain the introduction of the finger will be stopped. By reassurance of the patient and extreme care during examination contraction of the anus will be overcome and the examining finger can then be gently introduced to its full length. This is often aided by asking the patient to strain.

After the finger is fully introduced one can determine the tone of the muscle. The healthy sphincter muscle is in a state of constant contraction. The finger notes the firm, slightly yielding tone of the normal sphincter as compared to the spasm associated with acute or subacute inflammatory lesions around the anal margin. On the other hand, the nonspastic sphincter which relaxes under the digital examination and fails to grasp the finger easily, tiring rapidly into a state of relaxation, is often indicative of tabes dorsalis, syphilis of the central nervous system or tumor of the spinal cord. In the outpatient rectal clinic the first knowledge of tabes has often been gained through routine rectal examination.

The next observation to be made in the male is the consistency of the prostate. In the female, the firmness and movability of the cervix uteri and such pelvic organs as may come in contact with the finger should be noted. In virgins and in children the rectal finger aided by the abdominal hand permits excellent bimanual pelvic examination. The finger is now swept around the entire circumference of the rectum and before its removal, with the other hand placed over the coccyx, this bone is manipulated between the two index fingers placed over the coccyx, to determine fixation and possible pain on pressure. Referred pains at this site are often due to anorectal lesions. The examining finger then determines the movability of the rectal mucosa, the side of the rectal ampulla, the possibility of stricture, benign polyps, the presence of benign or malignant growths, the presence of a foreign body, impaction of feces or the general consistency of the stool. Fully 50 per cent of carcinoma involving the rectum can be diagnosed by the examining finger.

Direct inspection with an appropriate instrument is also an indispensable part of the examination in anorectal disease; both anoscope and proctoscope are necessary. The anoscope is an instrument used for the examination of the lower part of the rectum and anal region. It is a hollow metal tube 1.5 to 3 inches long and 0.75 inch in diameter, carrying an obturator with a tapering end which renders introduction easier. As a first step in the examination, the instrument is placed within the anal canal, again assuring the patient of gentleness, and slight pressure is made until the well lubricated instrument gently slides past the sphincter muscle. The obturator is now withdrawn. In the knee-chest position particularly, the internal viscera have a tendency to drop forward and the inrushing air dilates the inner rectum, allowing one to see well up towards the upper limits of the rectal ampulla. Carcinoma of the rectum, as well as benign polyps or other low-lying growths, can in this manner be seen. The lumen of a low rectal stricture can be thus determined. Hemorrhoids cannot be seen until the anoscope is withdrawn to the anorectal line.

With the sphincter thus held dilated, and aided by a slight straining upon the part of the patient, internal hemorrhoids quickly prolapse into the lumen of the anoscope and frequently drop outside the anal sphincter when the anoscope is withdrawn. A careful inspection through this hollow instrument under a direct light may reveal the internal opening of rectal fistulas and diseased rectal crypts, enlarged rectal papilla and all the various conditions common to the anorectal area.

The proctosigmoidoscope is a hollow metal tube from 9 to 10 inches in length with a tapering obturator to aid its passage. It carries a lighting apparatus to illuminate the interior of the bowel, an air pressure device to dilate the rectum and sigmoid, and to aid in the passing of the instrument, and better observation of the interior of the bowel. No attempt should be made to utilize this instrument in the diagnosis of lesions along the anorectal line. This may be accomplished far better with the anoscope. The proctoscope is a safe instrument when properly used, but dangerous when carelessly used. Every physician who treats anorectal lesions should be trained in the use of this instrument. Certain simple rules eliminate the danger and a definite routine assures one of discovering all that might be found through the use of this instrument. It is highly important to place the patient in the knee-chest position or on a modified table that permits the body to recline face down with the chest fairly dependent. For all general purposes the knee-chest position is adequate. The proctoscope should be completely and thoroughly lubricated. The attempt to pass this long metallic tube unlubricated, causes considerable pain and tearing of the anorectal skin and mucosa. The instrument should be introduced just past the sphincter muscle, or about 1.5 inches; at this point the obturator is withdrawn, and under electric illumination the first observation is made. At this time the appearance of bright red blood, blood clots, or excessive amounts of mucus should be noted, as well as the general appearance of the bowel mucosa. The lens or eye piece is now applied and air is forced into the instrument until the ampulla is well dilated. The instrument is now introduced under direct vision. This method is absolutely safe. Any blind introduction of a proctoscope increases the hazard of a perforation. With wide-sweeping circles the instrument is swung around to examine the mucosa of the entire bowel upward as far as possible. Every square inch of the mucosa should be observed and carefully noted. Each rectal fold, of which there are three prominent ones (valves of Houston), should be carefully examined; the proctoscope should be introduced beyond the valve, and gently withdrawn so as to make slight pressure, thereby flattening the folds of mucosa in order to observe both sides of it. Occasionally some difficulty is experienced on entering the sigmoid. If, in the hands of an inexperienced operator, any force is required to introduce the instrument into the upper reaches of the sigmoid, even under direct vision, it is advisable to stop because of the danger of perforation.

A majority of all cases of carcinoma involving the rectum and sigmoid can be observed under direct vision by means of the proctoscope. To confirm the diagnosis, a biopsy through the rectal sigmoidoscope can be performed which will give the pathologist a sufficient amount of tissue for microscopical examination. Only small pieces of tissue should be removed for biopsy. It is important to watch the site from which the biopsy is taken through the proctoscope until one is assured that no alarming hemorrhage is taking place. Through the proctoscope, scrapings and swabbings taken directly from the site of a rectal ulcer often lead to the diagnosis of amebic dysentery when stool examinations have proved negative. In withdrawing the proctoscope, the air pressure within the lumen is again increased if necessary, and the bowel mucosa again inspected as the instrument is withdrawn.

If blood and mucus are found in the ampulla of the rectum and the lower region of the sigmoid, and no lesion has been discovered to account for this bleeding, the next step is the use of the x-ray. The twenty-four hour x-ray film, taken to show the general appearance of the large bowel, and the barium enema are the only objective means of locating lesions of the remaining portion of the large bowel.

Hemorrhoids.—Commonly called piles, these lesions are probably the most common of all anal diseases. The pathology varies, but in general consists of a dilated venous channel covered by more or less redundant anal mucosa or skin. When visible externally they are called external hemorrhoids; when present in the inner anal canal they may not be evident except during defecation or on proctoscopic examination, and are called internal hemorrhoids. The dilated vessel may contain thrombosed blood, may be inflamed or ulcerated, and may be associated with proctitis or cryptitis. The pathogenesis of hemorrhoids is not always clear. When they develop after childbirth, as they frequently do, venous obstruction and stasis probably play a role. In other cases they may be induced by straining at stool induced by chronic fecal stasis and anal sphincter spasm. Undoubtedly, in many cases there is a congenital deficiency in the attachment of the rectal wall to the underlying fascia thus permitting the mucous membrane to be carried down into the anal canal during defecation. Clinically, internal hemorrhoids may become evident to the patient merely as a *protrusion,* noticed particularly after defecation and often associated with a mild degree of prolapse of the redundant mucosa. During defecation there may be *bleeding* which is usually slight, but may be persistent, and sometimes severe enough to lead to secondary anemia. *Pain* is not a characteristic symptom and is usually absent, except with infection, ulceration or thrombosis. Under such circumstances it is apt to be noted during and after defecation, which may leave a sense of soreness for many hours. In other cases the pain may be persistent and continuous, particularly when severe acute inflammation develops. Constipation is often present because of the associated chronic inflammation, anal spasm and fear of defecation. External skin tabs (external hemorrhoids) rarely produce symptoms unless acute inflammation occurs. *Thrombosis of an external hemorrhoid* is not infrequent; it produces localized pain which may be severe enough to lead to complete disability. The diagnosis is obvious on inspection. Tenderness over the indurated mass may be so excruciating as to preclude palpation; anoscopic examination will require complete anesthesia.

Treatment is operative and nonoperative. The latter measures include rest in bed, hot sitz baths, regulation of diet and mineral oil. If the patient presents a strangulated internal pile, the mass can often be reduced by manipulation with the well-lubricated gloved fingers, with considerable relief to the patient. Obviously, a thrombosed external hemorrhoid must not be mistaken for a strangulated internal hemorrhoid. Operation consists of the excision of the hemorrhoids along with redundant mucosa, and suture of the operative site to control hemorrhage and to promote adhesions to the underlying fascia during healing. The suture line of the

excised tissue should extend in the longitudinal axis of the anus and rectum, ending as high up as possible and starting just above the mucocutaneous margin.
When the hemorrhoids extend around the entire anus the danger of postoperative
anal stenosis can be avoided to a great extent by doing the operation in two stages.
When simple internal hemorrhoids with redundant mucosa are present, they may
be obliterated by the use of sclerosing solutions such as phenol, sodium morrhuate,
etc. Injection therapy may be carried out without hospitalization or disability
(Balch [28]).

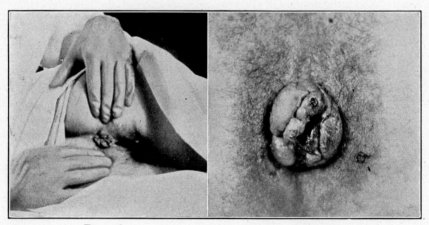

FIG. 428.   FIG. 429.

FIG. 428.—UNCOMPLICATED INTERNAL HEMORRHOIDS.

The lesion was invisible to inspection until an anoscope was inserted. The hemorrhoids
and redundant mucosa seen in the photograph appeared on withdrawal of the instrument. Symptoms consisted of the protrusion at each bowel movement, associated with pain and bleeding.
Hemorrhoidectomy was performed with complete relief of symptoms.

FIG. 429.—PROLAPSED INTERNAL HEMORRHOIDS.

The hemorrhoids became prolapsed two days previously and could not be reduced. Note
the ulceration, edema and inflammation. The pain was severe and required sedatives. The patient
was sixty-four years old and previously had very little difficulty reducing the "piles." Operation
was performed with excision of the redundant tissue.

External hemorrhoids rarely require treatment unless they become inflamed or
thrombosed. The acute pain accompanying a *thrombosed hemorrhoid,* which is
nearly always located in an external skin tab, may be completely relieved by incision
of the overlying skin and evacuation of the clot under novocain anesthesia. Such an
incision is not large enough to require suture. When the external hemorrhoid is the
site of simple inflammation, conservative local therapy is tried. If relief of pain
is not achieved excision under complete anesthesia will be necessary.

Prolapse of the Rectum.—Rectal prolapse occurs more commonly in infants
and children than in adults. If not reduced at once, manually or spontaneously,
the associated sphincter spasm may cut off the blood supply and lead to edema and
cyanosis, and in some cases to actual gangrene. In adults prolapse is prone to occur
in the very old without apparent cause. In healthy adults it is usually due to other
lesions; that is, hemorrhoids, polyps or any condition which is apt to lead to strain-

ing at stool. There is probably some congenital defect in the firmness of the fibrous attachments between the various layers of the rectum. Complete prolapse (procidentia), though rare, implies the extrusion of all layers of the rectum, which may be so extensive as to involve the rectosigmoid as well.

Treatment is simple replacement of the prolapsed mucosa manually or by elevation of the foot of the bed, aided by sedation or a preparatory hot sitz bath to relieve the sphincter spasm. The edema accompanying the prolapse, however, is relieved more efficiently by cold packs. In some cases relaxation may be achieved only by employing a general or sacral anesthetic. If the prolapsed mucosa is necrotic, excision will be necessary, but is not done in the presence of acute inflammation. After

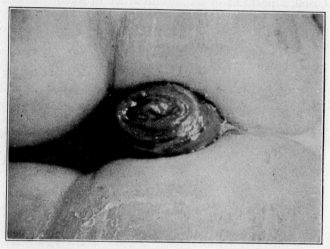

FIG. 430.—PROLAPSE OF THE RECTUM IN A FORTY-FIVE-YEAR-OLD WOMAN.

No strangulation is present; because of the repeated recurrence and extensiveness of the prolapse in spite of conservative care an abdominal operation was performed and the sigmoid anchored by sutures in order to prevent further prolapse. Other operations are also used including that of local amputation (St. Louis City Hospital).

reduction of the prolapse the underlying cause should be found and eradicated. Careful bowel habits and loose stools may prevent recurrence. In the simple cases, injection of a sclerosing substance at several points under the redundant mucosa will result in sufficient scar to prevent subsequent prolapse. For several days after injection, the buttocks must be strapped to prevent prolapse during the acute inflammation preceding the fibrosis. Persistent prolapse may require more radical procedure, such as actual resection of the redundant mucosa; occasionally an intra-abdominal operation will be indicated (Pemberton & Stalker [29]).

Cryptitis.—Inflammation of the tiny crypts (of Morgagni) which encircle the distal rectum just inside the anal canal at the pectinate line are of great importance in the pathology of fissure, fistula and ischiorectal abscess. Their location around the distal rectum makes them liable to trauma and irritation during defecation. These crypts should be observed during every anoscopic examination. Cryptitis itself may be responsible for anal spasm, vague pain on defecation, itching or frequent bowel movements. Dilatation of the sphincter and hot sitz baths may be beneficial. If the infection in the crypts results in abscess formation or is undermining the mucosa, incision with exposure of the cavity is indicated.

Fissure-in-Ano.—A frequent cause of itching, pain and bleeding on defecation is the presence of a break in the anal skin which may be quite superficial, but which fails to heal. In more marked lesions the ulcer or fissure connects with an infected crypt inside the sphincter and thus is a form of fistula. In the simple cases healing may occur only to be followed by recurrence. The pathogenesis is probably a combination of mechanical trauma and sphincter spasm, which produces a vicious circle; *i.e.,* the skin lesion produces a spasm which aggravates trauma during defecation, thereby preventing healing. Treatment in the simple cases consists of the ingestion of mineral oil, and adjustment of the diet in order to soften the fecal mass. Re-

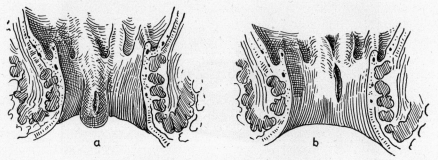

FIG. 431.—TWO TYPES OF FISSURE-IN-ANO.

A, associated with a sentinel pile, and *B,* due to an infected crypt with which it communicates through its base at the upper end.

peated dilatation of the sphincter by bougies of increasing size, or a single dilatation under general anesthesia is often effective in aiding spontaneous healing. Local applications of styptics, etc., are probably useless. Excision of the lesion may be necessary in protracted cases but the resulting wound should not be sutured but left open. When infected crypts are present they must be drained and sinus tracts opened.

Ischiorectal Abscess.—This is a common and painful type of infection which reaches the ischiorectal fossa from the rectum through a preëxisting though usually unsuspected lesion, located most commonly in the crypts and papillae just inside the anal canal. The inflammatory reaction leads to a tiny abscess in the crypt which then burrows under the mucosa and wall of the rectum into the loose areolar tissue where it finds little resistance and sets up an extensive cellulitis which soon suppurates. The resulting abscess may break into the rectum at another point higher up or through the outside skin with immediate relief of acute symptoms, but rarely does so until after the lapse of several days. The clinical manifestations consist of severe local pain and tenderness, which in most instances rapidly produce complete disability. There may be fever and prostration, generalized abdominal distress, distention, and thus be mistaken for an intra-abdominal infection or even a ruptured appendix. In most cases the localization of symptoms is much more definite and confined to the anal region. Excruciating anal pain may make defecation extremely difficult. The local tenderness is so pronounced that walking is almost impossible;

the patient prefers to lie on his side or abdomen. Leukocytosis and fever are present. On examination there may be an evident area of redness and induration characteristic of abscess, thereby leading to the correct diagnosis. When the abscess is deeper, there will be no external signs, but point tenderness will be elicited on deep palpation of the buttocks next to the anus. Rectal examination is often impossible because of the spasm and pain. An aspiration needle may be used in the detection of deep abscesses when the diagnosis is doubtful.

Treatment is that of an abscess anywhere. If pus is present, as it usually is when the patient is first seen by the doctor, incision for drainage should be performed. Because of the extreme tenderness, a general anesthetic is to be preferred. An adequate opening to expose all of the cavity is essential and is made in a radial

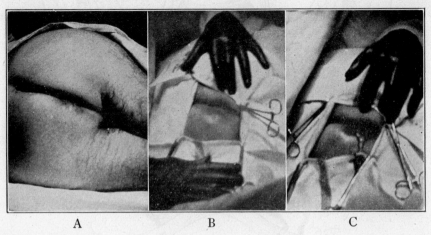

A   B   C

FIG. 432.—ISCHIORECTAL ABSCESS OF FOUR DAYS' DURATION IN A FORTY-YEAR-OLD MAN.

The local pain was so severe that defecation was impossible. After incision about 50 to 75 cc. of foul pus were evacuated. The cavity was adequately opened; it drained for four weeks and closed permanently. In a large majority of such cases a fistula-in-ano will develop. No communication between the abscess and rectum was apparent at operation. *A,* before operation; *B,* after being draped; *C,* after incision.

direction from the anus. The drain, preferably of soft rubber dam, should be gradually removed on the succeeding days to permit granulation from below. Regardless of adequate operative and postoperative care, in most cases the ischiorectal abscess does not heal completely, but leaves a draining opening which is then called a fistula-in-ano. The use of sulfanilamide after incision and drainage will probably aid healing and lower the incidence of fistula-in-ano.

Fistula-in-Ano.—The history of an initial acute abscess is nearly always obtainable. Frequently there is a history of spontaneous healing followed by reformation of an abscess. Occasionally the infection may spread throughout the tissues of the perineum and produce numerous fistulous openings, which communicate with each other. Even when only one opening is observed the tract may be long and tortuous. Some cases are associated with stricture of the rectum. The symptoms, aside from recurrent abscess formation, may consist of nothing more than a continuous discharge from the wound which thus requires constant dresssings. When the track drains inadequately, pain and systemic evidence of infection may occur. A slight difficulty in moving the bowels is often present, sometimes accompanied by pain.

The lesion itself varies greatly in extent and location. Sometimes the communication with the rectum is absent or microscopical. When no internal opening is present the term *blind fistula* is used. A *complete fistula* has two openings extending completely from mucosa to the skin at any level. The relation of the fistula to the external and internal anal sphincters is important. Some are distal to the sphincters; *i.e.*, entirely subcutaneous, and others pass between the internal and

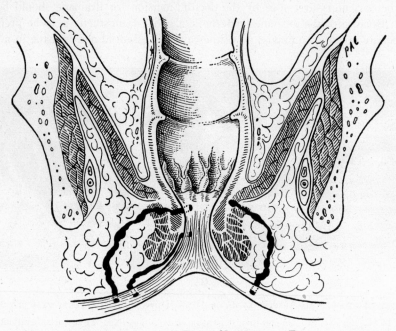

FIG. 433.—DIAGRAM SHOWING THREE VARIETIES OF FISTULA-IN-ANO.

The two on the left are complete and have two openings; one of the tracks opens above, and the other below the sphincter. The fistula on the right is "blind," in reality, therefore, only a sinus. It is believed, however, that an opening does actually exist, but is so small that it is not demonstrable.

external sphincters to enter the anal canal. *Internal fistula* is the result of an abscess which has broken into the rectum only (see Fig. 433). Variable, too, is the directness of the fistulous tract; nearly all are tortuous and burrow extensively, sometimes halfway around the circumference of the rectum, before they end. When more than one external opening is present they lead to tracks which are continuous. The chronicity of the lesion and its failure to heal in most cases is due to the continuous exposure to infection from the rectum. In other cases, when the opening is blind, other factors including especially insufficient drainage, may play a role; certain of them are tuberculous, and microscopic or cultural evidence thereof is obtainable, but when it is, most (77 per cent) of the patients are found to have demonstrable active or arrested pulmonary tuberculosis (Buie, Smith & Jackman[30]). A significant proportion of patients with pulmonary tuberculosis, moreover, suffer from anorectal infections (Chisholm and Gauss[31]).

Treatment is entirely surgical. Excision of the entire track is advisable. Division of the sphincter to lay the track open and to allow granulation from below is often necessary. Incontinence as an operative complication is not apt to occur following a single division of the sphincter, particularly if the operation in such cases is done in two stages (see also p. 714). The severe cases with multiple external openings, particularly when stricture of the rectum is present and there is extensive perirectal infection, may require a permanent colostomy for relief. Even if the lesion is tuberculous, cure may be achieved in a large percentage of cases provided careful, effective and radical surgery is carried out (Granet [32]).

Stricture of the Rectum.—This is a fairly common disease among Negro women. For a time it was considered of syphilitic origin, but most recent studies have shown that it is a manifestation of a venereal disease called lymphogranuloma venereum (see p. 99). The infection reaches the perirectal lymphatics through the venereal portal of entry and induces a mild type of proctitis which is evident by diarrhea, pain on defecation, and tenesmus. Ulceration may be seen at this stage. Slowly fibrous tissue is laid down, encircling the rectum and leading to a stenosis or stricture. Considerable infection above the stricture is usually present and pus is passed with each stool which is necessarily liquid in character. The infection may occasionally be responsible for the development of a perirectal (or ischiorectal) abscess which burrows through to the buttock and forms one or more fistulas which do not heal. Because of the many openings around the anus the term "watering-pot" is often applied. The

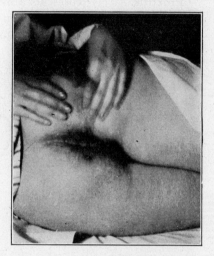

Fig. 434.—Fistula-in-ano of Two Years' Duration following Drainage of an Ischiorectal Abscess in a Thirty-year-old Woman.

The opening of the track can be seen in the skin just below the anus. Injection of methylene blue into the external orifice of the fistula failed to reveal an internal opening, nor was one demonstrated at operation several days later. The entire track was excised; its deepest point was at least one centimeter from the rectal wall. Healing was complete.

condition of such a patient is distressing indeed and the only hope for relief is usually the performance of a colostomy above the sigmoid with the formation of a permanent artificial anus on the abdominal wall. When the stricture alone is causing symptoms, progressive dilatation with the finger or rubber bougies of increasing caliber, affords considerable relief although a normal caliber cannot be regained.

Polyps.—These tumors occur in the rectum as well as in the colon and may be single or multiple. When in the distal colon or rectum, they may be seen through a proctoscope or sigmoidoscope. Polyps may also be detected in the rest of the colon, though with greater difficulty, by means of the x-ray following a barium meal or a barium enema. Clinical manifestations may be absent. When ulcerated, bleeding may be detected. A polyp near the anus may be mistaken for an internal hemorrhoid; when in the rectum it may be responsible for recurrent rectal prolapse. The greatest significance of polyps, however, is due to the fact that they are definitely precancerous lesions. Indeed, when polyps produce the signs of abnormal colonic function (diarrhea, obstruction) they are apt to be malignant (Swinton and Warren [33]). Treatment of the benign polyps consists of excision, when they can be approached from below. The malignant polyps are treated just as carcinoma of the colon or rectum.

Proctitis.—This represents a medical rather than a surgical problem, but produces symptoms which may be mistaken for other lesions. On proctoscopic examination, however, there are diffuse inflammatory changes in the rectal mucosa,

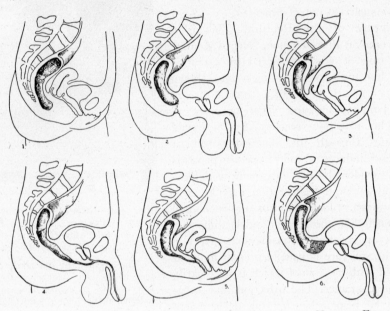

FIG. 435.—TYPES OF IMPERFORATE ANUS AND THE LOCATION OF THE VARIOUS FISTULOUS TRACTS FORMED.

1, absence of anus (proctodeum); *2,* fibrous cord attaching rectal pouch and proctodeum; *3,* perineal fistula; *4,* urethral fistula; *5,* rectovaginal fistula, and *6,* rectovesical fistula (From W. H. Cole, *Arch. Surg.,* 1931, 23:820).

including edema, multiple ulcerations, anemia or hyperemia. Such changes are usually the visible portion of more extensive lesions higher up in the colon. X-ray after a barium enema will reveal the extent of the disease above the rectum. Proctitis in Negro women is frequently due to lymphogranuloma venereum (see p. 99).

Pruritus Ani.—This is an annoying condition, the etiology of which in most instances is obscure. In children pin worms may be the cause of the itching. Careful proctoscopic examination of adults with pruritus ani will also lead to the discovery of these parasites in many instances. On other occasions food allergy appears to be the primary factor in the etiology. Fungous infection of the skin about the anus is commonly the cause of the disease. Troublesome itching may accompany fissure-in-ano or hemorrhoids, particularly the former. Treatment consists of removal of the cause if possible. If the cause is obscure, it may be wise to try applying an efficient fungicide, *e.g.,* resorcinol lotion or Whitfield's ointment.

Imperforate Anus.—This is a congenital defect due to maldevelopment of the lower alimentary tract; the various types are illustrated in Figure 435. It is evident soon after birth when the nurse attempts to insert a rectal thermometer. Otherwise, it may not be noticed for a day or two until distention, vomiting and absence of bowel movements proclaim the existence of some difficulty. Anatomically many vari-

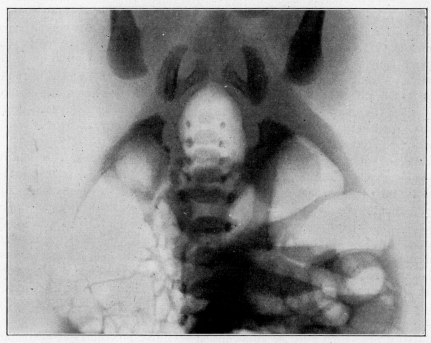

Fig. 436.—Roentgenogram of a Twelve-hour-old Infant with Imperforate Anus, While Being Held Head Down.

Note the air in the rectum which outlines its terminal end. Fluid levels in the dilated colon can also be seen. An incision was made in the perineum, the rectal pouch located and brought through the sphincter after which the rectal pouch was opened and the edges sutured to the cut edge of the skin.

ations exist. The lower rectum may be blind and often communicates with the bladder (in males) or the vagina (in females). In the former case it will lead to the passage of gas and feces through the urethra. The rectum itself may end high up in the pelvis or be separated from the outside by a single layer of skin and mucosa. X-ray with the infant upsidedown (Wangensteen) may show a bubble of gas at the termination of the rectum, thus locating its position accurately (Fig. 436).

Treatment depends on diagnosis of the type of anatomic defect present, but is in any case entirely operative. When the septum is thin the skin at the anal sphincter is incised and by inserting an instrument through the sphincter, the rectal pouch is located and opened; if possible the rectal mucosa is pulled out and anchored to the skin by interrupted sutures. Dilatation at frequent intervals is usually necessary to prevent serious stenosis. If the rectal pouch is high in the pelvis, preliminary colostomy is done and reparative procedures instigated later. In an excellent report by Crowell & Dulin,[34] a satisfactory result was obtained in 65 per cent of their cases with only a 17 per cent surgical mortality.

Foreign Bodies.—On rare occasions a sharp bone, toothpick or other object lodges in the rectum after being swallowed and passed uneventfully through the stomach, small and large intestine.

The history of swallowing the foreign body is helpful if it can be obtained. Acute local pain is the usual complaint; if the object is sharp it may lodge just proximal to the anus and produce an ulceration or abscess. Diagnosis depends on careful proctoscopic examination; treatment is that of the local infection. On rare occasions a foreign body such as a bottle may be introduced into the rectum by the patient himself in a demented state. Acute rectal symptoms will be present but the nature of the trouble will often be concealed by the patient. Rectal or proctoscopic examination makes the diagnosis. Removal of a large object usually requires a general anesthetic; when the object has been pushed up into the colon and is out of reach, a laparotomy may be necessary.

Anal Incontinence.—The normal tone of the anal sphincters must be inhibited before the expulsion of feces may be effected. Defecation, thus, is analogous to urination and is dependent on similar nerve connections, both voluntary and autonomic. Incontinence of feces (involuntary defecation) may be neurogenic or myogenic. *Neurogenic factors* comprise organic lesions in the spinal cord such as tabes dorsalis, injury, neoplasm, etc. Impaired cerebration by releasing the inhibitory mechanism may also result in incontinence; functional as well as organic disease of the brain may be responsible. *Myogenic factors* are produced by injury or disease which has resulted in a destruction of the integrity of the sphincters. Childbirth injury, extensive inflammatory disease, repeated or radical operative trauma, etc., are usually responsible for anal incontinence of this type. It is important to emphasize that special precaution must be taken during operative procedures about the anus in order to prevent injury to the sphincter which may lead to incontinence. This is particularly applicable to operations for fistula-in-ano; as already mentioned the sphincter can safely be severed at one point, especially in its lateral portion, but complete division at more than one point is usually followed by incontinence unless immediate adequate repair is effected or the operation is carried out in more than one stage. On many occasions the incontinence may be most prominent only when gas or liquid contents are present in the rectum.

Treatment depends on removal, if possible, of neurogenic factors, when present; frequently these factors are eliminated spontaneously, particularly when they are functional in type. The existence of extensive paralysis means a poor prognosis; careful nursing care is all that can be advised in such cases. When muscle is injured operative repair by suture of the divided sphincter is often effective in many instances. When the sphincter is irremediably damaged or permanent neurogenic factors are responsible, a plastic operation may be advisable in a few selected cases. Strips of fascia are utilized to surround the anus, and are attached to the gluteus muscles for voluntary control. This procedure is associated with the names of Wreden and Stone.[35]

Carcinoma of the Rectum.—Adenocarcinoma of the rectum constitutes a large part of malignant disease in the alimentary tract. It is about as frequent as cancer of the rest of the colon combined. It occurs anywhere between the rectosigmoid

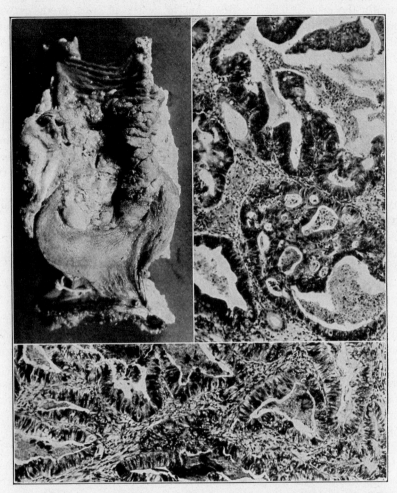

Fig. 437.—Carcinoma of the Rectum in a Fifty-four-year-old Woman Who Complained of Bleeding from the Rectum and Progressive Weakness for One Year.

Rectal (digital) examination revealed a large tumor mass almost filling the rectum. A biopsy confirmed the clinical diagnosis of cancer and a colostomy followed by a perineal resection of the rectum was performed. The gross specimen is illustrated above; microscopic section of the highest lymph node revealed no evidence of metastasis. The two photomicrographs are from the biopsy specimen and show the malignant character of the epithelium. The growth takes a glandular form with irregular, large, deep-staining cells; there is no basement membrane and the growth has penetrated deeply through the wall of the rectum.

junction and the anus. Cancer at the anal opening is, however, quite different, being of the squamous type; it is described separately. Adenocarcinoma grows from the surface of the rectum as a cauliflower growth or penetrates into its wall. In either case an ulcer forms which bleeds readily; in some instances the growth involves the entire circumference of the bowel, producing an annular tumor. Metastases occur by lymphatic spread posteriorly to the iliac nodes and into the colonic mesentery, or by the portal vein to the liver. The disease is twice as frequent in males as in females.

Clinically the growth may be silent, but in nearly all cases produces warning symptoms. *Bleeding* is common and is apt to be slight, but persistent; it may be the first symptom noted. Blood passed at stool varies in color, depending largely upon the length of time it remains in the rectum. Though bleeding is most commonly due to benign lesions—that is, hemorrhoids or fissure, this assumption cannot be made without adequate examination, *i.e.,* rectal palpation and proctoscopy. *Diarrhea* is also a prominent symptom due presumably to irritation and infection of the ulcerated lesion, but more particularly because the stenosis created by the tumor allows evacuation only by liquid stools. The stools in such instances may be frequent and contain mucus and blood. *Obstructive symptoms* may be the first manifestations, especially when the tumor encroaches upon the lumen of the rectum as a cauliflower growth. These symptoms start with increasing constipation or difficulty in moving the bowels, thereby necessitating catharsis. Pain of a cramping character in the left lower quadrant, and increasing distention also occur. Total obstruction is almost never seen in carcinoma of the rectum proper; when such symptoms arise the tumor is nearly always located at or above the rectosigmoid. *Change in bowel habits* in an individual past middle age, even if not marked, should be investigated. A sense of incomplete evacuation, looseness of the stool, the presence of blood or mucus, a more frequent desire for defecation have all been noted by patients who later develop the more evident signs of cancer. However, there are so many other benign and functional or transient disturbances which produce such symptoms that their value lies only in provoking a thorough examination of the rectum. Biopsy should be done when a tumor is present to confirm the diagnosis by microscopic study. *Late symptoms,* such as pain in the region of the sacrum, cachexia, and loss of weight are sometimes present even in operable cases; their development therefore is not always a hopeless sign. Ordinarily, however, they signify a far advanced lesion for which only palliative treatment is possible.

The *treatment* of carcinoma of the rectum is almost entirely surgical; it is still too early to evaluate the results of radium and x-ray.[36] Palliative procedures may relieve symptoms but will not prolong life; according to the extensive and excellent studies of Daland, Welch and Nathanson[37] the average survival without excision of the tumor is about 12 to 18 months. The operations designed for the relief and cure of carcinoma of the rectum are numerous; detailed descriptions may be found in the system of Pack and Livingston.[36] In nearly every case a colostomy (artificial or abdominal anus) is necessary. This operation is described and discussed on page 718. If an acute intestinal obstruction has been produced by the tumor a colostomy (or cecostomy) alone may be all that can be carried out at first in order to relieve the obstruction. If there is no acute obstruction the excision of the tumor may be planned according to a variety of methods with or without a preliminary colostomy (or cecostomy). In general, the excision is carried out from behind (posterior or perineal resection), or by a combination of the anterior and posterior routes (abdomino-perineal excision). Moreover, as already indicated, the operation may be carried out in one or more stages.

1. One-stage procedures were probably the earliest described; Kraske in 1885 performed a one-stage posterior resection of a carcinoma of the rectum, resulting in a perineal anus. It now has only an historical interest. The one-stage operation which is now frequently employed is that which was described by W. E. Miles in 1906 and consists of a combined abdominal and perineal approach enabling the surgeon to carry out an extensive excision *en bloc,* of the tumor together with most of the high-lying regional lymph nodes. These nodes, as shown by Gilchrist and David [38] and others, are the site of metastases in over half of all cases, and must obviously be removed if a cure is to be expected. In the Miles operation the superior hemorrhoidal artery is ligated and divided high so that the entire lymph node bearing area can be removed. The main disadvantage of the operation has been its high mortality, which, however, has fallen steadily because of better preoperative preparation, anesthesia and postoperative care, including the use of transfusions, and more recently, the prophylactic use of sulfanilamide and sulfasuxidine.

2. Two-stage procedures imply the performance of a colostomy (or cecostomy), at the first stage. The second stage, which follows within a week or two, varies. If the tumor is excised entirely from behind, the procedure is usually associated with the name of Lockhart-Mummery; it has the advantage of carrying a low mortality but is less effective in removing all possible lymph node metastases, for reasons already mentioned. If a combined abdomino-perineal resection is carried out at the second stage a variety of methods have been described, all modifications of the original Miles procedure; the names of D. F. Jones, Lahey, Rankin, and Coffey are associated with these variations. Of the two-stage procedures the methods described by Lahey,[39] and Rankin [40] are perhaps the most popular. In the Lahey operation, the sigmoid above the tumor is cut across transversely with the cautery, the proximal end brought out through the wound and the distal end brought out through a stab wound low in the midline. This allows through-and-through irrigation of the loop containing the tumor. This entire loop is removed at the second stage. In the Rankin operation, the sigmoid is likewise cut transversely with the cautery at the first stage, but the distal cut end is closed, leaving it inside the abdomen whereas the proximal loop is used for the colostomy. Dense fixation of the closed end of the distal loop may develop so far laterally that much time will be consumed in dissecting it loose at the second-stage operation. The name of Devine [41] should also be mentioned especially because he devised a transverse colostomy which is being used increasingly.

The main advantage of the two-stage procedure is its lower mortality. This is obvious in patients who are poor risks and especially in patients with acute obstruction in whom anything more than a colostomy is extremely hazardous. In patients with large and seemingly inoperable tumors, surgeons have noted after the colostomy has diverted the fecal stream for some time, that the tumor has become smaller and easily operable, due undoubtedly to subsidence of associated inflammation. This constitutes an additional advantage of the two-stage procedure. Otherwise it is obvious that the sooner the tumor can be removed the less likely distant metastases are to occur.

Carcinoma of the Anus.—Malignant disease visible at and involving the anal orifice is rare; it originates outside the muco-cutaneous margin and is therefore of the squamous-cell type similar in behavior to squamous cell carcinoma elsewhere (see page 302). It is a painful lesion, leads to early ulceration and metastasizes to the regional (inguinal) lymph nodes. Stenosis at the anal canal may occur. Treatment consists of surgical excision of the lesion including the regional lymph nodes or radiotherapy or a combination of both.

Colostomy.—This operation consists of creating an artificial anus in the anterior abdominal wall. In spite of the horror such a situation invokes in the minds of many patients and in a few doctors, the operation, properly carried out with adequate indication, has been responsible for the prolongation of life in relative

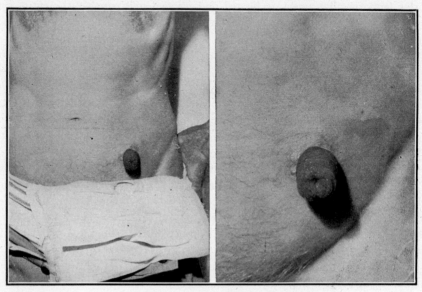

FIG. 438.—SINGLE BARREL COLOSTOMY.

A combined abdomino-perineal resection was performed for carcinoma of the rectum three years before. The patient, now 59 years old, works 12 hours a day without disability. In the left photograph above is shown the simple pad which is used to protect the colostomy; an elastic girdle is used to keep it in place. On the right is a close-up of the colostomy. This particular patient has a bowel movement every other day with the aid of a small enema, and has complete control in the interval with no escape of gas or discharge.

comfort and a minimum of disability. A colostomy may be placed in any of several sites. A most convenient colostomy is one which is located just below and to the left of the umbilicus; the bowel emerges through the retracted rectus muscle which tends to act as a sphincter. Many surgeons bring the colon out through a left lower quadrant (gridiron) incision as illustrated in Fig. 438. The Devine colostomy is higher in the epigastrium.[41] With adequate regulation of the diet a properly performed colostomy will act once or twice a day at a definite hour and remain dry during the interval, thus interfering very little with a normal active life. Obviously some type of dressing with a belt must be worn; the old-fashioned colostomy cup and bag is nearly always very inconvenient for the patient, and if prescribed is soon discarded. A detailed description of the care of a colostomy has been reported by an anonymous patient [42].

THE UMBILICUS

Since diseases of the umbilicus are rather rare they will be considered only briefly here. The details of these conditions may be found in the volume by Cullen.[43] The most frequent lesion is umbilical hernia which is considered on p. 797.

Embryology.—During early embryonic life there is an opening between the primitive gut and the yolk sac which is called the vitelline (omphalomesenteric) duct. This communication is a part of the primitive umbilical orifice which gradually closes by approximation of its margins to form the umbilicus (navel) of extrauterine life. In addition to the vitelline duct, the urachus and the umbilical vessels also traverse the umbilicus.

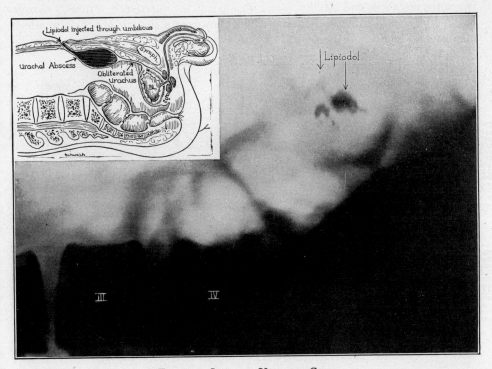

FIG. 439.—INFECTED URACHAL CYST.

The patient, a 19 year old boy, entered the hospital with a diagnosis of appendiceal abscess which seemed entirely correct except for the fact that the tender area was in the midline below the umbilicus rather than in the right lower quadrant. Several hours later a large amount of pus escaped spontaneously from the umbilicus with complete relief of all clinical manifestations. The illustration above is a print from the lateral x-ray film, made several days later, after the opening in the umbilicus had been injected with lipiodol. Note the detailed diagram in the upper left corner. The patient had no further symptoms. The infection apparently produced a necrosis of the epithelial cells lining the urachus thus allowing healing to occur.

The urachus in adult life is represented as an obliterated cord connecting the umbilicus with the dome of the bladder. It arises embryologically from the cranial part of the urinogenital section of the cloaca. The cloaca, which is a part of the hind gut, ultimately separates into a dorsal portion from which the rectum arises, and a ventral portion (urinogenital chamber) which divides into three parts: (1) the cranial part which is converted into the urachus, (2) an intermediate part giving rise to the bladder and (3) a caudal part which gives rise to the urethra, and in females to part of the vagina.

Anomalies.—There are a few congenital maldevelopments which produce lesions at the umbilicus; they are, however, quite rare.

Persistent Urachus.—If the urachus does not become obliterated completely it may give rise to a sinus which drains seromucoid material through the umbilicus; if it becomes obliterated at the ends only, a cyst may form which can be readily excised. However, cysts rarely produce symptoms unless they become infected. An infected *urachal cyst* produces manifestations of a localized intra-abdominal abscess which simulates an appendiceal abscess, except for its location in the midline between the umbilicus and bladder (see Fig. 439). If the infection is serious, drainage of the cavity will be the procedure of choice; however, a sinus is apt to form which may have to be excised later.

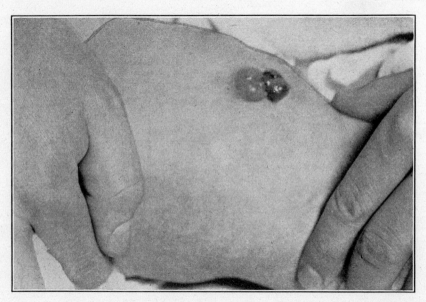

FIG. 440.—VITELLINE CYST IN A SIX-WEEKS-OLD INFANT.

Methylene blue injected into the cyst emerged from the rectum a short time later. Note redundant tissue as well as the cyst. Treatment was conservative; however, the infant died later of a paratyphoid infection (St. Louis City Hospital).

Vitelline (Omphalomesenteric) Cyst.—This anomaly is due to an incomplete obliteration of the terminal end of the vitelline duct, *i.e.,* that part of the yolk sac at the umbilicus; such a defect is noted at birth as a cystic mass at the navel. On some occasions these defects may be of a polypoid or adenomatous character; the greater portion of the solid tissue usually consists of structures resembling intestinal wall, particularly mucosa. On extremely rare occasions the vitelline duct remains open throughout its entire length so that an actual communication with the intestine exists, thus producing a fecal fistula.

Meckel's Diverticulum.—This anomaly is probably frequent but remains unrecognized unless it produces symptoms (see p. 679). It is in reality a part of the vitelline duct but represents the proximal or deep end which enters the primitive gut, and which fails to become obliterated completely, thus creating a permanent pouch or diverticulum in the distal portion of the ileum.

Infections.—The umbilicus may become infected after birth due to contamination and lack of cleanliness during delivery. More commonly the infections at the umbilicus occur in childhood or adult life as a type of *dermatitis*. The clinical manifestations include itching, slight pain and discomfort, and particularly a chronic discharge of mucopurulent material. Inspection of the depths of the orifice will usually reveal a low grade type of superficial skin infection, often associated with tiny ulcers. Treatment is usually effective in most cases and leads to prompt healing; simple cleanliness and daily irrigation of the umbilicus with diluted hydrogen peroxide or boric acid solution followed by careful drying of the invaginated skin, is all that is necessary. If such simple measures are not effective, the possibility of the presence of an anomaly should be considered. If a deep opening can be detected, injection with lipiodol may reveal the existence of a urachal sinus. Other anomalies have already been mentioned.

Neoplasms.—Primary squamous-cell carcinoma has been observed at the umbilicus and presents the characteristics of the disease in general. Benign tumors are usually associated with anomalies as already discussed.

BIBLIOGRAPHY

1. BLAIR, V. P., and IVY, R. H. *Essentials of Plastic Surgery,* C. V. Mosby Co., St. Louis, 2nd edition, 1936.
2. DAVIS, J. S. Incidence of Congenital Clefts of the Lip and Palate, *Ann. Surg.,* 80:363, 1924.
3. SHALLOW, T. A. Combined One Stage Closed Method for the Treatment of Pharyngeal Diverticula, *Surg., Gynec. & Obst.,* 62:624, 1936.
4. WOMACK, N. A. Esophagoplasty for Esophageal Achalasia, *Surg. Clin. N. Am.,* Oct., 1938, p. 1241.
5. CARTER, B. N., STEVENSON, J., and ABBOTT, O. A. Transpleural Esophago-gastrostomy for Caricinoma of the Esophagus and for Carcinoma of the Cardiac Portion of the Stomach, *Surgery,* 8:587, 1940.
6. CARTER, B. N. Resection of a Portion of the Thoracic Esophagus for Carcinoma, *Surg., Gynec. & Obst.,* 71:624, 1940.
7. BOLTON, C. Observations on Referred Pain, *Brain,* 57:211, 1934.
8. MASON, J. M., and GRAHAM, G. S. Ulceration of Aberrant Gastric Mucosa in Meckel's Diverticulum, *Ann. Surg.,* 96:893, 1932.
9. DRAGSTEDT, L. R., and MATTHEWS, W. B. The Digestion of Living Tissue by Gastric and Pancreatic Juice, *Am. J. Physiol.,* 105:29, 1933.
10. MATTHEWS, W. B., and DRAGSTEDT, L. R. Etiology of Gastric and Duodenal Ulcer, *Surg., Gynec. & Obst.,* 55:265, 1932.
11. STEINBERG, M. E., and STARR, P. H. The Factor of Spasm in the Etiology of Peptic Ulcer, *Arch. Surg.,* 29:895, 1934.
12. CANNON, W. B. *The Wisdom of the Body,* W. W. Norton Co., New York, 1932.
13. EMERY, E. S., and MONROE, R. T. Peptic Ulcer; Nature and Treatment Based on Study of 1435 Cases, *Arch. Int. M.,* 55:271, 1935.
14. SIPPY, B. W. Gastric and Duodenal Ulcer; Medical Cure by an Efficient Removal of Gastric Juice Corrosion, *J. Am. M. Ass.,* 64:1625, 1915.
15. LaDue, J. S. Therapy of Massive Hemorrhage Due to Peptic Ulcer, *J. Am. M. Ass.,* 113:373, 1939.
16. ALLEN, A. W. Acute Massive Hemorrhage from the Upper Gastro-intestinal Tract, *Surgery,* 2:713, 1937.

17. GAITHER, E. H. Gastric Carcinoma; Clinical Research; Pre-operative Course and Post-operative Results, *South. M. J.,* 28:107, 1935.

18. CROHN, B. B., GINZBURG, L., and OPPENHEIMER, G. Regional Ileitis, *J. Am. M. Ass.,* 99:1323, 1932.

19. WILKIE, D. P. D. The Etiology of Acute Appendicular Disease, *Canad. M. Ass. J.,* 22:314, 1930.

20. WANGENSTEEN, O. H., and DENNIS, C. Experimental Proof of Obstructive Appendicitis in Man, *Ann. Surg.,* 110:629, 1939.

21. IVANISSEVICH, O., and FERRARI, R. C. Todavía mueren cien mil apendiculares por año. El sindrome mínimo de la apendicitis aguda, *Semana Méd.,* 1:861, 1933.

22. SMITH, J. A., and BARTLETT, M. K. Acute Surgical Emergencies of the Abdomen in Pregnancy, *New England J. Med.,* 223:529, 1940.

23. KEYES, E. L., Jr. Death from Appendicitis; Mortality from Appendicitis and Causes of Death Following Appendicitis, *Ann Surg.,* 99:47, 1934.

24. FITZ, R. Perforating Inflammation of the Vermiform Appendix with Special Reference to Its Early Diagnosis and Treatment, *Am. J. M. Sc.,* 92:321, 1886.

25. STONE, H. B. Surgical Problems in Treatment of Chronic Ulcerative Colitis, *Arch. Surg.,* 41:525, 1940.

26. RANSOM, H. K. Carcinoma of the Right Colon, *Surgery,* 5:34, 1939.

27. STONE, H. B. Surgical Aspects of Carcinoma of the Large Bowel, *J. Am. M. Ass.,* 113:2282, 1939.

28. BALCH, F. G. Injection Treatment of Internal Hemorrhoids, *N. Eng. J. M.,* 212:57, 1935.

29. PEMBERTON, J. deJ., and STALKER, L. K. Surgical Treatment of Complete Rectal Prolapse, *Ann. Surg.,* 109:799, 1939.

30. BUIE, L. A., SMITH, N. D., and JACKMAN, R. J. The Role of Tuberculosis in Anal Fistula, *Surg., Gynec., & Obst.,* 68:191, 1939.

31. CHISHOLM, A. J., and GAUS, H. Anorectal Tuberculosis, *J. Am. M. Ass.,* 104:2067, 1935.

32. GRANET, E. The Therapy of Perianal Tuberculosis, *Ann. Surg.,* 112:440, 1940.

33. SWINTON, N. W., and WARREN, S. Polyps of the Colon and Rectum and Their Relation to Malignancy, *J. Am. M. Ass.,* 113:1927, 1939.

34. CROWELL, E. A., and DULIN, J. W. Congenital Anomalies of the Anus and Rectum, *Surgery,* 7:529, 1940.

35. STONE, H. B. Plastic Operation to Restore Voluntary Anal Control, *J. Am. M. Ass.,* 97:1205, 1931.

36. PACK, G. T., and LIVINGSTON, E. M. *The Therapy of Carcinoma and Allied Diseases,* Hober, 1940, Vol. III, p. 1451.

37. DALAND, E. M., WELCH, C. E., and NATHANSON, I. One Hundred Untreated Cancers of the Rectum, *N. Eng. J. M.,* 214:451, 1936.

38. GILCHRIST, R. K., and DAVID, V. C. Lymphatic Spread of Carcinoma of the Rectum, *Ann Surg.,* 108:621, 1938.

39. LAHEY, F. H. Two-Stage Abdominoperineal Resection for Removal of Cancer of the Rectum, *Surg., Gynec. & Obst.,* 51:692, 1930; LAHEY, F. H., and CATTELL, R. B. A Two-Stage Abdominoperineal Resection of the Rectum and Rectosigmoid for Carcinoma, *Am. J. Surg.,* 27:201, 1935.

40. RANKIN, F. W. Graded Perineo-abdominal Resection of the Rectum and Rectosigmoid, *Am. J. Surg.,* 27:214, 1935; RANKIN, F. W., BARGEN, J. A. and BUIE, L. A. *The Colon, Rectum and Anus,* W. B. Saunders Co., Phila., 1932.

41. DEVINE, H. B. Carcinoma of the Colon, *Brit. M. J.,* 2:1245, 1935.

42. MISCELLANY. Normal Life after Removal of Rectum, *J. Am. M. Ass.,* 115:1398, 1940.

43. CULLEN, T. S. Embryology, Anatomy, and Diseases of the Umbilicus Together with Diseases of the Urachus, W. B. Saunders Co., 1916.

CHAPTER XXV

THE PERITONEAL CAVITY

The peritoneal cavity is in reality only a potential space, but in disease or abnormal circumstances may be distended with many liters of fluid (ascites) or gas (pneumoperitoneum). The visceral peritoneum covers liver, intestines, etc., except at their points of attachment. In contrast to this visceral layer is its continuation inside the abdominal wall which is called parietal peritoneum. The lesser peritoneal space is a small potential cavity (lesser omental sac) which lies behind the stomach and lesser omentum, and normally communicates with the main peritoneal cavity by the foramen of Winslow.

PHYSIOLOGIC PROPERTIES OF THE PERITONEUM

The peritoneum is smooth and lubricated with a small amount of fluid, thereby allowing free motion of the intestines in their peristaltic function. The surface of the peritoneum is covered with endothelium. Beneath this, in the deeper layers of the peritoneum is an unusually rich network of potential blood vessels which probably function only in times of stress (e.g., inflammation). Lymphatic spaces are likewise abundant. Under normal circumstances hypotonic and isotonic fluids, and even microscopical foreign bodies, are absorbed by means of the capillaries of the portal system and the lymphatics, chiefly the former. Which of the two networks is the more important in the protection mechanism cannot be established. The physiologic properties of the peritoneum, as well as various clinical features, are discussed in detail in the excellent monograph by Hertzler.[1]

The peritoneum is highly resistant to infection, and bacteria coming in contact with it by operative contamination, etc., are rapidly destroyed. Phagocytosis by polymorphonuclear leukocytes is apparently the most important factor in this defense mechanism as shown by the studies of Coller and Brinkman [2] and others. This resistance is so pronounced that historically it actually served as a stumbling block to the acceptance of Lister's teachings, e.g., Lawson Tait and others used the argument that abdominal operations were seldom followed by peritonitis, even though no attention was paid to Lister's principles. We now know that this is true because the resistance of the peritoneum is so much greater than that of other tissues that contamination during an abdominal operation may result in a serious wound infection, but inflict no demonstrable harm within the peritoneal cavity. It must not be supposed from this statement that peritonitis is not feared; actually it is a most serious infection because of its high mortality. For this reason its virulence must be decreased as much as possible. Immunity of the peritoneum to infection may be augmented appreciably by repeated or continued exposures of a mild character. This is exemplified clinically by the decreased tendency for peritonitis to develop even following serious operations upon the large bowel when there has been an antecedent colostomy or some minor operation upon the intestine. Some surgeons introduce a vaccine of colon bacilli (colibactragen of Sternberg [4]) into the peritoneal cavity at the termination of colon operations, which are prone to be followed by peritonitis due to contamination, but in the light of experience their use is unnecessary and not worth while. Sulfonamide compounds, including sulfanilamide, sulfathiazole, and sulfadiazine, are now being used extensively (chiefly by the parenteral and intraperitoneal routes) as prophylactic therapy in abdominal operations where contamination from intestinal content, etc., has been significant. The intraperitoneal dose of sulfanilamide should not be greater than 5 grams because of the danger of hepatitis (Jackson and Coller [3]); with sulfathiazole and sulfadiazine the same limitation in dosage should be adopted, lest adhesions be formed because of the relative insolubility of the drugs (see also page 36). However, it should be emphasized that fatal peritonitis is less likely following a single contamination than it is from a continued soiling due to an enclosed leaking suture line.

The omentum, suspended from the greater curvature of the stomach and transverse colon, has often been spoken of as the "wandering policeman" of the abdomen because of its ability to locate and envelop foci of infection and prevent their spread. The omentum therefore plays a major part in the *defense mechanism* in the peritoneal cavity. It may even completely surround a perforation of the intestine and confine the process to a local area, thereby preventing a diffuse pritonitis.

Because of the peculiarities in the sensitivity of the peritoneum to painful and other stimuli, considerable confusion may be experienced clinically in localizing the source of the disease responsible for symptoms. The parietal peritoneum is sensitive to pain, but the visceral peritoneum is sensitive only to certain types of stimuli.

For example, pulling or tugging upon the mesentery of the intestine is painful, although the intestine itself may be cut completely across with a knife or cautery without the production of any pain. Increased tension in hollow organs may likewise produce pain. The early work of Ross [5] and Mackenzie [6] demonstrated that visceral pain of this type is often referred, the visceral stimuli passing into the spinal cord and being referred to corresponding skin fields. This pain is frequently localized to areas not overlying the lesion producing the pain, because the localizing quality of the central sensory mechanism with which the visceral (autonomic) fibers make contact, is poorly developed in comparison with localization by somatic nerve cells.

The mechanism of the production of the involuntary muscle spasm which appears early over an area of peritonitis is vaguely understood, but it is known to be an important protective mechanism. It may be explained as a reflex phenomenon arising from the inflamed peritoneum by way of the spinal cord (see Fig. 363).

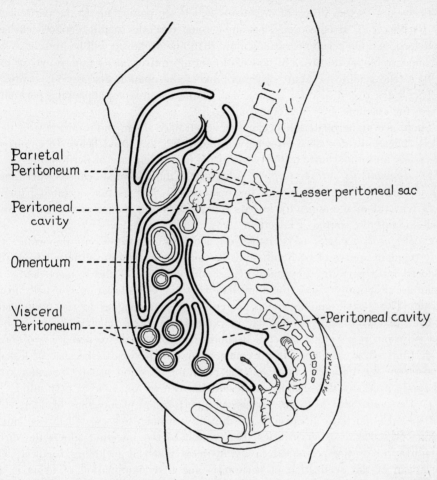

Parietal Peritoneum

Peritoneal cavity

Omentum

Visceral Peritoneum

Lesser peritoneal sac

Peritoneal cavity

FIG. 441.—LONGITUDINAL SECTION OF THE ABDOMINAL CAVITY IN THE ANTEROPOSTERIOR DIRECTION TO SHOW THE GROSS STRUCTURES, AND THE RELATION OF THE VISCERAL TO THE PARIETAL PERITONEUM.

ETIOLOGIC FACTORS IN THE PRODUCTION OF PERITONITIS

Any inflammation of the peritoneum, whether caused by infection, trauma or chemicals, may be classified as a peritonitis, but only that of bacterial origin is of much significance clinically, especially since the nonbacterial types heal so readily. Peritonitis of pyogenic origin, such as that produced by *Bacillus coli* and streptococcus, is serious and associated with a high mortality, especially if the infection becomes general. If the process remains local and is isolated from the rest of the peritoneal cavity by the omentum and adhesions, the systemic reaction is not so serious and recovery is to be expected. As stated on the preceding pages, the peritoneum is resistant to infection, but cannot repel the bacterial assault of a constant soiling, such as would be produced by an unrepaired rupture of the intestine. Under such circumstances the resultant infection in most instances would become diffuse and prove fatal.

There is a certain group of organisms which are pathogenic to the peritoneum, *i.e., Bacillus coli,* streptococcus, pneumococcus, tubercle bacillus, gonococcus and staphylococcus. On certain occasions more than one organism will be present as will be demonstrable by culture. This association of more than one organism may or may not be a true symbiosis. Many observers are of the opinion that various strains of gas bacilli are responsible for a great deal of the toxemia accompanying peritonitis caused, for example, by a perforated appendix.

There are numerous etiologic factors which may act in the production of peritonitis. These are described elsewhere in detail but are listed below to emphasize the variety and importance of the mechanisms in a given case of peritonitis:

1. *Appendicitis with perforation* is by far the most common cause of peritonitis and accounts for many deaths in the operated as well as non-operated patients. Early removal of the appendix lessens considerably the chance of a fatal outcome by eliminating the source of infection.

2. *Perforated peptic ulcer* either duodenal or gastric, is an important and fairly frequent source of peritonitis, but the mechanism is quite different from that produced by a perforated appendix. Since the contents of the stomach and duodenum are practically sterile, the immediate bacterial contamination is usually insignificant. The gastric and duodenal contents are so damaging to the peritoneum, however, that even slight contamination (unless immediate repair is done) is sufficient to result in a serious bacterial peritonitis in forty-eight to seventy-two hours.

3. *Gonorrheal salpingitis* is a frequent source of peritonitis because of leakage of pus from the Fallopian tube, but the resultant infection usually remains local, and rarely produces the serious manifestations seen in appendiceal peritonitis.

4. *Peritonitis due to trauma* (caused by perforation of intestine, bladder, etc.) is of special importance because of the difficulty in diagnosis created by the simultaneous presence of other injuries. Perforation of the intestine allows the direct contamination of the peritoneal cavity by fecal material including bacteria. The mechanism of the production of peritonitis due to contamination of urine is dependent upon chemical irritation with secondary infection.

5. *Peritonitis following laparotomy* is unfortunately an occasional complication of abdominal operations, much to be feared, but usually avoidable. Among the factors producing peritonitis of this type should be mentioned (*a*) leakage of an intestinal suture line, (*b*) contamination during operation, *i.e.,* faulty technic, including particularly *virulent streptococci from the nose and throat* of the operating room personnel, and (*c*) leakage of bile (bile peritonitis, see page 727).

6. *"Idiopathic" primary peritonitis* is a term frequently used to denote the fact that the pathogenesis of the peritonitis is obscure, although apparently blood-borne from a primary focus elsewhere. Streptococcus and pneumococcus peritonitis are types of peritoneal infection comprising this group.

7. *Tuberculosis* occasionally invades the peritoneal cavity, but is usually secondary to an active lesion in the lungs, mesenteric lymph nodes, Fallopian tubes, etc.

8. *Puerperal sepsis* occasionally breaks through the confines of the uterus and adnexae, resulting in a peritonitis. Not unlike the peritonitis produced by septic abortion, this complication is extremely serious and frequently fatal.

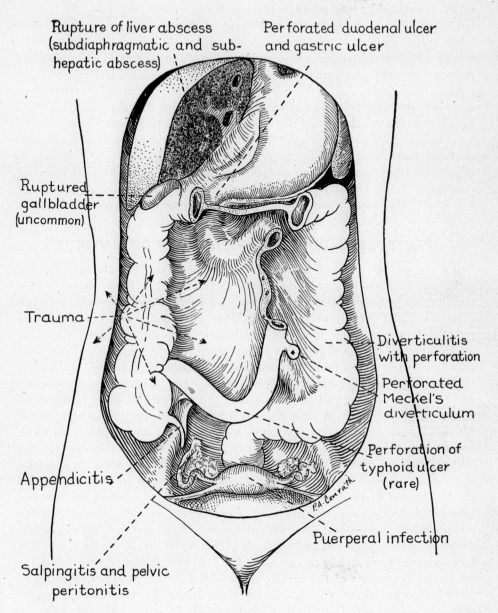

Rupture of liver abscess
(subdiaphragmatic and subhepatic abscess)

Perforated duodenal ulcer
and gastric ulcer

Ruptured
gallbladder
(uncommon)

Trauma

Diverticulitis
with perforation

Perforated
Meckel's
diverticulum

Perforation of
typhoid ulcer
(rare)

Appendicitis

Puerperal infection

Salpingitis and pelvic
peritonitis

P.A. Conrath

Fig. 442.—Schematic Drawing to Illustrate the Numerous Lesions Which May Give
Rise to Local or General Peritonitis.

9. There are numerous *miscellaneous lesions* capable of producing peritonitis which, when considered singly, are not of considerable importance because of their rarity. A gallbladder may perforate because of acute cholecystitis, and the resultant leakage of bile into the peritoneal cavity may produce a serious type of peritonitis. Diverticulitis with perforation (most commonly of the sigmoid) may produce a serious and fatal peritonitis unless operative repair is performed soon after perforation. Meckel's diverticulitis may also give rise to peritonitis because of perforation through the wall of the diverticulum. Perforation of a typhoid ulcer of the ileum will probably occur just often enough to demand that the surgeon acquaint himself with the possibility and the symptoms resulting therefrom.

Rarely, leakage of bile through traumatic rupture of the common duct, ulceration of the duct, etc., may result in *bile peritonitis*. The irritative action of bile on the peritoneum results in exudation of huge quantities of plasma-like fluid frequently resulting in shock. The local protective properties are reduced, resulting occasionally in a severe inflammatory peritonitis, which may become infected secondarily.

PERITONITIS DUE TO PERFORATION OF A VISCUS

Of the various types of peritonitis just enumerated, there are several whose pathology, manifestations and treatment are similar. In this group should be mentioned appendicitis with perforation, perforated peptic ulcer, traumatic perforation of intestine, postoperative peritonitis, etc. They are usually caused by the *Bacillus coli*. Rarely are they due to operative contamination, although unwise operative manipulation in the presence of an inflammatory intraperitoneal lesion may occasionally result in an extension of the infection to a general peritonitis.

Pathology.—The first evidence of peritonitis is a hyperemia and redness of the visceral as well as parietal peritoneum, which gradually loses its luster and assumes a grayish color. A clear fluid soon accumulates, but this exudate rapidly becomes cloudy and contains fibrin. On some occasions fibrin appears to be deposited without the accumulation of free fluid. Within two or three days the fluid thickens and becomes true pus. In the meantime the fibrin and omentum attempt to mat various loops of intestine together so that the infection will remain local and not be diffused everywhere throughout the peritoneal cavity. The attainment or failure of sealing of the perforated intestine or local lesion, with the development of a local abscess is dependent upon the rapidity of leakage, and to a less extent upon the resistance of the patient and virulence of the organisms. If the leakage is slow, adhesions may form rapidly enough to form a local abscess and prevent diffusion of the intestinal contents of the various parts of the peritoneal cavity. Most of the fibrin is absorbed as the process heals, but if the damage has been great, permanent adhesions may result. The pathologic processes, such as local abscess, adhesions, etc., are discussed in more detail under Complications. In addition to the changes mentioned, if the peritonitis is diffuse the entire bowel may become distended, paralyzed and filled with gas and fluid, a condition known as *paralytic ileus* (see p. 759). The systemic effects of inflammation in general are usually encountered. Because of vomiting and failure of absorption of fluid from the damaged intestine, marked dehydration may also be present. In general there are certain pathways by way of which infective fluid from perforative lesions may spread to other parts of the peritoneal cavity. For example, purulent exudate produced by a perforated appendix may reach the subphrenic space by way of the right external paracolic groove (see Fig. 446). Fluid escaping from a perforated peptic ulcer may spread from the right subhepatic space by overflowing anteriorly across the colon into the right infra colic space, thence into the pelvis or across the ascending colon to the right external paracolic groove, etc. (Mitchell [7]). Other details of the "watershed" of the peritoneum may be found in Mitchell's article.

Clinical Manifestations.—The clinical manifestations will depend largely on the stage of disease and the location, nature and severity of the primary or causative lesion. The manifestations produced by the causative lesion itself should if possible be distinguished from those of peritonitis; they are usually elicited by a careful history. The term "peritoneal irritation" is used to describe an early inflammatory lesion which so frequently precedes actual peritonitis. Obviously any diffuse peritonitis starts as a local process, but the term "local peritonitis" implies the confinement of the infection to a local area by such barriers as omentum, adhesions, adjacent organs, etc. Whether a local or general infection is present, will therefore depend not only on the lapse of time but also on the resistance of the patient.

Local Peritonitis.—Pain is the first complaint and is usually so severe as to confine the patient to bed. Local tenderness is demonstrable early and is located over the lesion, in contrast to the referred pain which may be experienced during the onset. Anorexia and nausea are almost always present, but vomiting is variable. Muscle spasm is constant over the lesion, but is not present over the entire abdomen. Tachycardia occurs early, but fever is seldom encountered for eighteen to twenty-four hours. After a few days the above symptoms lessen in severity, and as the muscle spasm decreases the local abscess may be palpable through the abdominal wall as a definite mass. Leukocytosis is rarely absent as long as pus remains undrained.

It is extremely important to discriminate between a true rigidity of the muscles of the anterior abdominal wall and voluntary muscle spasm which may be incited by rough palpation, cold examining hands, etc. A true muscle rigidity which is so pathognomonic of peritoneal irritation is of involuntary origin, may be elicited constantly, and cannot be eliminated by distracting the patient. When examining a patient for muscle spasm and local tenderness, the examiner must assume a reassuring attitude and be gentle during the examination. If pain is inflicted, voluntary muscle spasm is incited and the information gained may be inaccurate. For this reason it is usually wise not to palpate the area complained of until the rest of the abdomen has been examined.

Diffuse (General) Peritonitis.—Diffuse pain is one of the first symptoms to appear, but is usually secondary to the primary lesion as is exemplified by the severe pain and prostration produced by a perforated peptic ulcer. For example, there is little pain associated with peritonitis produced by a leaking suture line, except that produced by distention. A few hours after the onset of the diffuse infection, anorexia and nausea appear and are soon followed by vomiting. Localized muscle spasm, preceded by diffuse tenderness, is manifested early and after several hours may be sufficient to present a "board-like" sensation to palpation. Usually, however, the muscle spasm and tenderness, while diffuse, are more marked over the site of the perforation. Leukocytosis (10,000 to 30,000) is manifested early and usually persists. Tachycardia develops early, but fever is encountered only after eighteen to twenty-four hours. The pulse gradually becomes weak and poorly sustained, and is one of the most reliable means of estimating the physical condition

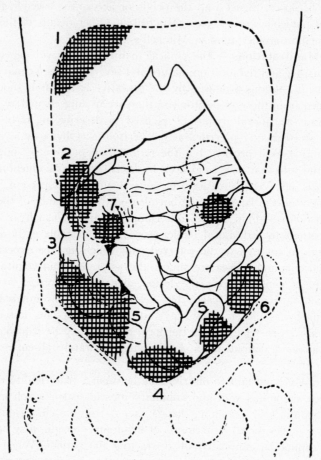

Fig. 443.—Common Sites for the Location of Intra-abdominal Abscesses.

1, above and behind the liver (subdiaphragmatic), commonly secondary to suppurative appendicitis. *2,* inferior surface of the liver (subhepatic) may follow suppurative appendicitis or acute cholecystitis with rupture of the gallbladder. *3,* right lower quadrant, the common site for an abscess following suppurative appendicitis. *4,* pelvis, may be secondary to appendicitis or acute pelvic inflammatory disease. *5,* tubo-ovarian region, secondary to salpingitis. *6,* region of the sigmoid, secondary to ruptured diverticulitis. *7,* about the lower pole of the kidneys (perinephric abscess).

of the patient relative to operability and prognosis. Distention, due to paralysis of the intestine (paralytic ileus) may appear within twenty-four hours, but rarely becomes pronounced for two or three days. This cessation of peristalsis, obviously resulting in constipation, is one of Nature's methods of preventing the spread of the infection. The dulness of free fluid may be demonstrable in the flanks. As noted previously, the clear fluid which forms first rapidly turns to pus, which at operation is observed to have a characteristically foul fecal odor if the infection is caused by the *Bacillus coli,* as is usually the case.

After a time the pain becomes less noticeable, but the vomiting (more often slight regurgitation) persists regardless of whether or not food or water is taken by mouth. Occasionally the vomitus is fecal, indicative of regurgitation from paralyzed ileum. Restlessness is pronounced and unless large doses of narcotics (morphine, etc.) are given, the patient will suffer physically from lack of sleep. After two or three days all the classical signs of peritonitis will be demonstrable. The Hippocratic facies, consisting of anxious expression, sunken and staring eyes, pinched nose and dusky pallor is pathognomonic of a diffuse peritonitis, but is of little value therapeutically, since it is a terminal manifestation. The patient retains consciousness until a short time before death.

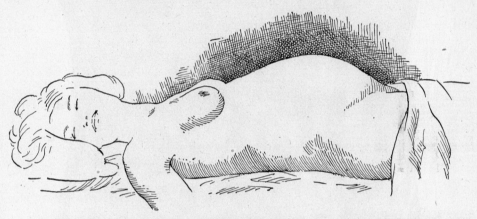

FIG. 444.—DISTENTION IS ONE OF THE MOST CONSTANT OF THE SIGNS OF PERITONITIS, BUT IS SLOW IN FORMING, USUALLY REQUIRING TWO OR THREE DAYS FOR ITS MAXIMUM DEVELOPMENT.

Part of the swelling is due to accumulation of exudate but most of it is due to paralytic ileus which is produced by the peritoneal infection.

Postoperative peritonitis produces manifestations which may be much more insidious. The abdominal pain, tenderness and muscle spasm are much less pronounced. Moreover, the pain produced by the peritonitis is apt to be mistaken for the abdominal discomfort incident to laparotomy. Vomiting and distention are quite constant. Frequently, tachycardia with a gradually weakening pulse, fever, distention and occasional vomiting are the only demonstrable manifestations, but the diagnosis should not be difficult, especially if other complications (such as wound infection, pneumonia, etc.) capable of producing a similar clinical picture are excluded.

The severity of symptoms is dependent upon many factors, among which should be mentioned etiology, virulence of the organism, age of the patient, type of treatment, etc. In children, peritonitis develops rapidly, usually presenting all of the classical symptoms and signs, whereas in the aged, progression of the infection may be slow and atypical which is also true of postoperative peritonitis. For example, pain, muscle spasm and even fever may be insignificant or absent. In the aged, even though few manifestations are exhibited, the prognosis is nevertheless poor and in fact worse than in children.

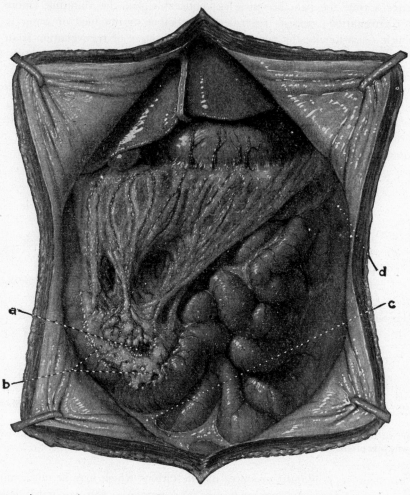

Fig. 445.—Autopsy Appearance of Diffuse Purulent Peritonitis Arising from a Perforated (and Therefore Neglected) Appendicitis.

a, Omentum adherent to appendix and adjacent coils of intestine; b, Yellowish green protective plastic exudate; c, Pus between coils of intestine; d, Cloudy fluid found at a distance from the appendix. (From Babcock, *Textbook of Surgery,* 1935, courtesy of W. B. Saunders Co., Philadelphia.)

Peritonitis is a prominent cause of death in gastro-intestinal surgery, accounting for about one-fourth the deaths in a series studied by Shambaugh,[8] but did not account for as many postoperative deaths as did pneumonia. Shambaugh also noted that fatal postoperative peritonitis was twice as frequent in operations on the colon as in operations on the stomach. Only one-fourth of the deaths could be attributed to soiling at the time of operation, thereby supporting the pre-existing knowledge that the peritoneum will overcome a tremendous lot of contamination; the remainder of the deaths were due to defective anastomoses, etc., thereby re-emphasizing the fact that continuous contamination from leaks due to careless placing of sutures is more serious than a single contamination at the time of operation. The most serious of the latter group is contamination sustained during operations on the colon.

Differential Diagnosis.—In no other group of diseases is it so necessary to make an early accurate diagnosis as it is in the diseases leading to peritonitis, because early operation is so often essential to the prevention of a fatal outcome. The number of diseases capable of simulating or producing peritonitis are innumerable, and at times offer serious diagnostic difficulty. In reality it is not necessary to establish accurately the cause of the peritoneal manifestations, but it is absolutely essential to make the correct decision as to whether or not an operation should be performed, since an error in this decision is serious and may lead to a fatality. In a consideration of differential diagnosis (see also pp. 726 to 728) it may therefore add to clarity to classify those diseases, which are discussed in detail later, into three groups: (1) diseases producing peritonitis for which operation is imperative; (2) diseases not associated with peritonitis, but for which operation is imperative or advisable; and (3) diseases not producing peritonitis and for which operation is detrimental or perhaps fatal.

1. *Diseases Producing Peritonitis and for Which Operation Is Imperative.*— A patient with a general peritonitis caused by a *perforated appendix* may present such diffuse tenderness and muscle rigidity that the source of the infection will be undetermined. The diagnosis can perhaps best be made by careful consideration of the history, supported by the fact that the maximum tenderness and muscle spasm will be located over the right lower quadrant. While the appendix is unperforated the pain is not diffuse, but usually located in the right lower quadrant. If the peritonitis is caused by a *perforation of a peptic ulcer* the point of maximum tenderness is more apt to be in the upper abdomen, but of more importance is the fact that the onset of pain, which is confined to the epigastrium, at least for a few hours, will be sudden and be of much greater severity than that produced by appendicitis. Moreover, the patient is invariably severely prostrated very soon after the perforation. An x-ray taken with the patient in a sitting posture will almost always reveal a collection of gas under the diaphragm, especially in the right side. The symptoms of peritonitis caused by perforation of an *inflamed diverticulum* of the sigmoid differs from the other types of peritonitis in so far as the pain at the onset practically always is confined to the left lower quadrant unless the peritonitis becomes general. Palpation of the abdomen will likewise reveal the tenderness and muscle spasm located to the greater extent at least, in this area. Perforation of a diverticulum occurs more commonly in elderly people than in young adults. An accurate diagnosis of an ulcerated or perforated *Meckel's diverticulum* may be difficult. About the only diagnostic feature, especially in its differentiation from peritonitis of appendiceal origin, is the location of maximum pain, local tenderness and muscle spasm which is usually demonstrable outside the right lower quadrant and frequently in the neighborhood of the umbilicus. Moreover, blood may at times be found in the stool. Early diagnosis of a perforation of a *typhoid ulcer* may be difficult because of the existence already of considerable abdominal tenderness and pain. The perforation may not be accompanied by severe pain, muscle spasm, etc., which are seen

in patients with rupture of a peptic ulcer, but the presence of the symptoms and signs of typhoid fever should of course prevent confusion with such conditions, the other more common sources of peritonitis requiring operation.

2. *Diseases Not Producing Peritonitis, but for Which Operation Is Imperative or Advisable.*—*Intestinal obstruction* because of distention may be difficult to differentiate from peritonitis, but an accurate consideration of the history, particularly as related to the onset and type of pain, will usually lead to the correct diagnosis. Fever, tachycardia, and leukocytosis are less common in complete intestinal obstruction. The pain of peritonitis is usually constant and confined to one area, whereas the pain associated with intestinal obstruction is intermittent and inconstant, coming on in cramping attacks, lasting a minute or two and subsiding for an equal length of time. Visible peristalsis will be demonstrable through the anterior abdominal wall, except in obese patients, and in the late stage when the intestine is paralyzed. Likewise, auscultation will reveal an unusual amount of peristaltic gurgling except in the late cases, in contrast to the silent abdomen of peritonitis. If a loop of gangrenous gut is present (strangulation) the pulse will be rapid and the patient will appear unusually ill considering the duration of his illness. If, through twisting of the mesentery or adhesions, large tributaries of the portal vein are obstructed in the base of the mesentery, the pain may be intense, but not of a cramping nature. It is important to note that intestinal obstruction is usually secondary to a preëxisting lesion such as tumor (*e.g.,* carcinoma of the colon), adhesions (produced by operation or inflammation) etc. In infants and young children, especially the former, *intussusception* is commonly observed and will present many of the manifestations of peritonitis, including vomiting and prostration. However, fever is not present; mild abdominal tenderness is noted in contrast to the acute tenderness and muscle spasm which accompanies peritonitis. A mass in the region of the ascending, transverse, or descending colon is practically always demonstrable. If the intussusception has been present for many hours there is practically always a history of bloody diarrheal stools, or the passage of pure blood. *Acute pancreatic necrosis* may produce symptoms and signs almost indistinguishable from peritonitis, but careful consideration will reveal certain important features. For example, at the onset of acute pancreatic necrosis, which is sudden, there is practically always a severe pain in the epigastric region which is completely disabling and will demand narcosis. The patient is in mild shock, the pulse rapid and weak. The level of blood amylase is elevated early in the disease but returns later to normal. The temperature for the first few hours is apt to be subnormal. Tenderness and muscle spasm may be diffuse, but is practically always most prominent over the region of the pancreas. Vomiting is variable but usually present. Leukocytosis is mild. At operation hemorrhagic necrosis of the pancreas will be noted and areas of fat necrosis may be found on the peritoneum, omentum and surface of the pancreas. *Acute mesenteric thrombosis* is a rather uncommon condition frequently associated with, but not responsible for, peritoneal suppuration except, perhaps, in the terminal stage of the disease. It may occur in supposedly healthy persons without antecedent peritoneal symptoms or obvious disease. The onset is dramatic with intense pain and is associated within a few hours with the major manifestations of shock. If the colon is involved the shock will be more intense than when the small intestine is affected.

Examination will sometimes reveal a tender tubular mass which represents the loop of intestine, the vessels to which are thrombosed. A mild bloody diarrhea is not uncommon. Regardless of the presence or absence of diarrhea, blood-stained fecal matter will usually be found in the rectum. Muscle spasm is usually not so pronounced as it is in peritonitis with equally toxic manifestations. On many occasions the intestine attached to the mesentery containing the involved vessels will become gangrenous, thereby making resection imperative. On the other hand, gangrene may not be produced (see p. 779) ; in that event, the condition should obviously be classified in group 3, below.

3. *Diseases Not Producing Peritonitis and for Which Operation Is Detrimental or Even Fatal.*—*Pyelitis* is frequently confused with lesions (*e.g.,* appendicitis) producing peritonitis, thereby leading to the performance of a needless laparotomy. Pyelitis occurs in patients of any age, but in children is most often confused with lesions demanding laparotomy. The disease is much more common in girls than boys, and may be ushered in insidiously with pain on one side of the abdomen, associated with abdominal tenderness, mild muscle rigidity, nausea and vomiting. Chills are not uncommon. Careful examination will rarely fail to reveal the fact that the most tender area is located posteriorly over the kidney. The presence of pus cells in the urine should lead one to the correct diagnosis of pyelitis. Obviously, if the left kidney is affected, localization of the pain, etc., over the left side of the abdomen should help eliminate acute appendicitis in the differential diagnosis. *Acute enteritis* due to "food poisoning," *i.e.,* caused by organisms of the colon and proteus groups, etc., may offer considerable difficulty because of the presence of nausea, vomiting and abdominal pain. The pain and tenderness, however, are usually poorly localized and are inclined to shift from one area to another. Moreover, nausea and vomiting are apt to precede pain, in contrast to the sequence in lesions leading to peritonitis. Muscle spasm of consequential degree is likewise rarely present. Leukocytosis usually does not occur. Frequently, a diarrhea is present, thereby issuing a warning that the diagnosis of early peritonitis must be quite definite before laparotomy is performed. *Acute salpingitis* is frequently confused with lesions (particularly appendicitis) for which laparotomy is indicated. If the tenderness and pain are limited to the left side there will, of course, be no confusion with appendicitis. The history of frequency and burning on urination (urethritis), vaginal discharge and positive findings on vaginal examination should lead to the correct diagnosis of salpingitis. In this disease, the severe manifestations of toxemia so characteristic of *Bacillus coli* peritonitis are absent. Peritonitis, limited usually to the pelvis, frequently results from acute gonococcal salpingitis and in that respect does not fit literally into this group, but operation is distinctly contraindicated regardless of whether or not the infection extends beyond the pelvis. *Acute cholecystitis* is a common disease ushered in almost invariably with severe pain in the right upper quadrant, radiating frequently to the tip of the scapula. Fever occurs early as does leukocytosis and a mild tachycardia. Jaundice may or may not be present. There is tenderness in the right upper quadrant along with muscle spasm. Some surgeons advise operation for acute cholecystitis; in that respect this disease may be classified in Group 1. Diffuse tenderness and muscle spasm, together with other evidence of a generalized peritonitis, may be present if a perforation of the

gallbladder into the free peritoneal cavity occurs, but such a complication is rare. Acute cholecystitis when it ruptures into the peritoneal cavity, may, therefore, be an exception to the classification and produce peritonitis for which immediate operation is indicated (see p. 733). In children *acute mesenteric lymphadenitis* is rather commonly observed and usually presents a clinical picture which is differentiated from early peritonitis with extreme difficulty. Abdominal tenderness, pain, nausea, vomiting, leukocytosis and even other signs of peritonitis may be present and develop acutely. About the only evidence which can be used to eliminate the diagnosis of peritonitis is found in the type of tenderness and pain. The pain and tenderness will usually not be localized to the right lower quadrant as it is in the most common disease (appendicitis) to be eliminated in differential diagnosis. The muscle spasm is apt to be diffuse and likewise located outside the limits of the location of the appendix (see p. 681). There is still another group of patients, including both children and adults, which offers serious difficulties in differentiating from peritonitis; this syndrome consists of abdominal pain and mild muscle spasm, which is presumably a *peritoneal irritation secondary to upper respiratory infections.* Anorexia and nausea are common, but vomiting is rare. Leukocytosis is usually absent, which is at least one reason which the surgeon has to justify conservative treatment. The presence of fever is variable, though usually present, and tends to support the decision to refrain from a laparotomy, especially if the manifestations are suggestive of a localized peritonitis and not a general peritonitis. The performance of a laparotomy in these individuals may, of course, be detrimental and damaging, and should be avoided at all costs if possible. *Ulcerative colitis ("idiopathic" or amebic)* may offer more difficulty in differentiation from the lesions necessitating operation. In the former instance there is practically always a history of preëxisting abdominal tenderness and pain. Vomiting is rarely present. Amebic dysentery of the acute type simulating peritonitis is usually accompanied by fever, diarrhea and blood in the stool. Differential diagnosis is extremely important in amebic dysentery since the erroneous performance of a laparotomy in this disease is very deleterious and often fatal. The pain in *spastic colitis* is usually mild and rarely localized. Nausea, vomiting and leukocytosis are rarely present. There are a few *miscellaneous diseases* which on rare occasions may produce pain and other peritoneal manifestations in the abdomen. Of this group angina pectoris and pneumonia should be mentioned particularly. Although the pain of coronary thrombosis and occlusion (angina pectoris) may occasionally be referred to the epigastrium and be accompanied by muscle spasm, it will rarely be difficult to differentiate the disease from peritonitis, because of the history of pain in the left side of the chest and left arm, and the relative infrequency of vomiting, leukocytosis, etc. It must be remembered, however, that vomiting may be present in acute coronary occlusion. When *pneumonia* occurs in a lower lobe there occasionally is sufficient diaphragmatic pleurisy to produce pain, tenderness and muscle rigidity of referred character in the upper part of the abdomen. The presence of pulmonary signs, such as increased respiratory rate, respiratory grunt, sharp limitation of abdominal signs to the upper abdomen, will rarely fail to differentiate the disease from a peritonitis. Occasionally *acute nephritis,* particularly if bilateral, will present generalized pain, tenderness and muscle rigidity over the abdomen, simulating peritonitis. Urinary findings should lead one to the correct diagnosis. The importance of establishing a correct diagnosis can be appreciated when one considers the fact that a laparotomy performed in any of the three diseases mentioned above (pneumonia, coronary occlusion, and acute nephritis) is apt to lead to a fatal outcome.

Treatment.—Prophylactic therapy in reality is most important in so far as peritonitis is secondary to other lesions or to contamination which, if prevented or treated promptly will eliminate infection of the peritoneal cavity. For example, when dealing with acute appendicitis appendectomy should be done as soon as possible after the diagnosis is made, hoping to remove the diseased appendix before it perforates and contaminates the peritoneal cavity. Likewise, closure of a perforation of an intestine should be done as early as possible after injury since the possibility of the development of a general peritonitis is dependent for the most part upon the length of time intervening between the injury and operative repair. The care with which the tissues are handled during the operation is also important. Rough handling may encourage the development of infection or even result in a tear or puncture of a loop of intestine, an accident which might lead to a fatal peritonitis unless repair is instituted.

Once a peritonitis is present the question of operation is dependent almost entirely upon (1) the source of the infection, and (2) the condition of the patient. If the peritonitis is diffuse and produced by a perforated appendix, opinions are divided as to the therapy to be followed. Some surgeons are of the opinion that the appendix should be removed immediately, as soon as dehydration and electrolytic imbalance can be corrected. On the other hand there are a number of surgeons who have presented evidence (mostly statistical) to indicate that a longer delay is justified in patients with peritonitis due to a *perforated appendicitis*. By treating the patient for diffuse peritonitis they hope that the entire process will subside or form a local abscess. In the latter instance incision and drainage can be carried out with lower mortality. If the process should subside completely, operation may be performed many weeks or months later as an interval appendectomy. Preliminary reports on the use of sulfanilamide in perforated appendicitis (see p. 739) are so favorable as to support the principle of immediate operation. It is therefore probable that conservative treatment will be employed less often, particularly since immediate operation has the distinct advantage of removing the source of the peritoneal suppuration.

It should be emphasized that the procedure of drainage in operations in peritonitis is often misunderstood; the insertion of drains does not drain the general peritoneal cavity. As shown by Yates[9] in 1905 drainage of the peritoneum affects only a local area and not the entire infected surface. Drains should therefore be used only to aid in evacuation of a definite abscess, or in exteriorizing a possible site of contamination or infection (*e.g.,* an insecure anastomosis); they should always be of soft material (*e.g.,* gutta percha) lest the intestine or other organs be injured by constant pressure of the drain.

To prevent spread of peritonitis the gastro-intestinal tract is put at rest by allowing the patient nothing by mouth. At least 3000 cc. of fluid must be administered, primarily by the intravenous and subcutaneous route. Glucose may be given by vein in 5 or 10 per cent solution but not faster than 300 to 500 cc. per hour. Winslow [10] has shown that 5 per cent glucose may be given at a rate of 500 cc. per hour with 98 per cent utilization and a 10 per cent solution at relatively the same speed with a 95 per cent utilization. Because of loss of chloride by vomiting, intestinal decompression, etc., physiologic saline should be given subcutaneously or intravenously with glucose in quantities up to 1000 to 1500 cc. per day depending upon the amount of fluid lost from the stomach. The administration of amounts greater than this for a period of days is very apt to lead to salt edema especially if hypoproteinemia is severe; in such a case urine output is small. As a routine, Wangensteen drainage by "nasal tube" is advisable in the attempt to decrease the harmful effects of peristalsis and distention although the results may be disappointing except in preventing gastric dilatation and its complicating effects, such as pressure on the heart and other important structures. Continuous gastric suction also serves to keep the intestine at rest by preventing entrance of fluid into the duodenum. If the fluid loss by the catheter or by vomiting is especially great, the patient will need more than 3000 cc. of fluid per day (see p. 151 for details of fluid balance). Transfusions of whole blood or of plasma are often indicated especially to correct hypoproteinemia which is aggravated by actual loss of plasma into the peritoneal exudate and wall of the intestine. Since patients with peritonitis are restless, it is extremely essential that they be given adequate doses of narcotics (morphine, etc.), especially at night, to encourage sleep. It is not sufficient that the patient rest, *he must receive a required amount of sleep daily* if his general resistance is to be maintained. Elevation of the head of the bed one or two notches will add to the comfort of the patient. It is thought by some that elevation of the head of the bed (Fowler's position) prevents absorption from the upper part of the peritoneal cavity and thereby lessens the severity of the disease. However, proof of this is not positive.

As has been shown by Puestow,[11] Orr [12] and others, morphine produces an increase in tonus of the intestine and should perhaps diminish some of the detrimental effects of distention induced by the peritonitis without resulting in enough intestinal activity to spread the infection. Attempts should be made to alleviate the distention by the insertion of a rectal tube. Every twenty-four to forty-eight hours a small enema (magnesium sulphate, glycerin and water) may be given to obtain expulsion of as much gas and fecal matter as possible. Results are frequently so poor that many surgeons give few enemas, but rely on rectal tubes to relieve distention. It has been suggested (Potter [13] and Brown [14]) that peristaltic stimulants such as pitressin, prostigmin, etc., be used to combat distention; however, as yet there is insufficient evidence to prove that the beneficial effects more than offset the damage sustained by activation of the infection by the increased intestinal activity.

The application of heat by a bake, electric pad, etc., is usually a source of comfort to the patient, and is to be preferred to cold applications. Bisgard [15] has shown that the application of heat over the abdomen decreases peristalsis whereas cold increases it. This fact may be utilized in the treatment as discussed in the preceding paragraph. When distention is prominent, Fine and associates [16] have reported reduction by having the patient breathe 95 per cent oxygen. An enterostomy in general peritonitis is not only a useless but an unnecessarily deleterious procedure; it rarely relieves distention as long as the bowel is paralyzed, whereas it is not needed as soon as the paralysis is corrected by the subsidence of the peritoneal infection.

Sulfanilamide has been found efficacious by Ravdin and associates [17] and others in the treatment of peritonitis associated with perforated appendicitis. The drug may be given parenterally or in a single dose directly into the peritoneal cavity and wound (Thompson, Brabson and Walker [18]). In certain types of peritonitis due to other causes it is also beneficial. The drug is being used very extensively in a prophylactic way following major operations on the intestine, particularly the large bowel where peritonitis is so apt to develop. Practically all surgeons using it in this way are convinced that the incidence of peritonitis is decreased sharply. A dose of five grams sprinkled in the peritoneal cavity or introduced as a suspension will produce a concentration of 8 to 12 mgm. per cent in the blood stream within three or four hours, but it rapidly recedes to 2 or 3 mgm. per cent within 24 hours. As much as 12 grams is introduced into the peritoneal cavity and wound by some observers,[18] but Jackson and Coller [3] warn against the use of large doses of the sulfonamides because of the danger of hepatitis. (See also page 724.)

Succinyl sulfathiazole [19] (sulfasuxidine), which is supplanting sulfanilylguanidine, is of great aid in the prevention of fatal peritonitis following operations on the intestine, particularly the colon. It is absorbed so slowly from the intestine that it can be given in doses (orally) as large as 12 or more grams per day. It is given for a few days before operation and reaches such a concentration in the bowel lumen that it decreases sharply the bacterial content therein.

Expert and attentive nursing care is essential to the recovery of patients with peritonitis and in many instances will be the deciding factor in their recovery.

Complications.—A large percentage of patients recovering from diffuse peritonitis develop complications of one type or another. Most of the complications are serious and in many instances will cause the death of the patient after he has apparently overcome the damaging effects of the peritonitis itself.

1. *Local abscess* may be single or multiple and is formed by the isolation of areas of infection by omentum, adhesions, loops of intestines, etc. They frequently form at dependent sites such as the pelvis and the concavities of the peritoneal cavity, early in the infection before adhesions are formed. Abscesses also develop between loops of intestine and their mesentery, and under the diaphragm. The persistence or recurrence of fever after the severe toxic symptoms produced by the peritonitis have subsided, is usually the first indication of the presence of an abscess. A mass may or may not be palpable, depending upon the size and location of the abscess. Consistent local tenderness over the abscess is usually present, but muscle spasm is absent in most instances. If the abscess is in the pelvis, rectal and vaginal examination will almost invariably yield positive information as to its presence. Such manifestations as fever, anorexia, failure to gain weight, weakness, restlessness, etc., usually accompany peritoneal abscess. Occasionally, after a variable length of time an abscess will rupture into a loop of intestine and in this way discharge its content. This is to be suspected when the local signs suddenly subside, and the fever suddenly drops. Occasionally, the pus will be seen in the feces if looked for, especially in abscesses which have broken into the rectum. Evacua-

tion by this means is usually as effective as incision, but unfortunately occurs only after the abscess has been present for many days or weeks. Incision and drainage is usually indicated, but may be delayed if definite regression is revealed after a day or two of conservative treatment; many abscesses will resolve without incision. If

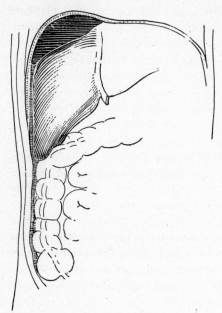

incision is resorted to, drains should, of course, be left in the wound and, if the cavity is large, should not be removed for four or five days or longer. A Penrose drain (tube of thin soft rubber), a rolled strip of rubber dam or a cigarette drain (rubber dam around gauze) represent the types of drains most often used.

2. *Subdiaphragmatic (subphrenic) abscess* presents features which are so different from those of other intraperitoneal abscesses that it is considered separately. An abscess may develop under the diaphragm as a complication of almost any infection within the peritoneal cavity. Inflammatory lesions of the liver and biliary passages, stomach or duodenum, and appendix account for about 60 per cent of the cases (Hochberg [23]). As would be expected, the majority of abscesses are on the right side. Dividing the right subphrenic space into posterior superior, inferior and anterior superior, Ochsner and associates [20] found the posterior superior space to be involved in 34 per cent of a large collected series. Next in frequency was the left anterior inferior

Fig. 446.—Subdiaphragmatic Abscess following Appendectomy for Perforated Appendicitis.

Cross-section to show the relationship to other organs. The shaded track along the ascending colon indicates the probable path of the infection in its migration to its present location. This pathway rapidly becomes sealed, however, with adhesions and scar tissue.

space (20.5 per cent). Not all subphrenic infections proceed to suppuration. Details of diagnosis may be found in the splendid article by Hochberg [23].

The existence of a subphrenic abscess should be suspected when the fever (produced by the initial lesion) which may have subsided somewhat, becomes more elevated and irregular. Systemic symptoms such as anorexia, weakness, sweating, malaise, nausea and occasionally vomiting may be present. Pain is insignificant and is rarely of any aid in the localization of the abscess which is presumed to exist. However, palpation may reveal slight tenderness over the twelfth rib posteriorly, or along the costal margin anteriorly (depending on the location of the abscess). It may therefore be of some aid in determining the location of the abscess; otherwise abdominal examination is usually negative. The leukocyte count is usually markedly elevated. When a subdiaphragmatic abscess is suspected, the limits of hepatic dulness should be observed closely by percussion from day to day. If, for example, the upper margin of dulness approaches the nipple line, it is advisable to establish by roentgenologic means, whether or not the leaf of the diaphragm is abnormally elevated. This observation is important since a subdiaphragmatic abscess rarely occurs without an elevation of the diaphragm. However, elevation of the diaphragm is by no means pathognomonic of subphrenic abscess, since it may be elevated by numerous lesions in the absence of pus. Absence of respiratory excursions of the diaphragm, as noted fluoroscopically, is an additional manifestation of diagnostic value. A positive diagnosis can be made by x-ray if gas exists in the abscess cavity and is revealed on the film by the presence of a fluid level. However, this situation will not be found in more than 20 per cent of cases. Aspiration should not be performed because of the danger of perforation of intestine, hemorrhage, etc. Pleurisy with sterile effusion on the affected side is the most common sequel and may be of diagnostic aid. Other complications such as rupture of the abscess into the pleural or free peritoneal cavity are serious, and are indicative of neglect.

The mortality rate varies considerably between 10 and 30 per cent, depending upon the type of therapy, resistance of the patient, complications, etc.

As soon as the diagnosis is made, drainage should be instituted provided the physical condition of the patient permits. Ochsner and associates [20] have emphasized the advisability of draining subphrenic abscesses extraserously, *i.e.,* without entering the pleural or .peritoneal cavity. Abscesses in the most common location, *i.e.,* in the right posterior inferior space, may best be drained by excising the twelfth rib and incising into the subphrenic space at the level of the spinous process of the first lumbar vertebra. If the abscess is located anteriorly it may be reached extraperitoneally by an incision along the costal margin, dissecting the peritoneum from the diaphragm upward until the abscess is reached. Only occasionally will it be necessary to drain through a lateral incision; in this case it will be necessary to suture the parietal to the diaphragmatic pleura at one stage, followed three or four days later by drainage through the area after adhesions have formed.

3. *Intestinal obstruction* resulting from contractions of fibrous adhesions is not at all unusual and if complete may demand immediate release of the obstructed loop. Obstruction may be produced in this manner as early as three to four days following the onset of the peritonitis, but usually occurs later (two to three weeks) and after the symptoms of the infection have become negligible. *Adhesions* which do not absorb are capable of producing obstruction, partial or complete, years after the attack of peritonitis. Except for intestinal obstruction, adhesions disclose little or no evidence of their presence. Details of intestinal obstruction are discussed in the following chapter.

4. *Pylephlebitis* or inflammation of the portal vein (accompanied usually by thrombosis) is an occasional and serious complication of peritonitis. The process may start in some of the extrahepatic tributaries of the portal vein and reach the major trunk by extension. One of the most reliable symptoms of pylephlebitis is the rather sudden occurrence of frequent chills along with an intermittent type of fever with sharp elevations and recessions. There may be few additional manifestations, perhaps icterus, tachycardia, slight abdominal tenderness and distention, enlargement of the liver and occasionally bleeding within the intestinal tract (see p. 596). The disease, however, is extremely serious, and frequently results in death.

5. *Pyogenic abscess* of the liver (see p. 602) may be encountered as a com-

plication of peritonitis and in most instances is probably caused by an extension of the infection by way of the portal vein into the small intrahepatic tributaries. In many instances the abscess formation will be multiple, in which case death almost always ensues. Suppurative cholangitis may likewise be responsible for multiple abscesses, but is associated only with infections of the biliary tract. Multiple abscesses may coalesce into one large cavity, but when a single abscess is present it is usually caused by amebic infection. Operation is indicated as soon as the diagnosis of pyogenic abscess is made in the hope that the abscess may be single and can be drained.

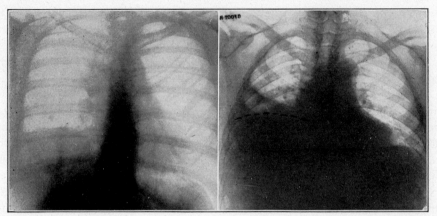

FIG. 447.   FIG. 448.

FIG. 447.—ROENTGENOGRAM REVEALING ELEVATED DIAPHRAGM (RIGHT) CAUSED BY SUBDIA-
PHRAGMATIC ABSCESS RESULTING FROM PERFORATED APPENDICITIS.

By far the majority of subdiaphragmatic abscesses occur on the right side.

FIG. 448.—SUBDIAPHRAGMATIC ABSCESS ASSOCIATED WITH PLEURAL EFFUSION.

The dotted line represents the level of the right diaphragm. The shadow above the elevated diaphragm is caused by fluid in the pleural cavity—a common complication. This fluid usually remains sterile unless treatment is delayed or neglected; perforation through the diaphragm occurs under such conditions.

6. *Gastric dilatation* is a frequent complication of peritonitis as well as of abdominal operations in general (see p. 678) ; if untreated it may produce damaging effects because of the mechanical pressure exerted upon the heart, lungs, and other viscera by the dilated stomach. The diagnosis should be suspected when there is frequent vomiting (or regurgitation) of small quantities of fluid. Gastric dilatation is in reality a part of the paralytic ileus which so constantly accompanies peritonitis and from a literal standpoint, perhaps should be considered as a manifestation and not a complication. Frequent gastric lavage or continuous "nasal suction" (see Fig. 457) should be instituted.

7. There are numerous *miscellaneous complications* which may develop, many of which are extremely serious. Death from peritonitis is usually attributable to the peritoneal infection with or without *septicemia*. As previously stated, *pneumonia* is a frequent complication of peritonitis, and commonly is a terminal feature. Myo-

cardial insufficiency, although secondary to other causes, is one of the main factors in the fatal termination.

OTHER VARIETIES OF PERITONITIS

Most of the clinical manifestations described in the previous pages of this chapter apply most specifically to peritonitis secondary to perforation or contamination and largely caused by the colon bacillus. The following types of peritonitis are caused by different organisms and may present different clinical manifestations and

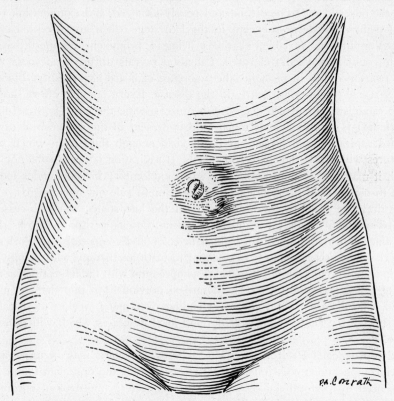

FIG. 449.—BULGING AT THE UMBILICUS IN PNEUMOCOCCUS PERITONITIS.

This is nature's attempt to effect drainage; indeed, in neglected cases perforation occurs here with subsequent evacuation of an abscess cavity. This phenomenon occurs very uncommonly in any other type of peritonitis; it is usually a late manifestation, but in this particular instance occurred on about the third day of the peritonitis.

therapeutic problems from the types of secondary peritonitis already considered. The infections produced by pneumococcus and streptococcus are the ones most frequently spoken of as primary or idiopathic peritonitis. In a series studied by Ladd and associates,[21] the streptococcus was encountered more than twice as frequently as the pneumococcus.

1. **Pneumococcus Peritonitis.**—This is a disease limited almost exclusively to children and occurs much more frequently in girls than boys. This latter feature has led some observers to conclude that the organism, on some occasions at least,

gains access to the peritoneal cavity by way of the genital tract (vagina, uterus and fallopian tubes). This must be considered only one of the etiologic mechanisms, however, since pneumococcus peritonitis occurs as a complication of such diseases as upper respiratory infection, pneumonia, pleurisy and nephritis, in which case it is blood borne. The length of time intervening between the onset of the original infection and the peritonitis varies from a day or two to many weeks, depending upon the severity and chronicity of the disease. Commonly one of the first evidences of this intra-abdominal infection is the development of a diarrhea. The symptoms and signs are similar to those produced by the colon bacillus, except that the pain even at the onset is apt to be diffuse and poorly localized, and examination reveals no local point of tenderness except in the late stage when an abscess may have formed. Vomiting is variable, at times being a prominent manifestation. The leukocyte count is markedly elevated. Palpation reveals diffuse tenderness with a doughy resistance, but in most instances absence of board-like rigidity. Blood culture may reveal the organism early in the disease. Every possible effort should be made to establish the correct diagnosis because specific therapy (with serum and sulfapyridine) is so effective. If much fluid is present in the abdomen, a carefully performed aspiration will be safe and will yield enough fluid from which smears and cultures will reveal the correct diagnosis. If aspiration is not feasible, or yields no fluid, it may be advisable to make a small exploratory incision under local anesthesia to obtain fluid for diagnostic purposes or to rule out appendicitis. Operation for drainage itself is not indicated until the late stages when abscesses are formed. The character of the exudate in pneumococcus peritonitis varies, but is usually thick, fibrinous, mucoid, greenish in color and comparatively odorless. As soon as the diagnosis is made it is essential to institute therapy with sulfapyridine and antipneumococcus serum. Intestinal decompression with the nasal tube, administration of saline and glucose, etc., as described previously in this chapter, may be indicated. The disease runs a course extending over many weeks; most patients, if they survive the acute stage, will develop local abscesses which will necessitate drainage.

2. **Streptococcus Peritonitis.**—This type of peritonitis may occur as a postoperative complication; occasionally the streptococcus is the organism found in the pus produced by perforated appendicitis; however, it is more often encountered as an associated manifestation of respiratory diseases of some sort. Occasionally no evidence of the original focus of infection can be found. The term "idiopathic or primary peritonitis" is therefore commonly applied to this type of infection as it is also to pneumococcus peritonitis, but perhaps correctly so only to the cases in which the portal of entry is not discernible, and is presumably blood borne. Except on occasions when streptococcus peritonitis is secondary to appendicitis or operative contamination, it is usually encountered only in children or infants (especially the latter). Regardless of the etiologic factor, the disease is serious and associated with a high mortality. The manifestations are fulminating, and include practically all those encountered in peritonitis caused by the *Bacillus coli*. Because of the beneficial effect of sulfanilamide, it is extremely important just as in pneumococcus peritonitis, that the diagnosis be made, resorting to a small exploratory incision only when necessary to make the diagnosis. In addition to massive doses

of sulfanilamide, the various therapeutic measures including parenteral fluids, gastric lavage, etc., as described previously, should be instituted as indicated. The mortality rate in streptococcic peritonitis will be higher than in the pneumococcic type.

3. **Gonococcus Peritonitis.**—This disease is confined entirely to females and is secondary to infection in the fallopian tubes from which site the exudate containing the organisms (gonococci) breaks into the peritoneal cavity, but rarely ascends above the brim of the pelvis. There are always localizing signs in one or both of the adnexal regions, a manifestation which in itself should be sufficient to make a diagnosis, especially if a vaginal examination is made. Occasionally, however, if only the right fallopian tube is involved the disease may be confused with perforated appendicitis. The peritonitis usually remains local and the patient does not appear as ill as in appendiceal peritonitis, even though there may be high fever and excruciating tenderness in the lower abdomen. The pulse rate is not as rapid and the face does not have the pinched, tired and flushed appearance that it does in peritonitis caused by *Bacillus coli*. Fatalities are rare. Occasionally generalized abdominal rigidity, tenderness and distention may be present which, however, subside spontaneously with the pelvic inflammation. Sulfanilamide, sulfathiazole and fever therapy are the most effective types of therapy available. Operations should not be performed in the acute stage, but months after the infection, it may be necessary to remove the fallopian tubes. Pelvic abscesses frequently develop and require drainage (see also Chap. XXXI).

4. **Tuberculous Peritonitis.**—The invasion of the peritoneum by tuberculosis is usually secondary to local lesions in the lungs, mesenteric lymph nodes, cecum, appendix or fallopian tubes. Occasionally it is a manifestation of acute miliary disease. In many instances it appears that organisms swallowed in sputum invade the intestinal wall (*e.g.,* cecum) escape by way of the lymphatics to the mesenteric lymph nodes, and in this way give rise to a peritoneal infection.

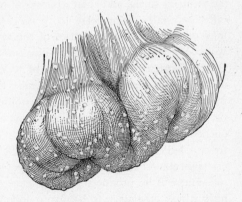

Pathologically, the peritoneal lesions are quite variable. On some occasions numerous tubercles (one-half to one millimeter in diameter) are scattered about the peritoneum which is reddened, but otherwise unaffected. On other occasions caseous masses are encountered and adhesions are present. Ascites is frequently noted, the fluid being clear and straw-

FIG. 450.—TUBERCLES UPON THE PERITONEUM.

(From Homans, *Textbook of Surgery*, 1935. Courtesy of Charles C. Thomas, Springfield, O.)

colored, turbid, or even thick and purulent. The fluid invariably has a high specific gravity (about 1.015). There is no definite relation of the type of lesion to the duration of the disease, except that the type associated with tubercles and mild ascites without adhesions is frequently encountered early in the disease, and the caseous masses with adhesions late in the disease.

The *clinical manifestations* are extremely variable both as to type and severity. Occasionally there is a rather acute onset with abdominal pain, nausea and vomiting. This type is frequently confused with appendicitis and at operation will reveal tubercles scattered diffusely over a slightly reddened peritoneum associated, perhaps, with a small amount of clear straw-colored fluid. However, usually the onset is insidious. Abdominal pain may or may not be complained of, but is rarely severe. Gradually the abdomen becomes distended because of the ascites. Anorexia and nausea, but rarely vomiting, are complained of. There is a gradual loss of weight and an associated anemia, weakness and malaise. Constipation or diarrhea may be present. Fever is extremely variable, but is usually moderately elevated in the afternoon and evening, receding to normal or subnormal by morning. The diagnosis is difficult and on most occasions is made only at operation. When found, exploration should be carried out for existence of an intraperitoneal primary source.

Treatment consists primarily of the hygienic principles advocated in tuberculous infections, but laparotomy does appear in many instances to have a mysterious curative effect regardless of whether or not a focus of the infection can be found and removed. For this reason alone, laparotomy appears justifiable in most cases, unless the presence of serious lesions elsewhere (*e.g.,* lungs) contraindicates operation. In any case diagnosis is thus made certain. However, patients with caseous areas and dense adhesions are rarely benefited by operation.

TRAUMA

Because of lawlessness, high speed automobiles and the mechanization of industry, injuries to the abdomen which lead to peritonitis are becoming important surgically, especially since delay in treatment or a mistaken diagnosis may result in a fatal outcome. Civilian injuries of the type mentioned will be discussed here. War wounds of the abdomen will be discussed in Chapter XXXIII.

1. **Rupture or Penetration of a Viscus.**—Accidents resulting in perforation of an intra-abdominal organ, especially the intestine and bladder, may be sustained in one of three ways. (*a*) A sharp object may penetrate the abdominal wall and perforate an intestine. Gunshot wounds of the abdomen are by far the most frequent example of this type of injury. Although the amount of bleeding resulting from a bullet wound of the abdomen is rarely sufficient to result in a fatal hemorrhage unless a major vessel is severed, in most instances a perforation of the intestine will be produced, which demands immediate repair because of the peritonitis which otherwise is bound to follow. (*b*) An intra-abdominal organ may be crushed and perforated, because of compression between two blunt objects, or between a blunt object and the spinal column. In such a case there may be no external evidence of an intra-abdominal injury or merely a slight contusion of the abdominal wall. (*c*) If a blow is sustained over the abdomen when the muscles are flaccid, there may be such a sudden and forceful expulsion of gas from one intestinal loop into another as to cause a rupture of the intestinal wall. Many instances of rupture of the colon have been reported in which workmen have jokingly released compressed air near the anus of a fellow workman. The collapse resulting from a rupture of this type is profound in spite of the fact that little hemorrhage is produced,

and most cases of this type are fatal, although operative therapy may be readily available and instituted.

The *clinical manifestations* of perforation or rupture of a hollow viscus, especially the intestine, are often overshadowed by the excitement of the occasion. How-

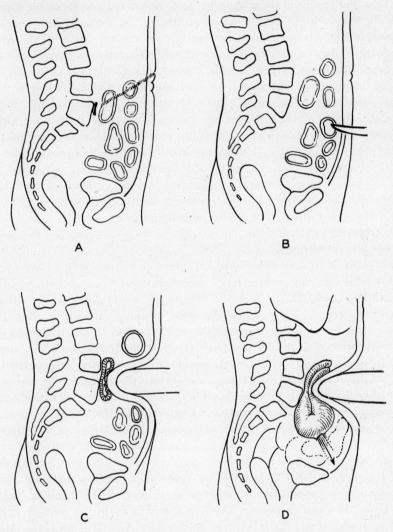

Fig. 451.—Common Mechanisms Producing Traumatic Intestinal Perforation.

A, gunshot wound; *B,* stab wound; *C,* laceration of the intestinal wall by compression against the vertebral column by a blunt object; *D,* rupture of the intestinal wall by sudden compression of gas within the lumen.

ever, severe pain is experienced immediately unless the patient is unconscious. A varying degree of shock including such manifestations as tachycardia, weakness, pallor, etc., will be produced, dependent largely upon the amount of hemorrhage accompanying the intestinal injury. Local signs may be minimal at first, *i.e.,* at a time when operation should be done. The most constant local signs are tenderness and muscle spasm which at first are confined to the injured area, but soon spread to the rest of the abdomen. Tenderness is rather constant at the outset but muscle rigidity may not be present for several hours. Nausea and vomiting will occur sooner or later, unless operative repair is instituted before vomiting takes place. An x-ray of the patient in the upright position may reveal gas under the diaphragm, a finding which is diagnostic of rupture of intestine or stomach. After a few hours the leukocyte count becomes elevated, but fever is not present until the peritoneal contamination takes on the features of peritonitis (eighteen to twenty-four hours). Of the signs mentioned above, muscle rigidity, if present to a significant degree, is one of the strongest indications for operative intervention, so long as one can eliminate voluntary spasm, rigidity due to injury of the abdominal wall itself, and reflex spasticity from skeletal fracture, especially of spine or ribs. It should be emphasized, however, that for several hours after perforation of a viscus, particularly gunshot wounds of the stomach and small intestine, there may be an almost complete absence of gastro-intestinal manifestation including vomiting, muscle spasm, etc.; frequently, they are overshadowed by the evidence of prostration or primary shock. For this reason, the clinical manifestations are not nearly as important in deciding the question of operation as is the location of the wound, which is then the chief factor leading to the decision as to whether or not the peritoneal cavity has been penetrated.

Perforation or rupture of the bladder, ureter or kidneys will present symptoms and signs similar to, but perhaps less severe than those mentioned above. Diagnosis can usually be made readily by examining the urine for gross blood. The inflammation of the peritoneum produced by urine escaping into the peritoneal cavity may be conducive to the development of peritonitis and this complication may be the most important factor in the cases terminating fatally, especially those not treated by operative repair. On rare occasions rupture of the base of the bladder or urethra may produce *extravasation of urine* into the subcutaneous tissues of the abdominal wall. This is a serious complication which may require expert judgment in its therapy; it is discussed in detail in Chapter XXXII.

The *treatment* of a ruptured viscus is, of course, surgical; it is well known that the earlier the operation is performed (assuming the patient's physical condition permits it) the more likely is it to be followed by success. Indeed, when a penetration of the peritoneal cavity is produced (gunshot or stab wound) laparotomy is performed without regard to the presence or absence of the manifestations mentioned above. If shock is present and is not due to injuries elsewhere it may be treated by transfusions, fluids, etc., while the operation is in progress. Any food or fecal material found free in the peritoneal cavity must be removed, and the wound in the intestine repaired. Exploration of the abdominal cavity must be thorough since *multiple injury to the intestine and other viscera is common,* regardless of the type of injury and its local manifestations. Treatment for shock, before, during and after operation is essential in all of these cases. It is rarely advisable to drain the peritoneal cavity. Occasionally, gunshot wounds of the abdomen are sustained without perforation of an intestine. The severity of the symptoms is much less pronounced in such instances, but the possibility of intestinal perforation is still so great that the surgeon deems it unsafe not to perform a laparotomy;

if the bullet has traversed any part of the peritoneal cavity in which a hollow viscus is normally present, an operation must be performed.

2. **Intraperitoneal Hemorrhage.**—In most instances intraperitoneal hemorrhage arises from rupture of an organ such as the liver or spleen, but in penetrating injuries, such as gunshot and stab wounds, any large vessel may be the source of the bleeding. Crushing injuries or direct blows sustained over the abdomen may produce a laceration of the capsule of the organ and the parenchymatous tissue as well.

The *clinical manifestations* of hemorrhage of the type described above may be identical to shock produced by any severe hemorrhage (see Chapter XIII). Pallor, tachycardia, weak and thready pulse, cold sweat and mental dullness are some of the important manifestations observed. If the hemorrhage takes place rapidly "air hunger" may also be present. In addition, there are usually at least a few of the symptoms and signs of peritoneal irritation. A diffuse tenderness is present which, as a rule, is no more pronounced over the organ injured than the rest of the abdomen. Muscle spasm is rarely as marked as it is when an intestine is perforated or ruptured. Likewise, nausea and vomiting are apt to be absent. Mild distention may develop and percussion may reveal a shifting dullness. If the abdominal findings are of such a trivial nature as to make the diagnosis of intra-abdominal injury appear unlikely, important information may be gained by hourly observation of the erythrocyte count, and hemoglobin determinations. If the hemorrhage is significant, within a few hours there will be a sufficient drop in the erythrocyte count and hemoglobin determination, to differentiate the condition from simple trauma and shock.

If the hemorrhage is of sufficient magnitude to produce symptoms of shock which are not improved in an hour or two by fluids, a transfusion, and other supportive measures, it is usually safe to assume that bleeding is still active. On such occasions immediate operation is usually indicated, treating the shock with constant transfusion during the operation. On many occasions the differentiation between hemorrhage and perforation of the intestine is so difficult that the latter possibility of itself will demand laparotomy. At operation any laceration of the liver or spleen should be repaired by suture. Occasionally if the spleen is badly lacerated it will be more feasible to remove it rather than repair it. If bleeding is severe and the condition of the patient precarious it will be necessary to begin a blood transfusion at the time when the operation is started, with the hope of preventing a serious collapse before the bleeding can be stopped.

3. **Retroperitoneal Hemorrhage.**—There are two common sources of hemorrhage of this type; namely, laceration of the kidney and fracture of, or severe injury to, the spine. Occasionally, injury to the soft tissues in the back may be sufficient to produce a retroperitoneal hemorrhage. The similarity of the symptoms produced by retroperitoneal hemorrhage and early peritonitis has been emphasized by one of us.[22] All of the manifestations of peritonitis including pain, muscle spasm, nausea, vomiting, leukocytosis, etc., may be produced by a hemorrhage of this type. It is difficult to explain the development of these symptoms in such an instance, but it seems apparent that the hematoma and the trauma located in this area may involve the nerves (sympathetic and somatic) which are important in the production of such symptoms. The surgeon may have ample evidence of damage to the

kidney or spine (*e.g.,* blood in the urine, x-ray of the spine showing fracture, etc.), but the symptoms may be so suggestive of intestinal injury that failure to perform an exploratory laparotomy is considered unsafe. However, in most instances

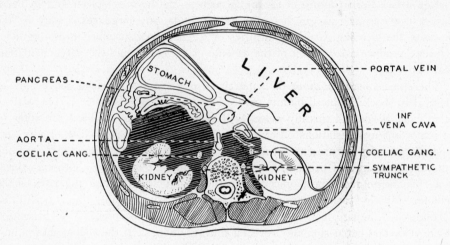

FIG. 452.—Two Common Sources of Retroperitoneal Hemorrhage.

On the left side is shown a blood clot arising from a lacerated kidney; on the right the hemorrhage is produced by a fracture involving the transverse process of the vertebra. In each case the clot infiltrates anteriorly. Note the close proximity of the blood clot to the numerous nerve trunks, ganglia and peritoneum of the posterior wall of the abdomen; this presumably accounts for the production of manifestations which are so similar to those produced by inflammation of the peritoneum.

differentiation can be made on the basis of severity and number of manifestations; in general, vomiting and tachycardia are less pronounced in retroperitoneal hemorrhage. Conservative therapy is obviously indicated in the absence of injury to a viscus or large vessel, thus avoiding the damaging effects of a laparotomy.

MISCELLANEOUS DISEASES ASSOCIATED WITH THE PERITONEUM

One of the most important of these is *malignant disease,* because it may occur in almost any organ within the abdomen and may involve the peritoneum secondarily. The invasion of the peritoneum by the tumor (*e.g.,* carcinoma) is noted as one or many tiny, irregular, hard nodules which become attached to the deeper tissue as they enlarge and likewise attach themselves to adjacent organs by malignant tissue or adhesions. The peritoneum may likewise become involved by extension of the tumor toward the periphery of the organ. Invasion of the peritoneum by extension or metastasis is accompanied by the development of free fluid which at first is clear, but rapidly becomes bloody. With a relatively few exceptions the presence of bloody fluid in the peritoneal cavity is quite pathognomonic of the presence of malignant disease involving the peritoneum.

Ascites.—This is encountered in many other conditions besides malignancy. It is associated, for example, with such diseases as myocardial insufficiency, nephritis and cirrhosis of the liver. In such instances, however, the fluid is practically always clear and being a transudate will have a low specific gravity. The presence of a large amount of ascitic fluid in the peritoneal cavity often produces a degree of distention which is occasionally differentiated with difficulty from the distention due to a tumor or even a slowly developing paralytic ileus. Ordinarily, however, palpation and percussion will reveal the true nature of the abdominal tumor. If the fluid is evacuated by a trocar (paracentesis abdominis) or by a laparotomy, much information may be gained by its physical characteristics. The most common lesions producing bloody ascites are carcinomatosis of the peritoneum, trauma, ruptured ectopic pregnancy, intestinal strangulation, volvulus, twisted pedicle of an ovarian cyst and acute pancreatic necrosis. In doubtful cases, a small incision under local anesthesia will not only evacuate and reveal the nature of the ascites, if present, but will also provide a view of the peritoneum and omentum; often a biopsy of diseased tissue can be obtained, thereby establishing the correct diagnosis. This cannot be achieved by simple aspiration, a procedure, moreover, which is apt to be damaging if distended bowel rather than ascites is the cause of the swelling.

Hernias.—With very few exceptions, hernias are associated with abnormalities of the peritoneum, are frequently secondary to congenital defects, and may be roughly divided into external and internal types (see Chapter XXVII).

Retroperitoneal Space.—Diseases and injuries of the retroperitoneal space are important because of the confusion with similar conditions in the peritoneal cavity. Most important is the kidney. Fortunately with the aid of pyelography (intravenous or cystoscopic) the kidney can be identified quite readily as the cause of disease. Occasionally serious tumors (lymphosarcoma) arise in the retroperitoneal lymph nodes. By the time they are discovered they are rarely operable. Benign tumors such as lipomas have been reported. Retroperitoneal abscesses may develop (from the kidney, spine and lymph nodes) and may present laterally or in the neighborhood of the inguinal ligament.

Diseases of the Mesentery.—No doubt the most common lesion affecting the mesentery is *lymphadenitis* of the nodes within the mesentery. These may obviously be pyogenic (as described on p. 681) or tuberculous. In either case, suppuration may take place and lead to peritonitis, adhesions, etc. Rarely, however, is there strangulation of the blood vessels. *Cysts* of the mesentery are encountered occasionally. They are located near the junction of the mesentery and intestine, and are frequently so intimately connected with the wall of the intestine that removal can be achieved only by resection of a segment of intestine. Occasionally, they compress the intestine so much that a partial obstruction is produced. When the cyst is so large and extends so far posteriorly that excision is not possible without injury to large vessels, marsupialization should be performed. *Cavernous lymphangiomas* have been encountered in the mesentery but are extremely rare. *Sarcomas* are likewise very rare, and will be operable only when encountered at an early stage.

Diseases of the Omentum.—Perhaps the most common lesion of the omentum is inflammation. Naturally, it may be affected secondarily when surrounding an inflamed appendix or other source of infection. Resolution without abscess formation in the omentum itself usually takes place. Occasionally, inflammatory masses develop in the omentum without an obvious primary lesion; they may produce abdominal pain, tenderness, nausea, leukocytosis and other symptoms of sufficient magnitude to lead the surgeon to a laparotomy. Resection is performed readily and relieves the condition. *Torsion of the omentum* is occasionally encountered as a complication of a hernia when the omentum is adherent to certain portions of the sac. More rarely it will be found within the peritoneal cavity, not associated with a hernia. In either case abdominal pain and other mild symptoms may lead to laparotomy. Resection of the portion of omentum involved is indicated. *Tumors* of the omentum may be cystic or solid; each group is rare. Of the solid tumors sarcomas (fibrosarcoma or lymphosarcoma) is most common. The only significant manifestation except in the terminal stage may be the presence of a mass. Resection may be possible. *Cysts* of the omentum, usually lymphatic in origin are encountered, but likewise are rare. Excision is simple and curative.

Chylous Ascites.—Although chylous ascites is somewhat uncommon, it may develop from numerous causes. Perhaps the most common is obstruction of the thoracic duct or upper portion of the cisterna chyli by tuberculous nodes, carcinoma, etc., thus giving rise to so much pressure in the cisterna chyli that rupture of the duct, or exudation of chyle takes place. Trauma, particularly of a penetrating type, may actually sever the cisterna chyli. Abdominal distention develops early. However, the condition is rarely diagnosed preoperatively; it is discovered at operation by the finding of milky fluid in the peritoneal cavity. If the condition is not relieved by development of collateral vessels, serious consequences including hypoproteinemia, malnutrition, etc., may develop. Treatment is not entirely satisfactory. Intravenous amino acids in addition to the oral food intake will be helpful.

Intra-abdominal Apoplexy.—Spontaneous hemorrhage from vessels in the peritoneal cavity is a rather uncommon emergency, resulting in typical manifestations of hemorrhage. It occurs most commonly in men in the latter decades of life; a great many of the patients will have hypertension or significant arteriosclerosis. Mild abdominal pain is complained of. Very little muscle spasm or abdominal tenderness will be found, but when the hemorrhage has occurred into the retroperitoneal space or mesentery, a hematoma may be palpable. Operation may be indicated because of the serious effects of the hemorrhage, but a correct preoperative diagnosis will rarely be made.

BIBLIOGRAPHY

1. HERTZLER, A. E. *Surgical Pathology of the Peritoneum*, J. B. Lippincott Co., Philadelphia, 1935.
2. COLLER, F. A., and BRINKMAN, H. Studies on the Reaction of the Peritoneum to Trauma and Infection, *Ann. Surg.*, 109:942, 1939.
3. JACKSON, H. C., and COLLER, F. A. The Use of Sulfanilamide in the Peritoneum, *J. Am. M. Ass.*, 118:195, 1942.
4. STERNBERG, B. A. A Rapid Method of Protecting the Peritoneum against Peritonitis, *Arch. Surg.*, 24:308, 1932; The Experimental Background and the Clinical Application of the Escherichia Coli Gum Tragacanth Mixture in Prevention of Peritonitis, *Am. J. Clin. Path.*, 6:253, 1936.
5. Ross, J. On the Segmental Distribution of Sensory Disorders, Brain, 10:350, 1888.
6. MACKENZIE, James. *Symptoms and Their Interpretation*, 4th ed., Shaw and Sons, London, 1920.

7. MITCHELL, G. A. G.   The Spread of Acute Intraperitoneal Effusions, *Brit. J. Surg.*, 28:291, 1940.

8. SHAMBAUGH, Philip.   Peritonitis as a Factor in the Mortality of Gastro-intestinal Surgery, Ann. Surg., 104:382, 1936.

9. YATES, J. L.   An Experimental Study of the Local Effects of Peritoneal Drainage, *Surg., Gynec. & Obst.*, 1:473, 1905.

10. WINSLOW, S. B.   Dextrose Utilization in Surgical Patients, *Surgery*, 4:867, 1938.

11. PUESTOW, C. B.   The Activity of Isolated Intestinal Segments, *Arch. Surg.*, 24:565, 1932; Intestinal Motility of the Dog and Man, *Univ. of Ill. Press*, 1940.

12. ORR, T. G.   The Action of Morphine on the Small Intestine and Its Clinical Application in the Treatment of Peritonitis and Intestinal Obstruction, *Ann. Surg.*, 98:835, 1933; Treatment of Peritonitis, *J. Am. M. Ass.*, 113:1489, 1939.

13. POTTER, P. C.   Acute Diffuse Peritonitis Following Acute Appendicitis with Report of Twenty-five Cases, *Surg. Clin. No. Amer.*, 14:479, 1934.

14. BROWN, H. P.   Peristalsis and Peritonitis, *Ann. Surg.*, 100:167, 1934.

15. BISGARD, J. D., and NYE, D.   The Influence of Hot and Cold Application upon Gastric and Intestinal Motor Activity, *Surg., Gynec. & Obst.*, 71:172, 1940.

16. FINE, J., HERMANSON, L., and FREHLING, S.   Further Clinical Experiences with 95 Per Cent Oxygen for Absorption of Air from Body Tissues, *Ann. Surg.*, 107:1, 1938.

17. RAVDIN, I. S., RHOADS, J. E., and LOCKWOOD, J. S.   The Use of Sulfanilamide in the Treatment of Peritonitis Associated with Appendicitis, *Ann. Surg.*, 111:53, 1940.

18. THOMPSON, J. E., BRABSON, J. A., and WALKER, J. M.   The Intra-Abdominal Application of Sulfanilamide in Acute Appendicitis, *Surg., Gynec. & Obst.*, 72:722, 1941.

19. POTH, D. O., and KNOTTS, F. L.   Clinical Use of Succinyl-sulfathiazole, *Arch. Surg.*, 44:208, 1942.

20. OCHSNER, Alton, and GRAVES, A. M.   Subphrenic Abscess, *Ann. Surg.*, 98:961, 1933; OCHSNER, Alton, and DeBAKEY, M.   Subphrenic Abscess, *Surg., Gynec. & Obst.* (Internat. Abst. Surg.), 66:426, 1938.

21. LADD, W. E., and BOTSFORD, T. W., and CURNEN, E. C.   Primary Peritonitis in Infants and Children, *J. Am. M. Ass.*, 113:1455, 1939.

22. COLE, W. H.   Retroperitoneal Hemorrhage Simulating Acute Peritonitis, *J. Am. M. Ass.*, 96:1472, 1931.

23. HOCHBERG, L. A.   Diagnostic Criteria for Subphrenic Abscess Based Upon a Study of 139 Cases, *Ann. Int. Med.*, 17:183, 1942.

CHAPTER XXVI

INTESTINAL OBSTRUCTION

Specific Lesions Producing Intestinal Obstruction

Intestinal obstruction is a serious surgical condition. While it produces an interruption to the passage of intestinal contents, the lethal symptoms and rapid death which sometimes occur are due to the secondary changes resulting from the obstruction. Before discussing specific lesions which produce intestinal obstruction or these secondary changes, definitions and terminology ought to be clarified and classifications presented.

DEFINITIONS.—*Ileus,* a commonly used term, is an old designation generally applied to intestinal obstruction of all types; it is somewhat loosely used in this country, at least, to define a remarkable condition which is seen in patients without actual organic obstruction but in which the intestinal content becomes stagnant just as if the lumen were occluded. Because this condition is due to a decrease of intestinal activity by one of several causes it is called paralytic or adynamic ileus. It will be described in more detail later. The term functional obstruction is also used to define ileus, to indicate the absence of an organic lesion producing obstruction. In contrast to functional obstruction are actual organic lesions producing intestinal obstruction comprising a great variety of conditions. Without defining them all, two general terms are often used which will form the basis for a classification as noted below. These two general groups are, first, *simple mechanical obstruction* in which only the lumen of the intestine is primarily occluded, and second, the group called *intestinal strangulation* in which there is primarily an occlusion of the mesenteric blood supply. Although bands and adhesions may produce either type, in many the causative lesion is characteristic. Such terms as mesenteric thrombosis, intussusception, volvulus, etc., are defined and described in detail later in the chapter.

High obstruction and *low obstruction* may be defined as indicating, as a rule, obstruction at high and low levels in the gastro-intestinal tract; these terms are relative, however, and are sometimes loosely used to indicate the rapidity of onset of symptoms, *i.e.,* obstruction at the high levels as the duodenum and pylorus is apt to be more acute than the more slowly developing onset in obstruction at a lower level. Low intestinal obstruction is considered by many to be limited to the large bowel; when this is meant it is best designated as *large bowel obstruction* as contrasted to *small bowel obstruction*. *Acute* (in contrast to *chronic*) intestinal obstruction is of much more importance surgically and most of the chapter will therefore be devoted to it. Acute intestinal obstruction is produced by a sudden cessation of the passage of intestinal contents whereas chronic obstruction results from partial or intermittent occlusions.

CLASSIFICATION.—In attempting to classify the various types of intestinal obstruction, difficulties are encountered as might be inferred from the many terms defined; actually it may be impossible to find clearly defined types because a combination of elements are often present in an individual case. Nevertheless, it is of considerable value to classify all cases of acute intestinal obstruction into the three types mentioned above because they really represent distinctive anatomic features, at least in the beginning of the disease. Of the following three types the first two are organic, the last functional: (1) mechanical obstruction to the lumen, (2) obstruction to the blood supply (intestinal strangulation), (3) paralytic ileus.

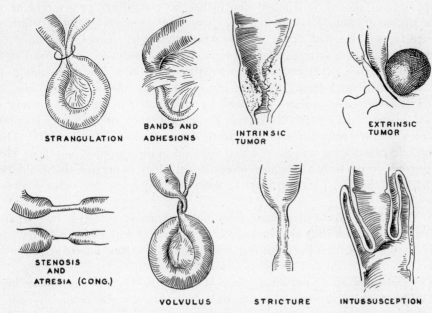

STRANGULATION   BANDS AND ADHESIONS   INTRINSIC TUMOR   EXTRINSIC TUMOR

STENOSIS AND ATRESIA (CONG.)   VOLVULUS   STRICTURE   INTUSSUSCEPTION

FIG. 453.—EIGHT COMMON CAUSES OF INTESTINAL OBSTRUCTION.

Note the various mechanisms producing occlusion of the lumen as well as blood supply. Though not indicated strangulation includes volvulus and intussusception; bands and adhesions may also produce strangulation.

The defects in this classification lie in the variability of response to the obstructive agent, in the presence of more than one factor in an individual case, and in that it does not indicate the sequence of events occurring after the onset of the obstruction. For example, the status of the intestine and mesentery is most important, and when it can be determined the condition may be more clearly defined in terms of local changes of which the most significant are the patency of the lumen of the bowel, the activity of the musculature and the integrity of the blood supply.

On an *etiologic* basis the various types of obstructing agents vary widely; a few are represented in Figure 453. Of those producing mechanical obstruction to the lumen (proceeding from above downward) are esophageal stricture and cancer, gastric carcinoma, pyloric stenosis, small intestinal bands, adhesions, enteroliths, large bowel cancer, adhesions and fecal impaction. Extrinsic agents such as tumors or abscesses may occlude the lumen at any level; the same is true of strictures of various kinds. In the group producing primarily an occlusion of the blood supply (intestinal strangulation) are such lesions as strangulation in hernias, intussusception, volvulus, mesenteric thrombosis, etc. The third group or paralytic ileus occurs in mild form after laparotomy and in a severe form in general peritonitis; it may also occur, presumably as a reflex phenomenon, after injury to the spine, after extensive skeletal trauma or in the course of certain serious extra-abdominal diseases.

INCIDENCE.—According to the statistical studies of McIver,[1] the most frequent organic cause of acute intestinal obstruction (exclusive of obstruction at the pylorus or above), is strangulation in hernias comprising 44 per cent of 335 cases studied by him. Next in frequency were postoperative adhesions which accounted for an additional 24 per cent, to which should be added 6 per cent due to other bands presumably congenital in origin. Neoplasms caused 10 per cent of the total, and intussusception and volvulus together 9 per cent. The remaining 7 per cent were distributed among the rare causes such as gallstones, enteroliths, etc.

PATHOLOGY.—The changes produced by intestinal obstruction, as already indicated, are secondary to the obstructing agent itself; they are the really important factors which are responsible for the acute symptoms and lethal outcome. These changes may be divided into those which are local in the intestines and those which are systemic in the body as a whole. Only the pathology of organic obstruction will be described herein; paralytic ileus is described separately for reasons already mentioned.

1. The *local effects* of organic intestinal obstruction comprise two separate mechanisms although both are often involved in varying degrees in any given case, as will be apparent from the following description. These local effects are occlusion of the intestinal lumen and occlusion of the blood supply.

(a) *Occlusion of the intestinal lumen* is one of the first effects of acute intestinal obstruction whatever the cause may be. Although the occlusion may be partial at first, it soon becomes complete because of local changes brought about by the vigorous attempts on the part of the bowel to force intestinal contents past the barrier. Wave after wave of peristalsis (accentuated by the ingestion of food and especially of cathartics) beat against the narrowed lumen and succeed perhaps in forcing contents through for a time. Soon, however, the bowel above dilates and bacteria multiply in the stagnant contents. The bowel wall becomes edematous which may make the partial obstruction complete or the weight of the fluid above the obstruction may kink the bowel, completely obliterating the lumen.

What happens from this point on depends on individual variations. In general, the accumulated obstructed bowel contents are increased in volume by swallowed air, intestinal secretions and the results of bacterial multiplication. The increased intra-intestinal pressure thus produced distends the bowel more and more. In certain cases this leads to regurgitation, the bowel emptying rapidly into the stomach, the contents then being vomited; the more this occurs the less the bowel dilates. On the other hand, if the distention is unrelieved and becomes great enough, the blood flow through the bowel becomes occluded and loss of viability and even necrosis, first of the mucous membrane and then of the entire wall, may occur. This necrosis produces many of the so-called toxic effects of intestinal strangulation, which is described next, and thus explains how, even in simple mechanical obstruction of the lumen, the local effects in neglected cases may be the same as those produced by strangulation.

(b) *Occlusion of the blood vessels,* often called *intestinal strangulation* occurs frequently in intestinal obstruction, developing quite rapidly in such lesions as intussusception, volvulus and obstructed inguinal hernia. Although such conditions are good examples of strangulation it should be emphasized that in all of them closure of the intestinal lumen is practically always present at the very outset and, indeed may precede by several hours occlusion of the blood supply. Conversely, as just described, simple occlusion of the intestinal lumen, if neglected and accompanied by severe distention, will impair blood supply and thereby produce the same effects as strangulation.

In complete strangulation of more than a few hours' duration, tissue injury develops rapidly and is soon followed by necrosis and gangrene. Since the bowel lumen contains many and virulent bacteria, infection rapidly sets in and the strangulated intestine then acts as any area of gangrene accompanied by a severe infection. Absorption of toxic material thus produced is most rapid when the gangrenous tissue is free in the peritoneal cavity as in a case of complete volvulus. Rarely is direct absorption prevented by walling off by the omentum; in strangulation by hernia the sac is usually so tight as to constitute an effective walling off of this sort. The gangrenous process may be so acute and rapid that the associated occlusion of the lumen, though nearly always present, is completely overshadowed by the effects of the strangulation.

2. The *systemic effects* of intestinal obstruction are, like the local effects, produced by two separate mechanisms which are frequently so closely associated as to be clinically indistinguishable. Their pathogenesis is so different, however, that they will be discussed separately; these two changes are dehydration from loss of water and electrolyte, and toxemia from absorption of infectious and other material in the strangulated bowel.

It should be emphasized that distention in itself produces many of the systemic effects regardless of the cause. Distention results not only from occlusion of the intestinal lumen, but also from inability of the musculature adequately to contract as well as other nervous and vascular factors. This is important because numerous workers have conclusively shown that animals or patients with completely occluded intestines may show no systemic effects if distention is prevented (in the absence of strangulation or high obstruction).

(a) *Dehydration* from loss of water and electrolyte is fairly well known and follows any extensive loss of gastro-intestinal secretions unless the loss is replaced.

Vomiting is a common cause for such loss and occurs frequently in intestinal obstruction and is nearly always associated with distention. Indeed, distention may result in vomiting from reflex action whether the lumen is occluded or not; this has been experimentally demonstrated by the abolition of vomiting through section of the nerves to the involved segment of bowel. The loss of water and electrolyte in the obstructed contents is, of course, increased by the excessive amount of secretions poured into the distended intestines. It should be emphasized, moreover, that dehydration follows such a loss of fluid into the distended bowel whether it is vomited or not; to this extent, therefore, the actual amount of vomitus may not give a clear indication of the total amount lost.

The systemic effects of dehydration are usually quite evident clinically. The severely dehydrated patient lies quietly, is prostrated, may be comatose, as if he were in shock. The skin everywhere is dry and inelastic, the mouth parched, the tongue coated and furred, the lips dark red in color. Examination of the blood will reveal a concentration of red cells which (if the count was normal before) may reach a value of 6 or 7 million per cubic millimeter; obviously such a finding should not be confused with a blood dyscrasia such as polycythemia. Blood chemical study will also reveal pronounced changes, e.g., loss of chloride (hypochloremia or dechlorination), alkalosis or acidosis, high nonprotein-nitrogen and urea, elevation of fibrinogen.

Dehydration, in general, is more common in high obstruction because loss of fluid by vomiting is so much more pronounced and persistent when the occluding lesion is at the pylorus. Indeed, unless an associated strangulation is also present, the changes due to dehydration account for most if not all of the systemic manifestations in patients with high intestinal obstruction. Most important is the fact that the blood and body tissues can be brought back to normal and the symptoms thereof relieved by parenteral administration of adequate amounts of fluids containing salts in isotonic concentration; such a solution is all that is needed to replace the elements lost in the vomitus. In other words, dehydration from loss of gastro-intestinal secretions can be rapidly and effectively cured (see p. 150).

(b) *Toxemia,* so-called, is the second systemic effect often seen in intestinal obstruction. Although always associated with impairment of the blood supply to the bowel wall, the pathogenesis in strangulation is not nearly so clear as that in dehydration nor is the treatment thereof so simple and direct. All that can be said is that the toxic symptoms are ascribed to the absorption of infectious material from the damaged bowel into the general circulation. It is known, of course, that absorption from any necrotic infected tissue tends to produce severe systemic reactions, and it is probable that absorption from strangulated intestine is no exception.

The toxic effects in strangulation vary considerably, dependent, no doubt, upon the extent and rapidity of the absorption. Clinical difficulty arises because of these variations. For example, the systemic effects may not be very clear-cut when absorption from the nonviable intestine is gradual; indeed in such cases the manifestations may often be scarcely differentiated from those due to dehydration. Much more definite are the systemic effects which follow *sudden* vascular occlusion such as occurs in volvulus, as will be described later. Such patients are severely prostrated, with a subnormal temperature, fast pulse and low blood pressure. Although there is in such cases both occlusion of the lumen of the gut as well as of the blood supply, the latter occurs so suddenly that the symptoms of shock are produced before dehydration from persistent vomiting and distention have had time to develop.

These considerations explain, in part, the difficulties which may occur in any individual case, *i.e.,* the systemic effects in severe intestinal obstruction varies with the local lesions. Besides variations in the degree and rapidity of toxic absorption there are the effects of dehydration, all of which add to the complexity of the pathogenesis. Nevertheless with the main outlines in mind it is remarkable how often the systemic effects can be evaluated in terms of pathology.

The *pathology of paralytic (adynamic) ileus,* as already mentioned, differs from organic obstruction in that the mechanism is a functional one. Although dehydration may occur in a similar way, toxicity depends on other factors, not connected with the bowel wall itself, which in spite of distention usually maintains

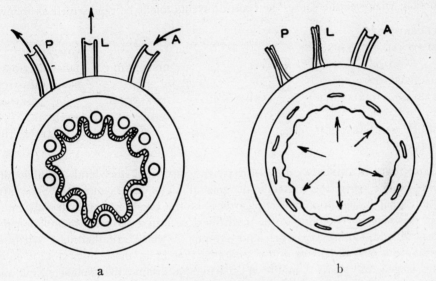

Fig. 454.—Diagrammatic Cross-section of Small Intestine.

a, under normal conditions; *b,* under the influence of increased intraluminary pressure produced by a simple mechanical obstruction. Note that the vessels in the submucosa are flattened by the pressure and that the flow into the portal vein (*P*) and the lymphatic vessels (*L*) are therefore interrupted. Arterial flow (*a*) is unimpeded. Because of the pressure the mucosa has been destroyed and is not represented. Absorption into the circulation from such a loop can only take place through the serosal surface, unless the intraluminary pressure falls sufficiently to permit a return of blood and lymphatic flow.

a fairly good blood supply in absence of complicating lesions. The four general conditions which nearly always precede paralytic ileus are: (1) Trauma inflicted during abdominal operations, *i.e.,* postoperative ileus, (2) General peritonitis during which the bowel is immobilized, presumably to put it at rest, (3) Skeletal, injury especially to ribs and spine, and retroperitoneal trauma which produce a reflex paralysis, (4) Extra-peritoneal infections or toxemia, *e.g.,* pneumonia, nephritis.

In paralytic ileus the fundamental derangement is the failure in propulsive peristalsis, undoubtedly due to interference with the nervous mechanism initiating and maintaining peristalsis or to a reduction in the capacity of the intestinal musculature to contract adequately. Another factor may be an interference in the blood supply following which the affected bowel becomes similarly paralyzed. Regardless of the mechanism, the reduction in effective peristalsis produces the same result, *i.e.*, stasis of intestinal content with distention and loss of fluid and electrolyte which is just as pronounced as if there were an actual mechanical barrier in the lumen arresting the passage of bowel contents. Once such stasis has supervened, distention ensues with its train of disturbances and blood chemical changes. The effects of distention in intestinal stasis due to peristaltic failure are just as severe as the distention from stasis produced from actual occlusion of the intestinal lumen.

If one were to summarize the gradually developing changes in intestinal obstruction, whatever the cause, the train of events might be represented as follows:

| OCCLUSION OF INTESTINAL LUMEN AND/OR EMBARRASSMENT OF INTESTINAL CIRCULATION AND/OR FAILURE OF INTESTINAL PERISTALSIS | → | STASIS OF INTESTINAL CONTENT | → | DISTENTION OF INTESTINAL LUMEN | → | VOMITING DEHYDRATION BLOOD CHEMICAL CHANGES TOXIC ABSORPTION |

CLINICAL MANIFESTATIONS.—First are considered the local or abdominal manifestations, then the systemic or general signs and symptoms. Soon after the intestinal lumen is occluded, regardless of the cause, four primary abdominal symptoms may develop, due to the mechanical occlusion *per se*. Strangulation produces, in addition, severe signs and symptoms which are described separately later. *Severe intermittent pain of a cramping type* is the most important; it occurs early, is generally located in the epigastrium or around the umbilicus, but may disappear as distention develops. There may be freedom of pain between attacks. Cramps may be especially aggravated by the ingestion of food or cathartics. Obvious *distention* appears in a day or two and increases gradually. Distention is more prominent the lower the obstruction. The abdomen is tympanitic due to the presence of considerable gas (tympanites). Distention must be distinguished from ascites which produces shifting dullness, from a mass which reveals itself by careful palpation, and from a distended bladder which disappears after catheterization. Occasionally the distended loops can be outlined as an intestinal pattern through the abdominal wall of thin individuals. On the other hand, it is often remarkable how much actual distention of the intestines may be present without much external evidence thereof, particularly in robust hyperesthetic individuals with thick abdominal muscles and in the obese. *Vomiting* is more common in high than in low obstruction. An early symptom, it is intermittent, usually follows eating or drinking and is practically or nearly *always preceded by pain*. The amount of vomiting varies greatly, and is usually inversely proportional to the degree of distention. Foul-smelling vomitus is apt to be observed when vomiting becomes persistent; fecal vomitus obviously originates from the lower ileum, thus pointing to an obstruction below this point. *Absence of bowel movements* while common in intestinal obstruction, is not necessarily pathognomonic thereof since it is possible to have bowel movements from retained feces below the obstruction or from a small amount of fecal material which has passed through a barrier not completely occluding the lumen. Another important sign is *visible peristalsis* which is especially observable in patients with thin abdominal walls, the waves being coincident with the cramping pain and with audible sounds apparent on auscultation. In infants with hypertrophic pyloric stenosis peristaltic waves crossing from left to right can often be seen in the upper abdomen. *Palpation* is usually negative unless a large tumor is causing the obstruction. In strangulation a tender mass or localized tenderness may be present. Incarcerated hernias can be felt except that a small part of the intestine may be strangulated in the femoral or inguinal ring without being apparent externally. Internal herniations are likewise not palpable externally but occur only rarely. Abdominal tenderness is, in general, absent except for localized tenderness over strangulated bowel; there may be diffuse tenderness in the paralytic ileus of general peritonitis.

X-ray of the abdomen is of considerable importance in the diagnosis of intestinal obstruction. A supine film may reveal the position and contour of dilated loops of bowel. In this way it is usually possible to distinguish large bowel from small as well as by the characteristic herringbone or "accordion" pattern seen in dilated small bowel due to the valvulae conniventi. An upright film may reveal the so-called "step ladder" effect or multiple fluid levels. Positive x-ray findings may be seen quite early in small bowel obstruction. When there is an associated strangulation the gas shadows may not be so easily found early; frequently the appearance of a small pocket of trapped gas suggests closed loop obstruction associated with volvulus and indicates the position of the obstructed loop. A barium enema is of considerable value in that it may reveal the site of or exclude obstruction of the large bowel. In high obstruction barium by mouth may be advisable in order to reveal the mechanism or completeness of the occlusion, especially when it develops soon after a gastro-enterostomy. However, barium should *never be given by mouth* in any case where its removal is not assured, because of the danger of increasing the obstruction.

The *systemic manifestations* in intestinal obstruction have been already discussed in part, under pathology (p. 758). In simple mechanical occlusion of two or three days' duration such symptoms may be surprisingly absent. If vomiting is profuse the picture of dehydration gradually develops as described on page 758. Occasionally systemic effects may be absent even though the distended bowel has developed necrosis. This is due to the fact that absorption from the nonviable tissue is prevented by the poor blood flow accompanying the distention. In such a situation general symptoms and signs of a profound infection (fast bounding pulse, restlessness and high fever) may rapidly follow *sudden release of distention*. This remarkable occurrence is explained (see Fig. 454) by the absorption of toxic material suddenly accelerated by the resumption of blood flow in the bowel wall due to the fall of intra-intestinal pressure. Another, somewhat different, example of this mechanism is the occasional fall of blood pressure and tachycardia which is seen during operation when the neck of the sac in a strangulated hernia is cut, the return of venous flow permitting the absorption of toxic materials from the damaged loop of bowel.

Strangulation gives rise to much more severe local as well as systemic manifestations than does a simple occlusion. Fortunately, it develops in a relatively small percentage of cases of simple occlusion; it is observed most commonly in hernias, volvulus and intussusception. When it develops the patient becomes more prostrated, the pulse is rapid, the temperature subnormal, and evidence of circulatory shock is shown by a low blood pressure, cold extremities and pale cyanotic skin. Pain becomes more severe, and is more constant. Local tenderness is increased, usually over the site of strangulation. A mass frequently becomes palpable. A variable amount of muscle spasm develops. Extremely important (particularly during nonoperative treatment), is the fact that damage to the bowel wall may

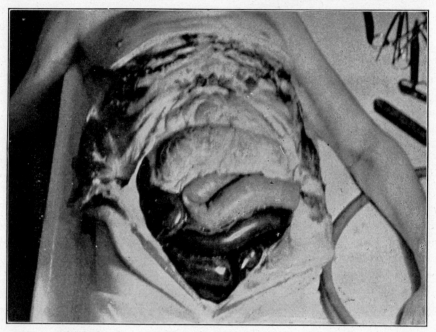

FIG. 455.—STRANGULATED, GANGRENOUS SMALL INTESTINE DUE TO AN EXTENSIVE VOLVULUS.

The lesion developed as a terminal manifestation in a patient with an extensive carcinoma of the lung. Nausea was present but no vomiting; severe prostration and circulatory failure developed shortly after the onset of abdominal pain. The photograph was made at the time of autopsy; note the striking difference in color between the normal viable gut, and the gut which is strangulated.

develop *at any time* during the course of the disease; indeed, occlusion of the lumen and of the blood supply may develop simultaneously. When these "toxic" symptoms develop in simple mechanical occlusion the cause, as already described, is probably the same as that occurring in cases of primary strangulation, *i.e.,* necrosis in the obstructed bowel wall produced in this case by the distention itself.

The clinical manifestations of *paralytic ileus* are confined in the main to distention, vomiting and absence of bowel movements. Pain is frequently absent except in general peritonitis and postoperative ileus. In the latter case the symptoms are usually transient and described as gas pains. It is important to emphasize that if pain is persistent or develops many days (a week or more) after operation, organic obstruction should be suspected. Tenderness is diffuse and more marked if peritonitis is present and is accompanied by muscle rigidity. Treatment of postoperative and posttraumatic ileus has been discussed in the section on post-operative care (see p. 167).

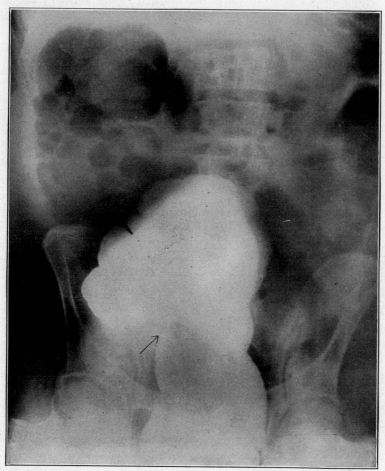

FIG. 456.—ACUTE INTESTINAL OBSTRUCTION: CARCINOMA AT THE MIDSIGMOID.

The patient, a fifty-six-year-old farmer, experienced gradually increasing lower abdominal pain and constipation for five weeks culminating in two days of vomiting and abdominal distension. A barium enema reached the midsigmoid but went no further; the exact point of obstruction (at the arrow) was seen under the fluoroscope in an oblique view, though not very evident in the film, a print of which is shown above. Note the dilated colon. At operation an annular constriction was found at the point of obstruction; the lesion was exteriorized and removed according to the Mikulicz technic. It proved to be adenocarcinoma. After closure of the double-barrelled colostomy the patient enjoyed normal health and bowel function with no evidence of recurrence (three years).

Laboratory study of the blood chemistry in any type of intestinal obstruction will show changes indicative of dehydration, but only when much fluid has been lost by vomiting or inadequate intake. The urine will also be concentrated and scanty, and is a fairly reliable clinical indication of the severity of the dehydration. The leukocyte count may be of differential value for it is usually normal in simple mechanical occlusion, whereas it may be elevated in the presence of strangulation even early in the process. A fall in plasma volume, due to loss of plasma into the affected bowel has been observed in distention from intestinal obstruction by Fine.[2] Such an effect can also be detected and in fact followed by observing progressive increases in the red cell count (hemoconcentration), and diminutions in the concentration of serum protein (hypoproteinemia).

Differential Diagnosis.—The list of acute abdominal diseases which simulate each other have been discussed previously (pp. 733 to 737); nearly all of them are considered in the differential diagnosis of acute intestinal obstruction. As indicated above, however, the surgeon must not only determine if intestinal obstruction is present but also must distinguish between functional and mechanical obstruction and particularly whether or not the intestine is strangulated.

Of especial importance in the diagnosis of intestinal obstruction is the identification of the cause. The demonstration of an incarcerated hernia, an abdominal scar from a previous operation, or an abdominal mass is obviously important. The causes of paralytic ileus are usually obvious and nearly always permit the surgeon to make such a diagnosis or exclude it as a possible cause of the clinical manifestations. *Cramping* intermittent pain followed by vomitus containing intestinal contents is especially significant. The x-ray is useful. Of greatest importance in diagnosis is the prompt detection of strangulation which demands immediate laparotomy.

Treatment of Acute Intestinal Obstruction.—Obviously, treatment in intestinal obstruction depends on the type of disease present. The question of operation is of immediate importance. To answer this question, the surgeon must first of all determine whether the clinical manifestations are due to functional or to organic obstruction, and if the lesion is organic, whether strangulation is present or not. Functional obstruction (paralytic ileus) is usually apparent from the history in most instances; treatment is in general conservative. Strangulation may be diagnosed, in most instances, on the general appearance of the patient, and the presence of a cause; treatment is, in general, immediate operation. Between these two extremes are the patients with simple mechanical obstruction. In the following description of treatment this type of disease will, in general, be considered. The discussion may be divided into prophylactic, nonoperative and operative treatment. An excellent summary of the various therapeutic considerations in acute obstruction of the small bowel is that of Crowley and Johnston.[3]

1. *Prophylaxis.*—Preventive measures concern both the surgeon and the general practitioner. For the surgeon, gentle and careful operative technic is essential to minimize the tendency toward postoperative adhesions and their resultant production of intestinal obstruction. A large percentage of cases follow gynecologic pelvic procedures; operations for perforated appendicitis are also prone to be followed by intestinal obstruction because of the excessive formation of adhesions due to the infection.

For the general practitioner two admonitions may be made, one concerning the administration of cathartics, and the other concerning the use of morphine in patients having intestinal obstruction. Nature often protects the patient when a cathartic is given because usually the medicine is promptly vomited. If it is retained it whips up a bowel already working hard to force contents through the small opening and, by increasing peristalsis and distention, aggravates the edema which finally makes the obstruction complete. The tendency of physicians to prescribe a cathartic over the telephone except when the diagnosis is known, is certainly a reprehensible one. Unfortunately it is most often the corner drug store attendant who is guilty of such well meaning, but potentially dangerous advice. The hypodermic of morphine does harm more certainly and insidiously when given merely to relieve pain. To be sure, it is occasionally useful early in strangulated hernia (*i.e.*, within the first hour or two), because the relaxation induced may allow reduction of the hernia, especially in children; but the patient must be in the hospital and ready for immediate operation if reduction is not effected. The usual circumstance under which it does so much harm is its use in the home, often after insufficient examination and certainly after incorrect diagnosis. The danger lies in the fact that the pathologic changes leading to necrosis of the intestinal epithelium go on under its apparent beneficent influence. The cramping pain is nature's warning call; the hypodermic stills this call effectively; the patient drops off to sleep and the family is grateful for the seeming miraculous therapeutic result. But after a short time the patient's pain returns, less severe now, less insistent, but still calling for relief. Distention now becomes more marked, dependent somewhat on the amount of fluid ingested and the amount vomited. By now the intestinal barrier of mucosa has perhaps been destroyed, thereby leading to a fatal outcome because of rapid absorption of toxic material through the unprotected wall.

2. *Nonoperative Treatment.*—Although the treatment of intestinal obstruction is primarily operative, a number of conservative procedures are of extreme importance, particularly in preparing the patient for laparotomy. Moreover, a few patients with simple mechanical obstruction, even in the late stages, will occasionally be saved from a lethal outcome and perhaps cured completely by nonoperative means alone; these measures consist of restoration of fluid loss, and particularly the effective use of gastro-intestinal decompression as will be described in detail later.

How long shall nonoperative therapy, particularly gastro-intestinal suction, be carried on before operation must be performed? This question is often difficult to answer but certain criteria are important:

(i) The presence or development of intestinal strangulation obviously calls for surgical intervention. When strangulation occurs as a primary event there is usually no difficulty in its detection, *e.g.*, in a strangulated hernia, or in volvulus. Indeed, operation is carried out as an emergency in such cases with no delay for conservative measures. Much more insidious is the type of vascular obstruction with resulting strangulation which may develop in a patient starting off with a mechanical occlusion of the lumen of the intestine, who becomes distended and whose distention then leads to nonviability of the bowel wall. Also insidious is strangulation which becomes superimposed upon a mechanical obstruction because of changes within the abdomen which permit bands to become tighter and occlude the vessels to a loop of intestine not previously involved. However, careful study of the patient at frequent intervals will practically always enable the surgeon to detect even these instances of gradually developing strangulation. Useful indications are the following manifestations: (1) increased pain and local tenderness, (2) increase in the pulse rate, (3) the appearance of either fever or subnormal temperature, (4) increasing leukocytosis, (5) the development of a palpable mass especially with associated local muscle spasm, (6) signs of even slight asthenia and prostration. It should be emphasized that one does not wait for all of the above signs, but only for one or more of them. For example, a small area of intestine may become strangulated by a band and be revealed only by a slight but distinct increase in local pain, perhaps more persistent in character and a rising pulse rate. Inasmuch as the dangers of strangulation are so great the surgeon should err on the side of radicalism, *i.e.,* operation should be carried out even if the presence of strangulation is merely, though strongly, suspected.

(ii) Treatment by gastro-intestinal suction drainage must not be continued if the patient appears to be losing ground. Inability to relieve the obstruction following *adequate decompression* is a strong indication for operation. Adequate decompression is shown by the evacuation of considerable gas and fluid from the intestinal tract, cessation of pain, decrease in distention and abdominal tenderness, passage of gas and stool per rectum, and obvious improvement in the patient's general appearance. It should be stated, however, that the greatest difficulty in obtaining adequate decompression is usually due to the fact that gastric suction alone is ineffective, and duodenal and intestinal intubation has been unsuccessful. Several hours may be utilized in trying to achieve adequate decompression but failure to do so for more than twelve hours in the hope of avoiding the necessity for operation is rarely justified.

(iii) In large bowel obstruction gastro-intestinal suction drainage should, at no time, be relied on as the sole method of treatment. In such cases a cecostomy, colostomy (or, rarely, a rectal tube inserted beyond the obstruction) is a simpler and more reliable means of decompression.

The nonoperative measures comprise the following:

(*a*) Rest in bed and nothing by mouth are primary orders which are so obvious that they need not be discussed.

(*b*) Parenteral fluids are necessary and often urgent in order to correct dehydration; the various methods have been described on page 150. Three important factors must be emphasized in fluid administration, whether they are given subcutaneously or intravenously. First of all, the amount must be adequate. It is usually insufficient to give 500 or 1000 cc. Ordinarily, at least 1500 to 2000 cc. must be given to bring the blood volume back to normal. In severely dehydrated patients as much as 5000 cc. may have to be given. In the absence of chemical analysis of the blood one may gain a fair idea of the adequacy of the amount of fluid given, by noting the color, volume, and specific gravity of the urine. As soon as a dilute urine is excreted below a specific gravity of 1.020 it is likely that the fluid balance has been restored. Such a result may often be achieved within relatively few hours.

The second important factor in giving fluid is that it contains sufficient electrolyte inasmuch as this is an important constituent of the fluid lost by vomiting. Glucose is added because of its advantage as a source of calories. It must be emphasized, however, that glucose solution alone, without electrolytes does more harm than good. While present in the blood stream the glucose solution is effective in diluting the concentrated blood but within a few hours the glucose itself is meta-bolized or stored; the situation then becomes the same as if plain distilled water had been administered. The blood, becoming thus hypotonic, provokes a rapid excretion of the water into the urine. During diuresis more salts are excreted, leaving the blood poorer in electrolyte and still more concentrated than before. Hyper-tonic glucose, when given without electrolyte, is even. more harmful since it with-draws fluid from the tissues and thus induces further loss of water as well as salts by the kidneys. The intravenous use of hypertonic solution of sodium chloride as a source of electrolytes is likewise inadvisable. Hypertonic salt acts, moreover, as an intestinal stimulant and while the bowel is obstructed its use is as dangerous as a cathartic by mouth.

The third factor is the frequent necessity of plasma transfusions to achieve fluid balance. Plasma may be lost in obstructed bowel and cause hypoproteinemia which is often aggravated if the patient has been chronically ill. Indeed, hypo-proteinemia may of itself produce nutritional edema of the intestinal mucosa and give rise to signs of intestinal obstruction (see p. 155). Obviously, if hypopro-teinemia is present the fluid injected intravenously must contain protein; plasma or whole blood transfusions are needed as much as saline and glucose.

(c) Procedures designed to aid in the passage of obstructed contents from below, if successful, are of value. While enemas are often used for this purpose a rectal tube placed well in the sigmoid with a proctoscope may be more effective and perhaps less dangerous. It should be emphasized that the obstructed intestinal contents are nearly always liquid in character; the evacuation of intestinal contents from *above* the obstruction is indicated by the passage of gas and of liquid stool. This is of particular importance after the institution of treatment in order to determine if progress is being made in the relief of the obstruction.

(d) Removal of fecal impaction when producing obstruction is an effective nonoperative treatment which is frequently overlooked, particularly when ab-dominal distention develops in older and debilitated patients. A rectal examination will nearly always make the diagnosis; manipulation of the fecal mass with the finger aided by oil and small enemas will usually result in relief, particularly if performed in several sessions.

(e) Gastro-intestinal decompression by the continuous removal of intestinal contents through a long catheter inserted through the nose, as advocated by Wangensteen [4] has revolutionized the treatment of intestinal obstruction and has been instrumental in saving innumerable lives. In certain instances operation is avoided entirely. The principle of this treatment lies in the fact that relief of distention, in absence of strangulation, alleviates symptoms, corrects many of the local changes at the obstruction, and permits more adequate study of the patient. Since the ordinary nasal catheter seldom passes into the duodenum, a balloon-tipped tube, described by Miller and Abbott,[5] may be necessary in certain cases in order to achieve decompression, because it can be passed directly to the ob-structed area. The balloon on the end of the tube acts as a bolus against which the intestine can contract, thus propelling the end of the catheter down the intestinal lumen. It is not always easy to pass a Miller-Abbott tube through the pylorus; a stylette in the tube and fluoroscopic visualization are helpful.

INTESTINAL OBSTRUCTION

Excellent detailed descriptions of the various manipulations may be found in other publications [6, 7]. The free end of the tube is fixed to the patient's cheek with adhesive and continuous mild suction exerted at the open end (see Fig. 457). The proper amount of suction is created by allowing water to flow out of a flask held about 6 to 8 feet above the floor; the vacuum thus created is just sufficient to aspirate

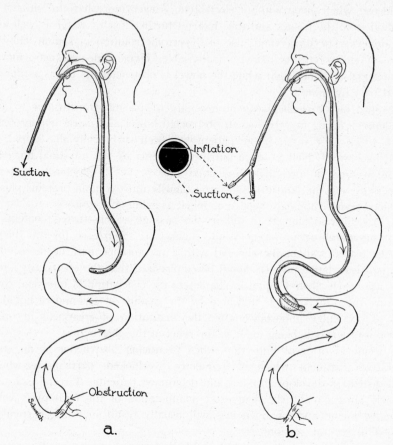

FIG. 457.—GASTRO-INTESTINAL DECOMPRESSION.

a, A single lumen long catheter will decompress the stomach and occasionally the duodenum but will rarely enter the jejunum. Only when regurgitation is active can this technic achieve complete deflation; b, The double lumen Miller-Abbott tube, because of the inflatable balloon, once it is in the duodenum, can be carried down to the point of obstruction (provided peristalsis is adequate) and thus achieve complete decompression. In each case mild suction is employed, *i.e.,* the equivalent of a column of water about six feet high. The apparatus must be constantly attended especially to remove plugs of food or mucus which tend to clog the lumen of the tube.

the stomach and intestines gently but efficiently. Whether the simple nasal catheter or the balloon-tipped tube is to be used depends upon the needs of the patient. Many patients respond well to the simple tube which aspirates the stomach and duodenum; others require a tube which is made to pass further into the intestine in order to be effective. In any case, the purpose of the procedure is to decompress the intestine; whichever is required to do so must be used. Detailed discussions of this form of treatment can be found in the report of C. G. Johnston.[7]

The success of continuous suction depends on removing enough gas and fluid from above the obstructed bowel to relieve distention, allow the local inflammation and edema to subside, and thus to permit passage of gas and fluid through a partly occluded lumen. That this actually happens has been amply shown.

Early postoperative adhesions sometimes become loosened in this way and obstruction relieved. Later postoperative adhesions are less likely to be freed and even if decompression relieves the obstruction operation is often necessary because of the tendency for recurrence. It should be emphasized again that decompression is not designed to replace operation since it does not correct the lesion producing it; nevertheless, its successful use, with limitations well in mind as already discussed, offers much aid in combating distention and thus making laparotomy less hazardous and the mortality much lower.

(f) Oxygen inhalations are often useful in combating the serious manifestations of strangulation, i.e., "toxic" symptoms, circulatory impairment, and anoxia; these may even persist after operative correction. Oxygen is also used to decrease distention (Fine).

3. *Operative Treatment.*—As already discussed, gastro-intestinal decompression and other conservative measures should be carried out whether or not operation is considered. Even the elimination of gastric distention, which is part of intestinal obstruction, will be advantageous particularly by minimizing aspiration if operation is done under general anesthesia. When the distention is so slight as not to interfere with surgical intervention, the safest procedure is early operation to correct the cause. Marked distention, on the other hand, always makes operation more hazardous and increases mortality because of the technical difficulties induced. Strangulation, when present, either primarily or as a complication, makes operation imperative as an emergency. However, even in such a case conservative measures, such as suction drainage and parenteral fluids, should be started while the patient is being prepared for operation, which, however, should not be delayed thereby.

In general, three operative procedures are available for the relief of acute intestinal obstruction; they are used either alone or in combination: (1) release of the obstruction; (2) enterostomy; and (3) resection and anastomosis. The details are to be found in works on operative surgery. When there is no evidence of damaged bowel or when relatively little distention is present the site of the obstruction is located by finding the junction between collapsed and dilated bowel. The band or bands are cut, or other causes eradicated. Deflation of the obstructed gut will follow correction of the cause. In the very ill patient operation may be confined to an enterostomy performed under local anesthesia. If intestinal strangulation is present and the involved tissue is definitely nonviable, resection and anastomosis are indicated. However, if the patient is very ill the gangrenous loop may be exteriorized (Mikulicz procedure) for removal, and plastic repair made later. Whether the obstructed or strangulated bowel is viable or not is an obviously important question at the time of operation; the manifestations of viability in strangulation are described on page 785.

The value of a laparotomy in *paralytic ileus* is in general confined to the relief of the primary lesion, i.e., eradication of the source of the peritonitis, such as drainage of abscesses, closure of perforations, etc. Although enterostomy has been advised and used in this condition, its efficacy is questionable even in relieving distention, for the drainage is ordinarily successful from only a short segment of bowel as long as peristalsis is absent. As soon as the gut becomes active such drainage is unnecessary since, in absence of organic occlusion, the peristalsis carries intestinal contents normally. The use of intestinal decompression is a direct ap-

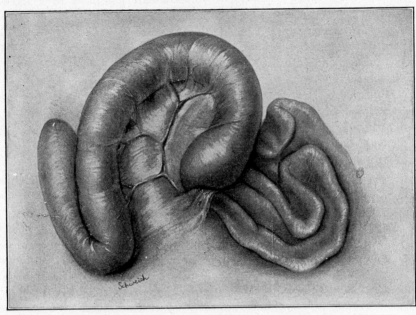

FIG. 458.—ACUTE INTESTINAL OBSTRUCTION (MECHANICAL OCCLUSION OF THE LUMEN).

Artist's drawing at time of operation; the dense adhesive band occluded the lumen completely. Note the marked distention of the proximal loop and collapsed distal loop; this obvious contrast was most useful at time of operation in locating the exact site of the occlusion which was corrected by cutting the band. The patient had had a hysterectomy two weeks previously; the pain, distention, vomiting, etc., were, at first, erroneously attributed to postoperative ileus. Recovery was complete.

proach to therapy in paralytic ileus, insofar as the tube will passively pass down the intestine. As the gut is decompressed activity may be resumed wholly or in part. Ordinarily, however, as mentioned above, paralytic ileus responds to conservative treatment and to measures which correct the primary lesion.

The treatment of intussusception and pyloric stenosis is described later in this chapter. The operative procedures used in high intestinal obstruction in general present no special problem inasmuch as strangulation of tissue so rarely complicates the lesion. The operations used have been described under the various diseases.

Chronic or Partial Obstruction.—Various lesions may produce chronic obstruction. Transient attacks of acute obstruction occur which subside only to recur; often, however, there may be only a progressive and insidiously developing abdominal distention with or without constipation. Besides the lesion causing the partial occlusion of the lumen, the intestine immediately above is thickened, dilated and hypertrophied. Prompt vomiting and cramps which follow acute distention of the normal bowel occur late if at all. It is remarkable that a chronically obstructed small bowel can become so tremendously yet insidiously distended. Early diagnosis is important not only because cancer may be present, but also because neglect of therapy will lead to progression of the intestinal changes. X-ray is of diagnostic value because the large, dilated, gas-filled loops of intestine show readily on the flat film. Unless its removal can be assured, barium should not be given by mouth lest it precipitate a complete obstruction. *Treatment* is in general surgical even if the lesion is benign. A diet confined to soft, well chewed or pureed non-bulky food may be tried, bearing in mind the danger of acute obstruction and progressive intestinal distention.

Chronic duodenal ileus is a term applied to a clinical syndrome consisting of anorexia, vomiting and severe loss of weight. It is supposed to be due to chronic, partial obstruction of the terminal duodenum at the ligament of Treitz as it crosses the bowel at this point. The diagnosis is usually made only by x-ray examination after a barium meal. If the presence of obstruction can be definitely established surgical treatment may be justified. Operation consists of an anastomosis around the occluding band, *i.e.*, duodenojejunostomy.

SPECIFIC LESIONS PRODUCING INTESTINAL OBSTRUCTION

Strangulated Hernia.—Perhaps the most common cause of intestinal obstruction is strangulated hernia; it is so frequent, in fact, that any patient with manifestations of intestinal obstruction should be examined for the possible presence of an inguinal or femoral hernia. The obstruction is nearly always complete. Any loop of intestine may be involved. Operation is of course imperative except when normal reduction is possible. A detailed discussion of strangulated hernia will be found on page 783.

Adhesions and Bands.—With a few exceptions, adhesions capable of causing intestinal obstruction are produced by a previous abdominal operation, or inflammation, particularly of pelvic origin. Operations commonly producing such adhesions are gynecologic, and those performed for perforated appendicitis. The obstruction may develop at almost any time following operation, but is perhaps encountered most frequently within several months following operation. When it occurs within the first two or three postoperative days, it is frequently associated with partial rupture of the abdominal wound, with or without the presence of wound infection. Diagnosis may be difficult at this time because of confusion with the manifestations of postoperative ileus which may include abdominal pain, nausea, vomiting, distention, etc. Since the adhesions producing obstruction so early after operation are friable and not dense, conservative therapy is usually safe and preferable (see p. 167). There is no doubt that a large percentage of patients with obstruction of this type will be relieved by gastro-intestinal decompression; this is particularly so because it relieves edema which is a prominent feature in the production of the obstruction and also because the friable adhesions may be loosened by the drag of peristalsis. However, when conservative therapy is ineffective operation may be necessary for the release of the obstructed loop, and should not be delayed if evidence of relief of the obstruction is not promptly obtained or if the patient does not show early improvement.

When the obstruction occurs months or years after operation, the adhesion or band is more apt to be tough and dense. The adhesion usually connects two peritoneal surfaces, and during the process of contraction, finally becomes tight enough to obstruct the lumen of the bowel, particularly when a secondary inflammation of the intestine and adjacent tissue with edema takes place. The adhesion may also strangulate a portion of the intestinal wall in the area compressed by the band; an entire loop of intestine may be strangulated by a circular band (see Fig. 453). Occasionally an obstruction is produced by attachment of a Meckel's diverticulum to an adjacent point with compression of the underlying loop. Even if the obstruction is relieved by conservative therapy, operation should be performed in order to cut the band and prevent the danger of recurrence or of chronic obstruction. The various procedures available for treatment of such patients have been discussed earlier in this chapter.

Neoplasms of the Intestine.—With few exceptions, the neoplasms of the intestine capable of producing obstruction are located in the colon and are malignant. It is true, however, that metastases to the serosal surface of the small intestine may obstruct the lumen because of an associated contraction of scar tissue deposited about the tumor. Carcinoma of the descending colon is more apt to result in complete obstruction than is carcinoma of the cecum and ascending colon. In the latter instance the manifestations may consist of frequent attacks of cramping pain associated perhaps with constipation and distention; there may be intervals of several days when symptoms are absent or insignificant. When the obstruction is complete, there will be only momentary relief of pain. Constipation will be complete and distention constant. Details of the clinical manifestations and treatment will be found where the specific lesions are discussed (Chap. XXIV).

Intussusception.—Invagination of a portion of intestine into an adjacent distal loop (intussusception) is a fairly common type of obstruction; it is rare in adults, and occurs most frequently in infancy and early childhood. This invagination occurs most commonly at the ileocecal valve, but may develop elsewhere in the small and large intestine, particularly in the terminal ileum and upper part of the descending colon.

The exact cause of the intussusception may not be demonstrable, but usually investigation will disclose one or more anatomical features which undoubtedly play an important role in the invagination. Filmy congenital bands, buckling the terminal ileum into the cecum, are occasionally found. On other occasions, a small Meckel's diverticulum may be the apparent cause of the invagination. Tumors, including polyps, aberrant pancreas, etc., may likewise be the instigating factor. The most frequent finding is an unusually long mesentery of the cecum and ileocecal region; in fact it is doubtful if intussusception can progress far without the existence of this long mesentery. On many occasions this is the only structural defect demonstrable which is capable of producing the intussusception. It is, therefore, possible that a long mesentery is an important prerequisite to the development of an intussusception. Strangulation of the vessels of the intussuscepted loop occurs at a variable time after onset. As this vascular compression increases, gangrene of the involved intestine develops, which leads to a fatal outcome unless the necrotic segment is sloughed into the lumen; this occurs but is extremely rare.

The *clinical manifestations* are remarkably constant and dramatic. One of the first symptoms noted is pain, which is presumably severe, as expressed by irritability of the child who screams and cries out frequently holding its abdomen. Shortly after the onset of the pain, nausea and vomiting are noted. Within an hour or two, manifestations of shock such as listlessness, weakness, prostration and pallor develop. The pulse rapidly becomes fast, weak and thready. There are two features of this shock which appear to be of particular diagnostic significance,

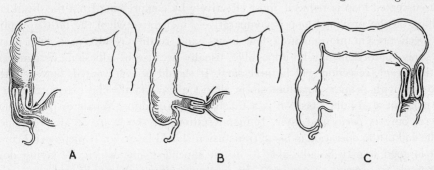

A   B   C

FIG. 459.—THREE SITES FOR INTUSSUSCEPTION.

The illustrations are diagrammatic and show only the initial step in the process. In most instances a far longer portion of the ileum or colon becomes involved by the time operation is performed. The arrows indicate the points at which the mesenteric vessels become obstructed by the intussusception. *A,* at the ileocecal valve; this is by far the most common location. *B,* at the terminal ileum; intussusception at this site is usually produced by a definite cause, such as an intestinal polyp, a Meckel's diverticulum, etc. *C,* in the descending colon.

namely the dusky color associated with the pallor, and the extreme prostration which develops so rapidly following onset. However, these features of shock may also be exhibited in infants with intestinal obstruction produced by other causes. Occasionally shock of the type just described will be one of the first manifestations; the child may exhibit none of the indications of pain (*i.e.,* screaming and crying), and the only indications of illness as noted by the mother will be listlessness, prostration and pallor. It is not uncommon for the infant or child to have a normal bowel movement shortly after the onset of pain. Following this, other stools will be passed, which at first contain mucus, later mucus streaked with blood, and finally pure blood, the color of which depends upon the location of the intussusception. A mass is usually palpable, first in the right lower quadrant, but moves progressively upward toward the epigastrium and across to the left side of the abdomen with the lapse of time. Muscle spasm and tenderness are rarely severe, if present at all. Peristaltic waves may or may not be visible. Distention usually occurs but is not a prominent feature until after twenty-four hours. Obstruction is usually complete soon after onset; an enema yields chiefly mucus and blood. On rare occasions the intussusception is relieved spontaneously or after an enema; this occurs only early in the disease and is apt to be followed by recurrence. Recurrent intussusception is probably the cause of certain obscure intestinal episodes in infancy.[8] Fever may be present, but usually only in the late stage of the obstruction. Leukocytosis may or may not be present. Rectal examination will reveal bloody mucus in the rectum; the mass may be palpable by the examining finger.

Treatment is obviously surgical and should not be delayed, after proper pre-operative therapy (including subcutaneous Ringer's and saline solution and perhaps intravenous glucose) has been instituted. Ether anesthesia will usually be necessary but if the child is in severe shock local anesthesia may be sufficient. A right paramedian incision should be made if no mass is palpable. However, if a mass is demonstrable, the incision should be made over it. At operation the intussuscepted loop is reduced, most effectively by compressing from the distal end. Pulling on the proximal loop is comparatively ineffective when the intussusception has been present more than a few hours, and readily results in a tear of the intestine. Reduction may be impossible, usually because of adhesions or gangrene. In this event, resection will be necessary. It should be emphasized, however, that resection with primary anastomosis is almost always fatal. The exteriorization of the mass in a Mikulicz fashion is a much safer procedure. Repair of the resultant enterostomy is performed later. If manifestations of shock are at all pronounced at the end of the operation, a blood transfusion should be given. If the general condition is good it may be advisable to do an appendectomy, which, by laying down scar tends to prevent recurrence.[8] An intussusception, when seen early and when the mass is still small, can occasionally be reduced under the fluoroscope by means of a barium enema which must be carefully given without too much pressure. However, this procedure has its limitations and, in any case, if used should not unduly delay operation which must be immediately carried out if the reduction by enema fails.

Proper postoperative feeding may be of extreme importance in the convalescence of these patients (most of whom are infants), particularly because of their tendency to vomit. A small quantity of water may be allowed three to four hours after operation and feedings resumed six to eight hours after operation, but must at first be small in quantity and not concentrated. The amount may be increased daily. Various types of feeding may be used, but the following formula appears to be particularly satisfactory: for a baby six to twelve months of age and of average weight, a mixture containing 30 cc. of evaporated milk, 20 per cent buffered solution * and water to which 4 cc. of Karo syrup is added, is given over a period of twenty-four hours in six feedings of 15 cc. each. The amount is increased daily so that the child gets 5 feedings of 150 cc. of a mixture of 355 cc. evaporated milk, 355 cc. of 1 per cent lactic acid and 45 cc. Karo. Other details of infant feedings may be obtained in special publications (Marriott[9] and others). If vomiting is troublesome during the first day or two, subcutaneous saline or intravenous glucose may be indicated. Frequently, gastric lavage with continuous drainage of the stomach for twelve hours will stop vomiting, and allow resumption of feedings. Occasionally, the administration of sedatives (*e.g.*, ⅛ to ½ grain sodium phenobarbital every four hours as indicated) will decrease or eliminate the vomiting;

---

* The concentrated (100 per cent buffered solution) is made up as follows: 150 cc. of U. S. P. lactic acid, 200 cc. of 10 per cent sodium hydroxide, and sufficient water to make up to one liter.

the use of sedation is obviously not considered if an actual mechanical obstruction is present.

Volvulus.—This type of obstruction consists primarily of a twist of a loop of intestine, and fixation in that position; occasionally, this fixation is maintained by adhesive bands, but more commonly is due to structural abnormalities. Volvulus (sometimes spoken of as torsion) occurs more frequently in the colon than small intestine. When it occurs in the small intestine, adhesions are very apt to be the inciting factor, or at least the factor responsible for maintenance of the twist. When it occurs in the colon the sigmoid is a common site for volvulus, apparently because of the long flexure in which the limbs of the loop are approximated so closely, and because of the long mesentery which exists so frequently at this point. Volvulus of the cecum and ascending colon, though rare, occurs nearly always in children, as a complication of malrotation of intestine as described later.

The clinical manifestations of volvulus are similar to those previously described for intestinal obstruction. If the blood supply at the mesentery is completely occluded the severe signs of intestinal strangulation as already described will rapidly develop. If the involved loop of intestine is in the colon, it becomes markedly distended with gas and fluid; this distended loop may be so prominent as to be palpable and thus lead to an accurate diagnosis. If strangulation exists, considerable fluid may be found in the peritoneal cavity at operation.

On rare occasions, when the volvulus is of short duration and located in the sigmoid, the torsion may be relieved by a barium enema; occasionally the torsion corrects itself spontaneously and a history of subsiding attacks may be obtained (recurrent volvulus). Unless promptly relieved, operation is the only curative procedure. If strangulation is not present, untwisting the loop may be sufficient to entirely relieve the obstruction. Any adhesive bands present should be cut. Occasionally it may be advisable to shorten the mesentery by plication, so as to minimize the possibility of recurrence. The sigmoid is the area most subject to recurrence of a volvulus. If strangulation with gangrene is present, excision of the involved loop will be necessary. Resection with primary anastamosis is usually preferable when the torsion involves the small intestine: in the sigmoid, exteriorization after the Mikulicz procedure, followed by anastamosis later, will usually be indicated.

Malrotation of the Intestine.—Anomalies of rotation of the intestine during embryonic life may be responsible for a number of different types of intestinal obstruction. Before the mechanisms of these types of obstruction can be understood, it is necessary to be familiar with the main features of intestinal rotation. Normally, the midgut recedes, from its position in the yolk sac, through the umbilical orifice into the abdominal cavity at about the tenth week of embryonic life. The cecum is the last portion of the intestine to enter the abdominal cavity and from its position in the left posterior portion of the yolk sac rotates 270 degrees on the axis of the superior mesenteric artery from the left upper quadrant in a counterclockwise direction to its permanent position in the right lower quadrant.

The most common anomaly of rotation is *incomplete rotation of the cecum.* When this occurs the cecum and part of the ascending colon are suspended with little or no mesenteric attachment, usually in the upper left quadrant; it is, therefore, freely mobile. Because the cecum is so freely mobile it is particularly prone to the development of obstruction, chiefly because of volvulus involving the terminal ileum, cecum and ascending colon. This obstruction may not occur for several years after birth; manifestations are similar to those of obstruction and volvulus as already described. In one type of incomplete rotation the obstruction occurs at the terminal duodenum because of a volvulus including all of the small gut. Cure may be effected by Ladd's operation.[10]

Occasionally, rotation takes place in the reversed direction (clockwise). In this case, the positions of the duodenum and colon with respect to the mesenteric artery will be reversed, *i.e.*, the duodenum will be anterior to the superior mesenteric artery and the colon posterior to the artery.

Details of the various features of malrotation of the intestine may be found in a publication by Dott.[11] Even in the absence of volvulus, symptoms of "chronic" intestinal obstruction may develop because of sharp angulations produced by anomalous attachments, particularly in the terminal portion of the duodenum. A correct diagnosis may often be made previous to operation by means of fluoroscopic and x-ray study with the barium meal. At operation, volvulus and most other factors producing an obstruction can be remedied, but the malrotation itself can rarely be corrected.

Congenital Stenosis and Atresia.—Partial or complete obstruction of the intestine may be produced by congenital stenosis (narrowing of the lumen) and atresia (complete obliteration of the lumen) of the intestine; such lesions are fortunately comparatively rare. More frequently, the stenosis is produced by a compression of the small intestine by a congenital band, located most commonly in the duodenum or terminal ileum. On other occasions, an obvious narrowing of the intestine itself will be present, thereby producing partial obstruction. More rarely, the intestine (particularly the duodenum and terminal ileum) ends blindly, *i.e.*, atresia (see Fig. 426).

In atresia symptoms of intestinal obstruction will be noted immediately after birth; important in the diagnosis is the absence of bile and food residue in the stools. If the obstruction is only partial, as produced by a stenosis or band, the child may be several weeks old before taken to a physician. In such instances, the persistent vomiting may resemble that of pyloric stenosis, but the presence of bile in the vomitus will invariably place the obstruction in the duodenum or beyond. If the obstruction is of sufficient consequence to disturb the child's nutrition, operation will usually be indicated. If a complete atresia exists, attempt should be made to perform a primary anastomosis; however, very few infants upon whom such an operation is performed will survive. The most favorable type of congenital obstruction, from the standpoint of mortality, is that produced by a band, particularly when the obstructing band may be severed with a minimal amount of operative trauma. Imperforate anus, another type of atresia requiring operative correction, is discussed on page 713. These and other abdominal lesions in infancy and childhood form the subject of an excellent monograph by Ladd and Gross [13].

Miscellaneous Lesions Producing Obstruction.—There are numerous miscellaneous lesions which are capable of producing either partial or complete obstruction; most of these are discussed in detail elsewhere. On rare occasions, the amount of inflammation occurring with a *diverticulitis* of the colon will be sufficient to produce obstructive symptoms (see p. 698). The inflammatory mass may be quite firm and resemble carcinoma. Occasionally the mechanical obstruction may be so slight that it is not detected with certainty even by the x-ray (*i.e.,* barium enema), yet the patient will complain of distention and cramping pain of a type quite suggestive of intestinal obstruction. Diagnosis will usually be made only at operation. If the obstruction is complete it may be necessary to perform a colostomy proximal to the lesion. If the obstruction does not disappear as the inflammation subsides, it may be necessary to resect the mass; the Mikulicz procedure will usually be most applicable.

Stricture formation (noncongenital) may occur in any part of the alimentary tract and may be sufficiently severe to produce a total obstruction. In the upper part of the digestive tract they occur most often in the esophagus and pylorus. Strangulation is rarely produced by this type of obstruction although dehydration from loss of fluid through vomiting may produce severe general manifestations, particularly in pyloric obstruction. Detailed descriptions will be found elsewhere. Stricture of the rectum due to lymphogranuloma venereum rarely results in acute obstruction (see p. 99). Occasionally *benign ulceration* of the intestine, produced by amebiasis, tuberculosis, etc., will result in a stricture; these lesions are usually located in the colon. Confirmatory evidence of obstruction will be noted by x-ray, but a diagnosis of carcinoma will usually be made. Operative correction will obviously be indicated in most instances. Two types of operative procedures are available: a primary anastomosis around the stricture can be performed, or the mass resected. If the latter procedure is chosen, the Mikulicz operation will probably be the most applicable.

Mesenteric thrombosis produces nearly all the manifestations of a complete obstruction (or adynamic ileus) because of the paralysis of the peristaltic mechanism in the involved area. More important is the effect of the thrombosis on the viability of the affected intestine, inasmuch as acute sudden manifestations, as described for intestinal strangulation, are produced thereby. The obliteration of the vessels may be due primarily to an embolus or thrombosis. The disease is encountered in patients afflicted with endocarditis, vascular disease, etc., but frequently develops in supposedly healthy people in whom no etiologic factor can be found. The effects are similar, in general, to those produced by intestinal strangulation, which has already been described (p. 761). Pain is severe, diffuse and constant; even large doses of morphine are often ineffective in relieving it. Nausea and vomiting are also present. Characteristic is the prostration and shock which rapidly develop; pallor, cyanosis and low blood pressure with rapid thready pulse may be noted. Mesenteric thrombosis involving the colon produces shock much more rapidly, and obviously is much more serious from the standpoint of prognosis. Examination of the abdomen reveals diffuse tenderness and muscle spasm. A tubular mass representing the involved intestine may be palpable. There is usually a marked leukocytosis. If a stool is passed, gross blood may be noted, which is of considerable diagnostic importance. The disease is apt to be fatal in spite of treatment which consists of immediate laparotomy with resection of the gangrenous bowel. There is a tendency for the thrombosis to extend after operation beyond the limits of the resection. Bloody fluid is commonly found in the peritoneal cavity. On rare occasions spontaneous resolution of the thrombosis occurs by gradual reëstablishment of collateral circulation.

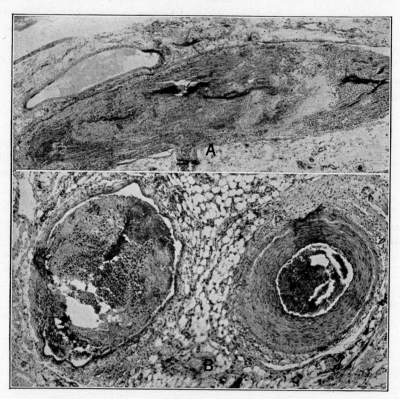

FIG. 460.—MESENTERIC THROMBOSIS. PHOTOMICROGRAPHS FROM A SECTION OF THE EXCISED INTESTINE, SHOWING OBSTRUCTED VESSELS.

A, is a thrombosed vessel in the intestinal wall and B, an occluded artery and vein in the mesentery. Note also the surrounding edema in A. The thrombosis in the mesenteric vein is obviously of longer duration than that in its accompanying artery. The patient was a thirty-seven-year-old housewife; two weeks previously she had been delivered of a normal infant and was enjoying a normal puerperium, when, two days before admission she was suddenly seized with generalized abdominal cramps which became severe and were accompanied by persistent vomiting; blood was noted in the stool. Prostration became quite pronounced. At operation, two and one-half feet of nonviable intestine was resected followed by a lateral anastomosis; recovery was uneventful.

Enteroliths are rare causes for intestinal obstruction. An obstruction of this type will be produced by the ulceration of a large gallstone through the wall of the gallbladder into the duodenum; the obstruction produced (usually in the ileum) is due to failure of peristalsis to dislodge the stone. The correct diagnosis will rarely be made except at operation. Removal of the gallstone, with a proper repair of the defect made in the intestine, will be indicated, and is associated with a comparatively favorable prognosis. *Fecal impaction* occurs frequently, but only rarely produces manifestations of acute obstruction.

Hypertrophic Pyloric Stenosis.—This disease has an interesting history which is well summarized by Mack [14]. It occurs in early infancy and is due to a pyloric obstruction produced by hypertrophy of the circular pyloric muscles but is probably associated with some spasm. The disease is much more common in males than females. The symptoms appear first at the second or third week of life and consist primarily of vomiting. At first the vomiting may be manifested merely as a regurgitation, but later becomes projectile. The child usually vomits after every feeding, and frequently the entire feeding. The vomitus never contains bile since the obstruction is proximal to the ampulla of Vater. Unless the child is fed again after vomiting, dehydration and loss of weight may take place rapidly. In spite of refeeding and extreme care in choice of formulas, etc., gradual loss of weight is the rule. Constipation is obviously and always present. Shortly after the onset of the disease peristaltic waves will be observed, beginning characteristically at the left costal margin and passing to the right, particularly after ingesting fluid (see Fig. 461). It may be

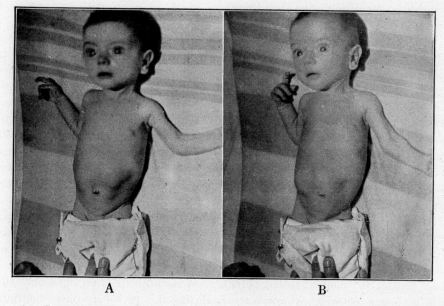

A   B

FIG. 461.—CONGENITAL HYPERTROPHIC STENOSIS OF THE PYLORUS IN A SIX-WEEKS-OLD INFANT.

The two photographs were taken a few seconds apart. *A*, note the peristalic wave beginning low in the left hypochondrium. In *B*, it has moved toward the right and downward; the trough of a second wave is also seen approaching the pylorus, above and to the right of the umbilicus. Pyloromyotomy (Fredet-Ramstedt operation) was followed by an uneventful recovery.

necessary to examine the child several times before significant peristaltic waves are demonstrable. A palpable tumor in the right upper quadrant of the abdomen can often be felt; it is about the size of a small olive and represents the firm area of hypertrophied pyloric muscle. However, palpation of a tumor is not essential for diagnosis. A roentgenogram will reveal merely a large dilated stomach. Fluoroscopy after a barium meal is often carried out and will indicate the degree and completeness of the pyloric obstruction; however, if barium is given, the part remaining in the stomach must be evacuated by a nasal tube when the roentgen examination is completed.

The *treatment* is primarily surgical, but it is of extreme importance that operation be performed only after dehydration is corrected. Treatment for dehydration consists of hypodermoclysis of 200 to 250 cc. physiological saline solution or Ringer's solution; intravenous administration of 20 cc. of 10 per cent glucose, per kilogram of body weight, once or twice daily should be used as indicated. If the infant is in especially poor condition a transfusion of 15 to 20 cc. of blood for each kilogram body weight may be advisable. Because infants with pyloric stenosis are prone to acquire infections of various types, particularly otitis media, frequent examinations must be carried out to detect their existence, especially if fever is present. Such infections in themselves are apt to produce vomiting. Proper therapy such as incision of an ear drum when indicated may be instrumental in the eradication or diminution of vomiting. In many instances it may even be advisable to remove the infant to its home within a day or two after operation in order to minimize the danger of acquiring such infections which are often much more prone to develop in hospitals than at home.

The operative procedure which is known as the Fredet-Ramstedt operation, instituted in 1912, consists of division of the dense, firm, hypertrophied, circular muscle fibers (pyloromyotomy) at the most bloodless point on the pylorus. Separation is continued until all fibers are broken and the submucosa pouts out into the wound in the pylorus. Extreme care must be taken not to perforate the submucosa because of the danger of a fatal peritonitis. This accident is most apt to occur at the duodenal end; if it occurs, the opening is repaired by one or two interrupted silk sutures taken in a diagonal longitudinal direction. Local or general anesthesia may be used. The former should be supplemented with a preliminary drug of some type, *e.g.,* seconal. Preoperative gastric lavage appears to increase the toleration for postoperative feeding.

The *postoperative care* is of particular importance, especially in regard to feeding. The tendency to force feeding in too large quantities during the first few days is harmful because the stomach is frequently unable to fully empty itself because of postoperative gastric atony and distention. According to observations by Faber and Davis [12] normal gastric peristalsis in such infants is regained only after 24 to 72 hours following pyloromyotomy. During this period overdistention must be avoided. Half an ounce of water may be offered as early as two hours after operation. Feeding may be started four hours after operation but on the first day should be limited to 15 cc. per feeding. A mixture * of 30 cc. evaporated milk, 30 cc. of 10 per cent buffered solution †, 30 cc. of water and 4 cc. Karo syrup is made up; this allows administration of six feedings of 15 cc. each. The individual feedings are increased in quantity 15 cc. each day so that the child gets six feedings of 30 cc. on the second day, 45 cc. on the third day and so on until a normal requirement of about 120 cc. is met. After several days the feeding should be concentrated slightly by prescribing a formula of two parts evaporated milk, two parts 1 per cent lactic acid and one part water; sufficient Karo

---

* As recommended by the pediatric service, St. Louis Children's Hospital.
† See footnote, page 774.

syrup is added to make a 6 per cent solution. Before the child is discharged from the hospital, the feeding should be concentrated still more to that of a normal intake, *i.e.*, equal parts of evaporated milk and water to which sufficient Karo syrup is added to make a 6 per cent solution.

If postoperative vomiting is troublesome, it may sometimes be diminished or eradicated by sedation such as phenobarbital gr. ⅛ every four hours or better still, by reducing the amount of feeding for reasons already mentioned. Gastric atony may also be combated by emptying the stomach once or twice every 24 hours for the first few days; favorable progress is indicated by the fact that the amount removed is progressively less than the amount ingested. Reoperation may then be postponed safely. Obviously if an obstruction remains because of an inadequate primary operation, these measures will be of no value and a second operation will be indicated, a rare necessity.

BIBLIOGRAPHY

1. McIver, M. A. *Acute Intestinal Obstruction*, P. B. Hoeber, New York, 1933.
2. Fine, J., Hurwitz, A., and Mark, J. A Clinical Study of Plasma Volume in Acute Intestinal Obstruction, *Ann. Surg.*, 112:546, 1940.
3. Crowley, R. T., and Johnston, C. G. Therapeutic Considerations in Acute Obstruction of the Small Bowel, *Surg., Gynec. & Obst.*, 73:1, 1941.
4. Wangensteen, O. H. *The Therapeutic Problem in Bowel Obstruction*, Charles Thomas, Springfield, Illinois, 1937.
5. Miller, T. G. and Abbott, W. D. Intestinal Intubation: a Practical Technique, *Am. J. Med. Sc.*, 187:595, 1934.
6. Leigh, O. C., Jr., Nelson, J. A., and Swenson, P. C. The Miller-Abbott Tube as an Adjunct to Surgery of Small Intestinal Obstruction, *Ann. Surg.*, 111:186, 1940.
7. Johnston, C. G. Decompression in the Treatment of Intestinal Obstruction, *Surg., Gynec. & Obst.*, 70:365, 1940. See also *Nelson's Loose Leaf Surgery*, Chap. XIV, p. 651, Vol. V, 1941.
8. Goldman, L. E., and Elman, R. Spontaneous Reduction of Intussusception in Children, *Am. J. Surg.*, 49:259, 1940.
9. Marriott, W. McKim. *Infant Nutrition*, C. V. Mosby Co., St. Louis, 1930.
10. Elman, R. Ladd's Operation for the Cure of Incomplete Rotation and Volvulus of the Small Intestine Producing Duodenal Obstruction in Infancy, *Ann. Surg.*, 112:234, 1940.
11. Dott, N. M. Anomalies of Intestinal Rotation, *Brit. J. Surg.*, 11:251, 1923.
12. Faber, H. K., and Davis, J. H. Gastric Peristalsis after Pyloromyotomy in Infants, *J. Am. M. Ass.*, 114.847, 1940.
13. Ladd, W. E. and Gross, R. E. *Abdominal Surgery of Infancy and Childhood*, W. B. Saunders Co., Philadelphia, 1941.
14. Mack, H. C. A History of Pyloric Stenosis and Its Treatment, *Bull. Hist. of Med.*, 12:465, 1942.

CHAPTER XXVII

HERNIA

Specific Types of Hernia

Definitions.—A *hernia* may be defined as a protrusion through an abnormal opening in the wall of a body cavity, particularly the abdomen. Through this opening such organs as intestine, omentum, etc., may pass. Most hernias are *reducible;* their contents can be replaced by manipulation into the cavity of origin, or may recede spontaneously when the patient lies down. When the mass cannot be reduced the hernia is spoken of as *irreducible*. An *obstructed hernia* is one containing intestine whose lumen becomes blocked by adhesions, angulation, volvulus, fecal impaction, etc. There is considerable difference of opinion as to the meaning of the term *incarcerated hernia*. Some authorities consider incarceration synonymous with irreducibility, whereas others use the term synonymously with obstructed hernia, but it appears more accurate to apply the term to permanent irreducibility. Occasionally only a portion of the intestinal wall is caught in a small hernial opening without obstructing the lumen of the intestine, thereby constituting what is called *Richter's hernia*. This type of hernia occurs most frequently in femoral and inguinal hernias. A *strangulated hernia* is one containing viscera whose blood supply is partially or completely blocked. In such an instance gangrene obviously follows, unless the strangulation is relieved within a few hours. The terms *true* and *false hernia* are sometimes used to differentiate between hernias having sacs (true hernias) and those not having sacs (false hernias).

Hernias are ordinarily classified according to their anatomic location. The most common types are those in the inguinal and femoral region. These and others are described in detail later in the chapter.

Etiologic Factors.—Although hernias are frequently considered traumatic in origin, it appears that the development of most hernias is associated with a preexistent weakness of the supporting structures at the point of herniation, and the existence of a preformed sac. It is true that workmen frequently give a definite history of sudden pain in the groin associated with the appearance of a hernial mass immediately following severe strain such as lifting, etc. In such instances it seems probable that the hernia is of congenital origin in so far as a preformed sac is present and that there is sufficient weakness at the external and internal ring to allow protrusion after trauma of a certain type. However, it should be stated that compensation boards usually consider trauma as being capable of producing hernias, and rarely fail to return a verdict in favor of the workman when the hernia appears following an accident or strain sustained during work.

Hernia may occur at any time during life, but an analysis by Watson[1] has revealed the fact that 15 per cent occur during the first year of life. Obesity, pregnancy and other conditions which predispose to relaxation and disuse of certain muscles are important secondary causes.

General Clinical Manifestations.—A hernia is usually noticed because of the appearance of a protrusion or mass, and is nearly always accompanied by a moderate amount of pain during the first few days. It may or may not be preceded by a history of undue strain, etc. The pain decreases so that after two or three weeks the symptoms complained of consist of nothing more than a mild feeling of discomfort. There is a tendency for the protruding mass to increase in size. Most hernias are reducible, especially so when they are of recent origin. The recumbent position facilitates the ease of reduction. After reduction of the mass one can usually feel the defect through which the hernia has protruded. Many hernias become irreducible, especially when the patient has been wearing a truss or other appliance, because of the adhesions produced between the sac and its contents. The mass is soft, semifluctuant and usually not tender. In contrast to hydrocele (see p. 1021) it does not transmit light. The surface is usually not so smooth or regular as that of hydrocele. If intestine is included in the contents of the hernia, percussion will usually reveal a tympanitic note. One of the most reliable diagnostic features of hernia is the impulse transmitted to the mass when the patient coughs; if a hernia is present but no mass presents, the impulse transmitted by coughing, when the finger is placed in the hernial opening, is of particular diagnostic value.

Frequently a patient presents himself with the history of having been examined by an industrial doctor who has found a dilated external ring with an impulse on coughing and has advised surgical treatment before employment will be recommended. Though an actual hernia is not demonstrable in these cases, operation may be indicated. On most occasions a tiny sac will then be found.

Pronounced and serious symptoms of hernia are produced when the contents become strangulated. This in itself is such a serious complication that it is considered first.

Strangulated Hernia.—The term strangulated hernia is frequently applied erroneously to obstructed hernias. With few exceptions, strangulation does not develop until several hours after the hernia becomes obstructed. Only in Richter's hernia does strangulation occur in the absence of obstruction. When obstruction occurs, symptoms will be identical to those described under simple intestinal obstruction, consisting of cramping intermittent pain, nausea and vomiting, followed by distention. Obstruction, and particularly strangulation, are most prone to develop when the ring (*e.g.*, external inguinal) through which the hernia protrudes, is small. The mechanism of strangulation consists first of compression of the veins, followed by edema, later by arterial compression, and gangrene.

When strangulation develops, symptoms become more acute (see Chap. XXVI). Tension within the mass increases, and there is less tendency to reducibility. Nausea and vomiting tend to become more pronounced. The pain usually increases and is so persistent that the patient seeks medical attention early. This pain at first is poorly localized, but soon becomes most prominent in the mass, radiating frequently into the depth of the abdomen. Within a few hours most of the other manifestations of intestinal strangulation, including prostration, severe tachycardia, etc., will be manifested. The temperature is normal or subnormal, but later becomes elevated. Occasionally the patient exhibits mild collapse with a cold, pale and moist skin, especially if a large amount of intestine is involved in the strangulation. Other manifestations of intestinal obstruction alone, including distention and tympanites, gradually develop (see p. 760). Enemas are ineffectual. The mass

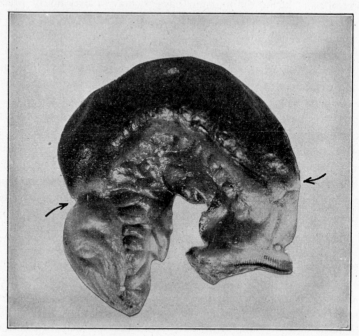

FIG. 462.—GANGRENOUS LOOP OF SMALL INTESTINE REMOVED FROM A STRANGULATED HERNIA.

The hernia had been present almost asymptomatically for a great many years. About twelve hours before admission the patient, aged forty-five, suddenly experienced severe abdominal pain, nausea and vomiting, and found that the hernia was irreducible. Marked prostration developed. At operation the entire loop of intestine constricted by the hernial sac was gangrenous; it was resected and a lateral anastomosis performed. The arrows indicate the points of constriction.

itself, if palpable, is usually moderately tense and tender. By percussion and trans-illumination of light, it may be possible to demonstrate the presence of both fluid and gas in the sac. The skin itself may become discolored but usually only after the strangulation has been present for a long time and gangrene has occurred. Spasm of abdominal muscles will be present if the hernia is intra-abdominal; if the hernia is scrotal, moderate spasm with pain may be noted in the lower abdomen.

On rare occasions, strangulation may occur in an internal hernia, and there will obviously be no demonstrable external herniation to account for the symptoms. In such instances the patient is usually operated on for intestinal obstruction, and the actual srangulation is not discovered until the time of operation. When the strangulated tissue consists solely of omentum, the pain is usually much less severe and vomiting frequently absent. The degree of tachycardia and prostration are likewise less prominent. Although strangulation of omentum is obviously followed by gangrene, this condition is not as serious as strangulated intestine. Occasionally the necrotic omentum becomes infected, which may eventually form an abscess and burrow through the skin.

The *treatment* of strangulation is of an emergency nature. If strangulation is recent or not yet present, gentle efforts at reduction may be attempted after giving a narcotic or placing the patient in a hot bath. However, if strangulation has been present for several hours, it obviously will be dangerous to manipulate the mass unduly because of the possibility of inflicting further damage, including rupture of a gangrenous loop. If possible, operation should be performed under local anesthesia because these patients do not tolerate general anesthesia well. When the hernial sac is opened a moderate amount of blood-stained fluid will usually be found within it, regardless of whether or not the contents consist of intestine or omentum. If the intestine is involved in the strangulation, color changes will be noted. In the early cases the intestine may be merely reddened or slightly cyanosed and the glistening luster of the serosa will be unchanged; in later cases the luster of the serosa will be lost, and the cyanosis so prominent that gangrene is obviously present. The viability of the intestines is determined to a great extent by the presence or absence of the glistening appearance of the serosa. If this is lost and is not regained after release of the obstruction, and application of warm wet packs for five minutes, it is usually considered unsafe to replace the affected portion of intestine. Resection of this gangrenous loop may be performed in one of several ways. If the patient appears to be in reasonably good condition and the strangulation of recent origin, it may be advisable to do a resection of the gangrenous loop with a primary anastomosis at the time of operation. On other occasions the patient may be so ill that a primary anastomosis will be inadvisable. In this case the so-called Mikulicz procedure should be carried out. According to this technic the gangrenous loop of intestine is brought out through the wound and clamps applied proximal and distal to the strangulation. The mass may or may not be removed at the time of operation. The wound is closed around the proximal and distal limbs of intestine which are anchored in approximation. In order to prevent soiling of the wound and peritoneal cavity with intestinal contents, clamps must be left on the loops for two to four days, or a rubber tube anchored in the lumen of the proximal loop to allow escape of intestinal contents. Anastomosis can be established at a later date by cutting the spur between these two double barreled loops by means of a special clamp which is applied for several days, followed several days later by a plastic repair. Such patients must be given adequate supportive treatment, including the administration of physiologic saline, Hartmann's solution, intravenous glucose, transfusion, etc., both as preoperative preparation, and postoperatively, as indicated (see Chap. VIII).

SPECIFIC TYPES OF HERNIA

Inguinal Hernia.—Hernias of this type may be either direct or indirect, but they can be more clearly discussed if the anatomic features of the *inguinal canal* are understood. This canal is an oblique passage about 4 centimeters long in the male, passing downward and medially from the abdominal (internal) to the subcutaneous (external) ring and is situated parallel to, and 2 or 3 centimeters above, Poupart's ligament. In the male it transmits the spermatic cord and vessels, the ilio-inguinal nerve and a branch of the genitocrural nerve; in the female the round ligament and the two nerves just mentioned. The roof of the canal consists primarily of the aponeurosis of the external oblique, and at the upper third, the fibers of the internal oblique. The posterior wall consists largely of the transversalis fascia. Poupart's ligament forms the lateral wall, and the arched fibers of the in-

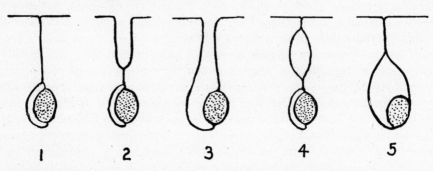

Fig. 463.—Relation of the Processus Vaginalis to the More Common Types of Hydrocele and Hernias.

1, normal obliteration of the funicular process; the distal end of the vaginal process remains at the tunica vaginalis. *2,* funicular hernia caused by the patency of the proximal portion of the process, *3,* complete patency of the process, resulting in the formation of a testicular hernia. *4,* hydrocele of the cord produced by patency of the central portion (and accumulation of fluid therein). *5,* hydrocele produced by the accumulation of fluid in the tunica vaginalis and lower portion of the funicular process; this is spoken of as a testicular hydrocele.

ternal oblique and transversalis muscle form the medial wall. The conjoined tendon is an important structure, particularly because its aponeurotic structure is useful in repair. It is a broad fascial band consisting of the union of the internal oblique, transversalis fascia and the anterior rectus sheath; it is attached to the tubercle of the symphysis pubis. The subcutaneous ring lies between the terminal portions of the conjoined tendon and Poupart's ligament; normally it is barely large enough to admit the tip of the finger. The abdominal ring cannot be palpated. The deep epigastric artery passes from its point of origin from the external iliac artery in the floor of the pelvis upward and inward toward the umbilicus from a point midway between the anterior superior spine and symphysis pubis. It lies between the peritoneum and abdominal muscles and is a landmark which determines (at operation) whether a hernia is direct or indirect; if the artery is lateral to the neck of the sac, the hernia is direct; if medial to the neck, the hernia is indirect.

Indirect (Oblique) Inguinal Hernia.—Hernias of this type in particular are usually due to a congenital defect which is presumed to be a patency of the upper end of the processus vaginalis, thereby accounting for the preformed sac into which the indirect hernia makes its entrance into the inguinal canal. This may be clarified by briefly reviewing the mechanism of the descent of the testicle. As the testicle descends from its embryonic retroperitoneal position it carries peritoneum along with it through the inguinal canal and into the scrotum. This potential sac is called the *processus vaginalis* and some time before birth becomes obliterated through its entire extent, except the part which surrounds the testicle. This portion becomes a closed potential cavity known as the *tunica vaginalis*. The part of the processus vaginalis which extends along the cord is called the funicular process. Normally the funicular process closes throughout its extent, but if this mechanism fails to take place before birth, there will be a direct communication from the peritoneal cavity down to the testicle, allowing the abdominal viscera to descend into the scrotum. This is called a *testicular* or *congenital hernia* and is usually manifested within the first year or two of life. The spermatic cord and vessels are imbedded in the wall of the sac and rarely can be separated from it. If the funicular process

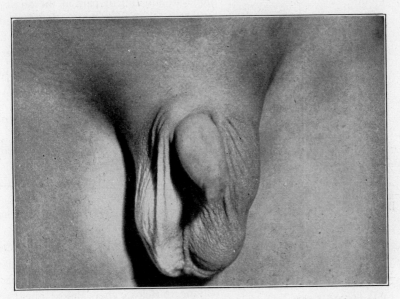

FIG. 464.—LEFT INGUINAL HERNIA IN A BOY SIX YEARS OF AGE.

Frequently more of the mass would descend into the scrotum than is shown in the photograph; however, aside from the mere presence of the hernia, very few symptoms were experienced

becomes obliterated only in its distal part, the portion persisting at the proximal end gives rise to a *funicular hernia* which is perhaps the most common type. The term *infantile hernia* is used to describe a hernia whose sac for some reason forms close to, but not into the funicular process. It is likewise common, but is differentiated with difficulty from the funicular type, even at operation. If the funicular process is obliterated at its proximal, but not at the distal end, fluid may accumulate in the latter portion of it and in the tunica vaginalis, thereby forming a hydrocele (see Fig. 463). Occasionally the process will be obliterated at each end, but will be open at some intervening portion; accumulation of fluid in such a sac is known as hydrocele of the cord. The *canal of Nuck* in the female corresponds to the processus vaginalis in the male and may be the source of herniation of the oblique (indirect) type of hernia. If the canal becomes obliterated everywhere except at one area near its midpoint, as it may do on rare occasions, a hydrocele of the canal of Nuck is formed.

Indirect hernias occur in young people, enter the abdominal (internal) ring and descend by way of the inguinal canal. There is a tendency for them to increase in size and progress in their descent, regardless of the type of congenital defect originally present. When the hernia descends past the subcutaneous (external) ring it is called *complete*. When it reaches the scrotum it is spoken of as *scrotal*. In the female the hernia may descend so far as to enter the labia majora, the homologues of the scrotum, and is called a pudendal hernia. The symptoms produced have already been described (p. 783) and consist chiefly of the appearance of a mass and a moderate amount of pain at the onset which gradually diminishes, but is supplanted by a feeling of heaviness and discomfort. The classical way to detect an inguinal hernia is to invaginate the skin of the scrotum up into the external ring of the canal with the index finger, and have the patient cough. If a hernia is present, an impulse is felt against the finger tip when the patient coughs.

Hernias are occasionally associated with undescended testicle. Conversely, most undescended testicles are associated with a hernia.

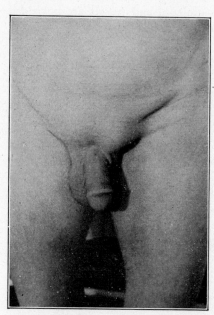

FIG. 465.—BILATERAL DIRECT HERNIA IN A FIFTY-FIVE-YEAR-OLD MAN.

The hernia on the right is not visible, but a definite impulse is made out upon coughing. Direct hernias are usually no larger than that observed on the left side; they strangulate infrequently and practically never descend into the scrotum.

Direct Inguinal Hernia.—These hernias are spoken of as acquired since there is no congenital preformed sac present. On the other hand, they depend upon the presence of a weakened transversalis fascia and oblique muscles. They almost always make their exit from the abdominal cavity at the "weak spot" in Hesselbach's triangle. This weak spot is located behind the lower fifth of the inguinal canal between the deep epigastric artery and the outer edge of the rectus muscle. As the herniation progresses anteriorly it practically always breaks into the inguinal canal, since this direction offers the least resistance. The sac presents through the external ring, is usually small and globular, and possesses a wide neck. It is, therefore, rarely the site of strangulation. Rarely does it descend into the scrotum. Direct hernia occurs practically only in men, and as a rule occurs later in life than does an indirect hernia; it is frequently bilateral. Aside from the protrusion and perhaps mild dull pain, it produces few symptoms.

Differential Diagnosis of Inguinal Hernia.—In the consideration of differentiation between inguinal hernia and other lesions in the inguinal region, the history of the development of the mass will frequently point to the correct diagnosis. For example, the history of reducibility is practically always present in hernias. They may become irreducible, but only on rare occasions do they fail to transmit an impulse upon coughing. This characteristic is almost pathognomonic of hernia. However, when a hernia becomes inflamed or strangulated it may be impossible to detect an impulse. In such an instance there will of course be a history of rather sudden onset of pain accompanying the inflammation or strangulation. Occasionally it may be difficult to distinguish between an inguinal and a femoral hernia, but an inguinal hernia always presents above Poupart's ligament, whereas a femoral hernia presents below the ligament, although the mass may extend upward and overlie it. Hydrocele may simulate inguinal scrotal hernia, but careful examination will rarely fail to make the correct diagnosis. When the mass is a hydrocele there will rarely be a history of reducibility, but there may be a gradual increase in size. An important feature is the shape. The hydrocele is pear-shaped, whereas the scrotal hernia is more cylindrical or globular. The percussion note over a hernia will be tympanitic, and peristaltic gurgling can frequently be heard by auscultation. On the other hand, the percussion note over a hydrocele is flat and no auscultatory sounds will be heard. If the hydrocele is small, it will be possible to demonstrate that the external inguinal ring is empty. There is, of course, no impulse over the hydrocele upon coughing, unless there is an associated hernia, which, however, frequently occurs. Light is transilluminated through a hydrocele, but not through a hernia. In a chylous hydrocele (containing cholesterol), light will not be transmitted.

Enlargement of the inguinal lymph nodes may occasionally be confused with a hernia of the irreducible type. A lipoma over or in the inguinal canal presents a similar difficulty. Again it is important to review the history of the development of the mass since reducibility is so constantly present some time or other in the course of a hernia. Acute inguinal lymphadenitis will usually be associated with pain and other inflammatory signs which, however, may also be demonstrable over a strangulated hernia. The sudden development of symptoms accompanying strangulated hernia is usually sufficient to establish a correct diagnosis (see p. 783). Occasionally a psoas abscess may present in the inguinal region and produce a bulging mass which resembles a hernia. In such a case the spine should be examined for the presence of Pott's disease.

Differentiation between direct and indirect hernia is of great importance at operation because of the difference in the surgical procedure required. As previously mentioned, the most important anatomic feature in the differentiation is the relation of the neck of the sac to the deep epigastric artery. An indirect hernia passes through the internal ring into the inguinal canal lateral to the deep epigastric artery, whereas a direct hernia passes into the lower portion of the inguinal canal medial to the deep epigastric artery. Unfortunately, this important feature can rarely be made out by external examination. At operation, however, this relationship of the sac to the artery is easily demonstrable. Moreover, in direct hernia the spermatic cord usually lies in front of and external to the sac, whereas in indirect hernia the cord usually lies behind and internal to the sac. As stated previously, direct hernia occurs more frequently in older people than does the indirect hernia, and rarely descends into the scrotum, whereas the indirect hernia frequently does. The shape of the sac of the direct hernia is significant since it is usually globular (not elongated); the defect in the abdominal wall is large, considering the small size of the hernia.

Treatment of Inguinal Hernia.—The treatment of inguinal hernia is confined in most instances to operative repair which, however, may not be advisable in infants and aged people. Inguinal hernia in infants can occasionally be cured by reducing the hernia and applying a yarn truss which, however, must be worn constantly for several months and must be tight enough to maintain reduction. After the age of one year, however, hernias in infants are rarely curable by this conservative treatment. In elderly people the question of operability presents itself.

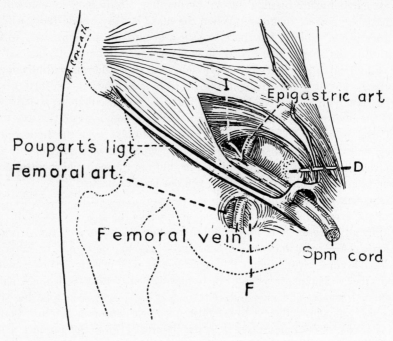

Fig. 466.—Diagram to Illustrate the Sites of Herniation of the Three Common Hernias Occurring in the Inguinal Region.

I, indirect; *D,* direct; *F,* femoral.

If the patient is no longer required to work, and the presence of a hernia produces only moderate symptoms, there may be no advantage in performing an operative repair. As a routine method of treatment, the use of a truss is unsatisfactory, but there are many instances when a properly fitted truss will be superior to other forms of treatment. For example, elderly people who live a sedentary life and who experience little pain or no inconvenience when their hernia is down, may be made comfortable by the use of a truss. A truss is likewise indicated in patients who are poor operative risks (*e.g.,* those inflicted with nephritis, myocarditis, etc.). At times there may be economic reasons for temporizing by using a truss instead of resorting to operative repair; this might be exemplified even in young patients when some defect such as amputation, blindness, etc., precludes muscular activity which is so apt to bring forth the disabling manifestations of hernia. It should be remembered that a truss cannot be worn on hernias which are not completely reducible; not only is pain produced by the truss in such instances, but strangulation may even be induced. It should likewise be emphasized that extreme pain and discomfort may be produced by wearing a truss that is applied while the hernia is not completely reduced. As a general rule, therefore, the patient is instructed to apply the truss while lying down, and after he has reduced the hernia. The growing tendency of various industrial corporations during recent years to hire no one who has a hernia (because of compensation responsibility) is frequently sufficient inducement for an unemployed person to have his hernia repaired.

On many occasions, the tendency for a hernia to become irreducible will be sufficient cause for advising herniotomy, because of the likelihood of strangulation as a sequel to irreducibility. Operation is particularly indicated if manifestations of obstruction or strangulation were present while the hernia was irreducible. A hernia in which the neck of the sac is small is more apt to strangulate than is a hernia with a large sac; this factor also affects the decision to operate.

The modern *operation for* the cure of inguinal hernia has many variations but its essential steps are first, opening the inguinal canal, second, careful dissection of and high ligation of the sac, third, closure of the canal. These features were first described independently by *Halsted* and by *Bassini* nearly fifty years ago. The variations in the operation are mainly concerned with the third step, *i.e.,* the method of closure of the canal after the sac has been eliminated. Halsted and Bassini both closed the canal after transplantation of the cord which normally passes through this structure. *Ferguson,* writing several years later (1899) condemned transplantation of the cord. It is important to note however that Halsted later described an operation in which the cord was not transplanted. Indeed, of the three names usually stated as originators of the modern operation (*i.e.,* Halsted, Bassini and Ferguson), Halsted is the only one who continued, after his original publication, to write about his experiences during which he made additional contributions to the subject. Thus it may be stated that he probably did more toward the gradual perfection of inguinal herniotomy than any other surgeon. The following description (cord not transplanted) is a brief composite one and is known by many surgeons as the Halsted technic, whereas others designate it as being a modified Ferguson operation.

An incision, parallel to and slightly above Poupart's ligament is carried through the external oblique aponeurosis, thereby opening the inguinal canal. The sac is then isolated, opened, its contents reduced, the neck ligated as high as possible, and excised distal to the ligature. Repair consists of the approximation of the conjoined tendon to the shelving portion of Poupart's ligament with interrupted sutures. An opening corresponding to the subcutaneous ring is left at the lower end near the pubic tubercle just large enough to transmit the cord. The external oblique is then closed. Transplantation of the cord, thus, is not practiced at the present time as a routine by most surgeons. However, in recurrent hernias or direct inguinal hernias most surgeons do transplant the cord either subcutaneously as originally described by Halsted or between the external and internal oblique fascia as described by Bassini.

Additional features include suture of the cremasteric muscle to the internal oblique for additional support which was recommended by Halsted in 1903. Halsted also suggested the use of a flap of the anterior rectus sheath in cases where the conjoined tendon was atrophied or weak. During recent years there has been an almost universal shift from the use of chromic catgut in the repair of hernias to the use of silk (as originally recommended by Halsted), or cotton. Unquestionably, the percentage recurrence will be reduced by silk. The use of fascia as an additional detail in the repair of hernia is mentioned below.

In the repair of any hernia it is extremely essential that the structures sutured in apposition consist largely of connective tissue. Its importance is demonstrated by the experimental work of Seelig and Chouke [2] who noted that suture of muscle to muscle, or even muscle to fascia, did not result in so strong a union as when both structures consisted of fascia. It is obvious then that when an inguinal hernia is repaired, the conjoined tendon instead of the internal oblique muscle should be sutured to Poupart's ligament if possible. Tension in suturing the structures in a repair should be avoided, since it is an important factor in the development of recurrence, particularly if catgut is used.

In an effort to prevent recurrences which are apt to follow even expert repair, McArthur [3] introduced the use of a fascial strip from the external oblique aponeurosis as a suture to increase the solidity and permanency of the repair. The authors wish to emphasize the importance of using a strip of fascia about one-half centimeter wide cut from the external oblique aponeurosis as McArthur originally described. By leaving the distal end attached at the pubic tubercle, a strip of ample length can be obtained to reinforce the suture line. This should be done on all hernias when the structures are weak, or when approximation by the sutures is obtained only by tension. Such a procedure is simple, done quickly and will certainly diminish the number of recurrences. This principle has been enlarged upon by Gallie and LeMesurier [4] who recommended the use of strips taken from the fascia lata removed from the lateral aspect of the thigh. The defect in large hernias may be so great that a satisfactory repair cannot be made without the use of these fascial strips which are used to reinforce the suture line, especially that approximating conjoined tendon and Poupart's ligament.

As stated previously, the development of strangulation makes immediate operation imperative. The decision as to the type of operation to be performed in such instances depends upon such factors as duration of strangulation, amount of intestine involved, condition of the patient, etc. Frequently, these factors will prevent the performance of a painstaking and orthodox repair; in fact, the patient's condition may be so precarious as to justify rapid closure without thought as to the possibility of recurrence.

Although herniotomy may be considered one of the simplest of the major operations, complications will appear in a surprisingly large percentage of cases. Very few complications will be encountered in patients under 20 years of age; after that age they increase in a direct ratio as the age increases. In a study of 2,000 herniotomies Beekman and Sullivan [5] noted an incidence of 8.5 per cent of respiratory lesions: the incidence of atelectasis was 2.3 per cent, pneumonia 0.7 per cent and pulmonary embolism 0.6 per cent. Although the incidence of pneumonia was greatest following general anesthesia, Beekman and Sullivan noted other respiratory lesions were decreased. For example, they found the incidence of all types of respiratory lesions to be 7.3 per cent following general anesthesia, 9.1 per cent following spinal, and 10.3 per cent following local anesthesia. The incidence of postoperative wound infection will vary from 1 to 5 per cent depending upon circumstances, but is observed by all surgeons to be much less following the use of silk or cotton. The mortality rate in inguinal herniotomy (exclusive of strangulated hernia), should be appreciably under one per cent.

During recent years the injection treatment of hernias (using a sclerosing substance) has been revived, but its application is extremely limited. Wernicke [7] and others have emphasized that only small indirect hernias should be subjected to this type of therapy.

Sliding Hernia.—Hernias of this type are in reality caused by a slipping of the posterior parietal peritoneum on the underlying tissue, thereby allowing the colon to descend as a herniation (usually inguinal, rarely femoral). The identification of such hernias is rarely made, except at operation. Sliding hernias on the right side usually contain the cecum and appendix; on the left side, sigmoid. In either case they are usually of the indirect type. If such hernias are small no sac may be present. As the mass enlarges a fold of peritoneum descends with the colon, forming a sac on the anterior portion of the mass. Sliding hernias descend so readily that a truss is rarely satisfactory in maintaining reduction. Operative repair is usually difficult. If the hernia is small, the lack of a sac may lead the surgeon into the error of mistaking the colon for the sac and opening it. After mobilization of the colon, and separation of adhesions between it and the sac, it is frequently advisable to anchor the colon to the posterior wall of the pelvis. Repair of the defect may be difficult because of the large size of the opening through which the mass herniates.

Occasionally, in direct hernias or in large indirect hernias with a widely dilated internal ring, the bladder becomes displaced and presents in the hernia. The amount of sac present varies with the size of the hernia. In operative repair it is extremely important to recognize the bladder as a part of the contents, because of the danger of injury. The surgeon should be warned by brisk bleeding from the vascular wall of the bladder and the appearance of the muscular wall, as contrasted to the areolar tissue adjacent to it. If through error, the bladder is opened, it should be closed promptly and a retention catheter inserted at completion of the operation.

Femoral Hernia.—This type of hernia occurs much more commonly in women than men (ratio about 3 to 1) and is confined almost entirely to adults, although it is slightly less common even in women than the inguinal variety. The hernia makes its descent into the femoral canal through the femoral ring, located in the floor of the peritoneal cavity. Weakness of Gimbernat's ligament, which bounds the femoral ring on the inner side is apparently the most important factor in the development of a femoral hernia. The fact that this ligament is more poorly developed in women than in men presumably accounts for the greater incidence of femoral hernia in women than in men. The *femoral canal* represents the narrow space between the femoral vein and the inner wall of the femoral sheath. Normally it is only about one-half an inch long and contains nothing more than a few lymphatic vessels and a little fat. As the hernia descends into the femoral canal it soon reaches the saphenous opening which offers little resistance, thereby allowing the hernia to appear in the soft tissues of the thigh. In general, these hernias are smaller than inguinal hernias and indeed may be present without a mass or other external manifestations. Strangulation is frequently encountered because of the narrow sac and the sharpness of the edge of Gimbernat's ligament. For the same reason, the femoral ring is perhaps the most frequent site for Richter's hernia, which is apt to produce a strangulation, but only of the small portion of the intestinal wall which is pinched in the neck of the sac. Cramping pain, perhaps of a disabling type, is present, even though the entire lumen is not blocked; other manifestations of strangulation are not apt to be present because the mesenteric vessels are not involved. In this type of hernia, the diagnosis may be extremely difficult because of the small size or absence of a hernial mass, and the lack of complete obstruction. Immediate operation, of course, is imperative because of the tendency for the rapid development of gangrene. In fact, any type of strangulation in femoral hernias is usually associated with the early development of gangrene on account of the narrowness of the ring.

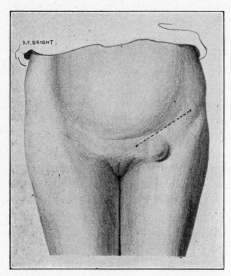

FIG. 467.—FEMORAL HERNIA IN A WOMAN.

Note that the mass which descends through the femoral canal is located below Poupart's ligament, which is indicated by the dotted line.

The *clinical manifestations* of uncomplicated femoral hernia are not unlike those described for hernias in general. However, because of their small size they are apt to contain only omentum, and therefore present so few symptoms and signs that they are frequently unnoticed by the patient. Such hernias may even strangulate and be unnoticed externally. However, if a loop of bowel is strangulated, the manifestations of intestinal obstruction will be so obvious that laparotomy is demanded.

If the omentum becomes adherent to the sac there may be a dragging type of dull pain. When intestines descend into the sac, the pain is apt to be more severe and be colicky because of the obstruction present. The hernial mass appears below Poupart's ligament at the saphenous opening and rarely attains a size larger than a hen's egg. At times the mass may extend upward over Poupart's ligament and thereby offer confusion in differential diagnosis between inguinal hernia, inguinal lymphadenopathy, etc. The similarity of a saphenous varix to a small femoral hernia should be emphasized because of the obvious difference in treatment. Although a saphenous varix is soft and compressible, as is a hernia, the varix disappears spontaneously when the patient lies down. When the patient coughs an actual impulse may be palpated over the varix, but a characteristic thrill can also be felt which is absent over a hernia. The skin over the varix may be bluish; frequently there are varicose veins on the extremity.

The *treatment* of femoral hernia is chiefly surgical because of the difficulty in obtaining a truss which will fit the patient and maintain reduction of the mass. If the mass protrudes beyond the truss, as it frequently does, strangulation is thereby encouraged. Even in the absence of many symptoms, if intestine protrudes into the sac, it is wise to repair the hernia for prophylactic reasons, since serious complications, such as strangulation and early gangrene, are so apt to occur.

Operative repair may be done by the femoral or inguinal route. When the femoral route is chosen, incision is made over the hernial mass extending upward above Poupart's ligament. The sac is dissected out, the contents reduced and the sac opened. It is then pulled down as far as possible so that the neck may be ligated high. The rest of the sac is then excised. Repair is carried out by approximation of Cooper's ligament to Poupart's ligament and the pectineal fascia to the falciform process of the fascia lata by interrupted sutures. Particular care should be taken to avoid injury to the femoral vein which is immediately lateral to the hernia. In operating on a strangulation, or even incarcerated femoral hernia, it is often necessary to enlarge the femoral ring. The edge of the ring should be nicked on the medial side in order not to injure the femoral vein. When the repair is made by the inguinal route, as was first recommended by Annandale in 1876, the incision is made from a point above the external inguinal ring extending downward over the femoral mass. The external oblique aponeurosis is split, the cremaster muscle and transversalis fascia likewise split, exposing the peritoneum at the neck of the femoral hernia. The advantage of this operation and the necessity of the use of Cooper's ligament in repair have been emphasized by Seelig and Tuholske.[6] The important feature in the repair is the approximation of Cooper's ligament (likewise Gimbernat's ligament) to the edge of Poupart's ligament by interrupted sutures. It is then necessary to repair the incision made in the inguinal region as described in the repair of the inguinal hernia. The cord may or may not be transplanted.

There is no doubt that the repair by way of the inguinal route as described above will be followed by fewer recurrences of the femoral hernia than any other type of repair available. However, this procedure adds tremendously to the intricacy of the repair and should not be attempted by the unskilled surgeon. There is likewise an added risk of paving the way for the development of an inguinal hernia. The results of repair of femoral hernias through the femoral route alone should be satisfactory except in the large hernias. When a laparotomy through the right rectus muscle has been performed for intestinal obstruction of unknown origin and a femoral hernia found, the repair of the sac after reduction of the mass is done by a simple purse-string suture.

Postoperative (Incisional, Ventral) Hernia.—This type of hernia is unfortunately common, but can be prevented to a great extent by careful aseptic technic and proper closure of abdominal wounds. Suppuration of the wound is conducive to the formation of hernias, but obviously infection of the wound cannot be avoided when intra-abdominal abscesses are drained. Thus, hernia is apt to follow operations for drainage of intra-abdominal abscesses (*e.g.*, appendiceal abscess). It is most common in the lower abdomen, partly because of the lack of a posterior rectus sheath. Postoperative hernias are also prone to occur in fat people. Any pulmonary complication which results in frequent coughing during the first five or six postoperative days may produce sufficient damage to pave the way for the development of a hernia, or even to produce a rupture of the wound which usually demands immediate closure. Certain types of incisions are less apt to be followed by herniation than others. The so-called "paramedian incision," made through the rectus fascia, retracting the muscle outward, is less apt to be followed by a hernia than are other incisions, because the rectus muscle falls over the line of suture and supports it when the wound is closed. Obviously, incisional hernias are nearly always abdominal, but on rare occasions may be located elsewhere (*e.g.,* transpleural hernia of the thorax).

If the fatty subcutaneous tissue is thick, the hernial mass may burrow for a considerable distance subcutaneously, especially downward, because of gravity. Rarely it may enlarge in a mushroom fashion until a large proportion of the con-

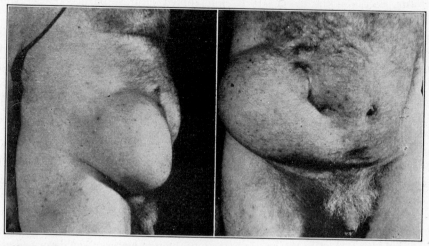

FIG. 468.—LATERAL AND ANTERIOR VIEW OF A POSTOPERATIVE (INCISIONAL, VENTRAL) HERNIA.

Although the hernia was irreducible the patient had had no obstructive symptoms since the onset, over twenty-five years previously.

tents of the abdominal cavity are contained in the sac. The omentum becomes adherent to the sac early, and if the sac becomes adherent to loops of intestine also, as it frequently does, the greater portion of the hernia may become irreducible. When the hernia first develops, the patient nearly always complains of a dragging pain arising in the neighborhood of the scar, but perhaps radiating deep into the abdomen. Early in the formation of the hernia, tenderness at the site of the defect is pronounced. When the hernia develops within a few days following laparotomy, because of partial rupture of the deep layers of the wound, the intestines herniating into the defect may at times become adherent and obstructed, thereby creating serious postoperative complications. Usually, however, definite evidence of a hernia is not demonstrable, subjectively or objectively, for several weeks or months following operation. Besides the dragging pain mentioned above, other symptoms, including constipation, anorexia, cramping pain, and even vomiting may develop. Strangulation is not usual because of the large ring.

The *treatment* depends to a great extent upon the size of the hernia and the condition of the patient, especially his age. If the hernia is reducible, the patient may be fitted with a large elastic belt or support which, in general, is unsatisfactory but may relieve the symptoms if applied correctly, *i.e.*, when the patient is lying down and the hernia is reduced. If the belt does not relieve the symptoms, or the patient is young and still active physically, operative repair will be indicated. At operation the contents of the hernia are reduced, and the sac, which is frequently multiloculated, excised; the peritoneum and fascia are then closed. When a large part of the abdominal viscera (ileum, colon, omentum, spleen, etc.) have become herniated, the resultant decrease in the size of the peritoneal cavity may make reduction difficult or impossible. The fascia must be dissected free from fatty tissue, overlapped and anchored with interrupted sutures of silk. If the defect is too large to allow satisfactory closure without undue tension, it may be necessary to resort to the use of strips of fascia lata as reinforcing sutures (Gallie and LeMesurier [4]).

For some unaccountable reason, repair of large hernias (incisional and others) occasionally results in a fatality of mysterious etiology; manifestations of prostration, including also respiratory difficulty, and an elevated blood pressure and temperature are usually present. It is possible that the cause of death is associated with the marked increase in intra-abdominal pressure incident to the reduction of the hernia and its repair. It is more apt to occur in obese people.

Umbilical Hernia.—With few exceptions hernias of this type are caused by a congenital defect of the abdominal wall at the umbilicus, and appear either in infancy or in late adult life. Normally, the umbilical ring closes after the ligation of the cord and its contents atrophy, resulting in scar tissue which forms a firm support at the umbilicus, covered by skin. Hernias at the umbilicus develop most commonly during infancy (up to two years) and are supposedly caused by an unusual strain causing rupture at a weak point, allowing a protrusion of a peritoneal sac, which is small and usually contains only omentum. The first evidence of a hernia will be evinced by a protrusion of the umbilicus when the child cries. Such a hernia rarely produces any demonstrable symptoms. Unless treated it may enlarge until intestine also protrudes into the sac. The neck of the sac is small (1 to 1½ centimeters in diameter) in children, but may attain a size two or three times as large. To be effective, treatment should be instituted as soon as the hernia is detected, but need not be operative. A strip of adhesive is placed transversely across the abdomen over the umbilicus tightly so that the skin folds inward. If desired, a small pad may be placed under the adhesive at the umbilicus. This treatment must be maintained for several months before closure of the defect may be expected. Frequently, the hernia is apparently eradicated by this type of fixation, but recurs years later. After the age of eighteen months, this type of conservative therapy will rarely be effective, regardless of whether or not it has been in use previous to this time. Cure can then be effected only by operation.

Umbilical hernias in adults occur usually in the latter part of life and are three or four times more common in women than in men. Relaxation of the abdominal muscles during pregnancy, obesity and debilitating diseases appear to be important etiologic factors. The herniation may take place directly through the umbilicus or a short distance to either side. Occasionally there are several openings. The omentum first protrudes into the hernia, but as the sac enlarges, intestine (usually colon) also is included. Adhesion of the sac to the omentum and intestine takes place early, and is usually so extensive that the hernial mass is lobulated or divided into compartments. The skin over the hernia is thin and very little subcutaneous tissue intervenes between it and the contents of the sac. For this reason, peristaltic movements are readily demonstrable if intestines are included in the sac. The symptoms of umbilical hernia in adults may not be pronounced, but include such complaints as constipation, dragging. pain and anorexia, especially if the hernia is large. The development of cramping pain, nausea and especially vomiting, indicate partial or complete obstruction. On account of the thin skin and the protrusion of the mass, the skin becomes traumatized readily and ulceration may develop. As the duration of the hernia increases, irreducibility becomes more pronounced. Strangulation is common.

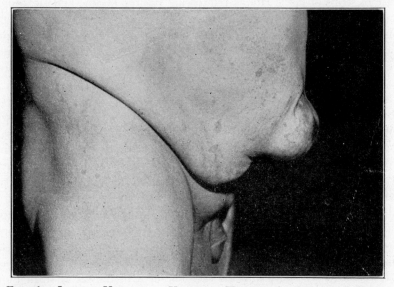

FIG. 469.—LATERAL VIEW OF AN UMBILICAL HERNIA IN A MAN, AGED FIFTY.
The mass had been present for fifteen years, had never been strangulated, but for many years had been incompletely reducible.

The *treatment* of umbilical hernia in adults is confined almost solely to operative repair. Elastic belts or supports usually fail to relieve symptoms and are usually harmful if the hernia is irreducible, which is usually the case, at least by the time the patient comes to the physician for relief. Operation consists of an elliptical incision made in a transverse direction (Mayo), excising a portion of the redundant skin and subcutaneous fatty tissue. This must be done with extreme care since the intestine in the dome of the sac usually lies immediately beneath the skin. After reduction of the intestine the adherent omentum is ligated and removed with the sac. The various layers of the abdominal wall, including the fascia, transversalis aponeurosis and peritoneum may be treated as one and overlapped, the upper flap over the lower after a slit is made laterally to the rectus muscle on each side to facilitate overlapping; the peritoneum must be removed from the internal surface of the external flap so as to encourage solid healing. Moreover, it is important to dissect off all fatty tissue from the sides of the flaps to be approximated. The sutures used to anchor the flaps in position should be interrupted silk. If it is possible to dissect the peritoneum from the fascia, it should be closed as a separate layer. Occasionally it may be advantageous to make the incision in a longitudinal direction. If the hernia is large, it may be advisable to use fascial sutures in its repair.

Diaphragmatic Hernia.—Diaphragmatic hernia is a protrusion of abdominal viscera into the thoracic cavity through an opening of the diaphragm. It is rare, occurring on the left side in 80 to 90 per cent of cases and usually is not associated with a true sac. There are three types of diaphragmatic hernias: (1) congenital

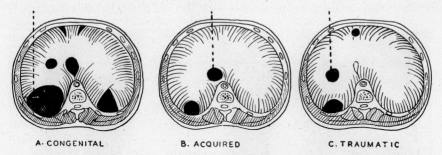

A. CONGENITAL   B. ACQUIRED   C. TRAUMATIC

FIG. 470.—DIAGRAMS ILLUSTRATING THREE TYPES OF DIAPHRAGMATIC HERNIA DESCRIBED IN THE TEXT.

Note the various defects through which such a herniation may occur. (Modified from Woolsey, *J. Am. M. Ass.*, 89:2245, 1927.)

hernias, usually present at birth; (2) acquired; and (3) traumatic. Of a series of 106 cases collected in 1927 by Woolsey [8] 50 were congenital, 28 acquired and 28 traumatic. The *congenital* variety is in reality not a true hernia, since an absence of a portion, or all of the leaf of the diaphragm, is the actual lesion present, thereby allowing the abdominal viscera to protrude into the thoracic cavity. The defect most common is a failure of fusion at the left pleuroperitoneal hiatus (foramen of Bochdalek). Most of the hernias of the *acquired* type are associated with a sac (71 per cent of Woolsey's series) and usually present through the esophageal hiatus. Most hiatus hernias are so small that the contents of the sac are limited to part of the stomach. It seems probable that many of the acquired type which are manifested in adult life are secondary to small defects in the diaphragm (usually at the esophageal hiatus) and that they are produced by a strain of some sort, which causes a protrusion of abdominal viscera through the weak spot. The *traumatic* hernias are caused by laceration due to a foreign body, or to a rupture resulting from a sudden change in pressure in the pleural or abdominal cavity, usually the latter; the dome of the diaphragm is the most common site. Obviously few of these hernias will be associated with a sac.

The *clinical manifestations* of diaphragmatic hernia are varied, and in many instances no symptoms exist. When the herniation is secondary to a *congenital* absence of a large portion of the diaphragm, symptoms are usually severe and are manifested soon after birth. These manifestations consist of dyspnea, cyanosis, tachycardia, constipation and occasionally symptoms of intestinal obstruction. Vomiting may be persistent. Hiccup is not uncommon. X-ray examination may reveal a displacement of the heart, thereby explaining the cardiac symptoms. Frequently, congenital hernias exist for years without producing any symptoms whatsoever.

The manifestations of the *acquired* type (Hiatus hernia) are rarely so acute as those mentioned above. Pain radiating upward into the shoulder or downward into the peritoneal cavity may be the first complaint. Digestive symptoms such as anorexia, nausea and vomiting or regurgitation without premonition, are not uncommon. Symptoms are so inconstant that they may simulate those of peptic ulcer, cholecystitis, heart disease, etc. Dysphagia, hemorrhage due to ulceration, and even cardiac symptoms due to pressure of the herniated mass may occur. Auscultation of the chest may reveal gurgling sounds over the left chest, but this may not be of

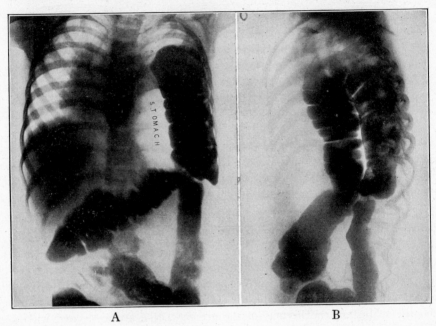

A   B

FIG. 471.—DIAPHRAGMATIC HERNIA IN A CHILD OF FIVE YEARS; ROENTGENOGRAM AFTER BARIUM ENEMA.

Note that the colon, as well as the stomach, has herniated through the defect in the diaphragm. *A,* anteroposterior view. *B,* lateral view.

great diagnostic aid, because of the transmission of such sounds upward from the stomach in normal individuals. A tympanitic note to percussion over the left chest should lead one to suspect diaphragmatic hernia. A roentgen examination, especially with the barium meal or enema, will usually lead to the correct diagnosis. When the hernia is small it may recede upon standing, and symptoms therefore become decreased. In such instances, the x-ray examination must be performed with the patient in the prone position, since gravity will pull the stomach downward while the patient is standing and thereby reduce the hernia.

On some occasions, it may be difficult to differentiate true diaphragmatic hernia from an *eventration of the diaphragm.* In the latter instance the diaphragm is elevated to an unusual height and is rarely mobile, thereby indicating that a disturbance in the innervation exists. A thorough discussion of eventration may be found in the publications of Lord,[9] Clopton [10] and others.

As stated, *traumatic* hernias are caused by injury of the direct or indirect type and may or may not be associated with symptoms at the time of injury. Obviously a sac is rarely present. Symptoms are dependent to a great extent upon the time and extent of herniation. The manifestations are similar to those described under the acquired type.

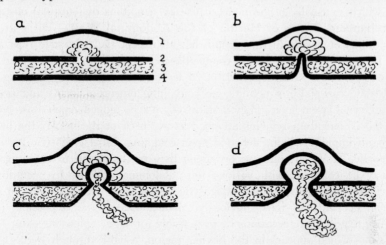

FIG. 472.—EPIGASTRIC HERNIA AND SUBSEROUS LIPOMA.

a, subserous lipoma, after breaking through sheath of rectus. *b*, subserous lipoma with some peritoneum pulled up into the fascial slit. *c*, subserous lipoma with a hernia sac containing some protruded omentum (epigastric fatty hernia). *d*, simple epigastric hernia, without lipoma. (Redrawn from De Quervain, *Clinical Surgical Diagnosis*, 3rd Eng. ed., 1922. Courtesy of Wm. Wood and Co., New York.)

The *treatment* of diaphragmatic hernias is surgical, but on many occasions, small hernias produce such few symptoms that repair is not necessary. Either the thoracic or abdominal route may be used in the repair. Usually better exposure is obtained through the thoracic route. If the hernia is large and the viscera adherent, reduction cannot be obtained through an abdominal incision. There is no more danger from ill effects of pneumothorax when operating through a thoracic incision than there is through an abdominal incision, since a pneumothorax is immediately produced in the latter instance as soon as the viscera are released from their position in the defect of the diaphragm. A positive pressure type of anesthesia is usually advisable. However, as Harrington[11] has pointed out, most hiatus hernias are most readily repaired through an abdominal incision. After the viscera are reduced, the defect in the diaphragm is repaired by suturing the edges together, and reinforced, if necessary, by fascial sutures. Crushing the phrenic nerve two or three days before the major operation will make the repair of the hernia much easier because the diaphragm will be elevated and its movements eliminated. In fact, in elderly debilitated patients, one may not be justified in doing more than this, since this procedure is apt to alleviate or eliminate symptoms in small hernias (Morton[12]). The stomach is sometimes sutured in place against the repaired diaphragm if the entire defect cannot be closed, but this procedure will seldom be found necessary if fascial transplants are used, either as woven strips or a segment of fascia lata.

Internal Hernia.—There are a number of fossae or depressions located chiefly on the posterior peritoneal surface of the abdominal cavity into which small loops of intestine may herniate on rare occasions. The most important of these are the duodenal (inferior, superior and paraduodenal) and cecal (ileocolic, ileocecal and retrocecal). Such hernias are not diagnosed clinically, but are encountered at operation, which is usually performed because of symptoms of intestinal obstruction.

Miscellaneous Types of Hernia of the Abdominal Wall.—There are many different kinds of hernia in this group, but all except the epigastric type are extremely rare. An *epigastric hernia* frequently consists of nothing more than a protrusion of properitoneal fat (properitoneal hernia) through a tiny opening in the linea albea. Occasionally, a definite sac containing omentum forms and protrudes past the external fascia layer. They may or may not be reducible; on most occasions a small tab of omentum remains attached at the neck of the sac. If the hernia is reducible, an impulse may be detected upon coughing. Most epigastric hernias are asymptomatic. However, on rare occasions they produce pain in the epigastrium which may be confused with various intra-abdominal lesions. In such instances repair will be indicated. A small epigastric hernia may occur without producing any visible or palpable signs; obviously, clinical diagnosis is impossible in such cases. They may on rare occasions be responsible for vague epigastric pain. *Lumbar hernia* is one which appears in the lumbar region, usually through Petit's triangle or the space of Grynfelt. An *obturator hernia* passes through the obturator foramen of the innominate bone, but usually presents no external manifestations. *Perineal hernias,* also extremely rare, occur usually in women and make their exit in the perineum at a variety of "weak points." *Sciatic hernia,* which is so rare as to be a surgical curiosity, passes out through either the greater or lesser sacrosciatic foramen.

BIBLIOGRAPHY

1. WATSON, L. F.   *Hernia,* C. V. Mosby Co., 2nd ed., 1938, St. Louis.
2. SEELIG, M. G., and CHOUKE, K. S.   Fundamental Factor in Recurrence of Inguinal Hernia, *Arch. Surg.,* 7:553, 1923.
3. McARTHUR, L. L.   Autoplastic Suture in Hernia and Other Diastases, *J. Am. M. Ass.,* 37:1162, 1901.
4. GALLIE, W. E., and LeMESURIER, A. B.   The Use of Living Sutures in Operative Surgery, *Canad. M. Ass. J.,* 11:504, 1921.
5. BEEKMAN, F., and SULLIVAN, J. E.   Analysis of Immediate Postoperative Complication in 2000 Cases of Inguinal Hernia, *Surg., Gynec. & Obst.,* 68:1052, 1939.
6. SEELIG, M. G., and TUHOLSKE, L.   The Inguinal Route Operation for Femoral Hernia; with a Supplementary Note on Cooper's Ligament, *Surg., Gynec. & Obst.,* 18:55, 1914.
7. WERNICKE, H. O.   The Injection Treatment of Hernia, *Surg., Gynec. & Obst.,* 68:1093, 1939.
8. WOOLSEY, J. H.   Diaphragmatic Hernia, *J. Am. M. Ass.,* 89:2245, 1927.
9. LORD, F. T.   Eventration of Diaphragm; Diagnosis and Treatment, *Arch. Surg.,* 14:316, 1927.
10. CLOPTON, M. B.   Eventration of Diaphragm, *Ann. Surg.,* 78:154, 1923.
11. HARRINGTON, S. W.   Esophageal Hiatus Diaphragmatic Hernia, *J. Thoracic Surg.,* 8:127, 1938-39.
12. MORTON, J. J.   Herniation Through the Diaphragm, *Surg., Gynec. & Obst.,* 68:257, 1939.

CHAPTER XXVIII

THE BREAST

Neoplasms
Infections
Miscellaneous Lesions

Even though the mammary gland is a superficial and readily observable organ, its pathologic conditions often offer considerable difficulty in early diagnosis, particularly in regard to neoplastic disease to which it is especially prone. Simple clinical examination, *i.e.*, inspection and palpation, is of particular importance and presupposes, of course, a definite knowledge of normal structures.

The Normal Breast.—In the female the breast, as one of the secondary sex organs, begins to develop with the onset of puberty when it rapidly undergoes enlargement due to a growth of the acinous (secreting or lactiferous) cells, the many collecting ducts, and particularly of the supporting framework, especially the hyaline connective tissue around the ducts. In addition there are numerous fibrous tissue strands which support this growing mass of tissue and which extend outward toward the nipple and the skin (suspensory ligaments of Cooper).

The size and consistency of the normal female breast varies considerably. It may be firm and elastic or soft and compressible, dependent largely on the relative amount of subcutaneous fat, and of hyaline connective tissue. The most important structure, however, is the parenchymatous tissue, *i.e.*, the acini and ducts. These are more readily palpable in the patient with a thin layer of subcutaneous fat; the parenchymatous tissue is distinctly firmer than the fatty and areolar tissue and normally imparts a slightly nodular sensation on palpation. Very commonly, one makes out a more grossly nodular or shotty character exhibited by the breast; this is usually described as chronic cystic mastitis, a condition which will be discussed later. Variations in size are normal unless true hypertrophy occurs to an extent embarrassing to the patient. The breast is often pendulous in elderly women and particularly after repeated lactation.

The nipple or teat is located in the center of the pigmented areola and is a rounded conical projection at the apex of which empty the twenty or more ducts which drain the lactiferous (acinous) tissue. The nipple is supplied with muscle fibers and is an erectile organ, responding often to mechanical stimulation, but frequently remaining retracted, particularly in young girls. This retraction is of no significance, except that it may interfere with nursing during lactation. Retraction of the nipple as a sign of cancer is discussed later.

The normal female breast, which at puberty develops in response to awakening endocrine activity, is also influenced by the cyclic variations in the production of

ovarian hormones which occur each lunar month with the appearance of menstruation. The same sex hormones (estrin and progestin) which are responsible for
changes in the uterus also provoke changes in the breast. The patient is often
aware of these changes, *e.g.,* fullness and pain in the breast. Microscopic study of
breast parenchyma has shown that the epithelium undergoes periodic hyperplasia
and involution of a nature analogous to that of the endometrium. A detailed study
of these histologic changes based on examination of human tissue during various

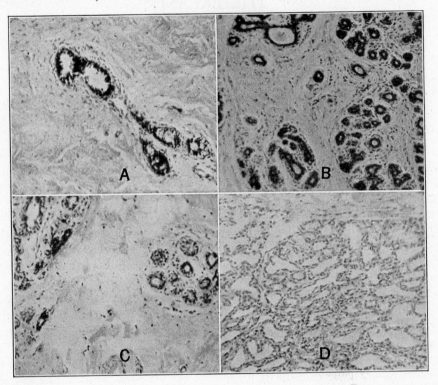

FIG. 473.—THE NORMAL FEMALE BREAST; PHOTOMICROGRAPHS OF THE PARENCHYMA UNDER
VARIOUS PHYSIOLOGIC CONDITIONS.

A, before the onset of puberty. *B,* the hyperplastic breast during menstruation. *C,* the resting
breast, showing the usual involution associated with the cessation of menstruation. *D,* the
lactating breast; note the absence of stroma and the many acini filled with milk.

stages of the menstrual cycle have been published by Lewis and Geschickter.[1]
During pregnancy the breast enlarges and becomes more vascular than normal.
With the approach of parturition the congestion becomes still more marked and is
due to the onset of lactation, the breast becoming filled with milk. The enlargement
may be so rapid as to provoke considerable pain. Involution occurs with subsidence
of lactation. At the menopause in most women the parenchymatous cells undergo a
gradual involution or atrophy. These changes are of special importance in considering the pathogenesis of nodular breast (chronic cystic mastitis).

In examining the female breast it is important to palpate the organ with the
patient in both the sitting and recumbent position. In the latter case the parenchyma

is felt against the anterior chest wall and pectoral muscle with the tips of the fingers; in the former case it is felt between the thumb and fingers of one hand or the fingers of both hands. Often a mass or nodule which might otherwise escape detection may be felt if the examiner stands behind the patient and palpates the breast with the palm of the hand. The skin over the breast is also examined, especially for retraction or attachment to the underlying parenchyma. No examination is complete without palpation of the axillary lymph nodes. Palpation is most accurate if the finger tips are inserted high into the axilla on the outer side of the axilla before pressing against the chest wall and palpating downward; by this maneuver the

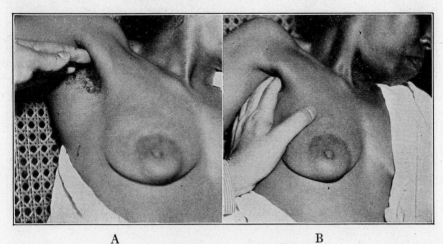

A   B

FIG. 474.—PALPATION OF THE AXILLARY LYMPH NODES.

A, the tips of the examiner's fingers are placed high in the axilla with the patient's arm abducted; the back of the hand lies along the upper end and head of the humerus. *B,* as the patient's arm is brought to the side the examiner's fingers are brought against the chest wall, palpating any nodes by rolling them between the pad of the finger tips and the ribs of the thoracic cage.

nodes are not pushed into the apex of the axilla before they can be palpated by the fingers. The axillary lymph nodes may be normally palpable as small shot-like structures. The lymph nodes above the clavicle are also noted because they become enlarged and palpable occasionally, especially in malignant disease.

Of the many diseases which occur in the breast, neoplasms are the most important. Second are the inflammatory lesions or infections. Finally a miscellaneous group will be considered. These conditions apply almost entirely to the female breast. The male breast, a tiny rudimentary structure composed of a few ducts and mostly connective tissue, is only rarely the seat of disease; inflammatory and neoplastic lesions occur, the latter not infrequently malignant. In any case they present similar features and in most instances require the same treatment as in females. An excellent book on diseases of the breast is that by Geschickter[18].

NEOPLASMS

Under this heading will be included not only the frankly neoplastic lesions, benign and malignant, but also the so-called chronic cystic mastitis which, in spite of its designation, is probably not an inflammatory disease at all, but secondary to hyperplastic changes, instigated by endocrine activity. Cysts in the breast though considered separately are usually a manifestation of chronic cystic mastitis, which because of its frequency will be discussed first. A detailed monograph on tumors of the breast is that of Cheatle and Cutler.[2]

Chronic Cystic Mastitis.—This designation, in reality a microscopic term, is applied clinically to the exceedingly common nodular breast. Other terms: cystic

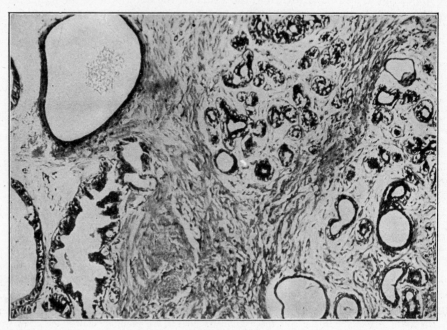

FIG. 475.—CHRONIC CYSTIC MASTITIS.

Photomicrograph (low power) of tissue in a lump removed from a forty-two-year-old housewife who first noted the tumor one year previously; there was no pain or increase in size. Examination revealed a lemon-sized nodular mass, freely movable but attached to and part of the parenchyma. Note the numerous cysts, some distended with fluid, others lined by hyperplastic epithelium; higher power magnifications are shown in Figure 476. Nowhere was malignant tissue seen although four blocks were cut from various portions of the lump. The periductile fibrosis and round cell infiltration were not marked (see Figures 477 and 492).

disease of the breast, Schimmelbusch's disease, chronic interstitial mastitis, chronic lobular mastitis, cobblestone breast, nodular breast, mastoplasia, mastopathia, cyclomastopathy adenosis, etc.

Pathology.—In spite of differences among pathologists as to the classification of the microscopic changes, the following basic alterations may be emphasized. They often occur simultaneously in the same specimen. (1) *Hyperplasia* of the ducts and acini, mostly the former. (2) *Fibrosis* around ducts or acini, the latter often called *adenofibrosis*. (3) *Cysts,* small and large, due to a combination of hyper-secretion and obstruction of the ducts. In addition, there may be varying degrees of round cell proliferation and cellular atrophy. The significant changes, of course, relating to the development of cancer, are the hyperplastic ones and this is discussed separately. The most frequent malignant change is that which follows hyperplasia of duct epithelium which takes the form of papillary ingrowths into the lumen of the duct (intraductal papilloma) or into the lumen of a cyst (intracystic papilloma) (see p. 810).

The pathogenesis of these changes in the breast, for a long time unknown, is now generally considered to be due to an abnormality in the reaction of the breast to the cyclic activity of the female sex hormones. Indeed, similar changes in the mammary glands of female rats have been induced by long continued estrogenic stimulation [8]. It would seem also that an essential feature of this disorder is the failure of normal involution, so that by repeated stimulation at each menstrual cycle, during pregnancy, and perhaps also by sexual excitement, the hyperplastic changes outstrip the hypoplastic or involutional process. It is especially important to discuss next the relation of the hyperplasia in chronic cystic mastitis to the development of malignant disease.

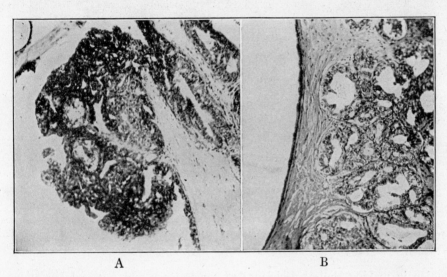

A   B

FIG. 476.—CHRONIC CYSTIC MASTITIS SHOWING THE WALLS OF TWO CYSTS.

Photomicrograph (high power) from the same specimen, represented in Figure 475. *A,* note the papillary ingrowth into the lumen of the cyst, *i.e.,* a beginning intracystic papilloma. *B,* note the hyperplasia of the small ducts adjacent to the wall of a dilated cyst; the cyst is filled with fluid and lined by flattened epithelium.

Relation of Chronic Cystic Mastitis to Cancer.—Since cancer is, after all, an abnormal growth of preexisting cells, it is but natural that the proliferating epithelium in chronic cystic mastitis was long suspected of being an early cancer. Indeed, the dividing line between benign hyperplasia and malignant neoplasia is not always a sharp one. This undoubtedly accounts for the varying estimates as to the frequency with which cancerous changes are observed in cystic disease of the breast. In a report of biopsies performed on 53 patients with nodular breasts, but with no clinical evidence of cancer, histologic evidence of malignancy was observed in 4 cases (Rogers and Nathanson [4]). This is a rather high incidence; others have reported much lower figures. For example, Lewis and Geschickter [5] followed 523 cases of adenosis and cystic disease of the breast for 5 years or longer and found but 4 of them (less than 1 per cent) developed cancer. In another report, Geschickter [6] found

3 cases of cancer among 271 similar patients followed over 5 years. On the other hand, Warren [7] detected 35 cases of malignancy in 1044 patients followed for an average of 9 years. An added and seemingly paradoxical feature of the Warren study was the greater incidence of cancer in women under 50 in contrast to those over 50; this would indicate that after the menopause cystic disease is less likely to become malignant (2.5:11.7) presumably because of the cessation of estrogen formation. This adds weight to the idea that estrogenic hormones are associated in some way with carcinogenesis (see p. 296).

These statistical studies, while they probably indicate a definite relationship between cystic disease of the breast and cancer must be used with the greatest

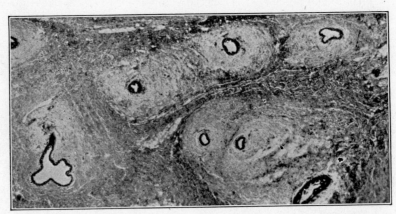

FIG. 477.—PHOTOMICROGRAPH FROM ANOTHER CASE OF CHRONIC CYSTIC MASTITIS SHOWING IN MARKED DEGREE THE PERIDUCTILE DEPOSITION OF HYALINE FIBROUS TISSUE.

This feature undoubtedly contributes in many instances to the nodular character of the parenchyma. In other parts of the section in this case marked epithelial hyperplasia and dilated cysts were made out.

caution in making clinical decisions lest unnecessary and repeated operations be advocated in these patients. It should be emphasized that the figures cited applied not to all women with nodular breasts but only to those who apparently exhibited sufficient deviation from the average to indicate operation. The data have no direct bearing on the incidence of cancer in women who have diffuse changes in the breasts and come to their physicians largely because of pain. The decision as to operation or as to the necessity for further observation is discussed in some detail on page 810. The important point is that each case must be judged on its own individual characteristics, and definite, unequivocal statements made to the patient, with special reference toward combating cancerphobia.

Clinical Manifestations.—It is of importance to realize that a great many women with chronic cystic mastitis will have no symptoms whatsoever. For example, the histologic changes in the breast already described were found in 15 of 17 patients coming to autopsy with a variety of diagnoses not connected with the breast (D'Abreu [8]). Moreover, the same author examined the breasts of 500 adult females of all ages and found that about 33 per cent of them showed some degree of nodularity, regardless of age. The only symptom referable to the breast was the presence of some degree of pain in two-thirds of those exhibiting the nodular breasts.

Of the many women who have chronic cystic mastitis, very few consult their physicians; those who do, complain of either a lump, or pain, or of discharge from the nipple. The *lump* may be single but if moderate in size is usually due to a large cyst; more often the lump is rather small and in reality represents merely a portion of a diffusely nodular breast which for some reason becomes locally more promi-

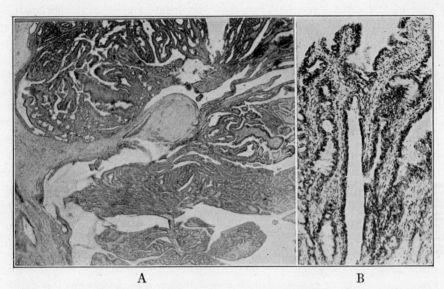

A   B

FIG. 478.—INTRACYSTIC PAPILLOMA IN A THIRTY-SEVEN-YEAR-OLD HOUSEWIFE.

The patient first noticed several months previously a discharge from the nipple which occasionally became blood-tinged but which never ceased. On examination a reddish discharge could be expressed from the nipple and a small tumor could be felt just below the areola. At operation the tumor was excised. *A,* photomicrograph showing a portion of the papillary growth as well as the stalk of the papilloma. The wall surrounding the tumor is only shown at the base of the stalk; it is probably the wall of a dilated duct rather than of a cyst. *B,* a high power view showing the character of the papillae and the hyperplasia of the cells. Despite this hyperplasia no evidence of carcinoma was found in any part of several sections, in this particular case.

nent or nodular than the rest of the parenchyma. In many cases, however, the patient believes she feels a lump, but on examination only a diffuse nodular parenchyma is made out.

The *pain* is usually slight and brings the patient to the doctor only because it has aroused a fear that such a symptom may be a sign of cancer, even though no lump may have been felt. Actually, of course, pain is not a manifestation of cancer except in the terminal stages when ulceration and infection have occurred. Indeed, severe pain is generally indicative of the presence of other lesions, such as acute mastitis, abscess, etc. The pain in chronic cystic mastitis is rarely constant, being worse at some period during the menstrual cycle, usually just before or during the flow. In a few patients, however, the pain may be severe enough to be disabling and demand relief; under such conditions it is called mastodynia (see p. 826). The breast parenchyma is tender to palpation and there is often an associated tenderness of the underlying pectoral muscle.

Discharge from the nipple in chronic cystic mastitis is relatively uncommon, being encountered in less than 10 per cent of cases. In a study made by Hinchey [9] the discharge was bloody in about half the cases, and serous or greenish-brown in the remainder. In duct papillomas the incidence of discharge is much higher and it is usually bloody: for example, Geschickter [6] noted a bloody discharge in 47 per cent of 204 cases studied. When duct papillomas are in or just beneath the nipple, they may be palpable, but when located in the depth of the breast, they are rarely palpable, because of their small size. A significantly large proportion of these lesions undergo malignant change, as will be discussed under treatment.

On examination of a breast which is the site of chronic cystic mastitis a diffuse nodular or shotty sensation will be encountered on palpation of the parenchyma. This will be particularly apparent in thin pendulous breasts in which palpation is not impeded by a thick layer of subcutaneous fat. Often the lateral margin of the breast parenchyma will be felt as a sharp firm edge. Both breasts are affected and frequently equally so. When a single lump is felt it is firmly attached to the rest of the breast parenchyma, and cannot be outlined as a separate tumor. In many patients, however, the differentiation between an actual tumor and a localized area of cystic mastitis may be made only after excision. On repeated examinations it will often be noted that the nodules vary in size, and in the degree of tenderness, at various periods during the menstrual cycle. In general the signs are most prominent before and during the flow, though not infrequently in the midperiod between menstruations.

Treatment.—Fear of cancer is quite common in women with even the slightest manifestations of chronic cystic mastitis. In many women, indeed, this fear is deeply rooted and may even assume a true *cancerphobia*. The importance of this fact in the treatment of these patients cannot be over-emphasized. Reassurance is, of course, essential but it must be definite and emphatic. Equivocation only increases the fear. Such reassurance can scarcely be justified or effective unless the surgeon can be *certain* of his statement that cancer is absent; to do so he must obviously be competent to make such a diagnosis either on clinical examination or with the aid of an adequate biopsy. When the pain is slight, reassurance and mild analgesics are usually sufficient. If the pain is more severe a supporting brassière, which relieves congestion in pendulous breasts by elevating them, will often achieve considerable relief. Endocrine therapy has also been used.[4, 5, 6] The pain in many women, however, undergoes spontaneous remissions. In a few patients past the childbearing age the pain may be so severe (mastodynia) and so resistant to conservative treatment as to necessitate total mammectomy.

When a localized nodular area is palpated as a definite lump, excision may be indicated, particularly to establish a diagnosis. Such an excision is important in women in the cancer age because of the possibility that malignant disease may be present (see p. 807). If there is some doubt as to the existence of a localized nodular area, the breast should be examined at frequent intervals. Detection of definite local growth may demand immediate operation, particularly if the patient is past thirty-five years of age. At operation, the excised tissue is bisected and searched for evidence of carcinoma; if malignancy is definitely noted, or if subsequent microscopic examination reveals it, radical operation will be necessary.

In the presence of significant bleeding from the nipple an immediate clinical diagnosis of intracystic papilloma is indicated; excision of the lump or nodule (if one is palpable), or mammectomy, is done promptly because of the frequency of carcinomatous change in this lesion. If such a change is apparent at operation a radical excision is carried out. In a few patients malignant disease will be detected only on microscopic section; in such an event a second operation for removal of pectoral muscles and the axillary lymph nodes will be indicated.

Cysts.—As already mentioned, cyst formation is one of the pathologic features of chronic cystic mastitis. These cysts are usually small and multiple, and often undetectable clinically, being noted only on gross or microscopic examination of the cut tissue. Occasionally, larger single cysts are encountered which are manifest clinically as a lump such as has already been described. Although their contents are serous they are under so much pressure that they are very firm and may be mistaken for a solid tumor, often imparting a hardness suspicious of carcinoma. The true diagnosis in such instances is made only by thoroughly examining the excised tissue by numerous sections. Occasionally the wall of large cysts of this type present a bluish translucent appearance when exposed at operation; the term "blue dome cyst" has been given to such a lesion by Bloodgood.

Another type of cyst is the so-called *galactocele,* or true retention cyst, due to a duct obstruction and containing retained milk. It is relatively rare and has little clinical significance because it usually empties spontaneously. If it does not empty, the contents will become inspissated; removal may then be indicated.

Benign Neoplasms.—The breast area may be the site of neoplasms found in skin and subcutaneous tissue anywhere, such as lipoma, fibroma, angioma, etc. In the parenchyma the most important benign tumor is the adenoma.

Adenoma (Adenofibroma).—This neoplasm varies somewhat in its histologic appearance, but usually contains a much greater proportion of fibrous than epithelial elements. Indeed, the adenomatous tissue may be so slight as to form single layers of epithelial cells surrounded by great masses of connective tissue, thus giving rise to the term *intracanalicular fibro-adenoma.* The fibromatous element may be diffuse connective tissue or hyaline periductile fibrous tissue which is more elastic and translucent. Mucoid degeneration may occur, imparting to the tumor the designation of *adenomyxoma.* Other variations have been described. The epithelial cells resemble those lining the ducts, although occasionally the acinous cells seem to give rise to the tumor. In any case, the tumor is clearly circumscribed and separated from the rest of the breast parenchyma by a loose layer of connective tissue, a characteristic which can often be made out clinically on palpation.

Recent investigations have shown that this tumor may have a similar pathogenesis to that of the adenomas noted in certain endocrine glands (*e.g.,* the thyroid). In this sense adenoma of the breast may be classed not as a neoplasm but as a result of endocrine stimulation. Its microscopic structure sometimes bears a resemblance to chronic cystic mastitis which is more definitely associated with endocrine activity (see Fig. 475).

Clinical manifestations are absent until a lump is discovered which is usually accidental. Pain is only occasionally present. In most instances the mass is felt while the patient is bathing, or is noticed on examining her breast after some slight trauma. This latter fact accounts for the frequent belief on the part of patients that the tumor followed an injury to the breast. Many women, however, now palpate their breasts regularly because of the lay propaganda conducted by the American Society for the Control of Cancer. All in all, therefore, many women now consult their physician simply because they have noticed a lump in the breast. His problem in general is one of differential diagnosis between a benign adenofibroma, cystic mastitis and cancer.

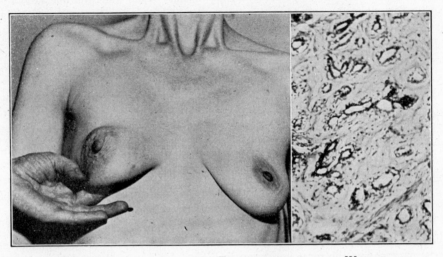

FIG. 479.—FIBRO-ADENOMA IN A TWENTY-SEVEN-YEAR-OLD WOMAN.

A lump had been noted two years previously; it had not increased in size but became slightly painful preceding each menstrual period. Note the lack of skin attachment although the tumor has been displaced by the examiner's fingers. At operation the tumor was not attached to the skin or parenchyma and shelled out very readily. Microscopic section of various parts of the tumor revealed features of adenoma, fibro-adenoma as well as of chronic cystic mastitis. The photomicrograph above shows this resemblance. (Compare with Figs. 475, 476, 492.)

Adenofibroma is largely a tumor of early adult life and is frequently encountered in young women and girls just after puberty. If the patient has known of the existence of the lump for a number of months or years, she may notice a definite, though slow, increase in size. Only rarely is the tumor multiple. Rapid growth may occur during lactation, due to the same stimulus which affects the rest of the breast; many women, indeed, first notice the lump during such a period. On examination a firm encapsulated tumor is felt, which is quite distinct from the rest of the breast parenchyma. The mass is usually much larger and more definite than the lumps noted in chronic cystic mastitis, except when a single cyst is present. However, in a good many cases a definite diagnosis cannot be made with certainty on palpation alone. A decision, therefore, must be made in each case as to the indications for operation.

Treatment may not be indicated if the tumor is not painful and is present in a young girl. However, since these tumors slowly increase in size, malignant degeneration is an ever-present, though fairly rare, danger. In general, surgical excision is indicated in most women over twenty-five years of age and in every woman over thirty-five. The operation is quite simple and healing should take place with a relatively insignificant scar. Excision enables a true diagnosis to be made, particularly if malignant disease is to be ruled out.

Malignant Neoplasms.—The importance of malignant disease of the breast may be realized from the fact that it accounts for nearly 9 per cent of all cancer

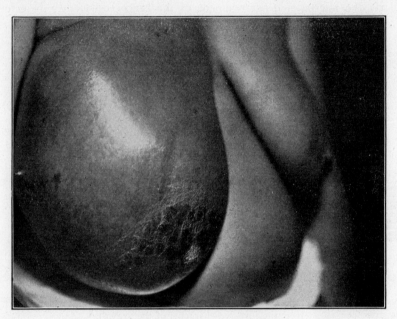

FIG. 480.—SARCOMA OF THE BREAST.

The patient, aged thirty-seven, had known of the existence of a small tumor in the breast since the age of thirteen. For the past year it has been steadily and rapidly growing to its present size. At operation the tumor was found attached to the pectoral muscle. It is important to remember that such a tumor does not metastasize to the axillary lymph nodes and for this reason a simple mammectomy is sufficient. The prognosis is good. This tumor, originating in a fibro-adenoma, is not to be confused with fibrosarcoma, which may also, though rarely, occur in the breast; its features have already been described.

deaths, including both sexes; it is estimated that there are constantly over 20,000 women with the disease in the United States alone (Olch). Nearly all of these tumors are of epithelial cell origin (*carcinoma*); sarcoma comprises but 3 to 5 per cent of them. The female breast is predominantly affected (100:1). As with carcinoma elsewhere, advancing age is the most predisposing clinical factor, few cases occurring before the age of 35. After this age the incidence rises sharply, half of all cases being noted beyond the age of 50. The etiology of cancer of the breast is unknown, except for the evidence already mentioned that the proliferative changes in chronic cystic mastitis may in a few cases lead to malignant growth. Indeed experimental cancer has been produced by repeated injections of estrin (see p. 296). The relation between skin irritation in Paget's disease and cancer is more definite; a detailed description of Paget's disease of the nipple will be found on page 821. Trauma and previous lactation have no proved etiologic connection with the disease, although cancer tends to grow quite rapidly when it occurs during lactation, due presumably to the abundant blood supply.

Pathology.—Various types of breast cancer have been described. They arise apparently from the duct epithelium, although some tumors seem to originate from acinous tissue. The various types of tumor are classified according to the relative proportion of fibrous and epithelial elements, the rapidity of growth, and particularly the microscopic arrangement of the cancer cells; *i.e.,* their tendency to form definite gland-like structures. In general, three main types are described:

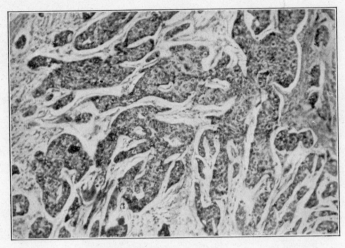

FIG. 481.—PHOTOMICROGRAPH OF A BREAST TUMOR SHOWING MEDULLARY CARCINOMA. Note the invasive character of the growth.

medullary, scirrhus and adenocarcinoma, but other lesser terms such as comedo-carcinoma and cancer cyst are also used to describe special tumors. *Medullary (encephaloid) carcinoma* or carcinoma simplex is a cellular and, in general, a rapidly growing tumor which often, however, exhibits periods of relatively slow progression. It is composed of an undifferentiated type of cell which does not form gland-like structures, is rather soft in consistency and occurs more often at an earlier age than the other types. The tumor is rather circumscribed and on cut section contains little scar tissue in contrast to the next type of tumor, scirrhus. *Scirrhus,* as its name implies, is composed largely of fibrous tissue with a paucity of epithelial elements. Indeed, the predominance of scar tissue, which often seems to be engulfing the cancer cells, gives one the impression that the body is attempting to overcome and strangle the tumor. The large amount of fibrous tissue also gives the tumor its characteristic "stony-hard" sensation on palpation. It is just about as frequent as medullary cancer, but is more slowly growing, metastasizes much later and occurs more frequently in women of more advanced age. *Adenocarcinoma* is so-called because its cells are arranged in the form of alveoli or acini. Many tumors of this group grow rapidly and metastasize widely within a year; others may be present for years before metastases occur. The tumor is more bulky than the scirrhus type, sometimes invades the skin and leads to extensive ulceration even before it spreads elsewhere. Colloid carcinoma is a form of adeno-carcinoma in which much colloid material is present. It is rare and exhibits even a lower degree of malignancy than adenocarcinoma. Comedocancer is a descriptive term applied to tumors in which tiny bits of material may be squeezed from the

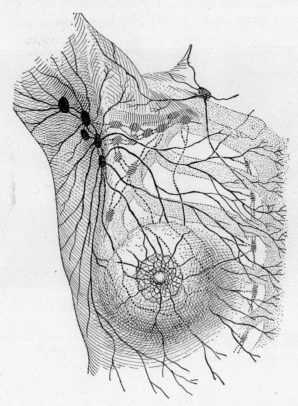

FIG. 482.—THE LYMPHATICS OF THE MAMMARY GLAND AND THE NODES INTO WHICH THEY DRAIN.

(From Homans, *Textbook of Surgery*, 1935. Courtesy of Charles C. Thomas, Springfield, O.)

cut surface of dilated ducts, many of which contain masses of tumor tissue. Cancer cyst is a term applied to a malignant tumor which on cut section is found to contain a cystic area due either to degenerative changes, to a dilated duct, or to an intracystic papilloma which has become malignant.

The spread of cancer of the breast occurs primarily, as first shown by W. Sampson Handley [10] many decades ago, by direct permeation into small lymphatic channels of the breast lobule and into the subcutaneous tissue, fascia, muscle and skin. When the tumor cells enter the skin lymphatics, they may be evident as small nodules just beneath the surface, giving to the skin an appearance similar to the studded breast-plates carried by the knights of old, to which it owes its name, *en cuirasse*. This is often noted in the late stage of cancer, but more commonly as a manifestation of local recurrence of a tumor which was removed surgically. Metastasis by way of the larger lymph channels occurs first to the regional axillary lymph nodes and occasionally the supraclavicular nodes. Spread also takes place in a diffuse manner, particularly along fascial lymphatics which penetrate the pectoralis muscles and the chest wall, as well as the sheath of the upper end of the rectus. Distant metastases occur by way of the blood stream, mainly to the liver and bony skeleton, particularly the spine and long bones.

The parasternal lymph nodes should also be mentioned as a site of cancer

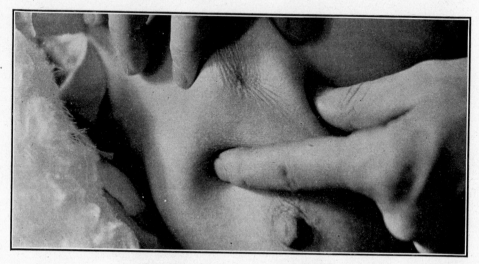

FIG. 483.—CARCINOMA OF LEFT BREAST.

Note retraction of the skin. The lump lay directly beneath the retracted area which was firmly fixed to the tumor. The patient was 65 years old and first noted the lump three months previously. No axillary metastases were felt or discovered at operation. The tumor proved to be a fibrosing type of adenocarcinoma.

spread. These nodes are particularly prone to become involved if the tumor is located in the medial half of the breast.

Clinical Manifestations.—If looked for, the first manifestation of cancer of the breast is the appearance of a lump. In some patients a gradual retraction of the skin or nipple will be their first intimation of disease, whereas in a few women nothing will be noticed, unfortunately, until the surface of the skin becomes ulcerated. *Pain is not a symptom* of cancer until late in the disease. In fact, the presence of pain is usually indicative of a benign (especially an inflammatory) lesion. The skin lesion in Paget's disease is described separately on page 821. In recent years women have become so educated to look for abnormalities in their breasts that the most frequent complaint is the presence of a lump which must then be examined by the physician in order to determine whether or not it is cancer. If he is uncertain he may repeat the examination at intervals. He should advise against examination by the patient herself. Massage is known to be dangerous in spreading cancer.

The clinical features of a malignant lump in the breast vary considerably as may have been inferred from the description of the various pathologic types. Nevertheless, certain general features may be listed as follows: (*a*) The cancerous mass arises from the breast parenchyma, but is palpable as a definite lump, although histologically and upon palpation, it is not circumscribed. (*b*) The tumor is usually hard, particularly if it is of the scirrhus variety, but so are some benign tumors.

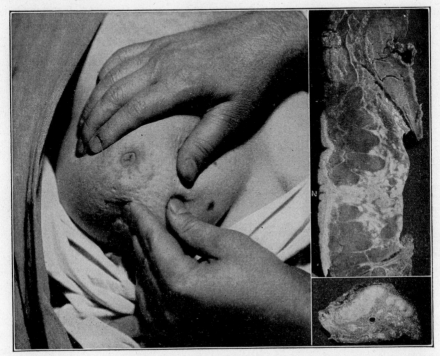

FIG. 484.—CARCINOMA OF THE BREAST IN A FORTY-YEAR-OLD WOMAN.

Note the retraction of the nipple and the dimpling of skin (orange-peel appearance) induced by relaxing the skin over the tumor. Note also the pitting edema. A tumor of the breast was first noticed four months previously but grew rapidly following daily massage of the lump, a procedure which was recommended to the patient by an irregular practitioner. A radical breast amputation was performed; parts of the block dissection are also represented. In the upper specimen are shown the strands of tumor attached to and retracting the nipple (N) and also includes part of the resected pectoral muscle; the lower specimen is a part of the axillary contents and shows the tumor tissue replacing the axillary lymph nodes surrounding a small vein.

(*c*) *Retraction of the skin* (*or nipple*) overlying the tumor is probably the most reliable early sign of cancer of the breast. It is due to the tendency for the carcinoma to become attached to and shorten the fibrous skeleton (Cooper's ligaments), thus producing a fixation to the adjacent tissue. Cooper's ligaments extend along the ducts, thereby accounting for the retraction of the nipple and are also attached to and similarly retract the skin. Retraction of the nipple, to be of significance, must be of recent origin and unilateral, for in many women both nipples are always retracted. Attachment to the skin is usually made more evident by relaxing the skin over the tumor (see Fig. 483). (*d*) The *"pig skin"* or *"orange peel"* appearance of the skin over a tumor of the breast is another important clinical sign of cancer often present together with retraction of the skin and like it made more prominent by relaxing the skin over the tumor. This sign probably is produced by a depression of the openings of many sweat glands and hair follicles, by a local edema of the skin overlying the tumor (see Fig. 484). (*e*) Edema may be present over an acute inflammatory tumor, but there is no difficulty in differentiating such an edema from that produced by cancer because of the lack of other signs of inflammation. (*f*) Still later in the course of the disease edema is followed by necrosis and ulceration, and soon a necrotic ulcerating mass is formed. This type of lesion is especially apt to develop if the patient has applied a cancer paste, which is nothing more than an

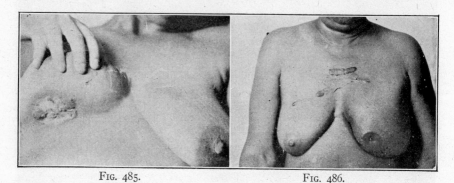

Fig. 485.　　　　　　　　　　　　　Fig. 486.

FIG. 485.—CARCINOMA OF THE BREAST WITH ULCERATION.

The patient, aged fifty-seven, noted a lump two years previously, which was recognized as malignant by her physician but operation was refused. The ulceration began one and one-half years later and progressed. A roentgenogram of the chest revealed pulmonary metastasis; a simple mammectomy was done, in order to excise the ulcer. The patient died sixteen months later.

FIG. 486.—CARCINOMA OF THE BREAST WITH PERMANENT RETRACTION OF THE NIPPLE.

A lump was noted eight months previously. Radical amputation was performed; axillary metastases were present. Note also the keloid of the chest, a sequel to a laceration sustained many years before.

escharotic. (*g*) Regional lymph node enlargement in the axilla or supraclavicular region is another late manifestation of cancer in that it indicates metastasis, except when the enlargement is secondary to an infection such as that associated with an ulcerating tumor. (*h*) Discharge from the nipple occurs in slightly less than 5 per cent of patients with carcinoma. Since the discharge in carcinoma of the breast is bloody in only about one-half of the cases (Hinchey [9]) it is important to remember that the presence of a serous discharge does not eliminate the diagnosis of malignancy. The discharge is more apt to be bloody in intracystic papilloma which is a frequent precursor of cancer as already mentioned.

A diagnosis of cancer must be seriously considered whenever a single painless lump is noted in the breast of a woman past the age of thirty to thirty-five years. Operation is advised if for no other reason than to establish or rule out such a diagnosis. The use of the frozen section of the excised tissue of doubtful malignancy, in order to reach a microscopic diagnosis in the operating room, has been highly extolled in order to aid the surgeon in the further treatment while the patient is still under the anesthetic. However, it should be emphasized that visual examination of the cut surface of the tumor and adjacent tissue will usually reveal an invasive appearance if the lesion is cancer. The firm consistency and the granular, somewhat friable sensation often imparted to the knife on bisecting the tumor is also indicative of malignancy. It has been noted, moreover, that in the really doubtful or borderline cases, even the frozen section may be unable to reveal the true diagnosis which is often made possible only when permanent sections are made. In such instances, therefore, it will be necessary to wait a day or two until such sections may be prepared from various parts of the tumor in order to determine definitely the presence or absence of cancer.

Treatment.—The only method of curing cancer is the total eradication of the malignant tissue by actual removal or by destruction. The former is achieved by surgical excision, the latter by radiotherapy (deep x-ray or radium). Frequently, both methods are used to insure complete eradication of the tumor. The

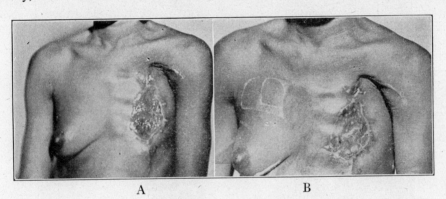

A   B

FIG. 487.—CARCINOMA OF THE BREAST REQUIRING REMOVAL OF A LARGE AMOUNT OF SKIN.

A, the skin defect two weeks after operation. *B*, two weeks later, following the application of a split graft.

operation consists of a radical *bloc* dissection of the entire breast and its surrounding lymphatic connections. The excision includes the axillary and, in some cases, the supraclavicular nodes, the pectoralis major and minor muscles, the upper end of the anterior rectus sheath and a good margin of normal skin and subcutaneous tissue surrounding the breast. Frequently skin defects are created by the excision. These may be allowed to heal by secondary intention or may be covered by primary or secondary skin graft. The technic of radical excision of the breast was described independently at about the same time nearly fifty years ago by Willy Meyer [11] and W. S. Halsted.[12] If the tumor is localized to the breast and has not involved the axillary nodes, a five-year cure will be achieved in about 65 or 70 per cent of the patients operated upon in this way. If, in the specimen removed at operation, the axillary nodes are found to contain cancer cells the probability of a five-year cure falls to about 30 per cent (Clopton [13]). Postoperative and preoperative radiotherapy may improve this percentage of cures slightly. Radium and x-ray are also used in late, inoperable cases as a palliative measure and over metastatic bone lesions largely to relieve pain.

Primary radiotherapy with interstitial radium (without surgical excision) has also been used, particularly by Keynes,[14] for over ten years. According to this method of therapy, needles containing radium are inserted into the breast and around the regional lymph nodes. This treatment was at first used by Keynes in

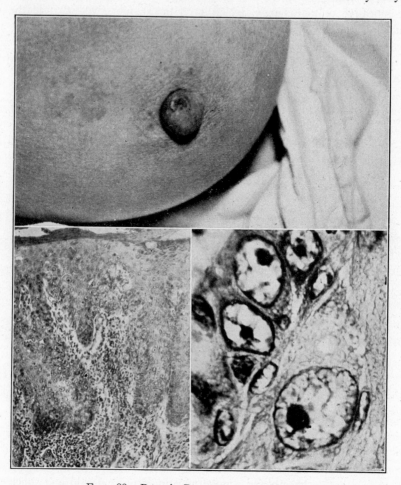

FIG. 488.—PAGET'S DISEASE OF THE NIPPLE.

This is a very early case in a fifty-eight-year-old woman. A tiny ulcer of the nipple, as shown in the photograph, first appeared four months previously; it healed at intervals, but always recurred. After operation several blocks of tissue were examined microscopically but no evidence of carcinoma was found, although the typical histologic picture of Paget's disease was noted in sections of the ulcer. This is shown in the low and high power photomicrograph as shown below the photo; note the characteristic appearance of the so-called "Paget cell."

late, advanced and inoperable cases and the results were so encouraging (over 30 per cent three-year cures) that patients with early lesions were treated in this way. The five-year cures in this early group compare favorably with the results of radical operation (71.4 per cent in patients with the disease confined to the breast itself; 29.3 per cent in those with axillary metastases). There were in addition 23.6 per cent of five-year cures in the inoperable group. A contrasting view of the value of primary interstitial radiation in operable cases may be obtained from the results reported by McKittrick.[15] Doubtless further study will reconcile these divergent observations.

When the diagnosis of cancer is doubtful at the time of local excision, the radical operation is not performed until permanent sections of the tumor are made and have revealed the malignant changes. This two-stage operation is to be avoided if possible, but it is doubtful if the trauma incident to the simple excision, and the delay of a day or two thus entailed between the time of the local excision and the radical removal, is sufficient to allow significant spread of the disease.

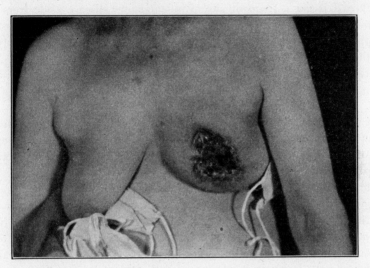

FIG. 489.—PAGET'S DISEASE OF THE NIPPLE.

This is an advanced case showing extensive destruction of the entire areola and underlying breast (Courtesy Dr. J. W. Gale).

Paget's Disease of the Nipple.—As already stated (p. 308) Paget's disease really consists of two lesions, a skin disease and a true carcinoma of the ducts of the breast. Since the skin lesion is observable early it should, whenever encountered, excite a suspicion of carcinoma being present. Most skin lesions of the nipple are simple and clear up in a few weeks with ordinary care, especially cleanliness. If the lesion is due to Paget's disease it will not heal but will progress and finally lead to a destructive ulceration of the entire areola (see Fig. 489). A biopsy is justified in doubtful cases in order to establish the diagnosis.

One of the distinctive histologic characteristics of Paget's disease of the nipple is the infiltration in the skin lesion of cells which are large and deeply staining, with sharp, round, vesicular nuclei and vacuolated cytoplasm (see Fig. 488). They are found under the epidermis and may extend outward, but remain in the superficial part of the lesion. It is believed by some observers that unless this peculiar cell (often called the "Paget cell") is present, a diagnosis of Paget's disease is unjustified. While this cell has a distinctly malignant appearance it is entirely unlike the disease process present in the deeper tissues; the latter consists of a duct cell carcinoma arising in the terminal portions of the lactiferous ducts.

Treatment in Paget's disease of the nipple is that of carcinoma of the breast in general, *i.e.,* radical mastectomy. The prognosis is particularly good in patients without obvious metastases, since many of these tumors are slow to metastasize. However, if the tumor has already extended and growth is active, the prognosis is no better than in the average case of carcinoma of the breast. Early removal of the lesion is, therefore, particularly important in this disease.

INFECTIONS

The breast is not a frequent site of inflammatory disease aside from the common infections similar to those present in the skin and subcutaneous tissue of any part of the body. A few infections, however, are characteristic of the breast itself in that they are located in the parenchyma of the organ.

Acute Mastitis.—This lesion starts as an acute cellulitis or lymphangitis, usually of one portion of the breast, and may be accompanied by evidence of systemic invasion. Its relationship to a condition known as "caked breast" is discussed later. In most instances the infection rapidly softens and suppurates, forming an *abscess of the breast.* The organism is frequently the *Staphylococcus.* Though it may occur in the nonlactating or virgin breast, acute mastitis is more common in pregnancy, particularly during lactation. Often the abscess forms at the site of a "caked breast" without definite acute cellulitis, unless one prefers to call caked breast a form of cellulitis (see p. 824). The infection enters the breast, probably through fissures or abrasions about the nipple, and travels along the lymphatics of the ducts to the depths of the gland. Heat, redness, local pain and tenderness rapidly develop; the pain is usually so severe that the patient seeks early relief. Less commonly the lesion is deeply seated and reaches the surface more slowly or may penetrate beneath the breast and form a submammary abscess.

Treatment is prophylactic is so far as cleanliness and protection of the nipple will prevent fissure and abrasions, and thus avoid a portal of entry. Once the infection is present the treatment is the same as that of acute inflammation elsewhere: heat, elevation and rest, followed by incision and drainage as soon as suppuration occurs. It is important that incision for drainage be made in a radial direction from the nipple in order to avoid cutting across the ducts. Incision must be carefully made, preferably under general anesthesia, and should be large enough to drain the cavity adequately. Since the abscess is apt to be multilocular, it is important to explore the ramifications of the cavity gently in order to insure complete drainage. Counter drainage is often necessary. The infection frequently burrows extensively, thereby accounting for its tendency to form a chronic draining sinus because of inadequate drainage or the presence of necrotic tissue. If the abscess is submammary, a more lateral circular incision may have to be made.

Chronic Mastitis.—A chronic draining sinus, which may be multiple, is usually the result of an inadequately drained abscess of the breast; a history of the acute process is often obtained. However, the possibility of tuberculosis or actinomycosis should always be considered, particularly from the history; it is often ruled out only by microscopic examination of excised tissue. If the lesion is actually due to a pyogenic infection heat, elevation and more efficient drainage may result in healing. Often, however, especially in the neglected cases, the destruction of tissue has been so great that total mammectomy may be indicated.

Tuberculosis.—Though a rare lesion, tuberculosis of the breast may be difficult to diagnose even if it is merely secondary to disease elsewhere. Adequate microscopic examination of the inflammatory tissue is usually necessary. The usual history is that of a painless lump of long duration which finally suppurates, opens

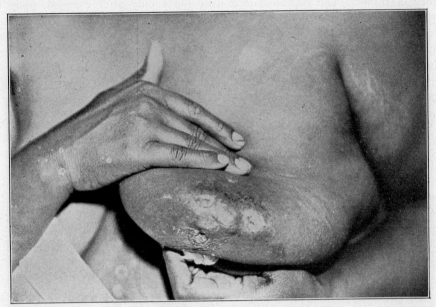

FIG. 490.—TUBERCULOSIS OF THE BREAST.

Note the ulcers which are the sites of draining sinuses which open and close at intervals. The patient, aged forty, had known of a lump for many years. Several years previously it became painful, was incised, and pus obtained. A second abscess appeared recently; pus was aspirated, showed no organisms on smear or culture, and gave an equivocal guinea-pig test (the animal died too soon). The diagnosis is based on the presence of tuberculosis elsewhere (lungs, tarsus). Excision of the breast with the diseased tissue has been advised; definite identification of the lesion can be established only by this means, or biopsy (aside from the tests already mentioned).

and results in one or more sinuses which fail to heal. If the pus is obtained before secondary infection has occurred, the organism may be found on smear; injection of pus into guinea-pigs should reproduce the disease. Otherwise, biopsy of the diseased tissue is the only certain method of diagnosis. Treatment consists of excision of the diseased breast. Preoperative radiation followed by cautery knife excision and post-operative radiation have also been recommended (McGehee and Schmeisser [16]).

MISCELLANEOUS LESIONS

Injury.—The breast is not infrequently the site of injury which in general presents no special problem in diagnosis or treatment. Often, however, a swelling is noted by a patient following some injury. In most instances the association is a coincidence, the lump having been present previously, but overlooked until the trauma caused the patient to palpate her breast. In some cases a true hematoma may be the cause of such a swelling; in a few instances the swelling may be due to fat necrosis. *Fat necrosis* of the breast is a definite lesion, especially in obese women, and produces a firm, palpable mass, frequently with skin retraction, and is, therefore, often mistaken for carcinoma. It does occur, however, without a history of trauma. The diagnosis is usually made only after excision, upon bisecting the tumor. The presence of an irregular mass of slightly reddened tissue in which are seen areas containing liquid fat, is characteristic. The microscopic section shows deposition of scar tissue and round cell infiltration, besides the necrotic fat. It has no etiologic relation to cancer.

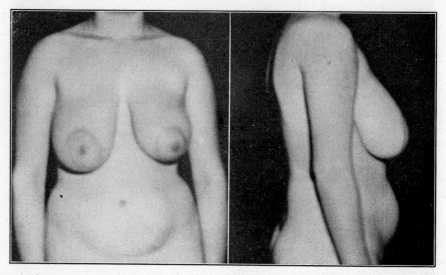

Fig. 491.—Simple Hypertrophy of Both Breasts in a Fifteen-year-old Girl.

The patient complained of severe pain which persisted in spite of medication but was somewhat relieved by an adequate supporting brassiere (Washington University Clinics).

"Caked Breast."—At any time during lactation one segment of the breast may become hard and somewhat tender, but without other signs of inflammation. The lesion is rather common and is generally called "caked breast." It usually subsides spontaneously, but may give rise to suppuration. The pathogenesis of the lesion is somewhat in dispute, but obstruction of the involved secreting parenchyma is generally considered to be an important factor. In addition to the local retention of milk, which produces an entirely different picture from a galactocele, infection is also supposed to play a role. The entrance of low grade organisms through the nipple is supposed to result in a local but mild type of mastitis, similar in nature to acute mastitis which has already been described. *Treatment* is directed toward relief of the lesion in order to minimize the danger of suppuration. A tight supporting bandage is usually sufficient, but massage and the use of the breast pump may also be indicated. In case suppuration develops the treatment is the same as for abscess of the breast.

Simple Hypertrophy.—The normal growth of the breast which occurs at puberty ordinarily ceases when the breast has reached a moderate size. In rare instances this growth stimulus does not cease and the breasts continue to enlarge until they attain such proportions as to interfere seriously with the comfort and even the health of the patient. Occasionally the enlargement is unilateral. If supporting bandages do not give relief, a plastic operation with partial amputation of the breasts may be necessary.

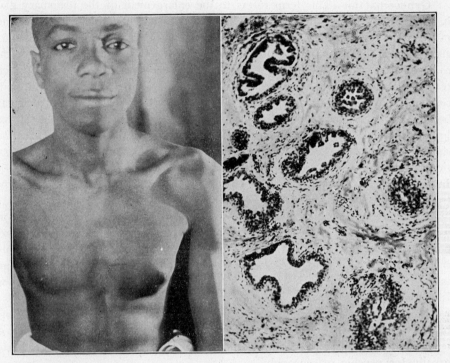

FIG. 492.—GYNECOMASTIA IN A SIXTEEN-YEAR-OLD BOY, AFFECTING THE LEFT BREAST AND DATING BACK ONE YEAR WHEN IT WAS FIRST NOTICED AFTER A TRAUMA TO THIS SIDE OF THE CHEST.

The chief complaints aside from the swelling were pain and tenderness. On the right is a photomicrograph of the tissue in the affected breast. Note the ducts lined by hyperplastic epithelium and the round cell infiltration. This lesion is similar to the physiologic changes often seen in the female breast to which the term cyclomastopathy has been given; it is presumably of endocrine origin.

On extremely rare occasions one breast will begin to enlarge prematurely in young girls before puberty because, presumably, of a precocious endocrine stimulus. There is often a history of trauma which brings the patient to the doctor; occasionally severe spontaneous pain occurs (puberty mastitis). The enlargement is rarely marked and causes no difficulty because of its size. Recognition of the nature of the swelling will enable a true diagnosis. Reassurance is usually all that is necessary. Surgical excision is obviously contraindicated; with the advent of puberty both breasts develop symmetrically, in most instances. In young boys, excision is indicated (see Gynecomastia).

Mastodynia.—This term applies to pain in the breast which is often of severe and disabling character. As already mentioned this symptom is nearly always due to an associated chronic cystic mastitis. Occasionally, however, palpation of the breast reveals little or no abnormality. Such cases have been called neuralgia of the breast and may be similar to other true neuralgias (see p. 556). Treatment is extremely unsatisfactory; mammectomy may be justified occasionally, especially in women past the child-bearing period.

Gynecomastia.—This term refers to the enlargement of the mammary gland in the male. When both breasts swell there may be endocrinologic cause (neoplasm of the testicle, etc.). More commonly the enlargement is due to inflammatory changes of a chronic type or to a cystic disease somewhat similar microscopically to chronic cystic mastitis in the female. If only one breast is affected a suspicion of neoplasm is aroused. Symptoms may be absent or consist of slight pain or discomfort. The unilateral tumors should be excised even if small in size, particularly because of the danger of cancer, which is a fairly frequent neoplasm in the male breast. If cancer is present, clinically or microscopically, a radical resection should be carried out. Simple excision is performed subcutaneously with preservation of the nipple. In young boys excision is often necessary for cosmetic reasons. In bilateral gynecomastia endocrine therapy with testosterone reduces the hypertrophy, but recurrence takes place when the therapy is stopped (Wernicke [17]).

Aberrant and Accessory Breast.—These congenital anomalies are rare and usually produce few clinical manifestations. The aberrant breast is a misplaced portion of normal parenchyma, located usually in the anterior axillary fold; unlike the accessory breast it is not associated with a separate nipple. It is usually mistaken for a benign tumor; excision may be indicated, particularly if carcinoma is suspected.

Accessory breasts usually consist merely of a more or less well-developed nipple without any secreting tissue. They occur along the "milk-line" which extends from the axillary to the inguinal fold. Simple excision is sometimes indicated, usually for psychic reasons only.

BIBLIOGRAPHY

1. LEWIS, D., and GESCHICKTER, C. F. Ovarian Hormones in Relation to Chronic Cystic Mastitis, *Am. J. Surg.*, 24:280, 1934.
2. CHEATLE, G. L., and CUTLER, M. *Tumors of the Breast,* J. B. Lippincott Co., Philadelphia, 1931.
3. EISEN, M. J. The Occurrence of Benign and Malignant Mammary Lesions in Rats Treated with Crystalline Estrogen, *Cancer Research,* 2:632, 1942.
4. ROGERS, H., and NATHANSON, I. T. Chronic Cystic Mastitis, *N. Eng. J. M.*, 212:551, 1935.
5. LEWIS, D., and GESCHICKTER, C. F. Endocrine Therapy in Chronic Cystic Mastitis, *J. Am. M. Ass.*, 109:1895, 1937.
6. GESCHICKTER, C. F. Mammary Tumors, *Surgery,* 3:916, 1938.
7. WARREN, Shields. The Relation of "Chronic Mastitis" to Carcinoma of the Breast, *Surg., Gynec. & Obst.*, 71:257, 1940.
8. D'ABREU, F. Chronic Interstitial Mastitis, *Brit. J. Surg.*, 22:456, 1935.
9. HINCHEY, P. R. Nipple Discharge, *Ann. Surg.*, 113:341, 1941.
10. HANDLEY, W. S. *Cancer of the Breast, 2nd ed..* Paul B. Hoeber, New York, 1922.

11. MEYER, Willy. Operation for Cancer of the Breast, *Med. Rec.*, 46:746, 1894.
12. HALSTED, W. S. The Results of Operations for the Cure of Cancer of the Breast, *Ann. Surg.*, 20:497, 1894.
13. CLOPTON, M. B. Cancer of the Breast, *Surg., Gynec. & Obst.*, 58:438, 1934.
14. KEYNES, G. The Place of Radium in the Treatment of Cancer of the Breast, *Ann. Surg.*, 106:619, 1937.
15. McKITTRICK, L. S. Interstitial Radiation of Cancer of the Breast, *Ann. Surg.*, 106:631, 1937.
16. McGEHEE, J. L., and SCHMEISSER, H. C. Tuberculosis of the Breast; Report of Eight Cases, *Am. J. Surg.*, 28:461, 1935.
17. WERNICKE, H. O. Gynecomastia, *Surgery*, 5:217, 1939.
18. GESCHICKTER, C. F. *Diseases of the Breast*, J. B. Lippincott, 1943.

CHAPTER XXIX

SURGICAL DISEASES OF THE CHEST

EVARTS A. GRAHAM AND BRIAN BLADES

In this chapter will be considered briefly some of those conditions involving the thorax which are now definitely considered to be of surgical interest. Lesions of the mammary gland, however, will not be considered here because they have already been discussed in Chapter XXVIII; this applies also to the esophagus which has been taken up in Chapter XXIV.

Thoracic surgery is one of the newest fields of surgical development; in fact, except for the surgical attack of lesions of the chest wall this whole new field may without much exaggeration be said to have been developed in the short period since the beginning of World War I. Occasional successful operations on the thoracic viscera were undertaken prior to that time by bold surgeons but the general feeling existed that, because of the normal negative pressure within the thorax, special apparatus was necessary which was so cumbersome as to preclude the possibility of making operations in this region really practical. Such, for example, was the now obsolete Sauerbruch negative pressure chamber. World War I, however, because of the large number of intrathoracic wounds, necessitated operations within the chest on so large a scale that many of the former fears of an intrathoracic surgical attack became dispelled. At the close of the last century the general idea was that intrathoracic operations, for example for the removal of a portion of the lung, were to be strongly condemned because of the necessarily prohibitive mortality which existed. Even if the mortality itself had been lower the diagnosis of intrathoracic diseases was so imperfect as compared with its present state that it would have been difficult to perform operations with the directness of attack and assurance which one can have now. The improvement in diagnosis has been due almost entirely to the improvement in x-ray technic and to the use of the bronchoscope. It has now been found possible to attack all of the intrathoracic viscera by surgical means. One of the pressing problems is to improve the technical aspects of intrathoracic operations so that the operative mortality will be constantly diminished. Advances in this new field are being made with such rapidity that in many respects the surgical procedures are revolutionized from year to year.

THORACIC CAGE

Malformations.—Many of the malformations are of no surgical importance because they produce no symptoms. There are some, however, which deserve attention. Occasionally there is a complete or partial absence of the anterior thoracic wall which may be associated with *ectopia cordis*. The overlying skin in such cases may or may not be absent. Sometimes this condition is severe enough to necessitate a plastic repair but it is, after all, rather rare. Another condition known as *funnel chest (pectus excavatum, Trichterbrust)* occurs, in which there is a more or less marked depression and concavity of the sternum. In most cases this condition is accompanied by no symptoms, but occasionally serious pressure effects on the heart and great vessels, the esophagus and even the liver may occur. This deformity is not always congenital but may result from trauma. When serious pressure effects are present it becomes necessary to perform an operative removal of the part of the chest wall which is causing the pressure. Usually this involves the resection of part of the sternum and of some of the costal cartilages.

Fractures and Dislocations of the Sternum.—These are very uncommon. Fractures of the sternum constitute less than one-half of one per cent of all fractures. After the fragments have been reduced as well as possible the thorax should be immobilized and the patient kept in bed for several weeks. Dislocations without fracture are still more rare and should be handled in the same manner (see also Chap. XVIII).

Inflammations of the Chest Wall.—Inflammations of the chest wall in a few respects have characteristics which distinguish them somewhat from inflammations of other parts of the surface of the body. Of the ordinary pyogenic infections *subpectoral* abscess and *subscapular* abscess are both worthy of special mention. The former arises from an infection which begins in the loose areolar tissue beneath the free border of the pectoralis major or minor muscles. It is sometimes secondary to an infection of the axillary lymphatics or to an abscess of the breast. When a swelling is apparent it is found under the outer border of the pectoralis major muscle. In many cases only a fullness is made out in that region without any local redness of the skin. Adduction and outward rotation of the arm are especially painful but in the severe cases any movement of the arm is painful. The constitutional symptoms are often very marked. The lesion is often overlooked and it is necessary, therefore, to bear the possibility of it in mind in connection with infections of the hand, arm or breast in which the constitutional effects persist after local drainage seems to have been adequately established. The treatment of the condition is to establish free drainage. For this purpose it is usually necessary to make an ample incision along the external border of the pectoralis major muscle and usually it is necessary to divide some of the fibers of that muscle. Chemotherapy may be used with surgery as discussed elsewhere.

Subscapular abscess is more rare than *subpectoral abscess*. It is often mistaken for a tumor of the chest wall, particularly of the scapula. Even when the abscess is produced by pyogenic organisms there may be practically no local evidences of inflammation except fluctuation. Few of these cases are tuberculous in nature. Ample drainage is imperative.

Osteomyelitis of the Sternum and Ribs.—Osteomyelitis of the sternum is fortunately rare because it is usually accompanied by a high mortality, generally estimated to be about 50 per cent. Primary osteomyelitis of the ribs is also rare but it occurs often enough to deserve some attention. When it occurs the best treatment is removal of the infected portion of the rib. Prompt recovery ordinarily follows this procedure. Secondary osteomyelitis is rather frequent, especially after operations for drainage of an empyema cavity at which a portion of a rib has been resected. In the great majority of cases healing occurs without any marked symptoms but sometimes small sequestra get into the abscess cavity and result in the establishment of a chronic fistula which runs the course of a typical foreign body infection with closure for a few weeks at a time followed by a recurrence of signs of local inflammation and a reopening of the fistula with the discharge of pus. In such cases it is often necessary to resect the involved portions of the rib.

A special type of osteomyelitis of the ribs and of the costal cartilages is that due to the typhoid bacillus. It is fortunately becoming more and more rare as the general incidence of typhoid fever is diminishing. This condition usually manifests itself by the formation of a fluctuant swelling over the site of the lesion. There are seldom any marked local signs of acute inflammation. A history of a preceding typhoid fever is ordinarily obtained but sometimes no such history is given and again the typhoid osteomyelitis may not manifest itself for years after the recovery from the attack of typhoid fever. One of the important features about the condition is to recognize it in order to prevent the infection of others with typhoid bacillus by failure to take proper precautions. The ordinary method of treating this condition is by surgical excision of the diseased bone or cartilage. The use of typhoid vaccines has also been found helpful. Winslow [1] has recently summarized the current knowledge of this condition.

Tuberculosis of the Sternum and Ribs.—Tuberculosis is the most common inflammatory disease of the ribs and sternum except for those which follow compound fractures. It occurs most frequently in middle life, is often secondary to tuberculosis of the pleura and the tuberculous abscess frequently travels a long distance to open spontaneously. It seldom discharges into the pleura. Like cold abscesses elsewhere the local evidences of inflammation are usually not marked. Frequently the first feature noticed by the patient is a soft swelling which fluctuates but is not red. If the swelling is aspirated the characteristic curdy pus will be obtained. If a sinus is already present necrotic bone can sometimes be felt with a probe. An x-ray examination, particularly after the injection of lipiodol into the sinus, is often helpful in making a diagnosis. If the disease is confined to a single rib its wide removal frequently results in satisfactory and complete healing. Heliotherapy and hygienic treatment are of great value as supplementary aids. If a costal cartilage is involved it is necessary to remove the entire cartilage.

Syphilis and actinomycosis of the bony chest wall occur but will not be given any special consideration here because of their comparative rarity.

Tumors of the Chest Wall.—Nearly all of the common benign tumors have been recognized as arising in the chest wall. The most important tumors, however, are those which arise from the bones. Simple osteomas have been described but nearly always cartilage is also present and, therefore, for the most part such tumors are really enchondromas. A large proportion of them are malignant. This is particularly true of the cartilaginous tumors which arise from the costal cartilages. Occasionally they arise in the scapula. They often become of enormous size even when they are benign and the symptoms which they produce for the most part are those of pressure against other structures, and visible deformities. They are usually hard, rounded and lobulated but frequently in parts of the tumor softening occurs from mucoid degeneration. Although they are slow to metastasize they show a marked tendency to recur after extirpation (see Fig. 181). The most difficult features of the diagnosis are the determination of the extent of the tumor and of whether or not it is malignant. Even when suspected of being benign and of limited extent the extirpation of these tumors should never be undertaken lightly because it is often necessary to remove large portions of the chest wall in order to get completely around the neoplastic tissue. The most frequent malignant tumor arising in the chest wall is a sarcoma. Practically all varieties of sarcoma have been observed in this region. It is noteworthy that many cases in which a diagnosis of simple chondroma has been made were subsequently proven to be sarcomas. In a series of 213 cases of tumors of the bony chest wall analyzed by Hedblom,[2] 131 were sarcomas. The usual origin is in the ribs. Carcinoma of the chest wall, exclusive of that which arises in the mammary gland or in the skin, is never primary. Pancoast[3] has described a tumor under the name of *Superior Pulmonary Sulcus Tumor* which is present at the thoracic inlet. He thinks that the tumor arises in the fifth pharyngeal pouch. It presents features of a carcinoma. The entity of this tumor is still in question. The present conception, however, is that the Pancoast tumors are merely bronchiogenic carcinomas which have arisen from a small bronchus in an upper lobe of the lung and have invaded the superior pulmonary sulcus. There is no good reason, therefore, to designate them by any special name.

Injuries of the Thorax.—For convenience the injuries of the thorax are usually classified as (*a*) nonpenetrating and (*b*) penetrating.

Nonpenetrating Injuries.—These are of importance chiefly because of the injury which may occur to important intrathoracic structures without any external evidence that such injuries have occurred. It is very common to find fractures of the bony cage without external evidence of injury to the skin. It is still more important, however, to realize that extensive injury of the intrathoracic viscera may occur without any fracture of the bony chest wall. Such a possibility is particularly prevalent in the elastic resilient thorax of a baby or a young child. There are three complications which deserve particular attention and should always be thought of. These are intrathoracic hemorrhage, a dangerous degree of tension pneumothorax and mediastinal emphysema. If a picture of shock occurs an hour or more after the injury the possibility of *intrathoracic hemorrhage* should be strongly considered. In lacerations of the lung hemoptysis usually, but not always, occurs. But intrapleural hemorrhage can occur from other vessels than those in the lungs, particularly intercostal arteries, the internal mammary artery, etc. Pneumothorax may occur alone or in association with a collection of blood. If the pneumothorax comes from a type of injury to the bronchial tree which permits the entrance of air into the pleural space but prevents its exit, very alarming symptoms of dyspnea may occur. This condition of *tension pneumothorax* requires prompt aspiration of the contained air in order to save the patient's life. *Mediastinal emphysema* usually occurs after a laceration of the trachea or of a main bronchus. It is not so likely to occur after a simple laceration of the lung. The air may travel from the mediastinum throughout the entire body. In a severe example of this sort all of the subcutaneous tissues may crackle even as far down as the feet, and marked swelling of the face is present. Ballon and Francis [4] showed experimentally that the air travels chiefly along the blood vessels (see also p. 843). Another complication is a laceration of the diaphragm which permits abdominal viscera to enter the thorax. The existence of this complication may not be recog-

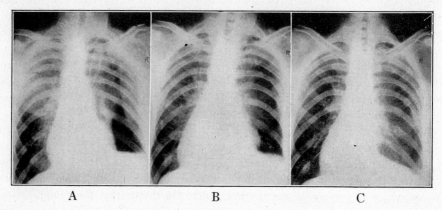

A   B   C

Fig. 493.—Hemopneumothorax due to Fractured Ribs following a Nonpenetrating Injury to the Chest.

The patient, aged forty-three, fell off a ladder. On admission was in mild shock, exhibited slight cyanosis and moderate subcutaneous emphysema; he recovered from these manifestations within twenty-four hours. Treatment consisted of immobilization of the chest with circular adhesive strips and rest in bed.

A, roentgenogram three days after injury; note the fluid level, the air in the pleural cavity and the collapsed left lung. The fractured ribs can be seen in the midclavicular line, X-ray taken in sitting position to show fluid level.

B, roentgenogram four days later, note the expanding edge of the left lung.

C, roentgenogram one month after injury; the lung is fully expanded and the fluid has disappeared as shown by the normal contour of the left diaphragm.

nized until some years later. Massive atelectasis also occasionally occurs. A severe type of nonpenetrating injury is seen as the result of a crushing injury in which much of one side of the chest wall may be pushed into the thoracic cavity. This condition is sometimes known as "stove-in chest." It is, of course, associated with multiple fractures of the ribs and usually extensive intrathoracic complications.

In the treatment of nonpenetrating injuries of the thorax consideration must always first be given to the immediate care of shock and to a careful examination of the patient for any evidence of injury to viscera, thoracic, abdominal or brain, and to the presence of multiple fractures. If, after a blood transfusion for the treatment of shock, a patient's condition improves and then grows worse again, the question of a continuing intrapleural hemorrhage should be strongly considered with the idea of opening the thorax to find the bleeding vessel. It is not necessary and in fact not always wise to remove by aspiration all of the blood from the pleural cavity, because the fluid, by keeping the lung collapsed, tends to minimize the amount of hemorrhage from that source. If, however, the fluid is withdrawn the same effect can be accomplished by replacing some of it with injected air. It is not wise to provide open drainage for a hemothorax because of the infection which will inevitably result. If there is evidence of injury to any of the abdominal viscera or to the brain they should be treated in accordance with the indications present. Fractures also should be treated according to the indications present. As a rule fractured ribs are more satisfactorily immobilized by placing adhesive straps entirely around the lower part of the chest than by the customary method of placing them only halfway around. Likewise, it is seldom necessary that the adhesive straps should be applied immediately over the particular fractured rib because satisfactory immobilization of the thorax can usually be accomplished merely by strapping the lower part of it. Massive pulmonary atelectasis should be treated by encouraging the patient to cough or to take a deep breath. Changing the position of the patient will often suffice for this purpose. Inhalations of carbon dioxide by stimulating deep respiration are also helpful; final resort may be made to the use of a bronchoscope if necessary.

Penetrating Wounds of the Chest.—Penetrating wounds differ from those which are nonpenetrating chiefly in the fact that the former are more likely to be associated with infection. In addition the element of open pneumothorax is likely to be added which in itself may be a very serious complication. Infection caused by penetrating wounds is often due not only to the direct introduction of pathogenic bacteria but also to the retention of a foreign body in the thoracic viscera with more or less destruction of tissue by the missile. All of the complications already mentioned for nonpenetrating injuries can occur after those which penetrate. The experience in World War I showed that the first and most important indication is to close a sucking wound of the chest after débridement of the edges. This procedure not only avoids the serious mechanical consequences of an open pneumothorax but it also tends to prevent the suction of bacteria into the chest and it prevents the rapid cooling of the body which ordinarily follows a sucking wound. Closure of a sucking wound is indeed an important first aid procedure and should be achieved by means of a firm occluding bandage (see page 1051). If a frank empyema develops it should be treated by adequate drainage as in the case of an empyema which arises as a complication of pneumonia. At all times after the wound is closed the patient should be carefully watched for the possible development of serious pressure effects from entrapped air under pressure or from too much fluid in the chest. Small missiles, such as rifle or pistol bullets, are usually comparatively innocuous even when retained in the lung. Large jagged fragments of metal, however, ordinarily should be removed and if there is positive evidence of retained particles of clothing which have been carried into the thorax these should also be removed. Under no circumstances should indiscriminate probing of the wound be carried out. Metallic foreign bodies can almost always be accurately localized with the x-ray. Splinters of bone driven into the lung may cause trouble later by being the focus of one or more pulmonary abscesses. If the fragments of bone are large enough to be detected with the x-ray it is usually better to remove them than to wait for an abscess to develop. Under no circumstances, however, should a thoracotomy be performed for the removal of foreign material until after the patient has recovered from initial shock following the injury. Various special technics were devised during the World War for the removal of retained projectiles in the chest. Special and more comprehensive works on thoracic surgery should be consulted for a description.

Hernia of the Lung.—This condition is rare and will not be extensively considered. Occasionally it is encountered as a congenital defect but more often it follows an injury of a sort which has permitted the lung to escape through an intercostal space. When the hernia is of any size it should be repaired by a plastic operation on the chest wall.

DISEASES OF THE PLEURA

Acute Empyema.—The most important surgical condition of the pleura is empyema, more properly designated as *empyema thoracis*. This is a condition in which pus is present in the pleural cavity and it is, therefore, an abscess of the pleura. It is most important to distinguish this condition from a collection of serous or serohemorrhagic fluid.

Empyema (suppurative pleurisy) is most often due to either the pneumococcus or streptococcus, although it may be due to any of the pyogenic bacteria. Tuberculous empyema is common and even such conditions as actinomycosis, streptothricosis and blastomycosis may be associated with an empyema caused by those specific organisms. It is practically always a complication of some type of pneumonia except when it occurs as the result of a penetrating wound of the thorax or more rarely by spreading upwards into the thoracic cavity of an abscess beneath the diaphragm. The type of pneumonia which precedes the development of the empyema may be different in different cases. For example, when due to a pneumococcus the empyema usually is a sequel of a lobar pneumonia; when due to a streptococcus it is most often a complication of a bronchopneumonia; when caused by other pyogenic bacteria it is usually a complication of some type of suppurative inflammation of the lung such as pulmonary abscess, bronchiectasis, etc. The pneumococcal and streptococcal varieties are more common in children than in adults.

Pathology.—The amount of exudate is subject to great variation. It is more common to find large exudates in cases of streptococcal empyema than in those due to the pneumococcus. The larger exudates are likely to be found earlier in the course of the disease. In the earlier stages during the formative period the pleural effusions may be serofibrinous, blood-tinged or distinctly hemorrhagic. Especially in the early stages of a streptococcal empyema will the fluid have those characteristics. Fibrin is deposited on both layers of the pleura and in chronic cases the pleura, especially the parietal layer, may become enormously thickened to the extent of 2 or 3 centimeters. Usually about ten days or two weeks are required for the transformation of the serofibrinous fluid into definite frank pus. A very important difference between pneumococcal and streptococcal empyema is the fact that in the former condition the pneumonia is usually in a stage of resolution before any collection of fluid is recognized in the pleural cavity and then it is nearly always frank pus. In the streptococcal cases, however, a large collection of pleural fluid may arise early but as a rule it will not become definite frank pus until after the pneumonia has cleared. The essential features of the streptococcal pneumonia are that there is a peribronchiolitis with patches of pneumonia; the walls of the bronchioles are infiltrated with inflammatory products and many of their lumina are plugged with masses of leukocytes, necrotic material, etc.; the obstruction of many of the bronchioles necessarily leads to the production of atelectasis which is often patchy but may be extensive. In some types of empyema one or more abscesses of the lung may be present. Bilateral involvement is not particularly rare but is much less common than unilateral involvement. A rare complication of empyema is a spontaneous perforation of the chest wall. This condition is known as *empyema necessitatis*. In chronic empyema not only is the pleura greatly thickened but the lung is frequently contracted into a much smaller mass than normal and Nature's attempts to obliterate the cavity spontaneously are clearly evident as shown by a narrowing of the intercostal spaces, often with overlapping of the ribs, an ascent of the diaphragm and a displacement of the mediastinal contents towards the affected side.

Symptoms and Diagnosis.—A suspicion of the presence of an empyema should always be aroused in any case of lobar pneumonia if the temperature comes down to normal for a day or two and then begins to rise. Formerly, many cases which illustrated this phenomenon were diagnosed as unresolved pneumonia. It is now, however, generally recognized that unresolved pneumonia is a comparatively rare condition and that nearly all cases which were formerly given that diagnosis are in reality examples of empyema. In not all cases of postpneumonic empyema does the temperature come down to normal before the empyema begins, but in the majority of pneumococcal infections such a phenomenon occurs. In the streptococcal cases this tendency is less evident. In any case of inflammation of the lung in which there is a sudden increase in the temperature with greater prostration of the patient the beginning of an empyema should be suspected. It is not always easy to be certain in such a case whether the increase in temperature is due to a spread of the pneumonia or to the beginning of an empyema. Evidence of a fresh involvement of the other lung is some indication that the condition is really a spread of the pneumonia. The ultimate diagnosis of an empyema, however, will depend upon an exploratory aspiration. Pain and tenderness are rarely present unless the chest wall itself is invaded. If the empyema has been produced by the spontaneous rupture of a pulmonary abscess, the signs and symptoms are usually much aggravated and often there will be air as well as fluid in the pleural cavity which may be recognized on an x-ray examination if the patient is placed in a suitable position to show a fluid level. Such a condition is often spoken of as *pyopneumothorax*.

The physical signs of an ordinary acute empyema are practically those which are found in connection with any collection of fluid in the pleural cavity. Occasionally in the acute cases if the effusion is large and if it has come on rapidly the affected side may show a bulging. More often, however, the affected side appears smaller and flatter than the other because of Nature's attempt to immobilize that side of the chest. In the early cases there may be a marked displacement of the mediastinal contents to the healthy side. In long-standing cases, however, the displacement of the mediastinum may be towards the affected side. In the acute streptococcal cases there may be extreme dyspnea and cyanosis because of the concomitant presence of extensive bilateral pneumonia. In the ordinary postpneumonic pneumococcal cases dyspnea and cyanosis are not extreme. In cases of encysted empyema the physical signs usually vary from those elicited when the empyema has originated in the free pleural cavity. In interlobar empyema the physical signs are often confusing and may be mistaken for a pulmonary abscess. In most cases of the latter type bronchial fistulas are present and therefore a fluid level with gas above it may be seen on an x-ray examination occupying the ordinary position of an interlobar fissure. Otherwise the x-ray examination in cases of empyema is not usually distinctive from the findings present in any pleural effusion.

The constitutional disturbances are essentially the same as with any other acute infection. In children the temperature is usually high (40° C. or 104° F.). As the empyema becomes more chronic, however, the temperature, which is of the septic type with remissions, generally has a lower daily maximum. A rather high polymorphonuclear leukocytosis is nearly always present. Clubbing of the fingers and toes is often seen in the subacute and chronic cases. Scoliosis is commonly present to a limited degree in children in subacute cases but may be extreme in chronic neglected cases.

Complications.—The most common complications of empyema are bronchial fistula, perforation of the thoracic wall (empyema necessitatis), suppurative pericarditis, peritonitis, blood stream infection, bilateral empyema, mediastinal abscess and various miscellaneous complications such as meningitis, brain abscess and multiple arthritis. The pneumococcal cases are much less likely to be complicated by other lesions than are the streptococcal cases. In listing the complications as has been done here the opinion is implied that empyema is a complication of pneumonia rather than that pneumonia is a complication of empyema. Likewise, when the empyema occurs in association with one of the acute exanthemata it is a sequel to the pneumonia which has complicated the main disease.

Treatment of Acute Empyema.—In the treatment of every case of acute empyema there are two fundamental considerations. One is to save life and the other is to prevent chronicity. It is unfortunate that the treatment of acute empyema has been clouded by strong advocacy of various detailed methods. In its true sense empyema is an abscess of the pleural cavity. When an abscess is present in that locality it should be treated like abscesses in other parts of the body, namely, by drainage. Much of the confusion in the literature about the treatment of empyema has arisen because a clear and precise discrimination has not been made between a fully developed abscess and one in its formative stage. In other parts of the body, drainage of infections which are destined to become abscesses is not considered until the abscess has actually developed to maturity. Experience has clearly shown that premature drainage of such infections is very likely to be accompanied by disastrous results to the patient.

In the case of infections of the pleural cavity a particular situation exists which makes it increasingly dangerous to establish wide free drainage before a definite abscess has been formed. The special reasons which obtain in the case of acute infections of the pleural cavity are concerned with the special physiology of the region involved. Since respiration is dependent upon the creation of a negative pressure in the thorax, at least at some time in the act of inspiration, it is apparent that any opening into a free pleural cavity is likely to result not only in embarrassment of the respiration but also of the circulation to some extent because of the dependence of the filling of the auricles of the heart, upon a negative pressure. During the formative period of an empyema the danger of interference with the normal intrathoracic pressure relationship is particularly great because at such a time the patient is usually suffering from a more or less extensive pneumonia and a consequent marked reduction in his vital capacity. If the patient is already cyanotic and orthopneic his vital capacity may be so low that it may approach the tidal air requirements. In other words, under such conditions, in spite of maximal inspiratory efforts the patient can take in scarcely more than enough air needed to carry on life even at rest in bed. There is, therefore, practically no reserve upon which he can draw to compensate for any further embarrassment of his respiration. Even a very small opening of the pleural cavity under such circumstances may be fatal because the effect of any opening in the pleural cavity is not confined to the lung of one side unless it is adherent to the chest wall or unless the mediastinal tissues are sufficiently stabilized by inflammatory thickening to prevent a shift of the mediastinum to the opposite side. On the other hand, a person with a normal thorax can withstand a much larger opening in his pleural cavity because he can compensate for the larger opening by drawing upon his respiratory reserve. In other words, in a thorax in which there are no adhesions and no stabilization of the mediastinum the size of the pleural opening which can be withstood by the patient depends largely upon that individual's vital capacity. During the formative period of an acute empyema there is not much stabilization of the mediastinum, and any adhesions which have formed are still delicate and easily broken, with the result that the creation of an open pneumothorax by establishing a free open drainage is equivalent to doing that in a thorax which has no protection against it. If, therefore, the vital capacity is very low because of the presence of an extensive pneumonia such an individual may die promptly of asphyxia if a free opening is made into his pleural

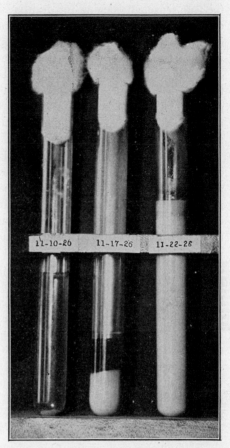

FIG. 494.—CHANGES IN THE EXUDATE IN A CASE OF STREPTOCOCCAL EMPYEMA.

The tube on the left shows a seropurulent exudate. In the middle tube will be seen one from the same patient obtained seven days after that in the first tube and the tube on the right shows exudate obtained twelve days after that in the first tube. The seropurulent exudate has become transformed into one that is frankly purulent. Open drainage of the first exudate would be very dangerous; of the second, less dangerous; of the third, practically without danger. (From Graham, Singer and Ballon, *Surgical Diseases of the Chest*, 1935. Courtesy of Lea and Febiger, Philadelphia.)

cavity which is allowed to communicate with the outside air. On the other hand, if the infection has developed into a definite abscess and has become an empyema in the true sense, an opening for drainage is accompanied by practically no respiratory disturbance. This absence of deleterious result is because of several features. One is that under such circumstances the opening is made into an abscess rather than into the free pleural cavity. There are, therefore, no serious pressure effects on either one or both lungs. Moreover, it happens that an empyema seldom becomes a true abscess until after the pneumonia has cleared to a considerable extent. The patient's vital capacity is, therefore, higher and even if there were pressure effects they would be of less consequence because the patient would be more able to withstand them.*

In view of the foregoing remarks it should be evident that the creation of an open pneumothorax by the establishment of free open drainage should never be undertaken unless definite frank pus has been demonstrated by aspiration. Experience has indicated that when definite frank pus is present there is no ascertainable difference in the results whether one uses an open drainage at that time or some method of drainage which will exclude the influence of the outside air. The principle involved in the latter method is known as closed drainage. Most of the discussion which has centered about the treatment of empyema in recent years has been concerned with the question of whether or not the pleural exudate should be drained either by aspiration or by closed drainage before it has become actual pus. As a part of the discussion on this point there has also been so much advocacy for particular methods of inducing closed drainage that the greatest possible confusion has resulted.

Any one particularly interested in this subject should acquaint himself with some of the old history of the treatment of acute empyema. If he does so he will find that aspiration was recommended as a sole method of the treatment of empyema more than a century ago and that for more than half a century there have been periodic revivals of the advocacy of treating empyema by various methods of closed drainage exclusively. One who attempts to take a somewhat judicial attitude towards the confused literature on this subject is forced to believe that it makes very little difference whether one treats an empyema during the formative stage by aspiration from time to time to relieve the pressure effects of too much exudate or by some method of continuous closed drainage. An important point that is often ignored is the well-established fact that the mortality rate ascribed to empyema is subject to enormous variation in different years. The mortality rates ascribed to empyema are approximately parallel to those which occur in pneumonia. For example, in some years one will have an experience in which there will be no deaths ascribed to empyema and in other years the death rate will be very high. This fact permits one to draw two very striking conclusions, one of which is that ordinarily the deaths in empyema occur because of the severity of the infection of the pneumonia of which the empyema is only a complication and in the

---

* For a more extensive discussion of these theoretical matters the reader should consult the article by E. A. Graham, "Alterations of Intrapleural Pressure and Their Significance," *Medicine*, 1924, 3:417; also an earlier article by E. A. Graham and R. D. Bell, "Open Pneumothorax: Its Relation to the Treatment of Empyema," *Am. J. Md. Sc.*, 1918, 156:839.

second place that too much false assurance should not be developed concerning any particular method of detailed treatment merely because the mortality for a year or two has been gratifyingly low. This remarkable variation in the mortality in different years probably accounts in large measure for the cycles of advocacy of treatment exclusively by aspiration on the one hand or by continuous closed drainage on the other which one sees all through the history of empyema. When a bad year follows a good one the author of a particular method is not so likely to be so enthusiastic about his method. It, therefore, falls into disuse for a period of years until essentially the same method is rediscovered and advocated with great enthusiasm by some other individual.

The obvious and most important conclusion to be drawn doubtless is that patients are not very likely to die of acute empyema itself. Many will die, however, from an injudicious operation if the surgeon *creates an open pneumothorax during the formative period of the empyema,* and in spite of whatever treatment is carried out many will die in bad years of other complications of the severe infection of which empyema is only one.

This brings us, then, to a consideration of how to treat an individual case of empyema.

The two most important principles to bear in mind are not to create an open pneumothorax during the time when pneumonia is present, and the second is to provide adequate drainage when it has been decided that drainage is necessary. A third principle is to attempt to maintain the nutrition of the patient. If, in a given case, an aspiration (thoracentesis) reveals only turbid fluid it is very unwise to create an open drainage. Instead the patient should be treated either by aspiration as often as seems necessary to relieve serious pressure effects or by some method of continuous closed drainage. The simplest procedure to accomplish the latter is the insertion of a catheter through a cannula passed through the chest wall. After the cannula is withdrawn the catheter, if it is of the same size, will fit snugly into the opening. The end of the catheter can be placed under water to prevent a free communication between the outside air and the pleural cavity, or gentle suction can be arranged so that the exudate will be constantly aspirated through the tightly fitting catheter.

If the aspiration of the pleural cavity reveals definite frank pus an open drainage can be performed immediately, either by an intercostal incision or by the removal of a segment of rib one or two inches long. If the patient is a baby it is desirable not to make the opening too large. If an intercostal drainage is made it must be expected that in a large number of cases a subsequent rib resection will be necessary. If the patient is very ill it is usually wiser not to make a large opening in the chest wall at first, despite the fact that the exudate may be thick frank pus.

After drainage has been established the question of irrigation arises. This, however, is a matter of minor importance although the use of Dakin's solution (neutral 0.5 per cent aqueous solution of sodium hypochlorite) is commonly employed for that purpose. The principal advantage of this chemical for irrigation is not so much because of its direct bactericidal power as because it loosens and dissolves necrotic tissue and thereby removes large numbers of bacteria. Mercurial antiseptics should not be employed as irrigants because of the danger of fatal mercury poisoning. The use of Dakin's solution occasionally results in bleeding from the wound and sometimes even from the lung. When that complication arises the irrigations should be promptly stopped. Likewise they should be stopped if violent coughing occurs, an evidence usually of a bronchial fistula.

Drainage should be maintained until the cavity is obliterated. The tube should not be removed until actual measurements have shown that the capacity of the cavity is approximately only 10 cc. An empyema should never be considered to be healed until there is positive evidence that the cavity itself is obliterated. In most cases of acute empyema complete healing should occur in a period of from five or six weeks after the exudate has become definitely purulent. In many cases healing will occur more promptly. In fact, in cases of pneumococcal empyema healing often occurs after one or two aspirations. One may expect that such an event will occur in from ten to 25 per cent of cases of pneumococcal empyema. This tendency is more evident in children than in adults.

Various methods of blowing against resistance are popular, based on the idea that the lung can be more readily expanded and the cavity thereby obliterated by such forceful inflation of the lung. There is no positive evidence, however, that such an event occurs; indeed, there is evidence that the use of such methods has no such result. Forceful blowing exercises, however, do prevent atrophy of the respiratory muscles on the affected side and are useful for that purpose.

The use of the sulfonamide drugs in empyema is discussed at the end of the chapter.

Chronic Empyema.—It has already been said that one of the primary objects in the treatment of acute empyema is to prevent chronicity. Chronic empyema is less common in children than in adults. One of the most frequent causes of the condition is the failure to provide adequate free drainage. The use, therefore, of methods of continuous closed drainage through small catheters should not be carried on too long in the treatment of an acute empyema because of the danger of permitting the condition to pass into a chronic state. It is important, therefore, that the drainage of an acute empyema should be at the most dependent portion of the cavity and that any tube used for the purpose should be of sufficient caliber to permit an easy exit of the pus.

Other important causes of chronic empyema are the presence of foreign bodies, communications with the lung or bronchial fistulas, cavities that cannot be obliterated spontaneously because of too much fibrosis of the lung and too much rigidity of the mediastinum, tuberculosis or similar infections.

Draining sinuses which persist after an empyema are not necessarily due to the presence of a chronic empyema. Such sinuses, for example, may lead to bronchial fistulas which are immediately beneath the chest wall but which have not closed spontaneously. Again the sinus may lead only to a necrotic portion of rib.

In establishing a diagnosis of chronic empyema it is desirable to determine not only the presence of a chronic empyema cavity but also to gain some idea of its size, location, and the possible cause of it. By the injection of a sufficient quantity of lipiodol through the external sinus, if one is present, some idea may be gained about the location and size of the cavity. If the case is one in which there is no external communication aspiration with the introduction of from 50 to 100 cc. of air will usually enable one to outline the cavity in a fairly suitable manner. The diagnosis of tuberculosis or other granulomatous infections can usually be made by the excision of a piece of pleura for microscopic examination.

Treatment.—Since, in the majority of cases of chronic empyema, the cause has been inadequate drainage, the treatment of a chronic case usually will be begun by the procedure of instituting adequate and satisfactory drainage in the most dependent portion of the cavity. This will often require the resection of segments of one or two ribs. In many cases even when the empyema cavity is of two or three years' duration, it will become obliterated within two or three months after the creation of satisfactory drainage. In nearly all cases the cavity will at least become greatly reduced in size even if it is not completely obliterated. At the time of such an operation the cavity is, of course, carefully explored for the possible presence of a foreign body. It must be borne in mind that the offending foreign body may be only a small piece of rib which is lying in the cavity. A piece of parietal pleura is also excised for microscopic examination, because in this way sometimes an unsuspected case of tuberculosis is recognized.

If, after the lapse of two or three months of adequate drainage, the cavity shows no signs of becoming obliterated, then some form of radical procedure for its obliteration must be considered. In such cases the failure of the cavity to become healed is due to the facts that the overlying chest wall is too rigid to be pulled downwards to the lung and that the lung is too rigid to be pulled to the chest wall by the contraction of the scar tissue. The obliteration of an empyema cavity always occurs by progressive formation and contraction of scar tissue from the periphery towards the center of the cavity. All of the radical surgical procedures used for the treatment of chronic empyema are based on a principle of freeing the rigid walls of the cavity to permit them to come together and unite by the formation of scar tissue. The original *Estlander operation* consisted in the removal of the overlying ribs. This procedure, however, is not usually adequate because the underlying parietal pleura is so greatly thickened that collapse of the chest wall will not occur unless it also is removed. The principle of the *Schede operation* is to remove the thickened parietal pleura. The principle of the *Delorme operation* is to remove the rigid coating of the visceral pleura from the lung to permit it to expand enough to help in the obliteration of the cavity. Various other modifications of these classical procedures have been proposed from time to time. For example, it is now recognized that it is not often necessary to remove the thickened parietal pleura but that by severing it from its attachments at the sides and lower part of the cavity, it can be utilized as a flap of living tissue with which to assist the obliteration of the cavity. Likewise, if the Delorme principle of satisfactory decortication of the lung cannot be accomplished the cross cutting of the thickened visceral pleura (Ransohoff) will be very effective, because it will permit the outgrowth of new capillaries through the cross incisions. In any operation for chronic empyema it is essential that the procedure should be sufficiently radical. Nothing is to be gained by halfway measures. It is essential that no overhanging edges of the empyema cavity should be allowed to remain. The cavity must be converted into a saucer with sloping edges in order to have it become satisfactorily obliterated by being filled up with soft tissues of the chest wall. Treatment of tuberculous empyema is discussed under pulmonary tuberculosis.

Rare Infections of the Pleura.—Actinomycosis, blastomycosis, streptothricosis and syphilis occur so rarely that they scarcely deserve a discussion in a textbook of this sort. The reader should refer to monographs on diseases of the lungs and pleura for information on these conditions.

Spontaneous Nontuberculous Pneumothorax.—Formerly it was a common belief that spontaneous pneumothorax was necessarily an indication of pulmonary tuberculosis. Now, however, it is well known that this condition often occurs in individuals who have no active tuberculosis. In such instances it is usually due to the rupture of an emphysematous bleb beneath the visceral pleura or to the rupture of a cyst in a case of congenital cystic disease of the lungs. Infections other than tuberculosis, such as pulmonary abscess, are sometimes associated with a spontaneous pneumothorax because of a rupture of the lesion into the pleural space. A complicating empyema almost invariably occurs in the latter case. However, in those cases in which the pneumothorax is the result of a rupture of a bleb or of a congenital cyst, an empyema or even a collection of sterile fluid does not necessarily follow. Ordinarily in such cases the air is gradually absorbed and the lung again fills the pleural space. Occasionally the air in the chest is under such pressure that it is necessary to aspirate it in order to relieve an impending asphyxia.

Tumors of the Pleura.—Tumors of various kinds, both benign and malignant, are found involving the pleura. One of the most frequent types is a metastatic carcinoma representing a spread from a carcinoma of the breast. Another malignant tumor which has caused much confusion in the literature is the so-called endothelioma. For many years this tumor was regarded as a primary tumor of the pleura. More recently, however, largely through the work of Robertson,[5] it is now generally recognized that this tumor usually, if not always, is a metastatic carcinoma originating in a carcinoma of a bronchus. True primary malignant tumors of the pleura represent various types of sarcoma such as round cell, spindle cell, fibrosarcoma, angiosarcoma, neurosarcoma, myxosarcoma and giant cell sarcoma. Various benign tumors have been described in this region such as fibroma, lipoma, angioma, chondroma, leiomyoma, etc.

Nearly all tumors of the pleura, regardless of whether they are benign or malignant, are sooner or later associated with a pleural effusion. In the case of malignant tumors, and occasionally in the presence of a benign tumor, the pleural fluid becomes bloody. In order to establish the diagnosis of a tumor of the pleura it is often necessary to resort to special means of examination and occasionally even to an exploratory thoractomy. The special means of examination which will be found helpful are the use of a diagnostic pneumothorax and an examination of the pleural fluid by the Mandelbaum method. The former procedure consists in the injection of about 100 cc. of air into the pleural cavity after an equivalent amount of fluid has been aspirated. By turning the patient in a suitable manner an x-ray examination will often then reveal an outline of the tumor. The Mandelbaum method of examining the pleural fluid has already been described (p. 879). In many instances an exploratory thoractomy will be found advisable.

There are other conditions which sometimes simulate tumors of the pleura.

Occasionally in pneumothorax cavities, fibrin bodies are formed which are roughly spherical in outline and often appear in x-ray films like tumors. Areas of calcification in the pleura may sometimes be mistaken for a new growth. Again various kinds of cysts of the pleura have been described, some of which are echinococcal in origin but others are due to congenital defects. In the latter instance it is more probable that many of the cysts thought to be primary in the pleura have actually had an extrapleural origin and are merely encroaching upon the pleura.

THE MEDIASTINUM

The various anatomical mediastina will be considered for practical purposes in this chapter as a single space. Conditions will, therefore, be described as involving the mediastinum without always exercising care to state which particular mediastinum is concerned. Roughly it will be regarded as that part of the thorax situated between the two lungs. The mediastinum is very important surgically because within that space are located the heart, the giant vessels, the trachea and its bifurcation, the esophagus and important nerve trunks. For practical purposes it is well to bear in mind the four anatomical divisions of the spaces, superior, anterior, middle and posterior, according to the relations which they present to the pericardium.

Mediastinal Emphysema.—It is important to realize that the persistence of a pressure less than that of the atmosphere is necessary for the proper functioning of many of the mediastinal structures. Serious elevations of pressure in the mediastinum, therefore, may result in physiologic disturbances which may be sufficiently extreme to cause death. One source of such an increased mediastinal pressure is the gradual accumulation of air within it, a condition known as mediastinal emphysema. This condition is nearly always the result of trauma and is directly due to the creation of an opening in the tracheobronchial tree of such a sort that air is permitted to pour outo into the mediastinal space. Usually the origin of the difficulty is an opening in one of the major bronchi. It may result to a less degree from lacerations of the lung itself. As the air accumulates in the mediastinum it comes upwards into the neck where it produces a swelling which crepitates on examination and is recognized as a subcutaneous emphysema. As the air increases in amount it tends to follow various fascial planes but in extreme cases the subcutaneous emphysema may involve the entire body from the feet to the head. The face becomes enormously swollen with the eyelids puffy and closed, crepitation may be elicited in any part of the surface of the body. Ballon and Francis [6] found experimentally that the air has a tendency to follow the course of large blood vessels. As the emphysema increases in amount the patient becomes more and more dyspneic and death will finally occur from asphyxia unless the increased mediastinal pressure can be lowered promptly and sufficiently.

In the treatment of serious mediastinal emphysema it is necessary to provide an outlet for the accumulated air in order to relieve the pressure as much as possible. Frequently an incision like one for thyroidectomy will suffice if the finger is introduced into the superior mediastinum and the edges of the wound are kept apart by loose packing. The use of constant suction by a pump has also been found helpful. It is seldom possible to operate and close the opening in the bronchus from which the air comes because of the critical condition of the patient at the time that the surgeon first sees him.

Mediastinitis.—Acute infections of the mediastinum as a rule represent the spread of an infectious process from the mediastinal lymph nodes. Probably most of the acute infections of the mediastinum occur as injuries to the esophagus. These result from the perforation of the esophagus by sharp foreign bodies which have been swallowed and also from perforations in association with benign stricture or carcinoma of the esophagus. The type of infection in such cases is usually a fulminating phlegmonous inflammation which in the majority of cases is fatal unless drainage is promptly instituted. Other cases are due to serious acute infections of the nasopharynx. An abscess of the mediastinum may often be recognized on x-ray examination by an undue prominence of the mediastinal shadow, particularly in the upper part. Since most of the mediastinal abscesses occur in the superior mediastinum the majority of them can be reached successfully for drainage through an incision in the neck. The location of such an incision will depend considerably upon the location of the abscess, especially whether it is in the anterior or posterior part of the mediastinum. Sometimes the usual collar incision for thyroidectomy will be adequate. In other cases, especially those due to a perforation of the esophagus, an approach along the anterior border of the sternocleidomastoid is preferable.

Chronic infections of the mediastinum are often tuberculous and they frequently originate from tuberculosis of the spine. They are, therefore, often in the posterior mediastinum. If secondarily infected they demand drainage usually through a posterior mediastinotomy incision. If they are not secondarily infected they should be aspirated and treated like tuberculous abscesses elsewhere. The possible connection with tuberculosis of the spine should always be borne in mind so that appropriate treatment will be given to that condition also.

A type of chronic mediastinitis which deserves special consideration is that which sometimes goes under the name of Pick's disease. As a result of a chronic nonsuppurative inflammation an extensive fibrosis of the mediastinal tissues may occur which may obstruct the large veins by scar tissue, and the pericardium may be transformed into fibrous tissue or may even become calcified. One of the serious results of such a condition, as Pick showed, is a pseudocirrhosis of the liver together with the development of ascites and other serious effects. This condition will be considered in a more detailed way in the part dealing with the surgical diseases of the heart. Syphilis and actinomycosis of the mediastinum occur as rare types of chronic infections.

Mediastinal Tumors.—With the development of thoracic surgery mediastinal tumors have become of increasing importance because of the possibility of extirpating many of them successfully. The most common effect of a mediastinal tumor, regardless of its type, is pressure on one or more important structures. In malignant tumors there may be in addition to pressure effects actual involvement of organs by extension or metastasis.

The most common result of increased mediastinal pressure caused by a tumor is dyspnea which is due probably not so much to compression of the air passages as to compression of the large veins. The vein which is particularly affected is the superior vena cava. Signs of obstruction of this large vein are usually present at some time in the case of any large mediastinal tumor. The specific signs of

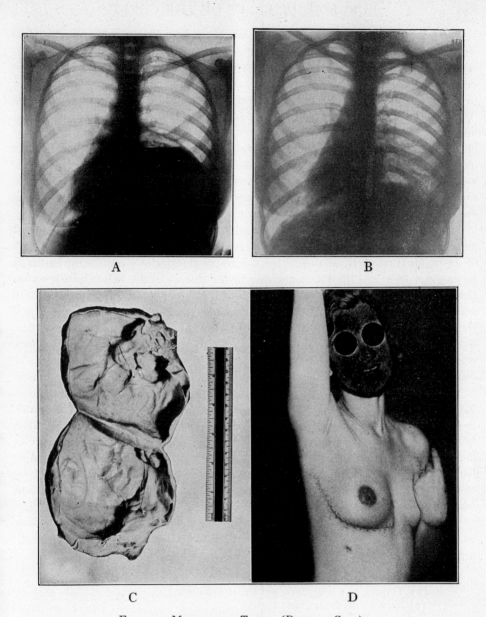

A   B

C   D

FIG. 495.—MEDIASTINAL TUMOR (DERMOID CYST).

The patient, aged twenty-five, presented a history of thoracic injury followed by dyspnea and nausea. Aspiration of a supposed area of encapsulated pleural fluid revealed nonpurulent gray material with a few cells and debris; this led to a suspicion of dermoid cyst. Operation (mediastinotomy) was performed and the tumor removed with an uneventful recovery. *A,* roentgenogram of the chest (in the upright position) after aspiration of 200 cc. of fluid with replacement of air; note the fluid level and the shadow of the cyst wall above it. *B,* chest film three months after operation showing practically normal conditions. *C,* photograph of the specimen which was removed at operation. *D,* photograph of patient soon after operation showing the submammary incision; note the absence of deformity and free motion of the arm. It is possible to remove most mediastinal tumors without the resection of ribs if, after making such an incision as illustrated, several costal cartilages are divided and the ribs are then spread out.

compression of the superior vena cava are cyanosis, orthopnea, dilatation of the superficial veins of the thorax and later, pulmonary edema, pleural and pericardial effusion. Determinations of the venous pressure in such cases show an increase. Subcutaneous edema of the head, neck and upper part of the thorax occur in the more severe cases of superior caval obstruction, likewise headache, vertigo, deafness, epistaxis, tinnitus and even loss of consciousness with epileptic convulsions may occur. The resulting effect depends somewhat upon whether the obstruction has occurred above or below the orifice of the azygos vein. If the obstruction is above the azygos orifice the symptoms are less severe than if it is below that point. The symptoms just mentioned may occur with any mediastinal tumor of sufficient size. In malignant tumors there will also be present signs and symptoms resulting from the development of metastases in other organs.

The diagnosis of the presence of a mediastinal tumor can now be made almost with certainty by an x-ray examination. It is important to determine the location of the tumor particularly as to whether it is in the anterior or posterior mediastinum because not only will the location give a better clue as to the nature of the tumor but it will also guide the surgeon as to the best approach for its removal. In adults the possibility of aneurysm should always be considered and the tumor should, therefore, be examined for pulsation fluoroscopically. In the case of dermoid and teratomatous tumors, nearly all of which are in the anterior mediastinum, it is desirable to examine the patient carefully by means of a Potter-Bucky diaphragm in order to see if teeth or bone can be recognized. In the case of tumors of the posterior mediastinum it is necessary to examine the spine for the possibility of the presence of an hour-glass communication between the origin within the spinal canal and the larger tumor which is present in the mediastinum. Most of the hour-glass tumors have their origin in the spinal or sympathetic nerves or their sheaths, or from the periosteum or ligaments of the vertebral canal. As might be expected, therefore, many of such tumors also give evidence of compression of the spinal cord. The most common tumor of the posterior mediastinum is one which has originated in the tissue.

The whole subject of mediastinal tumors is a very complicated one because of the large variety of conditions which may give rise to recognizable swellings in that region. A convenient and workable classification is as follows:

(a) Tumors of the thyroid (substernal)
(b) Tumors of the thymus, and hyperplasia, etc.
(c) Tumors of the nervous tissue
    Neurofibroma
    Sympathicoblastoma
    Hour-glass tumors
(d) Lipoma, fibroma, chondroma, myxoma
(e) Tumors of the trachea and esophagus
(f) Tumors of the lymph nodes
    1. Acute inflammation; tuberculosis (cold abscess)
    2. Hodgkin's (lymphogranulomatosis), leukemia, aleukemia, lymphosarcoma
    3. Metastatic tumor
(g) Cystic tumors
    Dermoids

Teratomas

Bronchial cysts

(h) Vascular tumors, aneurysms of aorta, aneurysms of heart

(i) Tumors of pericardium and heart, pericardial cysts, diverticula
of the pericardium

After having made a diagnosis of mediastinal tumor and after having located the tumor in either the anterior or posterior mediastinum the next question which arises is one concerning whether it is benign or malignant or an aneurysm. In most cases there is little difficulty about diagnosing a thoracic aneurysm by means of the pulsation seen either externally or with fluoroscopic examination together with other evidences of syphilitic vascular disease. The roentgenkymograph is often very helpful in the recognition of expansile pulsation. In order to differentiate between a benign and a malignant tumor we have found it to be a good practical rule to subject patients with anterior mediastinal tumors to x-ray therapy. If the tumor becomes greatly reduced in size one can be almost certain that it is malignant and of mesoblastic origin arising in the lymph nodes or remnants of the thymus. If, however, no visible response is obtained the chances are great that the tumor is benign. Posterior mediastinal tumors are seldom radiosensitive. Practically all malignant tumors of the mediastinum should be regarded as inoperable because the chance of removing the entire tumor if malignant is very small. On the other hand, most benign tumors should be removed. There are many reasons for recommending the removal of benign tumors in this region. Many of them are of a nature which will become malignant later. Especially is this true of the teratomas and the neurofibromas which arise in this region.

The operative removal of any mediastinal tumor should be regarded as an operation of the first magnitude. For those tumors situated in the anterior mediastinum the best approach in general is through an anterolateral incision in an intercostal space on the side towards which the tumor projects. The pleural cavity should be widely opened in order to get the best exposure of the tumor. For that reason it is important that the operation should be performed with intratracheal anesthesia. It is seldom necessary to remove any ribs even in the case of very large tumors. The costal cartilages can be cut through, the ribs spread apart and after the tumor is removed the cartilages can be sewn together again with catgut and the wound closed. In the case of women the scar can be completely concealed by making the incision in the fold of the breast and there may therefore be no later evidence of any kind that the patient has had a tumor removed.

In the case of tumors of the posterior mediastinum the approach is commonly made in one of two ways, either by dividing several ribs at their juncture with the transverse processes and thus entering the posterior mediastinum or else by making an intercostal incision traversing the pleural cavity and approaching the tumor in that manner.

The advance in thoracic surgery has made it possible now to remove even large mediastinal tumors with a minimum of risk and in many cases with no deformity whatever. Dermoid cysts should preferably be removed and not drained. The latter procedure is almost always unsatisfactory and with the use of modern technic it is accompanied by a higher eventual mortality than is the total removal of the cyst.

Mediastinal tumors of thyroid origin are usually best removed through the usual incision for thyroidectomy. The superior mediastinum can be entered in a generally satisfactory manner from that incision. Such thyroid tumors are usually adenomas which can be pulled upwards into the neck.

DISEASES OF THE HEART AND PERICARDIUM

The most common disorders of the pericardium of interest to the surgeon are those which are concerned with acute and chronic inflammations.

Purulent Pericarditis.—This condition is most commonly encountered as a complication of an infection of the lungs, although it may also occur as a complication of an infection elsewhere in the body. In severe streptococcal epidemic infections of the lung such as that which occurred in 1918, suppurative pericarditis of streptococcal origin is rather common. For example, Dunham [7] found in a total of 603 autopsies performed upon patients dying with streptococcal bronchopneumonia that 44 per cent showed pericarditis. Staphylococcal pericarditis is more likely to be a complication of an abscess elsewhere, particularly of osteomyelitis.

The chief signs and symptoms in addition to general evidences of infection are those of pericardial effusion, such as precordial discomfort and pain, dyspnea and a sense of oppression. Usually also the heart sounds are distant and muffled. There is an increase in the precordial dulness, often a pericardial friction rub, rapid pulse and frequently a palpable liver. On x-ray examination there may be noted an abnormality of the shape of the cardiac shadow which is altered by a change of position, a change in the shape of the angle formed by the posterior border of the heart, diaphragm and spine, and a faint or absent cardiac pulsation.

The serious features of purulent pericarditis are not merely those of a serious infection but they concern also the severe pressure effects of the accumulation of fluid in the pericardial sac. These effects are commonly spoken of under the collective term of *tamponade of the heart.* The normal adult pericardial sac can hold from 150 to 250 cc. of fluid without showing ill effects but when the amount greatly exceeds that figure the serious effects of tamponade become evident. The characteristic clinical picture is the complaint of pain in the region of the heart which extends to the left shoulder and often down the arm. There is dyspnea, anxiety, cyanosis, the pulse is usually weak and thready, the veins in the neck are full and dilated, and the upper abdomen may be tense. If the condition is severe enough death occurs with the picture of heart block.

The determination in a given case of whether the increased fluid in the pericardial sac is purulent or not will depend finally upon an aspiration. In many respects the condition from a diagnostic and therapeutic aspect may be regarded in a manner similar to that of an empyema. If aspiration reveals definite pus an operation for drainage of the pericardium should be advised. If it is not definite frank pus an open drainage should not be undertaken. The prognosis in any case of suppurative pericarditis is grave. In a series of 128 cases collected by Winslow and Shipley [8] only 55 per cent of patients recovered. Probably the actual percentage of recovery is very much lower than that figure because most of the successful cases are reported but the unsuccessful ones are not recorded in the literature. Use of the newer chemotherapeutic agents will probably reduce the incidence of purulent pericarditis and likewise the necessity of surgical drainage even when infection occurs. At present, however, there are no satisfactory statistics.

Tuberculous Pericarditis.—This fortunately rare lesion presents usually a very bad prognosis. In certain cases recovery apparently occurs after repeated aspiration of the pericardial sac followed by small injections of air.

Adhesive Pericarditis.—After an acute inflammation of the pericardium has healed, adhesions form between the visceral and parietal layers with the result that often the entire pericardial space is completely obliterated. At the same time the normal structure of the pericardium becomes transformed more or less completely into scar tissue and in places even calcification may occur. Sometimes the scar tissue extends into the heart muscle itself. Over a long period serious symptoms may develop consisting of evidences of myocardial decompensation and of a pseudocirrhosis of the liver with ascites, often known as *Pick's disease* or *Pick's cirrhosis of the liver*.

The diagnosis of *adhesive pericarditis* (*mediastinopericarditis*) can usually be made from the following evidence: (1) a clinical history of a previous attack of acute pericarditis, (2) ascites and edema associated with a small heart in which there is no evidence of alveolar involvement of the lungs, (3) cardiac hypertrophy not explained on the basis of aortic regurgitation or hypertension, (4) systolic retraction of the chest wall, (5) Broadbent's sign—systolic retraction of the tenth and eleventh intercostal spaces posteriorly, (6) inspiratory filling of the neck veins (Wenckebach), (7) fixation of the apex beat, (8) pulsus paradoxus (Kussmaul), (9) Dieuaide sign—an absence of a change in the form and amplitude of the electrocardiographic waves in shifting the patient from the right to the left side (probably of little value), (10) tugging of adhesions on the diaphragm with cardiac retractions and pulling on the pericardium with respiratory movements as seen fluoroscopically (Elsworth Smith). In any case of moderately severe cardiac decompensation in which digitalis proves to be of no value the possibility of chronic mediastinopericarditis should be considered.

Two kinds of operative procedures are performed for the relief of this condition. The original Brauer operation of cardiolysis consists of removal of three or four costal cartilages and segments of the ribs overlying the heart. The theory upon which the Brauer [9] operation is based is that because of adhesions to the chest wall each systolic contraction pulls upon the bony structure of the thorax which in time wears out the heart muscle because of the extra work involved. Thus the Brauer operation would be effective only in adhesive pericarditis. Delorme [10] had previously recommended that in such cases a decortication of the heart should be performed by the removal of much of the adherent parietal pericardium. This is obviously necessary if there is a constrictive pericarditis. Ordinarily now the procedure which is usually followed in such cases is to approach the heart through a curved incision which begins at about the level of the third left rib at the midclavicular line. It passes downward along the sternum and is extended laterally again at about the line of the seventh or eighth rib. The costal cartilages and anterior segments of the underlying ribs (usually three to five or three to six inclusive) are removed together with the periosteum and perichondrium. This procedure is essentially the operation recommended by Brauer. The operation should not be terminated, however, at this point. The pericardium should be incised and if it is much thickened and adherent to the visceral pericardium a considerable segment of the parietal pericardium should be removed. It is necessary, however, that if any pericardium is removed it should be a part of that which overlies the left ventricle as well as the right ventricle. It is dangerous to decorticate

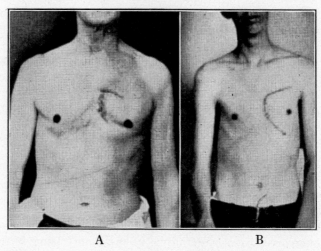

A   B

Fig. 496.—Two Patients Operated upon for the Surgical Relief of Pericarditis.

A, the Brauer operation (see text) for adhesive pericarditis was performed on this patient, fifty-five years old, who entered the hospital because of weakness, shortness of breath, swelling of the feet and ankles and palpitation of the heart. The most important sign in the examination was the finding of Broadbent's sign of systolic retraction of the intercostal tissues in the left posterior region corresponding to the tenth and eleventh intercostal spaces. Following operation recovery was rapid and uneventful; there has been no evidence of return of symptoms and the patient has been at work continuously for over ten years. *B*, the Delorme operation (see text) for adhesive pericarditis was performed on this patient, aged fifteen, who during the previous year had been examined and treated for a period of one year with a diagnosis of rheumatic fever, cardiac decompensation, adherent pericardium, mitral stenosis and insufficiency. Following operation much improvement in the general condition occurred so that the patient could walk as much as a mile a day; no symptoms were present save for dyspnea when he had to walk up a long flight of stairs. (From Graham, Singer and Ballon, *Surgical Diseases of the Chest*, 1935. Courtesy of Lea and Febiger, Philadelphia.)

only the thin-walled right ventricle for fear of overdistention of that part of the heart. In some cases there is so much scar tissue between the two surfaces of the pericardium that it is almost impossible to differentiate the two layers and to carry out a decortication without danger of seriously injuring the heart muscle. This danger exists particularly in cases of calcification of the pericardium. The wound in the chest is then closed without drainage.

Smith and Liggett [11] showed from a collected series of 107 cases that a properly performed operation for mediastinopericarditis has resulted in an improvement of the patient's condition in 84 per cent of cases. This would indicate that the operation probably should be performed much more often than it is because there are probably many patients who are allowed to go unrelieved who would be benefited by the procedure.

Wounds of the Heart.—Although wounds of the heart are primarily a condition of importance to military surgeons they occur frequently enough in civil practice to warrant some consideration. The overwhelming majority of cases occur in Negroes, and large series have now been collected by several of the southern surgeons; for example, the excellent report by Daniel C. Elkin (*J. Am. M. Ass.*, 111:1750, 1938). Wounds may occur in any part of the heart but obviously they most frequently involve either the right or the left ventricle. The mortality of such wounds has undoubtedly been greatly lowered and it would be still more reduced if the patient were seen early enough by a surgeon. The most serious complication is tamponade of the heart because of hemorrhage into the pericardium. This question has been previously considered under suppurative pericarditis and will not be discussed again here. Other immediate complications concern injury to other important structures especially to the internal mammary and the intercostal arteries. Penetrating wounds of the lung are also common.

There are several surgical approaches to the heart:

1. Incision and resection of the fifth costal cartilage and edge of sternum.
2. Resection of the sixth costal cartilage and adjoining sternum (Kocher).
3. Resection of the seventh costal cartilage.
4. The Delorme-Mignon-Kocher operation. A square flap of the soft parts is reflected outward. The fourth, fifth and sixth costal cartilages are removed, the internal mammary artery ligated, the triangularis sterni dissected away, and the edge of the pleura and lung retracted by gauze. The pericardium is then exposed.
5. The Spangaro operation or intercostochondral thoracotomy. Spangaro makes a long incision in the fourth interspace and then divides or disarticulates the fourth and fifth costal cartilages at their junction with the sternum. The fourth and fifth ribs are then forcibly drawn apart by a rib separator.
6. Median sternotomy of Milton.
7. Duval-Barasty operation. A paramedian incision is made from the level of the third cartilage to a point midway between the xiphoid and umbilicus. The abdominal cavity is opened and the diaphragm incised. The sternum is cut through below the third cartilage and split longitudinally for the rest of its length. The halves of the divided sternum are forcibly separated and a wide exposure of the pericardium results.

In a case of serious wound of the heart in which haste is necessary it is ordinarily desirable to use an approach which will permit access to the heart in the easiest and quickest manner. Either the Delorme-Mignon-Kocher or the Spangaro operation will ordinarily be found the most satisfactory. After the pericardium is opened the opening in the heart from which the blood is escaping can usually be plugged somewhat by lightly applying a finger over it until sutures can be placed through the heart muscle with which to close it. Beck [12] has advised the use of a suture through the apex for purposes of traction. It is usually desirable to close the wound in the pericardium and the chest wall without drainage.

Treatment of Angina Pectoris by Surgical Methods.—Various surgical procedures which have been recommended for treatment of angina pectoris have been based on different principles. The earlier operations were devised for the relief of pain. They consisted in the removal of the superior, middle and inferior sympathetic cervical ganglia. Although some patients were relieved of their pain by such procedures many were not. Moreover, there was never any sound physiologic basis for believing that such operations could be expected to relieve the pain. Various modifications of interruption of different nerve trunks have been carried out, the most recent of which is the paravertebral injection of alcohol in an effort to block the upper fifth or sixth pairs of white rami and the corresponding chain of dorsal sympathetic ganglia. An extensive discussion of the various methods employed to control pain cannot be entered into here. These are discussed at some length by Swetlow,[13] by J. C. White and P. D. White [14] and the various ideas are reviewed by Graham, Singer and Ballon.[15] On the whole, the results obtained by blocking nerve impulses have not been entirely satisfactory. At best, about all that could be expected of them was the relief of pain rather than any improvement in the fundamental condition of anoxemia of the myocardium (see also p. 587).

The next principle involved was an attempt to diminish the amount of work done by the heart. This principle was carried out by the total removal of the thyroid gland, a suggestion proposed by Blumgart, Levine and Berlin in 1933.[16] In certain cases this procedure has resulted in apparently a striking benefit to the patient but the procedure is too new to evaluate it properly. Not only does the removal of the thyroid gland reduce the total metabolism but it also seems to alter the response of the cardiovascular system to adrenalin. On the other hand some patients have not been pleased to substitute a condition of myxedema for the symptoms of angina pectoris.

The newest principle upon which a surgical treatment of angina pectoris has been based is that proposed by Claude Beck [17] which aims to improve the circulation of the heart muscle. Based on a large amount of experimental work on animals he has devised an operation by which a flap of pectoral muscle is placed around the heart. This procedure enables new blood vessels to grow into the myocardium from the muscle flap. In several cases he has reported striking results. Again, however, the procedure is too new to give it a proper evaluation.

O'Shaugnessy [18] has employed pedicled omental grafts placed against the myocardium to produce a new blood supply to the heart. Before his death in the Battle of Flanders he had given the method sufficient clinical application to demonstrate its feasibility. Heinbecker and Barton [19] have described an operation for producing collateral circulation to the heart in dogs which consists of creating a sterile adhesive pericarditis (a mixture of sodium morrhuate, aleuronat and lyonite is placed in the pericardium) and suture of the anterior parietal pericardium to the retrosternal tissues. After this procedure dogs have survived ligation of both branches of the left coronary artery near their origins at one operation. In human beings the operations of Beck and O'Shaugnessy have yielded encouraging clinical results.

Operative procedures for the relief of mitral stenosis have been devised by Allen and Graham [20] and by Cutler and Beck.[21] These procedures, however, while encouraging, have not met with a sufficient number of successful results to place the operation at the present time beyond the experimental stage.

Aneurysms of the Thoracic Aorta.—In some cases thoracic aneurysms can be greatly improved by introducing into them several feet of wire which coils inside the sac and then passing an electric current through the wire. The operation itself is simple. Under local anesthesia about ten feet of wire are introduced through a needle into the aneurysm sac. The positive pole of the battery is attached to the outer end of the wire and the patient lies upon the negative pole which must be in contact with the skin. The current should be between 50 and 70 milliamperes. It should be continued for about one hour. A type of wire must be used which is sure to coil in the sac after coming out of the needle. The chief advantage of this procedure is the remarkably sudden relief of pain which frequently occurs. A more detailed consideration of this subject will be found in the articles by Hare [22] and by Hunner [23] (see also p. 497).

Operation for Embolism of the Pulmonary Artery.—Operative removal of an embolus of the pulmonary artery was first proposed by Trendelenburg in 1908. It is only recently, however, that enough successful results have been accomplished to make the procedure seem to be of any practical value. Probably the best results have been obtained in the Swedish Clinics, notably by Giertz and Crafoord [24] at Stockholm and by Nystrom [25] at Upsala. The operation has not found general favor in this country and in other parts of Europe because of two great disadvantages. One of these is the difficulty of being sure that the patient has pulmonary embolism and that he will die if the embolus is not removed. The other disadvantage is that for the most part because of the sudden onset of the condition the operations must be performed by junior surgeons often without much actual operative experience. The question, therefore, inevitably arises whether more patients will be saved by the performance of this operation than will lose their lives as a direct result of it because of the difficulties already mentioned. It would seem out of place to go into this question with more thoroughness in a book of this kind. The interested reader may find more extensive descriptions in the articles by Giertz and Crafoord, and by Nystrom.

Ligation of the ductus arteriosus is discussed on page 494.

SURGICAL CONDITIONS OF THE DIAPHRAGM

The chief function of the diaphragm is to assist in the creation of a negative intrathoracic pressure by the enlargement of the thorax which is produced when it descends on inspiration. The diaphragm is also important because it separates the abdominal from the thoracic cavity. It is present only in mammals. A congenital absence of the left half has been reported on several occasions, a condition which does not seem to be incompatible with health and long life. Spasms of the diaphragm are responsible for the condition known as *hiccup* or *singultus*.

Eventration of the Diaphragm.—Normally the right leaf of the diaphragm lies about 1 centimeter higher than the left. In some individuals, however, one leaf, usually the left, is abnormally high. This constitutes the condition known as *eventration or insufficiency of the diaphragm*. Into the sac-like formation which results, one or more of the abdominal organs are likely to be displaced, especially the stomach, colon or spleen. The usual causes of such a condition when not produced by operations on the phrenic nerve, are congenital atrophy, neuromuscular degeneration following injury, neuritis or other involvement of the phrenic nerve, certain infectious diseases and changes in the musculature of the diaphragm in association with pseudohypertrophic lipomatosis and myositis. This condition is not incompatible with good health. Its chief importance lies in the possibility of confusing it with a true diaphragmatic hernia. It is recognized by the high position of the diaphragm and by the fact that the abdominal viscera are seen to be below it rather than above it. A small pneumothorax created for diagnostic purposes will often settle the diagnosis definitely between an eventration and a hernia of the diaphragm. Ordinarily the condition demands no surgical treatment.

Diaphragmatic Hernias.—These may be divided into the nontraumatic and traumatic. The nontraumatic hernias are essentially congenital and are due to the passage of an abdominal organ through one of the congenital openings shown in Fig. 470 A on page 799. The traumatic varieties may occur not only from penetrating injuries but also from a tearing of the diaphragm away from its attachments to the thoracic wall. Such hernias, for example, may occur after a severe automobile injury in which there has been no penetration of either the thorax or the abdomen. Another classification is that which comprises congenital, acquired and traumatic hernias (see p. 799).

The most common symptoms of diaphragmatic hernia are abdominal pain, vomiting relieved by a change in position, symptoms of intestinal obstruction, dyspnea, dysphagia, hemoptysis, cyanosis and pain in the left shoulder. Frequently abnormal tympany is found over the lower part of the thorax. Displacement of the heart to one side is also frequently noted. X-ray examination with a barium meal almost always reveals the true condition. The great danger of diaphragmatic hernia is that of strangulation. It is probably desirable, therefore, to operate on all cases, even if only mild symptoms are present.

Operative repair of this condition can often be performed through either an abdominal or a thoracic incision. In many cases it is helpful to make the approach through both incisions. It may be difficult to separate adherent intestine and to make a satisfactory reduction without the combination of both incisions. In any case, the operation will be made much easier if the diaphragm previously has been paralyzed on the affected side by crushing the phrenic nerve in the neck. Previous operation on the phrenic nerve ordinarily should be performed two or three days before the operation for the repair of the hernia. In some cases the repair is easy but in many it is exceedingly difficult. Especially is that true in those cases in which the diaphragm has been torn away from the anterior chest wall. In nearly all cases it will be found helpful to use sutures of living fascia obtained from the patient's own fascia lata. Ordinarily the lung rapidly expands to fill up the space formerly occupied by the herniated viscus.

Wounds of the Diaphragm.—Whenever recognized, penetrating wounds of the diaphragm should be promptly closed because of the possibility of the subsequent development of a diaphragmatic hernia.

Tumors of the Diaphragm.—Primary neoplasms of the diaphragm are so rare that they scarcely deserve mention. Binney[26] in 1931 in a careful review of the literature for the past fifty years could find but 4 instances of primary tumor of the diaphragm. One of these was reported as multiple fibromyoma, another one as fibromyosarcoma, another one as sarcoma and the fourth one as lipoma.

DISEASES OF THE TRACHEA

There are so few conditions involving the trachea which come to the attention of the general surgeon that in a book of this sort they need scarcely be discussed. Foreign bodies in the trachea are common but with the present excellence of bronchoscopic technic they are usually removed by that means without difficulty. Tracheo-esophageal fistulas are rare and for the most part they occur as a complication of advanced carcinoma of the esophagus. Attempts to close such fistulas are therefore practically never justifiable. Tumors of the trachea are very rare. The benign tumors which have been described include papillomas, fibromas, lipomas, intratracheal thyroid tissue, lymphomas, chondromas and chondro-osteomas. The benign tumors usually occur in the upper third of the trachea or in the region of the bifurcation. They can usually be best treated through the bronchoscope. Of the malignant tumors of the trachea, carcinoma is more than twice as common as sarcoma, but it is nevertheless comparatively rare. It usually arises in the lower third and is of the squamous cell variety. Coughing and hemoptysis are common symptoms to be followed later by severe dyspnea or pneumonia. Metastases usually occur late. Early perforation is to be expected from those malignant tumors which arise in the posterior wall. Malignant tumors in the upper part of the trachea are best treated by tracheofissure and diathermy. In other locations usually they must be treated by a combination of fulguration and radiotherapy. At best, the treatment of such tumors has been very unsatisfactory.

DISEASES OF THE BRONCHI

In considering surgical conditions of the bronchi it is essential to understand some of the specific effects of conditions which obstruct or cause inflammation of a part of the bronchial tree. Because of the relatively straight direction of the bronchus of the right lower lobe, foreign bodies which are aspirated are more likely to fall into that bronchus than into any other part of the bronchial tree. An obstructive lesion that is complete is almost always followed by an absorption of air in that portion of the lung to which the particular bronchus leads, with the result that the condition of atelectasis occurs. Recent work by VanAllen, Adams and Linkskog,[27] however, has shown that at least in the dog there is collateral circulation of air in different lobules and occasionally (Adams) even between different lobes of the lung. It would seem also that some evidence exists that in man similar collateral circulation of air occurs. In spite of this interesting fundamental physiological fact, clinically in the human being, atelectasis of a lobe almost always occurs as a result of complete obstruction of the bronchus of that lobe.

Inflammation of the bronchi of a suppurative character often produces purulent inflammations of the lung, especially if there is a more or less complete obstruction of the bronchus by a foreign body or by some other agent. Obstructive lesions are not always foreign bodies, they may be new growths or they may be scars resulting from severe inflammation of the bronchus. When destructive inflammation of the wall of a large bronchus occurs, the cartilage in the wall is more or less destroyed and the condition of bronchiectasis results. Only the large bronchi have cartilaginous walls.

It is important to emphasize the fact that the normal drainage from the lung is through the tracheobronchial tree. This is brought about chiefly by two mechanisms of which one is the expulsive action of the cilia of the epithelium lining the mucous membrane, and the other is the act of coughing. Likewise, it should be recalled that under normal conditions the bronchi are constantly changing their size and direction with each act of respiration (Heinbecker [28] and Francis [29]), that is, on inspiration the bronchi enlarge and become lengthened. This lengthening tends to make many of them in the lower lobes more perpendicular and corresponding changes occur in the direction of the bronchi in other parts of the lung. The movements just mentioned are dependent upon the action of the peribronchial muscle. It becomes apparent, therefore, that an inflammatory process or any other factor which alters the normal action of the bronchial muscle is likely to have some effects not only on the act of respiration itself, but also probably on the normal mechanism for the expulsion of secretions from the bronchial tree. Again consideration should be given to the fact that although coughing is one of the important mechanisms for the expulsion of products of inflammation of the bronchial tree, too violent coughing may be harmful because each act is necessarily preceded by a deep inspiration which may spread the products of inflammation into previously uninvolved alveoli of the lung. There is at the present time an insufficient amount of knowledge concerning the various points just discussed to permit one to be dogmatic.

Foreign Bodies.—Foreign bodies of various kinds are frequently aspirated by children into one of the large bronchi. When these are opaque they are readily recognized by x-ray examination. Many of them, however, are not opaque and therefore they cannot be recognized in that way. For example, peanuts, which are nonopaque, are frequently aspirated. Immediately after the passage of the foreign body into a bronchus, the child, as a rule, begins to cough violently, becomes cyanotic and gives evidence of more or less marked dyspnea. Cyanosis, as a rule, is not so marked as when the foreign body is lodged in either the larynx or the trachea. If the foreign body is not coughed up, the symptoms persist, and because of the violence of the coughing, together with an inspiration whoop, a diagnosis of whooping cough is often wrongly made. The serious consequences of a retained foreign body in the bronchus are the inflammation which occurs with more or less destruction of the cartilaginous wall and a resulting bronchiectasis. Often associated with that condition is a more or less extensive destruction of lung tissue with sometimes the formation of multiple abscesses. Peanuts are particularly likely to result in gangrenous changes in the lung because of the irritating fatty acids which are formed in their decomposition. A foreign body in the bronchus may cause either a partial or a complete obstruction of the lumen. In the case of a partial obstruction a diminished amount of air may pass in and out of the lung past the foreign body, or the latter may obstruct in such a way that the air which is inspired cannot be expired; in other words, it may act like a check valve. In such cases an obstructive emphysema of the lung may occur behind the obstruction. In the case of a complete obstruction, atelectasis will inevitably occur. These results are important to bear in mind in the interpretation of the x-ray film made of the patient who is suspected of having aspirated a foreign body. In any case in which a foreign body is suspected, even if its presence cannot be definitely proven, the patient should be examined with a bronchoscope. It is possible with modern improved technic for a skilled bronchoscopist to remove practically all

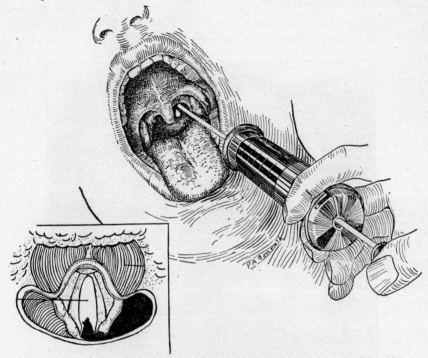

FIG. 497.—THE ASPIRATION METHOD OF INJECTING LIPIODOL (J. J. SINGER).

The method of introducing the iodized oil into the posterior pharynx while the patient breathes deeply; the inset shows how the oil collects in the interarytenoid fossae. It then trickles between the vocal cords and is aspirated into the bronchial tree. A roentgenogram obtained by this method is shown in Figure 498. In only 10 or 15 per cent of adults is it necessary to cocainize the pharynx. In little children the method can seldom be used; for them bronchoscopic injection of the lipiodol is preferable. (From Graham, Singer and Ballon, *Surgical Diseases of the Chest*, 1935. Courtesy of Lea and Febiger, Philadelphia.)

foreign bodies which may be present in the bronchial tree. Such attempts should always be made before the possibility of more radical surgery is seriously considered.

Bronchostenosis.—In the opening paragraph of this section some of the mechanical factors involved in bronchostenosis have already been discussed. The whole subject has recently been admirably and extensively discussed by Eloesser.[30] The symptoms and physical signs differ according to the location of the stenosis. The amount of dyspnea is naturally dependent to a great degree upon the amount of lung involved. As might be expected, therefore, a stenosis of the trachea or of both bronchi at the bifurcation results in more dyspnea than if the lesion involves the bronchus of only one lobe. Some degree of cough is usually but not always present. Inspiration is prolonged, difficult and wheezing. Expiration, as a rule, is much less difficult. Stridor is loud in stenosis of the trachea and of the bifurcation but it is usually absent in lesions lower down.

The physical signs of an obstruction of a bronchus are essentially those of atelectasis. Again those features vary depending upon the amount of lung involved. If a main bronchus is completely obstructed then the whole lung may show evidence of massive atelectasis. The patient complains of pain on the affected side, the intercostal spaces on that side are narrowed, there is more or less iimitation of respiratory movement and the heart and mediastinal contents are found to be drawn

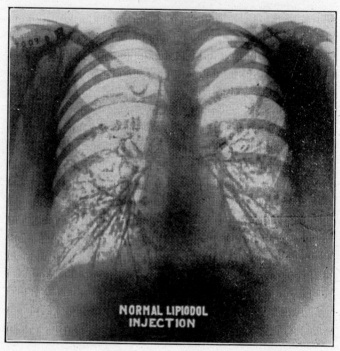

NORMAL LIPIODOL INJECTION

Fig. 498.—Roentgenogram of a Normal Chest following Injection of the Bronchial Tree with Lipiodol by the Aspiration Method.

(From Graham, Singer and Ballon, *Surgical Diseases of the Chest,* 1935. Courtesy of Lea and Febiger, Philadelphia.)

over towards the affected side. The diaphragm on that side is elevated, the breath sounds are usually absent or diminished and the percussion note is correspondingly dull.

The ordinary x-ray examination reveals an opacity in the region of the atelectasis, a deflection of the mediastinal contents towards the affected side and usually also a compensatory emphysema of the other lung. An x-ray examination, however, is not complete without the use of lipiodol. Again, although a lipiodol injection will usually clearly demonstrate the site of the stenosis, the whole examination should not be considered finished without the use of the bronchoscope. By the use of that instrument it is possible to determine whether the stenosis is due to a foreign bouy, an inflammatory stricture or to a tumor, or to ascertain whether the obstruction is due to pressure on the bronchus from the outside caused by perhaps a tumor of the mediastinum. If the tumor is found within the bronchus itself, a biopsy made at the time will reveal its character.

The treatment of bronchial stenosis will, of course, depend considerably upon the nature of the stenosis. If it is due to a foreign body the latter should be removed through a bronchoscope. Likewise benign tumors can often be removed in that way. If, however, it is due to a carcinoma of the bronchus then the treatment should be of a different sort which will be found discussed later in the part dealing with tumors of the lung. If the stenosis is due to an inflammatory stricture there will usually be an associated bronchiectasis which will require the sort of treatment discussed under that heading. If, on the other hand, it is due to the pressure of a mediastinal tumor upon the wall of a bronchus, appropriate treatment for the mediastinal tumor should be undertaken.

Bronchial Tumors.—Most tumors arising in the bronchi are carcinomas, discussed under Tumors of the Lung. Benign tumors also occur in the bronchi, mostly polyps or adenomas, arising from the bronchial epithelium. There is much confusion about which should be regarded as benign for many so-called benign adenomas are potentially malignant. Tumors of this type have rarely been completely removed through the bronchoscope by electrocoagulation and in other ways, and opinion is increasing that such limited removal is unsatisfactory. A lobectomy or a total pneumonectomy will give more assurance against a recurrence in cases in which malignant changes have occurred. A differentiation between a benign and a malignant tumor of the bronchus is not easy to make from a bronchoscopic biopsy.

Broncholithiasis (Lung Stones).—This condition is by no means as infrequent as a survey of the literature would indicate. We have noted their appearance in approximately 2 per cent of our cases of chronic pulmonary suppuration. The expectorated stones usually have about the same relative proportion of calcium phosphate and calcium carbonate that is contained in bone. They are usually multiple although occasionally they may be single. In one of our own cases the patient coughed up 126 stones during a period of six months. They vary in size from merely granular particles to stones which may weigh several grams. They are irregular in outline. They are often found in individuals with healed pulmonary tuberculosis but they may also be present with a variety of other conditions, such, for example, as all forms of pulmonary suppuration, tumors, cysts, actinomycosis and even with silicosis. Lerche [31] has suggested that in many cases broncholiths are concrements which have ulcerated through into a bronchus or into the lung from calcified tracheobronchial and bronchopulmonary lymph nodes.

Associated with the stones usually are frequent and severe attacks of coughing, sometimes with pain in the chest. Following the expulsion of the stone there may be blood in the sputum which occasionally is sufficient to be classed as a severe hemorrhage. The bleeding is probably due to the trauma of the mucous membrane produced by the sharp stone. Sometimes, if they are of sufficient size, the stones may be seen in an x-ray film, but usually they cannot be distinguished from calcified areas in the neighboring lymphatic nodes. Ordinarily the condition demands no special treatment. It is to be emphasized, however, that sometimes, because of the element of hemoptysis, such patients are wrongly diagnosed as having active tuberculosis. Occasionally bronchoscopic removal of broncholiths is indicated.

Bronchial Fistula.—Any abnormal communication between the bronchial tree and another surface or organ is termed a bronchial fistula. The most common site for such a fistula is between some part of the bronchial tree and the pleural cavity. Often, however, fistulas are noted in patients who have recovered from an operation for empyema or a lung abscess with the bronchial opening communicating directly with the skin. They naturally vary greatly in size depending upon whether they lead directly from a large bronchus or from some one of the finer divisions of the bronchus. They may be either acute or chronic. For the most part the small ones heal spontaneously in a relatively short period of time. It is only the larger ones which tend to remain chronic. Bronchial fistulas occur with any form of inflammation of the lung in which there is destruction of tissue. They are, therefore, especially likely to be found in cases of pulmonary suppuration of various kinds and also in pulmonary tuberculosis. The bronchial fistula may secrete mucus or mucopus or the product of the organ with which it communicates, as for example, bile in a bronchobiliary fistula. The character and the amount of the secretion from a bronchial fistula is considerably altered by the condition of the upper respiratory tract. When the patient develops a coryza or an acute infection of a nasal sinus, the mucous membrane of the fistula becomes congested and the secretion is greatly increased (Graham [32]).

One of the most serious features of a bronchial fistula is that hemorrhage, which may be severe, occurs from its mouth occasionally. In most cases, however, the chief complaint of the patient is the inconvenience caused by wearing a dressing and the impossibility of immersing the fistula under water because of the danger of drowning by the direct entrance of water into the lungs through the external opening.

There is a tendency for all bronchial fistulas to become healed spontaneously. When successful, this occurs as a result of the circular contraction of the peribronchial tissue and of scar tissue around the mouth of the fistula, as was shown experimentally by Bettman, James, Tannenbaum and Slobe.[33] If a large bronchial opening becomes adherent to the skin it is less likely to become closed than if it is situated deeply. It is well not to hurry too much in the ordinary closure of bronchial fistulas because the great majority of them will close spontaneously if an opportunity for them to do so is given over a period of several months. If, however, a decision has been made to close a fistula by surgical methods, the operation should be preceded by an attempt to make an exact diagnosis of the condition of the fistula. One should attempt to find out particularly its size, its extent and whether or not a foreign body is present within. All of this information can usually be obtained by injecting the sinus with lipiodol. Surgical closure of the fistula is based on the application of a variety of principles. In some cases repeated cauterizations of the mouth of the fistula are sufficient but usually not in the chronic cases in our experience. Another principle is to mobilize the lung from its attachments to the chest wall and to close the fistula with several rows of sutures after the mobilization has been effected. Such a procedure usually will permit the circular contraction of scar tissue, which is helpful in the closure. Another principle which is very effective is the transplantation of a vascular flap of muscle into the mouth of the fistula. This latter procedure is especially helpful in cases in which the bronchial fistula leads into a pulmonary cavity of considerable size. In some cases a partial resection of the lung will be necessary.

Bronchiectasis.—This condition has become one of extreme importance to the thoracic surgeon both because of its great frequency and because with modern methods it is now possible to offer hope of a cure to more than 90 per cent of properly selected patients.

In any case of bronchiectasis associated with expectoration of a large amount of sputum one must assume that a chronic infection is present. There is still some argument as to whether or not bronchiectasis may ever be congenital in origin. There is no doubt that congenital dilations of the bronchi occur even with the formation of cyst-like structures within the lung. The condition, however, does not produce the characteristic symptoms of bronchiectasis until after a chronic infection has set in. Although the presence of a sort of inflammation which destroys the cartilage of the bronchial wall is necessary for the development of bronchiectasis, another factor is often contributory, namely, a bronchostenosis due to any cause (foreign body, stricture, tumor, pressure from without, etc.). The type of inflammation which gives rise to bronchiectasis is that which is usually associated with bacteria which cause more or less extensive necrosis such as the anaerobic putrefactive organisms. Presumably, however, severe streptococcal infections alone can produce the condition. Pneumococcal infections rarely, if ever, produce it.

Various pathologic classifications have been made but probably on the whole they have not been of great practical value. It is important to realize that the condition of bronchiectasis once inaugurated is accompanied by more or less severe inflammation of the adjacent pulmonary tissue. In some instances there will be pulmonary abscesses of various sizes and in other instances there will be a minimum of parenchymatous change. More or less extensive atelectasis is common, due to a combination of stenosis of the principal bronchus to the part and the infection of the parenchyma of the lung with resulting fibrosis and contraction. The condition in general has a lobar distribution, in that ordinarily all of the larger bronchi of a lobe are involved in the process. Often, however, it is not confined to a single lobe but may involve the whole lung or even be bilateral. On external appearance the lobe which is the site of chronic bronchiectasis will usually be much smaller than normal; it will be cyanotic and firm. On cut section the dilated bronchi with thickened walls will be seen, the lumina of the bronchi will contain granulation tissue covered with mucopus often of a characteristic foul odor. A bronchial stenosis is not always demonstrated. Bronchiectasis is sometimes associated with pulmonary tuberculosis. In such cases it differs somewhat from that type which is not associated with tuberculosis. In the nontuberculous variety as a rule there is more thickening of the bronchial walls and more granulation tissue in the lumen. Moreover, the tuberculous variety is more likely to be present in the upper lobe than in the lower, in contradistinction to the nontuberculous variety.

The chief complaints of the patient are cough, expectoration, foul breath, hemoptysis and fever. The amount of sputum is variable but it may exceed 1000 cc. per day. It often has an odor due to putrefaction which is rather characteristic and which makes the patient with the disease often abhorrent to those with whom he is in contact. Characteristically, the sputum when collected in a glass vessel

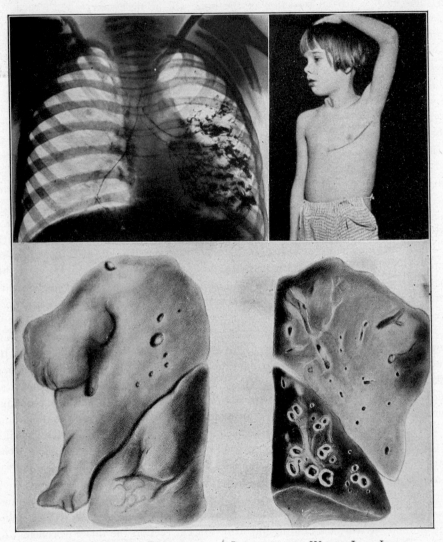

Fig. 499.—Extensive Bronchiectasis Involving the Whole Left Lung.

The patient is a child of ten years who had aspirated a peanut five years previously. Top left, roentgenogram of chest after injection of lipiodol. Top right, photograph of patient three months after total pneumonectomy. The wound is solidly healed and the patient is entirely free of her former symptoms. Below, drawing of lung after surgical removal (exterior and cut surface).

is seen to separate into three layers, the upper of which is nearly colorless or slightly greenish and contains air bubbles, pus and mucus. The second layer contains many of the products of the first layer but has less air. The third layer contains a greenish sediment which consists of pus cells, fat rests, Dittrich plugs and detritus. The expectoration of blood is frequent, sometimes it amounts to only a streaking of sputum but at other times it may be a severe hemorrhage. Fever, sweats and chills are common complaints. These occur intermittently and between such attacks the patient may feel reasonably well. They are probably due to repeated attacks of inflammation of the pulmonary parenchyma adjacent to the bronchiectasis. It is not uncommon for a patient with bronchiectasis to be required to go to bed with a bout of fever for a week or ten days at a time, at irregular intervals, two or three times a year.

Although one can diagnose the presence of bronchiectasis with a fair degree of accuracy merely on the fact that the patient has had a chronic cough with profuse expectoration of pus, such a diagnosis is far from satisfactory because it is incomplete. One should also attempt to diagnose the location of the disease (i.e., what lobe or lobes are involved), the size and distribution of the dilatations, the degree of fibrosis as evidenced by atelectasis and shift of the mediastinal contents, the nature of the process, whether tuberculous or not and the presence or absence of various local or systemic complicating features such as foreign body, pulmonary abscess, bronchial stenosis, carcinoma, empyema, brain abscess, amyloid disease, osteoarthropathy, etc. Such an examination often requires the employment of the following sources of information: (1) clinical history, (2) physical findings, (3) laboratory findings, (4) ordinary roentgenographic findings including fluoroscopy, (5) bronchography with lipiodol, (6) bronchoscopy, (7) diagnostic pneumothorax. Of the various forms of examination, ordinarily bronchography by the injection of lipiodol into the lungs and subsequent x-ray studies will be found to be the most useful procedure. By such means it will be possible not only to see the dilatations of the bronchi but also to locate them in the particular part of the lung involved. In that way it is possible to arrive rather accurately at a precise conception of the extent of the disease. Many patients with chronic bronchiectasis give evidence of clubbing of the fingers and toes, a condition usually known as *hypertrophic osteoarthropathy*. The sputum should be carefully examined to note the presence or absence of tubercle bacilli, spirochetal organisms of various kinds, etc. The bronchoscope is important because it may reveal a foreign body, a stricture or a tumor. The amount of atelectasis as determined by the shift of the mediastinal contents noted in the x-ray examination will also be important. In this connection it should be stated that often the left lower lobe when atelectatic is completely hidden behind the cardiac shadow and may not be recognized as the seat of bronchiectasis without a lipiodol injection. It is important also to diagnose if possible the presence of complications. The urine should be examined for the possibility of amyloid disease. The nasal sinuses should be examined because of the frequent association of chronic suppuration in those passages. Likewise the central nervous system should be carefully examined to detect if possible the presence of an abscess of the brain which is a complication in about 5 per cent of cases.

It has been well known for a long time that an intimate relationship exists between suppurative diseases of the nasal sinuses and bronchiectasis. Many patients with the more severe types of the latter disease have extensive suppuration in the upper respiratory tract. It is well, therefore, to examine all patients with bronchiectasis with reference to the nasal sinuses. Although a case of marked bronchiectasis cannot be cured in an anatomical sense by treatment of the nasal sinuses, the amount of sputum can often be reduced by correction of the disease of the sinuses. On a number of occasions we have seen bilateral cases improve by this means to such an extent that children have been able to go to school without being offensive to others. There is even some possibility that the progress of the disease may be somewhat arrested by proper treatment of the diseased nasal sinuses.

The *treatment* of bronchiectasis in recent years has become more and more surgical with the rapid development and improvement in technic of thoracic surgery. Nonsurgical methods for the most part have been ineffective. In making a decision as to whether or not a patient who has bronchiectasis should be subjected to radical surgical treatment, attention should be given to a number of considerations. In the case of a child there is a probability that the disease will become progressive. Again, if there is much atelectasis and parenchymatous involvement, experience indicates that eventually the disease is almost certain to be fatal. Moreover, the operative mortality in children and young adults is much less than it is after middle age. All of these considerations, therefore, justify one in giving more serious attention to the possibility of the radical procedure than is the case in an individual past middle age who perhaps has had the disease for many years and who is able to perform normal activities fairly well. More and more it is realized that permanent cures of severe cases are impossible without actual removal of the diseased tissue. In an occasional case it is possible that the condition becomes transformed into a so-called "dry" case, that is, one in which there is relatively little sputum. On the other hand, such a result can seldom be expected and one should not be led astray by the natural tendency of the disease to have remissions to conclude that any form of conservative treatment has really been effective.

Of the conservative methods of treatment the one which is perhaps the most effective is *postural drainage*. This is a procedure in which the patient by lowering his head and trunk induces a copious outflow of sputum. In many cases if the patient drains himself by this simple procedure in the morning upon arising and in the evening again before going to bed he will be bothered very little during the intervals by cough and sputum. The use of arsenicals has been extensively employed because of the frequent presence in the sputum of spirochetal organisms. This form of therapy often greatly reduces the number of such organisms in the sputum but it has not been found effective in improving the patient's symptoms to any considerable degree. Frequent bronchoscopic aspirations have been extensively employed but they probably have no great advantage over the more simple postural drainage. The use of artificial pneumothorax has been found in exceptional cases to cause some improvement in the patient's symptoms. It could hardly be expected, however, to cause any marked improvement except perhaps in very early cases. Moreover, in many cases the adhesions are so great that it is impossible to induce a pneumothorax. Other methods of inducing pulmonary collapse such as oleothorax, plombage, thoracoplasty and phrenicectomy have all been tried but in general the results have not been sufficiently satisfactory to give much encouragement to their use. Occasionally a patient may be made worse by a phrenicectomy because of the interference with the expulsion of the secretions by cough as a result of the paralysis of the diaphragm.

Of the more radical surgical measures, simple pneumostomy for external drainage was one of the earliest ones used. In probably the majority of cases in which such a procedure was successful, the condition was really one of pulmonary abscess rather than of bronchiectasis in the ordinary sense. It is impossible in a well-developed case of bronchiectasis to accomplish something approaching adequate drainage by a simple incision in the lung. The operation of lobectomy in recent years has been found to yield the most satisfactory results in the treatment of this disease. The former prohibitive mortality associated with this operation has been so much reduced that it is now not an unusual experience for trained thoracic surgeons to report a series of cases with less than 5 per cent mortality. Several methods of performing lobectomy have been described; some operators prefer a one-stage method, others prefer a multiple-stage method. The special tourniquets which have been devised for dealing safely with the hilus have done much to improve the operative mortality. For example, Churchill [34] reports 3.3 per cent mortality in 112 lobectomies, Edwards [35] has had only two deaths in his last 54 lobectomy cases, Graham and Blades [36] have had a successive series of 38 lobectomies for bronchiectasis with only one death (2.6 per cent), and many others have reported smaller series of cases with mortality rates of approximately five per cent. In a number of cases the whole lung has been successfully removed for this condition. There are certain cases in which the features of multiple abscesses predominate over that of a more ordinary bronchiectasis and in which the lung is so firmly adherent to the thoracic wall that it is impossible to mobilize it safely in order to perform a lobectomy. In such cases the author [37] has obtained satisfactory results in 70 per cent of a series of 80 cases by burning out the diseased lung tissue with an actual cautery in multiple stages. This operation at best is not entirely satisfactory; there is always the danger of fatal air embolism and occasionally there is danger of severe hemorrhage. On the other hand, the cases in which the method should be used represent the most serious types of the disease and they are of a kind for which the ordinary lobectomy is not feasible. Another accomplishment of the improved technic of thoracic surgery has made it possible to perform a lobectomy and even a total removal of the lung without removing ribs and therefore without any deformity of the thorax other than the scar of the incision. This is accomplished by making an incision at an intercostal space, dividing two or three costal cartilages, spreading the ribs apart, and later suturing the cartilages together again.

One of the most frequent postoperative complications after the removal of a lobe for bronchiectasis is the development of a localized empyema which usually makes its appearance in from seven to ten days after operation. Ordinarily it is due to an opening of the bronchial stump. As a rule, however, the bronchial fistula closes spontaneously within a few weeks and the empyema causes no further trouble. If the operation has been performed in multiple stages the empyema is likely to be more restricted because the remaining portion of lung is firmly adherent to the chest wall, and for that reason the amount of the pleural space liable to infection is greatly diminished. Improved operative technic, however, has made the incidence of bronchial fistula still less, regardless of whether the operation has been performed in one or several stages.

The high incidence of permanent closure of the bronchus in total pneumonectomy by individual ligation of each structure in the pulmonary hilum as suggested by Rienhoff [38] and others has stimulated study of the anatomy of the pulmonary lobes to determine the feasibility of separate ligation of each structure when lobectomy is performed. The anatomic and clinical studies by Blades and Kent [39] led them to the conclusion that in the majority of cases individual ligation technic for lobectomy has distinct advantages over mass ligation with a tourniquet, by insuring better bronchial closure. However, a detailed discussion of the more approved methods of suture of the bronchial stump is hardly suitable for a work of this kind.

Surgical intervention in bilateral bronchiectasis is feasible. Sixteen such patients have been operated upon at Barnes Hospital. In three cases all but the two upper pulmonary lobes (including the lingulas of the upper lobes) have been removed successfully.

DISEASES OF THE LUNG

Congenital Abnormalities.—Various abnormalities of the lung have been described. Occasionally an entire lung is absent. More frequently a condition has been described in which one lung has maintained its fetal state and has never expanded. From time to time variations are found regarding the locations of the

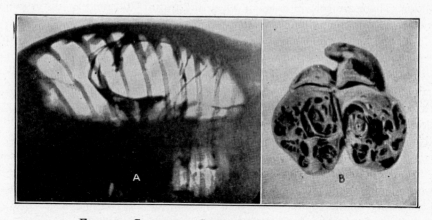

FIG. 500.—CONGENITAL CYSTIC DISEASE OF THE LUNG.

A, bilateral cystic disease of the lung in a child eighteen months old. The film was taken with the patient's left side up (after lipiodol injection), *B*, photograph of a specimen of true congenital cystic disease of the lung from a newly born infant. (From Graham, Singer and Ballon, *Surgical Diseases of the Chest*, 1935. Courtesy of Lea and Febiger, Philadelphia.)

interlobar fissures and even of the number of lobes in each lung. Incomplete interlobar fissures are not uncommon. This is a matter of considerable importance to the surgeon contemplating the performance of a lobectomy because he may find that the particular lobe to be attacked is not discrete or sharply separated from the rest of the lung. In recent years a congenital abnormality which has become of increasing importance is that known as *congenital cystic disease of the lung*. It is sometimes also known under the name of fibrocystic adenoma pulmonare. The cysts may be single, occasionally reaching such a size that almost an entire lobe is represented by a single cyst, or they may be multiple. They tend to be confined to a single lobe although frequently cysts may be scattered throughout an entire lung or even both lungs. When multiple, they are of various sizes, the largest of which may have an estimated capacity of 500 cc. and the smallest of which may be scarcely visible to the naked eye. They contain air and are, therefore, connected with the bronchial tree. They are lined by flattened cells which have ordinarily been considered to be epithelial in origin.

Congenital cysts of the lung are of clinical importance because of the complications which may arise. If a cyst is near the periphery of the lung, spontaneous rupture may occur easily into the pleural cavity with the formation of a pneumothorax. Undoubtedly many cases of nontuberculous spontaneous pneumothorax are due to the rupture of a congenital cyst. Especially is this true in cases of young children. The other important complication to which such cysts may give rise is that of infection. If a cyst does not rupture into the pleural cavity it may remain silent without causing any symptoms until adulthood or middle life, when some serious acute pulmonary infection may be the start of a chronic infection of the cyst. In such cases, because of the x-ray appearance of a walled-off region in the lung with a fluid level, and because the patient is expectorating pus, a diagnosis is often made of pulmonary abscess and the patient is treated as if he had an ordinary abscess of the lung. Apparently in most cases, when such a cyst has become once infected there is little likelihood of a spontaneous healing. Experience has indicated that in most of such cases it is necessary to remove the part of the lung which contains the cyst, and ordinarily this implies at least a lobectomy.

The diagnosis of congenital cystic disease of the lung is sometimes made with reasonable assurance by ordinary x-ray examination. Usually, however, it will be necessary to resort to the use of lipiodol to make the diagnosis certain. Sometimes, all that is necessary is to inject lipiodol in the ordinary way through the mouth into the larynx. In other cases it will be necessary to inject the lipiodol directly into a cyst through the chest wall. We have resorted to the latter procedure in a number of instances and have had no unfavorable results. It is very important to remember that the disease may not be confined to one lung. The examination, therefore, should not be stopped merely because evidence of the condition has been found present in one lung. It is essential that the lipiodol be allowed to spread around in both lungs and that the patient be placed in suitable positions to show both lungs in order to rule out the possibility of a bilateral involvement.

Since in most cases no symptoms are produced from the cyst until the occurrence of one of the complications just mentioned, it is unlikely that many cases will be recognized unless one of those complications is present. Any person who has congenital cystic disease necessarily runs the risk of more or less serious consequences at some time. Theoretically, therefore, if it is known that a patient has congenital cystic disease involving one lobe, it would probably be desirable to advise him to have that lobe removed before serious consequences may develop. The complicating pneumothorax in itself is not particularly serious unless it should result in an unrecognized acute tension pneumothorax, which might be fatal. In most cases, all that is necessary to do is to provide an outlet for the air under pressure in the pleural cavity, either by repeated aspirations or by some method of continuous closed aspiration which will keep the intrathoracic pressure down to safer limits. In most cases the rupture in the surface of the lung will heal spontaneously, the lung will come out to the chest wall where it will become adherent and the danger therefore of a repetition of a serious pneumothorax will be obviated. Sometimes, however, repeated attacks do occur because the adhesions between the lung and the chest wall are not sufficiently firm. If the patient has extensive bilateral disease, obviously nothing more can be done than to attempt to obliterate the two pleural cavities. The injection into the pleural cavity of a small amount (10 cc.) of the patient's own blood is often helpful in the obliteration of the pleural cavity. If the attention to the presence of the cysts has first been directed because of the presence of infection, it will usually be found necessary to establish external drainage until the acute infection has subsided and then to consider a more radical procedure, consisting of the removal of as much of the diseased lung as is necessary. Usually the cysts cannot be satisfactorily obliterated by the methods of collapse therapy which are so successfully employed in the treatment of tuberculous cavities in the lung.

Another congenital anomaly which deserves some mention is the *accessory lobe of the azygos vein (Wrisberg's Lobe)*. This condition occurs in somewhat less than 1 per cent of all people examined. It is of importance chiefly for diagnostic reasons because sometimes it is confused with other conditions. Various types of this abnormality have been described as follows:

(*a*) The fissure may cut the lung at any level from an oblique plane cutting the outer surface of the lung two inches below the apex, to a vertical plane cutting off a small tongue-shaped lobe from the mediastinal surface. Between these extremes is an intermediate type passing approximately through the apex of the lung. The first type is the commonest but a large number of cases may show about equal numbers of each.

(*b*) The azygos vein pursues a normal course from the aortic opening to the fifth thoracic vertebra, where it turns back and to the right to sink into the azygos fissure.

(*c*) The azygos vein empties into the junction of the two innominate veins, commencement of the superior vena cava.

(*d*) The fissure approaches the root of the lung and in some cases actually rests on the exposed medial branch of the eparterial bronchus.

A more extensive discussion of this question will be found in the book by Graham, Singer and Ballon.[40]

Pulmonary Abscess and Gangrene.—Formerly clinicians attempted to make a more or less sharp distinction between pulmonary abscess and gangrene. In recent times, however, the tendency to consider the two conditions together has become more and more pronounced. In either case, one is dealing with destruction of tissue. The reason why one individual develops an abscess and another does not is due chiefly to the fact that the former has manifested enough resistance to create a pyogenic membrane about the inflammatory region. Either condition can pass into the other one. An extensive gangrene of the lung can later become an abscess and in turn an abscess can spread to form a diffuse suppurative pneumonitis which may be essentially a massive gangrenous process. When the distinctive term of pulmonary gangrene is used it is ordinarily applied to a fulminating condition in which a whole lobe or even an entire lung becomes necrotic. Various factors which are important in determining whether or not a given inflammation is going to develop into either an abscess or an extensive gangrenous process are the nature of the responsible organism or organisms concerned, the natural resistance of the patient against an infection and finally whether or not the principal blood supply of the part is obstructed by a thrombosis resulting from the inflammation.

The various etiologic factors may be grouped under several headings: (1) surgical operations; (2) aspiration of foreign material; (3) pneumonia; (4) wounds of the lung; (5) carcinoma of the bronchus, lung and esophagus; (6) miscellaneous factors. Of the surgical operations, those performed in the mouth are especially dangerous. Particularly is this the case with the operation of tonsillectomy performed under general anesthesia, although actually, as was shown by Moore,[41] the chance of the development of a pulmonary abscess is only about 1 in 2500 to 3000 tonsillectomies. If the operation of tonsillectomy is performed under a deep general anesthesia the chance of developing pulmonary abscess is greater probably because there is likely to be aspirated into the lung a larger amount of blood and pus than if the normal swallowing and coughing reflexes are preserved. Although the possibility of the development of a pulmonary abscess from the aspiration of infected foreign material was seriously questioned, it has now been definitely shown experimentally that aspiration is an important factor. The pus from the gums in a case of bad pyorrhea is particularly effective in the development of an abscess when injected into the tracheobronchial tree, as was shown by Crowe and Scarff.[42] Duff Allen[43] showed that the experimental production of pulmonary abscess is easy if the pus from the human abscess is immediately injected into the tracheobronchial tree of a dog before an opportunity for cooling has occurred. The evidence is now overwhelming that aspiration of suitable material may result in the development of a pulmonary abscess. Again, it is well known that the aspiration of peanuts is likely to be followed by an extensive bronchitis (*arachidic bronchitis*) with the subsequent development of more or less extensive gangrene because of the irritating qualities of the fatty acids formed in the decomposition of the peanut. Pneumonia is often stated as a frequent cause of pulmonary abscess. This statement is mainly due, however, to the fact that any inflammation of the lung in its early stages is likely to be diagnosed under the inclusive term of pneumonia. The term pneumonitis would be preferable. Actually there is little evidence that ordinary lobar pneumonia is very often the precursor of pulmonary abscess. On the other hand, streptococcal pneumonia, especially that type which was present in the severe epidemics of 1917 and 1918, is often associated with pulmonary abscess. Wounds of the lungs seldom produce an abscess. Carcinoma of the bronchus is nearly always associated with single or multiple pulmonary abscesses at some time in its course. It is a matter of the greatest importance to bear this in mind because a pulmonary abscess in a person of middle age, which has come on with no apparent reason, is often due to a carcinoma. Miscellaneous factors of various kinds may also produce abscess of the lung, such as streptothricosis, actinomycosis, blastomycosis, etc.

Many different kinds of bacteria have been found in cases of pulmonary abscess. Besides the ordinary pyogenic bacteria, it is common to find various types of spirochetes and fusiform bacilli. Anerobic bacteria are also common. Burdon[44] and Varney[45] have emphasized the importance of *Bacterium melanino-genicum*. This organism is found in nearly all cases of pulmonary abscess. It is also frequently present in the pus in cases of pyorrhea and in some infected tonsils. It is strictly anerobic. It forms black pigment and it grows best in symbiosis with other organisms. When so grown, the cultures develop a foul odor resembling the breath of some patients with lung abscess. In pure culture it is not pyogenic but in symbiosis with other organisms it produces extensive necrosis of tissue regardless of where in the body it is injected.

The most common site of pulmonary abscess is in the right lower lobe. If a lung containing a true abscess is cut open a distinct pyogenic membrane will be seen. There will be numerous bronchial openings; fibrin and pus will be contained within the cavity, the lining of which is usually not smooth and is gray or brown in color. The term gangrene is applied to a condition in which a whole lobe or a whole lung is found to have undergone liquefaction necrosis without any sharp line of demarcation between normal and diseased tissue, and with a greenish black or brownish black appearance of the diseased tissue. During the formative period of a pulmonary abscess there is an extensive zone of edema and some extravasation of blood around the area. When the abscess is well developed there is a central cavity of considerable size, sometimes small and at other times very large, the wall of which is composed of more or less necrotic epithelial tissue. In more advanced cases of longer duration, the wall of the abscess cavity may be several millimeters thick and composed of dense fibrous tissue. Usually several smaller abscesses are present in the zone surrounding the main abscess. Blood-vessels are sometimes observed to cross through the cavity unsupported by epithelial tissue, giving the impression of ropes or cords which have been strung across. Sometimes they are thrombosed but when not they may give rise to the sudden massive hemorrhages which often complicate the condition of pulmonary abscess. The common varieties of lung abscess are often spoken of in the clinical literature as *putrid abscess*. More rarely, there occurs a condition known as *aputrid pulmonary necrosis*. It is thought that some of the cases of aputrid pulmonary necrosis have their origin in infarctions of a portion of lung tissue with subsequent infection by organisms which are not putrefactive. The condition has been described also as a rare complication of lobar pneumonia, presumably also because of the absence of putrefactive bacteria.

A common complication of pulmonary abscess is empyema from rupture of the abscess in the pleural cavity with the formation usually of pyopneumothorax because air also escapes into the pleural cavity. Brain abscess and meningitis, mediastinal abscess and suppurative pericarditis are all complications which occur with some frequency. Hemorrhage is sometimes severe enough to be fatal. Extension of the infection to other parts of the lung is a frequent cause of death in such cases. Clubbing of the fingers and toes and amyloid degeneration are complications seen with chronic pulmonary abscess, but seldom with the acute disease. In any case of chronic pulmonary abscess more or less marked bronchiectasis is probably always present.

The principal *symptoms* of pulmonary abscess usually occur in the following order of frequency: productive cough with the sputum often blood stained, fetor, fever, chills, sweats, pain in the chest, loss of strength and of appetite. The formative stage of pulmonary abscess usually has a duration of a few days to two or three

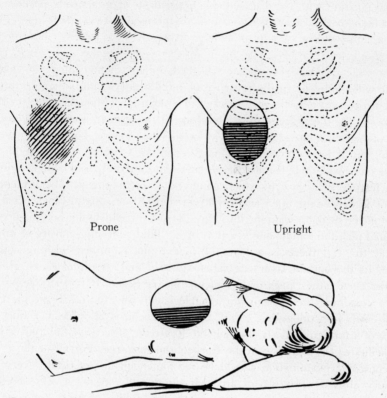

Prone   Upright

Fig. 501.—Diagram to Show the Advantage of Change in Position in the Demonstration of the Fluid Level in a Suspected Abscess Cavity by the Use of the Roentgen Ray.

(From Graham, Singer and Ballon, *Surgical Diseases of the Chest*, 1935. Courtesy of Lea and Febiger, Philadelphia.)

weeks. There may be no sputum during that time. As soon as a communication with a bronchus is effected foul expectoration occurs. In acute cases the patient is sometimes able to indicate the site of the abscess by the location of the pain. Empyema may complicate the picture early in the disease. Mediastinal abscesses and brain abscesses, however, are usually later complications. Clubbing of the fingers and toes is a complication of the chronic form of the disease. In the examination of the patient x-ray films are of paramount importance. Ordinary physical examination may reveal the presence of a large cavity but the accuracy of diagnosis is much greater with suitable x-ray examination. The use of lipiodol is not so helpful as might be expected because frequently the lipiodol fails to enter the cavity because of a stenosis of the bronchus leading into it as a result of edema. The most important finding in the x-ray examination is the presence of a fluid level within the lung field. In many cases, however, the fluid level cannot be demonstrated and in such cases only a region of induration will be detected. In searching for a fluid level it is of the greatest importance to have the patient in such positions as will demonstrate it. If the patient lies on the film either prone or supine, the level will almost certainly fail to be seen. It is necessary to have the patient either in a horizontal position with the diseased side uppermost, or in a sitting position. Films taken in both of the two latter positions are preferable to a single one. There is usually a leukocytosis of approximately 20,000 with a relative increase in the polymorphonuclear variety. The fever in the severe cases may reach 104° to 105° F. After drainage becomes established, either spontaneously or otherwise, the fever will diminish. In the presence of rapidly developing gangrene the symptoms of prostration may be very marked. The sputum, although scanty in the formative period of the abscess, may later become profuse. In some cases more than 500 cc. of pus may be expectorated in twenty-four hours. The color is not characteristic, but it is not uncommon for the sputum to show streaks of blood and sometimes a considerable hemorrhage occurs. An extremely foul odor is more likely to be a feature of a case in which gangrene is predominant. The presence of a foul odor is dependent upon active putrefaction. After standing in a glass vessel, the sputum is seen to separate into three layers in which the bottom one is the sedimented pus, the middle one is a thin turbid fluid consisting mostly of saliva and finally at the top there is a layer of foamy mucus mixed with mucopurulent material. In the bottom layer one can frequently find shreds of elastic tissue and sometimes even rather large masses of pulmonary tissue. It is desirable, of course, always to examine the sputum for tubercle bacilli and for other specific types of infection such as actinomyces, etc. The bronchoscope is of value in ruling out the presence of a foreign body. It also helps to locate the abscess and moreover it sometimes facilitates the drainage of the tracheobronchial tree. For all of those reasons a bronchoscopic examination should be recommended in practically every case of pulmonary abscess. The use of an aspirating needle in cases of suspected pulmonary abscess is dangerous because of the possibility of creating an empyema. It is seldom necessary to use a needle and therefore in most cases it should not be used. During and since World War I, many devices have been proposed to help in the localization of pulmonary abscess with the x-ray. It is seldom, however, that any of these special devices are necessary and for that reason they have not come into general use. It is always important to remember that the abscesses may be multiple and that consequently the localization of a single one does not necessarily complete the diagnosis.

The *treatment* of a case of pulmonary abscess will vary considerably according to the conditions which are present. All cases are certainly not surgical in the sense that they will require surgical drainage. Many patients recover merely by a spontaneous drainage created through the tracheobronchial tree. There is now a rather general agreement that the first consideration in the treatment of a relatively acute case is rest in bed supplemented by the drainage which may be effected by putting the patient into a suitable position to permit him to expel the pus in the easiest manner. This latter procedure is usually spoken of as *postural drainage*. It usually means that the patient's head and trunk are put into a position lower than the rest of the body. Gravity, therefore, assists in the expulsion of the pus after the flow has been started by coughing. With patients who are severely ill, postural drainage cannot be carried out for more than a few minutes at a time without causing distressing symptoms. When the procedure causes marked distress it should be stopped. The use of drugs is not particularly effective although in cases in which there are many spirochetes in the sputum the number of those organisms can be made to diminish by the use of arsenicals, such as arsphenamine, etc. Pneumothorax has been rather extensively tried and in many cases it has proven effective.

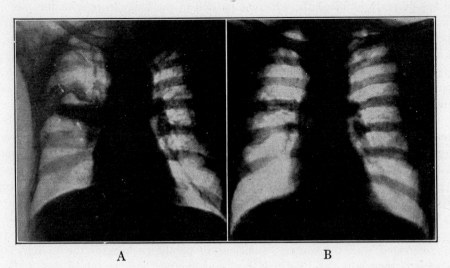

A   B

FIG. 502.—ABSCESS OF THE RIGHT LUNG (FOLLOWING TONSILLECTOMY).

A, before treatment. *B*, appearance of lung twelve weeks after the patient started postural drainage treatment; healing is complete (*Arch. Surg.*).

There are, however, certain dangers connected with its use, notably the risk of rupturing a peripheral abscess into the pleural cavity. Probably no more than 25 or 30 per cent of cases can be expected to improve greatly by pneumothorax treatment alone. Likewise other forms of compression such as is accomplished by operations on the phrenic nerve, by thoracoplasty and by the use of packing with gauze or rubber bags or paraffin plombes are not as a rule particularly effective. The more severe surgical operations for collapse and compression should be reserved for those cases which have become chronic. In most of such patients, however, some type of external drainage will be required.

In the majority of instances the cases in which no quick favorable response occurs from the more simple procedures of rest in bed and postural drainage will require the additional advantage of external drainage through an opening in the chest wall. A matter about which there has been much controversy has been the question of when to institute external drainage. There are many who think that an operation for drainage should not be performed until after the abscess has become essentially subacute or even chronic, in order to eliminate the danger of passing through a zone of edematous lung in order to reach the abscess. On the other hand, Neuhof [46] and his associates have been strong advocates of very early operation in these cases and their results are, on the whole, somewhat better than those which have been obtained by procrastination before operation. It is Neuhof's contention that adhesions between the lung and the chest wall in the great majority of cases are formed within ten days or two weeks of the beginning of the infection in the lung and that in practically all cases by careful examination of the patient, the site of these adhesions can be recognized. Therefore, almost as soon as the diagnosis is established he prefers to resect a rib, to find the pus with an aspirating needle after the resection of the rib, and then if he has properly localized the adherent portion of the lung, to remove the roof of the abscess cavity. If the site of adhesions to the lung is not found at the first operation, he searches again for the site of adhesions and continues the operation at another time. In carrying out such procedures he differs from others in several respects. The usual plan has been to operate only on those patients whose clinical course during the first four or five weeks has failed to show steady improvement after treatment with rest and postural drainage. It has been customary also when an operation for an acute abscess has been decided upon, to approach it at what has seemed to be the closest site, to resect a rib and to proceed to institute drainage if adhesions were present. If adhesions were not present it has been the custom to pack gauze, especially gauze containing some slightly irritant antiseptic such as iodine or iodoform, against the parietal pleura in order to create adhesions between the lung and the parietal pleura. Ordinarily about ten days are required by this method to produce firm adhesions. With the aspirating needle as a guide, the abscess is entered, preferably by means of an actual cautery and a large opening is created with the cautery, sufficient to permit packing of the cavity. The packing is then removed in a few days and another pack is substituted. Others have also carried out the procedure recommended by Neuhof of removing the roof of the abscess cavity. One or more bronchial openings are usually seen within the cavity at the time of its opening. Gradually, however, in favorable cases the cavity becomes completely obliterated with closure of the bronchial openings. The removal of the roof of the cavity is helpful in that not only does it provide more free drainage but also it removes actual diseased tissue. If, after such a procedure, the patient's cough and sputum do not almost completely disappear and if the temperature does not promptly return almost to normal, the presence of other pulmonary abscesses or of an empyema should be suspected. If an empyema is present it should be drained and treated like other forms of empyema.

The treatment of a chronic lung abscess with thickened fibrotic walls and much induration of the surrounding pulmonary tissue is often extremely difficult. Simple drainage and even removal of the roof will often be found ineffective. In some of such cases extensive removal of the diseased tissue will be necessary, either by the operation of ordinary lobectomy or by the operation of cautery pneumonectomy mentioned under the section on bronchiectasis. Extensive operative procedures on these cases are always difficult and dangerous. There is great danger from the development of air embolism of the brain because of the necessity of opening tributaries of the pulmonary vein which permit air to be carried directly to the brain. Schlaepfer [47] experimentally has shown conclusively that only a very small amount of air when introduced into a tributary of the pulmonary vein may produce a fatal cerebral air embolism. In many cases after the local treatment of the abscess, either acute or chronic, it will be necessary later to perform some plastic operation in order to close the open bronchial fistulas. Such operations are not to be carried out until after several months have elapsed because often the fistulas will close themselves spontaneously and, moreover, operations performed in the presence of acute infections are very likely to be unsuccessful. The common operative procedures employed for this purpose have already been discussed under the heading of Bronchial Fistula.

At best, a pulmonary abscess is a very serious disease and with present methods of treatment it is doubtful if we can expect to have more than 75 or 80 per cent of recoveries in patients in whom an abscess is positively diagnosed. Again, it should be recalled that many abscesses are merely complications of bronchiogenic carcinoma. In such cases treatment directed only at the abscess will necessarily be ineffective. The use of the sulfonamide drugs in pulmonary abscess is discussed at the end of the chapter.

Hydatid Disease (Echinococcus Cysts).—Because of its rarity in this country, no extensive discussion of this condition will be given here. Echinococcus infections have been discussed elsewhere in this book in more detail. From the standpoint of the thorax it is important to realize that next to the liver, the lung is the most frequent site of hydatid cysts, but they are much less frequent than in the liver, for example, the condition occurs with a frequency to the liver about seven times greater than in the lung.

Many pulmonary hydatid cysts produce no striking symptoms, even if they may be very large. Cough is perhaps the most common symptom produced, but unless the cyst is ruptured into a bronchus, the cough is not severe. It is intermittent and accompanied by very little expectoration. If, however, a rupture into the bronchial tree has occurred, the contents of the cyst will be expectorated in the sputum. Frequently also there will be hemoptysis of varying degrees. If the cyst is near the diaphragm, coughing is likely to be more pronounced even if it has not yet ruptured into a bronchus. The amount of dyspnea will be determined largely by the size of the cyst and the amount of pressure which it produces. The most common site of the cyst is in the right lower lobe. One of the principal dangers of rupture into the bronchial tree is that of severe allergy. This may be so severe as to cause death. According to Dew,[48] it is rare for a patient to become asphyxiated either by the sudden entrance of fluid into the lungs or by the impaction of a piece of membrane in the glottis.

The diagnosis of pulmonary hydatid cyst is made on the finding of a spherical shadow by roentgen examination and by the principal laboratory methods of diagnosis which have been discussed elsewhere, such as (1) the intradermal test of Casoni, (2) the complement fixation test of Ghedini-Weinberg, (3) the examination of the blood for the presence of an eosinophilia, and (4) the examination of the contents of the cyst and of the sputum for the characteristic hooklets, fragments of cyst membrane, etc. It is dangerous to aspirate a cyst because of the possibility of a severe allergic reaction from absorption by leakage into the lung or thoracic cavity.

Although it occasionally happens that cysts which have ruptured into the bronchial tree go on to a spontaneous healing, one cannot be assured that such a result will happen in a given case. Secondary infection of the cyst may result as one complication which may give rise to a condition somewhat resembling a pulmonary abscess. If the operation has been decided upon, one of two principles can be carried out. The first, which is the simpler one, is to marsupialize the cyst by sewing its edges to the chest wall after opening it to rid it of its contents and to allow for external drainage in that manner until the cyst has become completely obliterated. The other procedure is to undertake a radical removal of the diseased tissue. It is frequently necessary in performing a marsupialization operation to divide it in two stages, the first to create adhesions between the lung and the chest wall and the second to open the cyst and actually perform the marsupialization. Radical excision has been much less frequently employed in the past, but probably with the newer developments which have taken place in thoracic surgery this principle will be invoked more often in the future. It is always important to determine if possible whether the pulmonary cyst has originated in the lung or is merely an extension of the disease upward from the liver. In some cases it will be necessary not only to treat the cyst in the lung, but also that in the liver.

Pulmonary Actinomycosis.—This disease has been discussed more extensively on pages 96-99. When present in the lung it pursues the same tendencies as it does elsewhere in the body of ulcerating through to the surface, regardless of fascial planes or other barriers which ordinarily impede the progress of the more common pyogenic infections. A case of pulmonary actinomycosis, therefore, usually presents draining sinuses through the chest wall when first seen. Formerly it was looked upon as a nearly hopeless disease but by persistent use of operations for drainage of abscesses combined with x-ray therapy, opinion has changed and the condition is now not regarded as at all hopeless. Wangensteen [49] has been able to collect from the literature 19 cases including one of his own in which there has been an apparent recovery from thoracic actinomycosis. We have likewise had patients at the Barnes Hospital who have been well for over five years.

TUMORS OF THE LUNG

Perhaps nothing indicates more emphatically the development of thoracic surgery than the change of attitude regarding the treatment of pulmonary neoplasms. Formerly, even benign tumors were regarded for the most part as inoperable. More recently, however, the view has become accepted that not only is it possible to remove most benign tumors successfully but even many malignant ones can be removed safely with a reasonable prospect of a permanent cure.

The classification of pulmonary tumors has been much confused, partly by an uncertainty of the tissue of origin as well as by the use of a multiplicity of names based on the microscopic appearances. Although some of the benign neoplasms seem at times to have arisen in the substance of the lung parenchyma, perhaps by a process of metaplasia, yet in the light of the most recent evidence there is reason to believe that nearly all of the tumors roughly designated as primary pulmonary neoplasms actually arise in bronchial tissue. Certain tumors, however, sometimes found at the periphery of the lung (*e.g.*, myoma, fibroma) do possibly arise in the visceral pleura.

Much of the confusion which exists because of the multiplicity of names based on the microscopic appearances may perhaps be eliminated if the theory advanced by Womack and Graham [50] becomes generally accepted. They have called attention to the similarity between many of the tumors under discussion and those which, arising in the salivary glands, are well known to pathologists as "mixed tumors." Their study identifies as "mixed tumors" many of the hitherto unusual and unclassified neoplasms and places their pathogenesis, histology and clinical course on a firmer basis. These tumors, in accordance with the theory, represent fetal pulmonary tissue resulting from the failure of embryonic buds to develop into normal structures. When the mesoblastic elements predominate they become recognized as chondroma, sarcoma, etc. When, however, the epithelial elements predominate they become tumors which in the past have usually been termed adenoma, oat cell carcinoma, alveolar carcinoma, adenocarcinoma, etc. They are always potentially malignant. Although these epithelial tumors arise from fetal tissue, the mistake may easily be made, after they have become malignant, of thinking that they have arisen from adult bronchial epithelium. Thus autopsy studies made on advanced cases have often failed to reveal their true nature. These tumors, however, probably do not include the more common squamous cell carcinoma which seems in most instances to be a distinct type not due to the maldevelopment of fetal bronchial buds. Regardless of their origin, the tumors which are usually classified as benign are comparatively rare. The so-called bronchial adenoma is the most common and next in frequency is the chondroma.

Bronchial Adenoma.—These occur about equally in either sex and may appear at almost any age, from childhood to old age. The symptoms are chiefly those of bronchial irritation and of obstruction. These are discussed in a later paragraph on carcinoma. Although the presence of a bronchial obstruction can be diagnosed roentgenologically by the use of lipiodol a final diagnosis of bronchial adenoma can be made only by a bronchoscopic examination. A roughly spherical nodule projecting into the lumen usually will be seen which may be pink because of the large number of small blood vessels on its surface. A biopsy may reveal one of several more or less characteristic features, of which the most common is a collection of cells with small amounts of cytoplasm and relatively large nuclei. There is no characteristic arrangement although often the cells appear to be in cords and sometimes to have a glandular structure. For those reasons the tumors are sometimes designated as "round" cell, "oat" cell or "adeno" carcinoma. In the study made by Womack and Graham areas of cartilage, of bone and sometimes of fetal tissue, such as mesenchyme were found. The microscopic appearance often closely simulates that of fetal atelectatic lung. In those so-called adenomas which have become malignant, a tendency to invade the neighboring tissues is evident although no mitotic figures may be seen.

The treatment will depend on whether or not there is a suspicion of malignancy. Although it is our belief that these tumors are potentially malignant even when they reveal no definite evidence of such a change, some (notably by C. L. Jackson [51]) have been treated successfully by local removal through the bronchoscope. In many instances, however, a larger portion of the tumor is extrabronchial and only a small portion projects into the lumen. The tumor thus resembles an iceberg most of which is submerged and therefore invisible. Under such circumstances complete bronchoscopic removal is impossible and either lobectomy or total pneumonectomy becomes necessary to accomplish total eradication. In general, because of our belief in•the potential malignancy of these tumors, we prefer radical treatment, at least lobectomy, rather than the bronchoscopic removal, and we feel it is very strongly indicated in those cases in which there is a recurrence at the site of a previous bronchoscopic removal. The x-ray and radium have been notoriously ineffective in the treatment of bronchial adenomata.

Carcinoma.—By far the most important tumor of the lung is carcinoma. Statistical evidence indicates that its incidence has increased greatly in the past 25 years. It is known now to constitute between 5 to 10 per cent of all cancers. It is therefore in the same order of frequency as carcinoma of the colon. No satisfactory reason for its apparent increase exists. It is thought that perhaps occupations associated with the inhalation of large quantities of dust and other irritating substances are more likely to lead to this condition. For example, there has been an especially high incidence among the Schneeberg miners whose work consists in drilling hard rock with the production of large quantities of radioactive dust containing sharp angled particles with a high content of arsenic. Likewise the inhalation of gasoline products and cigarette smoke have been incriminated, but without convincing evidence.

Like cancer in other regions bronchiogenic carcinoma occurs most frequently between the ages of forty and sixty. It is four or five times more common in males. The squamous cell variety is almost exclusively a male disorder. The other, less clearly defined, types are possibly slightly more common in females and, for the most part, consist of those designated as "mixed tumors" by Womack and Graham [50].

All the evidence now favors the view that primary carcinoma of the lung really originates in a bronchus. The most common location is one of the larger bronchi, especially one with cartilaginous walls, although some arise in the smaller bronchi. Fried [52] has brought evidence that these tumors arise in the basal layer of the bronchial epithelium, a fact which he thinks is responsible for the variability of the morphology and arrangement of the cells composing the tumors.

A tumor arising in one of the larger bronchi, as a rule, produces bronchostenosis with the result that distal to the stenosis atelectasis occurs and subsequent infection takes place in the atelectatic area. This infection usually reveals itself as single or multiple abscesses. The local growth in the bronchus usually appears first as a tumor arising from one wall of the bronchus. It is not at first an encircling growth and it is attached by a broad base instead of by a pedicle. It spreads, as does cancer elsewhere, into the neighboring lymphatics and may travel either into the mediastinal nodes or outwards towards the periphery of the lung. The cartilages in the walls of the larger bronchi seem to offer the same amount of protection against the spread of the growth as does the cartilage in the larynx. There is, therefore, not an early extension through the wall of the bronchus unless the tumor arises in one of the smaller bronchi without cartilaginous walls. Tuttle and Womack,[53] in a study of the cases in the Barnes Hospital, showed that metastasis through the blood stream into distant organs occurs more often when the carcinoma arises in the smaller bronchi near the periphery of the lung than when it originates in one of the larger bronchi in the hilus region. Of particular importance in regard to the question of metastasis is the frequency of secondary deposits in the brain (about

25 per cent), in the adrenal (about 30 per cent) and in the kidney (about 25 per cent). In our own autopsy cases, the spleen showed metastasis in 10 per cent. Others have also noted the frequency with which bronchiogenic carcinoma metastasizes to the adrenal gland.

There are no symptoms which are pathognomonic of this condition. Any individual, however, especially a man past middle age, who has an unexplained chronic cough should be suspected of the possibility of a bronchiogenic carcinoma. The most frequent symptoms other than cough are pain or discomfort in the chest, dyspnea and sputum occasionally streaked with blood. The onset of symptoms is usually insidious. The physical findings are again of little assistance except that they may indicate the presence of bronchostenosis, atelectasis or a pleural effusion. Again, ordinary x-ray examination will usually reveal only an area of atelectasis and sometimes evidence of complications such as pulmonary abscess, pleural effusion, etc. In only a small percentage of cases does the x-ray examination reveal the tumor itself and then usually only in the more massive tumors which arise from the smaller bronchi at the periphery of the lung. Bronchography with the injection of lipiodol is sometimes helpful in locating the bronchial obstruction. The final diagnosis, however, will almost always depend upon a bronchoscopic examination with the removal of a piece of the suspected lesion for microscopic examination. In approximately 75 per cent of cases it is possible to establish the diagnosis with certainty by means of a bronchoscopic examination. In those cases in which the tumor has arisen in a smaller bronchus at the periphery it is not possible usually to make a satisfactory diagnosis by means of the bronchoscope. The same difficulty is experienced sometimes in cases originating from a bronchus in the upper lobe. In late cases with pleural effusion a positive diagnosis can often be made by examination of the pleural fluid by the so-called Mandelbaum method. This procedure consists in centrifugalizing a considerable portion of the fluid and then of fixing, imbedding and cutting the sediment like any piece of tissue. By such a method it is often possible to make a positive diagnosis of carcinoma when other means fail. Finally, in an occasional case it will be necessary to perform an exploratory operation. No examination of a patient should be considered complete without a consideration given to the possibility of metastases, because obviously, radical operative treatment will not be advised if the patient already has demonstrable metastatic growths.

In general the treatment of this condition has been in accordance with one of three general principles. One principle has been the direct attack on the tumor through a bronchoscope by means of cauterization with the electric current or in other ways. In some cases attempts at removal have been made with the use of snares and other instruments without necessarily the employment of coagulation. The second principle has been the attempted destruction of the tumor by some method of irradiation, either with radium or the x-ray. The third and most recent principle has been that of radical surgical removal. At the present time the treatment of this serious condition is somewhat confused by the fact that many inaccurate case reports are in the literature indicating that bronchiogenic carcinoma can be effectively treated by comparatively simple measures, either through the bronchoscope or by irradiation. Doubtless an occasional case of a true carcinoma has been cured by such methods, but an extensive experience has shown conclusively that such methods are unreliable and certainly are of no avail if the case is at all advanced. There can be little doubt also that some of the cases appearing in the literature as bronchiogenic carcinoma successfully treated without radical measures have in reality been benign tumors. On the other hand, since really radical surgery has been undertaken for this condition, the length of time which has elapsed has been too short to indicate what may be expected from the standpoint of a five- or a ten-year cure. However, in the first case of total removal of the lung for bronchiogenic carcinoma (Graham and Singer [54]) the patient, who had a squamous cell carcinoma is well and free from any evidence of recurrence ten years after his operation which was performed on April 5, 1933. In several instances local tumors which undoubtedly were carcinoma have been made to disappear by irradiation therapy (implantation of radium or radon seeds or the use of x-ray therapy or the combination of these various methods), but in every instance the patient has later died, and usually within a short time, from metastases.

If a *radical surgical removal* is contemplated, it is important to realize that from the work of Tuttle and Womack those cases are more likely to be operable in which the tumor has arisen from one of the large bronchi than are those which have arisen from one of the smaller bronchi. In other words, a tumor near the hilus which can be visualized by bronchoscopy is more likely to be operable than one situated at the periphery which cannot be visualized by bronchoscopy. The question naturally arises whether or not a simple lobectomy would be satisfactory. It would seem as if such an operation would not be sufficiently radical to give the best results. In this respect, the situation is probably no different from what it is in regard to cancer in other organs. The more simple operation of lobectomy is now being more and more supplanted by the total removal of the lung, often with removal of the tracheo-bronchial lymph nodes in the mediastinum. Up to the time of preparing this revision 51 patients of the writers had survived the operation of total pneumonectomy for carcinoma. Although in the early days the mortality was high it has gradually come down to a respectable level. For example, in 1942 in a consecutive series of 20 cases the mortality was 20 per cent, and in the first half of 1943 in 8 successive cases there was only one death (12.5 per cent mortality). The operation has now been performed often enough to establish it as a feasible procedure, but more time will be needed to determine the number of patients free from recurrences after a five- or ten-year period. In the authors' series, however, there are 5 patients who are well more than 5 years after the operation, one of whom is well more than 10 years later.

It is beyond the province of this book to discuss in detail such an operation as total pneumonectomy. Different incisions, different methods of removing the lung and different treatments of the remaining pleural space are in use. In general, however, it may be stated that individual ligation of the hilar vessels and a careful suture of the bronchus are now employed. Likewise, largely owing to the influence of Rienhoff, the older practice of obliterating the pleural space by a thoracoplasty performed at the time of the removal of the lung has been largely abandoned. In most cases a spontaneous obliteration occurs as the result of a combination of factors, the enlargement of the other lung and the moving over of it and the mediastinal structures into the empty space, the ascent of the diaphragm and the narrowing of the intercostal spaces on that side. Occasionally the marked deflection of the trachea and great vessels results in some dyspnea. Most patients, however, after recovery from a total pneumonectomy experience no more appreciable dyspnea after exertion than would be expected from an individual of that age group. Unfortunately in some cases an empyema develops necessitating open drainage eventually.

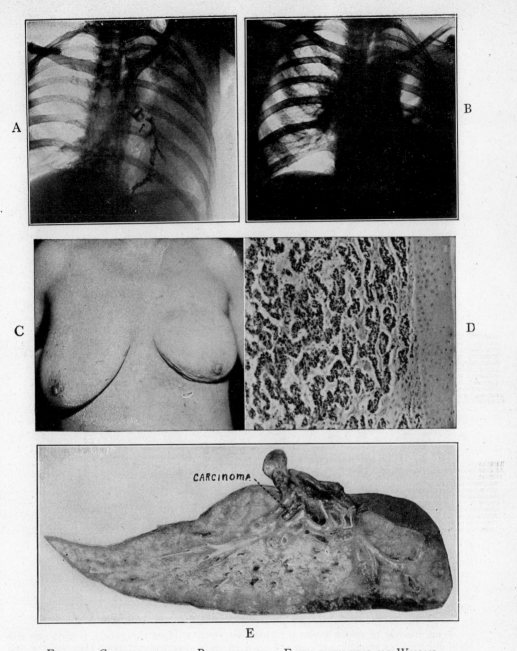

FIG. 504.—CARCINOMA OF THE BRONCHUS, IN A FORTY-SEVEN-YEAR-OLD WOMAN.

Symptoms began two years previously and consisted of a cough which improved during the summer but returned during the winter. For five months the patient has been bedridden because of a pneumonia; there have been several attacks of hemoptysis. *A*, chest film before operation (after lipiodol injection) showing the obstruction to the lower lobe bronchus (indicated by the arrow). *B*, chest film two months after total pneumonectomy; the pleural cavity is gradually becoming smaller and eventually will become completely obliterated, aided by the movement of the healthy side to the opposite side, and the ascent of the diaphragm. *C*, photograph of the patient showing the absence of deformity, the incision is hidden beneath the breast. *D*, photomicrograph of the tumor showing a histological picture resembling an adenocarcinoma, undoubtedly originating from bronchial epithelium. Note the typical glandlike formation. *E*, cut section of the removed lung, showing the carcinoma obstructing the lower lobe bronchus.

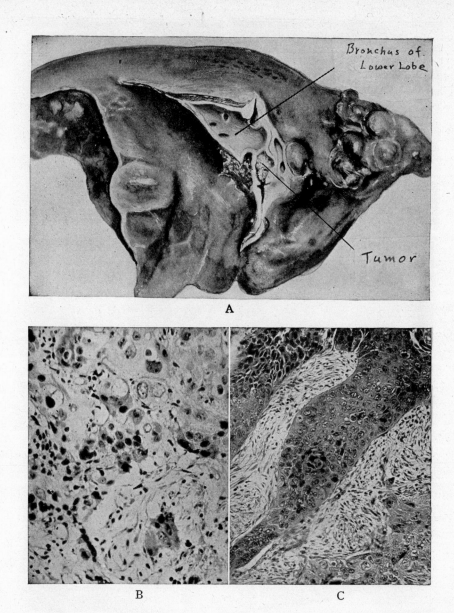

FIG. 503.—SQUAMOUS CELL BRONCHIOGENIC CARCINOMA OF THE LEFT UPPER LOBE.

Total removal of the lung was performed on April 5, 1933. The patient is well and free from any evidence of recurrence ten and one-half years after the operation. This was the first instance of total pneumonectomy for carcinoma. The patient, a forty-seven-year-old male, presented a history of repeated attacks of cough and fever with pain in the left chest for a period of seven months. The diagnosis of carcinoma was suggested by roentgenological studies, but was made certain by microscopic study of a biopsy removed through a bronchoscope. *A*, drawing of the excised lung showing mesial aspect, the tumor is seen projecting from the bronchus of the upper lobe. The main bronchus of the lower lobe has been split open. *B*, photomicrograph of specimen obtained during bronchoscopy. *C*, microscopic appearance of the tumor from a section of the growth obtained after pneumonectomy showing characteristic features of squamous cell carcinoma. No carcinoma was found in sections taken beyond the actual location of the tumor, *i.e.*, no evidence of metastases or extension of the tumor was made out. (From Graham, Singer and Ballon, *Surgical Diseases of the Chest*, 1935. Courtesy of Lea and Febiger, Philadelphia.)

In such an event the large size of the cavity together with the resultant thickening of the mediastinal pleura present serious obstacles to the spontaneous obliteration of the empyema cavity. A thoracoplasty may therefore be required. These considerations have led to the belief that perhaps the convalescence could be greatly shortened if a thoracoplasty were performed more often at the time of the pneumonectomy. This is a matter of technic which is not yet settled. In general, one of two incisions is employed for the operation of pneumonectomy. An anterior incision made under the fold of the breast and without the removal of a rib gives the best cosmetic result in the case of a woman but often the exposure is inadequate. Our own preference is the posterolateral incision of Crafoord [55] with the removal of the entire fifth rib because of the excellence of the exposure obtained.

SURGICAL ASPECTS OF PULMONARY TUBERCULOSIS

It is remarkable that so rational an idea as the employment of surgical measures for the treatment of pulmonary tuberculosis should have been so long in establishing itself. As far back as 1820, James Carson of Liverpool proposed the use of artificial pneumothorax. Apparently, however, the first actual use of artificial pneumothorax in this disease was made by Carlo Forlanini in 1888. Even then the method did not become of general use until it was popularized in the early part of this century by Brauer.

Pulmonary tuberculosis is a disease characterized by the formation of cavities within the lung. Nature's process of obliteration of any cavity in the lung is by immobilization and more or less collapse of the affected side of the chest by drawing the ribs together, by pulling up the diaphragm and by pulling the mediastinal contents over to the affected side. When these phenomena can occur to a satisfactory degree the cavity will often be spontaneously obliterated. There are many cases, however, in which Nature's efforts fail because the structures to which the lung is attached by adhesions are sufficiently unyielding to prevent the spontaneous collapse of the cavity. The basis of all surgical methods used in the treatment of pulmonary tuberculosis is the theoretical assistance given to Nature by overcoming some of the resistance to the spontaneous contraction of the lung. These methods, therefore, are commonly spoken of under the general term of *collapse procedures*. The simplest one is the creation of an artificial pneumothorax. Gradually, however, as the utility of that procedure became more and more realized, other procedures were devised for the purpose of promoting an adequate collapse of the lung. Thus, ribs were removed from the chest wall in order to make the wall more yielding and therefore more likely to be pulled in by subsequent contraction of scar tissue. Also, operations were devised based on the principle of interrupting the phrenic nerve so that the diaphragm on one side would become paralyzed and ascend readily into the thorax, thereby assisting in the collapse of the lung. As these procedures became more developed it became apparent that in certain cases more was necessary than mere collapse, and that on the contrary an amount of definite forceful compression was necessary to obliterate a thick-walled cavity. Operations were therefore devised which have sometimes been designated as *compression operations* as distinguished from collapse procedures. In order to accomplish compression, artificial pneumothorax is sometimes increased to the point of keeping the pressure constantly positive. Likewise the various operations of removing ribs have in certain cases been extended to a point where all of the ribs on one side throughout their total length have been removed and firm compression binders or other devices have been employed in order to squeeze the chest wall forcibly against the lung. Likewise the use of firm packing with such substances as gauze and paraffin has been introduced to exert pressure more or less directly against the wall of a cavity.

Tuberculosis is a disease not only characterized by the frequent occurrence of cavities within the lung but also by the development of empyema. In the latter instance, of course, the condition is again one of cavity although the cavity is pleural instead of pulmonary. Many of the principles, therefore, of collapse and compression which are useful for the obliteration of pulmonary cavities are likewise useful for the treatment of tuberculous empyema.

As experience with collapse methods of treatment became more extensive, it was realized that such methods were applicable not only to cases in which they were demonstrable pulmonary cavities but also that many patients improved after such methods of treatment even when demonstrable cavities were not present. Now it is well known that the immobilization and shrinkage of the lung produced by methods of collapse therapy diminish the toxic absorption from the active lesions in the lung by diminishing the circulation of lymph (Dolley and Wiese [56]), and also produce a chronic passive hyperemia of the lung. These two factors result in limitation and demarcation of the affected areas of lung tissue and also in the proliferation of connective tissue. An exudative process is, therefore, converted into a productive one. Moreover, collapse therapy also facilitates and increases the amount of expectoration which is the natural method of drainage of the débris from the cavities in the lung.

Artificial Pneumothorax.—Artificial pneumothorax is being used more and more widely and the indications for its use are being extended more and more over what they were a decade ago. The decision in a given case as to whether or not to attempt pneumothorax should preferably rest with someone who has experience in the handling and treatment of patients with tuberculosis. There is some controversy as to how soon after the appearance of the disease pneumothorax should be induced. The general opinion is that this form of treatment should not be undertaken until after a period of rest in bed under proper sanitarium care. In general, also, its use is restricted to those patients in whom the disease is generally unilateral. More and more, however, it is being cautiously used in certain cases of bilateral tuberculosis. A particular indication for its use is the presence of hemoptysis associated with a unilateral lesion. The age of the patient makes no appreciable difference. Children withstand pneumothorax as well as adults. In many patients it is impossible to induce pneumothorax because of obliteration of the pleural cavity by adhesions. It is interesting that the total percentage of tuberculous patients considered to be proper subjects for pneumothorax has increased greatly in recent years. Fishberg,[57] in 1932, gave the figure as 10 per cent, which at that time was estimated to be high. At the present time, however, this figure is not considered especially high and in many institutions a much larger percentage of patients are subjected to pneumothorax.

Formerly it was judged advisable to inject a large quantity of air into the pleural cavity, as much as 1000 to 1500 cc. Nowadays it is customary to use much smaller amounts of air (250 or 300 cc. at each injection) and not to resort to the creation of a positive intrapleural pressure unless special indications demand it. In the ordinary case artificial pneumothorax is, therefore, a collapse rather than a compression procedure. It is necessary that pneumothorax should be continued for a considerable period of time. Ordinarily because of the absorption of the air which is introduced, it will be necessary to make refills about every week or ten days. The satisfactory results from pneumothorax treatment can be well appreciated by the table prepared by Rist in 1927.

TABLE 10

PERCENTAGE OF RESULTS IN 759 CASES OF ARTIFICIAL PNEUMOTHORAX *

	Number of Cases	Per Cent	
Healed	51	6.5	
Clinically well, symptom-free, working, but still under treatment	336	45.5	52
Condition unchanged	33	4.0	
Bilateral (alive)	99	13.4	48
Deceased	240	30.5	
Total	759	100	100
Condition of Controls (Adhesions) (Rist) Able to work	8	8.5	
Living in institutions (unable to work, condition unchanged or worse)	35	37.2	
Deceased	51	54.2	91.4

* Rist, *Am. Rev. Tuberc.*, 15:294, 1927.

The relationship of the duration of the pneumothorax to the final results is well seen in the statistics compiled by Roloff.[58] He, in a series of 1128 cases, found that the best results were obtained when the pneumothorax treatments were carried out for at least two years. Thus in his series of cases 253 patients were subjected to pneumothorax treatment for less than one-half year. There were only 9.1 per cent clinical cures in this group. Eighty-eight patients were subjected to pneumothorax treatment for one-half to one year. There were 22.7 per cent clinical cures in this group. One hundred and twenty patients were subjected to pneumothorax treatment for a period of one to two years. There were 50 per cent clinical cures in this group and of 54 patients who received pneumothorax treatment for over two years, 68.5 per cent could be considered as clinically cured.

The principal complications of pneumothorax treatment are the formation of effusions which sometimes develop into tuberculous empyema, air embolism and tearing of the lung with the creation of a tension pneumothorax.

There are many forms of apparatus used in the creation of an artificial pneumothorax. The most essential requirement in all of these various types of apparatus is that a manometer should be attached to enable one to know the intrapleural pressure at any time. We have found the most convenient and satisfactory appa-

ratus to be that devised by Dr. J. J. Singer at the Barnes Hospital, which is manufactured by Phillips of St. Louis. The technic of creating a bilateral pneumothorax
is not essentially different from that of the unilateral one, but much greater caution
is necessary in recommending the use of it in a bilateral case.

Intrapleural Pneumolysis.—Many patients are prevented from getting satisfactory results from pneumothorax treatment because of the presence of adhesions
which prevent the desired collapse of the lung. In order to make it possible to sever
such adhesions and thereby to complete therapeutic collapse of the lung, operations
of two kinds have been performed. The first type is an operation in which an
incision is made into the thorax and the adhesions which are present are cut between
ligatures. This is the so-called open operation. The other type of procedure was
originally devised by Jacobaeus.[59] This consists of the introduction through an
intercostal space of a special instrument known as a thoracoscope, by which it is
possible to see the adhesions and to cut them. The advantage of this procedure is
that no incision is required and therefore the chances of introducing a secondary
infection and also the chances of failure of the incision to heal because of a tuberculous infection of it are reduced to a minimum. Since the introduction of this
principle by Jacobaeus, various modifications in technic have been proposed; for
example, nowadays some form of electrical coagulation through a thoracoscope is
ordinarily employed. An extensive review of this whole question has been done by
Ralph C. Matson.[60] One of the principal dangers of the older methods of operation,
namely, that of hemorrhage from the severing of the vascular adhesions, has been
greatly reduced by the newer methods. The advantage claimed by Matson for his
use of electrical coagulation is not only less hemorrhage, but less exudate of various
kinds. In 206 cases Matson states that of those patients in whom the operation was
technically successful 86 per cent were returned to normal work. The complications
of the operation are listed by him as follows:

TABLE II

Postoperative Complications of 206 Cases of Intrapleural Pneumolysis

Complication	Number	Per Cent
Serous exudate	60	29.1
Purulent exudate	40	19.4
Hemorrhagic exudate	26	12.6
High fever	7	3.4
Severe hemorrhage	3	1.4
Pulmonary fistula	4	1.9
Spontaneous pneumothorax	1	0.4
Severe postoperative vomiting	1	0.4

Oleothorax.—In certain selected cases, oil is injected into the pleural cavity.
The preparation that is commonly used is paraffin oil to which gomenol has been
added in a strength varying from 1 to 10 per cent. Gomenol is a volatile oil obtained by distillation of the leaves of myrtle trees growing in the region of Gomen,
New Caledonia. This is somewhat antiseptic. It is said to be especially effective in
destroying the acid-fast group of bacilli. Oleothorax is used in certain cases to

attain the effects of pneumothorax without the necessity of frequent refills of the chest with air. It is also used as a means of disinfection in the treatment of empyema which occurs after pneumothorax, and finally it is used as a method of producing more compression against the lung than is obtained by pneumothorax. It is injected with a needle through an intercostal space. An extensive review of the use of oleothorax will be found in the section on that subject by Ray W. Matson in *Surgical Diseases of the Chest* by Graham, Singer and Ballon.

Operations on the Phrenic Nerve.—The purpose of the operations on the phrenic nerve is to paralyze the corresponding half of the diaphragm. Because of the paralysis which occurs, the diaphragm, unless held down by adhesions, ascends into the thorax and permits more or less collapse of the lung on that side, depending upon the amount of its ascent. The effect of a paralysis of one leaf of the diaphragm, therefore, is not merely a compression against the lower part of the corresponding lung but it may also be even upon the apex of the lung. Occasionally, therefore, operations on the phrenic nerve will have a beneficial effect on apical lesions although generally they will be found most useful in cases in which the lesions are in the lower part of the lung. When the diaphragm ascends high into the thorax as a result of its paralysis, the effect is similar to that of an artificial pneumothorax, although not nearly to the same degree. By some, the operation is employed instead of artificial pneumothorax because of its simplicity and because it removes the necessity of refills with air and finally also, because the complications on the whole are less than those of pneumothorax. On the other hand, beneficial results of operations on the phrenic nerve are not so good as are those of pneumothorax. The operation is probably chiefly used in cases in which pneumothorax has been impossible to accomplish because of obliterating adhesions and in which for various reasons a decision has been made against immediate performance of a thoracoplasty. In some cases a combination of pneumothorax and paralysis of the diaphragm will be found effective in closing pulmonary cavities because of the relaxation of adhesions permitted by the ascent of the diaphragm. Formerly it was customary to initiate a paralysis of the diaphragm before performing a thoracoplasty. There is less tendency now, however, to make an operation on the phrenic nerve a routine preliminary to thoracoplasty.

In general there are two types of operation on the phrenic nerve. The principle of one type is to make the paralysis of the diaphragm only temporary so that there will be no permanent effect upon the lower part of the lung, and the other type of operation is to make the paralysis permanent. In the first type of operation, the phrenic nerve in the neck is only crushed. This procedure usually produces a paralysis which will continue for about six months before regeneration of the nerve occurs. In the permanent type of operation, the phrenic nerve, after exposure in the neck, is twisted out of its bed in an effort to attain the entire length of nerve from within the thorax. So often is there an accessory phrenic nerve that experience has shown that a permanent paralysis of the corresponding half of the diaphragm is likely not to occur unless the nerve is actually avulsed. By the procedure of avulsion the accessory nerve is nearly always removed along with the main nerve. There are many variations in the anatomy of the nerve, and in certain cases it is very difficult to be sure whether all the nerve fibers to the diaphragm have been interrupted. If they have not all been interrupted, the diaphragm may continue to move sluggishly but will not be paralyzed on the corresponding side and will therefore not show the characteristic paradoxical movements which one sees with the fluoroscope after successful paralysis of one-half of it.

Scaleniotomy.—The scalene muscles are accessory muscles of respiration which by their effect on the first and second ribs play a role in the respiratory movements involving the upper part of the thorax. Many workers individually suggested the advantages of cutting the scalene muscles in cases of apical tuberculosis in order to assist in the process of immobilization of the lung. In this country Gale and Middleton [61] were the first to use the procedure extensively. It is a simple matter to combine the division of the scalene muscles with an operation on the phrenic nerve because of the normal position of that nerve on the anterior border of the scalenus anticus muscle. The usual procedure is to divide the scalene muscles with a cautery knife in order to prevent bleeding. It is necessary, of course, to exercise care not to injure the brachial plexus. In some cases the vital capacity can be diminished almost 10 per cent by division of the scalene muscles, an amount which is indicative of the degree of immobilization effected by the procedure. This operation should probably be regarded as only an accessory one or as one of the many surgical methods which are now employed in the treatment of pulmonary tuberculosis. By itself, it is not nearly so effective as artificial pneumothorax, operations on the phrenic nerve or thoracoplasty.

Plombage.—This procedure consists in the direct application of pressure exerted on the parietal pleura against a cavity in order to assist in its obliteration. Although packs of gauze, inflatable rubber bags and other agents have been used for this purpose, the one which is now most commonly employed is paraffin, which solidifies at body temperature. The details of preparing the paraffin and the methods of using it will not be described in this book. The interested reader can find them in modern books on the treatment of tuberculosis and recent books on thoracic surgery. Occasionally the operation is of great value but there are many dangers connected with the use of paraffin plombes, the chief one of which is ulceration of the plombe into the pulmonary cavity.

Extrapleural Thoracoplasty.—Of all the surgical procedures for pulmonary tuberculosis the operation of thoracoplasty, next to the creation of pneumothorax, is the most effective and the most important. The modern present day operation of thoracoplasty has gone through a period of evolution starting with operations for the collapse of cavities by the removal of ribs. Because of the extensive accumulation of experience with this operation, it is now possible to state rather dogmatically that the operation is not usually effective unless considerable portions of the upper ribs are removed. The modern operation is entirely extrapleural. It is divided into stages separated by intervals usually of at least two or three weeks and it is carried out through a posterior incision. One of the essential requisites that has been learned is that to be effective in collapsing the upper part of the lung, it is necessary that there should be a dropping downwards of the pulmonary apex. This cannot be expected to occur unless large segments amounting usually to practically the entire lengths of the first and second ribs are removed. If such an operation is performed, ordinarily it is not so necessary that very long segments of the lower ribs be removed, although it is customary in a case of complete unilateral thoracoplasty to remove the lower ribs from the corresponding transverse processes to at least the posterior axillary line and often to the anterior axillary line. It is customary also in most cases to begin the operation with the removal of the first two or first three ribs. This constitutes the first stage. Two or three weeks later, three or four more ribs are removed and two or three weeks after that, the remaining ribs including the 10th and sometimes even a portion of the 11th ribs are removed. In other cases in which the tuberculosis is limited to the upper part of the lung, a total thoracoplasty is much less commonly performed than formerly because it is recognized now that often removal of the upper 3 or 5 ribs is often sufficient to accomplish the desired result. This procedure leaves the function of the lower part of the lung relatively uninterrupted. The operation is not disfiguring to the patient to any considerable degree.

The indications for this operation are gradually being more and more extended. The best results, however, are obtained in cases in which there has already been a demonstration of a resistance against the disease. Such a resistance is shown by the development of scar tissue, the relative absence of moist râles in the affected lung and the subsidence of fever. The function of scar tissue is shown by the pulling of the mediastinal contents to the affected side. The operation, therefore, probably finds its greatest field of usefulness in patients who have a unilateral cavity or cavities in the upper part of the lung but are free from fever and who have developed a pull of the mediastinal contents to the affected side. But many patients without demonstrable cavities are benefited by the operation. Ordinarily it is not performed until after a period of sanitarium treatment and pneumothorax have been tried for at least several months or a year and preferably longer. It is especially important to realize that patients with unobliterated demonstrable cavities seldom live more than five years. If such patients can have their cavities obliterated by the operation of thoracoplasty, they have a greater chance of becoming arrested cases. Moreover, the absence of sputum containing tubercle bacilli makes them no longer menaces to their families and intimate associates.

The principal dangers associated with the operation of thoracoplasty, in addition to those attendant upon any operation, are the dangers of a spread of the tuberculous process to other parts of the lung. Presumably this is accomplished in some cases by the sudden squeezing out of the cavity of débris containing large numbers of living tubercle bacilli. In other cases, it would seem as if death occurs following the operation because of excessive tuberculinization of the patient as a result of squeezing into the circulation large amounts of tuberculin and other products of the tubercle bacilli. No surgeon should decide on performing an operation of thoracoplasty for tuberculosis unless he has had extensive experience with tuberculous patients or unless the operation has been recommended by someone who is thoroughly familiar with pulmonary tuberculosis and the effects of thoracoplasty. In occasional cases a bilateral apical thoracoplasty is justifiable.

As for the results to be obtained by thoracoplasty, it is probable that somewhere between 50 and 70 per cent of patients who would otherwise die of their disease can be restored to normal activity as arrested cases by this operation. The operative mortality varies greatly, depending upon how radical the operation is and upon how carefully the patients have been selected for operation. In the best risk cases the operative mortality is practically zero. As one widens his indications to go into groups of patients in which the risk is greater, the operative mortality will necessarily be higher.

In certain cases in which the ordinary posterior extrapleural thoracoplasty has been ineffective in obliterating cavities, the result can sometimes be improved by supplementing the posterior operation with an anterior one in order to remove

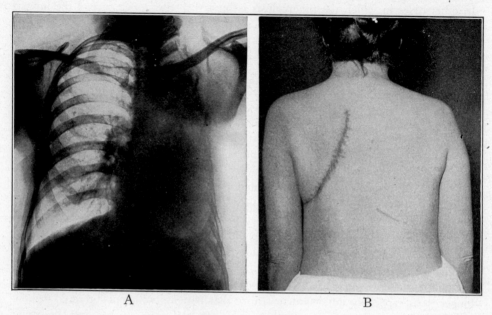

A   B

FIG. 505.—EXTRAPLEURAL THORACOPLASTY FOR UNILATERAL TUBERCULOSIS IN A THIRTY-EIGHT-YEAR-OLD WOMAN.

A, chest film after operation; note the marked narrowing of one side of the chest with resulting collapse of the lung. *B*, photograph of the patient, showing the healed incision. The visible deformity is very slight. The patient has been completely relieved of cough and sputum and is apparently perfectly well.

the entire length of all of the ribs. Some surgeons also prefer to remove the transverse processes of the vertebrae in order to prevent the cavity from falling into the paravertebral gutter and thereby escaping the pressure which the thoracoplasty would ordinarily exert upon the cavity. Occasionally also supplemental pressure is added by the use of tight bandages, the application of weights, etc., to the operated side.

Tuberculous Empyema.—Tuberculous empyema is essentially of two varieties, one in which there is a pure infection of tubercle bacilli and the other in which there has been added to the tuberculous infection another one due to some pyogenic organism. In the latter type of case it is usually necessary to establish open drainage and later, after the toxic symptoms have subsided, to consider the possibility of some more radical procedure if necessary to obliterate the pleural cavity. In such cases, however, it is desirable to make the drainage somewhat anterior (preferably in the anterior axillary line) in order to leave the back uninfected for a later thoracoplasty. On the other hand, if the case is one of pure tuberculous infection, open drainage should not be instituted. Some of such cases can be adequately cared for by repeated aspiration followed by the injection into the pleural cavity of an equivalent amount of 10 per cent gomenol in paraffin oil. In other cases an extrapleural thoracoplasty will be required in order to obliterate the pleural cavity. The extent of the thoracoplasty will depend upon the size of the pleural space to be obliterated. Often a complete unilateral thoracoplasty with the removal of prac-

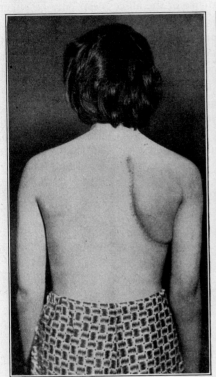
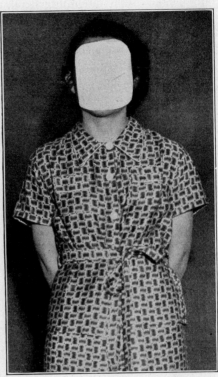

FIG. 506.—SCAR AFTER THORACOPLASTY FOR UPPER LOBE TUBERCULOSIS WITH THE REMOVAL OF THE FIRST FIVE RIBS.

For cosmetic reasons this incision has advantages over one which reaches to the neck.

tically the total lengths of all the ribs will be necessary. The operation of thoracoplasty has enormously improved the prognosis in tuberculous empyema.

Sulfonamides in Thoracic Surgery.—When introduced, there was naturally great hope that the sulfonamides would be effective in the treatment of empyema thoracis and pulmonary abscesses. There is ample evidence that their use decreases the incidence of postpneumonic empyema [62, 63]. However, once an empyema has developed, the fundamental principle of adequate drainage must be observed. The inhibiting action of the pus against the sulfonamides is sufficient to prevent any appreciable therapeutic effect. Surgical drainage of the abscess therefore becomes necessary. In those cases in which empyema has developed in spite of the use of chemotherapy during the pneumonia there is a greater tendency for the formation of multiple pockets of pus which may require separate incisions for drainage.

The sulfonamide drugs are also of value during the formative stage of a lung abscess. The rationale of their use is, of course, to decrease the severity of the infection by destroying or crippling those organisms which are vulnerable to the drugs during the invasive stage. On the other hand, there have been few actual cures recorded in the literature, and in these cases the predominant organism in the sputum was the hemolytic streptococcus [64, 65]. No definite beneficial effect has been noted in any case of true putrid pulmonary infection. As is the case in the treatment of empyema, and suppuration in general, a cure of the abscess can only be effected by evacuation of the pus [66].

As to their prophylactic use, the sulfonamides have been used extensively at the Barnes Hospital both preoperatively and postoperatively, in an attempt to decrease the incidence of empyema following lobectomy and pneumonectomy. Not only have the drugs been given by mouth and parenterally, but sulfanilamide crystals have been placed in the wounds and in the pleural cavity, sometimes without drainage. None of these measures has prevented putrid empyemas when the bronchus has opened following amputation of a lobe or the entire lung. There may have been some benefit in lessening the severity of infection and delaying its appearance.

BIBLIOGRAPHY

1. WINSLOW, N. Typhoidal Osteomyelitis, *Ann. Surg.*, 77:319, 1923.
2. HEDBLOM, CARL A. Tumors of the Bony Chest Wall, *Arch. Surg.*, 3:56, 1921.
3. PANCOAST, H. K. Superior Pulmonary Sulcus Tumor, *J. Am. M. Ass.*, 99:1391, 1932.
4. BALLON, H. C., and FRANCIS, B. F. Consequences of Variations in Mediastinal Pressure; Mediastinal and Subcutaneous Emphysema, *Arch. Surg.*, 19:1627, 1929.
5. ROBERTSON, H. E. "Endothelioma" of Pleura, *J. Cancer Research*, 8:317, 1924.
6. BALLON, H. C., and FRANCIS, B. F. *Loc. cit.*
7. DUNHAM, E. K. The Medical Department of the U. S. Army in the World War, Vol. II, Part 2, Section 1, 1924.
8. WINSLOW, N., and SHIPLEY, A. M. Pericardiotomy for Pyopericardium, *Arch. Surg.*, 15:317, 1927.
9. BRAUER, L. Die Kardiolysis und ihre Indikationen, *Arch. f. klin. Chir.*, 71:258, 1903.
10. DELORME, E. Sur un traitement chirurgical de la symphyse cardiopericardiaque, *Gaz. d. hop.*, 71:1150, 1898.
11. SMITH, E. S., and LIGGETT, H. S. Cardiolysis for Chronic Mediastinopericarditis, *Proc. Interstate Postgraduate Medical Assembly of North America*, p. 489, 1928.
12. BECK, C. S. Wounds of the Heart: The Technique of Suture, *Arch. Surg.*, 13:205, 1926.
13. SWETLOW, G. I. Paravertebral Block in Cardiac Pain, *Am. Heart J.*, 1:393, 1926.
14. WHITE, J. C., and WHITE, P. D. Angina Pectoris; Treatment with Paravertebral Alcohol Injections, *J. Am. M. Ass.*, 90:1099, 1928.
15. GRAHAM, E. A., SINGER, J. J., BALLON, H. C. *Surgical Diseases of the Chest*, Lea and Febiger, Philadelphia, 1935, p. 319.
16. BLUMGART, H. L., LEVINE, S. A., BERLIN, D. D. Congestive Heart Failure and Angina Pectoris: The Therapeutic Effect of Thyroidectomy on Patients Without Clinical or Pathologic Evidence of Thyroid Toxicity, *Arch. Int. Med.*, 51:866, 1933.
17. BECK, CLAUDE. Further Data on the Production of a New Blood Supply to the Heart by Operation, *J. Thoracic Surg.*, 5:604, 1936.

18. O'SHAUGNESSY, L. Surgical Treatment of Cardiac Ischaemia. *Brit. J. Surg.*, 23:665, 1936. *Lancet,* 1:185, 1937.

19. HEINBECKER, P., and BARTON, W. A. Operation for Development of Collateral Circulation to the Heart. *J. Thoracic Surg.*, 9:431, 1940.

20. ALLEN, D. S., and GRAHAM, E. A. Intracardiac Surgery, New Method, *J. Am. M. Ass.*, 79:1028, Sept. 23, 1922.

21. CUTLER, E. C., and BECK, C. S. The Present Status of the Surgical Procedures in the Valvular Disease: Final Report of all Cases, *Arch. Surg.*, 18, 2:403, 1929.

22. HARE, H. A. Three Cases of Aortic Aneurysm Treated by Wiring and Electrolysis, *J. Am. M. Ass.*, 73:1865, 1919.

23. HUNNER, G. L. Aneurism of the Aorta Treated by the Insertion of a Permanent Wire and Galvanism (Moore-Corradi Method), *Bull. Johns Hopkins Hosp.*, 11:263, 1900.

24. GIERTZ, K. H., and CRAFOORD, C. On the Thromboembolic Disease and Its Surgical Treatment, *Acta. Chir. Scandinav.*, 64:121, 1928.

25. NYSTROM, G. Experiences with Trendelenburg Operation for Pulmonary Embolism, *Ann. Surg.*, 92:498, 1930.

26. BINNEY, H. Tumors of the Diaphragm, *Ann. Surg.*, 94:524, 1931.

27. VANALLEN, C. M., and ADAMS, W. E. Mechanism of Obstructive Atelectasis, *Surg., Gynec. & Obst.*, 50:385, 1930.
VANALLEN, C. M., and LINDSKOG, G. E. Obstructive Atelectasis; Problems of Pathogenesis and Clinical Management, *Arch. Surg.*, 21:1195, 1930.
Collateral Respiration in the Lung: Role in Bronchial Obstruction to Prevent Atelectasis and to Restore Patency, *Surg., Gynec. & Obst.*, 53:16, 1931.

28. HEINBECKER, P. A Method for the Demonstration of Calibre Changes in the Bronchi in Normal Respiration, *J. Clin. Invest.*, 4:459, 1927.

29. FRANCIS, B. F. Changes in the Shape and Size of the Tracheobronchial Tree Following Stimulation of the Vagosympathetic Nerve, *Arch. Surg.*, 19:1577, 1929.

30. ELOESSER, L. Bronchial Stenosis, *J. Thoracic Surg.*, 1:194-270-373, 485, 1931.

31. LERCHE, W. Infections of the Lymph Nodes of the Bronchial Tree, *Arch. Surg.*, 16:338, 1928.

32. GRAHAM, E. A. Observations on the Reaction of Bronchial Fistulas to Acute Infections of the Upper Respiratory Tract, *Am. J. Surg.*, 14:382, 1931.

33. BETTMAN, R. B., JAMES, W. A., TANNENBAUM, K., and SLOBE, E. Further Studies on Closure of Bronchi in Lobectomies; Experimental Work, *Surg., Gynec. & Obst.*, 46:602, 1928.

34. CHURCHILL, E. D. Resection of the Lung, *Surgery*, 8:961, 1940.

35. EDWARDS, A. T. Modern Principles of Treatment in Bronchiectasis, *Brit. M. J.*, 1:809, 1939.

36. GRAHAM, E. A., and BLADES, B. (unpublished data).

37. GRAHAM, E. A. Treatment of Pulmonary Suppuration, *Ann. Surg.*, 86:174, 1927.

38. RIENHOFF, W. F., Jr. Pneumonectomy, *Bull. Johns Hopkins Hosp.*, 53:390, 1933.

39. BLADES, B., and KENT, E. M. Individual Ligation Technic for Lower Lobe Lobectomy, *J. Thoracic Surg.*, 10:84, 1940.

40. GRAHAM, E. A., SINGER, J. J., and BALLON, H. C. *Surgical Diseases of the Chest,* p. 776, Lea and Febiger, Philadelphia, 1935.

41. MOORE, W. F. Pulmonary Abscess, *J. Am. M. Ass.*, 78:1279, 1922.

42. CROWE, S. J., and SCARFF, J. E. Experimental Abscess of the Lung in the Dog, *Arch. Surg.*, 16:176, 1928.

43. ALLEN, DUFF. Etiology of Abscess of the Lung, *Arch. Surg.*, 16:179, 1928.

44. BURDON, K. L. Bacterium Melaninogenicum from Normal Pathological Tissue, *J. Infect. Dis.*, 42:161, 1928.

45. VARNEY, P. L. Bacterial Flora of Treated and Untreated Lung Abscess, *Arch. Surg.*, 19:1602, 1929.

46. NEUHOF, HAROLD, and WESSLER, HARRY. Putrid Lung Abscess—Its Etiology, Pathology, Clinical Manifestations, Diagnosis and Treatment, *J. Thoracic Surg.,* 1:637, 1934-35.

47. SCHLAEPFER, K. Collateral Circulation in Chronic Obstruction of the Pulmonary Veins and Its Relation to Air Embolism in Following Various Diagnostic and Therapeutic Procedures, *Surg., Gynec. & Obst.,* 37:510, 1923.

48. DEW, H. *Hydatid Disease,* Sydney, The Australasian Medical Publishing Company, Ltd., 1928.

49. WANGENSTEEN, O. H. Actinomycosis of the Thorax with Report of a Case Successfully Operated Upon, *J. Thoracic Surg.,* 1:612, 1932.

50. WOMACK, N. A., and GRAHAM, E. A. Mixed Tumors of the Lung; So-called Bronchial or Pulmonary Adenoma, *Arch. Path.,* 1938:26, 165.

51. JACKSON, C. L., and KONZELMANN, F. W. Bronchoscopic Aspects of Bronchial Tumors, *J. Thoracic Surg.,* 1937:6, 312.

52. FRIED, B. M. Primary Carcinoma of the Lung, *Medicine,* 10:373, 1931.

53. TUTTLE, W. M., and WOMACK, N. A. Bronchiogenic Carcinoma—A Classification in Relation to Treatment and Prognosis, *J. Thoracic Surg.,* 4:125, 1934.

54. GRAHAM, E. A., and SINGER, J. J. Successful Removal of an Entire Lung for Carcinoma of the Bronchus, *J. Am. M. Ass.,* 101:1371, 1933.

55. CRAFOORD, CLARENCE. On the Technic of Pneumonectomy in Man. *Acta Chir. Scandinav.* 81, Suppl. 54, Stockholm, 1937.

56. DOLLEY, F., and WIESE, E. R. Effects of Large Closed Bilateral Pneumothorax on Thoracic Lymph Flow, *Arch. Surg.,* 18:542, 1929.

57. FISHBERG, M. *Pulmonary Tuberculosis,* Philadelphia, Lea and Febiger, 1932.

58. ROLOFF, W. Dauererfolge der Lungenkollapsbehandlung; Statistischer Bericht über 1128 Fälle aus den Jahren 1918-1928, *Beitr. z. Klin. d. Tuberk.,* 78:495, 1931.

59. JACOBAEUS, H. C. Cauterization of Adhesions in Pneumothorax Treatment of Tuberculosis, *Acta. Chir. Scandinav.,* 53:293, 1921.

60. MATSON, RALPH C. Surgical Diseases of the Chest by Graham, Singer and Ballon, Philadelphia, Lea and Febiger, 1935, p. 880.

61. GALE, J. W., and MIDDLETON, W. S. Scaleniotomy in the Surgical Treatment of Pulmonary Tuberculosis, *Arch. Surg.,* 23:38, 1931.

62. HURWITZ, S., and STEVENS, H. B. Empyema in Children, *J. Pediat.,* 14:11, 1939.

63. THOMPSON, L. D., EDWARDS, J. C. and HOAGLAND, C. L. Experiences in Treatment of Lobar Pneumonia, *Ann. Int. Med.,* 13:738, 1940.

64. HUI, F. A. Sulfanilamide Therapy of Lung Abscess: report of a case, *Chinese M. J.,* 56:153, 1939.

65. MURPHEY, F. B., JR., and FRERE, J. M. Acute Streptococci Lung Abscess Treated with Sulfanilamide, *South. M. J.,* 31:1136, 1938.

66. NEUHOF, H., and TOUROFF, A. S. W. Acute Putrid Abscess of Lung; Surgical Treatment and Results in 86 Consecutive Cases, *J. Thoracic Surg.,* 9:439, 1940.

CHAPTER XXX

THE ENDOCRINE GLANDS

Thyroid
The Parathyroid Glands
The Adrenals (Suprarenal Glands)

Pancreas
Pituitary (Hypophysis)
The Gonads

During the past few years so many important physiologic and pathologic features of the various glands of internal secretion have been discovered that this phase of medicine is becoming a science or specialty of its own—endocrinology. Already it has been discovered that the treatment of many of the diseases of these glands is primarily surgical. It is not improbable that as more knowledge accumulates in this field, still more surgical procedures will be adaptable in treatment of diseases of these organs. However, the complexity of certain of the endocrine glands interferes considerably in the diagnosis and the application of the various therapeutic procedures. Many of the glands contain more than one type of secreting structure, such as the medulla and cortex of the adrenal and the anterior and posterior lobe of the pituitary gland. Many of them seem to be directly affected in their activity by impulses carried by the autonomic nervous system. Finally the endocrines have an intimate relationship to each other, reacting in a balanced antagonistic or synergistic manner. The demonstration by Loeb and Bassett [1] (1929) that administration of an extract of the pituitary gland to animals would produce a hyperactivity of the thyroid gland is an example of the influence of the secretion of one organ over the function of another. The pituitary, anterior lobe particularly, is known to exert important controlling influences not only over the thyroid, but also over the adrenal cortex, the gonads, the parathyroids and the pancreas. Because of the close interrelationship of the various endocrine glands to each other, it appears appropriate to combine the discussion of them into one chapter.

THYROID

Although the thyroid gland is not absolutely essential to life, the organ normally performs important fuctions, the most significant of which is the maintenance of a metabolic rate at a level compatible with good health and efficient function. The active principle of the thyroid is a tissue catalyst; it was isolated and named thyroxin by Kendall [2] in 1914 and synthesized a number of years later by Harington.[3] It has been estimated (Kendall) that there are about 14 milligrams of thyroxin in the human body. Plummer [4] has made a detailed study of the physiologic effects of thyroxin; he concluded that "the daily discharge of this agent from the thyroid is approximately 0.75 milligram." In normal persons the administration of thyroxin

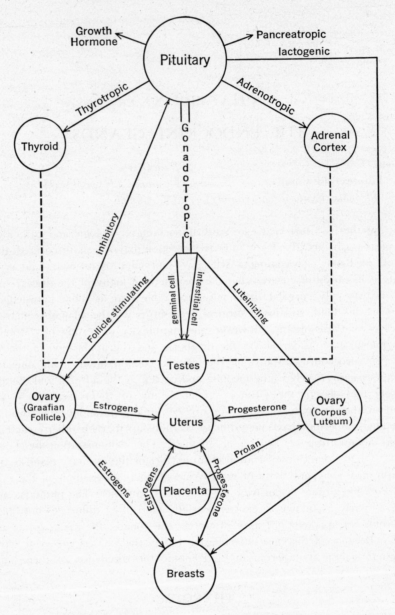

FIG. 507.—DIAGRAM OF ENDOCRINE RELATIONSHIPS.

The chart aims to show some of the interrelationships between the various endocrine glands. Note the prominent place occupied by the pituitary (largely anterior lobe). The broken lines represent relationships which exist but are not direct. Because of the present intense activity in endocrine research the above chart must obviously be not only incomplete, but may have to be changed soon on the basis of newer knowledge.

to the point of physiologic effect produces tachycardia, weakness, loss of weight, increased appetite and other manifestations (except exophthalmos) noted in toxic goiter (hyperthyroidism). Diminution or deprivation of the active principle of the thyroid gland in children produces a syndrome known as *cretinism,* in which stunted growth, dulled mentality, coarse features, etc., are prominent manifestations. An absence of thyroid secretion in adults produces *myxedema,* important manifestations of which are physical and mental lethargy, thick skin, loss of hair, etc. (see p. 915).

The *classification of the diseases of the thyroid gland* has always been a stumbling block to a clear understanding of the various diseases, especially because many authorities use different terms to designate a particular disease. It is important, then, that an effort be made to standardize the classification in order to eliminate confusion which may arise by use of such a varied number of terms for one particular disease. The classification (excluding tumors, thyroiditis and hypothyroidism) recommended by a committee [5] appointed by the American Society for the Study of Goiter appears to be simple and adaptable as far as terminology is concerned: diffuse nontoxic goiter, nodular nontoxic goiter, diffuse toxic goiter and nodular toxic goiter.

Diffuse Nontoxic Goiter.—Although this type of goiter (frequently called simple colloid goiter) is the most prevalent of the various kinds encountered, it is the least serious from the standpoint of the effects on the patient. The chief gross pathologic features of diffuse nontoxic goiter are a slight but generalized and symmetrical enlargement and hypertrophy of the gland associated with the presence of an excess amount of colloid secretion as noted on cut section. Microscopically, the acini are larger than normal and the cells flattened. However, numerous areas of hyperplasia, consisting of heightening of the cells with layering and plication, are usually noted here and there throughout the gland. This lesion is encountered in animals as well as human beings and is commonly seen in the human at the age of puberty and during pregnancy. In these latter two instances the goiter is caused, to a certain extent at least, by excessive demands made by the body on thyroid function.

Etiology.—The etiology of this type of goiter is still obscure, in spite of the fact that an enormous amount of work has been done on this phase of the disease. Although numerous contributory causes of this type of goiter have been discovered, the primary cause is probably still unknown. For many decades it has been known that a deficiency of iodine in the drinking water and food was associated to some extent with the development of goiter. The relationship can be readily appreciated when one bears in mind the fact that in the United States goiter occurs most commonly in the northern states (exclusive of New England, but including particularly the northwestern and Great Lakes region) where the iodine content of the water is low, that is, lower than one or two parts per billion (McClendon and associates [6]).

The early work of Marine and Lenhart [7] and McCarrison [8] proved, however, that other factors (contaminated food, infection, etc.) were capable of producing simple goiter. Likewise, Cole and Womack noted that certain types of infection, toxemias and chemicals might produce goiter in animals (sometimes accompanied

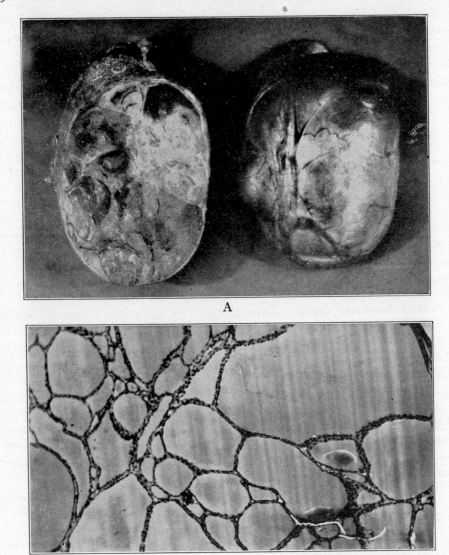

A

B

FIG. 508.—NODULAR GOITER REMOVED FROM A PATIENT WITHOUT EVIDENCE OF HYPERTHYROIDISM.

A, cut and external surface of a large nodule which represented an entire lobe on one side. Note the lack of hemogeneity of the cut surface; this is produced by the profuse deposition of scar tissue and the large acini or cysts containing colloid. In its gross appearance, such a goiter can scarcely be differentiated from a toxic nodular goiter. *B,* microscopic section reveals flat acinous cells, scanty interstitial tissue, and large acini containing colloid. Such a gland is frequently spoken of as a colloid goiter.

by hyperplasia), particularly if the food and water were low in iodine content. Hellwig[9] has noted that a diet high in calcium will produce experimental goiter and is inclined to minimize the importance of iodine deficiency in the etiology of goiter. In addition to iodine lack, certain positive factors such as cyanide (as such or in cabbage, Brussels sprouts or cauliflower [10]) will cause experimental goiter. Tissue oxidation is diminished and the demand for thyroid hormone is increased.

Clinical Manifestations.—The clinical manifestations of diffuse nontoxic goiter are really very few. The most important is enlargement of the neck produced by the hypertrophied thyroid gland. This enlargement is never very marked; rarely does it constitute a cosmetic blemish, and in many instances is noticeable only on careful examination. The basal metabolism is normal or even lower than normal. There is no tachycardia, tremor of the fingers or exophthalmos. Rarely does the thyroid of this type of goiter become so large as to produce pressure symptoms related to breathing and deglutition. However, if present in a pregnant woman this type of goiter, if untreated by iodine, etc., may lead to the production of cretinism in the offspring.

Treatment.—Treatment is not of special importance, because symptoms are rarely produced by this disease, but more particularly because a mild hypertrophy appears as a normal physiologic phenomenon during puberty, pregnancy, etc. However, there appear to be definite reasons for prophylactic therapy in goitrous regions by the routine administration of iodine. This favorable effect of iodine on the disease was first definitely demonstrated by Marine and Kimball [11] when they reported the eradication and prevention of goiter in the school children of Akron, Ohio, through the administration of iodine in the drinking water. No more than a few milligrams of iodine (either as the free element or as iodides) per day is necessary. When given prophylactically, administration of this quantity of the drug over a period of a few days, three or four times a year is all that is required over a long period of time since it is believed by some observers that occasionally a simple goiter may be converted into a toxic one by prolonged use of the drug. Another indication for treatment lies in the fact that mild myxedema occasionally develops when a diffuse goiter has been present for a long time. It is especially important that the goiter not be allowed to exist in women throughout the childbearing period since there are definite hereditary tendencies in the transmission of simple goiter, frequently with an associated cretinism in the offspring. Rarely does iodine fail to effect at least a significant decrease in the size of diffuse nontoxic goiters. With few exceptions, iodine will prevent the myxedema which is occasionally seen in this type of goiter, but of more importance is the fact that the drug, when given to a goitrous pregnant woman, will rarely fail to prevent the development of goiter in the child. Surgical excision in diffuse nontoxic goiter of recent duration is distinctly contraindicated since the enlargement is to a great extent physiologic, *i.e.,* caused by the demand for increased thyroid secretion. In "goiter belts" diffuse nontoxic goiter frequently persists beyond the period of physiologic strain (puberty, pregnancy, etc.). Not uncommonly it becomes nodular and takes on the characteristics of nodular nontoxic goiter as described below.

Nodular Nontoxic Goiter.—The occasional transformation of diffuse nontoxic goiter to nodular nontoxic goiter as just described might lead one to the assumption that the latter is simply an advanced stage of the former; whether or not this is true in all cases cannot be determined.

The pathogenesis of nodular nontoxic goiter can best be understood by first outlining its *pathologic features*. Grossly, there is an asymmetrical enlargement of the gland with nodules distributed diffusely throughout. On cut section the nodules are found to consist of tissue containing a large amount of glairy, gelatinous material which is called colloid; hence, the frequent use of the term colloid goiter. Occasionally, these nodules contain a thin brownish fluid (cystic goiter). Less frequently, areas of hemorrhage are encountered. If the goiter has been present for several years, areas of calcification may be found in the fibrous tissue between the nodules. Microscopically, the acini are found to be widely dilated. It is apparent that the largest acini or cavities containing colloid, are formed

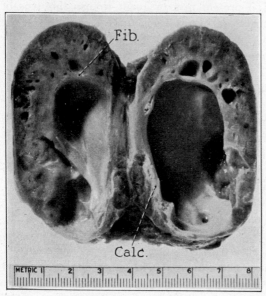

FIG. 509.—CYSTIC ADENOMA.

Note also fibrous tissue and calcification. Patient had no symptoms of hyperthyroidism.

by the rupture of the walls of numerous smaller acini with consequent coalescence. The acinous cells are flat or cuboidal. Throughout the gland, however, will be found areas of hyperplasia where the cells are columnar and plicated, the acini small and devoid of colloid. Areas of lymphocytic infiltration are not uncommon.

Of more importance than the degenerative processes (cysts, calcification, etc.) mentioned in the preceding paragraph, are the hyperplastic changes which may take place. The development of hyperthyroidism (toxic nodular goiter) and carcinoma are not uncommon.

The *pathogenesis* of nodular nontoxic goiter is similar to that of diffuse nontoxic goiter, in so far as lack of iodine and physiologic strain upon the thyroid are important etiologic factors. The presence of nodules of nontoxic nodular goiter constitutes an important difference and may be a later stage of the disease as previously mentioned. Clinical and experimental proof of the supposition that development of the numerous nodules throughout the gland in nodular nontoxic goiter is dependent upon frequent remission and exacerbations of the hyperplastic process (as brought about by physiologic need and strain) has been offered by Marine,[12] Rienhoff,[13] and others. When the urgency for an increased function is passed the gland involutes into a resting stage with flattened cells lining the acini, which become filled with colloid. The hyperplastic and involutional changes are largely confined to focal areas throughout the gland. These areas become circumscribed and surrounded by varying amounts of fibrous tissue which may encapsulate them; such nodules, which are often called *adenomas* (but perhaps erroneously), may be solitary, but usually are multiple. However, there is one type of adenoma, *viz., fetal adenoma* which is generally believed to be of actual neoplastic origin. Such nodules are sharply circumscribed, usually solitary, grayish or white on cut section, contain very little colloid and are of more solid consistency than the involutional type of adenoma already described. Microscopically, the acini are very small and interstitial tissue is profuse in amount, resembling as the name implies fetal thyroid tissue.

Clinical Manifestations.—The clinical manifestations of nodular nontoxic goiter are in reality few. The patient may have an asymmetrical enlargement of the thyroid for years without any symptoms. Occasionally there is a history of the

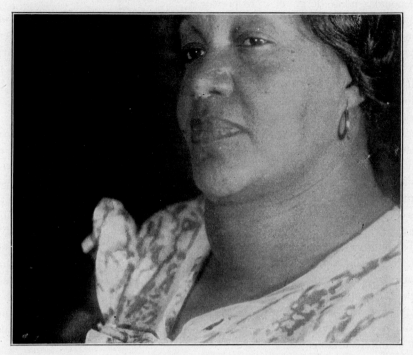

FIG. 510.—PHOTOGRAPH OF A COLORED WOMAN AGED THIRTY-TWO WITH A NODULAR NONTOXIC GOITER.

This patient had no symptoms whatsoever. To inspection and even palpation the gland may appear smooth (particularly so in this patient) thereby resembling a diffuse nontoxic goiter. However, when such glands are removed the nodular characteristics are obvious on examination of the specimen.

presence of a diffuse, symmetrical, nontoxic diffuse goiter during puberty, pregnancy, etc., for a few months before the asymmetrical nodular enlargement is noted. Although nodules or part of a lobe not infrequently descend behind the sternum or clavicle (see p. 914), they usually enlarge outward in the direction of least resistance, sometimes producing a tumor so unsightly as to lead the patient to request its removal merely for cosmetic reasons alone. As the goiter enlarges there is an increasing tendency for the production of pressure symptoms consisting of difficulty in deglutition and breathing. The respiratory difficulty usually consists of such symptoms as coughing, a slight transitory "smothered" sensation, or attacks of actual orthopnea. Symptoms referable to the esophagus are rarely severe. The pressure may be caused by the thyroid encircling or compressing the trachea or esophagus, or by intrathoracic extension. Patients afflicted with nodular, nontoxic goiter over a period of years are apt to develop mild symptoms of myxedema which may require therapy with desiccated thyroid or thyroxin. On the other hand, thyrotoxicosis occasionally develops in the presence of nodular nontoxic goiter, particularly in the third and fourth decades of life. For some unknown reason thyrotoxicosis of this type develops most commonly in the United States and only infrequently in goitrous regions such as Switzerland, where nodular nontoxic goiter is so prevalent.

Upon examination the nodules are moderately firm except that cystic nodules are fluctuant. The mass is not movable vertically, but can be displaced to either side with the trachea. When the patient swallows the goiter moves with the larynx. This characteristic is particularly valuable in differentiating goitrous tumors from various other masses in the neck. X-ray of the neck may show definite compression of the trachea by the thyroid, particularly if two views are taken.

Treatment.—The treatment of nodular nontoxic goiter is preventive and surgical. The nodular, as well as diffuse type of nontoxic goiter, may be prevented at least to a great extent by the administration of iodine in childhood and early adulthood. Furthermore, it has been shown in Switzerland [14] that the administration of iodine to expectant mothers with nodular nontoxic goiter decreases the incidence of goiter in the children. Throughout the endemic areas of the United States (Great Lakes region and northwest) it is customary to administer iodine to young people and pregnant women at regular intervals either as iodized salt, Lugol's solution by mouth, or by addition of some form of iodine to the drinking water. Iodine, however, cannot be expected to cure nodular goiter, but is valuable from a prophylactic standpoint and to a less extent in prevention of progressive growth. It should not be administered over a long period of time to patients with nodular nontoxic goiter, because of the slight possibility of inciting the gland to hyperactivity. However, proof of the production of thyrotoxicosis by this means is not definitely established.

Once this type of goiter develops, surgery offers the only means of eradicating it. Various indications for excision may be enumerated, the most important of which are: (1) relief of tracheal or esophageal obstruction; (2) danger of development of a toxic goiter or carcinoma; and (3) cosmetic reasons. Operative treatment consists of the removal of the greater part of the diseased gland. To prevent myxedema, a small portion of the most normal appearing thyroid tissue is left. In young people the posterior capsule of the gland must be left undisturbed; otherwise, tetany may develop through loss of the parathyroid glands. Particular care must be exercised in removal of large goiters lest the recurrent laryngeal nerves be injured.

Diffuse Toxic Goiter (Graves' Disease, Basedow's Disease, Exophthalmic Goiter, Hyperthyroidism).—*Etiology.*—This is a disease occurring more commonly in women than men (ratio 4 or 5 to 1) and in young adult life, apparently produced by the secretion of an excessive amount of the thyroid principle, thyroxin. Some authorities are of the opinion that the etiologic factor producing the disease is not normal thyroxin, but a toxic and chemically distorted substance secreted by the diseased thyroid, but evidence supports the theory that most of the symptoms, at least, are caused by a true hypersecretion of the active principle. Up to the present time, however, there are a number of possible explanations for this excessive secretion. One is that it is presumably brought about by the stimulative action of some other endocrine gland. Knowing that the administration of certain extracts (hormones) of the pituitary gland (Loeb and Bassett[15]) produce hyperplasia of the thyroid gland of animals with many of the manifestations of hyperthyroidism, including exophthalmos (Loeb and Friedman[16]), it would appear that the hyperplasia of toxic goiter might be due to an excessive secretion of this

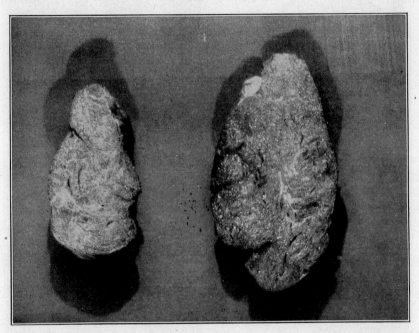

Fig. 511.—Two Examples of the Thyroid (Cut Surface) of Two Patients with Diffuse Toxic Goiter (Graves' Disease).

Each specimen has the typical beefy, somewhat homogeneous appearance, but the lobe on the left contains considerable scar tissue which is not present on the right.

pituitary (thyrotropic) hormone. Although this hormone has been given to human beings on numerous occasions for various reasons, the authors are not aware of the production of hyperthyroid symptoms in any instance. Another explanation is the evidence offered from time to time that a specific bacterium of some type is responsible for the production of toxic goiter, but confirmation is always lacking. However, there is ample proof as has been shown by Roger and Garnier,[17] Cole and Womack[18] and others that infections and toxemias may be instigating factors in the production of hyperplasia of the thyroid in animals. This feature has been illustrated recently by Anderson[19] who noted that administration of alkaline extract of anterior pituitary when given to a rat intraperitoneally with a killed suspension of staphylococci, would always produce a hyperplasia of the thyroid, whereas the administration of anterior pituitary alone would produce hyperplasia only occasionally. A surprisingly large percentage of patients with toxic goiter, especially of the diffuse type, date their symptoms from an acute respiratory infection from which they "did not completely recover." Less frequently, psychic shocks have been known to precipitate symptoms of toxic goiter. The factors just

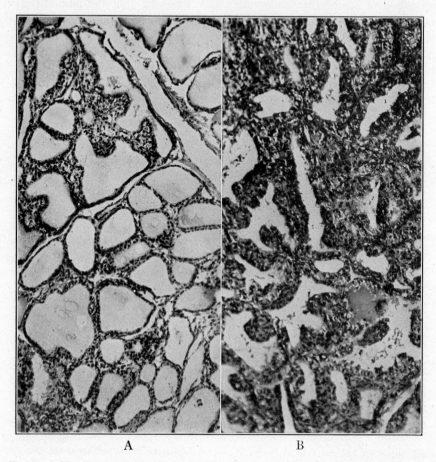

A   B

FIG. 512.—MICROSCOPICAL APPEARANCE OF THE THYROID IN GRAVES' DISEASE (DIFFUSE TOXIC GOITER).

The sections were taken from two patients with approximately the same degree of toxicity; operation after twelve days preoperative treatment with iodine. *A,* this section reveals the typical response of the gland to iodine therapy. The acinous cells in general are columnar, but not high; the acini are large and contain considerable colloid. Numerous small areas are found, however, where the cells are high columnar, plicated and layered, indicative of a hyperactive gland. *B,* this section exhibits practically no response to iodine. The acini are small and contain no colloid; the cells are high, plicated and layered. Patients with glands of this type are slightly more apt to suffer recurrence of the goiter than patients whose thyroid responded to iodine.

mentioned should be considered contributory in the development of toxic diffuse goiter; the exciting cause is as yet undiscovered.

Iodine Metabolism.—It has long been known that the thyroid is the only organ in the body containing iodine in any significant quantity and that the iodine content of the organ is decreased in toxic goiter. Unquestionably, lack of iodine is of some importance in the development of toxic diffuse goiter, because, as in the non-toxic types just described, the disease is most prevalent in "goiter belts" where the iodine content of water and food is low. Curtis and associates [20] have shown that in both types of toxic goiter there is a negative iodine balance, *i.e.*, more iodine is being excreted than is ingested. The blood iodine is usually slightly above normal. Perkins and Lahey [21] have found that in the group of patients with toxic diffuse goiter having a normal blood iodine prior to operation, there is a higher incidence of recurrence than in patients with an elevated level. Although it is thought that in certain localities (*e.g.*, Michigan) the use of iodized salt has decreased the incidence of toxic goiter, there is no confirmation thereof in the Chicago goiter area where iodized salt is used but perhaps to a less extent.

Pathology.—The thyroid gland in toxic diffuse goiter is friable, extremely vascular and usually but not always enlarged. Because of the lack of colloid the cut surface is beefy instead of glairy. Microscopically the acini are columnar instead of cuboidal and are layered as well as plicated within the lumen of the acinus. If the patient has received iodine for more than a few days the friability of the gland is lost and the normal glairy appearance of the cut surface is regained in part; furthermore, the columnar cell becomes cuboidal, the acinus larger and contains more colloid. If the disease has been present for a long time, cardiac hypertrophy may develop. The glycogen content of the liver is greatly reduced and in fatal cases of hyperthyroidism considerable destruction of hepatic cells may be noted microscopically. The exophthalmos, which frequently accompanies the disease, is apparently due to an edema and swelling of the retrobulbar structures including the muscles.

Clinical Manifestations.—One of the first symptoms is the gradual development of a nervous irritability. The patient is restless and is reluctant to remain quiet for any length of time. Changes in personality are common in so far as the patient becomes angered or upset emotionally without due provocation. Household cares and the demands made by children may be so irritating to women afflicted with the disease as to be almost unbearable. The mind may be very active, and frequently the patient plans more activities than she is capable of performing. Fatigue occurs readily and weakness is complained of. The appetite is not decreased, but on the contrary may be sharply increased, although loss of weight is usually noted in spite of the increased caloric intake; the weight loss may be pronounced. Increased sweating is usually complained of. Palpitation may be present. Intolerance to heat and tolerance to cold are commonly noted. Difficulty in sleeping is almost a universal complaint, especially if the disease is severe. In highly toxic individuals diarrhea and occasionally vomiting occur.

The patient is apt to have spontaneous remissions so that symptoms may disappear almost entirely. These remissions may last for weeks, but with few exceptions symptoms return and are frequently so intense as to be designated as thyroid "crises." If the disease is severe or has been present for a long time, symptoms of cardiac disease, such as dyspnea and edema may appear.

Examination reveals a restless patient. The thyroid gland is usually diffusely enlarged, but severe toxicity may be present without any demonstrable enlargement whatsoever. Exophthalmos is present in many, but by no means all patients with diffuse toxic goiter. With the exophthalmos a widening of the palpebral fissure is demonstrable (Stellwag's sign). There may be a lag of the upper lid as the eye follows the finger downward (von Graefe's sign). Difficulty in convergence (Moebius sign) as evinced when the patient looks at close objects may be demonstrable. A fine tremor of the fingers is noted, particularly when they are extended and abducted. The skin is warm and moist, particularly that on the palm of the

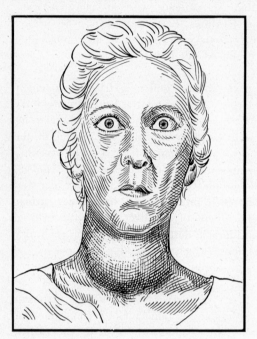

FIG. 513.—PATIENT WITH APPEARANCE TYPICAL OF EXOPHTHALMIC GOITER.

Note the exophthalmos, apprehensive expression, and diffuse swelling in the neck.

hands. The face may be flushed and an anxious expression which has been described as "frozen terror" may be noted. Tachycardia, which is increased sharply by mild stimuli, is a reliable sign. Auricular fibrillation is only rarely present; it is more common in toxic nodular goiter. If the gland is appreciably enlarged a thrill may be palpable over it or the vessels entering the gland, and a bruit heard by auscultation. A pulsation of the expansile type is usually palpable over the gland. The systolic blood pressure is usually elevated and the pulse pressure distinctly high.

One of the most reliable signs of toxic goiter is an increase in the basal metabolic rate. In severe cases this may be elevated as much as 60 to 90 per cent above normal. A rise of greater than 10 or 15 per cent above normal is considered indicative of the disease unless another cause for the elevation can be found. Numerous observers have noted that in most instances there is a decrease in the blood cholesterol in hyperthyroidism and an elevation in hypothyroidism; the test has, therefore, been recommended as an auxiliary test for thyroid disease.

In the absence of such obvious signs as exophthalmos and enlargement of the thyroid, the diagnosis may have to be made by such features as increased metabolic rate, excess appetite, difficulty in sleeping, excess sweating, loss of weight, increased appetite, tachycardia and increased pulse pressure. Because of the loss of weight, sweating, and weakness, many of these patients are erroneously diagnosed as tuberculosis suspects; when the mental symptoms are pronounced a manic psychosis is simulated. It is probable that not infrequently mild cases of thyrotoxicosis masquerade as neuroses of various types. When cardiac manifestations are prominent they may lead to a mistaken diagnosis of primary myocardial disease.

Treatment.—It is now generally agreed that thyroidectomy is more efficacious in the treatment of toxic goiter than medical treatment, although the latter procedure may be adopted in the mild atypical cases with slight enlargement of the thyroid. X-ray therapy has been recommended, but is associated with a very high incidence of failure; it is sometimes useful in decreasing the toxicity in patients who are not safe subjects for operation because of severe toxicity. However, several weeks are required for the maximum benefit to be attained from irradiation.

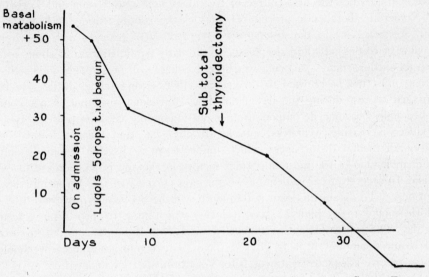

Fig. 514.—Basal Metabolic Curve in a Patient with Exophthalmic Goiter Exhibiting Typical Response to Iodine Therapy and Subtotal Thyroidectomy.

Thyroidectomy has been made a much less dangerous procedure by the preparatory administration of iodine practiced many decades ago, but reinstituted and popularized by Plummer [22] twenty or twenty-five years ago. By using iodine the operative mortality has been reduced from 4 to 6 per cent to 0.5 per cent, and the operation has been made easier and complications fewer. The iodine may be given in any form (*e.g.,* Lugol's solution Min. V. or X, t.i.d.), but with few exceptions should not be given except in preparation for operation and for a period of a few weeks or months following operation. The period of maximum benefit following iodine therapy is usually ten to fourteen days after beginning treatment, but frequently operability will continue to improve for many days following this period, particularly in severely toxic patients. Although it is doubtful if the continued use of iodine ever increases the symptoms of hyperthyroidism, there is no doubt that there is a period as mentioned above when the beneficial effects of iodine are maximal and that if iodine administration is prolonged beyond this point (*i.e.,* a few weeks) its therapeutic effect is rapidly lost and a return of symptoms is observed. For this reason it is particularly desirable to limit its use to preoperative therapy. If given continuously as part of a purely medical regimen, an acute severe exacerbation of symptoms may develop for which it may be highly desirable to have in reserve a highly efficient method of treatment, such as that afforded by iodine. Many authorities, moreover, believe that patients receiving iodine continuously may become refractory to the drug, thereby making it necessary to withdraw the iodine for three to four months before it may be given again with benefit. This is an added argument against the use of iodine except as a pre- and postoperative measure. However, the authors are of the opinion that this conception of refractoriness to iodine has been exaggerated because satisfactory results frequently occur from a second period of iodine therapy even though no more than ten to fifteen days have elapsed since the first course of treatment (see also Means and Lerman [23]).

Numerous therapeutic procedures, besides the administration of Lugol's solution, are necessary in the *preoperative preparation* of patients with toxic goiter. In view of restlessness and sleeplessness, the daily administration of some sedative such as phenobarbital (particularly in the evening) will be strongly indicated. The patient must not be allowed to do manual labor, except trivial duties. He is encouraged to rest during the day (including afternoon naps) but is not confined to bed unless cardiac decompensation or an impending crisis is present. Bed rest produces increasing weakness, muscle atrophy, etc., and thereby lowers operability. All mental disturbances which might serve as psychic trauma should be eliminated. One of the most important factors in therapy is an increase in caloric intake. In severely toxic patients a weight gain *must be elicited* before operation is considered. To obtain this gain it frequently will be necessary to increase the daily caloric intake to as high as 5000 calories which may require 4 or 5 feedings per day. The appetite is so ravenous that rarely will these patients fail to consume the required amount if it is offered them. Any complication present should of course receive adequate treatment before operation is contemplated.

Unquestionably, the greatest cause of a high mortality in surgery of toxic goiter patients is inadequate preoperative preparation or a poor choice of time for operation. Of such great importance are these two factors that it is imperative to outline certain *precautions or prerequisites* which are to be met before operation is considered: (1) Except in mildly toxic patients, a gain in weight must be attained before operation is performed. (2) The pulse rate must be lowered to a safe level; in general, a resting rate below 110 may be considered safe from the operative standpoint. (3) The basal metabolic rate should be below 50. Although the basal metabolic rate is frequently in error and may be a very misleading gauge of the degree of toxicity, it is still true that operations done in the presence of rates above 50 are associated with a high incidence of complications including crises, etc. (4) When toxicity is more than slight, the patient must have been on iodine therapy for at least 15 days and should have shown a favorable response. A beneficial response is splendid evidence of confirmation of the diagnosis. Moreover, patients with toxic diffuse goiter who show but little benefit, are apt to have a stormy postoperative convalescence, supposedly because of low utilization of iodine. (5) There must be a freedom from complications such as uncontrolled diabetes, or from symptoms of severe toxicity including jaundice, diarrhea, nausea, vomiting and undue restlessness or apprehension.

When the above precautions are met, bilateral subtotal thyroidectomy is usually safe. If they are not met by routine measures, the operation is done in two stages (removing one lobe at a time) or postponed for continued treatment, watching the patient for a remission. In view of the negative calcium balance which occurs in hyperthyroidism, as shown by Aub and associates [24] and by Curtis and associates,[25] calcium and vitamin D therapy is advisable in prolonged thyrotoxicosis.

Thiourea and thiouracil, which inhibit thyroid function (Astwood [80]), may prove very useful in therapy, probably in preparation of patients for operation, since symptoms recur after cessation of therapy.

At operation the posterior capsule and 2 or 3 gms. of tissue are preserved. Special care is taken not to injure the parathyroids or recurrent nerve.

Postoperative care is likewise important in lowering the mortality rate. Perhaps the most important single procedure is the administration of intravenous glucose. No less than 3000 cc. of 5 per cent solution should be given the day of operation. Water and liquid diet is allowed almost immediately but should be supplemented with intravenous glucose depending on toxicity, etc. In severely toxic patients, oxygen (by nasal tube or tent) is essential for a day or two postoperatively. Sedatives should be given in large enough quantities to promote an adequate amount of sleep. The wound should be watched closely for postoperative hemorrhage or infection. If hemorrhage develops, it usually manifests itself within 2 to 10 hours following operation. The presence of respiratory stridor demands immediate inspection of the wound. If a blood clot is causing the stridor, the wound must be opened immediately, the clot evacuated, and the bleeding controlled. If cyanosis remains after evacuation of the clot, tracheotomy may be necessary. If the stridor is due to recurrent laryngeal nerve paralysis tracheotomy will likewise probably be necessary. If the paralysis is due to pressure from edema or mild trauma, the tube can usually be removed in a few weeks; if both nerves have been cut the tracheotomy will probably have to be permanent unless the nerves can be successfully resutured. The operation designed by King [26] (attaching the arytenoid to the thyroid cartilage, with consequent widening of the aperture between the cords) promises to allow removal of the tracheotomy tube in bilateral nerve paralysis.

When considerable myocardial damage (as evidenced commonly by auricular fibrillation) is present, the need for oxygen will be more acute. Intravenous fluids must be given more slowly and in smaller quantities. Digitalis is used before operation in patients with cardiac decompensation. Its postoperative use may become necessary if pulmonary congestion and other signs of heart failure appear.

A disturbing complication of thyroidectomy is the rare occurrence of so-called thyroid "crises" which develops during the first day or two following operation. This complication is characterized by extreme tachycardia, fever, marked excitability and occasionally delirium. Treatment consists of intravenous sodium iodide, oxygen therapy, and heavy doses of narcotics. The patient must be kept cool, utilizing electric fans, wet towels or an air conditioned room in warm weather. Intravenous glucose is essential. Blood transfusions may also be given. Additional data on pre- and postoperative care may be found in a publication by one [27] of us.

Recurrence of thyrotoxicosis after thyroidectomy is usually indicative of an incomplete operation; *i.e.*, that an insufficient amount of thyroid tissue had been removed. This conclusion as to cause is more accurate when the hyperthyroidism persists (perhaps with less intense symptoms) following operation, than if operation resulted in cure for a few years. However, in spite of adequate removal of glandular tissue and proper postoperative care, recurrences will occur occasionally (2 to 8 per cent of cases) and again disable the patient. The treatment of recurrent goiter is not much different from that already described, except that when operation is performed attempt is made to be more radical in excision of thyroid tissue. When exophthalmos is so severe as to threaten loss of sight through ulceration of the cornea and papilledema, decompression of the orbit as suggested by Naffziger [28] may be indicated. This is particularly the case when thyroidectomy has failed to produce sufficient recession of the eyes; failure of recession is not infrequent; in a few cases, indeed, exophthalmos may become more pronounced in spite of an adequate thyroid operation (see Fig. 515).

Nodular Toxic Goiter (Toxic Adenoma).—For years there has been considerable discussion as to whether or not this disease was etiologically different from toxic diffuse goiter. Although the main symptoms of toxicity are similar, there are a few prominent differences, namely, that the symptoms of toxic nodular goiter are milder, and exophthalmos much less common than in toxic diffuse goiter. Moreover, the nodular disease occurs ten to fifteen years later in life than the diffuse type.

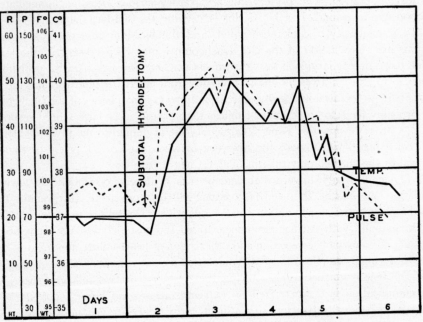

CHART 8.—TEMPERATURE AND PULSE OF PATIENT WHO SUSTAINED A "CRISIS" FOLLOWING SUBTOTAL THYROIDECTOMY.

In typical cases the temperature and pulse rate begin to rise a few hours after operation, reach their maximum twenty-four or more hours following thyroidectomy, but recede in two or three days. Reactions of this type may be fatal, but are extremely uncommon at the present time due to preoperative iodine therapy.

Pathologically, the gland in toxic adenoma is nodular and asymmetrical. The adenomatous changes may be localized to one area (presenting as a nodule), but are usually diffused throughout the gland. Small areas of hyperplasia are almost always demonstrable at various points in the gland. The gland may encircle or compress the trachea and esophagus and produce obstructive signs. Occasionally, a large adenomatous nodule descends and is located behind the clavicle or sternum (see p. 914). Rarely, the entire gland descends into the thorax so that nothing more than the upper margin is palpable in the suprasternal notch. On cut section the gland reveals globular masses of colloid containing tissue surrounded by a

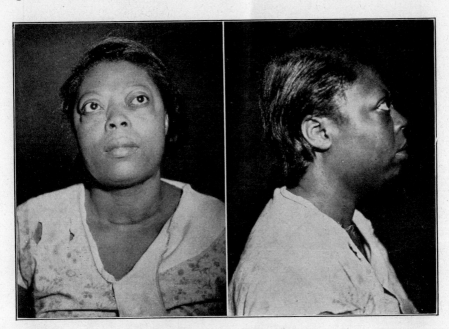

FIG. 515.—PERSISTENT EXOPHTHALMOS.

The patient, a Negro woman aged thirty, had exophthalmos at the time of operation two and one-half years ago. The exophthalmos receded slightly within a few months following operation, but during the past year has increased slightly. There is no evidence of recurrence of the hyperthyroidism. Exophthalmos usually recedes following operation, but in many patients it persists indefinitely.

fibrous capsule. Dense deposits of fibrous tissue may occur at any point throughout the gland. In addition there may be areas of beefy tissue resembling the gland seen in toxic diffuse goiter.

Clinical Manifestations.—The disease is not greatly unlike toxic diffuse goiter. However, it occurs in persons ten or fifteen years older, is a milder disease, develops more insidiously and rarely is accompanied by exophthalmos or any other eye signs. Crises are rarely encountered. Usually there is a history of the presence of a nodular enlarged thyroid for years before toxic symptoms develop. "Nervousness," weakness and unusual susceptibility to fatigue are early symptoms. Irritability and emotional instability are likewise apt to be present. Difficulty in sleeping is also a fairly common complaint.

There is a greater tendency for the development of symptoms of cardiac decompensation in toxic nodular goiter than in toxic diffuse goiter. This may be due in part to the fact that the manifestations in the former disease are so insidious that they may exist for years before the patient is aware of symptoms; but a more logical explanation would appear to be in the fact that patients with nodular toxic goiter are older, and therefore have hearts with less reserve. This myocardial dam-

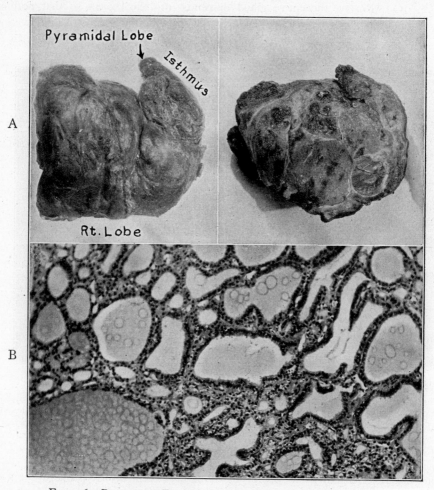

FIG. 516.—PATHOLOGIC FEATURES OF THE THYROID IN TOXIC ADENOMA.

A, external surface and cross section of a nodular goiter removed from a patient with toxic adenoma. The lobulations circumscribed by fibrous tissue are readily discernible in the cross section; *B,* photomicrograph of tissue removed from *A.* Large acini filled with colloid are numerous, but here and there are scattered areas where the acini are small, the cell tall columnar, plicated and layered, indicative of hyperactivity.

age may be uncomplicated or be associated with auricular fibrillation. In either case shortness of breath, orthopnea, weakness, swelling of ankles, etc., may be complained of.

Examination reveals a nodular enlarged gland with or without a thrill and bruit. Frequently, the nodular enlargement is confined to one lobe; occasionally, the only abnormality made out in the gland is the presence of a solitary nodule.

Exophthalmos or other eye signs are rarely encountered. Restlessness and irritability are usually demonstrable and a fine tremor of the fingers upon extension and abduction is always present. The palms of the hands are unusually moist. Tachycardia is noted and if auricular fibrillation is present there will be an irregularity of the pulse with a pulse deficit. There is usually an elevation of the pulse pressure. The basal metabolic rate is elevated (15 to 50 per cent above normal), but not as high as in toxic diffuse goiter.

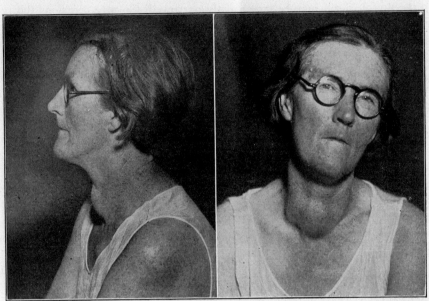

FIG. 517.—TOXIC ADENOMA.

Note the absence of exophthalmos. The patient aged fifty-one had a basal metabolism rate of plus 43 on admission; after six days of iodine therapy (at the time the photograph was taken) the B.M.R. had dropped to plus 29.

Treatment.—Patients with toxic nodular goiter are treated similarly to those with toxic diffuse goiter. The response to iodine may not be so spectacular as it is in toxic diffuse goiter, but this is probably due to the fact that the toxicity is not as great, and to morphologic changes which have taken place in the gland. Although several years ago it was thought that iodine was harmful to patients with toxic nodular goiter, the experience of recent years offers strong evidence to the contrary. Toxic nodular goiter responds even less favorably to x-ray therapy than does toxic diffuse goiter. Surgical treatment, *i.e.,* subtotal thyroidectomy, is especially efficacious because recurrences are seldom encountered; the resection, therefore, need not be so radical. Moreover, unless severe myocardial damage has been sustained the symptoms of heart failure are usually relieved and the heart will be restored to a fairly normal function.

The same precautions used in the operative treatment of toxic diffuse goiter must be exercised in nodular goiter, except that even more care must be taken not to injure the recurrent laryngeal nerves, because of the distorted anatomic relations.

Substernal or Retroclavicular Goiter.—Occasionally, large masses of thyroid tissue (toxic or nontoxic adenomas) are encountered behind the sternum. The mechanism of the development of a retrosternal goiter is dependent to a great extent upon the downward growth of the enlarged gland. It should be emphasized that goiters of this type are at first retroclavicular in type; most of them remain so permanently. If growth of the gland persists, the mass is apt to descend, moving toward the midline behind the sternum. The pedicle connecting these adenomas with the thyroid itself may become greatly narrowed. On rare occasions the retrosternal mass may have no connections with the thyroid because of its development in an aberrant thyroid or because of atrophy of the pedicle.

Clinical Manifestations.—The clinical manifestations of the substernal goiter are varied, but are primarily due to the effects of pressure. They may be a source of considerable discomfort and be serious because of obstruction to the trachea and esophagus. There is apt to be a sensation of tightness or fullness in the upper portion of the chest, but more frequently the first symptom complained of by the patient is dyspnea or orthopnea. The dyspnea is, of course, caused by pressure on the trachea which may progress to such an extent as to produce an audible stridor. Occasionally, mild dysphagia is present. Periodic short attacks of choking, terminating in coughing, are quite common, particularly at night while the patient is asleep. There may be dilatation of the veins of the neck or of the upper part of the chest due to compression of the thyroid on the jugular and subclavian veins. A fullness of the neck or in the suprasternal notch may or may not be visible. Deviation of the trachea, or even of the larynx from the midline is an important diagnostic sign and can be demonstrated by the x-ray. X-ray, moreover, may show an abnormal shadow in the superior mediastinum which may be suggestive of a retrosternal goiter. If the substernal mass is sufficiently large, it may be demonstrable because of dullness to percussion. Differential diagnosis is frequently difficult because of the confusion with such lesions as aneurysm, thymoma, dermoid cyst, Hodgkin's disease, etc. The expansile type of pulsation noted fluoroscopically in an aneurysm should identify this lesion. X-ray therapy may be useful at times in establishing a diagnosis since nearly all the primary malignant tumors occurring in this region are remarkably sensitive to radiation; roentgenologically, a rapid and marked diminution in size will be noted following x-ray therapy in contrast to a slight or no decrease in size of a substernal goiter. Dermoid cysts will, of course, not be altered in size by radiation.

Substernal thyroids producing no symptoms need not be removed. If either obstructive or toxic symptoms are produced, excision is advisable. This may be done in most instances through an ordinary thyroid incision and the mass removed by blunt dissection with the finger. If the tumor cannot be dislodged with the finger it may be necessary to split the sternum. Removal by any method must be done with care because of the proximity of the recurrent laryngeal nerves and the danger of injury to them.

Acute Thyroiditis.—Pyogenic infection of the thyroid is a rare disease. It is usually seen in young adults secondary to a primary focus elsewhere, such as acute pharyngitis, etc., and is usually confined to the lower portion of one lobe. Tenderness over the affected lobe is perhaps the first manifestation noted and may be excruciating. Fever and pain usually are present. In hyperplastic glands, which are affected more often than normal glands, the infection rarely proceeds to suppuration, but subsides spontaneously within a few days. When infection does take place in a normal gland, redness of the skin may appear, and shortly thereafter, fluctuation. When suppuration develops the infection is treated by incision, just as it is in an ordinary abscess. If evidence of acute infection should develop in a hyperplastic gland (toxic goiter), treatment should be conservative, consisting of bed rest and symptomatic therapy since suppuration in such glands is uncommon. Obviously, thyroidectomy in such instances should not be performed for many days following subsidence of the inflammatory manifestation.

Riedel's Struma (Ligneous Thyroiditis, Chronic Thyroiditis).—Many years ago Riedel described a rare type of disease characterized by woody hardness of the thyroid gland, but associated with no known etiologic factor. However, it now appears that the disease is caused by a nonbacterial perithyroiditis (De Courcy[44]) with a constriction of surface blood vessels. The fact that dense adhesions are always present, and that the pathologic changes are more noted in the periphery of the gland supports this view. Mild cases are becoming more frequent. Microscopically, there is a diffuse deposition of scar tissue with a diminished number of alveoli of irregular shape and size scattered about the gland. There is usually an extensive lymphocytic infiltration. The gland becomes so adherent to the surrounding tissue, and the parenchyma so fibrosed that frequently it is impossible to identify the margin of glandular tissue. Mild symptoms of obstruction to the trachea and esophagus may be produced. Myxedema may be present, but hyperthyroidism rarely accompanies the disease. If tracheal or esophageal obstruction is present and persists, operation will be indicated. Since a large percentage of patients with Riedel's disease will develop myxedema following operation (33 per cent in Clute and Lahey's series [29]) it is usually advisable to remove no more thyroid tissue than is necessary to correct the difficulty in swallowing or breathing.

A similar disease, *struma lymphomatosa,* has been described (Hashimoto[30]) in which a bilateral enlargement of the lobes with a firm consistency was noted. Microscopically, numerous lymph follicles with germinal centers, fibrosis and atrophy or hypertrophy are encountered. Opinions differ as to a possible relationship to Riedel's disease. The fact that about half the cases are not associated with adhesions (McSwain and Moore[31]) suggests that the diseases are not related.

Myxedema.—Although a severe degree of hypothyroidism may result from the removal of too much thyroid tissue in the treatment of toxic goiter, rarely is it comparable to the idiopathic myxedema. The idiopathic disease may rarely follow an attack of toxic goiter or acute and chronic thyroiditis, but in most instances there is no history of antecedent thyroid disease. The gland is small and microscopically a sharp diminution of acinar tissue with increase in amount of fibrous tissue is noted.

Clinical Manifestations.—The development of clinical manifestations is so insidious that the disease may be far advanced before the patient is aware of its presence. The patient becomes mentally dull, the speech slow and "thick," as if the tongue were too large for the mouth. Constipation is rarely absent. The appetite is poor. Early in the disease the patient notes that he is very sensitive to cold, and requires an unusually large amount of sleep. A gain in weight is the rule. The temperature is subnormal and the pulse rate slow. There is a mask-like expression of the face, the features of which are enlarged as if swollen. The skin and subcutaneous tissue over the entire body is thickened. Sweating is diminished. The hair is dry and thin. Diagnosis is readily confirmed by a basal metabolic test which will reveal a metabolic rate 20 to 40 per cent below normal. However, many patients with a low B.M.R. do not manifest symptoms of myxedema. Reference has already been made to the value of the blood cholesterol as an aid in the

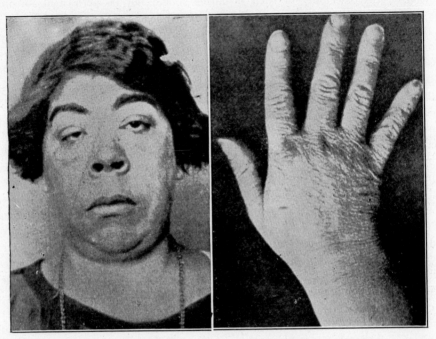

FIG. 518.—CHARACTERISTIC FACIAL APPEARANCE IN MYXEDEMA.

Note the thickening and puffiness of the eyelids and the coarseness of all the features. (From Graham, *Surgical Diagnosis,* Vol. II, 1930. Courtesy of W. B. Saunders Co. Philadelphia.)

diagnosis of hyperthyroidism and hypothyroidism. A reciprocal relationship seems to exist between the decrease in basal metabolism in thyroid deficiency and a rise in blood cholesterol. If the determination is carefully made, a blood cholesterol of 250 mg. per cent or more in the absence of other causes for hypercholesterolemia (nephrosis, nephritis, diabetes, etc.) is suggestive of hypothyroidism.

Treatment.—The treatment consists almost entirely of administration of desiccated thyroid or thyroxin. It usually requires 30 to 60 grains of desiccated thyroid given over a period of several weeks to bring the patient's basal metabolism up to normal; the amount necessary for maintenance of a normal metabolism is determined by the effect on the heart rate and basal metabolic rate. A dose of 2 to 4 grains daily is usually sufficient. Treatment should be begun with small doses and increased very slowly since it will take several weeks for the full effect of desiccated thyroid to become manifested. After it is determined how much is required to maintain a normal metabolic rate, it is usually necessary to maintain this dose or a slightly smaller one indefinitely.

Cretinism.—This is a disease of childhood consisting physiologically of a diminution or absence of thyroid secretion. Cretinism may be endemic, *i.e.*, occurs in localities where goiter is prevalent, or may be encountered in the sporadic form, a type in which the child is born of healthy parents and in a region where goiter is not prevalent. In many instances pituitary deficiency is no doubt an important etiologic factor in the development of the disease. Cretinism is apt to develop in a child when the mother has been suffering from diffuse nontoxic goiter during pregnancy. The glandular defect is no doubt present at birth, but so long as the child is breast fed manifestations of the disease do not appear.

The child grows at a slower rate than average and appears stupid and unusually placid. The skin is dry. The face is large, appears bloated and the nose broad and flattened. The tongue, which is presumably too large for the oral cavity, protrudes through a thick-lipped mouth. Talking and walking are delayed and teeth are slow to appear. The temperature may be subnormal. The basal metabolism is below normal. If the disease is severe dwarfism may result. Cretinism slightly resembles rickets, but is more apt to be confused with achondroplastic dwarfism, a disease characterized by short pudgy extremities and premature ossification of the epiphyses.

Treatment.—The treatment must be instituted early in childhood if mental apathy or idiocy is to be prevented. Growth responds fairly well to the administration of desiccated thyroid, but correction of the mental dullness or idiocy is much more difficult to obtain, particularly if treatment is not started within the first year or two of life.

Malignant Tumors of the Thyroid.—Malignant tumors of the thyroid offer perhaps more difficulty in diagnosis than in any other organ; this is true even after microscopic examination of the excised tissue. Previous to the work of Allen Graham,[32] many benign adenomas were no doubt erroneously classified as malignant tumors. Graham has emphasized the importance of the presence of invasion of the blood vessels of the gland with tumor cells before a diagnosis of malignancy can be made. Other evidences of malignancy are invasion beyond the capsule, recurrence after excision, and metastases. The microscopic appearance of the cell is not very helpful in determining whether a given tumor is malignant or not, since the hyperplastic cells in toxic goiter closely resemble malignant cells. Of a group of 65 tumors of proved malignancy Allen Graham classified 55 as malignant adenomas, 8 as papilliferous adenocarcinoma and 2 as scirrhous carcinoma. He is of the opinion that 90 per cent of malignant tumors of the thyroid arise in preexisting adenomas. Carcinoma of the thyroid is not very common, but it is estimated at 1 to 3 per cent of all thyroids removed at operation are malignant. It occurs slightly more commonly in women and in goitrous regions; its appearance in people under the so-called cancer age is comparatively common.

In a splendid survey of malignant neoplasms of the thyroid, Ward [33] has called attention to the fact that the incidence of carcinoma of the thyroid in patients operated on for goiter varied from 6.5 to almost 10 per cent in endemic areas (*e.g.*, Switzerland), whereas, the incidence will be no higher than 1 or 2 per cent in areas where goiter is not endemic. He noted that papillary carcinoma was the least malignant of all types and was least common in endemic areas.

Clinical Manifestations.—The clinical manifestations of carcinoma of the thyroid are no different from those of a benign adenoma in the early stage. The history usually reveals the fact that an adenoma which had been constant in size for many months or years suddenly starts to grow. The growth of the gland is usually asymmetrical and ultimately progresses to a point where it is fixed to the skin and adjacent tissue. Pain in the neck is a not uncommon symptom. As the tumor develops, it may compress the trachea and esophagus, producing difficulty in breathing and swallowing. Hoarseness of the voice, produced by pressure on the recurrent laryngeal nerves or actual invasion by the tumor may be present. Occasionally, hyperthyroidism, but rarely hypothyroidism accompanies carcinoma of the thyroid. The general condition of the patient usually remains unaltered until metastases occur. As would be expected from the tendency to invade blood vessels, the most common site for metastases is the lung. Bones are also commonly affected and may be the seat of spontaneous (pathologic) fractures.

Treatment.—The treatment consists of excision if possible. Any adenoma which suddenly begins to increase in size should be removed. Unfortunately, by the time a definite diagnosis is possible, there is rarely any hope of completely removing the tumor by operation. Not infrequently, tracheotomy will be necessary, particularly in the later stages of the disease. Irradiation either with x-ray or radium is helpful and should be resorted to in all cases, regardless of whether or not operation is performed. Although carcinoma of the thyroid is a serious disease, it is by no means the most fatal of the carcinomas. In an analysis of the patients observed at the Mayo Clinic, Pemberton and Dixon [34] noted that of 323 patients with carcinoma of thyroid treated during a twenty year period, 43.9 per cent lived five years or longer after treatment was first instituted.

Miscellaneous Diseases of the Thyroid.—Tuberculosis, syphilis, and even actinomycosis of the thyroid occur, but are so rare as not to justify discussion here. Primary sarcoma of the thyroid is exceedingly rare, if it occurs at all. Aberrant thyroid is relatively rare; it occurs as a lingual thyroid, but more commonly in the neck as single or multiple nodules, above and lateral to the thyroid lobe. These nodules tend to become malignant, and should be removed when encountered.

THE PARATHYROID GLANDS

The parathyroid bodies are tiny glandular structures, usually four in number (occasionally more), located in most instances on the posterior capsule of the thyroid gland. Their function in body metabolism is so important that excision of all parathyroid tissue is followed by death or severe tetany (see p. 921). The control of calcium metabolism is the most important function of the parathyroids. Hyperparathyroidism and tetany (hypoparathyroidism) which are the two most important diseases attributed to the parathyroids are associated respectively with an elevation and diminution of calcium in the blood. Calcium is found in the blood serum in two forms: (1) ionizable calcium, and (2) calcium bound to protein. McLean and Hastings [35] have emphasized the importance of the fact that the ionizable calcium is the type which is altered by hyper- and hypoparathyroidism. The symptoms are evidently dependent chiefly upon this disturbance in the blood calcium level.

Hyperparathyroidism.—This disease may be produced by a generalized hyperplasia of all the parathyroid glands or by a definite adenomatous enlargement of one of the parathyroids (rarely more than one); in either case excess production of the active principle of the gland is the factor responsible for the disease. Careful study has revealed the fact that the disease is identical with so-called osteitis fibrosa cystica (von Recklinghausen's disease [36]) (see p. 327). Although the relationship of parathyroid hyperplasia to osteitis fibrosa was probably first noted by Askanazy,[37] the successful removal of an adenoma was not reported until 1926 by Mandl.[38] Since the report by Barr and associates [39] numerous publications relative to this disease have appeared in this country. Consideration of the effect of the active principle of the parathyroid gland (parathormone) as isolated by Hanson [40] and Collip [41] on the calcium metabolism readily explains the pathologic findings in the bones (diffuse decalcification with formation of cysts) and other organs. In fact, these changes can be produced in animals, at least in part, by administration of parathyroid extract (Jaffe and Bodansky [42]).

Clinical Manifestations.—The earliest symptoms noted by the patient are apt to be muscular weakness, pains in the extremities and back, and polyuria. In a group of cases reported by Churchill and Cope,[43] a surprisingly large percentage of them complained first of weakness, pains in the legs and thighs (particularly upon walking) backache, and difficulty in walking as produced by disturbance in gait. Occasionally a spontaneous ("pathologic") fracture through a cyst or decalcified bone is the first manifestation noted. Tumors (with or without associated tenderness) may be noted on the surface of the bones (humerus, mandible, radius, ulna, etc.). Deformity, such as kyphosis, shortening of the spine, flatfoot, etc., created by actual softening of the bones may occur and may therefore be readily confused with Paget's and other diseases of the bone. Lassitude, undue fatigue and constipation are usually complained of. Polyuria and polydipsia, presumably attributed to the increased excretion of calcium and phosphorus are commonly noted. Not infrequently renal colic and manifestations of infection in the kidney are the most prominent manifestations of the disease. Rarely is the parathyroid tumor palpable. In 5 to 10 per cent of cases there will be two adenomas present, a fact the surgeon must keep in mind.

X-ray examination of the bones is of great aid in arriving at a correct diagnosis. With few exceptions there is a generalized decalcification (osteoporosis) of the bones which is revealed in the roentgenogram as a diffuse atrophy and moth-eaten appearance throughout the skeleton. Localized bone defects, particularly noted in the long bones and mandible, may be one of two kinds: (1) bone cysts containing thin brownish fluid, or (2) benign giant cell tumors (osteoclastomas). These cysts or tumors are usually multiple, as are shown by the x-ray. It is difficult to differentiate the cyst from the solid tumor roentgenologically, except that the solid tumors reveal more bony trabeculations through the defect. Renal calculi, containing large amounts of calcium, are commonly noted, may be bilateral and fill the entire pelvis of the kidney.

Laboratory data, particularly determination of the amount of calcium and phosphorus in the blood, are perhaps the most reliable means of establishing a diagnosis. Typical findings consist of the elevation of serum calcium from a normal of about 10 to a level varying from 12 to 18 milligrams per 100 cc. of serum, and

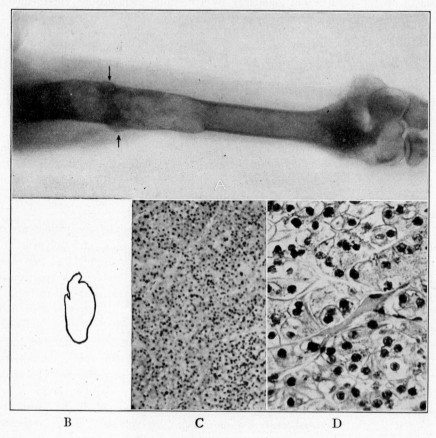

B   C   D

FIG. 519.—HYPERPARATHYROIDISM.

The patient came to the hospital because of a fracture of the humerus, sustained after only slight exertion. X-ray revealed a fracture at the site of a cyst in the shaft of the bone; numerous cysts were found in other bones. Serum calcium was 13.3 milligrams per cent, but dropped to 9.8 the day following removal of the parathyroid tumor. A renal calculus was revealed by x-ray; it did not disappear following operation (observed for five years). A, x-ray of humerus showing cystic defects in the bone and the healed fracture (several months after admission). X-rays three or four years later revealed deposition of calcium in these defects; B, actual size of the parathyroid tumor removed; C, low power photomicrograph and D, high power photomicrograph of the tumor (Courtesy of Dr. I. Y. Olch).

a depression of the serum phosphorus from a normal of about 4 down to 1.5 to 3.5 milligrams per 100 cc. There is usually a negative calcium balance, *i.e.*, more calcium is excreted in the urine and feces than is ingested in the food. The plasma phosphatase level which is dependent largely upon the amount of bone change may be elevated from a normal of 2 to 4 Bodansky units to 30 to 40.

The disease may be present for years and is rarely fatal except through infection or destruction of the kidney. Severe renal impairment and bony deformities are usually late manifestations; fracture may be the first manifestation.

Treatment.—Excision of the tumor offers the only hope of relief. X-ray therapy has been successful in a few cases. If the tumor is not readily found, it will be necessary to conduct a very thorough exploration of the neck, because the tumor, in many instances, will be located in an aberrant position. For example, in 58 adenomas found in 54 patients, Cope [43] reported that 11 were found in the anterior and 5 in the posterior mediastinum. Intratracheal anesthesia aids considerably in doing a thorough exploration. If possible, all the parathyroids (4 or 5) should be inspected since occasionally more than one will be the seat of disease. Symptoms rapidly disappear following removal of the tumor and the serum calcium drops to normal (within twelve to twenty-four hours). Following removal of the tumor the bone lesions of the giant cell type disappear after a few months, but the bone cysts usually remain much longer. The small rarefied areas become recalcified. The renal calculi cease to enlarge, but do not disappear spontaneously. They are treated as are other kidney stones. Removal of the parathyroid tumor is occasionally followed by severe but transient tetany which is treated by parathyroid extract injections, intravenous or oral calcium, vitamin D or dihydrotachysterol (A.T.10) as in tetany following accidental parathyroid injury or removal in thyroid operations. However, postoperative hypoparathyroidism tends to diminish and disappear.

Tetany (Hypoparathyroidism).—Before parathyroid tetany is discussed, attention should be directed to the fact that there are other types of tetany whose pathogenesis is not associated with the parathyroids. For example, the tetany observed so frequently in children with rickets is apparently caused by the lowered blood calcium level associated with an elevation of the phosphorus content of the blood, and is not related to parathyroid deficiency. The symptoms and signs of tetany produced by over-breathing (with resultant alkalosis) as first described by Grant and Goldman [45] is occasionally seen in patients in the operating room during induction of anesthesia. Gastric tetany caused by depletion of the acid of the stomach contents by persistent vomiting is likewise a manifestation of alkalosis.

Parathyroid tetany is most commonly observed following subtotal thyroidectomy (for toxic goiter) in which the parathyroid glands were inadvertently removed with the thyroid or deprived of their blood supply. The disease in such instances is manifested usually within twenty-four or forty-eight hours after operation, but may not appear until two or three weeks later. In the latter instance it is assumed that fibrosis resulting from excessive trauma associated with the operation is the cause of the tetany, whereas in the former instance the disease is caused by removal of the glands or severe direct trauma to them. The blood calcium drops from its normal level of about 10 milligrams per 100 cc. of serum to a content of only 4 or 5 milligrams per 100 cc. Symptoms are rarely produced if the serum calcium is 8 or above. Headache, restlessness, tachycardia, irritability and twitchings of the muscles, particularly of the upper extremities, are early manifestations. Pain associated with spasm of the muscles may be noted in the extremities and is apt to radiate downward, particularly in the arms. Diagnosis is certain when the typical carpopedal spasm, consisting of flexion of the fingers at the metacarpophalangeal joints with adduction of the thumb develops. The wrist and forearm are likewise apt to be flexed. Occasionally, spasm of the laryngeal muscles will be sufficient to produce respiratory difficulty. The muscular spasm of the hand may be induced by pressure on the nerves, such as that produced by a tourniquet (Trousseau's sign). Irritability of the muscles may be so pronounced that tapping over the nerve may instigate a spasm. This is particularly true when the face is lightly tapped over the facial nerve (Chvostek's sign).

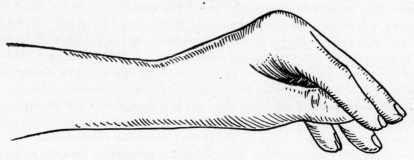

FIG. 520.—TYPICAL POSITION OF HAND IN PARATHYROID TETANY.

Treatment.—Since the epochal discovery by Hanson [40] and Collip [41] of an active extract of the parathyroid gland, the treatment of acute parathyroid tetany is much more logical and efficient. Parathyroid extract should be given in all severe cases, particularly the acute cases following thyroidectomy and in most instances will elevate the serum calcium level and effect a marked improvement in the patient's symptoms. If a fatal outcome can be prevented during the first few days after operation, the disease rarely terminates in death. For the severe symptoms of acute tetany intravenous calcium chloride or gluconate gives prompt relief but the effect is transient. Parathyroid extract exerts its maximum effect 4 to 6 hours after intramuscular injection and most of its calcium-elevating action is spent in 24 hours. Unfortunately, continued daily use of parathyroid extract leads in most patients to a gradually diminishing response until the hormone finally becomes ineffectual. Calcium lactate by mouth taken as a powder well stirred in water or milk, in doses of 5 grams two to four times daily is advisable. The addition of large doses of vitamin D to the oral calcium is effective in many chronic cases. Most effective of all in the treatment of chronic parathyroid deficiency is the oral use of dihydrotachysterol (A.T.10) and calcium as described by MacBryde [46] and others.

THE ADRENALS (SUPRARENAL GLANDS)

Although in 1855 Addison described a clinical syndrome associated with destructive disease of the adrenals, it was not until 1894 when Oliver and Shafer demonstrated some of the properties of extracts of the medullary portion of the gland that the first significant physiologic data regarding the function of the adrenals was available. A few years later Abel and Takamine, working independently, isolated the active principle of the medulla and named it epinephrin and adrenalin, respectively. The physiologic effects of epinephrin, including elevation of the blood pressure, vasoconstriction, tachycardia, etc., are well known. The adrenal cortex is essential for life. In 1928, Hartman and associates,[47] and Rogoff and Stewart,[48] independently announced the prolongation of life of adrenalectomized animals by the injection of adrenal cortex extracts. A number of physiologically active steroids have been isolated from the cortex. Of these, desoxycorticosterone has proved of greatest value in the treatment of adrenal insufficiency. It has a marked effect in restoring to normal the disturbed electrolyte metabolism. Corticosterone, another of these crystalline steroids, has less effect upon the electrolytes, but is more active in causing gluconeogenesis, in raising the blood sugar and increasing the body's glycogen stores. The normal adrenal likewise produces both male and female sex hormones. Numerous fractions not yet isolated are important in the maintenance of life and muscular strength. Details of normal and abnormal physiology may be found in an article by Cahill and associates [81].

Adrenocortical Insufficiency.—This may be acute or chronic and is characterized by: (1) a loss in sodium ion, chiefly through the urine, resulting in chloride loss, water loss, hemococentration and a fall in blood pressure; (2) an increase in the blood potassium, associated with a decrease in the excretion of potassium; (3) serious disturbance in carbohydrate metabolism, resulting in lowered blood sugar and a greatly reduced glycogen content of liver and muscle. Acute adrenocortical insufficiency can be produced in many species by bilateral adrenalectomy and is followed by death in a week or two. In the human being, removal or destruction of both adrenals will result in death within 24 to 72 hours. Delirium may develop, with lapse into unconsciousness with a very low blood pressure, rapid weak pulse and hyperpyrexia. Anuria is common and muscular weakness is pronounced. Chronic adrenocortical insufficiency produces manifestations first described by Thomas Addison in 1849, and the disease is now generally given his name. The chief symptoms of Addison's disease are brownish pigmentation of the skin, weakness, loss of appetite, low blood pressure and frequently vomiting and diarrhea. In most cases tuberculosis of the adrenal glands is responsible, while diffuse atrophy is the next most common cause. Rarely carcinoma, sarcoma or adrenal hemorrhage is present. The treatment of acute severe adenocortical insufficiency such as occurs in the crises of Addison's disease consists primarily of the administration of large amounts of adrenal cortex extract, and the parenteral administration of solution of sodium chloride and glucose. Maintenance therapy consists usually of a high sodium chloride intake and the intramuscular injection of adrenal cortex extract or desoxycorticosterone acetate.

Surgery finds a place in the therapy of Addison's disease through the subcutaneous implantation of pellets of desoxycorticosterone acetate as suggested by Thorn and his associates [49] in 1939. The required maintenance dose of desoxycorticosterone acetate when administered by intramuscular injections in oil is first ascertained. One pellet is then implanted for each 0.5 mg. daily required by injection. The pellets weigh between 100 and 150 mg. each and are usually implanted in the infrascapular region. The necessary number of pellets (usually between 2 and 10) may be inserted radially from a single small incision, a small forceps and a nasal speculum being useful for this purpose. The absorption per pellet per day varies from 0.3 to 0.9 mg. A store of the hormone is thus established which will last for many months. The appearance of hypertension, headaches, edema, rapid

weight gain or cardiac symptoms suggests hormone overdosage and may necessitate removal of some of the pellets.

Surgical procedures, especially when accompanied by the administration of a
general anesthetic, are apt to precipitate crises in patients with adrenocortical insufficiency. Whenever possible patients with Addison's disease should be spared
the risk of surgery. Urgent surgical procedures may be performed if appropriate
preoperative and postoperative measures are observed. These consist primarily of the
administration of adrenal cortex extract, and sodium chloride and glucose solutions.

In surgical shock desoxycorticosterone therapy has been suggested for both
prophylaxis and treatment. To prevent shock it has been suggested that large
amounts of the synthetic hormone and of sodium chloride solution be administered
for several days before operation. This procedure would increase blood volume
and might place an increased burden of serious nature upon the circulatory system.
Other cortical hormones such as corticosterone may prove more effective than
desoxycorticosterone; certainly these two sterols in spite of their chemical similarity, exert markedly different physiologic effects which may have a decisive bearing on their use in the treatment of shock. There are also other fractions in the
adrenal cortex whose action is as yet incompletely known. For this reason, in
the treatment of shock, cortical extracts may be superior to synthetic products.
Experimentally it is agreed that cortical extract is effective in the prevention and
treatment of shock.[50] Most investigators (Selye and associates, and Weil and associates [50]) obtained favorable effects in the treatment of shock with cortical extract,
but not with desoxycorticosterone acetate which is most effective in maintaining
life in adrenalectomized animals. Selye and associates found that corticosterone is
effective in shock in animals and think it may be the active principle in cortical
extract. Further chemical and experimental investigations are urgently needed in
exploring this gland which is indeed a chemical manufactory of many active physiological compounds.

Hyperfunction of the Adrenals.—This condition may be due to simple hyperplasia of the adrenals, or to a tumor (usually the latter), the symptoms of which
vary tremendously, depending chiefly on the age of the patient and to a less extent,
the sex. The excessive hormone manifests itself largely by its effect on the sexual
characteristics of the patient. A pseudohermaphroditism may be produced if the
increase in adrenal function is effective *in utero*. If the hyperfunction occurs before
puberty, the child may develop prematurely from the standpoint of sex characteristics. Growth may be active and the child's strength may be above normal. The
external genitalia develop rapidly. In girls the labia hypertrophy and menstruation
begins at an unusually early age. In boys the voice changes and the penis develops
an adult appearance. Axillary and pubic hairs develop early. If the hyperfunction
begins after puberty a different set of symptoms appear, among which virilism and
hirsutism are prominent; these manifestations in females, lead to the development
of male characteristics. Since the cause of the hyperfunction during this (adult)
period of life is usually a tumor (excluding hypernephroma*) which may be re-

___

* Very few cases of true hypernephroma produce any of the manifestations described under
"hyperfunction of the adrenal." In fact, no symptoms at all may be noted until metastases are
evident (see p. 999).

moved, these manifestations have an especial surgical interest and will be described below.

Tumors of the Suprarenal Cortex.—Most of the neoplasms of the adrenal cortex producing endocrine symptoms (suprarenal cortical syndrome) are of the adenoma-

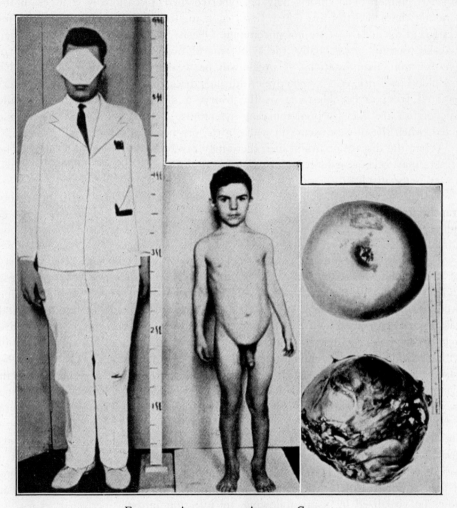

FIG. 521.—ADENOMA OF ADRENAL CORTEX.

Patient is a boy aged four years and eleven months; note the adult-size genitalia and pubic hair. A slight mustache is developing. On the right, encapsulated tumor removed successfully from the left adrenal; an apple is illustrated for comparison. As stated in the text, males are affected infrequently. (From Lisser, *Transactions of the Association of American Physicians,* Vol. 48, 1933.)

tous variety, but are usually malignant; they are very rare. Cortical tumors are much more common than tumors of the medulla. Many are associated with basophilic adenomas of the hypophysis (Walters *et al* [51]). Very commonly the manifestations are similar to those of basophilic adenomas of the hypophysis. Women are more frequently affected than men; the patients may be of any age, but more commonly they are past the age of puberty. The most common manifestations are virilism and hirsutism. The growth of hair may be noted all over the body, but is most prominent over the chin, upper lip, chest and back. Occasionally the strength of the patient appears to be increased. Amenorrhea or irregularity in menstruation is very common. The clitoris may be hypertrophied. Occasionally changes in the patient's characteristics are noted (*e.g.,* egotism, irritability, etc.). Superficial infections of the acne type are not uncommon. Obesity of the face, trunk and abdomen may be present. Occasionally, the symptoms of hyperfunction change to those of hypofunction, manifestations of which will be weakness, emaciation, melancholia, low blood pressure, etc., as noted in Addison's disease. The disease must be differentiated from arrhenoblastoma of the ovary, a disease in which hirsutism and amenorrhea are likewise predominating symptoms. As Walters and Kepler [52] have noted, when the disease occurs in young girls, precocious puberty usually develops.

When the disease occurs in men there may rarely be heterosexual changes. The breasts may become enlarged and painful and the areola more pigmented. Sexual power is usually lost. Obesity is common.

Patients presenting symptoms as noted above should be explored, preferably transperitoneally [81]. Perirenal air injection (see below) will aid in diagnosis. A tumor, if found, should be removed. If merely a hyperplasia or hypertrophy of one adrenal is noted, it should be removed if the other is normal.

Tumors of the Medulla (Chromaffin Cell Tumor).—Tumors of this type may be either benign or malignant and are sometimes classified as pheochromocytoma and pheochromoblastoma respectively. Neither is common. The clinical syndrome produced by such tumors is known as the suprarenal sympathetic syndrome and has been summarized by Belt and Powell.[53] The most significant symptoms are hypertension and tachycardia which are of a paroxysmal type, fluctuating usually within a wide range. Periodic attacks of flushing and pallor of the skin caused by vasodilatation and vasoconstriction may be observed. Headache is a prominent symptom. Nausea and vomiting may be present; dyspnea and a sensation of choking may be complained of. At autopsy, pulmonary edema and cardiac hypertrophy are notable findings. It can readily be discerned that the manifestations of the disease are similar, if not identical, to those which would be produced by continuous administration of epinephrin. Moreover, Belt and Powell noted that the tumor of a patient reported by them contained a large quantity of epinephrin. Treatment consists of excision. Either type of adrenal tumor (*i.e.,* cortical or medullary) may at times be visualized by x-ray following air injection into the perirenal spaces, as introduced by Carelli in 1921. The technic may be found in a report by Roome [54] and many others.

PANCREAS

The pancreas, like most other organs of the body, may be the seat of various diseases including inflammation, cysts, tumors, etc., which are discussed in Chapter XXIII. They concern, however, the part of the pancreas which produces the external (digestive) secretion, *i.e.,* the acinar tissue.

Disturbances in the endocrine function (internal secretion) of the pancreas are perhaps more important than the diseases just mentioned, particularly because of the severity of the symptoms produced and greater threat made upon life. The islets of Langerhans secrete insulin and are therefore presumably affected in diseases which are dependent either upon diminished secretion of insulin (diabetes, hypo-insulinism, hyperglycemia) or increased secretion (hyperinsulinism, hypoglycemia). Only the latter disease (hyperinsulinism) which may be caused by adenomas or carcinoma of the islets will be considered here since diabetes is a disease primarily of medical importance.

Although the most serious cases of hypoglycemia are caused by tumors (adenoma or carcinoma) of the islets, such patients comprise only a small number of

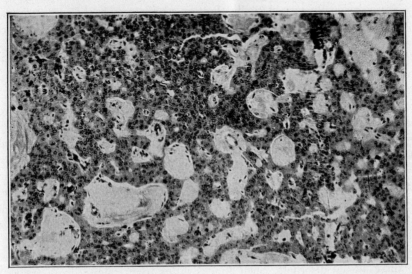

FIG. 522.—PHOTOMICROGRAPH OF ADENOMA OF PANCREAS WHICH WAS PRODUCING TYPICAL SYMPTOMS OF HYPOGLYCEMIA, AND WAS SUCCESSFULLY REMOVED.

The cells which are similar to the so-called beta cells of the islands of Langerhans are arranged in sinuous cords. Dense connective tissue separates the cells into imperfect lobules.

those actually suffering from hypoglycemia. Hepatic insufficiency may be a direct cause of hypoglycemia. Deficiency in the secretion of the anterior lobe of the pituitary body may likewise result in hypoglycemia, which may be produced experimentally by removal of the anterior pituitary, but may be alleviated by pancreatectomy. Hypoglycemia may be a prominent feature in adrenal cortex deficiency (Addison's disease). In the absence of a tumor, hypoglycemia has also been attributed to a diffuse hyperplasia of the islets, but it appears more logical to explain the hypoglycemia in such cases by a mechanism similar to that just described (*i.e.,* pituitary or adrenal hypofunction) particularly because microscopical proof of actual hyperplasia is only rarely demonstrable.

Hypoglycemia Due to Tumors of the Islets.—It has only been during the past few years that the dramatic syndrome produced by hypoglycemia has been recognized and understood to the extent that treatment may be conducted on a logical basis. The work of Harris [55] on hypoglycemia has to a great extent paved the way for the development of many of the facts regarding tumors of the islets. The first case of hyperinsulinism due to a tumor of the pancreas was reported by

Wilder and associates.[56] This patient suffered from a carcinoma of the islets which rapidly metastasized and caused death.

Microscopically, it is difficult to determine whether a tumor of the islets is benign or malignant. However, from the clinical standpoint it is apparent that most of them are benign. The first histologic study of a series of cases, as reported by O'Leary and Womack,[57] indicates that the adenomas are tumors with cells "closely allied to the beta cells of the normal islets of Langerhans." The microscopic structure of an adenoma may resemble that of a normal islet, *i.e.*, cuboidal and pyramidal cells in columns adjacent to capillaries or rosettes of cells around a capillary. Occasionally, the cells are arranged in a duct-like structure. Mitotic figures are occasionally seen. Usually the tumors are completely encapsulated, are commonly small (1/4 to 2 centimeters in diameter) and are of a bluish-pink color. They are readily identified except for a slight resemblance to lymph nodes.

Clinical Manifestations.—The symptoms of hypoglycemia due to tumor are dramatic, but extremely variable. The most common manifestations are attacks of weakness, lassitude, and mental confusion occurring several hours after meals, particularly in the morning before breakfast. Between attacks the patient may complain of being unusually hungry and not infrequently has a craving for sweet food such as candy, etc. Occasionally, the patient will make the discovery that partaking of food between meals, particularly at night, will prevent the development of symptoms. The patient fatigues readily and for that reason is unable to perform much manual labor. Profuse sweating and trembling of the extremities are not uncommon. The type of mental change varies from mild confusion to attacks of unconsciousness with convulsions and is frequently erroneously diagnosed as idiopathic epilepsy, brain tumor, etc. The mild attacks may closely resemble the petit mal attacks of epilepsy. The patient rarely has any recollection of incidents happening during these mental disorders. Such attacks differ from epilepsy in so far as they are not accompanied by aura (unless hunger, weakness and malaise are considered as such). The intravenous administration of glucose rarely fails to relieve the patient of his mental symptoms if they are caused by a true hypoglycemia. If the attacks of mental disorder persist over a long enough time, an actual mental deterioration may develop. Speech may be slurred and tremulous; occasionally, there is a hesitation in speech as if there were a mild aphonia. Rarely are any neurologic signs other than a positive Babinski present. The patient may die in an attack.

Laboratory data are of extreme value in arriving at a correct diagnosis. The fasting blood sugar is below normal and may be as low as 30 or 40 milligrams (true sugar) per 100 cc. of blood, or lower during attacks; in children the blood sugar may be as low as 20. The carbohydrate tolerance is usually increased (see Fig. 523). The subcutaneous administration of epinephrin and pituitrin in patients with islet tumors usually produces only a mild elevation in the blood sugar level, but with alleviation of the symptoms mentioned above. The administration of 5 units of insulin to fasting patients with islet cell tumors usually produces an appreciable fall in the blood sugar level and may precipitate the patient's symptoms in a severe form.

Treatment.—If there is a reasonable possibility that the hypoglycemia is caused by an adenoma of the pancreas, an operation is usually indicated (unless there are physical contraindications), because excision of adenomas of this type has been remarkably successful. The likelihood of an adenoma being the cause of the hypoglycemia is increased by exclusion of other causes by careful study as discussed further under the next heading. Obviously, if the hypoglycemia is caused by generalized carcinoma of the islets, operation will be of no value. Fortunately, such tumors are much less frequent than adenomas. The pancreas is most readily exposed by making an incision through the gastrocolic omentum. Any neoplastic growths encountered should be excised. Although most tumors are located in the tail or body

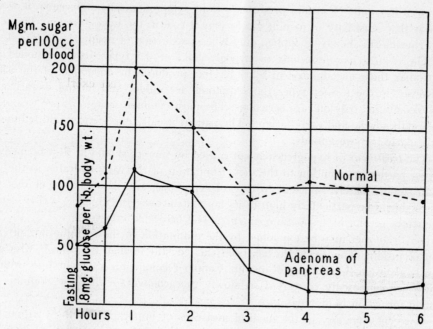

Fig. 523.—Comparative Sugar Tolerance Curves of Normal Individual and Patient with an Adenoma of the Pancreas Producing Symptoms of Hypoglycemia.

The blood sugar level in the patient with the adenoma (solid line) does not rise as high as the level of the normal individual (dotted line).

of the pancreas the entire organ must be inspected because of the variability in location of the tumors.

A more detailed description of this disease may be found in publications by Graham and Womack,[58] Whipple and Frantz [59] and others.

Hypoglycemia Not Due to Tumors of the Islets.—Harris [55] has largely been responsible for the development of our knowledge regarding so-called idiopathic hypoglycemia, i.e., not produced by adenoma of the islets. This type of hypoglycemia is in reality much more common than that caused by adenomas. As has been demonstrated by Gray and Feemster,[60] a few of these are due to actual hypertrophy and hyperplasia of the islets. In the majority of instances, however, the hypoglycemia is probably due to hepatic insufficiency or to disease of the adrenal or pituitary glands. Detailed accounts of these types of hypoglycemia may be found in the monograph by Sigwald [61], and the article by MacBryde [64]. Differential diagnosis and the use of insulin tolerance tests is discussed by the latter author. Occasionally, hypoglycemia develops as an aftermath of diabetes.

Various mechanisms may result in spontaneous hypoglycemia not due to islet cell tumor. There are two possible explanations for its development, viz.: (1) insulin may be produced in such large quantities that it cannot be utilized; or (2) there is a diminution below normal in insulin resistant factors, thus making the patient more sensitive to insulin and its effects. Insulin tolerance tests should be of considerable aid in determining which mechanism is at fault. When the administration of a few units of insulin produces serious symptoms of hypoglycemia, it would appear that sensitivity to insulin would play a role in the hypoglycemia. The term hyperinsulinism should be applied only when production of insulin is increased.

The *clinical manifestations* of hypoglycemia of the types just mentioned are not unlike those encountered in hypoglycemia produced by adenomas of the islets. However, in the former types the symptoms are milder and mental disturbances are encountered only on rare occasions. The most common symptoms are weakness, malaise, headache and early fatigue. The patient usually experiences undue hunger, particularly for sweet foods.

The *treatment* of hypoglycemia not caused by tumors should at first be medical, paying particular attention to the diet. Limitation of the carbohydrates in the diet to an amount barely sufficient to control symptoms, and maintenance of this diet which should be particularly high in its fat content over an extended period of time frequently results in a spontaneous cure. The favorable effect exerted by the low carbohydrate diet may be explained by the diminution in the stimulus for production of insulin. This principle has been carried still further by John,[62] who cautiously gives small quantities of insulin. Conn [63] recommends a diet high in proteins which are supposedly converted so slowly to carbohydrate that the stimulus for insulin formation is minimal.

A recent summary of the medical measures of importance in the treatment of the various types of hypoglycemia with discussion of the use of diets is given by MacBryde.[64] Frequently, it is impossible to exclude the possibility of a pancreatic adenoma, particularly if the symptoms are severe and *not relieved by appropriate medical treatment*. In such instances, laparotomy should be performed. If no tumor is found, subtotal pancreatectomy may be indicated. In a review of patients treated by this procedure, Whipple and Frantz noted, however, that complete relief of symptoms following subtotal pancreatectomy for this type of hypoglycemia was obtained in only one-third of the cases.

PITUITARY (HYPOPHYSIS)

The pituitary gland is a small structure connected by a slender stalk to the base of the brain and isolated in a protected manner by its position within the sella turcica. The gland is composed of an anterior and a posterior lobe. The anterior lobe (pars anterior) is composed of chromophil cells with protoplasm containing granules which stain with acid or basic dyes and chromophobe cells whose protoplasm contains very few granules and stain feebly. The posterior lobe is composed of several structures, including the pars nervosa and pars tuberali. The pars intermedia is usually considered to be a separate independent structure.

In spite of Marie's observations on acromegaly (1886) and Frölich's description of a tumor of the hypophysis associated with adiposity, etc., the medical profession has been slow in accepting the importance of the hypophysis in the pathogenesis of disease. This is partly due to the fact that the organ is too inaccessible to allow thorough experimental, pathological and clinical study, but more especially because of the assumption that an organ so small and attached to the brain by such a slender pedicle could hardly be of great physiological significance. Recent discoveries have proved beyond doubt that the hypophysis elaborates a large number of hormones, many of which are necessary for the maintenance of health and perhaps even life itself. The early experimental work of Cushing [65] on the effects of partial or total removal of the hypophysis has to a large extent been responsible for the recent development in our knowledge of the functions of the organ.

The *function* of the hypophysis is concerned chiefly with the secretion of hormones of which there are at least five: (1) the action of the growth or somatotropic hormone (Evans [66]) is clearly illustrated by the production of gigantism following experimental administration of an extract of the anterior lobe and by the dwarfism which follows hypophysectomy in young animals. (2) The presence of a gonadotropic hormone was suggested independently in 1926 and 1927 by P. E. Smith [67] and Aschheim and Zondek.[68] The latter authors noted that a gonadotropic substance similar to extracts of anterior pituitary was present in large quantities in the urine of pregnant women, a fact which they made use of in developing a test for pregnancy (see page 972). In view of recent work it appears that there are two urinary gonadotropic hormones, one of which has been designated as the "follicle stimulating hormone" (prolan A) and the other, "luteinizing hormone" (prolan B), the latter of which may be of placental origin ("chorionic gonadotropin"). The gonadotropic hormone also acts as a stimulus to the growth of the male organs. (3) Experimental evidence of the thyrotropic hormone was discovered independently by Loeb [69] and and Aron [70] in 1929. When given to animals a marked hyperplasia of the thyroid results. (4) The anterior lobe of the hypophysis also elaborates a lactogenic hormone (prolactin) which stimulates the secretion of milk by the mammary gland (Riddle [71]). (5) The anterior lobe of the hypophysis also secrets a diabetogenic substance which, when injected into hypophysectomized animals, will produce hyperglycemia and glycosuria. Proof of the secretion of this substance is offered by the fact that the diabetes produced by experimental pancreatectomy is greatly diminished by hypophysectomy (Houssay [72]). This substance is therefore important in carbohydrate metabolism and to a certain extent has an action antagonistic to insulin.

There are several miscellaneous functions [73] of the hypophysis, most of which are chiefly related to the activity of other organs. For example, administration of pituitary extracts to hypophysectomized dogs produced a hyperplasia of the adrenal. Various authors have noted a similar effect on the parathyroid glands following administration of pituitary extracts. Burn and Ling [74] have described a pituitary extract which is of significance in fat metabolism in so far as it produces an increase in excretion of ketone (acetone) bodies. The three substances just mentioned are known respectively as adrenotropic, parathyrotropic and ketogenic principles.

Most of the functions already discussed are performed by the anterior lobe. However, one of the first substances known to be elaborated by the hypophysis is that extractable from the posterior lobe. This is a pressor substance used to produce certain physiologic effects, such as elevation of the blood pressure, contraction of uterine muscle, increase in intestinal peristalsis, etc., and is commonly designated as pituitrin. It is not a pure hormone, however, since two (or more) products (*e.g.*, pitressin having pressor and antidiuretic properties, and pitocin, having oxytocic properties, stimulating uterine contraction) with separate physiologic effects have been isolated from posterior pituitary extracts.[75]

The pars intermedia secretes a hormone possessing chromatophoric properties which is capable of producing a darkening of the skin of cold blooded animals by expansion of the melanophores (Zondek [76]). This chromatophorotropic principle has been called intermedin.

Pituitary Insufficiency, Pituitary Cachexia, Simmonds' Disease.—Most of the symptoms of pituitary insufficiency were originally described by Simmonds.[77] If the hypofunction develops in childhood before normal stature is obtained, dwarfism will result. The bones fail to grow, and ossification of the epiphyseal cartilages is delayed. Normal sexual development does not take place in either sex (sexual infantilism). The skin remains smooth and of a fine texture. There may not be much retardation in the mental development. If the disease occurs at the time of puberty the male skeleton may assume a feminine appearance, consisting particularly of a broad pelvis and genu valgum; the fingers are apt to be narrow and tapering. Hair on the face, pubis and axillae is scanty or absent.

If the disease develops after puberty, there will usually be a gradual diminution of sexual activity with impotence. In women, sterility and amenorrhea are quite constantly observed. Drowsiness and somnolence are common manifestations. Polyuria and a high carbohydrate tolerance are not uncommon. The body temperature may be lowered considerably, as is also the basal metabolism. In the neuro-hypophysial syndrome, probably due to hypothalamic as well as pituitary disturbance, sex dystrophy occurs and obesity is a common manifestation; in men the fat is apt to be deposited in such a way as to simulate a feminine physique. Hypotension is observed not uncommonly, and along with the extreme weakness complained of, presents a picture very similar to Addison's disease. Convulsions, attacks of unconsciousness, and mental changes of varied types may be present.

In complete pituitary failure there is the appearance of premature senility, with loss of hair, emaciation, wrinkling of the skin and progressive severe cachexia. The pathologic processes responsible for the development of pituitary cachexia are extremely varied and include such lesions as carcinoma, cysts, syphilis, tuberculosis and embolism.

From the surgical standpoint, the most important feature in therapy is the determination as to whether or not a tumor is present. Removal of the tumor would obviously halt progression of the disease and may be followed by considerable improvement. Medical treatment is at present unsatisfactory because of the lack of a potent pituitary extract which is capable of producing all the effects of the pituitary. Administration of the various hormones of the pituitary may be recommended, depending upon indications. Administration of extracts and hormones of other organs (*e.g.,* adrenal cortex extract and desiccated thyroid) may also be indicated.

Neoplasms (Adenomas) of the Pituitary.—Neoplastic growths of the pituitary may give rise to various symptoms referable to disturbance in the secretions of the gland, most of which can be classified roughly into those produced by hyperfunction or hypofunction. However, as in the case in diseases of most other endocrine glands, the explanation of symptoms is by no means simple since many of the manifestations cannot be attributed to increased or decreased function of the gland *per se.* Most of these tumors in-

volve primarily the anterior lobe. Manifestations of increased intracranial pressure may be produced by these tumors, but are not as pronounced as those due to other brain tumors. Manifestations due to pressure on adjacent structures ("neighborhood symptoms") are often characteristic; the most important of these symptoms is disturbance in vision, because of pressure upon the optic tracts at or near the chiasm.

Chromophile Adenoma.—Tumors involving the chromophile cells (those taking an acidophilic or basophilic stain readily) are usually associated with symptoms of hyperfunction. For example, an adenoma containing acidophilic cells results in certain growth manifestations, thereby substantiating the supposition that the acidophilic cells elaborate the growth hormone. If the tumor manifests itself in young people before the epiphyses close, *gigantism* results. This in reality is the explanation for the famous giants in history. In most instances the disease affects the male. The eunuchoid features so frequently encountered in these patients are presumably due to a deficiency of testicular hormone, the secretion of which may be inhibited by the overproduction of an anterior pituitary hormone. The bone and muscular tissue resulting from this growth

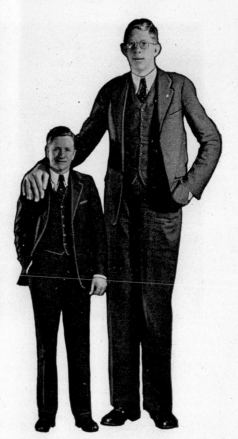

FIG. 524.—GIGANTISM.

The patient, sometimes known as the Alton giant, was 22 years old at the time of his death. He was 8 feet 9½ inches tall and weighed 491 pounds; he wore a size 36 shoe (Courtesy of Peters Shoe Company).

stimulus appear to have a normal gross and histologic appearance, but patients afflicted with this disease do not possess a corresponding muscular strength and are very susceptible to complicating diseases, particularly infections. Surgical treatment (partial hypophysectomy) is followed by uncertain results. Testosterone propionate should be tried in males and estrogens in females when hypogonadism is present.

The patient must receive careful medical attention, since often his nutrition is poor and he is apt to be afflicted with various diseases. X-ray therapy has been advised in an attempt to diminish the growth of the adenomatous cells.

Acromegaly is produced when the adenoma manifests itself after the epiphyses have closed. It develops insidiously and slowly; the first manifestation noted by the patient usually lies in the observation that larger shoes, hats and gloves are required to fit him. The head becomes large, and the lips and tongue thickened. The lower jaw protrudes so far that the teeth of the upper and lower jaw do not approximate

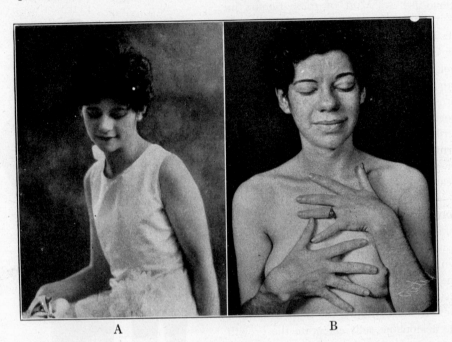

A   B

FIG. 525.—ACROMEGALY.

A, photograph of patient before development of the disease. *B*, patient is twenty-three years of age; three years before this photograph was taken patient noted beginning thickening of the lips and coarseness of facial features. Recently, her hands and feet have enlarged; headaches are very troublesome, and amenorrhea has been present for the past nine months. During the past several months, vision has become blurred. Visual fields reveal a bitemporal hemianopsia. See Figure 527 (Courtesy of Dr. Ernest Sachs).

(prognathism). The brow and nose are prominent. Hypertropic changes in the skin associated with wrinkling are noted, particularly about the face.

In almost all instances of gigantism or acromegaly, examination by the x-ray reveals an enlargement of the sella. There is usually an accompanying erosion of the sella which is manifested by a thinning, but rarely a roughening of its bony wall. The hands are broad and roentgenograms reveal a thickening of the phalanges with prominent exostoses. The bones of the head are likewise thickened and massive.

Subjective symptoms may be slight. Headaches, however, are common. At first there may be an actual increase in sexual power and desire, but usually these characteristics are gradually lost. There may be secondary changes in other endocrine glands. The thyroid may be enlarged and hyperthyroidism, as evinced by an increase in the basal metabolic rate, may be present. Polyuria and mild glycosuria are not uncommon. True diabetes occurs in about 25 per cent of cases. Occasionally the tumor may progress upward so that there is compression against the optic chiasm, thereby producing defects in the visual fields. These defects are usually not noted by the patient until they are far advanced. Examination by perimetry will reveal variable defects, but usually bitemporal hemianopsia.

The treatment of acromegaly may or may not be surgical. If the adenomatous growth is so large as to produce an impairment of vision by pressure against the optic chiasm, removal of at least a part of the tumor is indicated. If the tumor is

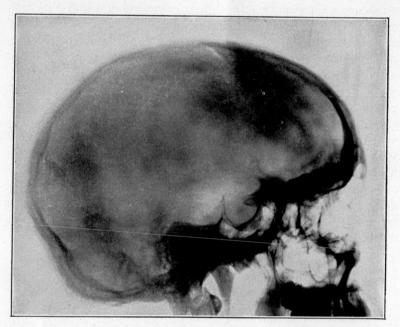

FIG. 526.—X-RAY OF SKULL SHOWING MARKED ENLARGEMENT OF THE SELLA TURCICA IN A PATIENT AGED NINETEEN, WITH A CHROMOPHOBE ADENOMA OF THE PITUITARY.

There is mild thinning and erosion of the posterior clinoid process. The patient had poor vision and headaches of six and four months' duration respectively. He also complained of a poor memory during the past few months. Visual fields revealed a bitemporal hemianopsia (Courtesy of Dr. Ernest Sachs).

large and has eroded the floor of the sella, an intranasal route may be preferable; if there is very little enlargement of the sella a transfrontal approach will be indicated. The tumor is best removed by suction. Even in the absence of visual impairment operation may be advisable because of prominent symptoms, especially headache. Resection of a large part of the tumor usually relieves the symptoms, but no improvement in the bony changes can be expected. X-ray therapy frequently will be found helpful as a substitute for operation in many cases, and should be given postoperatively, especially if symptoms recur.

Basophilic Adenoma.—This type of tumor is usually nothing more than an abnormally large collection of basophilic cells (originally described by Teel[78] and

Cushing [79]), and is spoken of as pituitary basophilism. The growth of these cells occurs in the anterior lobe but in most instances is not sufficient to produce a gross enlargement of the hypophysis. It is possible that the disease is secondary to a dysfunction of some other gland of internal secretion, particularly the adrenal.

The disease is much more common in women. One of the first significant features is the development of obesity, confined to the face, neck and torso. The skin is dry and the growth of hair increases in women to the extent that the face actually becomes bearded. Amenorrhea develops early in the disease. Purplish striations frequently develop on the abdomen. There may be a definite decalcification of bone, as shown by x-ray. Compression of vertebrae has been noted. Hyperglycemia and hypertension are not uncommon. Death may ensue within a few years after onset of symptoms. There is usually so much doubt as to the actual existence of an adenoma in these patients that operative procedures are inadvisable. Treatment is therefore limited to symptomatic care of the patient. X-ray treatment to the pituitary has been recommended.

As yet, it is not generally agreed that the hyperplasia of basophilic cells is the major primary factor in the production of the disease. In many patients with manifestations of the type described, adrenal tumors have also been found.

Chromophobe Adenoma.—This type of tumor is more common than the chromophile type which causes acromegaly and attains a much larger size, usually breaking through upward toward the brain. For this reason "neighborhood" symptoms are more common than in acromegaly. The most frequent and significant of these neighborhood symptoms is defective vision of the same type encountered in acromegaly, and is produced by pressure on the optic chiasm by the tumor. Headaches are common. Adults are afflicted much more often than children.

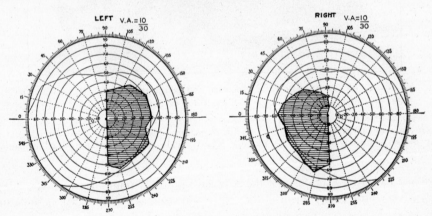

FIG. 527.—VISUAL FIELD REVEALING A BITEMPORAL HEMIANOPSIA (SAME PATIENT AS IN FIGURE 525).

The fields for a normal individual are outlined on the charts with a continuous line.

Because of the destructive feature of the tumor many of the manifestations are in reality those of pituitary insufficiency as described on page 932. The manifestations of this group which are encountered most frequently may be briefly enumerated as follows: There is usually a diminished sexual power and desire, beginning shortly after onset of growth of the tumor, produced perhaps by pressure of the tumor on the basophilic cells. In women amenorrhea is usually present. The patients are usually sluggish physically and a tendency toward somnolence is not uncommon. The basal metabolic rate is frequently low and the temperature subnormal. There may be a high carbohydrate tolerance. Examination reveals a soft, pale, smooth skin with loss of hair, particularly in the pubic and axillary region. In men the hair on the face becomes finer and grows slowly so that shaving is necessary only at infrequent intervals. All patients become obese. Affected males develop feminine characteristics, with fat pads in the breast regions and mons veneris, knock knees, tapering fingers and soft, smooth, hairless skin. The genitals are atrophic. The x-ray usually reveals a greatly enlarged sella turcica.

With few exceptions, treatment is surgical only when the eyesight is threatened. Under this circumstance the removal of the greater part of the tumor prevents progression of the visual defect and in many instances results in restoration of vision. Since many of the manifestations of the disease are in reality a hypofunction of the gland, surgical removal of the pituitary would obviously exert an unfavorable effect except for the relief of symptoms caused by local or general pressure of the tumor.

Cystic Tumors.—Several types of cysts are encountered about the pituitary, only a few of which are actually intrasellar. Most of them are suprasellar or retrosellar. They are thought to be of congenital origin, arising in "cell rests," misplaced during the neurobuccal development of the pituitary gland. A variable amount of solid tumor tissue may accompany the cyst. Many of the symptoms, as in chromophobe adenomas, are referable to pituitary hypofunction. Such cysts develop early in life and usually are recognizable in childhood by the manifestations produced. However, many are present for years without producing symptoms.

Dwarfism or stunted growth is usually the first feature noted. The genitals remain infantile. The skin is soft and pale and there is a slight tendency toward obesity. The child may develop mentally in a normal manner unless pressure manifestations occur. These pressure symptoms are extremely variable in type and may be either local or general; they are similar to those encountered in chromophobe adenomas. If the cyst encroaches upon the third ventricle, compression of vital centers in this region may lead to a fatal outcome. The foramen of Monro is occasionally blocked, resulting in hydrocephalus. After the tumor has been present for many years, calcium becomes deposited in the wall of the cyst, thereby enabling a diagnosis to be made readily by the x-ray.

Unless symptoms are absent or mild, the treatment is obviously surgical. On account of the extreme variability in the location of the tumor and its attachment, operation in these cases is not only difficult, but accompanied by a high mortality. Exposure of the cyst through a transfrontal approach by removing an osteoplastic flap and aspirations of its contents usually relieves the pressure symptoms, but is not curative since the cyst refills.

THE GONADS

Although detailed discussion of the ovaries and testes will be found in the chapters on gynecology and genito-urinary diseases, respectively, certain features of these organs which are primarily of endocrine importance are considered here.

Ovaries.—Certain ovarian disorders may result in endocrine abnormalities and require surgical attention. *Granulosa cell neoplasms* are composed of cells which secrete large amounts of estrogenic hormone. When they occur in young girls they produce precocious puberty with development of breasts, hair growth and other adult secondary sex characteristics, including menstruation, either cyclic or irregular. When such tumors appear in women past the menopause, there is a return of menstruation, which is apt to be irregular and excessive. The treatment is surgical removal of the neoplasm. *Arrhenoblastoma* is an ovarian neoplasm composed of testicular type cells developing from embryonic rests within the ovary. A male type hormone similar to or identical with testosterone is secreted, and masculinizing effects are produced. Menstruation ceases, the face becomes bearded and body hair becomes more abundant and changes to the male type. The breasts atrophy and body contours become masculine. These symptoms resemble those associated with neoplasms of the adrenal cortex but differ chiefly in the absence of obesity, hypertension and hyperglycemia, which are apt to occur in the latter. Surgical removal will lead to complete cure. *Follicle cysts* occur because of failure of ovarian follicles to rupture and may result in prolonged absorption of large amounts of estrogenic hormones, leading to menorrhagia and metrorrhagia. When hormone therapy is unsuccessful in such patients removal of the cyst or the whole offending ovary may prove necessary.

Testes.—Certain tumors of the testes, particularly the group called teratoma, may secrete hormones, curiously enough, which are similar to the chorionic gonadotropins (prolan) produced in the placenta of the pregnant female. These patients may exhibit positive tests for prolan (see p. 1019). Other endocrine disturbances in the male associated with the sex hormones such as gynecomastia have been discussed elsewhere (p. 826). The discovery and use of testosterone, one of the male hormones, promises much in the treatment of various types of testicular deficiency, and in certain menstrual disorders, particularly menorrhagia.

BIBLIOGRAPHY

1. LOEB, L., and BASSETT, R. B.   Effect of Hormones of Anterior Pituitary on Thyroid Gland in the Guinea Pig, *Proc. Soc. Exper. Biol. & M.*, 26:860, 1929; Comparison of Effects of Various Preparations of Anterior Pituitary Gland on Thyroid of Guinea Pig, *Proc. Soc. Exper. Biol. & M.*, 27:490, 1930.
2. KENDALL, E. C.   The Isolation in Crystalline Form of the Compound Containing Iodin which Occurs in the Thyroid, *J. Am. M. Ass.*, 64:2042, 1915.
3. HARINGTON, C. R.   Chemistry of Thyroxine: Constitution and Synthesis of Desiodothyroxine, *Biochem. J.*, 20:300, 1926.
   HARINGTON, C. R., and BARGER, G.   Chemistry of Thyroxine: Constitution and Synthesis of Thyroxine, *Biochem. J.*, 21:169, 1927.
4. PLUMMER, H. S.   Interrelationship of Function of the Thyroid Gland, *Oxford Med.*, 13:839, 1921.   *J. Am. M. Ass.*, 77:243, 1921.

5. VanMeter, S. D., Shivers, M. O., and Simpson, W. P.   Report of Committee on
   Classification of American Association for Study of Goiter, *Western J. Surg.,*
   39:947, 1931.
6. McClendon, J. F., and Williams, A.   Simple Goiter as a Result of Iodin Deficiency, *J. Am. M. Ass.,* 80:600, 1923.
   —— The Distribution of Iodine with Special Reference to Goiter, *Physiol. Rev.,*
   7:189, 1927.
7. Marine, D., and Lenhart, C. H.   Colloid Glands (Goiters): Their Etiology and
   Physiological Significance, *Bull. Johns Hopkins Hosp.,* 20:131, 1909.
8. McCarrison, R.   Fats in Relation to the Genesis of Goiter, *Brit. M. J.,* 1:178, 1922.
   —— *The Simple Goiters,* London, Bailliere, Tindall and Cox, 1928.
9. Hellwig, C. A.   Geographic and Experimental Studies on the Etiology of Goiter,
   J. Kansas M. Soc., 34:389, 1933.
   —— Experimental Goiter: Functional, Chemical and Histological Studies, *Arch.
   Path.,* 19:364, 1935.
10. Chesney, A. M., Clawson, T. A., and Webster, B.   Endemic Goiter in Rabbits:
    Incidence and Characteristics, *Bull. Johns Hopkins Hosp.,* 43:261, 1928.
11. Marine, D., and Kimball, O. P.   The Prevention of Simple Goiter in Man,
    J. Am. M. Ass., 77:1068, 1921.
12. Marine, D.   On the Occurrence and Physiological Nature of Glandular Hyper-
    plasia of the Thyroid (Dog and Sheep) Together with Remarks on Important
    Clinical (Human) Problems, *Bull. Johns Hopkins Hosp.,* 18:359, 1907.
    —— and Lenhart, C. H.   The Pathological Anatomy of the Human Thyroid
    Gland, *Arch. Int. M.,* 7:506, 1911.
13. Rienhoff, W. F., Jr.   Involutional or Regressive Changes in the Thyroid Gland in
    Cases of Exophthalmic Goiter, *Arch. Surg.,* 13:391, 1926.
14. Foreign Letters.   Iodine Prophylaxis and Endemic Goiter, *J. Am. M. Ass.,*
    107:2064, 1936.
15. Loeb, Leo, and Bassett, R. B.   *Loc. cit.*
16. Loeb, Leo, and Friedman, H.   Exophthalmos Produced by Injection of Acid Ex-
    tract of Anterior Pituitary Gland of Cattle, *Proc. Soc. Exper. Biol. & M.,*
    29:648, 1932.
17. Roger, H., and Garnier, M.   La sclerose du corps thyroide chez les tuberculeux,
    Comp. Rend. Soc. de Biol., 50:873, 1898.
18. Cole, W. H., and Womack, N. A.   Thyroid Gland in Infections: Preliminary Re-
    port, *J. Am. M. Ass.,* 90:1274, 1928.
19. Anderson, E. M.   The Production of Hyperplasia of the Thyroid with Hyper-
    thyroidism in the Albino Rat, *Canad. M. Ass. J.,* 28, 23, 1933.
20. Curtis, G. M., Cole, V. V., and Phillips, F. J.   The Blood Iodine in Thyroid
    Disease, *West. J. Surg.,* 42:435, 1934.
21. Perkin, H. J., and Lahey, F. H.   Level of Iodine in Blood, *Arch. Int. Med.,*
    65:882, 1940.
22. Plummer, H. S.   Results of Administering Iodine to Patients Having Exophthalmic
    Goiter, *J. Am. M. Ass.,* 80:1955, 1923.
23. Means, J. H., and Lerman, J.   The Action of Iodine in Thyrotoxicosis: With
    Special Reference to Refractoriness, *J. Am. M. Ass.,* 104:969, 1935.
24. Aub, J. C., Bauer, W., Heath, C., and Ropes, M.   Calcium and Phosphorus Meta-
    bolism: The Effects of the Thyroid Hormone and Thyroid Disease, *J. Clin. Inves-
    tigation,* 7:97, 1929.
25. Puppel, I. D., Klassen, K. P., and Curtis, G.   Calcium Metabolism in Thyroid
    Disease. *The 1939 Transactions of the Amer. Assoc. for Study of Goiter,*
    p. 221.
26. King, B. T.   A New and Function Restoring Operation for Bilateral Abductor
    Cord Paralysis, *J. Am. M. Ass.,* 112:814, 1939.

27. Cole, W. H. Precautions in the Treatment of Thyrotoxicosis, *Ann. Surg.*, 113:752, 1941.

28. Naffziger, H. C., and Jones, O. W., Jr. The Surgical Treatment of Progressive Exophthalmos Following Thyroidectomy, *J. Am. M. Ass.*, 99:638, 1932; Naffziger, H. C. Progressive Exophthalmos Associated with Disorders of the Thyroid Gland, *Ann. Surg.*, 108:529, 1938.

29. Clute, H. M., and Lahey, F. H. Thyroiditis, *Ann Surg.*, 95:493, 1932.

30. Hashimoto, H. Zer Kentniss der lymphomatösen Veränderung der Schilddrüse (Strumalymphomatosa), *Arch. f. klin. chir.*, 97:219, 1912.

31. McSwain, B., and Moore, S. W. Struma Lymphomatosa, *Surg., Gynec. & Obst.*, 76:562, 1943.

32. Graham, A. Malignant Epithelial Tumors of the Thyroid, *Surg., Gynec. & Obst.*, 39:781, 1924.
——— Malignant Tumors of the Thyroid, *Ann. Surg.*, 82:30, 1925.

33. Ward, Robertson. Malignant Goiter, A Survey of Geographical Types, Read at the Annual Meeting of the American Association for the Study of Goiter at Salt Lake City, *Western J. Surg.*, 43:494, 1935.

34. Pemberton, J. de J., and Dixon, C. F. Summary of the End Results of Treatment of Malignancy of the Thyroid Gland and the Colon, Including the Rectum and Anus, *Surg., Gynec. & Obst.*, 58:462, 1934.

35. McLean, F. C., and Hastings, A. B. Clinical Estimation and Significance of Calcium-Ion Concentration in the Blood, *Am. J. M. Sc.*, 189:601, 1935.

36. von Recklinghausen, F. D. Die fibröse oder deformuende ostitis, etc., *Festschrift f. Rudolf Virchow, zu seinem 71 geburststag*, Berlin, 1891, p. 1.

37. Askanazy, M. *Beitrage zur Knochenpathologie*, quoted by Moore, J. J., and Lorimier, A. A. Roentgenographic Studies of Parathyroid Deossification, *Am. J. Roentgenol.*, 31:496, 1934.

38. Mandl, F. Therapeutischer Versuch bei einem Falle von Ostitis Fibrosa Generalista Mittels Exstirpation eines Epithelkörperchentumors, *Zentralbl. f. chir.*, 53:260, 1926.

39. Barr, D. P., Bulger, H. A., and Dixon, H. H. Hyperparathyroidism, *J. Am. M. Ass.*, 92:951, 1929.

40. Hanson, A. M. Hormone of Parathyroid Gland: Changes in Blood Serum Calcium of Thyroparathyroidectomized Dogs Modified by Bovine Hydrochloric Acid, *Minn. Med.*, 8:283, 1925.

41. Collip, J. B. The Extraction of a Parathyroid Hormone Which Will Prevent or Control Parthyroid Tetany and Which Regulates the Level of Blood Calcium, *J. Biol. Chem.*, 63:395, 1925.

42. Jaffe, H. L., and Bodansky, A. Experimental Fibrous Osteodystrophy (Ostitis Fibrosa), in Hyperparathyroid Dogs, *J. Exper. M.*, 52:669, 1930.

43. Cope, O. Surgery of Hyperparathyroidism: The Occurrence of Parathyroids in the Anterior Mediastinum and Division of the Operation into Two Stages, *Ann. Surg.*, 114:706, 1941.

44. De Courcy, J. L. A New Theory Concerning the Etiology of Riedel's Struma, *Surgery*, 12:754, 1942. Churchill, E D., and Cope, O. Parathyroid Tumors Associated with Hyperparathyroidism: Eleven Cases Treated by Operation, *Surg., Gynec. & Obst.*, 58:255, 1934.

45. Grant, S. B., and Goldman, A. A Study of Forced Respiration: Experimental Production of Tetany, *Am. J. Physiol.*, 52:209, 1920.

46. MacBryde, C. M. The Treatment of Parathyroid Tetany with Dihydrotachysterol, *J. Am. M. Ass.*, 111:304, 1938.

47. Hartman, F. A., Griffith, F. R., and Hartman, W. E. Observations upon Adrenalectomized Cats Treated with the Cortical Hormone, *Am. J. Physiol.*, 86:360, 1928.

48. Rogoff, J. M., and Stewart, G. N. Studies on Adrenal Insufficiency in Dogs:

Influence of Adrenal Extracts on Survival Period of Adrenalectomized Dogs, *Am. J. Physiol.,* 84:660, 1928.

49. THORN, G. W., ENGEL, L. L., and EISENBERG, H. Treatment of Adrenal Insufficiency, *Bull. Johns Hopkins Hosp.,* 64:155, 1939.

50. SWINGLE, W. W., and PARKINS, W. M. Comparative Study of Effect of Trauma on Healthy Vigorous Dogs with and without Adrenal Glands, *Am. J. Physiol.,* 111:426, 1935; SELYE, H., DOSNE, C., BASSETT, L., and WHITTAKER, J. On the Therapeutic Value of Adrenal Cortical Hormones in Traumatic Shock and Allied Conditions, *Canad. M. A. J.,* 43:1, 1940; WEIL, P. G., BRAM, R., and BROWNE, J. S. L. The Reduction of Mortality from Experimental Traumatic Shock with Adrenal Cortical Substances, *Canad. M. A. J.,* 43:8, 1940.

51. WALTERS, W., WILDER, R. M., and KEPLER, E. J. Suprarenal Cortical Syndrome with Presentation of Ten Cases, *Ann. Surg.,* 100:670, 1934.

52. WALTERS, W., and KEPLER, E. J. Adrenal Cortical Tumors and Their Treatment, *Ann. Surg.,* 107:881, 1938.

53. BELT, A. E., and POWELL, T. O. Clinical Manifestations of the Chromaffin Cell Tumors Arising from the Suprarenal Medulla, *Surg., Gynec. & Obst.,* 59:9, 1934.

54. ROOME, N. W. Visualization of the Adrenal Gland by Air Injection, *J. A. M. A.,* 112:196, 1939.

55. HARRIS, S. Hyperinsulinism and Dysinsulinism, *J. Am. M. Ass.,* 83:729, 1924.
   ────── Hyperinsulinism, a Definite Disease Entity, *J. Am. M. Ass.,* 101:1958, 1933.
   ────── Nomenclature of the Disorders of Insulin Secretion: Diabetes Mellitus, Hyperinsulinism and Dysinsulinism, *Ann. Int. M.,* 7:1084, 1934.

56. WILDER, R. M., ALLAN, F. N., POWERS, M. H., and ROBERTSON, H. Carcinoma of the Islands of the Pancreas: Hyperinsulinism and Hypoglycemia, *J. Am. M. Ass.,* 89:348, 1927.

57. O'LEARY, J. L., and WOMACK, N. A. Histology of Adenoma of Islets of Langerhans, *Arch. Path.,* 17:291, 1934.

58. GRAHAM, E. A., and WOMACK, N. A. The Application of Surgery to the Hypoglycemic State Due to Islet Tumors of the Pancreas and to Other Conditions, *Surg., Gynec. & Obst.,* 56:728, 1933.

59. WHIPPLE, A. O., and FRANTZ, V. K. Adenoma of Islet Cells with Hyperinsulinism, *Ann. Surg.,* 101:1299, 1935.

60. GRAY, S. H., and FEEMSTER, L. C. Compensatory Hypertrophy and Hyperplasia of the Islands of Langerhans in the Pancreas of a Child Born of a Diabetic Mother, *Arch. Path.,* 1:348, 1926.

61. SIGWALD, J. *L'hypoglycémie,* Paris, Gaston Doni et Cie, 1932.

62. JOHN, H. J. Further Observations on the Treatment of Hyperinsulinism with Insulin, *Endocrinology,* 19:689, 1935.

63. CONN, J. W. The Advantage of a High Protein Diet in the Treatment of Spontaneous Hypoglycemia, *J. Clin. Investigation,* 15:673, 1936; The Spontaneous Hypoglycemias, *J. A. M. A.,* 115:1669, 1940.

64. MACBRYDE, C. M. Hypoglycemia and Hyperinsulinism, in *Modern Medical Therapy in General Practice* (Barr), Williams and Wilkins, Baltimore, 1940.

65. CUSHING, HARVEY. *The Pituitary Body and Its Disorders,* Lippincott, Philadelphia, 1912.

66. EVANS, H. M., and LONG, J. A. The Effect of the Anterior Lobe Administered Intraperitoneally upon Growth, Maturity, and Oestrus Cycles of the Rat, *Anat. Rec.,* 21:62, 1921.
   ────── Clinical Manifestations of Dysfunction of the Anterior Pituitary, *J. Am. M. Ass.,* 104:464, 1935.

67. SMITH, P. E. Hastening Development of Female Genital System by Daily Homoplastic Pituitary Transplants, *Proc. Soc. Exper. Biol. & M.,* 24:131, 1926.

68. ASCHHEIM, S., and ZONDEK, B. Hypophysenvorderlappenhormon und Ovarialhormon im Harn von Schwangeren, *Klin. Wchnschr.,* 6:1322, 1927.

69. LOEB, LEO, and BASSETT, R. B.   Effect of Hormone of Anterior Pituitary on Thyroid Gland in the Guinea Pig, *Proc. Soc. Exper. Biol. & M.*, 26:860, 1929.

70. ARON, M.   Action de la prehypophyse sur la thyroide chez le cobave, *Compt. rend. Soc. de biol.*, 102:682, 1929.

71. RIDDLE, O., BATES, R. W., and DYKSHORN, S. W.   A New Hormone of the Anterior Pituitary, *Proc. Soc. Exper. Biol. & M.*, 29:1211, 1932.

72. HOUSSAY, B. A., and BIASOTTI, A.   *Endocrinology*, 15:511, 1931.

73. COLLIP, J. B.   Diabetogenic, Thyrotropic, Adrenotropic and Parathyrotropic Factors of the Pituitary, *J. Am. M. Ass.*, 104:916, 1935.

74. BURN, J. H., and LING, H. W.   The Effect of Pituitary Extract and Adrenalin on Ketonuria and Liver Glycogen, *Quart. J. Pharmacol.*, 2:1, 1929.

75. KAMM, O., ALDRICH, T. B., GROTE, I. W., ROWE, L. W., and BUGBEE, E. P.   The Active Principles of the Posterior Lobe of the Pituitary Gland. I. The Demonstration of the Presence of Two Active Principles. II. The Separation of the Two Principles and Their Concentration in the Form of Potent Solid Preparations, *J. Am. Chem. Soc.*, 50:573, 1928.

76. ZONDEK, B.   Chromatophorotropic Principle of the Pars Intermedia of the Pituitary, *J. Am. M. Ass.*, 104:637, 1935.

77. SIMMONDS, M.   Ueber Hypophysisschwund mit tödlichem ausgang, *Deutsche med. Wchnschr.*, 40:322, 1914.
    _____ Zwergwuchs bei Atrophie des Hypophysisvorderlappens, *Deutsche med. Wchnschr.*, 45:487, 1919.

78. TEEL, H. M.   Basophilic Adenoma of the Hypophysis with Associated Pluriglandular Syndrome, *Arch. Neurol. & Psychiat.*, 26:593, 1931.

79. CUSHING, H.   The Basophil Adenomas of the Pituitary Body and Their Clinical Manifestations (Pituitary Basophilism), *Bull. Johns Hopkins Hosp.*, 50:137, 1932.

80. ASTWOOD, E. B.   The Treatment of Hyperthyroidism with Thiourea and Thiourcil, *J. Am. Med. Ass.*, 122:78, 1943.

81. CAHILL, G., MELICOW, M. M., and DARBY, H. H.   Adrenal Cortical Tumors, *Surg., Gynec. & Obst.*, 74:281, 1942.

CHAPTER XXXI

GYNECOLOGY

Malformations and Malpositions   *Miscellaneous Conditions*
Injuries of Childbirth   *Endocrine Disturbances*
Infections   *Diseases of the Vulva and Vagina*
Neoplasms

Concerned as it is with disorders of the female genital organs, gynecology represents a rather well demarcated anatomical specialty. Its relationship to obstetrics is natural and obvious, and to surgery important, though acquired. Historically, surgery owes much to gynecology inasmuch as the first systematic abdominal operations were performed for ovarian cyst. Much of the development of surgery, though made possible by antisepsis and anesthesia in the last half of the nineteenth century, was accelerated by the epoch-making successful ovariotomy performed in 1809, by Dr. Ephraim McDowell on Jane Todd Crawford in Danville, Kentucky. In spite of its many advances during the last century, especially through the work of J. Marion Sims, and its growth during the present century, particularly through the efforts of H. A. Kelly, gynecology has been only partly successful in maintaining itself as an independent specialty. Gynecology has been somewhat facetiously compared to a shy maiden who is being constantly wooed on the one hand by the persistent obstetrician and on the other hand by the enterprising general surgeon. Each has been successful in various sections of the country.

From the point of view of surgery, the female genital organs are frequently involved in lesions which are similar to nongynecological disease. This is particularly true of lesions in the pelvis which, after all, is but a part of the general peritoneal cavity. Moreover, through the vagina one may by examination gain much information of lower abdominal disease, even when there is no pelvic lesion. The more external and obvious manifestations of gynecological disease, finally, are so common that a fundamental knowledge of them should be possessed by all practitioners whether or not they specialize in surgery, obstetrics or gynecology. No attempt is made in this chapter to cover the field of gynecology, but only to call attention to the aspects of more general interest. There are a number of single volume works on gynecology which can be recommended: Crossen,[1] Kelly,[2] Curtis,[3] Miller,[4] and Graves.[5]

Definitions.—*Normal menstruation* * (catamenia, monthly flow, monthly sickness, period, menses, being "unwell") begins at puberty which occurs usually about the fourteenth year, but varies between the eleventh and sixteenth year. Its onset is accompanied by other manifestations of sexual maturity, both external

---

* A brief discussion of the physiology of menstruation has been reported by Allen.[6]

(growth of pubic hair, breasts and external genitalia) and internal (growth of ovaries, uterus and vagina). Although normal menstruation varies, the average flow lasts three to five days and consists of 40 to 50 cc. of fluid blood mixed with cervical secretion and uterine débris. The intermenstrual period varies somewhat between twenty-seven and thirty-one days, the average being twenty-eight days or one lunar month. Normally there is hardly any pain associated with menstruation. Changes in the breasts, external genitalia, uterus and ovaries occur and are often noticed by the patient; other symptoms of a neurovascular nature are also present in some individuals. Menstruation occurs normally (except during pregnancy) from puberty to the *menopause* (climacteric, "change of life"). The menopause may be sudden, but is usually gradual, taking several months to years, and normally develops at about the age of forty-five, although great variations exist; in 68 per cent of women it occurs between the fortieth and fiftieth year. Symptoms may be absent, but are frequently severe enough to demand medical aid. Functional disturbances, such as nervousness, "hot flashes," and general irritability may hardly be classed as pathologic unless very pronounced and persistent. These functional disturbances are apt to be more severe when an *artificial menopause* has been produced by bilateral oophorectomy (excision of ovaries) and may require substitution therapy (administration of ovarian hormones). *Dysmenorrhea* indicates the presence of severe pain during the menstrual period. Though definitely an abnormal manifestation, it is so frequent among many otherwise normal women that the cause is often difficult to determine. In the severe cases medical aid is sought; in such patients a cause should be detected if at all possible by thorough investigation. Inflammatory, mechanical, neoplastic, neurogenic, allergic and other factors have been described. *Amenorrhea,* or absence of menstruation, is normal before puberty, during pregnancy and after the menopause. Otherwise it may be due to maldevelopment, inflammatory or neoplastic disease, or operations (hysterectomy). *Oligomenorrhea,* or scanty menstruation, is normal preceding menopause. It may be due otherwise to endocrine deficiencies. *Menorrhagia* refers to an excessive amount or duration of the menstrual flow. Since individual variations are great, menorrhagia is said to be present only when a change develops which is greater than normal for the particular patient. The presence of clotted blood may in some cases be significant. *Metrorrhagia* indicates the presence of bleeding between menstrual periods. Although spotting may occur with ovulation, metrorrhagia is nearly always abnormal and even if slight demands investigation, particularly with the possibility of malignant disease in mind.

Leukorrhea refers to an abnormal vaginal discharge. Normally there is a slight mucoserous discharge at the vaginal opening which keeps the parts moist. It is increased in amount during sexual excitement. It is also apt to be prominent for a few days after menstruation. When the discharge is profuse and continuous, or is of an abnormal character, it is generally an indication of inflammatory or other disease. Leukorrhea usually consists of a whitish, colorless or yellowish vaginal discharge. If brownish the presence of blood is almost certain. Often the discharge is definitely purulent in nature or thick and mucinous. It may be profuse and cause intense irritation to the surrounding skin. *Dyspareunia* refers to painful sexual intercourse. It may be due to anatomic causes or to psychic incompatability.

Methods of Diagnosis.—As a rule, gynecological diseases do not offer as much difficult in diagnosis as many other surgical conditions, except for the group of diseases involving disturbed ovarian secretion.

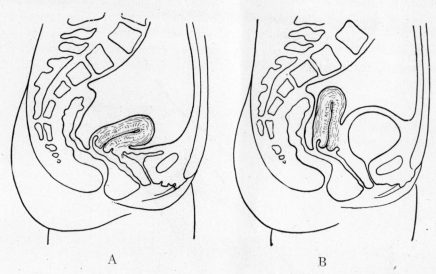

FIG. 528.—LONGITUDINAL SECTION OF THE ADULT FEMALE PELVIS.
A, the normal relative positions of the various organs. *B,* the effect of a distended bladder.

History.—This is of special importance in gynecology because the symptoms are frequently characteristic. Inquiry into the menstrual and marital history is obviously important and should be detailed. Urinary symptoms, such as frequency, burning and pain on urination are present in many gynecological diseases. The number of complaints referable to disease of the genital organs are relatively few, but the degree of disability or the severity of the pain, especially of backache or other symptoms, may be either exaggerated or minimized. Careful evaluation of social, personal and sexual factors are often of great significance in the history. Much care and tact are necessary in eliciting these factors, but when important they should be obtained.

Examination.—A routine physical examination is of course always important. Too often, treatment is ineffective because of an incorrect diagnosis. Frequently this is due to an incomplete or inadequate examination, particularly of the genital tract. It must be emphasized that gentleness and avoidance of pain are necessary in order to obtain as much information as possible. Judicious persistence, however, is often necessary in order to make sufficiently complete observations.

Of special importance in gynecology are abdominal, pelvic and rectal examinations, alone or in combination, and direct inspection of the cervix. On special occasions other examinations are indicated. These include cystoscopic and proctoscopic study, x-ray visualization of the uterus and tubes by iodized oils, determination of their patency by injection of air and finally, examination of urine and blood for hormones (Aschheim-Zondek test, etc., for pregnancy). In some patients biopsy of cervical tissue or of endometrium (after curettage) may be necessary to arrive at a proper diagnosis.

It should be emphasized, of course, that physical examination of adult females, whether it includes the pelvis or not, should if possible be carried out in the presence of a nurse or other witness. An excellent description of the various methods of gynecological examinations is that of Kelly.[7] *Abdominal examination* will frequently reveal much information by excluding disease outside the pelvis. However, acute pelvic inflammation often produces abdominal tenderness, rigidity and

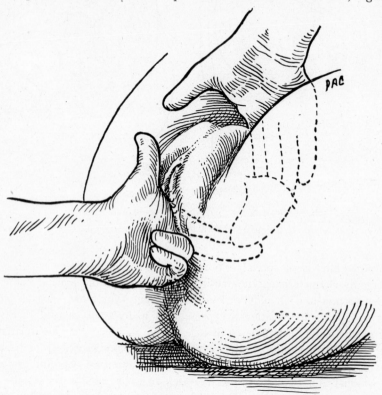

FIG. 529.—DIGITAL EXAMINATION OF THE VAGINA AND CERVIX.

Note also the manner in which a bimanual palpation of the uterus, tubes and other pelvic structures may be carried out. The term pelvic examination is also applied to the bimanual technic.

muscle spasm which is usually bilateral; but may also be located in the midline if an endometritis is present. A mass is rarely palpable. A full bladder is often a source of confusion and should be borne in mind as a possible explanation of pelvic tumor, of lower abdominal dulness and even distention. Any tumor mass arising from the pelvis can be palpated abdominally after it attains a certain size (2 to 4 inches in diameter, depending on location and attachments). Thus, a pregnant uterus or large myoma can be felt as a prominent suprapubic enlargement. Ovarian cysts are often detected on examination of either or both sides of the abdomen. *Inspection of the external* genitalia will often reveal evidence of inflammation, ulcers, chancre, condyloma, cystic or other swelling, congestion and redness about the opening of the urethra. Other abnormalities to be searched for include cystocele, rectocele, uterine prolapse, vaginal discharge, congenital malformations, etc. The presence of a hymen may at times be an important factor in eliminating certain types of pelvic disease.

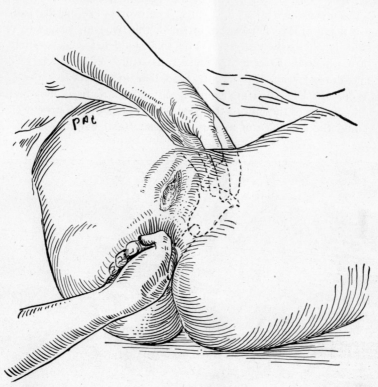

FIG. 530.—BIMANUAL EXAMINATION OF THE PELVIS WHEN A VAGINAL EXAMINATION IS NOT CARRIED OUT.

With the index finger in the rectum, gross abnormalities can usually be made out with a fair degree of accuracy. This method of palpating pelvic and lower abdominal structures is used in virgins and in children.

Digital vaginal examination is ordinarily not performed during menstruation or at any time on virgins. During late pregnancy it should not be done unless necessary, and then only with special precautions in order to avoid the danger of infection. Much information as to form and consistency of the cervix is obtainable by palpation with the tips of the fingers. The direction in which the cervix points indicates the position of the uterus; its shape and consistency is noted; tenderness on manipulation of the cervix is often significant. A soft mass or bulging behind the cervix is frequently an important indication of fluid or inflammation in the cul-de-sac. The cul-de-sac is the peritoneal reflection between the posterior wall of the uterus and the anterior wall of the rectum, often called Douglas' pouch. Digital pressure over the urethra when applied from above downward may reveal on inspection a purulent discharge emerging from the urethral orifice, or from Skene's ducts.

Bimanual examination is probably the most important method of pelvic examination, because with two fingers in the vagina and the other hand on the lower abdomen, the entire pelvis can ordinarily be palpated and much information obtained. In normal sized women the tip of the examining finger reaches well up on the wall of the uterus and broad ligaments. The ovaries are usually palpable, but the tubes are not normally felt except in small, thin women. Complete relaxation of the patient is obviously necessary. For this, gentleness, coöperation and reassurance are essential. In obese patients satisfactory examination is often impossible. The dorsal position is usually used, but in some cases the knee-chest posture is useful. In a few patients examination under anesthesia may be indicated. The size and position of the uterus, the condition of the adnexal structures (ovaries and tubes) and the existence of masses, tenderness and induration are especially noted.

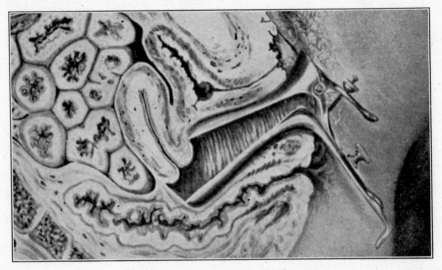

FIG. 531.—INSPECTION OF THE CERVIX.

Bivalve speculum in place. Sectional view, showing relations of speculum and exposure of the cervix and vaginal vault by opening the blades. (From Crossen, *Diseases of Women*, 1930. Courtesy of C. V. Mosby Co., St. Louis, Mo.)

Rectal palpation should be part of the routine gynecological examination, but in virgins it is used in place of the digital vaginal examination in order to palpate the pelvis bimanually. In children especially, the entire pelvis can be palpated with great facility by bimanual recto-abdominal examination. In the later stages of pregnancy or during menstruation, a rectal instead of vaginal examination is often done. The cervix can easily be felt through the thin rectovaginal wall.

Inspection of the cervix is often important and requires the introduction of a speculum to separate the walls of the vagina and a strong light to visualize the cervix. The dorsal position is usually advisable. The patient is sometimes placed on her side with the knees flexed (Sim's posture). In young girls and adult virgins the cervix may be visualized with a tiny speculum without injuring the hymen.

MALFORMATIONS AND MALPOSITIONS

Malformations.—Congenital malformations of the genital tract, though present at birth, may not produce symptoms until puberty or later during active sex life. They are due to defects in embryonic development. In the external genitalia there may be enlargement of the clitoris and a rudimentary scrotum and vagina which is characteristic of a hermaphrodite. In some cases it may be difficult to tell whether a child is male or female unless the gonads are examined histologically. Such abnormalities are extremely rare. Exstrophy of the bladder and epispadias are analogous in development to similar anomalies in the male (see pp. 1002 and 1021).

Imperforate hymen produces no symptoms until puberty when menstruation begins. The uterine blood accumulates and distends the vagina (hematocolpos) which produces definite symptoms. No menstrual blood appears, but each month there occur the other manifestations of menstruation, called molimina, which consist of pelvic heaviness, engorgement of the breasts, etc. Since no blood can escape, the discomfort and pain in the lower abdomen becomes more and more marked as more blood accumulates, until the uterus becomes distended (hematometra) and a tender mass appears above the symphysis pubis. On examination there is no vaginal opening, but merely a distended, fluctuating membrane. Rectal examination reveals the extent of the mass. Treatment consists of adequate incision or excision of the hymen and evacuation of the old blood under scrupulous aseptic precautions to avoid infection.

Atresia of the vagina (*gynatresia*) is most commonly due to an imperforate hymen (see above), but may be due to a thin septum in the canal or to a congenital absence of more or less of the entire vagina. There is in such patients an associated malformation of uterus, tubes and ovaries, which can often be determined by recto-abdominal examination. Many instances of atresia are acquired and are really due to a stenosis produced by injury or infection. The clinical manifestations of atresia are rarely due to hematocolpos, but usually are produced because of the associated lack of development of the uterus (amenorrhea) or because of the obstacle offered to normal sexual intercourse. Treatment depends on the local conditions present and on the problem presented by the individual case.

Double vagina is due to the presence of a longitudinal septum which divides the vagina into two canals. Symptoms may be absent. Dyspareunia may be produced by the lesion and interference with normal labor may occur. Division of the septum is easily performed.

Bicornate uterus usually produces no obvious symptoms of disease and is often detected accidentally, especially during pregnancy or during x-ray study after injection of lipiodol. When one horn is associated with a stenosis at the cervix, hematometra may form, due to accumulation of menstrual blood.

Malposition of the Uterus.—Displacements of the uterus may be congenital but are usually acquired. Backward displacements are spoken of as retrodisplacements and include retroversion (tipping of the entire uterus backward) and retroflexion (tipping of the upper part of the uterus backward). The clinical manifestations and treatment of these two types are so similar that they will both be discussed under Retrodisplacement.

Retrodisplacement.—In retrodisplacement the uterus may be tipped so far backward that it rests on the rectum; it is very common. In some patients it is due to a weakness and relaxation of the various supporting ligaments of the cervix. In many the malposition is associated with pelvic inflammatory disease. In most cases, however, retrodisplacement is one of the results of childbirth and will be discussed under that heading. It should be emphasized, however, that pelvic lesions are frequently multiple, retrodisplacement being associated with cervicitis, chronic pelvic inflammation, etc. The symptoms produced by retrodisplacement are various and include backache, pain and discomfort in the pelvis aggravated by exercise, constipation by rectal pressure, sterility, and repeated miscarriage, particularly at the fourth month. In many cases these symptoms are due to associated lesions. Diagnosis is made by vaginal or rectal examination combined with abdominal examination (bimanual palpation).

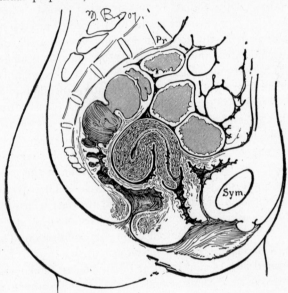

Fig. 532.—Acute Retroflexion of the Uterus. (After Kelly.)

Treatment of retrodisplacement depends on many factors, particularly its cause. In many patients in whom symptoms are not due to the malposition, no treatment may be indicated. The use of pessaries is indicated in some patients, not to correct a malposition, but to maintain the normal position which has been achieved by manual manipulation; its use, however, is contraindicated in many individuals. The operative procedures for the correction of retrodisplacement are described under treatment of childbirth injuries.

Anteflexion.—This is uncommon and rarely produces symptoms, except when the lumen of the uterus is kinked by the malposition. It is usually congenital. Symptoms include dysmenorrhea, especially cramplike pain during menstruation, sterility and dyspareunia. Treatment consists of eradication of other associated lesions and of dilatation of the cervical canal to overcome the uterine stenosis. Pessaries are sometimes useful.

INJURIES OF CHILDBIRTH

Many gynecological diseases, inflammatory or otherwise, are due directly to the process of childbearing. The lesions considered under this heading are those produced mechanically by the tearing or permanent stretching of the pelvic structures during passage of the fetus. Infections due to pregnancy are considered separately.

Relaxation and Laceration of the Perineum.—The mechanical changes produced during labor vary from a simple dilatation of the vaginal opening to complete tearing of the perineum into the rectum (third degree tear). Various types of fistulas may be produced by childbirth (*e.g.,* rectovaginal and vesicovaginal). In most patients, the external laceration is the most common injury, but is often associated with tearing of the deep pelvic muscles and fascia, particularly the levator ani, so that there is a marked weakness and relaxation of the pelvic floor. Through the wide vaginal opening the posterior vaginal wall with the adjacent rectal wall may bulge (*rectocele*); the anterior wall with the adjacent urinary bladder may also protrude (*cystocele*). Frequently, the uterus itself may slip down into the dilated vagina so that the cervix presents at the outlet (*prolapse*). If the prolapse is extreme, so that the entire uterus protrudes outside the vagina, which is thus really turned inside out, the term *procidentia* is used. Though prolapse and procidentia are nearly always the result of injuries sustained during childbirth, they have been known to occur in rare cases in women who have not borne children.

Clinical Manifestations.—The symptoms produced by cystocele, rectocele and prolapse are generally described by the patient as a sense of "bearing down" or pelvic pressure, associated with considerable fatigue after standing or walking. Backache and dragging pain are often frequent complaints. Occasionally, bladder symptoms such as frequency, burning, etc., may be present. In many cases the lacerated cervix may become reddened and inflamed, and occasionally ulcerated. In severe cases (prolapse) the difficulty in maintaining satisfactory position of the uterus is usually so pronounced that operation is advisable unless contraindications exist.

Treatment.—First of all, treatment should be preventive by careful supervision of the second stage of labor; the performance of an episiotomy (De Lee) and adequate postnatal rest and care will lessen remarkably the incidence of relaxation of the pelvic floor and its various manifestations. Conservative treatment consists of the use of pessaries, rest, vaginal douches, etc. Operation is frequently indicated and may be abdominal, vaginal or both. Abdominal operation has as its object the support of the uterus, thus preventing its descent into the vagina. The procedures consist of shortening the round or uterosacral ligaments. These suspension operations are numerous and are associated with the names of Baldy, Webster, Crossen, and a great many others. Vaginal operations are particularly indicated for rectocele and cystocele and consist of repair of the pelvic floor (colporrhaphy) through posterior (and often anterior) vaginal incisions. Repair of the lacerated cervix is often done at the same time. Fixation of the uterus may also be achieved through the vaginal route by interposing it below the bladder and is sometimes

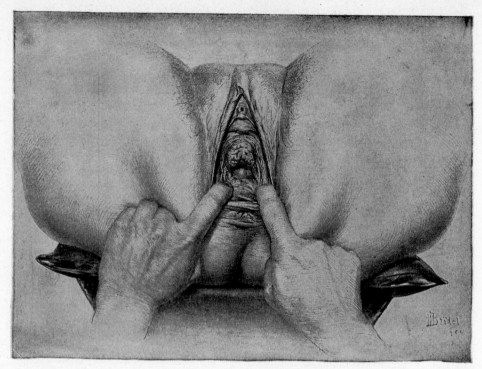

FIG. 533.—METHOD OF DEMONSTRATING RELAXED VAGINAL OUTLET.

The fingers are hooked in the vagina on both sides and pulled outward and backward. Note the protrusion of the anterior vaginal wall (cystocele). (After Kelly.)

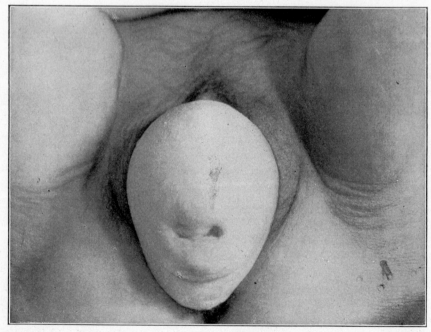

FIG. 534.—COMPLETE PROLAPSE OF THE UTERUS IN A SIXTY-YEAR-OLD WOMAN WHO HAS BORNE MANY CHILDREN (ST. LOUIS CITY HOSPITAL).

useful in older women well past the menopause. It is called the interposition operation and is associated with the name of Watkins.

Laceration of the Cervix.—This lesion is nearly always present after childbirth. It is of significance only when it does not heal, leading thus to erosion of the cervical mucosa, hypertrophy, cyst formation and ulceration, all of which are manifestations of chronic infection (chronic cervicitis). Diagnosis is often possible by palpation, but is made certain only by inspection of the cervix by means of a vaginal speculum. Clinically, the patient may suffer only from a profuse vaginal discharge originating in the inflamed cervix. Treatment is often indicated to relieve this leukorrhea or because the lesion suggests the existence of cancer. Moreover, the presence of chronic infection of this sort is supposed to encourage the development of malignant disease. Electrocoagulation or actual excision of the diseased tissue is the most effective treatment. The latter method permits microscopic study of the tissue. Conservative care, notably frequent vaginal douches and topical applications to the cervix are sometimes effective in allowing healing to occur (see Chronic Cervicitis).

Fistula.—Fistulas which occur after childbirth are due to communications between the rectum and vagina (rectovaginal fistula) or between the bladder or urethra and vagina (vesicovaginal fistula). The opening may, on rare occasions, be into the uterus itself or into the cervix, rather than into the vagina. Unfortunately, these lesions sometimes occur after vaginal operations or application of radium; malignant neoplasms are occasionally the cause. The distressing lack of control of feces and urine may lead to serious invalidism. Operative repair is difficult. Though silver wire is seldom used now, its introduction by Marion Sims in the middle of the last century for the operative cure of these lesions was an important step in the development of surgical technic. Each case requires its own type of operation.

INFECTIONS

On the basis of the etiologic organism, infections of the female genital tract may be classified into four groups: those due to the gonococcus, tubercle bacillus, spirochete pallida and the pyogenic group. The first and last mentioned organisms are the most important. The manifestations of each type, however, are variable, depending on which of the several organs are involved to the greatest extent. In many instances, however, all of the pelvic structures are obviously the site of an infective process and the term pelvic inflammatory disease is used. In the acute stage, diagnosis may be made very easily, but when chronic infection is present, differentiation on the basis of the causative organism may be fairly difficult. Since the chronic manifestations produced by the various organisms are so similar, they will be considered together in more detail under the heading of chronic pelvic inflammation (p. 961).

Gonorrhea.—This is a veneral disease transmitted only by coitus (except in juvenile vaginitis). Gonorrhea in the female is a prevalent disease largely because of sexual promiscuity, transmission being especially common by prostitutes. In this way innocent women are infected by their husbands who at the time of marriage consider themselves free of the disease which may have been contracted months previously. It may require six months or years after a male acquires gonorrhea before such a danger is past (see p. 1014). It is important to realize that infectivity in women may last for several years. The seriousness of the disease in the female is due to the duration of the disease, and the frequency and ease with which it produces complete disability of the procreative and even the endocrine function of the genital organs. General disability due to chronic or recurrent infection is also common. The gonococcus, though a fragile organism, once it gains a foothold, spreads rapidly, usually along the surface and between the cells of the mucous membranes; it soon reaches all the pelvic structures and sets up a severe, acute, inflammatory process. Extreme variations of severity exist. The acute manifestations usually last from one to several weeks and are followed by the chronic stage

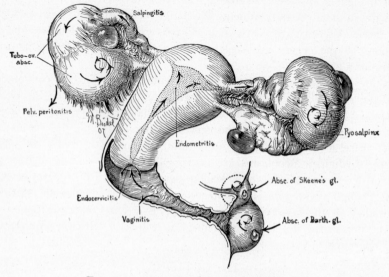

FIG. 535.—CHIEF LESIONS OF GONORRHEA.

The whorled arrows mark the common sites of infection. All lesions are those of adult women, except the vagina which is infected primarily only in childhood (juvenile vaginitis) (After Kelly).

which often lasts indefinitely and is subject to recurrent exacerbations of acute nature from time to time.

Acute Gonorrhea.—The disease is usually manifested within a few days after exposure as a dry, burning pain in the external genitalia, followed by a yellowish vaginal discharge, frequency of, and pain and burning on, urination. These initial symptoms may be severe or may be so mild as to escape the patient's notice. The urinary symptoms are due to associated urethritis, the leukorrhea to the presence of vulvovaginitis and endocervicitis. Other lesions are frequently present, or develop during the course of several days or weeks. Thus, infection of the Bartholin's glands on either side of the vaginal opening often leads to abscess or cyst formation. Skene's glands which are located on each side of the urethral meatus are also infected, and may lead to periurethral or suburethral abscesses. The inguinal lymph nodes are usually enlarged. In most patients the process sooner or later extends into the pelvis, producing an acute salpingitis or commonly an extensive inflammatory reaction of all pelvic structures. The terms pelvic cellulitis, pelvic peritonitis or acute pelvic inflammatory disease are often used to describe the extensive nature of the swelling, edema and tenderness. Such an extension is particularly prone to develop when the infection takes place during or near the menstrual period. Of special importance to the surgeon is the fact that the lower abdominal pain, fever and leukocytosis which accompany pelvic cellulitis may lead to a mistaken diagnosis of ruptured acute appendicitis. Important in the differentiation (see also p. 686) is the absence of toxic symptoms such as prostration, even when the fever is high. The bilateral localization of the tenderness and muscle spasm, particularly when located in the lower abdomen over the adnexal regions, is characteristic of gonorrhea. The presence of vaginal and urethral discharge is, of course, important and should be looked for. Palpation of tender masses on both sides of the pelvis on bimanual examination, and tenderness on manipulation of the cervix are nearly always noted. Occasionally, however, only one tube is affected, at least for a short time during the course of the disease. If the affected tube is on the right side, extreme difficulty in the differential diagnosis from appendicitis may be experienced. The demonstration of gonococci (intracellular, gram-negative diplococci) in stained smears of material obtained from the cervix is of obvious significance. Unlike acute appendicitis, gastro-intestinal symptoms such as nausea and vomiting are generally absent. It has been reported that the sedimentation time of the erythrocytes is prolonged in acute appendicitis, but rapid in acute gonorrhea, the difference being of diagnostic value particularly during the first twenty-four to forty-eight hours, at a time when such a differentiation is most needed (Smith, et al.[8]). If a mistaken diagnosis is nevertheless made and the patient is operated upon, it is important that no operative procedures be carried out on the acutely inflamed organs in order to insure against extension of the infection.

Other diseases which may offer diagnostic difficulty are tubal pregnancy, infected dermoid cyst, ovarian cyst with a twisted pedicle, etc. These conditions are discussed later.

In a few patients, pelvic cellulitis will be accompanied by distention, tenderness, pain in the entire abdomen, and may produce vomiting, so that the picture of general peritonitis or intestinal obstruction is suggested. This is especially prone to occur in Negresses. In spite of these abdominal symptoms, the absence of toxic manifestations and the detection of pelvic cellulitis on palpation generally give the true clue to the diagnosis. These abdominal manifestations may be due to invasion of the general peritoneal cavity by the gonococcus, but are most likely due to an extension of the pelvic edema to the parietal peritoneum, or perhaps to a partial intestinal obstruction produced by adhesion of a loop of intestine to the inflammatory mass; spontaneous subsidence in a few days is the rule. On rare occasions the inflammatory mass becomes sufficiently adherent to such a loop of intestine as to produce complete occlusion.

Treatment of acute gonorrhea in the female should be specific, symptomatic and hygienic. Cleanliness and a large fluid intake is important, and isolation, in order to prevent contagion as much as possible should be assured. Local treatment is impossible because of the pain and tenderness and is, moreover, unimportant. The introduction of chemotherapy with the sulfonamide compounds has revolutionized the treatment of gonorrhea in both the male and female. A general discussion of the sulfonamide drugs including a list of their toxic and other effects will be found on p. 35. As in other infections sulfanilamide was the first drug extensively used in the treatment of gonorrhea but was later replaced by sulfapyridine. However, the effectiveness of sulfathiazole is so much more pronounced that this last drug will probably be the one finally adopted in combating the gonococcus. When given in doses of 1 gram every six hours for five days sulfathiazole has been reported as curing as high as 90 per cent of acute cases. It should be emphasized, however, that although this treatment may eliminate the organisms from the smears and alleviate all local symptoms, it does not relieve any symptoms resulting from permanent damage to the tubes and ovaries produced by the infection.

In stubborn and refractory cases the employment of artificial fever therapy is strongly indicated either alone or in conjunction with chemotherapy. Artificial fever should be given, however, only by those expert in its use and by carefully controlled methods; details may be found in special reports.

Complications of acute gonorrhea are generally included under the term chronic gonorrhea, although the dividing line between acute and chronic infection may be difficult to draw. Complications may be entirely absent; occasionally the infection subsides without leaving any residual pathologic changes. More commonly, the acute invasion leaves permanent and *serious disease* as an aftermath. In some patients these after-effects seem to develop insidiously with few or slight clinical manifestations at the time of invasion. Recurrent attacks of acute infection are not uncommon during the chronic stage. Other complications such as gonorrheal arthritis are discussed elsewhere.

Chronic Gonorrhea.—This term is applied to such lesions as persistent infection of the cervix (endocervicitis), a localized abscess in the uterus (pyometra) and tubes (pyosalpinx), a pelvic abscess in the pouch of Douglas, a tubo-ovarian abscess, or to extensive adhesions and scar tissue in and about the various pelvic organs. Other lesions include chronic infection of Skene's and Bartholin's glands.

Bartholin's gland abscess is obvious on inspection as a rounded tender mass in the posterior portion of the labia. Pain is severe, especially on walking. It usually demands incision and drainage to relieve pain. The pus usually fails to show gonococci. *Infection of Skene's glands* generally subsides spontaneously or responds to simple local treatment. Occasionally they form tiny abscesses which may have to be incised for adequate drainage. Excision is sometimes necessary.

Endocervicitis is diagnosed with certainty only on inspection. Swelling of the cervix with ulceration and erosion at the os are typical findings. The causative organism, however, can rarely be found in the discharge except during the acute stage. However, the presence of a tenacious, mucopurulent exudate is said to be characteristic. It presents the same therapeutic features as chronic cervicitis due to other causes and is discussed in detail separately on page 959.

Chronic pelvic infection due to gonococcus comprises a variety of lesions, particularly chronic salpingitis and ovaritis, and is manifested by such various symptoms as bearing down pains, especially during the menstrual periods, backache, menorrhagia, dysmenorrhea and general malaise. The diagnosis depends on thorough physical, and particularly bimanual pelvic examination. On palpation the uterus is often in a retroverted position and adnexal masses or an abscess in the cul-de-sac are demonstrable. The findings depend on the stage and extension of the disease. Great variations exist. The entire pelvis may be the site of a solid mass of granulation tissue and adhesions, in the midst of which may be an abscess. Frequently the tubes alone are involved, either as dilated structures containing pus (pyosalpinx) or in the latter stages as sterile cysts due to the disappearance of the organisms (hydrosalpinx).

On many occasions a chronic pelvic infection due to gonorrhea is of diffuse nature and can be distinguished with difficulty from the disease produced by pyogenic infections. This type of infection may be quite disabling, resist conservative therapy, and thereby require surgical treatment; it is described on page 961 with similar infections not due to the gonococcus.

The *treatment* of gonorrhea in its chronic stage is at first conservative except for the incision and drainage of superficial abscesses as already mentioned. Conservative treatment consists of hot douches, rest and general hygiene. However, the use of the sulfonamide drugs, especially sulfathiazole, has revolutionized the treatment of chronic gonorrhea just as it has the acute infection, as discussed on page 956. The problem of operation is discussed in detail under chronic pelvic inflammation (p. 961). In younger women conservation of structures is important, but in older women radical excision of diseased tissue is often indicated. Cul-de-sac abscesses, though not common, are usually due to secondary infection, *e.g.,* anerobic streptococcus and B. coli; they may frequently be drained by a vaginal incision posterior to the cervix.

It is important to realize the infectivity of these chronic lesions, even when the patients have no symptoms. A large percentage of prostitutes are thus permanent carriers of gonococci which remain hidden in the various occult lesions about the cervix, vagina and urethral glands; they thus explain the constant dissemination of the disease.

Acute Gonorrheal Vaginitis of Children.—This lesion represents a clinical entity which follows inoculation of fresh gonococci on the external genitalia, usually by contact or contamination from an infected adult or another child with the disease. It is seen most commonly among children living in squalid, unhygienic and crowded quarters and is most prevalent in Negroes. Its contagiousness make it an especially dangerous disease in institutions caring for large numbers of little girls. The symptoms produced are usually confined to the development of a persistent, profuse, creamy, vaginal discharge which contains the organisms, and often irritates the vulva and skin of the thigh. It differs from adult gonorrhea in the absence of inguinal adenitis, gonorrheal arthritis, and the rarity of salpingitis. Occasionally, however, the abdominal signs seen in adults are produced, thereby simulating closely the picture of general peritonitis from a ruptured appendicitis. These abdominal manifestations subside rapidly, however, without any special treatment and are not accompanied by the severe nausea and vomiting and prostration which are so characteristic of a *B. coli* peritonitis, and therefore offer no serious diagnostic problem, provided the vaginitis is noted.

In the *treatment* of gonorrheal vaginitis isolation from other children is required until the discharge shows an absence of the organisms on three successive examinations. Various types of douches and antiseptics have been advocated, but it is probable that simple cleanliness is all that can be achieved by such local treatment. The disease may run its course in about eight to twelve weeks, but a great many cases persist for longer periods or enter a chronic stage with recurrent infection which lasts indefinitely. Lewis [10] has reported relatively rapid healing of gonorrheal vaginitis in children following the injection of the ovarian hormone theelin. However, vaginal suppositories containing estrogens (TeLinde [11]) are very effective, widely used, and much better than injections of the hormone. That a deleterious effect on the ovaries results from the use of this hormone in young children has apparently been disproved by the experiments of Allen and Diddle.[12] Moreover, the use of suppositories containing estrogens has become so extensive that it is probably fair to state that this form of therapy is without danger.

Tuberculosis.—This infection attacks the Fallopian tubes most frequently, and though relatively rare, is found most commonly in younger women. It is supposed to originate either as a hematogenous infection or by extension from an adjacent tuberculous peritonitis. The latter lesion was present in two-thirds of the 200 cases reported from the Johns Hopkins Hospital (Greenberg [13]). The uterus and ovaries are secondarily involved, but the cervix is seldom, and the vagina rarely, affected.

The *clinical manifestations* develop insidiously and vary remarkably, resembling in this respect tuberculosis of the peritoneum (see p. 745). Abdominal pain, fever, gastro-intestinal symptoms, disturbed menstruation and urination, leukorrhea, backache and sterility have been described as important symptoms. Bimanual examination reveals only the evidences of chronic pelvic inflammation, indistinguishable from those produced by chronic gonorrhea which, when it can be excluded, especially by the history, helps in establishing the diagnosis of tuberculosis. Often, however, the diagnosis is first made at laparotomy.

Treatment consists of general and hygienic care with plenty of good food and sunshine; surgical excision of the diseased tissue may be advisable. As in the case of tuberculous peritonitis, many patients seem to improve after laparotomy alone without drainage.

Syphilis.—Syphilis produces local lesions in the female external genitalia which are similar to the primary and secondary lesions in the male, though more often occult, because they are hidden in the vagina, and hence not easily seen unless careful inspection is carried out. The chancre, inguinal adenitis, mucous patch and condyloma latum are usually similar, but may be overshadowed by a coincident gonorrheal invasion. The vulva is, however, the site of other lesions which are not syphilitic and are discussed later (p. 978). Syphilitic disease of the uterus, tubes and ovaries is rare and of no special significance, except that the cervix is reported to be frequently the site of the chancre; however, it is probably often overlooked. Syphilis is also a common cause of spontaneous abortion.

Diagnosis is based on the appearance of the local lesions, the visualization of the treponema by dark field illumination, the manifestations of the disease elsewhere, and by the Wassermann or Kahn reaction.

Pyogenic Infections.—These organisms include a number of bacteria which produce a great variety of pelvic disease. By excluding the gonococcus which has already been considered, nearly all of the acute infections are of puerperal origin and follow pregnancy or abortion. Chronic inflammatory disease may follow such an acute invasion; more commonly, however, the chronic lesions develop insidiously, presumably through portals of entry created or induced by childbirth injury. Other less obvious factors also play a role; in general, therefore, chronic pyogenic infection always offers a difficult problem in diagnosis, as far as determining the causative organism as well as the portal of entry is concerned.

Acute Infections.—Puerperal infections develop either as an aftermath of a presumably normal delivery or following a criminal abortion. This represents a large and serious group of acute pelvic infections and each year accounts for thousands of fatalities. These infections are of two types, exogenous and endogenous. The former are due to contamination usually of B. coli, streptococci and staphylococci and represent infections which should be almost entirely avoidable. Endogenous infection, due to various types of anaerobic streptococci (Schottmueller) which the patient harbors herself, presents a more difficult problem (Schwarz and Dieckman [14]). Even when the infection is not fatal it often results in complications which are the cause of serious and persistent disability. Puerperal infections are also of surgical interest because of their historical association with the development of aseptic technic (see Chapter III). The too frequent occurrence of the exogenous type in modern days is probably just as clearly due to contamination as it was in the time of Oliver Wendell Holmes. The clinical manifestations are those of general septicemia as well as of pelvic inflammation, and are described in detail in obstetrical texts.

When pelvic infection follows a criminal abortion, the manifestations of general septicemia are accompanied by acute abdominal signs and symptoms which are often mistaken for a general peritonitis from a ruptured appendicitis, especially since a correct history is often difficult to obtain from these patients. The presence of a foul bloody discharge, the profound toxic appearance of the patient, and the evidence of extensive pelvic inflammation on bimanual palpation are ordinarily sufficient to make the diagnosis. The treatment is an obstetrical problem.

Chronic Pyogenic Infection.—As already mentioned, chronic infections of the genital tract in general are frequent, even if gonorrhea is excluded. Although acute pelvic cellulitis of puerperal origin is often responsible for these chronic lesions, many result from obstetrical injury which has permitted an insidious secondary invasion. In many patients the source of the infection may be difficult to determine. Invasion of this type may be classified into infection of the cervix (chronic cervicitis) and infection of the pelvis (chronic pelvic inflammatory disease).

Chronic cervicitis (endocervicitis) produces symptoms largely because it is the source of leukorrhea which may become irritating to the patient. Such symptoms as backache, dragging pelvic discomfort and pain over the sacrum are often present, but frequently are due to associated lesions, particularly chronic pelvic inflammation and various pelvic lacerations and uterine malpositions which have already been described. Regardless, however, of whether the disease has been produced by gonorrhea, unhealed lacerations or other causes, the symptomatology, pathology and treatment are similar.

On inspection the cervix is hypertrophied, eroded or ulcerated, and may show many cysts and polyps, particularly in the canal from which a mucopurulent discharge appears. Various terms such as cervical catarrh, glandular endocervicitis, cystic disease, inflammatory hypertrophy, etc., are used to describe the lesion. The existence of chronic cervicitis is especially important in older women in whom such a lesion may be a precursor of cancer. The chronicity is due to the presence of the organisms deep within the mucous glands adjacent to the cervical canal, and of obstruction to the glands producing cysts. In a few women polyps are present in the cervical canal and become infected, leading to exudation which contributes to the chronic irritation. Chronic purulent discharge from deeply infected

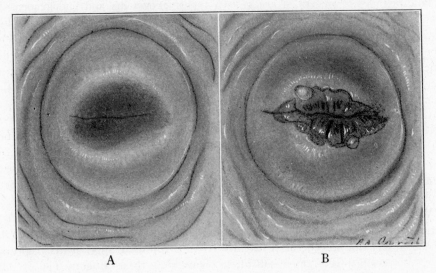

A   B

FIG. 536.—CHRONIC CERVICITIS AS VIEWED THROUGH A VAGINAL SPECULUM.

A, mild type, consisting of slight erosion, associated with a linear laceration. *B*, more severe type, consisting of definite ulceration and cyst formation. This type, if present for years, is believed to be a lesion which is a precursor of cancer.

cysts also plays a similar role. Only rarely is bacteriologic study of any value since secondary invaders nearly always predominate, even if the primary organism is present. A mixed flora is therefore found.

The decision as to the type of *treatment* in chronic cervicitis depends on the age of the patient, the amount of discharge and the presence of other disease. Therapy may be carried out according to a variety of methods which consist of (1) conservative care such as vaginal douches, cleanliness and topical applications; (2) electrocoagulation of the diseased tissue, or (3) excision and plastic repair of the cervical canal which contains the cystic infected glands and crypts (trachelorrhaphy). One type of operation is called conical excision, and is usually associated with the name of Sturmdorf. More recently, excision (conization) is carried out with a cautery wire so that bleeding is minimized, and yet the coagulation is so slight that sufficient tissue is obtained for microscopic study.

Chronic Pelvic Inflammatory Disease (*Chronic Pelvic Cellulitis, Parametritis*). —This lesion presents a diagnostic problem not only because of the variety of agents capable of producing it (gonococcus, tuberculosis, puerperal infections, etc.), but also because other lesions are so often confused with it, such as myoma of the uterus and other tumors, tubal pregnancy, ovarian cysts, etc. Its pathology is variable and may be confined to a diffuse fibrosis or induration, or it may consist of the presence of one or more abscesses, small or large, located in various parts of the pelvis. Malposition of the uterus is often associated. On pelvic examination induration or extreme hardness is felt very low in the pelvis, especially on either side of the cervix. A mass may be made out and, if tender and fluctuant, suggests the existence of an abscess.

The *clinical manifestations* as well as the physical findings often give no clue as to the etiology of the disease, which produces in general such nonspecific symptoms as backache, pain in the lower abdomen, tenderness in the pelvis and various menstrual disturbances. Leukorrhea alone may bring the patient to the physician. The disability, however, may occasionally be severe enough to provoke rest in bed. Frequently, no symptoms are produced except that the patient comes to the doctor because of sterility. In other patients evidence of chronic, long standing infection may be present, such as fever, emaciation, anemia, etc.

Differential diagnosis is of special importance in order to carry out effective therapy. The diseases to be considered (modified from Crossen[15]) are as follows: (a) *Chronic endometritis* is rare except when due to polyps, abortion, functional bleeding or malignancy. It is a cause of leukorrhea (when the cervix is normal), and of vaginal bleeding; it can often be diagnosed only by the examination of endometrial tissue obtained by curettage. The lesion is sometimes due to abnormal hyperplasia (fungous or polypoid endometritis). Treatment consists of removal of the primary lesion. (b) *Myoma of the uterus* produces symptoms of gradual onset; there is no fever or history of pelvic peritonitis; the mass is hard and not tender or fixed, and is a part of the uterus (see p. 963). (c) *Tuberculosis* is of gradual onset and there is no history of acute infection. The presence of tuberculosis elsewhere as well as general malaise and loss of weight is often suggestive. Encysted ascites is sometimes detected. (d) *Syphilis,* though rare, is suspected when syphilis is present elsewhere and the Wassermann reaction is positive. Occasionally, gonorrhea may also be present in these patients as an associated disease. (e) *Ovarian and broad ligament tumors* produce symptoms of gradual onset, there is no fever or much menstrual disturbance or history of pelvic infection. The mass is lateral and while fluctuant is not tender. (f) *Tubal pregnancy* besides its other features (see p. 972) is associated with a positive Aschheim-Zondek test; however, this is true in only 50 per cent of cases. (g) *Other conditions,* such as chronic appendicitis, mucous colitis, bladder and rectal disease, neurasthenia, etc., nearly always can be excluded by the absence of tenderness and other local signs, and by the manifestations characteristic of these conditions as noted elsewhere in the text.

Treatment of chronic pelvic inflammation, whatever the cause, may be conservative or operative. In many women satisfactory relief of symptoms may be achieved by nonoperative therapy, which consists of a number of palliative measures, such as bed rest, local applications of heat and general hygiene, including good food, plenty of fluids, and care of fecal stasis. In some patients the presence of pus low in the pelvis, especially in the cul-de-sac, will necessitate incision and drainage through the vagina.

The question of *abdominal operation* in these patients is less easy to answer. The presence of a tender mass obviously containing pus may require transperitoneal drainage in certain cases, *i.e.*, in patients with puerperal infections in whom a general septicemia from absorption is feared, and in whom vaginal drainage is impossible or inadequate. The danger of inducing a general peritonitis was greatly feared in the past, but this should not develop if the infection is well walled off, which usually occurs after a week or two, just as it does in appendiceal abscess. On the other hand, if abdominal operation is carried out for a tubo-ovarian

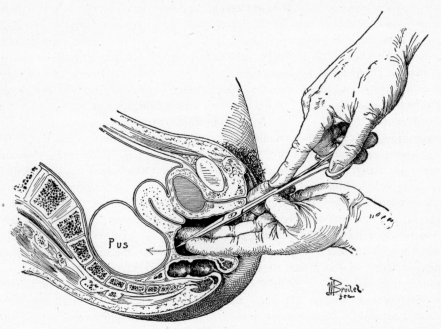

FIG. 537.—PELVIC ABSCESS; A COMMON LOCATION IN THE CUL-DE-SAC.

The drawing also shows the manner by which such an abscess may be drained (After Kelly).

abscess of nonpuerperal origin, complete removal of the inflammatory mass, rather than incision and drainage, should be done. Each patient, however, must be considered individually in making a decision as to the time for and the type of operation.

In absence of pus, as shown by the physical findings and clinical manifestations, the indications for abdominal operation in chronic pelvic inflammation are also often difficult to determine. A few general principles may be mentioned. If the infection is due to the gonococcus, conservative treatment is generally advisable, especially chemotherapy and artificial fever therapy which promise to supplant most of the older methods and to minimize the need for operation. Operation for removal of diseased tissue is only indicated after the lapse of several months or years, and even then only when the mass is clearly the source of symptoms which have not been relieved by conservative care. On the other hand, if the infection has followed a pregnancy, it is often due to the streptococcus, which in general contraindicates abdominal operation, even after the lapse of some time, unless specific lesions are mechanically producing the symptoms. Careful history and study of each patient should be carried out to determine the etiologic organism if possible. In any case, the avoidance of radical pelvic operations should be emphasized, particularly in younger women in whom sufficient ovarian tissue should be preserved to maintain its endocrine function, and enough of the Fallopian tube to make pregnancy possible. For the same reason the uterus should not be removed unless absolutely necessary. The tendency for promiscuous pelvic evisceration, particularly in younger women, is to be seriously condemned; plastic operations are often sufficient to relieve symptoms; conservative nonoperative care is frequently satisfactory.

NEOPLASMS

Tumors of the female genital organs comprise benign and malignant growths. They are best classified as they affect the various organs, uterus, ovaries, Fallopian tubes and vagina. Detailed discussion of pelvic tumors may be found in the monograph by Meigs.[16]

Uterus.—The most common benign tumors of the uterus are the myomas. (Endometriosis is described here since it may start in the uterus.) The malignant tumors are carcinoma, which is common, and chorio-epithelioma and sarcoma, both of which are rare.

Myoma (Fibroid Tumor, Fibromyoma).—This is the most common pelvic tumor (aside from pregnancy). It is essentially a benign neoplasm of the smooth muscle of the uterine wall, but nearly always contains a variable amount of fibrous tissue, hence its name. In some patients endometrial cells are found scattered through the tumor; the term adenomyoma is used in these cases (see also Endometriosis). Myomas may be single or multiple; they are nearly always encapsulated and can be easily shelled out when in the uterine wall, where they begin their growth (interstitial or intramural myoma). Their growth is slow and progressive, requiring years before they reach an appreciable size; when they grow toward the peritoneal surface, they are called subperitoneal myomas which comprises 20 to 30 per cent of all myomas. If they grow out still further, they may become pedunculated or even become attached to other structures, and lose their connection with the uterus (wandering or parastic myoma). If the tumor grows inward toward the lumen of the uterus, it is called a submucous myoma which also may become pedunculated; if it pushes into the broad ligament, it becomes an intraligamentary tumor. Only rarely (5 per cent) is myoma located in the cervix. Secondary changes which may occur in large myomas are necrosis, due to inadequate blood supply, hyaline changes and liquefaction, hemorrhage into the mass, sarcomatous degeneration, infection, suppuration and calcification, etc. Associated effects are due to attachments with or pressure on neighboring structures. In this way the ureters may be occluded, thereby producing urinary obstruction; the vessels or nerves to the lower legs may be compressed, producing various effects; the intestines may be involved in associated adhesions with the resultant production of intestinal obstruction.

Clinical manifestations may be absent when the tumor is small, or may be confined to menorrhagia, dysmenorrhea and slight leukorrhea. However, bleeding may be profuse and lead to secondary anemia. As the tumor grows, pressure symptoms develop which are often indefinite at first. Bladder irritability is common. Pain is a late symptom, but pelvic discomfort and backache, particularly on exer-

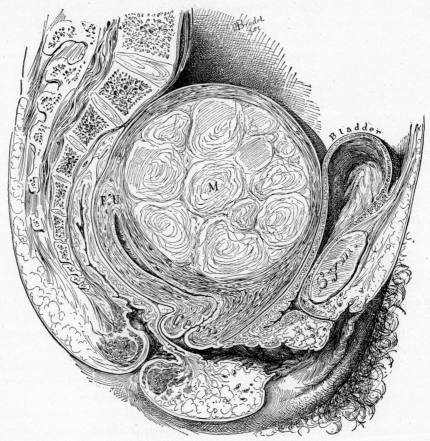

Fig. 538.—Large Globular Myoma Choking Pelvis, Compressing Rectum and Bladder and Forcing Bladder up into the Abdomen.

Note the retroflexion of the uterus (After Kelly).

tion, is not uncommon. Some women with the complaint of sterility are found to harbor a myoma. In a great many patients, however, the first manifestations of the myoma is the detection of a firm lower abdominal mass presenting usually just above the symphysis.

Diagnosis is made fairly easily by bimanual palpation of the pelvis. Examination should not only reveal the existence of the tumor, but also its location, extent and type. The tumor is to be differentiated from a normal pregnancy, cyst of the broad ligament, ovarian tumors, pelvic inflammatory disease and malposition of the uterus. Repeated examinations at reasonable intervals may furnish evidence as to the rate of growth and the development of secondary changes.

Treatment may not be indicated when the tumor is not producing symptoms. The diagnosis in these cases is usually made accidentally. However, if the tumor is in the cervix, removal is indicated for prophylactic reasons (Crossen). When the tumor is producing definite symptoms, treatment consists of palliative measures, operative removal and radiotherapy. Palliation is only indicated for temporary relief of symptoms, or when curative procedures are refused or impossible. Uterine astringents (ergot, etc.), vaginal douches and such measures are ineffective. Excision of the tumor by abdominal operation is a curative procedure, although in many instances when the myoma is large, adherent, or the site of secondary changes, the technical difficulties may be great. Excision is the form of treatment which is much to be preferred. Radiotherapy, however, is effective in certain selected patients. A thorough study has been reported by Corscaden,[17] who achieved satisfactory results in over 95 per cent of a series of cases comprising 30 per cent of his patients with myoma. In general, radiotherapy is used only in patients at or near the menopause, when the tumor is not too large, when there is no adnexal disease, and when symptoms, especially bleeding, require treatment. It should be emphasized, however, that in the presence of bleeding a diagnostic curettage must precede therapy in order to rule out malignancy.

Endometriosis (Endometrial Cyst).—This lesion is really not a neoplasm at all, but a cystic swelling which forms because endometrial tissue is implanted, misplaced or develops (by metaplasia) at various sites outside the uterus; secretions are formed at each menstrual period and may accumulate with a resultant gradual increase in size of the cyst. The bloody contents of the cyst change with time to a brownish color, giving rise to the term *chocolate cyst*. For a long time the pathogenesis of this tumor was unknown until the brilliant observations of Sampson [18] revealed its true mechanism, at least in those implantations occurring in the ovary and pelvic peritoneum. Endometrial tissue may penetrate the wall of the uterus by direct extension (adenomyosis), may escape through the tubes and become implanted anywhere in the pelvis or peritoneum; it may likewise spread by mechanical (operative) means, or by way of lymphatics and veins, or be displaced during embryonic life. The process of endometrial transplantation is often called endometriosis. The most frequent site of endometrioma is the ovary, but it has been found in the tubes, rectovaginal septum, rectum, sigmoid, broad ligament, round ligament, appendix, and even in the wall of the small intestine.

Clinical manifestations depend somewhat on the site of the cyst. Endometriosis is far more common than is generally suspected. Pain during and after menstruation is characteristic in most cases. Atypical pain which occurs only during the menstrual period should always excite a suspicion of endometriosis. Many cysts which are located on the right side are operated on with a diagnosis of acute appendicitis. Sudden rupture of the cyst into the peritoneal cavity may occur with transient collapse. Adhesions from partial rupture may produce intestinal obstruction. A correct diagnosis, however, is usually made only at operation, but even then only if the chocolate colored or bloody contents of the tumors are noted. In some cases only on microscopic study is the true nature of the lesion revealed.

Treatment consists of excision, taking precaution to prevent further implantation.

Carcinoma of the Uterus.—Uterine cancer is a common carcinoma, comprising 14 per cent of the deaths due to malignant disease of both sexes. It occurs more commonly in the cervix than in the body or fundus (5:1).

In the *cervix,* carcinoma produces ulceration and destruction of tissue, forming a fungating growth which invades by direct extension into the parametrium, and through the lymphatics into the iliac nodes, and through the blood stream to distant

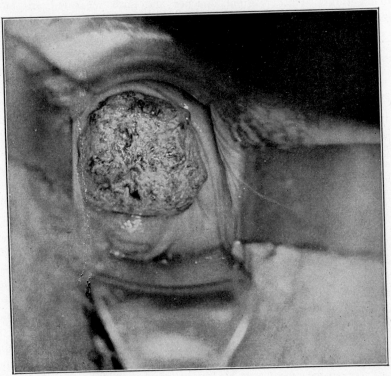

FIG. 539.—SQUAMOUS CELL CARCINOMA OF THE CERVIX.

Photograph of the view obtained by retracing the vaginal walls. The cervix is entirely replaced by malignant disease. The patient, aged thirty-two, had had leukorrhea for some time but only for a few months had it become, first brownish, and later red, in color. Biopsy confirmed the clinical diagnosis. Radiotherapy was instituted with satisfactory conversion of the diseased tissue to extensive scar. Complete destruction of the tumor, however, was probably not achieved (St. Louis City Hospital).

organs, including the lungs. There are two types, the squamous cell and the adenocarcinoma. The former arises from the vaginal portion of the cervix or the extension of the squamous epithelium just inside the external os; the latter arises from the cylindrical cells lining the glands in the cervical canal. Squamous-cell carcinoma is far more frequent (8:1).

Clinically, the first and most important manifestation is abnormal bleeding. The vaginal hemorrhage may be small in amount, not more than a mere "spotting," occurring between periods or it may be present as a menorrhagia. Recurrence of menstruation in women after the menopause is always a suspicious symptom and demands examination. Next in importance is leukorrhea, which may be overlooked by the patient until it becomes foul, profuse or blood-tinged, which occurs later. As indicated above, leukorrhea is most often due to chronic cervicitis; the role of such chronic irritation in the etiology of cancer, particularly of the squamous-cell type must be considered at least in older women in whom cancer of the cervix is common. Pain and other local manifestations of malignant disease of the cervix are usually present only in the terminal stages.

Diagnosis depends upon a careful direct visualization of the cervix by means of a vaginal speculum. Lesions which are not cancer usually respond rapidly to treatment. Chronicity, persistence and failure to heal are general features of malignant ulceration; progression of the lesion is often characteristic. However, delay in diagnosis is unjustified if there is any suspicion of cancer. Biopsy will lead to a definite diagnosis. The danger of spreading the malignant cells by biopsy is remote. Hyperplastic or deeply ulcerating lesions, particularly those which bleed easily when touched with an applicator, are considered cancerous. The presence of induration is also suggestive of malignant disease. However, in most cases, microscopical study of excised tissue is necessary, particularly if diagnosis is doubtful.

In treatment, radical excision (panhysterectomy) used to be advised, but was followed by a high mortality. In recent years the use of radium applied to the cervix, and deep x-ray therapy given through the lower abdomen and pelvis, has achieved a percentage of five-year cures which varies between 20 and 50 per cent; it is now the treatment of choice.

In the *body of the uterus* adenocarcinoma is fairly common, particularly after the menopause. At or before the menopause cervical carcinoma is more frequent but after the cessation of menstruation malignancy is about equally divided between the body of the uterus and the cervix. Any vaginal bleeding occurring at this period is always suggestive of malignant disease of the uterus. Diagnosis, however, depends on microscopic examination of tissue obtained by curettage. In the presence of a normal cervix (myoma and periuterine disease being excluded by palpation) chronic endometritis may produce bleeding and discharge which may be mistaken for carcinoma. This lesion, however, responds rapidly to conservative treatment in most cases. If bleeding persists, curettage should be performed for the purpose of diagnosis. Treatment of carcinoma of the body of the uterus consists of complete hysterectomy preceded and/or followed by radiotherapy. Excellent results have been obtained by radiotherapy alone in patients who are poor operative risks.

Chorio-epithelioma (*Deciduoma Malignum*).—This is a rare but exceedingly rapid-growing and fatal tumor of the uterus. It arises from the fetal cells covering the chorionic villi, and hence may occur weeks or months after normal delivery or miscarriage. It is especially likely to follow hydatidiform mole, a degenerative neoplasm related to the growth of the placenta which is well described in obstetrical texts (Williams). It produces persistent bleeding and early pain. Diagnosis is made only after curettage. The Aschheim-Zondek test is almost always positive; the test is always carried out in patients, delivered of hydatidiform moles. *Treatment* consists of complete hysterectomy, radiotherapy or both.

Sarcoma.—Sarcoma of the uterus may occur spontaneously, but usually forms at the site of a myoma. Rapid growth in a myoma should always suggest the development of malignant change. Sarcoma sometimes grows slowly. Diagnosis is often made only on section of the tumor. Treatment is surgical excision.

The Ovaries.—The ovaries are the site of a great variety of tumors, 95 per cent of which are cystic. A complete but brief classification is that reported by Gardner and Trout.[19] Besides the true neoplasms (both epithelial and mesodermal) which include benign and malignant groups, retention cysts occur commonly, and teratomas uncommonly, in the ovary. Inflammatory cysts (abscesses) have already been considered under chronic pelvic inflammatory disease. The pathology and clinical course vary in each type of cyst; but there are two complications which may occur in many of them: rupture of the cyst and rotation (torsion or twisting) of the pedicle.

Simple Retention Cysts.—These nonproliferating cysts comprise a variety of types. Among them are Graafian follicle cyst (due to failure of the follicle to rupture), corpus luteum cyst (due to failure of normal luteal absorption), and tubo-ovarian cyst (union of ovarian cyst and tube, usually of inflammatory origin). These cysts are small, rarely larger than an egg, and produce no special symptoms, except, on occasion, abnormal bleeding. They are noted during laparotomy most commonly, and are frequently resected leaving as much normal tissue as possible.

Cystadenoma (Ovarian Cyst, Proliferating Cyst).—Cystadenoma represents a benign epithelial neoplasm which is the most common of the true ovarian tumors. There are several types: the small unilocular type is called simple serous cystoma which is rarely larger than an infant's head; the larger multilocular type is called pseudomucinous cystadenoma and represents the classical ovarian tumor whose removal really established gynecology as a specialty, and paved the way for other abdominal operations. Many cysts contain proliferating epithelial masses, and represent a special group which are called papillary tumors or papillomata. Some are pedunculated; a few are located in the broad ligament. Para-ovarian cysts originate in the tubular remains of the embryonic Wolffian body and account for 10 per cent of excised cystic tumors of the ovary. Most cysts of the broad ligament are paraovarian in origin. The pathology of the various tumors is fairly complex and a great many variations have been described. Many grow to a large size if untreated, because of the accumulation of serous or pseudomucinous fluid within the cystic areas. They occur at any age, but are most common between the twentieth and fiftieth year. The small serous cysts are usually bilateral.

Clinical manifestations are dependent on the size of the tumor; when sufficiently large it produces mild symptoms of pelvic discomfort which brings the patient to the doctor for examination. The small serous cyst may remain stationary and produce few manifestations; the proliferating cysts grow slowly, usually taking several years to reach an appreciable size, but never cease growing. In the late stages the large amount of fluid contained in the cyst may be mistaken for ascites. In many patients the growth of the tumor simulates a normal pregnancy; menstrual disturbances are not infrequent. Bimanual pelvic examination usually suffices to make the diagnosis. The pedunculated cysts, however, are so freely movable that the origin from the pelvis may be difficult to demonstrate except at operation. On rare occasions gradual rupture of a cyst may occur, thereby resulting in adhesions to neighboring structures. Sudden rupture may produce the picture of an acute abdominal emergency; more commonly torsion of the pedicle is responsible for acute symptoms. Torsion of the pedicle which is more common in the smaller cysts, including the retention and simple serous cysts, produces severe lower abdominal pain, nausea, vomiting and leukocytosis, provided the twist is sufficient to interfere with the blood supply. If gangrene occurs, the patient may become prostrated and develop true shock. In a few instances the twisted pedicle occludes small intestine, thereby producing the manifestations of acute intestinal obstruction. The palpation of the mass may be sufficient to make the diagnosis.

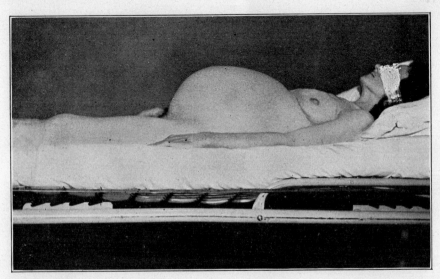

FIG. 540.—OVARIAN CYST; LARGE MULTILOCULAR, PSEUDOMUCINOUS TYPE.

Note the characteristic manner in which the swelling rises sharply from the symphysis; this is not present in abdominal distention and ascites. The patient, a forty-eight-year-old housewife, eight months previously, noted a small tumor just above the pubis; it grew steadily to its present size. Edema of the feet and ankles developed more recently. At operation a large cystadenoma was removed as well as a myomatous uterus and the opposite adnexa. Recovery was uneventful (Gynecological Service, Barnes Hospital).

Differential diagnosis in the small ovarian cysts includes consideration of tubal swellings which are due to inflammatory disease (salpingitis, pyo- and hydrosalpinx), tubal pregnancy, myoma, retroverted pregnant uterus and broad ligament cyst. In the larger cysts, such conditions as abdominal distention (paralytic ileus), obesity, ascites, pregnancy, degenerated cystic myoma, and abdominal tumors (hydronephrosis, hydrops of the gallbladder, etc.) are to be considered. Ascites, however, is often associated with malignant ovarian tumors which are described on page 971. In a few cases the nature of the tumor will not be recognized until laparotomy.

When acute torsion of the pedicle of an ovarian cyst occurs, the differential diagnosis demands consideration of acute appendicitis, rupture of ovarian cyst or pus tube, renal or gallstone colic, acute intestinal obstruction with strangulation, ruptured ectopic pregnancy, mesenteric thrombosis, etc.

Treatment of ovarian cyst is urgent when torsion of the pedicle or acute rupture occurs, and consists of immediate laparotomy with excision of the tumor. Under ordinary circumstances removal of the smaller ovarian cysts is indicated in order to prevent further growth, the danger of torsion, and finally because of the danger of malignant degeneration. The small bilateral cysts which produce little or no symptoms rarely justify laparotomy, but if they are resected, all of the remaining normal ovary should be left, particularly in younger individuals.

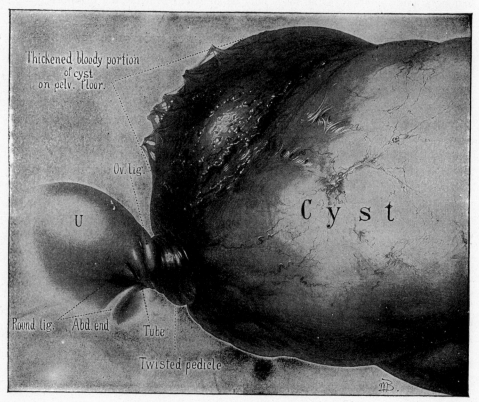

FIG. 541.—ACUTE TORSION OF AN OVARIAN CYST.
The pedicle includes also the uterine tube, ovarian and round ligaments (After Kelly).

Dermoid Cysts.—While dermoid cysts may produce symptoms similar to those already mentioned, they are quite different pathologically. They occur at any age, and are in reality *teratomas* in which the skin elements predominate. They are more likely to become infected than other cysts, and being more adherent are often more difficult to excise. They seldom undergo malignant change. Treatment consists of excision of the tumor, preserving ovarian tissue, if possible.

Solid Tumors.—Solid tumors comprise the remaining neoplasms of the ovary. They are extremely rare, comprising but 5 per cent of all neoplastic diseases of the ovary which come to operation (Crossen). The benign growths are the *fibroma* and *myoma* which are usually small and are diagnosed only at operation or by microscopic section. *Granulosa cell tumors,* because of their endocrine effects are discussed in Chapter XXX.

Carcinoma of the ovaries may rarely develop as a primary solid tumor, usually of the medullary type. Most frequent is the carcinoma which forms in a cystadenoma possessing papillary ingrowths. This type is called malignant papillary cyst, and presents the same clinical manifestations as a cystic tumor of the ovary. The true diagnosis is often made only on microscopic study of the excised cyst. A third group comprises tumors which occur in both ovaries, but which are secondary to cancer elsewhere in the peritoneal cavity, most commonly in the uterus or intestines. When they assume a scirrhous form, they are associated with the name of Krukenberg. Sarcoma has also been observed in the ovary and is important in children, in that it comprises nearly one-half of ovarian neoplasms in early life.

Early diagnosis in malignant disease of the ovaries is nearly always difficult if not impossible on clinical grounds alone, unless operation is performed, at which time the true nature of the tumor can often be ascertained by gross inspection. Frequently, however, the existence of malignant disease becomes evident only after study of the microscopic sections, especially in the case of cystic tumors which have become malignant. In the late cases the presence of severe pain, extensive masses, or marked ascites is frequently noted. Treatment consists of excision; radiotherapy is also used.

The Fallopian Tubes.—Tumors in this location are exceedingly rare and are usually mistaken for the various neoplasms which originate in the ovaries, uterus or broad ligaments. The small cysts or hydatids of Morgagni are seen at the fimbriated end of the tube, but have no clinical significance.

The Vagina.—Solid tumors are so rare as to require no special consideration. Malignant disease is usually secondary to that of the cervix, although primary carcinoma occurs, usually on the posterior wall. Squamous-cell carcinoma is seen in the vulva (see p. 980). Cystic tumors are not so rare, and comprise epithelial inclusion (epidermoid) cysts which form in the scar following lacerations or perineal operations; cysts arising in the glands of the vaginal wall are rare; congenital cysts due to embryonic inclusions are likewise uncommon. Bartholin's gland cyst at the vaginal outlet is not infrequent and is described under diseases of the vulva.

MISCELLANEOUS CONDITIONS

Normal Pregnancy.—Though the main concern of the obstetrician, normal pregnancy not infrequently is encountered by surgeons because it may simulate acute abdominal disease. In some instances the patient may not herself be aware of the true diagnosis; in a few women, such knowledge is withheld in the hope that an operation may be performed which will result in abortion. Abdominal pain, vomiting, local tenderness, muscle spasm and leukocytosis may lead to a diagnosis of acute appendicitis. Even if the history is unreliable, bimanual examination will rarely fail to establish the true state of affairs.

If the diagnosis is not urgent, any doubt may be dispelled by the Aschheim-

Zondek test which consists of the injection of the patient's urine (or blood) into a young immature female rat, which is killed eighteen to forty-eight hours afterwards. If the patient is pregnant, characteristic changes will be seen in the ovaries. In the Friedman test, a modified Aschheim-Zondek procedure, a rabbit is utilized. A positive test will be obtained even in the early weeks of pregnancy. A negative test (especially when repeated) rules out pregnancy in 85% of cases.

Ectopic (Extra-Uterine) Pregnancy.—When a fertilized ovum lodges and grows outside the uterine cavity, the patient suffers from an ectopic pregnancy which obviously cannot result in a normal delivery. In nearly every instance serious symptoms develop within a few weeks or months after conception because of bleeding which arises from erosion of the vessels by the trophoblast or from rupture of the tube due to distention. The hemorrhage may be either sudden

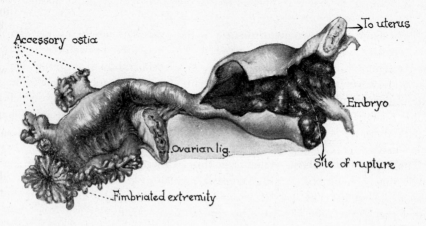

FIG. 542.—ECTOPIC (TUBAL) PREGNANCY; SPECIMEN REMOVED AT OPERATION.

Inside the ruptured blood clot, the tiny embryo could be made out on careful gross inspection. The patient, aged fifteen, was suddenly seized with acute abdominal pain in the right lower quadrant, thirty hours before admission. The pain remained severe and was referred to the upper abdomen and under the shoulder blades; prostration, shock and pallor developed rapidly. The erythrocyte count was 1,500,000. At operation the peritoneal cavity contained a great deal of clotted blood.

and profuse, slow and persistent, or encapsulated. The ovum is most commonly lodged in the Fallopian tube (tubal pregnancy) but may develop in the peritoneal cavity (abdominal pregnancy) or in the broad ligament. The etiology of ectopic pregnancy is nearly always mechanical, of a type which interferes with the passage of the fertilized ovum through the tube into the uterus. Inflammatory adhesions are often thought to be the most common cause, though careful work has shown that various malformations (diverticula) play the most important role (Mc-Nalley [20]). The pathology varies with the location of the fetus as well as its viability. When the mass ruptures but remains encapsulated in the tube, the sudden symptoms will subside, and a local mass will form (tubal abortion). A localized hematoma in the broad ligament or cul-de-sac or a tubo-ovarian hematoma may form in a similar manner. Not infrequently, rupture into the peritoneal cavity occurs, thereby causing a sudden intra-abdominal hemorrhage with collapse and manifestations of surgical shock. If the patient recovers, or the bleeding is slow, a marked secondary anemia develops. It is rare for ectopic pregnancy to proceed to term without rupture, but when this occurs, it is usually an abdominal pregnancy.

Clinical Manifestations.—As indicated, the clinical manifestations vary with the pathologic and physiologic changes. Before rupture occurs, the patient may be asymptomatic, or note only the signs and symptoms of early pregnancy, *i.e.,* amenorrhea, slight pelvic pain, increasing nausea, pain in the breasts, general malaise, etc. In some patients there will be a history of previous pelvic inflammatory disease. Bimanual examination will often be diagnostic, not only in detecting a mass, but also in revealing a soft, succulent cervix and a uterus which is slightly enlarged. However, because of the paucity of symptoms, it is rare for a patient to consult a physician with an unruptured tubal pregnancy. In most instances acute rupture of the growing ovum produces sudden and severe manifestations which are the first indication of disease; the diagnostic accuracy of the Aschheim-Zondek test is unfortunately of little practical value in such cases because it requires too much time to carry out when an immediate diagnosis is necessary.

Acute rupture often occurs after some exertion, but may develop spontaneously. The clinical manifestations in the severe cases are of dramatic suddenness, the patient falling to the ground in profound collapse. Unlike the collapse following rupture of a peptic ulcer, there is evidence of circulatory shock of the type due to severe hemorrhage. The pulse is rapid and weak, the blood pressure low, the extremities are cold and moist, the skin extremely pale, and air hunger is present. Nausea and vomiting are frequent because of the peritoneal stimulation by the blood. The abdomen is tender to palpation and may be distended with fluid. Pain is, of course, severe, but usually unilateral. Pelvic examination reveals the presence of a bulging, boggy mass in the cul-de-sac; an adnexal tumor may also be palpable. A bloody vaginal discharge is often present. Aspiration of pure blood from the cul-de-sac is often of considerable diagnostic aid.

In less severe cases, the patient recovers rapidly from the initial collapse because of cessation of bleeding and the efficient encapsulation of the blood clot. In many patients recovery is slow and accompanied by signs of marked secondary anemia. Occasionally there may be no acute manifestations of rupture, the patient gradually becoming weaker and more anemic. In these patients an erroneous diagnosis of tuberculosis or cancer may be made. The Aschheim-Zondek test is of especial value in this type of patient, provided that the fetus is still viable.

Differential diagnosis in acute rupture rests between the following diseases: (*a*) Ruptured peptic ulcer is extremely rare in women and is not accompanied by circulatory shock. (*b*) Abortion has a similar history, but the pain which consists of intermittent cramps is localized to the region of the uterus and gradually increases in intensity. Vaginal bleeding may be present in either abortion or ectopic pregnancy, but is much more profuse in the former condition. Pelvic examination is obviously important. (*c*) Acute exacerbation of chronic salpingitis is accompanied by little or no prostration and no circulatory collapse; the pain is usually bilateral. (*d*) Acute appendicitis is accompanied by no pelvic signs and produces characteristic gastro-intestinal symptoms and signs. (*e*) Torsion of an ovarian cyst is apt to be confusing, but the history is different; there is no anemia, and pelvic examination reveals a normal cervix and uterus, as well as the location of the mass, which is higher in the pelvis than is an ectopic pregnancy.

Treatment.—If the diagnosis is certain, patients with an unruptured tubal pregnancy should be subjected to laparotomy and the mass excised. In this way the almost certain danger of rupture is avoided. When rupture has resulted in an encapsulated hematoma, further bleeding may stop provided the embryo has ceased growing. However, even though bleeding has ceased, laparotomy is usually necessary in order to remove the placenta and other tissue so as to prevent hemorrhage at a later date. In the acute cases laparotomy is indicated as an emergency procedure in order to prevent death from shock. Treatment of the shock is carried out at once and is continued during and after the operation; the intraperitoneal blood may be used as soon as it is obtained (autotransfusion), provided, of course, it is not clotted. The most difficult cases technically are those in which the placenta is attached to the peritoneum rather than to the tube.

ENDOCRINE DISTURBANCES

The most important advance in gynecology in recent years has been the investigations of the hormones which govern the activities of the genital organs. These studies which were to a large extent initiated by Born, Fraenkel and Leo Loeb, and recently developed by Edgar Allen, Doisy, Corner, Evans and others, have explained much regarding the mechanism of menstruation and the changes following conception and pregnancy. Moreover, it is now recognized that many conditions, previously ill-understood or attributed to organic disease and uterine malposition, are in reality due to endocrine disturbances. Many of these patients can be satisfactorily treated by administering the hormone which is absent. Diagnosis is obviously important, but extremely difficult in most instances. Direct analysis of blood or urine to determine the amount of hormones is possible, but laborious. There is no test as simple as the basal metabolism test which determines the presence of hypo- and hyperfunction of the thyroid. Great strides in the identification of conditions caused by ovarian dysfunction will no doubt be made within the next few years. The clinical evidences of abnormal endocrine function are only partly useful. The menstrual flow itself is only one manifestation of ovarian hormone activity. Changes in the endometrium are useful, but are detectable only by curettage. In the mammary gland, endocrine effects can be determined only to a slight extent by palpation; accurately, only by biopsy. Thus, much of the status of our knowledge of endocrine disturbances is incomplete and complicated, because of intrinsic difficulties in measuring their clinical manifestations. A few general principles, however, have been established and these will be briefly described. Further details may be found in publications by Allen [21] and others. The chapter on endocrines should also be consulted, especially page 896.

The ovary, as the essential female sex gland, has two functions, the maturation of the germ or ovum (ovulation) and the production of hormones. The latter function is responsible for the development of secondary sex characteristics, and governs the periodic changes in the uterus (menstruation), in the mammary glands and other organs. This periodicity (roughly twenty-eight days) is one of the important features of ovarian activity. The stimulus to the ovary is the presence of gonadotropic hormones produced periodically by the pituitary which is thus often referred to as the "motor of the ovary." A delicate balance exists between the hormones of the ovary and pituitary which is described below. Other endocrine glands, such as the thyroid and adrenal, also exert important, though lesser influences on the ovary and pituitary. Indeed there is growing evidence that a balance exists between many if not all endocrine glands—an interesting general phenomenon which is made still more complicated by the influences exerted on them by the autonomic nervous system.

In gynecology the cyclic production of ovarian hormones, controlled in turn by the pituitary, are responsible for the periodic changes in the uterus and breast. The mechanism is somewhat complicated but fairly well understood. Before explaining this mechanism it may be useful to enumerate a few of the hormones, many of which have been isolated in crystalline form and indeed synthesized. The pituitary hormones which activate the ovary are two in number, one of which is a follicle-stimulating hormone, the other a luteinizing hormone. The ovaries also produce two hormones, one of them comprising a group called estrogens which originate from the Graafian follicles and the corpus luteum, the other is progesterone which originates in the corpus luteum alone. Progesterone (formerly called progestin) was first isolated in pure crystalline form in 1934 by Wintersteiner and Allen.[22] The important part of the mechanism of these two groups of hormones, as far as their cyclic behavior is concerned, is the reciprocal relationship they bear to each other by which the pituitary stimulates the ovary to produce hormones which in turn inhibit the pituitary thus setting at rest (for a while) the stimulus to ovarian activity. The consequent fall in the production of ovarian hormones then removes the inhibition from the pituitary, which begins to act again and the ovary is then stimulated, completing the cycle.

Thus the cyclic changes in the uterus and breast are due to the periodic increase and decrease of the ovarian hormones governed in turn by the reciprocal stimulation and suppression of pituitary activity. Of the changes in the uterus, vascularization and hyperplasia are stimulated by the estrogens whereas secretion of the uterine glands are due to the presence of progesterone. These changes cease with the fall in the hormone concentration which also corresponds with the appearance of the menstrual flow; the onset of menstruation has been shown to coincide with the diminution of the ovarian hormones. The ebb and flow of the ovarian and pituitary hormones thus accounts for the regular cycles which occur in normal females. It is obvious that with this cycle the hyperplastic changes in the uterus and breast are succeeded by involution or regression back to the resting stage. In the breast, absence of this regression or hypoplasia may result in a nodular condition of the parenchyma, usually called chronic cystic mastitis (see Chap. XXVIII). When pregnancy occurs, the cycle is temporarily upset and under these conditions the large amounts of gonadotropic hormone are produced by the placenta. This hormone, called prolan, should really be referred to as "human chorionic gonadotropin." This secretion begins immediately after conception, and because the presence of prolan can be detected easily by its effect on the ovary of an immature rat (Aschheim-Zondek test), the diagnosis of pregnancy can be made by analyzing a specimen of blood or urine in this way. As pregnancy proceeds, the amount of prolan excreted in the urine increases, reaching its maximum by the second month and then recedes but continues to be large.

The difficulties in applying this knowledge to gynecologic disturbances are due not only to the number of hormones involved, but particularly to their balanced relationship. Thus we may consider not only the effects of overactivity and under-activity of the ovaries, but also an imbalance between the pituitary and ovaries. These factors make diagnosis more difficult. Therapy is complicated, too, by the delicacy of the threshold for these hormones; a certain dose will produce one effect whereas a larger dose quite a different one, dependent partly upon the stage of the cycle in which they are given, but also on other factors, such as their effect on the activity of other organs. By analyzing the urine and blood for the content of ovarian and pituitary hormones over a long period of time, Frank and his co-workers have produced evidence of over- and underfunction of the ovaries which seems of definite value in correlation with the clinical symptoms present. An excellent discussion of endocrine therapy in gynecology is that of Hamblen.[23]

Ovarian Underfunction.—Diminution of ovarian function may be produced by x-ray or radium therapy to the pelvis, or by diseases such as chronic infections or undernutrition. It may likewise be due to congenital underdevelopment. Ovarian activity is abolished of course after surgical extirpation (artificial menopause), and normally tapers off during the normal menopause. Underfunction may be due to primary pituitary disease. The important clinical manifestations of ovarian underfunction are sterility (including certain types of miscarriage), amenorrhea (including oligomenorrhea and dysmenorrhea) and the menopause.

Sterility.—Underfunction of the ovulating mechanism may be responsible for sterility in that mature ova are not produced; if produced, they may not be discharged because of failure of the Graafian follicle to rupture. These patients may present no other clinical evidences of underfunction; menstruation may be normal. This type of underfunction may be due to hypofunction of the thyroid, but is also due to insufficient pituitary stimulation; the latter, however, is difficult if not impossible to determine.

It must be emphasized, therefore, that sterility is due to many causes, which must be considered and evaluated by thorough study before diagnosis and treatment are possible. On the other hand, many instances of miscarriage may be due to progesterone deficiency which is readily replaced by daily administration of the hormone. Since the placenta produces considerable quantities of progesterone after the third month such therapy is not necessary after this time.

Dysmenorrhea.—Painful menstruation may be produced by any of several causes. Stenosis of the cervix and malposition or the uterus are important factors. In other instances it may be due to ovarian underfunction; if this is definitely determined, treatment with the missing hormone, ovarian or pituitary is indicated. Dysmenorrhea, however, may be present with excessive menstruation which is usually considered to be due to abnormal function of the ovaries (see p. 977). In a number of patients with dysmenorrhea the etiologic factor has been allergic; relief has followed elimination of substances to which the patient is sensitive.

Amenorrhea.—Lack of menstruation is a symptom which, in itself, should produce no disability. It occurs normally during pregnancy and in many nonpregnant women, without interfering with general health. Similarly, oligomenorrhea or scanty menstruation may be present without clinical significance unless the patient is concerned about it psychologically; in sterility, of course, it assumes considerable importance. Amenorrhea may be due to ovarian insufficiency of ovarian origin (maldevelopment), debilitating systemic disease, or to the absence of pituitary hormone; however, other causes, inflammatory, neoplastic and operative (hysterectomy), must obviously be excluded before a diagnosis of endocrinopathy can be considered. Treatment obviously depends upon which condition is responsible; detection of the cause should be established, if possible, by thorough study. Clinical manifestations of ovarian activity such as changes in the uterus, breasts, etc., occurring in spite of complete amenorrhea, are grouped together and called *molimina;* they consist of engorgement of the breasts, pelvic heaviness and periodic leukorrhea. Evidence of the cyclic production of ovarian hormones has been found in these patients.

Other symptoms may accompany amenorrhea which occurs at the menopause, especially when an artificial menopause has been tragically and often needlessly produced in young women by gynecological *furor operativus.* These clinical manifestations consist of a variety of neurovascular, psychic and other disturbances which are frequently severe enough to demand therapy. Obviously pituitary medication is useless. True substitution organotherapy is indicated. This was attempted decades ago by H. A. Kelly, who gave such unfortunate young women sandwiches spread with minced hog ovaries obtained from an abattoir close to the Johns Hopkins Hospital. It is now known, of course, that such attempts at replacement therapy of missing hormones were entirely useless because the dose was completely inadequate. To be effective ovarian hormones must be given in sufficiently large amounts, and this is now done by administering them in relatively pure form. In treating menopausal symptoms the estrogens are most useful and widely employed. Stilbesterol, a new compound, synthesized by Dodds and his co-workers, has also been found to exert therapeutic estrogenic effects, although its toxicity is still the subject of some disagreement (MacBryde and associates [24]).

Functional Uterine Bleeding.—Abnormal bleeding from the endometrium, due to disturbances in ovarian function occurs frequently during adolescence and the climacteric. The bleeding may be prolonged and profuse. The endometrium usually shows no progestational change [26]. In most instances the ovaries contain numerous graafian follicles, but no corpora lutea, indicating that the abnormal bleeding is associated with a failure of regular periodic ovulation and corpus luteum formation. The bleeding is almost invariably painless, especially in young individuals, can be interrupted and the cycle restored to normal by the use of progesterone [27, 28]. On rare occasions, excessive production of estrin may be due to *granulosa cell tumors* of the ovary which is discussed on page 938.

DISEASES OF THE VULVA AND VAGINA

Identification of diseases of the vagina and vulva is, as a rule, more simple than is the case with the diseases of the internal pelvic organs, chiefly because the lesions are external and are easily examined by direct inspection. Many of the diseases have already been considered in detail. An excellent discussion of diseases of the vulva is that of Taussig.[25]

Vulvovaginitis.—The vulva and vagina are rarely subject to primary inflammation, although they are frequently the site of secondary lesions. Redness of the external genitalia, edema, pain and heat are similar to the cardinal signs of acute inflammation anywhere in the body, although the signs are more superficial, rarely involving the deeper structures. The symptoms of pain and burning, when present, are usually aggravated by walking. Many of these patients, whether adults or young girls, will present such manifestations because of a *gonorrheal infection* as already described. The inflammation is due to invasion by the gonococcus only in the primary stages of the disease; in the later stages the manifestations are due to the irritant effect of the vaginal discharge which originates in most instances not from the vagina but from the cervix. Indeed, any irritating vaginal discharge, whether of gonorrheal origin or not, is apt to be the main factor in producing a vulvitis. In some cases irritating urine is apt to be an important cause. In many instances vulvitis is secondary to other irritating mechanisms, such as pediculosis, masturbation, chafing, uncleanliness, etc. Skin lesions of various sorts may be present in the external genitalia and set up an acute inflammatory reaction; some are secondary to the acute exanthemata. Treatment consists of local care, but particularly removal of the cause.

Simple vaginitis is a term used to describe a primary inflammation of the vaginal mucosa, and is actually a rather rare disease. Inspection reveals the reddened, inflamed, vaginal wall; the etiology may be apparent. Occasionally an injury, a foreign body or irritating douches may be the cause of the inflammation. In many patients a flagellated protozoa (*Trichomonas vaginalis*) has been found in the discharge; in these instances the term *trichomonas vaginitis* is used. The etiologic role of this organism has not been scientifically established; while many observers attribute to it a primary etiologic importance, others claim that it is a secondary invader. The vaginal discharge in these cases is particularly profuse and is thin and watery in character. Various forms of local therapy (cleanliness, vaginal douches, antiseptics, etc.) are advocated; it is generally agreed, however, that persistence and a long period of time are necessary before the organism can be permanently eradicated. As in every disease, the exciting factor in the production of the lesion should be searched for and eradicated when possible.

In older women the vagina becomes atrophic. Occasionally the walls adhere to each other; the term *adhesive vaginitis* is applied to this condition.

Injuries.—Trauma due to childbirth has already been described. In the vulva, lacerations are nearly always located in the perineal body or located in the posterior part of the vaginal outlet. Other injuries are encountered following rape or from penetrating or lacerating wounds which children sustain in climbing trees and fences. They present the same problems of treatment as wounds sustained in other parts of the body.

Ulcers.—As in the extremities and elsewhere, ulcers are found in and about the vulva; they present a similar and often a complicated diagnostic problem, except that circulatory factors are generally absent (see Chap. VII). *Simple ulcers* are usually due to trauma or pyogenic infection, and heal rapidly on removal of any irritating factors. Frequently, simple ulcers are produced at the vaginal outlet because of excessive and irritating vaginal discharge. Ulcerations due to *chancroidal* infection and lymphogranuloma venereum are also encountered; in either instance the lesion may be single or multiple. The ulcer of a chancroidal infection is apt to be large, deep and undermined, whereas the ulcers produced by lymphogranuloma are small (see p. 99). Ulcers due to syphilis may be primary or secondary, *i.e.,* the *chancre* and *flat condyloma.* In both, the causative organism may be demonstrated in dark field illumination of the discharge from the lesion. The chancre has a hard indurated base and is single.

The flat condyloma (condyloma lata) represents multiple rounded elevations with a flat plateau surface, grayish and moist. When in the vagina, it is called a mucous patch, similar to the lesion of the mouth in secondary syphilis. The Wassermann and Kahn reaction is positive at this stage. It is easily distinguished from the condyloma acuminatum, which is described below. It should be emphasized, however, that most of the perineal lesions which are called condylomas (except the flat syphilitic type described above, and the venereal warts described below) are in reality due to *lymphogranuloma venereum,* which has been described in Chapter VI.

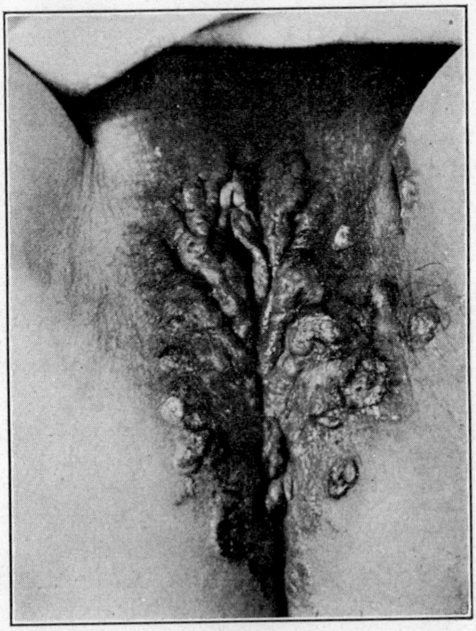

. A type of chronic ulceration which is associated with an overgrowth of skin and subcutaneous tissue is called *chronic hypertrophic ulcerative vulvitis.* It is probably due to chronic lymphangitis and is therefore a type of *elephantiasis,* a term, however, which is used only when the overgrowth of tissue becomes tremendous.

FIG. 543.—CONDYLOMA LATUM.

Secondary luetic lesions of five weeks' duration, around the vulva, in a thirty-five-year-old housewife followed a definite history of exposure; severe itching was the only complaint. The Wassermann reaction was positive. The lesions disappeared within a few days after intensive antiluetic therapy (St. Louis City Hospital).

Treatment depends on the symptoms produced by its size; surgical excision may be indicated. *Granuloma inguinale* also occurs about the vulva and is considered in detail elsewhere (p. 105).

Condyloma acuminatum (venereal wart) is a papillary and hence conical (rather than flat) skin lesion which is single or multiple, and consists of an overgrowth of the epithelial layer of the skin; unlike the true wart or verruca vulgaris, it does not penetrate the layers of the skin, but extends out from its surface. It is usually associated with lack of cleanliness and the presence of an irritating leukorrhea, especially that due to gonorrhea. Superficial ulcers may form which cause some discomfort; otherwise the warty overgrowths produce no symptoms. Local cleanliness and treatment of the discharge is all that is needed in the way of treatment in many cases. Others, however, are more resistant and require local excision, electrocoagulation or chemical cauterization.

Kraurósis is a term frequently used to describe a lesion in the vulva which in reality should be called *leukoplakic vulvitis,* which has a definite histology and clinical appearance (Taussig). As mentioned below it is to be considered as a definite precursor of carcinoma. Hyperplasia of the outer skin layers is supplanted later by atrophy. Most of these patients suffer from pruritus; dyspareunia also occurs. Treatment consists of excision of the diseased skin (vulvectomy); this is particularly important in order to prevent the development of carcinoma.

Neoplasms and Cysts.—All the various benign tumors, such as fibroma, lipoma, hemangioma, etc., have been found in the vulva and even in the vagina. Malignant disease is confined to squamous-cell carcinoma.

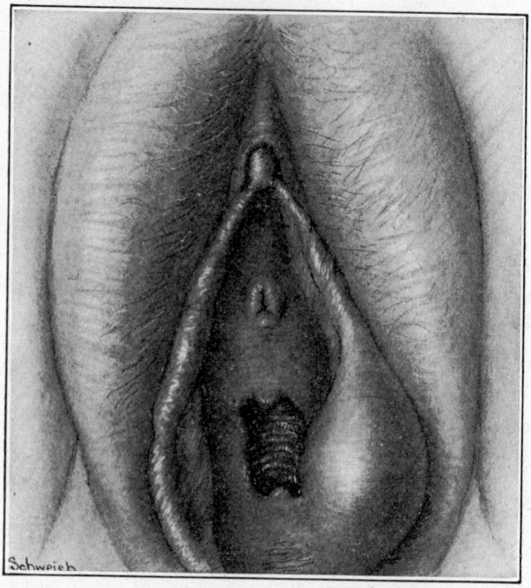

FIG. 544.—BARTHOLIN'S GLAND ABSCESS.

Note the characteristic location. The patient, a twenty-three-year-old housemaid, contracted gonorrhea several weeks previously, but suffered very little disability until severe pain, aggravated by walking, developed with the appearance of a tender mass in her vulva several days before. Incision and drainage resulted in immediate relief; the causative organisms were found in the pus.

Carcinoma of the vulva is an important though rare type of squamous cell tumor and occurs usually only in older women; occasionally it is of the adenocarcinoma type. It is so often preceded by leukoplakia, that early diagnosis should be relatively easy. Excision of the vulva is thus advisable in all cases of leukoplakia or kraurosis in order to eradicate the lesion before it undergoes malignant change (Taussig). Treatment of the lesion when definitely carcinomatous should include excision of the regional lymph nodes, as well as radiotherapy.

Cysts are nearly always confined to Bartholin's glands which are located on either side, just inside the posterior portion of the labia. Bartholin's glands normally produce a mucoid secretion which lubricates the inner labial surfaces; they are not infrequently the site of infection, forming abscesses which produce the usual acute manifestations and often require incision or open spontaneously. These abscesses are nearly always associated with acute gonorrheal infections. If the opening of one of Bartholin's glands becomes occluded because of inflammation, or if an acute abscess subsides without drainage, a Bartholin cyst may develop. Such a tumor is rarely of large size, but may cause sufficient discomfort to demand excision.

A soft swelling which is present in the labia may really be due to a *pudental hernia* or to a hydrocele of the canal of Nuck. These lesions have been described

PRURITUS VULVAE

981

elsewhere (see p. 788). Swellings due to varicose veins are also seen, particularly during pregnancy.

Pruritus Vulvae.—Itching of the vulva presents somewhat the same problem as pruritus ani (see p. 712). The severity varies greatly, but often assumes serious proportions. Detection of the cause is obviously important and a thorough history and physical examination is a *sine qua non*. Pruritus is not a disease, but only a manifestation of a disease, the nature of which may require much study before it is detected. In many patients the cause will be found in the presence of irritating vaginal discharge or of irritating urine, especially in diabetics. Skin diseases of various types, such as eczema, leukoplakia, or kraurosis may be present. Lack of cleanliness, foreign bodies, fungus infection and many other factors are sometimes of importance. Treatment consists of the eradication of the cause and the application of soothing lotions and cleanliness; fungicides may be indicated in some cases. Persistent cases may require more radical therapy.

BIBLIOGRAPHY

1. CROSSEN, H. S. *Diseases of Women*, C. V. Mosby Co., St. Louis, 1930.
2. KELLY, H. A. *Gynecology*, D. Appleton & Co., New York, 1928.
3. CURTIS, A. H. *Textbook of Gynecology*, 2nd ed., W. B. Saunders Co., Philadelphia, 1934.
4. MILLER, C. J. *Introduction to Gynecology*, C. V. Mosby Co., St. Louis, 1931.
5. GRAVES, W. P. *Gynecology*, W. B. Saunders Co., Philadelphia, 1923.
6. ALLEN, EDGAR. Menstruation, *J. Am. M. Ass.*, 104:1901, 1935.
7. KELLY, H. A. *Loc. cit.*
8. SMITH, C. T., HARPER, T., and WATSON, A. Sedimentation Time as an Aid in Differentiating Acute Appendicitis and Acute Salpingitis, *Am. J. M. Sc.*, 189:383, 1935.
9. DESJARDINS, A. U., STUHLER, L. G., and POPP, W. C. Fever Therapy for Gonococci Infection, *J. Am. M. Ass.*, 104:873, 1935.
10. LEWIS, R. M. Study of the Effects of Theelin on Gonorrheal Vaginitis in Children, *Am. J. Obst. & Gynec.*, 26:593, 1933.
11. TeLINDE, R. W. The Treatment of Gonococcal Vaginitis with Estrogens, *J. Am. M. Ass.*, 110:1633, 1938.
12. ALLEN, EDGAR, and DIDDLE, A. W. Ovarian Follicular Hormone Effects on the Ovaries, *Am. J. Obst. & Gynec.*, 29:83, 1935.
13. GREENBERG, J. P. Tuberculous Salpingitis; a Clinical Study of 200 Cases, *Johns Hopkins Hosp. Reports*, 21:97, 1921.
14. SCHWARZ, O., and DIECKMAN, W. J. Puerperal Infection Due to Anaerobic Streptococci, *Am. J. Obst. & Gynec.*, 13:467, 1927.
15. CROSSEN, H. S. *Loc. cit.*, p. 690.
16. MEIGS, G. V. *Tumors of the Female Pelvic Organs*, The Macmillan Co., New York, 1934.
17. CORSCADEN, J. A. Failures Following the Treatment By Radiation of Cases of Benign Uterine Bleeding and Fibromyomata, *Am. J. Roentgenol.*, 45:661, 1941.
18. SAMPSON, J. A. Perforating Hemorrhagic (Chocolate) Cysts of the Ovary, *Arch. Surg.*, 3:245, 1921.
19. GARDNER, G. H., and TROUT, H. F. In Kelly's *Gynecology*, *loc. cit.*
20. McNALLEY, F. P. The Association of Congenital Diverticula of the Fallopian Tube with Tubal Pregnancy, *Am. J. Obst. & Gynec.*, 12:303, 1926.
21. ALLEN, EDGAR. *Sex and Internal Secretions*, Williams and Wilkins Co., Baltimore, 1932.

22. WINTERSTEINER, O., and ALLEN, W. M.   Crystalline Progestin, *J. Biol. Chem.,* 107:321, 1934.

23. HAMBLEN, E. C.   *Endocrine Gynecology,* C. C. Thomas, Springfield, 1939.

24. MACBRYDE, C. M., FREEDMAN, H., LOEFFEL, E., and CASTRODAL, D.   The Synthetic Estrogen Stilbesterol, *J. Am. M. Ass.,* 115:440, 1940.

25. TAUSSIG, F. J.   In Curtis' *Obstetrics and Gynecology,* Vol. 3, W. B. Saunders Co., Philadelphia, 1933.

26. BURCH, J. C. and PHELPS, D.   A General Concept of the Etiology of Functional Menstrual Disturbances, *South. Med. Jour.,* 35:150, 1942.

27. ALLEN, WM. and HECKEL, G. P.   The Effect of Progesterone in Young Women in Functional Uterine Bleeding, *Am. Jour. Obst. & Gyn.,* 44:984, 1942.

28. JONES, G. E. S. and TELINDE, R. W.   An Evaluation of Progesterone Therapy in the Treatment of Endometrial Hyperplasia, *Bull. Johns Hopkins Hosp.,* 71:282, 1942.

CHAPTER XXXII

THE GENITO-URINARY SYSTEM

Kidney	*Epididymis*
Bladder	*Testicle*
Prostate	*Penis*
Seminal Vesicles	*Miscellaneous Lesions of the*
Urethra	*Genito-urinary System*

The early use of operative procedures (cystostomy for stone) and mechanical instruments (crude sounds and catheters for urinary obstruction) in ancient times represented greater accomplishment in the treatment of surgical diseases of the genito-urinary organs than of any other organ. However, the physician's ignorance of physiologic principles, and the poor results obtained, allowed even the sound principles to be discarded. Without special instruments the inaccessibility of the urinary organs naturally made progress slow. However, the invention of the cystoscope by Nitze [1] in 1889, and the perfection of the technic of ureteral catheterization by Albarran,[2] as introduced a few years previously by numerous independent workers, were the means of instigating rapid development in the knowledge of the diseases of the urinary system and their treatment.

Methods of Examination.—Because of accessibility of the organs of the genitourinary system and their simplicity of function, numerous procedures for examination have been devised. These methods of examination have been largely responsible for the exactness of diagnosis which exists in genito-urinary surgery to a greater degree, perhaps, than in most other specialties. A definite routine, however, should be adopted and carried out methodically in steps as follows:

1. History and physical examination.

2. Urinalysis: In the male the "two glass" test is made. The first glass contains enough urine to wash accumulated pus from the urethra whereas the second glass contains only bladder urine (plus any excessive amount of urethral pus); a comparison of the two glasses often enables a differentiation between urethritis and cystitis and the degree of each. If urinalysis is necessary in an acute emergency and the patient cannot void, catheterization may be justified. In the female catheterization is always indicated for microscopic examination especially in the presence of a vaginal discharge; otherwise a voided specimen may be used for routine urinalysis.

Unless urine is examined when fresh, inaccurate and often misleading results may be obtained particularly in the search for bacteria, because many types of organisms may multiply sufficiently in an hour or two, to give the erroneous impression of a massive bacteriuria. The routine urinalysis includes the staining of sediment, determination of pH (*i.e.,* acid or alkaline), search for pus cells, albumin, etc.

3. Rectal examination: The tone of the sphincter is estimated in male or female. In the male the size and shape of the prostate and seminal vesicles are noted and prostatic fluid is expressed and examined at this time. If the rectal examination precedes the routine urinalysis, microscopic blood may be found and prove confusing.

4. Measurement of residual urine: In certain cases it is necessary to know how much urine is left in the bladder after voiding. This is known as "residual" and is drawn off by catheterization which, however, must be done within a minute or two of voiding, particularly if the patient has recently drunk considerable fluids.

5. Cystoscopic examination: The introduction of cystoscopic (retrograde) pyelography consisting of the passage of small catheters through the cystoscope into the ureter and kidney followed by the injection of radiopaque solutions (Voelcker and Lichtenberg[3]) has been very helpful in the diagnosis of renal lesions. Sodium iodide and bromide (Cameron[3]) were originally used but have been largely supplanted by organic compounds of iodine as mentioned below.

Cystoscopic examination includes the visual inspection of the bladder and ureteral orifices, collection of fractional urines, excretory (phenol red) tests, and a variety of roentgenograms, in different positions.

6. Intravenous pyelography: The discovery by Von Lichtenberg and Swick[4] that uroselectan (a compound containing 42 per cent iodine by weight), when injected intravenously, is secreted so rapidly by the kidney as to make the urine impervious to the x-ray has to a great extent displaced cystoscopic pyelography, because of the pain produced by the instrumentation of cystoscopy and the occasional reaction (fever, chills, etc.) produced by it. Various types of organic compounds of iodine, including diodrast, neo-iopax, and hippuran are used for intravenous pyelography. The adult dose of the three drugs is 7, 15, and 15 grams respectively. Although the intravenous method is used as a routine, the retrograde method may be necessary when accurate detail in the pyelogram is needed, *e.g.,* the early stages of tuberculosis and neoplasms of the kidney.

KIDNEY

In general there is a clearer understanding of the surgical diseases caused primarily by the kidney than those caused by practically any other organ, because the function of the kidney is limited to one important process, namely, excretion of urine. The amount of kidney tissue necessary to carry on the normal excretory function is no greater than one-half of one kidney, but the reserve amount of renal tissue is of extreme importance in combating the effects of disease. The amount of urine excreted depends upon the amount of fluid ingested, but on certain occasions a diminution of the amount excreted may definitely signify acute renal impairment. Especially is this true when comparisons of the amount secreted by each kidney is made by ureteral catheterization. The phenosulphonphthalein excretion test (Rowntree and Geraghty[5]) may be of great value in detecting certain types of disease. Normally the two kidneys should excrete 40 per cent of 1 cc. of a 6 per cent solution of phenosulphonphthalein within an hour after intramuscular injection. This test is of even greater value in determining the extent of renal damage when the dye is given intravenously with ureteral catheters in place. Normally the dye should appear in the urine from each kidney two to six minutes after injection; at the end of fifteen minutes about 15 per cent of the total amount should have been excreted by each kidney. When renal insufficiency exists in each kidney, there may be a suffi-

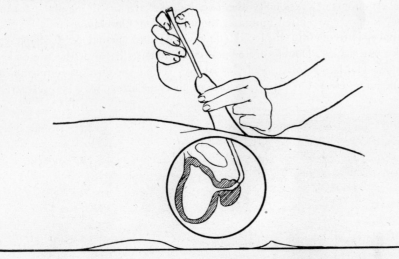

FIG. 545.—TECHNIC OF CATHETERIZATION IN THE MALE.

Note the sharp curve made by the membranous and prostatic urethra; this angulation adds to the difficulties of catheterization, particularly when enlargement of the prostate is present.

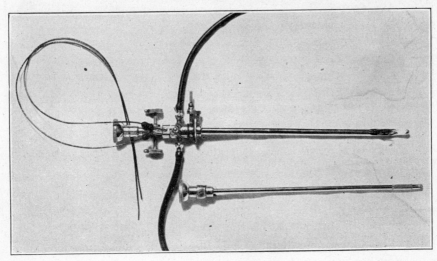

FIG. 546.—PHOTOGRAPH OF A CYSTOSCOPE WITH URETHRAL CATHETERS IN PLACE IN THE INSTRUMENT.

cient retention of nitrogenous compounds (urea, creatinin, uric acid, etc.) to produce a demonstrable increase in the blood stream. An elevation of the nonprotein-nitrogen in the blood (normal of 35 to 45 milligrams per 100 cc. of blood) is an accurate method of detecting bilateral renal damage, or a urinary retention, especially the common type produced by prostatic hypertrophy. The nitrogen retention in such instances may be merely an expression of urinary retention in the absence of permanent renal damage, but is a good criterion for the determination of operability, etc.

Anomalies.—Congenital anomalies of the kidney are very common and often produce symptoms. Occasionally the two kidneys are fused together, forming a horseshoe kidney, most often united at the lower pole. One kidney may be small or rudimentary, is frequently displaced (downward) and anomalous in shape (round or mushroom shape). Double ureter and congenital stricture of the ureter are not uncommon. The latter condition is, of course, serious because of its complications (pain, infection, etc.). On rare occasions an aberrant artery may be present and by

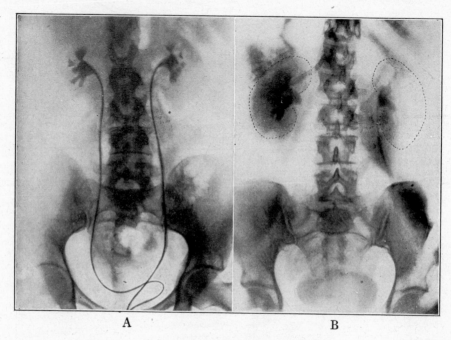

A   B

FIG. 547.—NORMAL PYELOGRAMS.

A, after injection of sodium bromide through ureteral catheters (retrograde pyelography);
B, after intravenous injection of 6 grams of diodrast (brand of iopyracyl).

pressure produce a kink of the ureter. Frequently nephroptosis (movable kidney) is present at birth; on other occasions there is apparently sufficient deficiency in the structures supporting the kidney that the organ becomes displaced downward later in life (see p. 997). Many of these anomalies produce few or no symptoms and may therefore not be detected except at autopsy or at operation performed for other conditions. Of the manifestations produced by anomalies, pain and urinary infection are perhaps most frequently encountered. Treatment is therefore determined by the symptoms produced; on rare occasions conservative measures fail, and it may be necessary to resort to such radical procedures as nephrectomy. Obviously, nephrectomy should never be performed until it has been established definitely that another kidney is present and is functioning adequately.

Injuries of the Kidney.—Although the kidney lies in a protected position adjacent to the vertebral column and above the margin of the lower ribs, it is injured frequently. On most occasions the injury is of a crushing type, although not infrequently it is of a penetrating type (*e.g.,* gunshot injury). There may be no external evidence of injury in the former case, but a history of a blow over the region of the kidney can usually be elicited. The type of injury sustained by the kidney varies from a microscopic tear in the organ to complete division, laceration or maceration. Degree of destruction, subsequent scar, and urinary leakage are the important points.

The *clinical manifestations* are dependent upon the extent of the injury, and upon whether the peritoneal cavity has been entered. Hematuria is the most constant symptom. Microscopic tears may produce no manifestations except hematuria and slight tenderness over the kidney. When the injury is extensive, the patient may present all the manifestations of shock, including tachycardia, low blood pressure, pallor, weakness, etc. Hemorrhage is no doubt the most important factor in the production of these symptoms. Extravasation of urine of significant amount occurs rather infrequently and adds to the severity of the early symptoms. If the injury to the kidney is associated with a tear through the posterior peritoneum, the symptoms and signs are apt to be more acute because of the increased amount of hemorrhage and the peritoneal irritation. On most occasions, even in the absence of a rupture of the peritoneum, there will be definite manifestations of early peritonitis, including localized abdominal tenderness, muscle spasm, nausea, vomiting and leukocytosis. These manifestations appear to be caused primarily by direct irritation of important nerves by the retroperitoneal hemorrhage, and not because of the urinary extravasation, because identical findings are encountered frequently in hemorrhage associated with fracture of the spine. (See also page 749.)

X-ray examination after the intravenous injection of one of the organic iodine compounds mentioned on page 984 will frequently be of value in revealing the site and extent of injury provided significant escape of urine is taking place.

The *treatment* is likewise dependent upon the extent of the injury. In the absence of severe manifestations operation is not necessary; the patient may be treated by bed rest alone, even though considerable hematuria is present. The spontaneous reparative process in the kidney is considerable, provided the injury is not too severe and has not involved the peritoneum. However, if hematuria is accompanied by marked signs of peritoneal irritation or by a progressive development of shock, it is safe to assume considerable injury to the kidney has been sustained; an operation will therefore be indicated to prevent further bleeding and serious peritoneal extravasation, as well as to repair anatomic defects, *i.e.,* lacerations. An incision through the anterior abdominal wall may be advisable because of the likelihood of simultaneous injury to other organs within the abdomen. Simple lacerations should be repaired by interrupted sutures, whereas severely injured kidneys should be removed. Drainage through a stab wound in the loin should be established to prevent accumulation of urine or bloody fluid. Failure to operate in the serious cases may allow the development of a perinephric abscess, or if the peritoneum is ruptured, a fatal peritonitis. As long ago as 1903 Watson [6] noted that in patients with a severely damaged kidney the mortality was remarkably lower in those operated upon than it was in those treated conservatively without operation. On the other hand, in the lesser injuries the patient will recover completely with rest in bed alone. Therefore, the decision as to operation depends on the extent of the injury as indicated by the manifestations presented by each individual patient.

Infections (Nontuberculous) of the Kidney.—The various infections of the kidney may be classified into (1) *pyelitis,* (2) *pyelonephritis,* (3) *pyonephrosis,* and (4) *carbuncle* of the kidney; but such a division is arbitrary and inaccurate since these diseases, with the exception of the latter, on most occasions merely represent various stages in one infectious process, and are usually associated with obstruction to the urinary flow. For example, a persistent pyelitis practically never

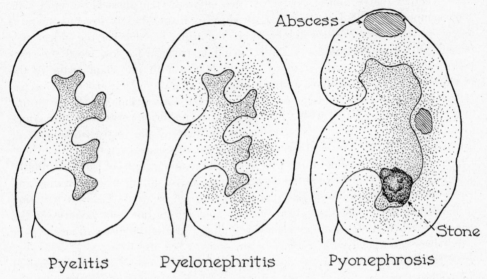

Pyelitis   Pyelonephritis   Pyonephrosis

Fig. 548.—Drawing to Illustrate the Three Common Types of Nontuberculous Infection of the Kidney.

From the drawing it appears that the three diseases represent increasingly severe grades of the same process; this, indeed, is true in a large percentage of cases. The term pyelitis is confusing because a certain degree of parenchymal infection undoubtedly exists in most instances of pyelitis, but is of insufficient degree to impair function. In pyelonephritis and pyonephrosis, infections in which the parenchyma is significantly damaged, function may be severely impaired. Stones may or may not be present. A variable amount of hydronephrosis accompanies pyonephrosis.

exists without also a pyelonephritis, except on occasions when the infection is induced by ureteral catheterization. The accompanying pyelonephritis may be slight and limited to the central portion of the kidney adjacent to the pelvis. The term pyonephrosis is applied to that type of infection associated with ulceration about the calices, abscesses in the parenchyma, and a thinning of the cortex due to hydronephrosis. The function of the kidney is least disturbed if the infection is limited primarily to a pyelitis and impaired to the greatest extent in pyonephrosis in which the loss of function may be complete and permanent. The colon bacillus is the causative organism in over three-fourths of the patients. The streptococcus and staphylococcus account for most of the remaining cases.

Infection may gain access to the kidney in one of *three* ways: (1) the blood stream, (2) by ascending infection, or (3) by way of the lymphatics. Since most of the infections are produced by the colon bacillus it would appear that on most occasions the organisms are carried to the kidney by the lymphatics which surround the ureter, or by anastomotic channels between the colon and kidney. However, it is probable that an additional factor, *i.e.,* urinary stasis due to obstruction, is necessary before an actual infection develops.

Urinary obstruction, thus, may be responsible for the development of the three main types of infection; obstruction may be produced in various ways: (1) Calculous obstruction of the ureter (usually at the ureterovesical orifice), or of a calix in the pelvis of the kidney, is one of the most common causes of obstruction. (2) Congenital stenosis at the ureterovesical orifice is a frequent anomaly. (3) A kink may be produced in the ureter by nephroptosis. (4) Anomalies such as double ureter, bifid pelvis, aberrant renal artery, etc., may result in obstruction to the normal flow of urine. (5) Abdominal masses including neoplasms, pregnant uteri, abscesses, etc., may press directly upon the ureter.

The experimental production of hypertension by renal ischemia by Goldblatt [7] and associates has placed an additional responsibility upon the urologists. Numerous clinical reports (Nesbit and Ratliff [8]) are now available of cures of hypertension following removal of a kidney affected with chronic sclerosing pyelonephritis, proving that renal ischemia was undoubtedly produced by the lesion. Obviously, operative therapy is feasible in such cases only when examination reveals a normal kidney on the other side.

Clinical Manifestations.—There is no uniformity in the early symptoms produced by the infections designated as *pyelitis, pyelonephritis* and *pyonephrosis.* Frequently the onset is sudden with a chill, fever, nausea, vomiting and severe pain in the region of the kidney, but radiating downward to the thigh or genitals. On other occasions the onset is insidious with fever, lassitude, weakness, anorexia, loss of weight, etc. In either case there is a tendency for the infection to persist along with the symptoms unless eliminated by proper therapy. The urine contains bacteria and pus cells, usually early in the disease and in large numbers. Frequently, red blood cells are found. Albumin is rarely present in more than slight amounts. Pyelitis is extremely common in young girls. When the infection involves the right kidney and is associated with pain, it may simulate appendicitis; extreme care must be exercised to arrive at a correct differential diagnosis. However, as stated in more detail below, the presence of pus cells in the urine and tenderness over the loin will usually lead to a correct decision. In most instances pyelitis subsides without the development of more than a trivial infection in the kidney parenchyma, and with very little residual change.

If the infection persists, regardless of treatment, and a hydronephrosis occurs, the cortex gradually becomes destroyed and thinned out and very little urine is excreted. This process may continue until all function ceases and an *autonephrectomy* is established, *i.e.,* the infected organ becomes encapsulated to a great extent by scar tissue and little absorption from the infection takes place. When the function is destroyed to the extent that little or no urine is excreted, pus cells but no bacteria may be found in the urine.

Diagnosis.—Examination of the urine is perhaps the most reliable method of establishing a diagnosis. Bacteria and pus cells will be found except in the instances mentioned above. It must be remembered, however, that bacteria and pus cells may be found in various other diseases, including prostatitis, urethritis, etc. A leukocytosis is usually present. Tenderness, and in acute cases, muscle spasm will be demontrable over the infected kidney. Cystoscopic examination including inspection of the ureteral orifices, ureteral catheterization and a search for bacteria in a stained smear of urinary sediment from each kidney obtained by centrifugation may be of great value in establishing the diagnosis. The amount of urine obtained from the infected kidney and the excretion of phenolsulphonphthalein will be diminished late in the disease, when considerable renal damage is present, for example, pyonephrosis or severe pyelonephritis.

Occasionally when a complete block of the ureter occurs, the infected urine cannot enter the bladder; only the clear urine from the other kidney will then be voided. Sooner or later, however, the escape of pus will lead to its detection in the urine; repeated urinalysis is often necessary, therefore, before making a negative diagnosis of infection.

When considerable pain is present, differential diagnosis between infections of the kidney and such intra-abdominal lesions as appendicitis may be difficult. There are several features, however, which should allow one to make the correct diagnosis. For example, the pain associated with a renal lesion usually radiates downward toward the thigh or genitals and the tenderness is confined posteriorly. Fever is present much earlier in the onset of the disease than it is in appendicitis. The presence of fever alone, especially if associated with a chill, will rule out many of the intra-abdominal lesions of alimentary tract origin since they are usually associated with pain, and few have chills.

Treatment.—One of the most important features in the treatment of renal infections is *chemotherapy,* a procedure extremely valuable in the treatment of urinary infection of all types because these drugs are largely excreted by the urinary route. Of the group of drugs used at the present time, sulfathiazole and sulfadiazine are most commonly used, sulfathiazole being slightly more effective (Helmholz [33]). Sulfadiazine produces less systemic reactions of the type including headache, vertigo, nausea, etc., but is more apt to result in renal complications such as hematuria and ureteral obstruction by precipitation of crystals. Administration of sodium bicarbonate is recommended by Herrold [9] and others to increase the solubility, and therefore decrease the precipitation of crystals. The intake of a copious amount of fluids (*e.g.,* 3000 cc. per day) will decrease the precipitation of sulfadiazine crystals. The dose should be about 70 grains the first day, but need be no more than 45 to 60 grains per day thereafter. Details of therapy may be found elsewhere [9, 10, 36]. Neither drug is very effective against the streptococcus fecalis. When the infection is resistant to sulfonamides, mandelic acid may be tried.

Occasionally, changing the reaction of the urine appears to be effective in relieving bladder irritation. It may be made alkaline by small doses of sodium bicarbonate (1 to 3 grams daily), or acid with acid sodium phosphate (1 to 2 grams daily) or ammonium chloride. In combination with either of the latter two drugs, methenamine in doses of 2 to 3 grams daily is frequently given because of its effect as a urinary antiseptic. The degree of acidity or alkalinity of the urine can readily be determined by testing the color reaction with selected dyes.[9]

When the infection is acute and associated with ureteral obstruction, the insertion of a ureteral catheter is extremely effective in its elimination by establishing drainage. It is frequently difficult to determine whether significant obstruction is present, yet its presence or absence must be determined since ureteral catheterization performed in the absence of obstruction may aggravate the symptoms as well as the infection. Sudden onset of fever and other symptoms, accompanied by severe pain, usually signifies the presence of a urinary obstruction at some point (usually in the ureter). Diagnosis is confirmed if ureteral catheterization reveals a retention of more than a few cubic centimeters of urine in the pelvis of the kidney. Occasionally, it will be advantageous to leave the ureteral catheter in place for two or three days. Bed rest, care of the bowels, and other symptomatic treatment is employed as indicated. Operative treatment is justified only when the function of the kidney is jeopardized or destroyed. If no function remains, nephrectomy is performed after acute symptoms have subsided. If adequate drainage cannot be established by ureteral catheterization and the infection is so fulminating as to threaten destruction of the kidney, nephrostomy may be a wise procedure.

Carbuncle of the kidney is the fourth type of nontuberculous infection, is commonly of hematogenous origin and pathologically resembles a cellulitis. There is usually a history of a furuncle or carbuncle on the skin several days preceding the onset of symptoms. As would be expected, the causative organism is usually the staphylococcus. In a small series of 8 cases, 7 of which developed a perinephric abscess (see below), Lazarus [11] was able to isolate a staphylococcus from the pus in every instance. The manifestations are much less variable than those of the other types of renal infection already mentioned. Symptoms are insidious and consist primarily of fever, malaise, anorexia and mild, dull pain in the region of the kidney. Tenderness over the kidney posteriorly is a fairly constant finding and is therefore significant diagnostically. Leukocytosis is usually present. Urine examination may reveal pus cells and erythrocytes, but is commonly negative at the onset. The absence of pus cells in the urine is frequently of considerable aid in differentiating this from other types of infections in which pyelitis is the predominating lesion. Treatment is limited to the nonoperative therapy as described above, except when a perinephric abscess is present. Exploration of the kidney may be justified when a carbuncle of the kidney is suspected, on the assumption that an abscess in the kidney or perinephric space exists.

Perinephric (Perirenal) Abscess.—Infection of the perirenal space may be produced by any of several mechanisms, but perhaps the most frequent source is a "carbuncle" of the kidney which in its invasion throughout the cortex finally breaks through the capsule. Frequently it appears that a small abscess, resulting from suppuration in a carbuncular infection, or from a tiny infected embolus, breaks through the cortex. Less commonly the infection perhaps arises from infected emboli lodging initially in perirenal tissue, or results from rupture of a pyonephrosis through the thinned cortex.

The pain associated with a perinephric abscess is variable, is usually located posteriorly in the region of the kidney, but may be so mild as to escape detection by the patient. The pain may be aggravated by bodily movements; the patient and even the physician may thus be led to interpret the pain as originating in the spine. Because of the muscle rigidity, a diagnosis of spinal arthritis or tuberculosis of the spine may erroneously be made. Tenderness posteriorly over the kidney associated with spasm of the lumbar muscles is quite constant, and is significant because of the lack of positive abdominal findings. Fever develops early, is variable in amount, but may be associated with a chill at the onset. Leukocytosis is usually pronounced. Examination of the urine rarely reveals any pathologic findings, and is of no diagnostic aid. After the abscess has been present for some time, many systemic manifestations become prominent. Anorexia and nausea are usually pres-

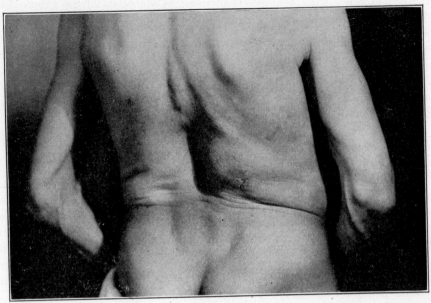

FIG. 549.—PERINEPHRIC ABSCESS ON THE RIGHT.

Note the bulging abscess which has perforated through the deep fascia and is "pointing" posteriorly. The patient, a forty-year-old-male, complained of pain in the back, anorexia, fever, and increasing weakness of three months' duration. No urinary symptoms were present and urinalysis was persistently negative. Incision and drainage were carried out with uneventful recovery; the staphylococcus was isolated from the pus.

ent, but vomiting is not so common. The patient becomes weak and pallid, complains of lassitude and rapidly loses weight. If the abscess increases in size, induration of the deep tissues over the kidney may be demonstrable. On rare occasions the abscess may eventually present anteriorly, thereby masquerading as an appendiceal or liver abscess. The pus may burrow through a small defect in the deep fascia posteriorly and present superficially as a bulging mass. When this happens, fluctuation is demonstrable, but rarely before; in reality, such a superficial mass is a part of a collar button abscess.

The *treatment* of a perinephric abscess is drainage by operation posteriorly over the kidney as soon as the diagnosis can be made. One or two large cigarette drains are placed in the wound and left in place for five or six days until the abscess cavity is largely obliterated, and drainage insignificant. Diagnostic aspiration, if carefully carried out, is occasionally justified in doubtful cases. If possible, the operator should explore for an associated renal carbuncle.

Nephrolithiasis.—Kidney stones may be composed of any of the urinary components; uric acid, calcium oxalate and calcium phosphate are common, xanthine and cystine less so. Usually solitary and ovoid, the stone, when large, tends to assume the shape of the pelvis and calices. Small stones less than 1 cm. in diameter frequently find their way into the ureter and pass into the bladder.

Little is known of the actual cause of renal calculi, except that on most occasions stasis and infection appear to be important. One type, which is called a "primary stone" (commonly composed of uric acid, calcium oxalate or urates) occurs in children or young people apparently in the absence of infection or stasis; they are perhaps of metabolic origin. Also metabolic are the large stones, which may be bilateral, seen in hyperparathyroidism (see page 919). The so-called "secondary stones", commonly composed of calcium phosphate, are apt to be associated with stasis or infection and may be deposited around a primary stone as a nucleus. That calcification of pre-existing lesions of the renal papillae may be the cause of stone is the conclusion of Randall and associates [30], who studied 609 autopsies and found calcium plaques in the papillae in 22.9 per cent, and small stones attached to the papillae in 8 per cent.

Clinical Manifestations.—The manifestations of renal calculi are extremely variable. In many instances stones are carried in the kidneys for years without producing any symptoms (see Fig. 550). More commonly, a mild infection develops in the pelvis about the stone and gradually involves the cortex of the kidney until a severe pyelonephritis develops. If the stone is large, or several are present, the infection may progress to a pyonephrosis, resulting in the ultimate destruction of the kidney. Mild fever, pain, malaise and anorexia are usually present. Pus, casts and a variable amount of albumin are present in the urine. Frequency of urination and mild burning pain usually accompany infection of this type. Diagnosis can almost invariably be made by plain x-ray film since practically all of these stones contain sufficient calcium to be radiopaque.

The most dramatic manifestation of renal calculi is that spoken of as *renal colic* which is brought about by the entrance of a stone into the ureter and its passage downward to the bladder. The pain is most excruciating and usually radiates toward the thigh or genitals. The stone may pass rapidly into the bladder, often within a few hours, occasionally in two or three weeks, or become permanently lodged near the kidney or at the ureterovesical orifice. Hematuria is a constant finding and is an important sign, but is not diagnostic because it is frequently present in such diseases as purpura, hemophilia and vitamin C deficiency, as emphasized by McKenna and Birch [12]. If the stone is not passed rapidly, infection may develop and pus as well as bacteria will be found in the urine. At least a mild degree of frequency of urination and burning is present. Fever is absent except when obstruction has been present long enough to allow the development of infection. Regardless of the size of the stone, an obstruction to the flow of urine develops at the onset because the impaction produces a total ureteral occlusion. However, as the ureter dilates, the urine may pass around the stone, even though it remains lodged in the ureter. In either case hydronephrosis develops almost invariably, and if the obstruction to the flow of urine is complete, may be serious because of infection, the development of which is encouraged by urinary stasis. If this condition is not relieved, the hydronephrosis and back pressure in themselves may become so marked as to permanently destroy the function of the kidney. On rare occasions the stone produces sufficient ulceration in the ureter during its passage as to lead to stricture formation later on after healing takes place. Differentiation of renal colic from other acute abdominal conditions can usually be made readily by history, urine examination and X-ray.

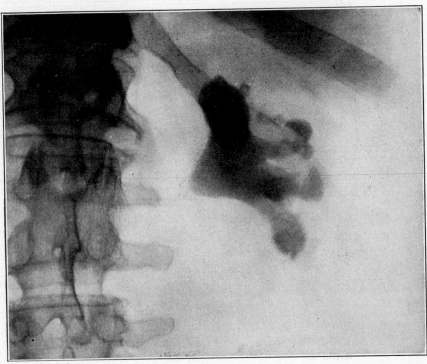

Fig. 550.—Roentgenogram, Revealing a Renal Calculus Filling the Entire Pelvis.

In this patient the finding was an incidental one; the film was taken only because of a supposed acute injury to the spine. Such stones produce variable manifestations; not infrequently no symptoms whatever are present. Hyperparathyroidism, though a rare disease, is frequently accompanied by stones of this type.

Treatment.—Unless the renal stone is "silent," treatment should be directed toward its removal. Most stones which have entered the ureter will pass spontaneously into the bladder by the institution of conservative treatment such as forcing fluids, sedation, etc. During the attack of colic enormous quantities of morphine may be required to control the pain. If, after many days, there is no evidence of progression in the descent of the stone, ureteral catheterization may be instrumental in dislodging it. Occasionally, dilatation of the ureter with a bougie, or several ureteral catheterizations will result in spontaneous passage of the stone. On rare occasions an operation (usually extraperitoneal with incision into the ureter) will be necessary to remove the stone. Large stones in the kidney cannot be passed by way of the ureter and if symptoms are produced, may necessitate operation. This is best done by a posterior incision in the loin, and removal of the stone by incision into the pelvis (pyelotomy). The opening in the pelvis is then repaired and the wound closed around a drain. On rare occasions when a ureteral stone has produced a complete urinary obstruction and thereby threatens to produce permanent damage to the kidney, it may be necessary to perform an emergency nephrostomy or a pyelotomy, and suture a small soft rubber tube in place for drainage. The stone in the ureter can then be removed at a later date. If the function of the kidney is permanently destroyed, nephrectomy is usually indicated after acute infection has subsided. If the stones are present in both kidneys it is usually preferable to operate first on the kidney with the poorer function, since the operation may produce a temporary anuria; if the better kidney is the one operated on first, and this complication (*i.e.,* temporary anuria) results, a fatal outcome may ensue.

Higgins [13] has reported a method of dissolving or breaking up renal calculi by giving the patient an acid ash diet with a high vitamin A content. This diet consists of certain fruits, including oranges, lemons, grapes, etc., large quantities of butter and cream, and vegetables high in acid ash. If this diet does not maintain the pH of the urine down as low as 5, sodium acid phosphate or ammonium chloride must be given in addition. However, other observers (Oppenheimer and Pollack [14]) have not been able to obtain favorable results.

Hydronephrosis.—Although the dilatation of the kidney pelvis or calices in hydronephrosis is usually caused by obstruction to the urinary flow, it is a fact that in many instances infection appears to be a responsible factor even in the absence of demonstrable obstruction. Prostatic hypertrophy and stricture of the urethra may produce hydronephrosis, but the damage inflicted by infection in these instances is more significant than the hydronephrosis. However, in ureteral obstruction "no distensible bladder intervenes to distribute the pressure, and infection is often entirely absent; so that the aseptic dilatation of kidney and ureter progresses rapidly and unobscured" (Keyes [15]). The obstruction may be ureteral and be produced by a variety of causes: (1) stones, tumor or trauma, (2) kink of the ureter due to nephroptosis, congenital malformation (megaureter with or without stricture), and (3) extrinsic pressure (aberrant vessels or tumors).

As the hydronephrosis progresses the cortex becomes thinned and function impaired, but not to a degree proportionate to the thinning of the cortex. On many occasions the cortex may be nothing more than a mere shell; yet there may be few if any demonstrable manifestations of impairment of renal function. A sudden complete obstruction produced by a stone or by accidental ligation of the ureter may diminish the function to zero and produce irreparable damage in as short a time as one week, whereas a partial obstruction may exist for months or years with little impairment of function.

The *clinical manifestations* of hydronephrosis are variable. On many occasions a pronounced dilatation of the ureter and kidney pelvis may develop before sufficient symptoms are produced to bring the patient to a doctor. Mild pain in the region of the kidney, radiating downward along the ureter is a common complaint. Tenderness over the kidney posteriorly is usually present. The dilated kidney may or may not be palpable anteriorly. Fever may or may not be present, depending largely upon the amount of infection. If the obstruction is sudden and complete, or nearly so, acute symptoms (renal colic) as described previously in this chapter will be produced. Diligent effort must be made to find the cause of the hydronephrosis. Ureteral catheterization, pyelography, x-ray, examination of the prostate and urethra, etc., should be carried out until the source of the obstruction is found.

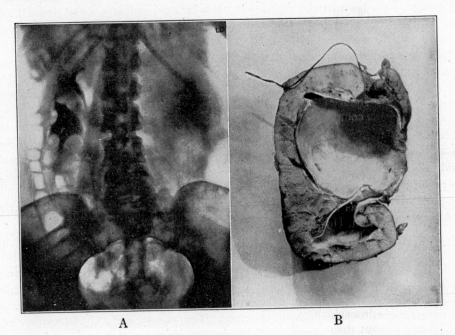

A   B

FIG. 551.—HYDRONEPHROSIS.

A, on the patient's right a dilated pelvis with double ureter is noted (after intravenous pyelography). On the left a shadow of a large mass may be observed, but none of the diodrast is passing through the kidney, thus indicating that the function on this side is almost, if not completely, destroyed. Lack of function was corroborated later by intravenous phenolsulphonphthalein with a ureteral catheter in place. B, longitudinal section of the excised kidney. Note the thinned cortex and the hydronephrosis which was produced by a congenital stricture at the ureteropelvic juncture (Courtesy of Dr. J. H. Sanford).

Treatment should be directed to release of the obstruction which, if acute and complete, demands immediate relief. If the obstruction is produced by a stone in the ureter, such procedures as ureteral catheterization or actual operation are available to remove the calculus, if it is not dislodged spontaneously. Ureteral strictures may be kept open by such a simple procedure as occasional dilatation by ureteral catheterization and bougies. Kinks produced by nephroptosis may be eliminated by correction of the nephroptosis. Extrinsic pressure due to a tumor may be corrected by excision of the mass. When the hydronephrosis has progressed to the point that function of the kidney is destroyed, nephrectomy may be indicated, particularly if symptoms are manifested.

Nephroptosis.—Ptosis of the kidney occurs most frequently in women, almost always on the right side and may be caused by a number of factors. Narrowness of the paravertebral niche, a decreased amount of perirenal fat, emaciation, weakness of the abdominal wall, etc., may be mentioned as prominent etiological factors. As stated previously, if the ptosis is sufficient to produce a kinking of the ureter, a hydronephrosis, perhaps with an associated infection, will develop.

Only a small percentage of patients with nephroptosis have symptoms of ureteral obstruction. The most common symptoms are those spoken of as renal colic, consisting of pain in the region of the kidney and perhaps radiating down the ureter toward the thigh or genitals. This pain may not be severe but is usually aggravated by jolting as sustained by riding in automobiles, streetcars, etc. Frequent and painful urination is not uncommon. Palpation usually reveals tenderness over the kidney. When the patient changes from the recumbent to the sitting position, it is usually possible to demonstrate a shifting in position of the organ downward. If there is doubt about the demonstration of an abnormal amount of mobility, pyelographic examination should be resorted to, and roentgenograms of the kidney taken in the recumbent and standing position. If distention of the kidney pelvis by retrograde pyelography reproduces the pain complained of, it is reasonably presumptive that the kidney is the cause of the pain. If replacement of the kidney to its normal position by recumbency and maintenance there by a "kidney belt" relieves the pain, the evidence is still more conclusive that renal ptosis is the cause of the patient's complaints.

Treatment should be directed toward improvement in the general health. It is important that the patient gain weight so as to increase the amount of perirenal fat. Frequently, correction of faulty posture will shift the abdominal organs so as to make more room for them in the upper abdomen. A wide abdominal support or elastic belt (with or without a "kidney pad") frequently relieves all symptoms, because of the support given the abdominal organs. Nephropexy, that is, fixation of the kidney in its normal position by operative means, is performed occasionally with variable success.

Tuberculosis of the Kidney.—Tuberculous infection of the kidney is a disease of early adult life and is primarily unilateral, but in 10 to 25 per cent of the cases both kidneys are affected. The organisms reach the kidney by way of the blood stream. Usually a primary focus can be found elsewhere, most often in the lungs, but frequently no primary lesion can be demonstrated. The infection starts usually at the base of the papilla in the lower or upper pole of the kidney and may spread by the lymphatics so that several foci will be produced within the organ. A toxic nephritis of the parenchymatous type may develop in the opposite kidney as well as the diseased organ. The large amount of albumin and casts found so frequently in the urine collected from each ureter is explained by this complicating lesion. As the disease progresses and involves the bladder, the opposite kidney may become infected, usually by ascending infection.

The lesion progresses slowly, healing by scar tissue in isolated areas. This scarring gradually produces a shrinking of the kidney and a contraction of the pelvis. The infection may spread by caseation or cavitation until ulcers appear in the pelvis after which the ureter is obviously exposed to the disease. Sooner or later the infection becomes implanted in the ureter. Peristalsis is lost early. Ulceration leads to scarring of the wall of the ureter, thereby producing strictures at numerous points and a shortening of the ureter. If the fibrosis in the kidney progresses to the point that the arteries become obliterated, an autonephrectomy will be produced.

Clinical Manifestations.—The symptoms produced by tuberculosis of the kidney are so insidious that the disease may be present for weeks or months before the patient is aware of it. Frequently, systemic symptoms such as fever, malaise, anorexia and loss of weight are the first noted. On other occasions, frequency of urination caused by secondary invasion of the bladder is the first complaint. Sooner or later, in untreated cases the bladder becomes infected. When this occurs, troublesome symptoms, such as frequency of urination and severe dysuria, are apt to develop. The urine becomes cloudy because of the pus contained in it, and frequently is smoky or red because of hemorrhage in the pelvis. Pain in the region of the kidney is not uncommon and is occasionally colicky, but never severe. Mild tenderness over the kidney may or may not be present. Examination of the urine reveals pus in large quantities, a variable amount of red blood cells, albumin and casts. Cystoscopic findings, including ulcers in the bladder, reddening, ulceration and retraction of the ureteral orifice, are fairly diagnostic of the disease. Pyelograms reveal irregularities in the shadows of the calices with narrowing, or clubbing, and a contraction of the pelvis with irregular constrictions and dilatation of the ureter. The excretion of phenolsulphonphthalein by the affected kidney is diminished, but not early in the disease.

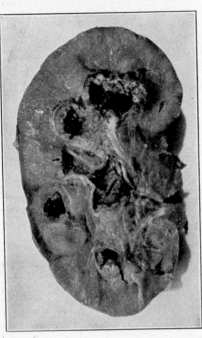

Fig. 552.—Tuberculosis of the Kidney (Longitudinal Section after Operative Removal).

Note the ulceration surrounding the calices. Abscess formation is common and may at times destroy practically the entire cortex (Courtesy, Dr. D. K. Rose).

Treatment.—The most effective method of treatment of tuberculosis of one kidney is surgical excision of the organ, which is especially indicated since the lesion rarely heals, but descends to the bladder and tends to spread to the other kidney and to the genitals. Before nephrectomy is done, it must be established (by pyelography, etc.) that the opposite kidney is sufficiently healthy to sustain life. It is always important to examine the patient carefully for the possible existence of an active lesion elsewhere (particularly lung and bone). Nephrectomy should not be performed if such an active lesion is found. Removal of the kidney may be technically difficult because of the large amount of dense perirenal scar tissue. On account of the involvement of the ureter it is usually advisable to remove all of it, even though it may be necessary to do it through another incision at a later date. Partial nephrectomy is rarely advisable. The ulcerations in the bladder heal rapidly following nephrectomy unless the remaining kidney is infected. Hygienic measures such as rest, large amounts of wholesome food, etc., are important in the convalescence.

Tumors and Cysts.—The great majority of the neoplasms in the kidney are malignant; few are benign. An enormous amount of confusion exists as to their classification. Some authorities are inclined to classify most if not all as hypernephroma (arising in adrenal rests), whereas others deny the occurrence of malignant adrenal rests in the kidney and classify the tumors as carcinoma of the kidney. However, most observers agree that these two designations represent in reality two different types of tumor: hypernephroma and carcinoma of the kidney. Diagnostically there is no necessity for drawing a sharp distinction since the symptoms produced by carcinoma and hypernephroma are identical, and the treatment relatively the same. They are described separately because of histologic and pathologic differences.

Hypernephroma.—In 1883 Grawitz made the suggestion that many of the malignant tumors of the kidney arise from adrenal rests within or rarely without the kidney. The cells in this tumor are quite large, have pyknotic nuclei, are characteristically arranged in sheets or cord-like structures, and are large and "foamy." The cytoplasm is clear, profuse in quantity, and contains lipoid globules and glycogenic granules. Grossly the tumors are characteristically yellow except for occasional areas of brownish mottling due to hemorrhage. Because of the paucity of fibrous tissue, these tumors are very friable. Contrary to the opinion of many authorities, Rose [16] has concluded that hypernephroma is distinctly less malignant than carcinoma arising from kidney tubular cells.

Hematuria, although not constant, is the most common symptom and is manifested early when present. It is usually sufficiently severe to be detected by the patient. The bleeding is painless unless it occurs in such large quantities as to form clots and produce renal colic. Mild pain in the region of the kidney may be present, but is rarely noted before a tumor is palpable. The function of the kidney is rarely impaired until the terminal stage. Except in rare instances, pyelography reveals an abnormal "filling defect" in the x-ray. Occasionally the tumor remains small and produces such few symptoms that metastases (usually to the brain, lungs or bone) may occur and produce symptoms before the local tumor does.

Nephrectomy is the treatment of choice unless metastases are present or the opposite kidney is severely diseased. X-ray therapy may be beneficial in reducing the size of the tumor preparatory to nephrectomy; if the tumor is inoperable, x-ray therapy is likewise indicated.

Carcinoma of the Kidney.—Tumors of this type may be classified as (1) papillary adenocarcinoma or (2) alveolar carcinoma. Microscopically the cells in the former growth are arranged around strands of fibrous tissue presenting a papillary appearance. Like hypernephroma, papillary carcinoma may be yellow in color and microscopically it contains clear cells. The cells in the alveolar type of tumor usually resemble the tubular structure of the renal cortex so closely that confusion with other tumors is not likely. The malignancy of these tumors varies, but metastases occur in a manner quite identical to hypernephroma except perhaps more rapidly. The symptoms produced and the treatment indicated are no different from those described under hypernephroma.

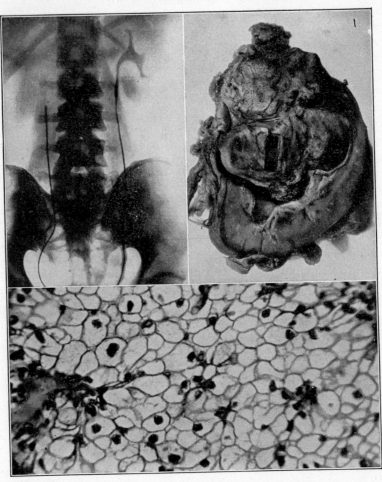

FIG. 553.—HYPERNEPHROMA.

Upper left, pyelogram (per ureter) of the left kidney shows elongation and narrowing of the upper calyx, thus indicating a tumor in this portion of the kidney. The patient had pain in the region of the left kidney, and hematuria of four months' duration. Upper right, photograph of a longitudinal section of the kidney after operation. The tumor involves the entire upper portion of the kidney and has filled the pelvis much more than the pyelogram indicates. Below, high power photomicrograph of the tumor, revealing the "foam" cells with very little connective tissue stroma (Courtesy, D. J. H. Sanford).

Epithelial Tumors of the Renal Pelvis.—These tumors are usually of papillary type and may be either benign or malignant. In either case the papillary or warty growth may grow profusely and completely fill the pelvis and even extend down into the ureter. Hematuria is the predominating symptom. Nephrectomy should be performed if possible.

Embryoma of the Kidney (Wilm's tumor).—This tumor is sarcomatous in type, but contains many embryonal structures including connective tissue, cartilage, muscle, abortive renal elements, etc. Spindle and polyhedral cells along with epithelial tubules, usually constitute the major cellular elements. It is encountered only in children, rarely after the age of ten. The tumor attains a huge size, has a greater tendency to remain encapsulated than most malignant tumors, but may metastasize through lymphatics as well as the vascular system (including the wall of the renal vein). Like other renal tumors, the only early symptom is hematuria. Since this is less apt to be detected in children than adults, the tumor is usually very large before it is detected. If metastases have not taken place and the size of the tumor permits, nephrectomy should be performed. The tumor is so sensitive to x-ray therapy that many supposedly inoperable tumors are made operable. However, Ladd and Gross [37] advise against this, on the basis that metastases may take place while waiting for radiation effect. Prognosis is poor.

Polycystic Kidney.—Multiple cysts of the kidney are usually bilateral and are presumably of congenital origin, although symptoms may not be produced until late in adult life. They appear to be hereditary as suggested by the fact that frequently more than one member of the family is affected. The cysts contain thin or gelatinous amber-colored fluid, not urine. There is usually a large amount of fatty tissue deposited about the organ. Surprisingly little renal tissue is demonstrable, even on cut section.

Except for hematuria, which may be present early in the disease, the symptoms are those of nephritis, although the patient may live a life of average duration with few if any symptoms. Albumin and casts are demonstrable in the urine. Polyuria may be present. One kidney usually increases in size faster than the other and may or may not be palpable. Diagnosis can be confirmed readily by pyelography because of the lengthening and distortion of the calices.

Since both kidneys are usually involved, treatment is rarely surgical. Occasionally suppuration develops within the cysts, thereby demanding drainage or nephrectomy.

Solitary Cyst of the Kidney.—Such cysts are practically always unilateral, but may attain considerable size. The fluid within the cyst is clear and amber colored or hemorrhagic, but not urinous. Mild pain in the region of the kidney may be complained of when the cyst becomes large. Frequently they may attain a size large enough to be palpable through the abdominal wall without producing any symptoms. Treatment consists of excision of the cyst with repair of the defect; rarely is nephrectomy indicated.

BLADDER

Reference has already been made (p. 983) to surgical procedures performed upon the bladder (cystostomy for stone) in ancient times, but a clear understanding of the physiology of the bladder and the types of disease affecting it was not possible until the invention of the cystoscope. The bladder is innervated by autonomic fibers comprising two separate nerve tracts: (1) fibers from the second dorsal to the third lumbar anterior roots constitute the sympathetic innervation and permit filling of the bladder by maintaining contraction of bladder neck and relaxation of the wall; (2) pelvic nerve fibers arising from the second and third sacral roots constitute its parasympathetic innervation and are important in emptying the bladder since stimulation of this group of nerves causes contraction of the bladder wall and relaxation of the bladder neck. In 1927 Rose [17] introduced the use of the cystometer, an instrument designed to measure bladder pressure and capacity, and their relation to pain, desire to void, etc. This instrument opened up an entirely new field for the study of the physiology of the bladder and the diseases affecting it.

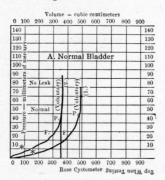 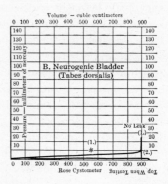

FIG. 554.—DIAGNOSTIC CHARTS OBTAINED WITH THE ROSE CYSTOMETER.

A cystometrogram is obtained by introducing sterile water through the cystometer into the bladder of the supine relaxed patient. The graphs, as exemplified above, record pressure changes against volume and also the sensations of the patient, e.g., first desire to void is indicated by an asterisk (*), a sense of fullness is shown at "F" and of pain at "P." Note that two consecutive superimposed graphs are obtained at each examination in order to stimulate the stretch reflex and to measure the strength of the bladder wall (Modified from Rose, D. K., J. Urol., 46:257, 1941).

Congenital Anomalies.—*Exstrophy of the bladder* is an exceedingly distressing congenital deformity in which exposed bladder mucosa lies open on the anterior abdominal wall. It occurs most often in males, but fortunately is rather rare. The defect is explained by a failure of the symphysis pubis and the abdominal wall just above it to unite in the midline. The roof of the bladder is absent; the floor of the bladder including the trigon protrudes outward. The penis and scrotum are small. The prostate and seminal vesicles are atrophic or absent. The escaping urine must be drained into a special type of cup or be absorbed by dressings. Sufficient urine escapes, however, to produce irritation and maceration of the skin about the defect. The floor of the bladder becomes infected and presents a red beefy appearance. Infection ascends readily up the ureters and is instrumental in causing the death of two-thirds or three-fourths of these poor unfortunates before they attain the age of eighteen or twenty.

The most successful treatment consists of the transplantation of the ureters into the sigmoid, preferably in two stages (one ureter at a time). This operation meets with the most success if not performed before the age of seven or eight. The technic as originally outlined by Coffey [18] has been adopted with modifications. The ureters are transplanted obliquely through the wall of the sigmoid so that a valve-like action is produced. The rectum acts as a bladder and life becomes bearable, except that the danger of renal infection is always imminent.

A *diverticulum* is a common defect thought by some to be congenital in origin, but in reality is usually associated with urethral obstruction (especially prostatic) of some type (Keyes [19]). Diverticula may vary in size from a tiny saccule, which is not visible on the exterior of the bladder, to a defect which is larger than the bladder itself. They occur most often on the posterolateral wall, and as they increase in size may pull the trigon into the defect. There may be no symptoms of the diverticulum itself; however, frequency or burning on urination, difficulty in urination, etc., may be present because of the obstruction and infection. The infection may be secondary to stagnation of urine in the diverticulum or to the urinary (*e.g.,* prostatic) obstruction. Treatment is directed toward eradication of the infection by irrigation of the bladder and relief of the urethral obstruction. If the diverticulum is large, it is usually advisable, however, to remove it surgically, because of the liability to reinfection. This is not a simple and innocuous procedure, and should not be attempted by one not skilled in urologic surgery; postoperative care, including the use of a retention catheter, etc., is likewise important.

Injuries of the Bladder.—Because of the protected position of the bladder within the pelvis, injury is uncommon except when produced by fracture of the pelvis or penetration by bullets. When a patient sustains a severe fracture of the pelvis, the jagged bone edges may tear or perforate the bladder. A moderate blow over an overdistended bladder may cause a rupture, but spontaneous *rupture of the bladder* because of overdistention is exceedingly uncommon. Traumatic rupture is occasionally associated with fractures of the pelvis; it occurs most frequently when the bladder is full, and therefore is relatively more common in drunken people. Unless the patient is drunk or unconscious there is invariably considerable pain at the time of rupture. On the other hand, since sterile urine often excites only mild irritation of the peritoneum, very few symptoms and signs may be manifested, and the diagnosis will be missed. Peritonitis due to associated infection is apt to occur ultimately (unless prevented by early repair) and adds greatly to the seriousness of the situation. Mild shock may be present because of associated hemorrhage. Tenderness over the bladder is constant, but variable in intensity. Diffuse abdominal tenderness, muscle spasm and other signs of peritoneal irritation, such as nausea and vomiting, may be present. Of most diagnostic importance is the inability to void. If rupture of the bladder is suspected, catheterization (using strict aseptic technic) should be performed; if perforation exists, rarely will more than a few cubic centimeters of bloody urine be obtained. Diagnosis is further confirmed if after instillation of 20 or 25 cc. of sterile saline through the catheter into the bladder, only a few cc. are procurable by aspiration.

Treatment is obviously surgical, consisting of laparotomy with repair of the laceration as soon as the diagnosis is made. To prevent leakage at the suture line because of distention, it is necessary to insert a retention catheter and leave it in place for several days.

Cystitis.—The term cystitis correctly used refers to an infection of the bladder, usually but not always accompanied by dysuria, *i.e.,* frequency and pain on urination. On the other hand, the term cystitis is often used, perhaps incorrectly, in patients with the same symptoms, due not to infection of the bladder itself but to other causes, *e.g.,* Hunner ulcer, urethritis, etc.

Infection of the bladder occurs as a primary disease: also it is secondary to infections of the kidney. Of the other factors which may be responsible for cystitis, the following should be mentioned: prostatitis, residual urine, hyperplastic epithelial changes, tumors and contamination from catheterization. The bacillus coli, tubercle bacillus, staphylococcus, streptococcus and proteus bacillus are the organisms most commonly responsible for infection. The disease occurs in either the acute or chronic form. The bladder mucosa is reddened and edematous. Ulcers are not uncommon.

Because of the danger of production of infection by catheterization, such a procedure should be performed only when necessary, and only with strict aseptic technic. Especially is this true when a residual urine, tumor of the bladder, hypertrophy of the prostate, calculus or neurogenic lesion is present. Cystitis in the presence of such lesions is apt to be especially serious.

Clinical Manifestations.—The most significant symptoms are frequency and burning on urination. There may be severe pain at the end of urination because of the excessive contracting efforts of the bladder to empty itself. Pus cells are always found in the urine, frequently in such large quantities as to make the urine cloudy; red blood cells are not uncommon. Cystoscopy will reveal a reddened edematous mucosa perhaps with ulceration.

In tuberculous cystitis the depression of the ureteral orifice ("golf ball ureter") noted in cystoscopic examination may be the most diagnostic finding. The edema and redness are most commonly found in the trigon where the ulcerations produced by the miliary tubercles are likewise most frequently encountered. The symptoms and urinary findings in tuberculous cystitis are similar to those just mentioned except that with proper technic the tubercle bacillus can frequently be found in the urine.

The *treatment* of cystitis consists primarily of elimination of the primary source of the infection, an achievement which often can be accomplished only when a urinary obstruction is relieved. Rarely does a cystitis fail to subside readily when the offending focus is removed, regardless of whether or not the infection is tuberculous. Fluids should be given in large quantities. Sedatives may be necessary because of the pain, especially in tuberculosis. When the urine is highly acid, the burning and frequency on urination may sometimes be relieved by the administration of alkalis such as sodium bicarbonate or citrate. Irrigation of the bladder once or twice daily with a 1:5000 solution of potassium permanganate, or a 3 per cent solution of boric acid will accelerate healing. Instillation of a few cubic centimeters of 10 or 20 per cent solution of argyrol after irrigation of the bladder may be helpful. Chemotherapy (see pp. 36 and 990) will be very helpful.

Bladder Calculus.—Stones in the bladder usually occur singly, but may be multiple. Most of them are comprised chiefly of urates (descending from the kidney), but uric acid, phosphate and oxalate stones are also encountered. There is usually sufficient calcium present to make the calculi impervious to the x-ray. Vesical stones are encountered most commonly in men, less frequently in children, but rarely in women except in hyperparathyroidism. The size is variable; on rare occasions they may be 2 inches or more in diameter. Frequently, stones originate from small calculi from the kidney as well as form primarily in the bladder; they may develop around a foreign body.

The *symptoms* include burning and frequency on urination, but the type of pain occurring in the perineum, radiating to the head of the penis and accentuated by activity of the patient, is more diagnostic. Pain is frequently severe at the end of urination when a few drops of bloody urine are occasionally observed. On rare occasions the stream is stopped suddenly by the stone lodging in the prostatic urethra. Infection is a frequent accompaniment of stones.

The *diagnosis* may frequently be made by contact of the stone with a sound, but the x-ray and cystoscope constitute much more reliable means of making a diagnosis. The urate stones, however, are occasionally radiotranslucent so that diagnosis cannot be confirmed by x-ray.

The *treatment,* of course, consists of removal of the stone. If the calculus is small, it may frequently be removed readily by litholapaxy; *i.e.,* crushing with a lithotrite introduced through the urethra, and removing the fragments by irrigation. If the stone is large or too hard to crush, or if obstruction due to urethral stricture or prostatic enlargement prevents the passage of the instrument, it will be necessary to open the bladder in order to remove the stone. The bladder is frequently left open to drain through the suprapubic opening, but rarely is it unsafe to close it, providing a retention catheter is placed in the urethra and allowed to remain for a few days.

Foreign Bodies in the Bladder.—It is not uncommon to find foreign bodies such as hair pins, pieces of rubber, catheters, etc., in the bladder, introduced by sexual perverts. Not only do these foreign bodies produce infection, but with few exceptions they act as the nucleus for the formation of stones. On rare occasions the foreign bodies (broken tip of ureteral catheter, broken needles, etc.) are obviously introduced by accident during operative procedures. If the objects are small, they are usually removable by the cystoscope; if not, it will be necessary to resort to suprapubic incision into the bladder.

Tumors.—Neoplasms of the bladder may be either benign or malignant, but with few exceptions can be classified into one of three types.

Benign Papilloma.—Benign papillomas are encountered most commonly in males, previous to the age of forty-five. They appear usually in the base of the bladder and may be single or multiple. The tumor grows insidiously and no doubt is commonly present months or years before symptoms are produced. Frequently, the growth is responsible for the development of an infection (cystitis). On rare occasions calcareous encrustations are found on the papillomatous strands. Ulceration is not common. Perhaps the most common manifestation is hematuria, occurring usually at the end of urination. Such tumors are best treated by fulguration through a cystoscope. On rare occasions it may be necessary to resort to excision by cystotomy.

Malignant Papilloma.—This tumor is not unlike the benign papilloma in appearance, but occurs for the most part in older people (usually males). It arises most commonly in the trigon, but there is a greater tendency toward multiplicity of foci or implantation of growth than in the benign tumor. The microscopic appearance of the base of the tumor is the determining factor in the differentiation between the benign and malignant growths. Metastasis occurs slowly. Ulceration is more common in the malignant tumor, as is also cystitis and calcareous encrustation. Hematuria may be the only symptom except for burning and frequency of urination incited by infection. On rare occasions, bits of tumor break off and are passed in the urine or actually produce urethral obstruction. Fulguration, implantation of radium seeds or needles, and x-ray therapy constitute the chief procedures in the treatment, and are fairly efficient in effecting a local disappearance of the tumor. Because of the involvement in the base of the bladder, resection of the bladder is rarely indicated since transplantation of the ureters into the colon (a formidable procedure in these patients) must also be done.

Carcinoma.—In addition to the malignant papilloma there is another type of malignant growth designated as carcinoma, which is a squamous-cell tumor, appearing as an ulcerating, elevated thickening of the bladder wall. The symptoms encountered are similar to those produced by the papillomatous tumors. Diagnosis can best be made with the cystoscope. Except when the tumor is local in the dome, treatment should be limited to fulguration, radium implantation and x-ray therapy and not resection of the growth.

A procedure recently recommended by Rose [20] utilizing x-ray therapy (through a suprapubic opening) in the treatment of malignant tumors of the bladder without obvious metastases, gives promise of being much superior to the various types of therapy previously used, with the exception perhaps of excision in the early cases. Rose performs a cystotomy and subjects the tumor directly to the x-ray. In this way he is able to treat the tumor with several times the average dose, since it is not necessary to penetrate the skin, which has always been a serious obstacle in the treatment of tumors with heavy x-ray dosage.

Retention of Urine.—Urinary retention occurs most commonly as a complication of operations, particularly those about the pelvis and perineum.

The difficulty in urination is made more acute by the recumbent position of the patient. Before resorting to catheterization, all possible effort should be made to assist the patient in voiding, particularly because repeated catheterizations may lead to cystitis. Such simple procedures as a warm water douche of the genitals, and the psychic effect of turning on a water faucet in the patient's room, may enable the patient to void. Enemas are frequently effective in inducing sufficient relaxation of the urinary sphincter to allow the patient to void. When discomfort exists and attempts to void are unsuccessful, it will be necessary to resort to catheterization. In general catheterization should not be delayed until the bladder distention is pronounced, since only rarely is the patient able to void when distention with pain has been present longer than a hour or two. Moreover, a bladder which has been subjected to considerable distention is much more liable to become infected. In any event, extreme care, utilizing perfect aseptic technic, must be exercised during catheterization; no part of the catheter which is to be inserted beyond the meatus should be touched except with a sterile instrument or the sterile gloved hand. Gentleness is likewise important. Following catheterization the patient should be encouraged to void in a few hours, before sufficient urine has accumulated to produce pain. If difficulty is still experienced in voiding, catheterization should be repeated in eight or ten hours, because the normal mechanism is usually regained more rapidly than it is if one waits until distention develops to the point of pain.

Following certain operations, *e.g.*, resection of the rectum, retention of urine may persist for many days; it is assumed in such instances that the retention is not due to simple reflex spasm, but to actual division of the pudic nerve which supplies the bladder. Numerous other conditions produce retention of urine in addition to other disturbances in bladder function; the term neurogenic bladder is applied to such cases.

Neurogenic Bladder.—The term neurogenic bladder refers to disturbances in urinary function which are not due to disease of the urinary tract but to disease, injury, or abnormal function of the nerves supplying the bladder. The disturbances produced by neurogenic factors vary greatly, and are often associated with or complicated by other lesions, inflammatory or neoplastic. Strictly speaking, any variation in bladder function from the normal is classified as neurogenic when the primary factor lies in the central nervous system. When the abnormal function is secondary to changes in the bladder wall, induced by trauma, prostatic or other obstruction, etc., the term myogenic bladder is used.

The disturbances in bladder function which are of neurogenic origin, may be either hypotonic or hypertonic. Of the first group the etiologic factor is usually tabes, or occasionally trauma; reflex causes following rectal and pelvic operations especially are frequently responsible for a hypotonic bladder. In the hypertonic type, irritative lesions play a great role, such as neuritis, some spinal cord tumors, spinal meningitis, etc. To understand the mechanism of production of these types of bladder disturbances it is necessary to have a clear understanding of the physiologic mechanism of the bladder.

The function of the bladder is divided into that exerted by the bladder wall (expulsive force) and that due to the sphincter control (the "lock"). The latter mechanism is made up of the internal sphincter, which is but a thickening of the circular muscle layer of the bladder wall, and the external sphincter, which consists of the muscle in the urogenital trigon, and is influenced in its action by the anterior part of the levator ani. When the posterior roots of the spinal cord are diseased as in tabes dorsalis, an atonic bladder results; in diseases such as spina bifida, in which both anterior and posterior roots may be damaged, marked retention with low intravesical pressure and increased bladder capacity is apt to be present.

The autonomic nerve supply to the bladder contains both sympathetic and parasympathetic fibers from the standpoint of function; however, this is difficult to demonstrate anatomically. Actually, all three types of impulses (pain, stimulation and inhibition) are carried by the autonomic nerves supplying the urinary bladder. These fibers are carried in the parasympathetics of the second and third sacral roots, and in the sympathetics arising from the second dorsal to fourth lumbar roots. This wide distribution explains the imperfect results when merely the presacral nerve is resected in attempt to relieve pain in the bladder and to decrease its capacity. The occurrence of pain in itself may be primarily responsible for inhibition of normal contraction of the bladder wall, and thus produce retention of urine. Such cerebral inhibition is, of course, a normal impulse; in neurogenic bladders, however, it has a great clinical importance since suddenly impaired cerebration (organic or functional) may cause its release and thus produce incontinence. On the other hand, augmentation of this inhibitory influence as by fear, etc., may produce urinary retention (psychic retention). Postoperative retention is intimately tied up with inhibition, being partly due to the fear of initiating the act of voiding, particularly in pelvic and rectal operations; reflex spasm of the sphincter is probably also important.

Clinical Manifestations.—The manifestations produced by a neurogenic bladder vary considerably with the type of disease responsible for it. As already indicated, two groups of disturbance are recognized, hypotonic and hypertonic; both types, however, may play a part in the symptomatology in a particular patient. *Incontinence* (involuntary urination) is an important clinical manifestation and implies an inability of the patient to control the voiding act. When it occurs during sleep, it is called enuresis. It may be associated with a retention of urine, *i.e.,* the bladder may be dilated to capacity and small amounts of urine will dribble through the urethra constantly; however, this is an undesirable situation because of the increased danger of infection. *Frequency* of urination is most often due to organic disease (*e.g.,* urethritis and cystitis), but may also be due to abnormal impulses carried by the autonomic nerves. *Pain* is present when retention is associated with a hypertonic state of the musculature. *Inability to void,* whether associated with pain or not, is likewise most often due to organic obstruction (enlarged prostate, etc.) ; if due to neurogenic factors, it is produced by either a paralysis of the expulsive power of the bladder or a failure of the sphincters to relax. *Lack of desire to void* is distinctly a manifestation of a neurogenic bladder and is associated with marked *retention of urine.* Retention of urine is objectively manifested by the demonstration of increased bladder dullness, but more certainly by catheterization. If other lesions are present, or if catheterization has induced an infection, the manifestations due to neurogenic factors will obviously be complicated. The data furnished by the cystometer (Rose and others) give considerable information as to the type of neurogenic disturbance which is present; thorough physical and especially neurological examination will usually reveal the true nature of the disease responsible for the urinary abnormalities.

Treatment.—Obviously, therapy depends on the type of disturbance present. Retention of urine due to reflex causes has already been considered. When tabes dorsalis is responsible for the retention, catheterization is used as necessary; on account of the low intravesical pressure little damage to the kidney due to the pressure is sustained. Hence, bacterial contamination is less likely to lead to serious infection of the kidney. In the hypertonic bladder with retention, however, catheterization is less permissible because of the likelihood of the production of infection.

In the case of spinal cord injuries the problem of treatment is more difficult because of the sudden development of the disturbance which is in most cases due to an inability to void, incontinence or retention. It may be difficult, moreover, to estimate accurately the seriousness of the cord damage.

In general there is much disagreement among urologists as to the treatment of this group of neurogenic bladders, sustained, for example, by injury to the spinal cord. It is agreed, however, that attempt should be made to produce an "automatic" bladder by effecting evacuation through the mechanism of massage of the bladder at regular intervals, four to eight times per day. In a large percentage of cases an automatic bladder, which will empty itself fairly completely with stimulation or effort on the part of the patient, will be developed. If this fails, tidal irrigation arranged in a manner similar to that described by Munro,[21] utilizing a mild antiseptic such as 1½ per cent boric acid, may be instituted. Less preferable is a retention catheter. Most urologists believe that a retention catheter or a suprapubic cystostomy is preferable to frequent catheterization.

If infection develops with the conservative methods, a retention catheter or suprapubic cystostomy may be necessary. However, sulfonamide therapy will be very useful in the treatment of infections, and will minimize the necessity for radical therapy. Additional data on neurogenic bladder may be found in an article by Evans [26].

PROSTATE

The prostate is a gland composed of a framework of elastic and connective tissue in which are secreting glands. These glands empty into the posterior urethra through a series of small ducts.

Acute Prostatitis.—Acute infection of this organ is due for the most part to gonorrheal infection arising from the urethra. Infection may likewise result from nonspecific urethritis, or from trauma due to instrumentation. The infection produces pain in the perineum which is accentuated by walking. Burning and frequency of urination, and occasionally terminal dysuria are usual symptoms. The systemic reaction may be quite severe, consisting of fever and its allied symptoms. Rectal examination reveals a tender and swollen prostate. On rare occasions an abscess forms with accentuation of the manifestations just mentioned.

Treatment.—Chemotherapy, rest in bed, application of local heat, and symptomatic care represent useful therapeutic agents. There must be complete abstinence from sexual excitement. Prostatic massage is strictly contraindicated. Any abscesses which form usually rupture into the urethra, but may demand drainage through the perineum.

Chronic Prostatitis.—A chronic infection of the prostate may develop insidiously or be the result of an acute prostatitis. Mild pain in the perineum, and burning and frequency of urination, are common symptoms. A mild urethral discharge containing shreds and pus cells is usually present; such shreds and pus cells are readily found in the urine. Rectal examination will reveal a large, boggy prostate, frequently with soft fluctuant areas. Massage of the prostate expresses the purulent "shreddy" material into the urethra from which smears may be made for the establishment of the type and severity of the infection.

The *treatment* consists of prostatic massage at intervals of five to seven days, followed immediately by urination to wash out the infective material. Mild antiseptics such as 10 or 20 per cent solution of argyrol may be used for instillation. Chemotherapy should be utilized, but in chronic infection of this type may not be very efficacious.

Prostatic Hypertrophy.—Until recent years, hypertrophy of the prostate was thought to be caused by infection. The profession is now beginning to realize that this disease is in reality due to an endocrine abnormality. Lower and Johnston [22] explain the mechanism of development of the disease upon the fact that the testicular tubules which utilize anterior pituitary hormone become atrophied, thereby allowing an excess amount of hormone to accumulate and act upon the prostate and seminal vesicles, resulting in their enlargement. The hypertrophy is noted particularly in the lateral lobes, but, as noted by Randall,[23] probably arises in submucosal glands of the prostatic urethra. The enlargement is due to an adenomatous hypertrophy, although at times there may be considerable fibrosis scattered throughout the gland. The disease occurs only in late adult life, rarely before the age of fifty or fifty-five.

Clinical Manifestations.—One of the first evidences of the disease is frequency of urination, particularly at night. The patient usually has difficulty in starting the stream and when through voiding frequently has the sensation that the bladder has been incompletely emptied. The stream is weak; dribbling at the end of urination is characteristic. As the hypertrophy increases, the amount of urinary retention in the bladder increases until even the patient may be aware of the mass produced by the distended bladder. The constant presence of a distended bladder produces deleterious effects upon the kidney, consisting primarily of hydronephrosis, atrophy of the cortex, and, if infection is present, pyelonephritis or pyonephrosis. The renal impairment may be serious, regardless of whether or not infection is present, resulting at times in uremia. Any or all of the symptoms of uremia including a clouded sensorium, delirium, weakness, headache, anorexia, vomiting, etc., may be present. The nonprotein nitrogen content of the blood will be elevated. Acute retention of the urine is commonly experienced and frequently demands catheterization before relief is obtained.

Infection (cystitis) may be present early in the disease, but usually does not take place until catheterization has been instituted. With infection, other symptoms including burning and pain upon urination become prominent. Fever and its allied symptoms are apt to be present. The infection ascends readily to the kidney and may be instrumental in the development or exacerbation of the symptoms of uremia.

Examination of the patient will usually reveal a distended bladder. The amount of retention is useful in estimating the severity of the obstruction and may be determined by measuring the amount of urine obtained by catheterization immediately after voiding (residual urine). A rectal examination rarely fails to reveal a large prostate with firm lobes, but occasionally considerable obstruction may be present due to enlargement of the median lobe with only mild increase in size of the prostate itself. Cystoscopic examination is a reliable method of confirming the diagnosis. If infection is present, pus cells will obviously be found in the urine. If much renal damage is present, albumin will likewise be present. The degree of renal impairment may be estimated by the degree of elevation of the nonprotein nitrogen content of the blood.

Treatment.—Unless the disease is severe enough to demand operative treatment, catheterization and cystoscopic examination should be avoided. When it becomes necessary to resort to the two latter procedures, extreme care as to aseptic technic and gentleness must be utilized. Large quantities of water should be taken at all times. Urinary antiseptics as mentioned on page 990 will be helpful in minimizing infection. It is thought by many that a distended bladder of the type encountered in prostatic hypertrophy should not be decompressed (by catheter) suddenly, *i.e.*, not all the urine should be removed at one time, on account of damage which may be inflicted upon the kidneys by the sudden change in the pressure against which the kidney is accustomed to excrete. However, this danger has no doubt been greatly exaggerated.

Although operative removal of the prostate offers great relief to patients afflicted with this disease, urologists have learned that such procedures cannot be done without adequate preoperative treatment. In addition to proper decompression of the bladder over the course of at least two or three days, the bladder must remain empty or nearly so for several more days, perhaps best accomplished by an indwelling catheter. Observations on the nonprotein nitrogen content of the blood and the phenolsulphonphthalein excretion of the kidneys must be made at intervals to determine the patient's progress; such tests should approach normal values before operation is resorted to. Fever is likewise a manifestation which strongly contraindicates operative procedures. Bed rest is desirable. It is of course essential that adequate caloric intake be maintained during the preoperative period. Fluids must be forced.

Prostatectomy may be performed by (1) the suprapubic, (2) perineal or (3) transurethral method. The former method consisting of removal of the gland by a suprapubic cystostomy was originally the most popular. It is usually performed in two stages (with an interval of several days for bladder drainage), but in patients who are good risks or have little urinary infection, may be performed in one stage. Transurethral resection is performed without a skin incision, by passing a resectoscope (McCarthy [24]) through the urethra. It is most adaptable in patients with small bars, contractures or small middle lobes but is used by some urologists in nearly all cases of prostatic hypertrophy.

Carcinoma.—Malignant tumors of the prostate are commonly encountered, occurring as a rule, however, at a later age than does prostatic hypertrophy. Apparently the tumor originates in the posterior lobe which is not as a rule affected by prostatic hypertrophy. Because metastases occur early, and patients come to the physician late, the prognosis is extremely poor.

Frequency of urination is the most common early symptom. Hematuria may be present at times. After the growth has extended throughout the gland, acute retention is frequently encountered. Occasionally the first symptoms will be severe pain in the back and pelvis caused by metastases, although the original tumor in the prostate may be proved at autopsy to be confined to only a small nodule. Diagnosis can usually be made by rectal examination by the stony hard nodular surface, except in these instances when the initial growth remains small. Cystoscopic examination may not be of much diagnostic aid, but portions of the gland removed by the "punch" may reveal malignant tissue. Elevation of acid phosphatase is of little value diagnostically unless the level exceeds 10 King-Armstrong units.

Treatment of prostatic cancer is rarely curative unless early detection permits complete removal by perineal prostatectomy. Palliation with radio-therapy may relieve pain; transurethral resection relieves obstruction. Remarkably, Huggins [25] has found that castration is followed by recession of the growth (including metastases) in 75 per cent of the cases. Herbst [27] has demonstrated that estrogen (stilbestrol) is very efficacious in controlling carcinoma of the prostate; at Washington University it is always used before advising castration (Rose).

Prostatic Calculi.—Calcareous deposits occasionally develop in the dilated prostatic alveoli and may produce the symptoms of prostatitis. Removal may be accomplished by the urethroscope or by prostatectomy.

SEMINAL VESICLES

Acute vesiculitis is no doubt a frequent disease, and in most instances is secondary to gonococcal infection of the posterior urethra. It is difficult to differentiate accurately the symptoms produced by acute prostatitis, acute posterior urethritis and those manifested by acute vesiculitis. It is agreed, however, that the pain in the latter disease is frequently localized to the region of the rectum. Rectal examination reveals tender and distended vesicles, from which may be expressed a large amount of tenacious material containing large numbers of pus cells. It is probable that this suppurative process rarely progresses to the state of abscess formation. The treatment is symptomatic, but includes complete abstinence from sexual excitement. Expression of the purulent material by gentle massage rectally, followed by urination, is probably helpful, but is dangerous because of the danger of production of acute epididymitis.

Chronic vesiculitis in most instances is the result of acute vesiculitis, but may develop without any evidence of preëxisting acute infection. It is apparent that in the latter instance, the streptococcus on many occasions is the etiologic factor. Symptoms are extremely variable, consisting primarily of mild pain in the perineum and along the rectum, but may be absent altogether. Ejaculation may be painful. A mild urethral discharge may be present. The disease is occasionally discovered by rectal examination performed as a part of a complete examination made, perhaps, in an effort to discover a cause for a chronic arthritis. When chronically infected, the walls may be palpated as being thickened and roughened.

Careful massage of the vesicles every five or ten days may be an effective method of treatment. Injection of 5 to 10 per cent argyrol into the vesicle through the vas deferens, at times is considered by many urologists as being effective in relieving the pain of certain types of arthritis which are due to focal infection in the seminal vesicles. Vesiculectomy may be done but advisability is doubtful.

On rare occasions the seminal vesicles may be the seat of *tuberculosis* in which instance vesiculectomy may be indicated providing the diagnosis can be made.

URETHRA

Wounds.—Injury to the urethra is not uncommon and may be produced by direct laceration or by a crushing injury such as that sustained by falling astride a fence or similar object. When there is an obvious laceration of the urethra, repair should be performed by interrupted sutures over a soft rubber catheter.

Occasionally rough catheterization results in abrasion, and even a complete tear through the wall. Althought strictures may result from injuries as well as infections (gonorrheal), the immediate effect of rupture or laceration of the urethra is the escape of urine into the surrounding tissues.

Extravasation of Urine.—Leakage of urine takes place readily through tears in the urethra into adjacent tissue, and, because of the concomitant infection associated perhaps with gangrene, may be so dangerous as to threaten life. It is now evident that the urine acts as a vehicle to disseminate infection; urine in itself, unless the extravasation is large and continuous, is not a necrotizing agent. With the advent of the sulfonamides extravasation of urine, therefore, carries less risk because the infection can be controlled. If the injury is located in the penile urethra, the extravasation will usually be limited to the shaft of the penis; if in the deeper part of the urethra, but still in front of the triangular ligament (urogenital diaphragm), the extravasation may extend into the scrotum and anterior abdominal wall. In lacerations behind or posterior to the triangular ligament, the urine may infiltrate into the posterior perineum around the neck of the bladder and the deeper portion of the anterior abdominal wall. The tissue affected by the extravasation rapidly becomes swollen and edematous. Tenderness is variable but is increased in the presence of infection which is prone to develop in the involved area. The skin may become reddened; if the condition is neglected, areas of gangrene may develop. Malaise, prostration and fever, with its accompanying manifestations, are commonly observed. The toxemia resulting from extravasation of urine is profound; death is apt to ensue unless adequate and early treatment is resorted to.

Treatment consists of immediate and numerous incisions to prevent fatal spread of infection which is so prone to develop in the tissue where extravasation has occurred. It is usually necessary to perform a suprapubic cystostomy, unless a retention catheter can be inserted into the bladder through the urethra.

Foreign Bodies in the Urethra.—Foreign bodies encountered in the urethra include objects inserted by the patient, or stones arising usually in the kidney or bladder. The symptoms of pain and difficulty associated with urination usually disappear after removal of the foreign body.

Urethritis (Nonspecific).—Mild acute urethritis not of gonorrheal origin caused by the *Bacillus coli, Streptococcus, Micrococcus catarrhalis,* etc., is relatively frequent, and may cause the patient (male or female) considerable worry because of the similarity of the symptoms to gonorrhea in the early stages. It may also be produced by instrumentation or chemicals injected for prophylactic reasons. Mild frequency and burning on urination, and urethral discharge are common manifestations. Most of them subside spontaneously after a few days, especially if effort is made to drink a large amount of water and to void frequently. Unless the infection is of chemical or instrumental origin, chemotherapy or the injection of 1 per cent protargol two or three times a day for two or three days is usually effective in eradicating the infection.

Gonococcal Urethritis (Gonorrhea).—Gonorrhea * is a venereal disease contracted with few exceptions only by sexual contact, and is first manifested as an anterior urethritis after an incubation period of four to six days. The first symptom is a burning or stinging pain in the anterior urethra upon urination. A slight discharge of turbid, sticky secretion is noted which becomes thick, purulent and profuse within a few days. The meatus is reddened and swollen. Frequency of

* Infection in the female is discussed on page 954.

urination is always present, but is not severe during the four to eight days while the infection is limited to anterior urethritis. Unless effective treatment is instituted early, posterior urethritis develops in nearly all patients and is manifested by a pronounced exacerbation of symptoms. Mild fever is commonly present. The pain experienced during urination (especially at the beginning and end) becomes severe. The patient may be awakened frequently at night by a painful erection with curvature of the shaft (chordee). After six to eight weeks the symptoms, as a rule, decrease, the discharge lessens and convalescence is well under way, although a cure is not expected for many months.

A mild chronic urethritis exists for a time, but on the average no manifestations remain after five or six months except perhaps the morning drop (slight urethral discharge noted in the morning upon arising). The chronic stage of the infection usually represents a residual infection of the mucous glands along the urethra or residual infection of the periurethral tissue. On many occasions, however, the chronic stage of the disease, as manifested by mild burning and frequency of urination and slight urethral discharge, are produced by complications such as prostatitis and seminal vesiculitis. The patient is usually infectious as long as a urethral discharge is present.

The *diagnosis* of the acute stage is readily made by examination of the urethral discharge. Gram-negative intracellular and extracellular diplococci are present in large numbers. The intracellular characteristic of the organisms is extremely important diagnostically because extracellular gram-negative diplococci are normal inhabitants of the urethra, and may be found in nonspecific or chemical urethritis. Urinary shreds arising from the posterior urethra are diagnostic of the chronic disease. The two glass test (see p. 983) may be helpful in determining the presence of posterior urethritis, since there will be no turbidity of the first glass if the bladder or kidney is the seat of the infection. The confirmation of the termination of the disease may be important, particularly from the standpoint of infectivity. If the disease is still present, though symptoms are few or absent, the inflammation can usually be relighted by strenuous exercise, sexual excitement or insertion of a urethral sound.

Complications.—The development of prostatitis and seminal vesiculitis in association with posterior urethritis is not uncommon. In the acute stage of gonorrhea the symptoms are increased in severity by the development of prostatitis and seminal vesiculitis, but can be differentiated only with difficulty from acute posterior urethritis. An acute epididymitis may be secondary to acute posterior urethritis and seminal vesiculitis, and frequently results from errors in treatment such as instrumentation, excessive treatment, strenuous exercise, etc. The manifestions are described on page 1016. Acute balanoposthitis (inflammation of the glans penis and prepuce) is not a common complication; it occurs usually only in the presence of phimosis. Acute arthritis (see p. 472) occurring six to twelve weeks after the acute onset of the urethritis is not uncommon. Periurethral and prostatic abscesses are uncommon, but may add considerably to the severity of the symptoms. They may break spontaneously into the urethra, but on many occasions require incision from the exterior. Acute lymphadenitis due to a Ducrey infection is not an uncommon complication of gonorrhea, but is fortunately not a serious one although it may suppurate. Swelling and tenderness of the inguinal lymph nodes may also be produced by secondary pyogenic infection. The lymphadenitis due to the gonococcus does not suppurate, but if secondary pyogenic infection is present (*e.g.,* balanoposthitis) the lymph nodes may become acutely inflamed, fluctuant and require incision.

Urethral stricture occurs usually in the bulbomembranous urethra, results from periurethral infection, but rarely develops earlier than eighteen to twenty-four months following the acute gonorrheal infection. It is much more common in Negroes than whites, and is frequently multiple as contrasted to the solitary strictures which follow trauma. Early manifestations consist of the appearance of slight urethral discharge, mild burning upon urination, and decrease in size of the stream. The stricture may progress to the point that the stream is reduced to a dribble. Acute retention may develop. Because of the ulceration which frequently develops proximal to the stricture, urinary extravasation or even fistulas may develop.

Treatment is most effective if started early before serious narrowing is produced, and consists of dilatation of the urethra every four to six days with as large a sound as possible. No sounds smaller than 16F or 18F should be used because of the danger of injury to the urethral wall. The size of the sound should be increased at each successive treatment until a size 28F can be passed. Any dilatation which is followed by the escape of more than a small drop of blood is harmful in that it indicates injury; thus the deposition of more scar tissue is encouraged. Unfortunately, even this amount of dilatation is not permanent and the patient should be instructed to return every six months or a year for further dilatation to prevent serious contraction. If the stricture is so pronounced as not to allow the passage of a size 18F sound, it is usually wise to pass a filiform bougie which is then threaded on to a small sound and pushed into the bladder ahead of the sound. Rarely is urethrotomy (incision of the scarred area) indicated. Resection of the narrowed part of the urethra may occasionally be performed satisfactorily when the stricture is traumatic, but is not feasible in gonorrheal strictures because of their greater extent.

Treatment of Gonorrhea.—Since gonorrhea can be prevented, even after exposure, the most important feature in the treatment is prophylactic. Evidence is accumulating that sulfonamide compounds are effective in the prophylactic treatment of gonorrhea as well as after the disease has developed. On the day of exposure 80 to 90 grains of sulfathiazole should be given and a daily dose of 60 grains continued for 6 to 8 days. Prophylaxis by local means was known to be effective long before the introduction of sulfonamides; distention of the urethra for 5 minutes with 2 per cent protargol up to eight hours following exposure, rarely failed to prevent the disease in men. It appears logical then that local treatment combined with chemotherapy might be advisable in the prophylactic treatment. In actual practice, however, prophylactic therapy is difficult to carry out, except in the Army and Navy where compulsion is effective.

Sulfonamide therapy has displaced local treatment with silver or other chemicals. Originally, sulfanilamide and sulfapyridine were used; however, it is now obvious that sulfathiazole is superior, although sulfadiazine is perhaps as effective. With the latter two drugs systemic reactions are much less common, particularly since it has been discovered that the dose need not be maximal. A dose of one gram 4 times a day for 5 to 7 days will result in cure of the infection in about 90 per cent of the cases. During treatment the patient should abstain from alcohol, sexual excitement, and excessive exercise. Details of the sulfonamide treatment may be found in the monograph by Herrold [9].

It must be emphasized, however, that patients treated with sulfonamide compounds may still harbor gonococci in their urethra for some time after symptoms have disappeared. For that reason careful smears, cultures and examination of urine sediment must be made before patients are discharged as cured. If one sulfonamide compound fails to produce a favorable effect in a few days another may be tried, or therapy with the original drug repeated after a few days' cessation of treatment. If the sulfonamides fail, fever therapy as reported by Carpenter and associates,[28] and Bromberg [29] and others should be used and may in fact be effectively combined with chemotherapy.

EPIDIDYMIS

Acute Epididymitis.—Acute infection of the epididymis is usually gonorrheal in origin and is a common complication of untreated gonorrhea. Since it develops only in the presence of posterior urethritis, it rarely is encountered earlier than three weeks following onset of the infection. Ordinarily, abstinence from sexual excitement, limitation of exercise and careful supervision of treatment will prevent acute epididymitis.

The most important manifestations are tenderness and pain which develop with swelling of the epididymis and are roughly proportionate to it. A moderate amount of fever may be produced by epididymitis, regardless of its cause, but is obviously more pronounced in the acute infections. The pain and tenderness may be so severe as to be completely disabling. Rarely does the process proceed to suppuration, regardless of the cause.

The most important feature in the *treatment* is bed rest. However, if bed rest is impossible, the application of a suspensory for the scrotum will be very helpful. Even while in bed, the pain will be greatly relieved if some sort of suspensory is applied so as to prevent dependency of the scrotum. The application of heat or cold will aid in relief of the pain. Ordinarily the pain disappears and the swelling recedes within a few days after institution of bed rest, but if the above treatment does not afford relief, a short incision into the distended epididymis is frequently efficient in eliminating the pain, although it may not shorten the convalescence to a very great extent. The fluid obtained by such a procedure may be turbid, but is rarely thick and purulent.

On many occasions acute epididymitis is not of gonorrheal origin. Especially is this true in elderly men who may develop the disease in the absence of a significant posterior urethritis, which ordinarily must be present before acute epididymitis develops. Vigorous instrumentation such as that associated with frequent cystoscopic examinations is not infrequently followed by acute epididymitis. Ligation of the vas deferens prevents epididymitis, and for that reason is frequently done

before urethral instrumentation is performed, especially in elderly men. The non-specific type of epididymitis is more apt to suppurate than the gonorrheal type and may require incision. Otherwise the treatment of the two types is largely the same; sulfonamide therapy is obviously important in either type.

Chronic Epididymitis.—Acute epididymitis usually resolves into chronic infection of the organ, which may remain enlarged permanently, though produce no symptoms. Recurrent attacks are not uncommon, but may be prevented to a certain extent by treatment of any existing urethritis, and having the patient wear a suspensory. The amount of pain and tenderness is extremely variable. Sterility results much less often than would be expected. Occasionally it may be necessary to excise the epididymis.

Tuberculous Epididymitis.—Tuberculous infection of the epididymis is usually secondary to tuberculosis of the kidney or seminal vesicle. It begins in the globus minor, spreads to the entire organ and may involve the testicle. The invasion is usually insidious, producing a slow, gradual enlargement without pain. There is a tendency for fluctuant areas to develop which may break down and form permanent sinuses. Because of the failure of response to conservative treatment, excision is usually indicated as soon as the diagnosis is made, providing there are no contraindications.

Spermatocele.—Occasionally a collection of cloudy fluid containing spermatazoa collects about the epididymis, but does not invade the testis. Such a cystic swelling is called a spermatocele. Very few symptoms are present, but the lesion may be confused with chronic epididymitis or tuberculosis of the epididymis.

TESTICLE

Undescended Testicle (Cryptorchidism).—The testicles descend during the latter months of fetal life, but cryptorchidism is noted in about 15 per cent of babies at birth. The testicle may lie within the abdominal cavity, but more frequently is present in the inguinal canal. Descent of the testicles will occur, however, in a large percentage of these infants within a year or two after birth. The main cause of the lack of descent usually appears to be shortness of the blood vessels of the vas; abnormalities of the inguinal canal, may also exist. In view of the effect of antuitrin therapy the primary cause appears to be hormonal imbalance.

It is essential that cryptorchidism be treated sometime during childhood, since it has long been known that the increased temperature in the abdominal cavity over that in the scrotum is sufficient to inflict serious damage to the spermatogenic function of the testicle, which develops at puberty. Patients with bilateral cryptorchidism are usually sterile. Many observers have reported a greater incidence of malignancy in undescended testes than in descended testes, but there is not agreement on this point.

Treatment.—During recent years the gonadotropic hormone of pregnancy urine (antuitrin S) has been used with varying results in the treatment of cryptorchidism, but on account of frequent recurrence and damage to the testicle [31] it is being abandoned by many physicians. Operative correction, preferably between the ages of 8 to 12 years, is again becoming the procedure of choice. A hernia is usually present along with the undescended testicle and should be repaired at the same time.

Operation consists of opening the canal, finding the testicle, dissecting away the short fibrous tissue strands connecting the tortuous vessels, freeing the vas, and anchoring the testicle to the fundus of the scrotum (Bevan) or to the subcutaneous tissue of the thigh (Torek). The latter procedure requires a minor operation several weeks or months later to separate the attachment to the thigh.

Torsion of the Spermatic Cord.—Because of a weakened gubernaculum associated with maldescent, the testis may be suddenly pulled upward by the cremaster

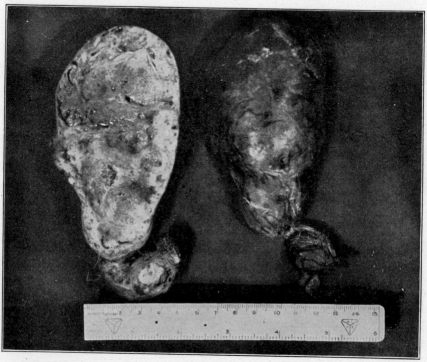

Fig. 555.—Teratoma of the Testicle in a Man, Aged Twenty-eight.

Enlargement of the testicle was first noted four months previously. The Aschheim-Zondek test was positive; two weeks after operative removal of the tumor it was negative.

muscle in such a manner as to allow twisting of the cord. This rarely occurs in children. The blood supply may be completely strangulated, in which case gangrene of the testis occurs, terminating either in an abscess or atrophy of the testis or both. The pain associated with torsion of the cord is intense. Nausea, vomiting and mild shock may be present. Unless reduction can be attained within an hour after development of the torsion, operation (orchidectomy) is advisable.

Miscellaneous Diseases of the Testis.—As a tertiary manifestation, *syphilis* may affect the testis either as an interstitial orchitis or as a gummatous degeneration. The swelling is insidious and associated with no pain or inflammatory signs. Autiluetic treatment produces a retrogression of the swelling.

There are a few diseases among which mumps is the most important which may be associated with *orchitis*. During the acute process the testis may be swollen and tender, but atrophy later develops. *Tuberculosis of the testis* may be encountered in association with tuberculous epididymitis, but is a rare lesion; orchidectomy will usually be strongly indicated.

Tumors of the Testis.—With the exception of a few benign tumors such as fibroma, etc., most tumors of the testis are malignant. Ewing is of the opinion that all malignant tumors of the testis (which comprise less than one-half of 1 per cent of all malignant disease) can be classified as teratomas. They arise from the sex cells, but contain many different types of tissue including muscle, cartilage, fat, etc. They occur in young adults, are very malignant, grow rapidly and metastasize to the lumbar chain of lymph nodes as well as to the nodes in the retroperitoneal portion of the upper abdomen. Reference has already been made to the relation of malignant tumors to cryptorchidism. It should be mentioned that tumors of the testicle frequently develop insidiously, the patient being entirely unaware of its presence. Even if he consults a physician, the enlargement may be passed up. In a few instances a relatively small tumor may metastasize and produce manifestations of epigastric enlargement before the patient is aware that there is anything wrong with his testicle. The anterior hypophyseal sex hormone (prolan A) is present in the urine of patients with malignant tumors of the testicle in such large quantities as to be demonstrable by the Aschheim-Zondek test (Zondek[32]).

Treatment.—As soon as the diagnosis is made, orchidectomy should be performed unless metastases are obvious and growing so rapidly as to threaten life within a very short time. Dissection of lymph nodes at the time of the orchidectomy does not appear to increase the chances of a cure. However, according to the studies of Cabot and Berkson[34] radiotherapy is effective in certain types of neoplasms of the testis. Regardless of the type of therapy used, five year cures are not common.

PENIS

Phimosis.—Frequently, the orifice of the prepuce is congenitally too small to allow retraction behind the glans (phimosis). This allows accumulation of smegma which may be the source of considerable irritation. This irritation may at times be associated with considerable infection of the glans and prepuce (balanoposthitis). Adhesions between the glans and prepuce are frequently present. If the preputial orifice is large enough to allow retraction, these adhesions may be separated readily in children without resorting to operative procedures.

Circumcision is strongly indicated in all instances when there is an actual phimosis and is advisable when the prepuce is redundant. It may be performed at any age. Local or general anesthesia may be used, depending upon the age of the patient. A dorsal slit is made backward to within 0.5 centimeter of the sulcus. Excision of the prepuce is carried forward on each side with a scissors until the incisions meet in front of the frenum on the ventral side. A generous amount of skin must be left on the ventral side near the frenum so as to prevent deformity of the penis during erection. All bleeding points must be carefully ligated. The cut edges are then approximated with interrupted sutures of 000 catgut.

Paraphimosis.—When the prepuce is tight and becomes retracted, it is occasionally difficult or impossible to reduce it because of the edema which rapidly develops. The prepuce distal to the line of constriction becomes very edematous. The glans may be cyanotic and painful; if the constriction is complete enough to block all circulation, gangrene will develop. Reduction should be attempted, but not until the edema of the glans and prepuce distal to the constriction has been squeezed out by digital compression. If this can be accomplished, reduction may be possible. However, if reduction is impossible, and necrosis of tissue seems imminent, it is advisable to cut across the constricted prepuce in a longitudinal direction on the dorsal surface, and treat the patient by bed rest and local irrigation until the edema subsides. After the edema and inflammation subside, circumcision may be performed in a routine manner.

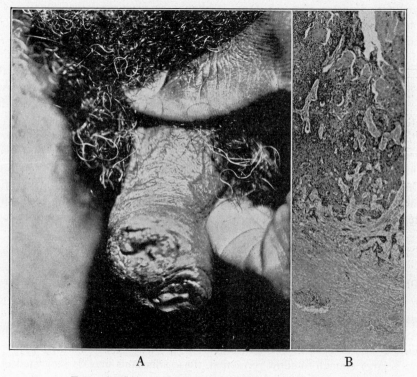

A   B

Fig. 556.—Squamous Cell Carcinoma of the Penis.

A, appearance of the lesion six months after onset; *B*, low power photomicrograph from a section of the excised specimen; note that the hyperplastic epithelial growth is invading the subcutaneous tissue.

Carcinoma of the Penis.—Rarely indeed is carcinoma of the penis encountered in a patient who has been circumcised, suggesting that in this instance irritation is an important factor in the development of the tumor which usually appears on the unexposed surface of the prepuce. The tumor is of the squamous cell type and metastasizes slowly to the inguinal lymph nodes.

The type of treatment required depends upon the size of the carcinoma. If small, it may be excised locally, and after a dissection of the inguinal lymph nodes has been performed, x-ray therapy should be given over the penis and groins. If the tumor is large, amputation is advisable. Since these tumors are of the squamous-cell type, they usually recede favorably after x-ray therapy.

Congenital Anomalies.—Very few of the anomalies of the penis are common unless phimosis, as already discussed, is considered to be congenital. An abnormally small urethral meatus is, however, fairly frequent.

Hypospadias.—This lesion, consisting of the location of the urethral meatus on the *ventral* surface of the penis, proximal to its normal position, is in reality just as much an anomaly of the urethra as the penis. There are three types: (1) balanic, in which the meatus is located at the junction of the glans and shaft, (2) penile, in which the meatus is located at the penile-scrotal angle, and (3) perineal in which the meatus is located just in front of the triangular ligament. A downward and backward curve of the urethra, noted particularly upon erection (chordee), is usually present because of an atrophy or absence of the corpus spongiosum and the presence of a fibrous band along the ventral surface of the shaft.

Treatment is operative and is usually confined to the penile type because treatment is not very necessary in the balanic type and is relatively unsuccessful in the perineal type. Innumerable operations have been devised to correct the anomaly. The urethra is constructed by skin grafts of various types taken from the thigh, prepuce, or scrotum. McKenna [35] has called attention to the necessity of eliminating the deformity by excision of the scar tissue on the ventral surface of the penis and by establishment of a long urethra.

Epispadias.—This anomaly, consisting of the location of the urethral orifice on the dorsal surface of the penis is less common than hypospadias. The defect which represents a cleft, may extend through the entire length of the shaft and even be associated with exstrophy of the bladder.

Herpes Progenitalis.—Single or grouped blisters may arise on the glans penis or skin and a few days after onset the blisters may rupture, after which infection frequently occurs. This lesion is seen frequently and is often ushered in with considerable pain which disappears as soon as the vesicles appear. Treatment consists of cleanliness and dusting powders.

MISCELLANEOUS LESIONS OF THE GENITO-URINARY SYSTEM

Hydrocele.—There are different varieties of hydrocele (see Fig. 557), most of which are congenital in origin. A few appear to be caused by infections or by operative procedures. The vaginal type of hydrocele (fluid in the tunica vaginalis) is said by many observers to be the most common, but the fact that most hydroceles extend so far upward along the cord suggests that patency of the distal cord of the funicular process exists at least to a slight degree in most instances.

There is usually a history of a slowly growing mass in the scrotum which, with the exception of the congenital hydrocele, is irreducible. They are pear or oval shaped and may attain an enormous size, containing several hundred cubic centimeters of fluid. The mass is dull to percussion. No impulse is noted over the mass upon coughing except when a hernia is also present and projects downward against the apex of the hydrocele. The mass transmits light except in the rare instances when a chylous hydrocele (containing shimmering cholesterol crystals) is present. The fluid contained in the sac is usually clear and straw colored, but may be colorless and opalescent.

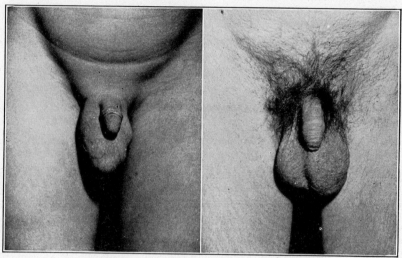

FIG. 557.   FIG. 558.

FIG. 557.—HYDROCELE IN A BOY, AGED FIVE.
The swelling was first noted two years previously.

FIG. 558.—HYDROCELE IN A MAN, AGED FIFTY-FIVE.
The swelling was first noted six months previously. All of the fluid was removed by aspiration three weeks previously, but, as is usually the case, reaccumulated rapidly.

Treatment.—The mass may be reduced readily by aspiration, but fluid always reforms. Injection of irritating and sclerosing substances has been recommended and may be indicated in certain cases. There are two types of operative procedures: (1) The bottle operation consists of making a small incision in the apex of the sac and inverting the testicle through the hole in the sac. This is a simple procedure quickly done, but is occasionally followed by a tender mass which may have to be excised later. (2) Excision of the hydrocele sac along the margin of its attachment with the testis and cord probably results in a greater percentage of cures than other procedures. On account of the delayed tendency for the tiny vessels on the cut surface of the sac to stop bleeding, it is essential that a running suture of fine catgut be taken along the cut edge to prevent postoperative hemorrhage, which is a serious complication from the standpoint of obliteration of the blood supply to the testis with resultant atrophy.

Varicocele.—Dilatation of the spermatic veins is a common anomaly and is probably of congenital origin. It is usually located on the left side because the left spermatic vein has no valves, and empties into the vena cava at right angles.

Standing for long periods of time and strenuous exercise are probably secondary etiologic factors. The dilated veins are tortuous and rarely associated with tenderness or pain. Occasionally mild discomfort in the scrotum is complained of, but this is usually relieved satisfactorily if the scrotum is supported with a suspensory. Excision of the varicose veins will rarely fail to relieve the symptoms, but is not often indicated.

BIBLIOGRAPHY

1. NITZE, MAX. Lehrbuch der Kystoskopie, Ihre Technik und klinische Bedeutung, Weisbaden, 1889, J. F. Bergmann.
2. ALBARRAN, J. The Lever Principle in Ureteral Catheterization, *Bull. Acad. Med.*, 37:384, 1897.
3. Quoted by *History of Urology*, Vol. 11, p. 210, Williams & Wilkins Co., Baltimore, 1933.
4. VON LICHTENBERG, A., and SWICK, M. Klinische Prüfung Des Uroselectans, *Klin. Wchnschr.*, 8:2089, 1929.
5. ROWNTREE, L. G., and GERAGHTY, J. T. The Phthalein Test: An Experimental and Clinical Study of Phenolsulphonephthalein in Relation to Renal Function in Health and Disease, *Arch. Int. Med.*, 9:284, 1912.
6. WATSON, F. S. Subparietal Injuries of the Kidney, *Boston M. & S. J.*, 149:64, 1903.
7. GOLDBLATT, H., LYNCH, G., HANZAL, R. F., and SUMMERVILLE, W. W. The Production of Persistent Elevation of Systolic Blood Pressure by Means of Renal Ischemia. *J. Exper. Med.*, 59:347, 1934; GOLDBLATT, H. The Production of the Malignant Phase of Hypertension, *J. Exper. Med.*, 67:809, 1938.
8. NESBIT, R. M., and RATLIFF, R. K. Hypertension Associated with Unilateral Nephropathy, *J. Urol.*, 43:427, 1940.
9. HERROLD, R. D. *Chemotherapy of Gonococcal Infections*, C. V. Mosby, St. Louis, 1943.
10. CULVER, H., and SEIFERT, W. F. Urinary Antiseptics: Collective Review, *Surg., Gynec., and Obst.*, 70:574, 1940, Internat. Abst. Surg.
11. LAZARUS, J. A. Carbuncle of the Kidney, *Am. J. Surg.*, 25:155, 1934.
12. McKENNA, C. M., and BIRCH, C. L. Hematogenous Hematuria, *J. Urol.*, 42:171, 1939.
13. HIGGINS, C. C. Production and Solution of Urinary Calculi, *J. Am. M. Ass.*, 104:1296, 1935.
14. OPPENHEIMER, G. D., and POLLACK, H. Attempted Solution of Renal Calculi by Diuretic Measures, *J. Am. M. Ass.*, 108:349, 1937.
15. KEYES, E. L. *Urology*, D. Appleton & Co., New York, 1928.
16. ROSE, D. K. Hypernephroma and Carcinoma of the Kidney: a Comparative Study, *Arch. Surg.*, 10:943, 1925.
17. ROSE, D. K. Cystometric Bladder Pressure Determinations: Their Clinical Importance, *J. Urol.*, 17:487, 1927; Clinical Application of Bladder Physiology, *ibid.*, 26:91, 1931.
18. COFFEY, R. C. Transplantation of Ureters into Large Intestine by Submucous Implantation; Clinical Application of Technic, *J. Am. M. Ass.*, 99:1320, 1932.
19. KEYES, E. L. *Loc cit.*, p. 399.
20. ROSE, D. K. An Immobilizing Retractor Which Allows Direct Exposure of Bladder Carcinoma to X-ray Therapy, *J. Urol.*, 33:664, 1935.
21. MUNRO, D. In the *Practitioners Library of Medicine and Surgery*, Vol. 5, p. 795, D. Appleton & Co., New York, 1934.
22. Lower, W. E., and JOHNSTON, R. L. Further Studies on Experimental Work on Probable Cause of Prostatic Hypertrophy, *J. Urol.*, 26:599, 1931.

23. RANDALL, A. *Surgical Pathology of Prostatic Obstruction,* Williams & Wilkins Co., Baltimore, 1931.

24. McCARTHY, J. F. A New Apparatus for Endoscopic Plastic Surgery of the Prostate, Diathermia and Excision of Vesical Growths, *J. Urol.,* 26:695, 1931.

25. HUGGINS, C., STEVENS, R. E., JR., and HODGES, C. V. Studies of Prostatic Cancer; Effects of Castration on Advanced Carcinoma of Prostate Gland, *Arch. Surg.,* 43:209, 1941.

26. EVANS, J. P. The Physiologic Basis of the Neurogenic Bladder, *J. Am. Med. Ass.,* 117:1927, 1941.

27. HERBST, W. P. Biochemical Therapeusis in Carcinoma of the Prostate Gland, *J. Am. M. Ass.,* 120:1116, 1942.

28. CARPENTER, C. M., BOAK, R. A., MUCCI, L. A., and WARREN, S. L. Studies on Physiologic Effects of Fever Temperatures; Thermal Death Time of Neisseria Gonorrheæ in Vitro with Special Reference to Fever Temperatures, *J. Lab. & Clin. M.,* 18:981, 1933.

29. BROMBERG, LEON. Artificial Fever Therapy; Report on Three Years' Clinical Experience, *J. Missouri M. A.,* 36:24, 1939.

30. RANDALL, A., EIMAN, J. E., and LEBERMAN, P. R. Studies on the Pathology of the Renal Papilla, *J. Am. Med. Ass.,* 109:1698, 1937.

31. EISENSTAEDT, J. S., APPEL, MAX, and FRAENKEL, MAX. The Effect of Hormones on the Undescended Testis, *J. Am. M. Ass.,* 115:200, 1940.

32. ZONDEK, B. Versuch einer biologischen (hormonalen) Diagnostik beim malignen Hodentumor, Chirurg. 2:1072, 1930.

33. HELMHOLZ, H. F. The Bacteriostatic Action of Sulfadiazine, Sulfathiazole, Sulfacetimide, and Sulfapyridine on Bacteria Isolated from Urinary Infections, *Proc. Staff Meet. Mayo Clinic,* 17:529, 1942.

34. CABOT, H., and BERKSON, J. Outlook for Patients with Malignant Tumors of Testis Associated with Massive Metastases, *Proc. Staff Meet., Mayo Clin.,* 14:377, 1939; Neoplasms of Testis, Study of Results of Orchidectomy with and without Irradiation, *New England J. Med.,* 220:192, 1939.

35. McKENNA, C. M. Hypospadias, *J. Am. M. Ass.,* 113:2138, 1939.

36. Review of Urologic Surgery, *Arch. Surg.,* 44:1126, 1942.

37. LADD, W. E., and GROSS, R. E. *Abdominal Surgery in Infancy and Childhood,* W. B. Saunders Co., Philadelphia, 1941.

CHAPTER XXXIII

WAR AND CATASTROPHE SURGERY

War and catastrophe always offer a challenge to surgical therapy; in the present world-wide conflict a number of changes, already evident, have so affected modern warfare as to present many new diagnostic and therapeutic problems. Moreover, they have influenced the care of the injured during civilian catastrophes occurring either as a result of war or of accidents.

Of the larger wars in the present century, the Boer war and the Russo-Japanese war were still characterized by injuries due largely to bullet wounds alone, the treatment of which was fairly simple and in general conservative. In World War I the use of high explosives on a large scale made it necessary to revise completely the treatment of wounds because of the extensive tissue damage produced by shell fragments and shrapnel. The non-operative treatment of these wounds was soon found to lead to disastrous infections. Radical wound excision, therefore, became adopted as the definitive form of treatment. The Spanish Civil War of 1936-1938, however, was the first real rehearsal of modern warfare and ushered in the newer aspects of injury as produced by increasingly severe explosive force especially from aerial bombs as well as problems created by rapid mechanized warfare. The injuries occurring in this conflict are well described by Jolly [1], Trueta [2], Eloesser [3] and others. Injuries in the present world war are considered in a number of publications that have already appeared and can be recommended [4, 5].

Before discussing these new problems, the intensity and magnitude of modern total and global war must be emphasized. These potentialities have not materialized as yet, as far as we in the United States are concerned. Thus, during the first 19 months of the present conflict the number of wounded suffered by the American army, navy, marines and coast guard has been relatively slight, *i.e.,* up until December, 1943, the total dead (29,317), wounded (40,917), missing (32,131) and prisoners (28,733) was but 131,098 *, or an average of 57,940 per year. When we compare these figures with the deaths from automobile accidents alone (*e.g.,* 39,643 in 1937) we realize that war is not the only mechanism involved in the useless, massive sacrifice of human beings. Although the number of deaths sustained by United

---

* Release from Office of War Information, November 30, 1943.

States military forces from action in the present conflict cannot be determined accurately (because of the unknown status of the missing) it is quite obvious that up to date they are much less than the deaths from automobile accidents alone for a similar period before the war. On the other hand, the British losses (dead, wounded and missing) totaled 514,997 up to June 1, 1943. The climax of modern land and air warfare, however, has already been reached on the Russian front where the casualties on both sides have unquestionably reached many millions. In view of the fact that the tempo of land action will undoubtedly be increased, we may expect, therefore, a peak of casualties when our forces participate in a European invasion.

Modern warfare has another feature of importance to the surgeon and that is the relative absence of any definite "front". This is partly due to the extreme mobility of motorized equipment. But it is also due to the fact that the airplane has brought destruction to life and property far beyond the lines of combat. This involvement of the civilian population presents problems similar to those due to great catastrophes, which occur infrequently during peace time. In this country the organization of communities for aerial attack has already demonstrated the value of such preparation for the care of wounded resulting from any type of catastrophe such as fires, explosions, floods, etc.

Wounds due to high explosives, particularly those resulting from aerial bombs, are a special feature of present day warfare; this fact deserves particular comment. In previous wars explosive missiles were fired almost entirely from mortars or cannon. To withstand the propelling force, these shells are made with rather thick casings; thus, when they explode the fragments are relatively large, but traveling at less velocity than fragments resulting from the explosion of aerial bombs. Aerial bombs have a relatively thin casing since they have to withstand merely the friction of the air after being dropped from the airplanes. This difference is of extreme importance in the production of wounds because the extent of the wound inflicted is directly proportional to the energy possessed and dissipated by these fragments as they enter the tissues. This energy is expressed by the well-known physical law of inertia.

$$E = \frac{1}{2}MV^2$$

It will be noted in this formula that while the energy, *i.e.*, destructive property, is directly proportional to the weight of the fragment, it is directly proportional to the *square* of its velocity. Thus relatively small fragments from an aerial bomb travelling at terrific speed, which at the time of explosion often reach the incredible figure of 4000 feet a second, will produce tremendous destruction of the tissue after entering, even though a trivial wound of the skin is produced. On the other hand, the fragments are so small that their destructive force is quickly lost. Indeed, relatively slight protection is sufficient to prevent their penetration or at least to minimize their devastating effect.

Aerial bombs produce wounds which have other important characteristics. Their location is unusual. Whereas bullet wounds or even wounds from artillery projectiles strike the anterior surface of the soldier, fragments from aerial bombs more frequently enter the back, shoulder and buttocks. This war has sometimes been called therefore "the war of the crouching soldier". Moreover, the wounds produced by aerial bombs are very apt to be multiple inasmuch as the tremendous explosive force produces a large number of tiny fragments. Finally, by the very nature of the explosion, much of the injury will be due to flying splinters of glass and masonry and crushing injuries due to falling timbers, etc. The extensive use of explosives in modern warfare has also led to recognition and understanding of serious internal injuries in the absence of any external evidence thereof. These injuries fall under the designation of "blast" and will be discussed in detail later in this chapter.

Rapid movement and the increasing use of mechanized equipment is another feature of modern warfare which presents important problems in regard to the transportation of the wounded and in the fact that thermal injury from burning gasoline is much more frequent.

In presenting the details of war and catastrophe surgery in this chapter, discussion will be confined to the new and unusual features, including particularly features in war which are different from those in civilian surgery. Therefore, much of the material will supplement that on the same subjects in the body of the text. A few of the subjects are quite new, *e.g.*, blast injuries and crush syndrome, and have not been described previously in this book.

PRIORITIES IN TREATMENT

Under ordinary civilian conditions there is little or no priority in treatment of injured patients inasmuch as there is usually sufficient time and facilities to treat all of them. Following violent combat, or during extraordinary civilian catastrophe, the number of injured may be so great as to demand a definite and prearranged system of priorities based upon the well known democratic principle of doing the most good to the greatest number. Under such conditions the most severely injured with very little chance of recovery may have to be passed by in favor of those in whom the prognosis is better. Again, those severely injured and requiring relatively simple therapy may receive priorities over those requiring much more time. Hard and fast rules cannot, of course, be laid down, and meticulous judgment must be exercised by those in charge. At the front line hospital is a group of surgeons called the *triage team* whose function it is to exert this judgment. Decisions will obviously be based upon such considerations as the available personnel, the amount of supplies, the extent of transportation facilities, and of course, above all, the exigencies of the military situation, which in general supersedes other considerations, since it is more directly connected with the immediate aims of warfare and the protection of the healthy fighting forces. In establishing priorities in treatment, first aid and transportation play an important part and will be discussed in detail. To this will be added a section on special features of catastrophe management.

Importance of First Aid Treatment.—The first to reach the injured must be prepared to administer first aid [41] treatment. To a large extent, first aid treatment consists of preparing the injured for transportation to a dressing station where medical assistance is available. This point should be emphasized, inasmuch as a good deal of the details concerning first aid treatment disseminated among lay individuals carries with it a possibility of doing more harm than good. This refers not only to the use of the tourniquet, but also to the use of splints, each of which in untrained hands may produce unnecessary damage. Even in the hands of trained personnel a tourniquet may be responsible for grave results (see Crush Syndrome). Indeed Jolly [1] has stated "More limbs and lives are lost at the front from the improper use of the tourniquet than are saved by its proper use." The control of hemorrhage as a first aid measure is of obvious importance, but should rarely involve anything more than the elevation of the extremity or the application of local pressure. A compression dressing utilizing resilient material such as cotton waste as recommended by Gallagher [6] is an effective way of stopping hemorrhage without the dangers so frequently associated with the constriction of a tourniquet. Artificial respiration is important when indicated, but aside from drowning, can probably seldom be given by untrained personnel.

The trained personnel of the medical corps administering first aid become quite efficient and actually carry out much work ordinarily carried out by physicians. The bravery and courage of these men deserve special mention particularly because they suffer a high incidence of injury themselves. For this reason sufficient numbers of trained reserves are essential for replacement, as emphasized by the British in the North African campaign.

First aid treatment may now be considered to include plasma transfusions inasmuch as such treatment is administered by non-medical personnel at the front lines. The first use of the sulfonamides may likewise be placed under first aid care but is discussed in detail elsewhere. Relief of pain is obviously important and may often be given by first aid personnel. In most cases pain is relieved by a hypodermic of morphia which may be injected intravenously in urgent cases. Another method for momentary relief of pain especially during the process of extricating wounded from tanks is the inhalation of a few drops of chloroform or ethyl chloride. Ampoules containing enough of these anesthetic agents are used in both the American and Russian armies for brief but complete relief of pain, especially when a painful procedure must be carried out.

In contrast to fist aid the term *definitive* or *full* treatment is used to describe the procedures, including operations, carried out by medical officers and nurses.

Transportation of the Injured.—Of greatest importance, of course, in transportation, is the element of time inasmuch as the complications become multiplied the longer the period elapsing between sustaining of the injury and the arrival of the soldier at the first station where treatment may be started. This time-lag not only increases the incidence of shock, but also the likelihood of infection. It is this more or less inevitable delay in treatment of war injuries which in general makes it difficult to achieve as good results as may be expected in civilian practice.

Transportation in general, however, is poorly borne by many severely injured individuals, particularly over poor roads and where movement and rough handling is inevitable. Under these conditions it may be advisable not to move certain types of patients. For example, it has already been noted that severely burned patients stand transportation poorly between 8 hours and 4 days after the burn. If they can be transported before or after this interval, deterioration in their general condition is less likely to occur. A similar principle applies to other severely injured soldiers with certain types of injury, *e.g.*, cranial and intra-abdominal, or in which slowly developing shock may occur. Repeated movements of the injured is just as deleterious as repeated dressings. Transportation from the field of battle is obviously urgent; as soon as possible thereafter a definite decision must be made in order to avoid repeated trips from one station to another.

During a successful offensive with rapidly advancing troops, evacuation of the wounded becomes relatively simple. However, during a retreat it may become impossible. On the other hand, when movement is at a standstill, the existence of casualties presents a problem of delay insofar as the wounded can be evacuated only under cover of darkness. Under such conditions, the injured may suffer a delay of 12 hours or more before they are even reached by medical personnel. An important departure from this policy has been achieved by the Russians who have devised a method of evacuating the injured from the field of battle under actual combat conditions by means of field nurses who single handed carry the wounded on their backs or by means of canvas ground sheets to the first dressing station. By this method the injured may be treated by the medical corps within a few hours after sustaining their injury [7].

Litter bearers should, of course, confine their activities to those requiring transportation in the horizontal position. This applies generally to those in severe shock, those with serious lung or abdominal injuires and those with fractures of the lower extremities. Most injuries of the upper extremities and head do not require stretchers, but may be transported as ambulatory patients under their own power, thus saving personnel and equipment for more seriously injured. However, the existence of blast and other injuries of the lung due to war gases or thermal injury requires transportation in the horizontal position; medical personnel must bear this in mind even though there is very little or no external evidence of injury. Any movement in the upright position by those with lung injuries is apt to precipitate severe respiratory difficulties or uncontrollable anoxia.

Motorized ambulances have accelerated greatly the speed of transportation of the wounded and the use of the airplane has already achieved remarkable results in carrying injured soldiers far behind the lines where more complicated definitive treatment can be given. In severely shocked patients and in those with pneumo- and hemothorax, however, the danger of anoxia at altitudes above 5000 feet may prove deleterious. The airplane already has been used by the American forces in various parts of the world. In North Africa for example, 13,000 wounded were transported by airplanes which had arrived at the front carrying various material of war [8].

The organization of the American army for evacuation of the wounded follows the classic method of graded stations beginning with the battalion first aid station close to the front line. Up to and including the divisional units apportionment of personnel and supplies is rigidly fixed. Inevitably, therefore, the work and supply requirements of an individual unit may vary from intense 24 hour activity to lulls when there is little to do. To some extent this variation is inevitable but fortunately applies less to the larger units. Thus above the level of the division, *i.e.,* in the corps or army organization, considerable flexibility is possible thus permitting much elasticity in assigning surgical hospitals, evacuation hospitals and various other units to any other part of the front where needed. Indeed, attached to general headquarters are special surgical teams, shock teams, splint teams, maxillo-facial teams, gas teams, research teams, etc., which may be sent to any part of the front as indicated.

This flexibility is, of course, of extreme importance in shortening the period between injury and definitive treatment and in avoiding unnecessary and repeated movements of the wounded. Such elasticity of organization has been recognized to a greater extent in the Russian army in that they have loosened the rigid divisional organization, as seems evident from the following quotation [9].

"Formerly every division had its hospitals. If the division was in the rear or in reserve, its hospital remained inactive, while at some part of the front there might have been more wounded than could be taken care of. Even at the front some divisions, with light losses, would have idle facilities while other division hospitals would be overburdened. The centralized administration of the medical services is directed by the chiefs of the given army, not the individual division. It is the duty of the medical chiefs to maneuver the facilities at their disposal to the best advantage. . . . Centralization has proved its value. It has saved a great deal of manpower and equipment by economical handling, and it has spread the burden more equitably over the entire army medical corps."

Special Aspects of Catastrophe Management.—In the management of civilian catastrophies, one of the important elements in priorities is the immediate elimination of the dead, inasmuch as their presence impedes the care of the living. At some convenient place a physician should be placed in order to segregate the fatalities, so that they may be transported away from the field of active treatment. If possible, this physician should be present at the scene of the accident in order to avoid an unnecessary load on the transportation facilities. A lay person, being unable to distinguish between the seriously injured living and dead will obviously transport both to the hospital, thus creating an unnecessarily difficult problem. If this separation cannot be made at the scene of the accident, it should be done immediately as the bodies are received at the emergency station and before they have been admitted to the actual receiving room for treatment.

The Office of Civilian Defense in this country has been responsible for setting up excellent organizations of hospital staffs to handle the injured resulting from possible enemy action from the air or by sabotage. While such events have as yet not transpired, the advantages of this prearranged organization in civilian catastrophe due to accident has already been demonstrated. Important in this organization is the availability of large stores of plasma and intravenous sets for the administration of transfusions to a large number of individuals at one time. Adequate supplies of other sorts such as splints are also important in order to handle a sudden influx of injured. Surgeons not directly assigned to the care of patients have proved most valuable because by viewing the over-all clinical picture they will recognize special aspects and developments which may be overlooked by those immediately concerned with the emergency treatment.

WAR WOUNDS: GENERAL CONSIDERATIONS

War wounds in general are much more serious than civilian wounds and are much more likely to be accompanied by surgical shock and are particularly prone to infection. The reasons are to be found in the following 3 factors which also alter therapy considerably in military as contrasted to civilian wounds:

1. Delay between injury and treatment is much longer and inevitable in war wounds.

2. War wounds contain much more foreign material imbedded deeply in the tissue.

3. Destruction of tissue is much more extensive due to the devastating effect of bomb fragments.

In spite of the fact that the wounds in the present conflict are more severe, the death rate is much less than in World War I. Thus the death rate in evacuation hospitals during World War I was 15 to 18 per cent, compared to 2½ to 3½ per cent (Kirk [10]) in the North African campaign of 1943 (exclusive of Northern Tunisia). The mortality is greatest in wounds of the peritoneal cavity, thorax and brain.

War wounds may be inflicted in numerous ways, and therefore differ greatly in type. As already stated, wounds made by modern high explosives will be associated with massive destruction of tissue, and will contain more foreign bodies. Bayonet wounds are also serious because of the massive laceration of tissue beneath the skin. Crushed wounds, which are commonly produced by walls of crumbling buildings, are, of course, serious, and may be fatal without an actual open wound. The military surgeon rapidly learns that the external wound bears little relationship to the amount of damage inflicted inside the body. This is particularly true of wounds produced by thin bomb fragments which may enter the body lengthwise, producing a slight skin laceration, yet result in massive laceration because of rotation of the foreign body as it passes through the tissues. On the other hand, bullet wounds in general produce much less tissue damage. Bullet wounds sustained at close range have a relatively small wound of entrance, but a much larger wound of exit; while there may be considerable local trauma at the site of entrance, the shock of the impact is so great that the victim falls or is hurled to the ground. The force of this impact decreases inversely with the range from the gun and with the velocity of the bullet. At long range the impact may be so trivial that the soldier himself is unaware of being wounded. Under such circumstances, the wounds of entrance and exit are relatively small. The percentage of seriously injured has been much larger in the present than in any previous war. This is due undoubtedly to the increasing destructive power of modern implements of war and particularly the use of larger bombs and increasing explosive forces, particularly in aerial attacks. Thus the proportion of injured to dead in World War I was about 4 to 5 to one, whereas in the present conflict it tends to approach equality.

Surgical Shock.—As might have been expected, the incidence of surgical shock has been very great among the injured in the present world conflict. The extensive use of large amounts of plasma, however, has already demonstrated the great value of and more than fulfilled the promise originally made for this new method of increasing blood volume in soldiers with peripheral circulatory failure due to surgical shock. The noteworthy efforts of the Red Cross and the response of the civilian population have made it possible to provide pooled plasma in dried (lyophilized) form which has facilitated transporting this material to all the far-flung theatres of action. The effectiveness of plasma transfusions confirms the fact that most cases of surgical shock are indeed due to a fall in blood volume and that its correction with a fluid exerting a colloidal osmotic pressure is true replacement therapy. It should be mentioned, however, that in *severe hemorrhage red cells are also important* and transfusion of whole blood *cannot be dismissed as an old fashioned procedure* (see page 155). However, there have been a number of instances in which neither the use of plasma nor whole blood has proved effective and this, among other considerations, has again raised the question of the existence of other factors which may play a part in the pathogenesis of shock.

Extensive study has already and is being made particularly in surgical shock not accompanied by actual hemorrhage. These studies have indicated in general that two mechanisms (mentioned below) not directly producing a loss of blood or plasma may play an important role in precipitating surgical shock, particularly in certain types of injury. These two mechanisms had been mentioned and studied in the past, but most surgeons considered them as rarely responsible for surgical shock in patients.

1. The existence of a "toxic" factor associated in nearly all cases with tissue damage of a severe sort leading to death and autolysis particularly of muscle appears very possible. This mechanism is probably responsible for many of the signs of surgical shock in soldiers suffering extensive crushing injuries of muscle or indeed extensive damage to muscle from bomb fragments, which, as discussed in the beginning of this chapter, are capable of producing death of large masses of muscle tissue often through relatively tiny openings in the skin. This aspect of surgical shock has been discussed in some detail separately under the heading of Crush Syndrome.

2. Neurogenic factors probably play a role in the initiation of shock at least, and may even be responsible for many of the manifestations which persist after the time of the injury. This mechanism has been investigated particularly by Phemister [11] in this country and by workers in Russia. The most easily available of the latter data has been published in English by Lena Stern [12].

While the most frequent cause for surgical shock is undoubtedly the actual loss of blood or plasma by hemorrhage, tissue trauma or burns, it must be admitted that devitalized muscle tissue as well as neurogenic factors may both play a role in many instances and indeed be of primary importance in a few cases. In combating surgical shock, therefore, the surgeon should bear in mind the possibilities of a crush injury and of neurogenic factors. As far as treatment is concerned the importance of early excision of necrotic tissue is discussed separately. The influence of neurogenic factors is a little more difficult to treat except that it emphasizes the importance of eliminating pain and of the necessity of careful and complete anesthesia during surgical procedures. These factors are discussed separately.

A third important though more obvious factor in the production of shock is the existence of dehydration and malnutrition in the wounded soldier. Victims of torpedo sinkings set adrift for days or weeks, and men lost in jungles, or exposed to the elements, are obviously more likely to suffer surgical shock; these considerations play an obvious part in the preparation of the injured for operative repair.

Regardless of these additional mechanisms in the production of surgical shock, it should be emphasized again that one of the important factors in its control is the element of time, *i.e.,* the promptness with which the injured soldier is treated not only for his local lesions but for the earliest systemic manifestations of shock. The availability of plasma which can be given directly on the battlefield has already proved the importance of this fundamental concept. Even more important are advances made in the efficient transportation of the injured to stations where this form of treatment can be given more effectively, as well as definitive therapy for the local lesions can be carried out. The details of transportation are discussed under another heading.

Preoperative Factors.—Treatment of war wounds and the results of treatment are decisively influenced by numerous preoperative factors many of which have already been mentioned but are now discussed in detail. The *"time-lag"* or the interval elapsing between injury and definitive treatment is extremely important, as already intimated. If there has been considerable delay and infection of the wound has developed, thorough débridement cannot be done, although removal of foreign bodies and incisions for adequate drainage are permissible. As already mentioned mortality rates increase sharply in direct ratio to the length of this "time-lag". Other factors are also important.

The *kind of transportation* used to bring the wounded to the hospital will affect the physical condition of the patient. If he has been carried by stretcher over long mountain trails or by ambulance over rough roads, various factors such as persistence of pain, increasing extravasation of plasma into wounded areas, and recurrent hemorrhage, combine to increase shock and lower general resistance to operation.

The *physical condition of the soldier* at the time of injury often determines his resistance to trauma and thus influences mortality. It has been known since World War I that a soldier who has been fighting for two or three days with inadequate water and food tolerates a wound poorly. Under such conditions operative treatment of a rather trivial injury with an anesthetic may be followed by surprisingly severe shock. It, therefore, becomes an important duty of the medical attendant to ascertain the degree of hardship undergone by the wounded during the days preceding injury, so that prophylactic measures may be instituted. Similarly the type and availability of *first aid,* as already discussed, is also of importance in evaluating the physical condition of the patient. For example, the *administration of plasma,* being now considered first aid treatment, and performed by medical attendants at the front line, will be responsible for saving many lives.

Early *sulfonamide treatment* may actually be considered a first aid procedure and, from the information available at the present time, is very important in the prevention of infection. The American soldier carries an envelope in his first aid pouch containing 4 grams of sulfadiazine which he is instructed to take by mouth. The local use of sulfanilamide in the wound has been discontinued as a first aid procedure in the army.

The *triage team* at the front line hospital is a very important group in determining the fate of wounded men. This group makes decisions regarding operation or observation and priorities, *i.e.,* which wound is to be treated first. Since decisions must be made rapidly, such men should be mature surgeons whose judgment is of the best.

The *types of work* done by the surgeons themselves obviously will be important. During a heavy "drive", it will be necessary for the surgeons to maintain great speed in operative work. However, it should be emphasized that speed alone is not the sole requirement; careful technic is also essential since more harm than good can easily be done by reckless and careless work. Jolly[1] has very appropriately warned that the surgeon must have rest, lest his judgment become so impaired as to jeopardize the life of his patient.

The *facilities available* to the medical personnel will naturally be an important factor in determining results. For example, the availability of an x-ray machine will aid tremendously in discovery and removal of foreign bodies. Adequate lighting and sterilizing equipment are obviously important.

Anesthesia.—Many of the principles and methods of anesthesia in the armed forces are fundamentally the same as those in civilian life; others are markedly different. These differences are noted chiefly at the front and are largely dependent upon (1) type of patient, (2) type of injury, (3) urgency and volume of cases, (4) scarcity of personnel and experience of personnel, (5) limitation of equipment, (6) peculiarities of accommodations, etc.

The patients are mostly young husky individuals, although some may be in shock, anemic from hemorrhage or debilitated from sepsis. Having gone through the emotional stress of battle they have a high nervous tension and, as pointed out by Kaye[13], are prone to show severe excitement during induction. A rapid smooth induction is therefore indicated. In suitable cases pentothal may be used for induction to avoid this complication. It may easily be followed by nitrous oxide but is less satisfactory when preceding ether anesthesia.

In military hospitals near the fighting zones there are apt to be periods of inactivity alternating with periods of intense activity. When numerous casualties are admitted in a short time, anesthesia and operation must be accomplished in the shortest possible time. Here again, especially for short or simple operations, or for induction to be followed by inhalation anesthesia, pentothal has an advantage. Spinal anesthesia can also be accomplished quickly but has the disadvantage of increasing the danger of shock by producing a fall in blood pressure. An ether induction is apt to be slow, but the use of a little ethyl chloride or chloroform followed by ether can reduce the time required. Local and block anesthesia are time consuming. Local anesthesia, however, will be most suitable for minor procedures. Recent experiences at and near the front indicate that sodium pentothal and ether are in general the most adaptable.

The lack of adequate personnel in busy periods has an important influence on anesthesia. Since adequate post anesthetic care may be impossible, it is important to use agents and methods which will result in the rapid recovery of patients. Basal narcosis and excessive sedation should be avoided. Gas anesthesia, or gas combined with a little ether, results in a more rapid recovery than deep ether anesthesia. Recovery from a short pentothal anesthetic is rapid but if the anesthesia has been long the recovery may be slow. Regional anesthesia has the advantage that the patient is awake when he leaves the operating room.

When it becomes necessary to call upon corps men or other nonmedical assistants to give many anesthetics only simple and relatively safe methods should be approved. Open drop ether is probably the best. One anesthetist may have to administer more than one anesthetic at a time by himself. Local anesthesia administered by the surgeon may relieve the anesthetist in some cases. Patients under spinal anesthesia should be watched throughout the operation, but if necessary the anesthetic can be administered by the anesthetist and the patient subsequently watched by a nurse or corps man. This is particularly true of low spinals. Spinal anesthesia for upper abdominal work is apt to result in more serious complications and the patient may require more skilled attention.

Near the front where most of the emergency surgery must be done the dearth of mechanical equipment including gas machines, gas tanks, etc., will limit the methods of anesthesia, and in fact will call for greater skill than need be exercised under more normal circumstances. The anesthetist will have to be versatile. Facilities for regional anesthesia, intravenous anesthesia and open drop inhalation anesthesia should be available wherever major procedures are undertaken. Sometimes, however, the anesthetist will have to get along with very limited or improvised equipment as happened when an American anesthetist worked for days with only chloroform borrowed from the British.

The physical accommodations of military hospitals in war zones involve inconveniences. Pavilions may be separated by considerable distances to avoid offering a good bombing target. Patients may have to be transported from one pavilion to another. This is another reason why a quick recovery in the operating room is important. Another physical feature to be considered is the means of lighting the operating room. Where open flames are required the danger of ignition of inflammable anesthetics is serious. Intravenous and regional anesthesia avoid this hazard. Chloroform and nitrous oxide are not inflammable. Ether is inflammable; if its use is unavoidable one should remember that the vapor is heavier than air and, barring air currents, will drift towards the floor. Lamps should, therefore, be placed high above the level of the patient.

A patient operated on near the front lines and *transported immediately* to the rear should make a quick recovery from the anesthetic so that he will not have respiratory difficulties. Anesthetics which lead to nausea and vomiting should be avoided both for the patient's own comfort on the trip and for the comfort of others with him. Local or block anesthesia would be the best choice. Spinal anesthesia would not be suitable unless its effects would be completely worn off before the trip started. Gas anesthesia would be suitable. Ether would be a poor choice. Local or block anesthesia may even be used to provide pain relief during the trip.

In the presence of *surgical shock,* local anesthesia is best if it will provide suitable working conditions. Its use has definite limitations such as lack of abdominal relaxation. Injecting of more than 100 to 125 c.c. of one per cent procaine is undesirable. Spinal anesthesia produces good relaxation but is contraindicated in cases of shock because it may cause still a greater fall in blood pressure. Spinal anesthesia is particularly dangerous in the presence of blast shock, and even in patients subjected to blast but revealing no manifestations of shock. Deep pentothal anesthesia may cause a fall in blood pressure, but a short light anesthetic with pentothal might be satisfactory. Intravenous sodium pentothal was used by Americans during the Pearl Harbor attack, but was given up because of toxic effects. However, the British are using it a great deal in the acutely injured, and find it satisfactory. It would appear to have its greatest usefulness in the reduction of fractures in patients who are not in shock, or who have none of the signs of impending shock. It should be stated, however, that this anesthetic should not be used unless the anesthetist can devote his entire attention to the patient, so that oxygen can be administered when indicated, and the airway be maintained if vomiting, obstruction and other complications develop. Although deep ether anesthesia may cause a fall in blood pressure it may be the best choice if other methods are inadequate or unsuitable. An intercostal or abdominal wall block may be used for abdominal relaxation and if necessary supplemented with nitrous oxide or pentothal.

Operations for certain types of injuries will require utilization of special methods in anesthesia. For example, *intrathoracic operations* should be dealt with by special technics if suitable facilities are available. It has been noted that patients with chest injuries tolerate operations better than the average civilian requiring an intrathoracic operation because the patient has not been debilitated by a protracted pulmonary disease. Shock and hemorrhage are apt to be common but adequate replacement therapy and relief of pain can do much to overcome these. The anesthetist should try to choose an anesthetic which will have the least tendency to increase shock. Patients in shock are usually easily anesthetized with a low concentration of the agent. They require high oxygen in the inspired atmosphere. Nitrous oxide with ample oxygen would be satisfactory but adequate anesthesia may not always be achieved without reducing the oxygen. Ample premedication or the addition of a little pentothal intravenously or a little ether in the mixture may help.

Anesthesia in *abdominal operations* in the presence of shock will be a serious problem. In general, ether is not satisfactory; neither is spinal anesthesia safe. The English find that nitrous oxide and oxygen combined with local infiltration or intercostal block are safe and effective. The use of one of the gases, combined with block anesthesia (*e.g.*, procaine) would, therefore, appear to be the most practical. If there is no evidence of shock, ether is permissible and may be the anesthetic of choice.

In *head injuries* there will be less indication for a general anesthesia because muscular relaxation is not necessary; in fact, general anesthesia may be extremely dangerous because of the depressant effect. Local anesthesia will, therefore, be the agent of choice.

It should be emphasized that the anesthetist must exercise care in proper cleansing of masks, etc., between cases; urgency for saving time, and the lack of facilities are apt to discourage proper aseptic care. The equipment should be washed thoroughly with soap and water (if available) and when indicated, attempts made to sterilize it in some way. Metal pieces can be boiled. For rubber pieces soaking in a 1 to 8000 solution of biniodide has been found practical by at least some of the British units. Lysol or other coal tar products should not be used on rubber as they are absorbed by the rubber and may subsequently cause a burn.

As in all anesthesia, the choice of agent and method (if a choice is available) may depend largely on the preferences and experience of the anesthetist. Any anesthetic well given will do the patient less harm than a more suitable anesthetic badly administered.

Operative Treatment.—In spite of delay and shock most war wounds require operative therapy. The decision regarding the *type of anesthesia* is important and is discussed in some detail in the preceding section. To a great extent the choice will largely be determined by the agents and facilities available. At the front line the anesthetist will probably be limited to intravenous sodium pentothal, procaine for local anesthesia and ether for open-drop anesthesia.

Débridement remains as one of the most important procedures in the operative treatment of war wounds. Débridement has a much different meaning in military than in civilian surgery. In war wounds débridement is an operation of excision rather than of cleansing. The reasons for excision are many, though perhaps the most important is the fact that there is so much necrotic tissue to be removed, particularly muscle. But more than obviously necrotic tissue must be excised. A thin shell of all of the contaminated surface is excised with sharp dissection including a narrow edge of skin. This is a much more rapid way of eliminating contamination than meticulous cleansing and requires fewer supplies. Extensive incisions are also important in order to expose deep tissue which is so often extensively injured through a tiny wound of entrance. Deep fascia is also incised or excised to expose damaged muscle for removal. However radical the process of débridement may be, important structures such as vessels and nerves are meticulously preserved. Irrigation is not used not only because of the added supplies and time it requires but also because of the danger of spreading contamination in these extensive wounds. War wounds, in general, are not closed; there are a few exceptions as intracranial wounds, wounds of the peritoneal and thoracic cavities, and wounds of large joints. The importance of the open wound method in preventing gas gangrene is exemplified by the experiences after the Pearl Harbor attack; in the 11 cases of gas gangrene all occurred in wounds which had been closed after débridement (Halford [14]).

As to *chemotherapy* it must be emphasized that the use of the sulfonamide drugs cannot take the place of adequate débridement. At most the proper employment of the sulfonamides permits a less radical excision of contaminated tissue although it will not detract from the necessity to remove all of the necrotic tissue. After débridement the wound is sprinkled with *sulfanilamide*, and a dressing of vaseline gauze applied to the surface of the wound. The gauze should be fine-mesh so that granulation tissue will not grow through it.

Under certain circumstances a *plaster cast* may be applied over massive soft tissue wounds. When the patient is to be transported soon after operation such immobilization with plaster is one of the most important factors in the healing of the wound. Unless there is a fracture a thick wide plaster slab mold is just as effective for immobilization as a circular cast. On the other hand, a circular plaster cast has the additional advantages of exerting mild pressure in the face of subsequent swelling and also of insuring infrequent dressings.

Postoperative Care.—A booster dose of *tetanus toxoid* should be given to all wounded men who have been actively immunized; otherwise tetanus antitoxin must be given. There is slight disagreement as to the necessity of giving *gas gangrene antitoxin,* although there is a growing tendency to recommend the use of large doses in prophylaxis as well as in the treatment of the infection itself. *Sulfonamide therapy* must be continued for at least several days after operation to help minimize the possibility of severe infection. The kind of drug and method of administration will vary with circumstances. However, if the oral route is permissible, there is a growing tendency to employ sulfadiazine, 50 to 60 grains a day, being careful that sufficient water is given to prevent renal complications; if the oral route is not permissible, the drug is given intravenously as the sodium salt.

Antiseptics themselves in the treatment of wounds, have been discussed on page 26 and in Chapter X. Although they have little or no place in civilian wound therapy, there is evidence of their value in war wounds. For example, many military units in North Africa (as reported by Mitchell and Buttle [15], and others), have used proflavine sulphate in a dose of 2 grams or less in infected wounds with excellent results. Clark, Colebrook, Gibson and Thomson [16] have obtained promising effects with the local application of penicillin and a new drug, propamidine. Fresh solutions (under 6 months old) of both proflavine dihydrochloride (1-1000) and 2 per cent aqueous solution of iodine (U.S.P.) may be considered safe and fairly effective surface antiseptics.

Infrequent dressing, in the postoperative care of war wounds, is an important principle which is too often forgotten. Dressings should not be changed, once properly applied, unless definitely indicated because each dressing inflicts trauma and pain, and introduces a great danger of secondary contamination. Indeed Jolly [1] has expressed the importance of the principle of infrequent dressings by writing "Innumerable sufferers in every war have been bandaged into their graves at the hands of over-enthusiastic dressers." When dressings are done the surgeon and personnel should wear efficient masks. Gloves are important and should be washed in soap and water after each dressing. To minimize air contamination an interval of two hours must elapse after sweeping and dusting before dressings are done; windows should be closed and the traffic through the wards stopped. These precautions are more necessary in military than in civilian hospitals because the larger area of the exposed wounds are more prone to possible contamination.

Postoperative *nutrition* is extremely important and includes not only the necessity of *maintaining fluid and electrolyte* balance in the form of saline but also energy, protein and vitamin requirements. These factors have already been discussed on page 151 and will be mentioned again under convalescent care in the next section.

When *transportation* is inevitable the patient must be prepared for the ordeal. As already stated, a plaster cast or splint may be advisable for large wounds even though they involve only the soft tissues. Skin casts should not be used, but if necessary because of lack of supplies, must be split and spread the entire length to allow for swelling. Adhesive tape should not be placed over hair because it produces tremendous discomfort. Bandages must be securely fixed because transportation tends to loosen them and expose the wounds. The presence of drains should be indicated on the plaster cast or dressings lest they slip into the wound and escape detection. Records, including the dose of medication and time given, should be kept (*in legible handwriting*) and forwarded with the wounded man.

Much of this data can be written on the surface of the plaster, a method which eliminates the danger of loss of the patient's record.

Specialized care must be emphasized such as will be possible only in a *general hospital*. This includes the application of skin grafts and plastic procedures, correction of deformities, etc. During this period the patient must be watched carefully for the possible development of complications which must be treated as early as possible to avoid serious defects.

Convalescent Care.—Postoperative care of the wounded must not be limited to short periods during which acute complications are apt to occur but should include full convalescence. Indeed the aim should really be one of complete rehabilitation as rapidly as possible. Moreover, the surgeon may have to perform secondary operations and these may be impossible unless the convalescent care following the first operation has been adequate. Both psychic factors such as maintenance of morale as well as purely medical procedures will insure better and more rapid convalescence. The British, for example, have emphasized the necessity of so-called *luxury care* in the convalescence of the wounded soldier. This includes such items as moving the patient to a porch for sun baths, ample reading material, music, entertainment, and especially expert nursing care which is of extreme value in swinging the balance toward rapid recovery.

Usually overlooked but of primary importance in convalescence is *adequate nutrition*. Physicians and nurses are too prone to rely on the patient's appetite to insure an adequate dietary intake. Yet it has been demonstrated beyond doubt that many normal individuals, due to ignorance or poverty, subsist on inadequate diets. Malnutrition is frequent, though its manifestations may be subclinical, among civilians in many walks of life. True enough, the soldier soon becomes well nourished after several months of army food and he may be assumed to harbor no nutritional deficiencies at the time of his injury. However, within a short time, deficits begin to accumulate, due somewhat to the added demands imposed by the injury, by operation and particularly by infection. These added needs are correctable by increasing the dietary intake, except that anorexia is pronounced and is commonly associated with the injury and its aftermath of disability and infection.

Nutritional deficits in the injured soldier include largely proteins and vitamins and both must be considered in the care of the convalescent soldier. Loss of weight is a sure indication that nutritional defects are present but deficits may be lurking even when the patient seems relatively well padded with adipose tissue. Unless this aspect of convalsecent care is realized and studied, nutritional deficiencies will be corrected slowly or not at all, thus leading to slow recovery with permanent invalidism as a serious danger. Moreover, the malnourished soldier is less able to throw off infections, to conquer disability, and to withstand formidable surgical procedures necessary for his rehabilitation than those adequately nourished. Even if reconstructive procedures are carried out, healing may occur poorly or not at all in the presence of nutritional deficits.

Besides adequate vitamins and calories it is often necessary to increase the daily protein intake to combat hypoproteinemia which is common in the convalescent soldier. The ordinary protein intake of the normal adult is usually placed at 75 to 100 grams per day; this must be increased to 150 to 250 grams a day if severe protein deficits are to be corrected rapidly. Hypoproteinemia of nutritional origin cannot be permanently corrected by plasma transfusions (see page 151); if the oral intake is inadequate it may be wise to supplement the diet by the intravenous injection of an appropriate amino-acid mixture of hydrolyzed protein as already discussed.

WAR WOUNDS: SPECIFIC TYPES

In spite of careful preparation and attempts to provide excellent equipment for the care of the wounded, it must be emphasized that war wounds more frequently than not must be treated under relatively primitive circumstances. Aside from the large units in the rear, it is impossible at the front to expect the conditions available in a well equipped hospital. These factors are of extreme importance because they necessitate tremendous simplification in the methods of treatment and an ability to improvise. The frequency of relatively primitive conditions is not only due to the difficulty in transporting modern equipment to the battle fronts, but also because of inevitable shortage of supplies, the necessity of concealing activity from the enemy, and the frequent impossibility of movement of the wounded and supplies quickly, often under cover of darkness. Indeed, supplies are as likely as not to be scanty or wanting entirely, either because they cannot be brought up, or because they have been destroyed. Water particularly is apt to be scanty. For these reasons the surgeon must often improvise and alter his methods of therapy to meet conditions of the moment.

These considerations as well as the likelihood of a sudden influx of large numbers of wounded make it necessary for surgical procedures to be simple and rapid and require a minimum of material. This is one of the reasons why the irrigation cleansing of wounds which is practiced in civilian life cannot be carried out under war conditions. In its place, the procedure of débridement consists merely of extensive incisions and excision of contaminated and necrotic tissue. Moreover, all supplies, especially dressings, must be used with great economy. Similarly, simple plaster splints are preferable to elaborate fixation apparatus.

Thermal Burns.—The present war has shown a remarkable increase in the incidence of thermal burns. Much of this increase is due to the extensive use of mechanized equipment motivated by gasoline which increases the hazard of flame, particularly in inclosed vehicles such as tanks. Widespread use of incendiary bombs in aerial warfare has also played its part. Naval personnel are particularly susceptible to thermal injuries from escaping steam as well as burns from flaming oil and gasoline; in battle they are susceptible to flash burns from exploding bombs. Indeed, many reports of naval casualties at sea have shown that a majority of the injured exhibited varying degrees of thermal burns.

The newer developments in the treatment of burns are based on the principles discussed in the chapter on burns, but the details have aroused considerable discussion and differences of opinion. In the still prevalent problem of infection, two primary principles have been emphasized as of particular importance.

1. The recognition that infection in burns is largely due to contamination during the hours after the injury, largely by careless technic during the dressings;

adequate masking and meticulous aseptic precautions must therefore be scrupulously maintained.

2. Frequent dressings often lead to an increased danger of contamination especially by cross infection from other infections in the ward. Infrequent dressings, therefore, have come to assume just as important emphasis in the principles of the care of burns as in the care of compound fractures. Indeed, the use of the plaster cast is definitely of value particularly since it introduces immobilization as well as infrequent dressings.

As in civilian life intravenous administration of plasma remains as one of the most important therapeutic procedures, and requires rigid priority in treatment, preceding local care of the burned surface. Depletion of the supply of plasma will justify transfusion of whole blood, although whole blood is undesirable in burns unless anemia develops. According to British experience, it exerts such beneficial results that the deleterious effect of the red blood cells in the presence of hemo-concentration is more than neutralized. The danger of toxicity from sodium citrate must always be kept in mind in patients with extensive burns receiving large quantities of plasma.

Flash burns were prevalent in World War I as cordite burns from the back-flash down the ammunition shafts of fighting ships; these have now been eliminated [17]. However, flash burns are still frequent though due to other causes. The injury, as now seen, is due to the momentary exposure of the skin to explosions of incendiary bombs, to the sudden combustion of inflammable gases, to widespread ignition of a large sheet of gasoline or to the actual explosion of gasoline when suddenly ignited under favorable conditions. Sudden blasts of superheated air or steam may also be responsible for momentary thermal injury of this sort.

Flash burns are characterized by a very short lasting but intense thermal injury and thus are quite superficial; yet the thin layer of skin which is involved is destroyed. Notable is the fact that only exposed skin is involved in flash burns. The thinnest of clothing protects the body against such an injury. Flash burns are therefore only sustained over the face and hands, and on the legs of personnel in the tropics because they wear shorts. The burns of the face, while intense and often followed by tremendous swelling, usually heal without very much difficulty. Flash burns of the hands or indeed any burns of the hands are more serious because of the well-known liability of the hands to atrophy by disuse. These injuries of the hands are particularly important in the air force, whose personnel require long periods of time for training and whose loss is very serious. Efforts toward shortening the period of disability in the treatment of burns of the hands are therefore of great importance. Over the rest of the body flash burns present no new problems other than those already mentioned in the chapter on burns.

Treatment of flash burns is that of any other first and second degree burn. Prophylaxis is more important inasmuch as these burns can be averted by covering the exposed skin; the difficulty has been to insure that it is done. Anti-flash clothing is supplied to most personnel likely to be exposed to severe flashes or flame.

Lung injuries in burns have been observed sporadically whenever there was inhalation of smoke and were usually described as pneumonia. However, it was not until the Cocoanut Grove tragedy in Boston on November 28, 1942, that the true nature and importance of this lesion was fully realized[18]. The possibility that the lungs may be involved in any patient suffering from thermal injury must be recognized inasmuch as the treatment is decisively influenced thereby.

Involvement of the lung together with thermal burns of the skin is apt to occur from inhalation during sudden explosions or rapidly burning material such as gasoline, particularly when the accident occurs in a relatively closed space. In civilian life lung injuries have been observed in burns following accidental explosions when gasoline or kerosene has been poured into a fireplace or stove in order to rekindle a fire. It is probably present with most flash burns, inasmuch as a flash burn of the face is frequently present in patients with pulmonary involvement.

Pulmonary injury in a thermal burn should be suspected in any individual who has sustained a flash burn of the face, or in any case in which the burn has occurred in a closed space and in which there has been an actual flame or tremendously superheated air. The development of hoarseness in the patient should also suggest the existence of a pulmonary injury. Edema of the larynx may be observed by direct examination within an hour or two of the accident. Inspection of the nostrils may show singed hairs or actually burned turbinates. Examination of the tongue may also reveal a superficial burn of its mucous membrane. These lesions are probably due to the inhalation of actual flame or certainly of super-heated air. More important, however, are evidences of injuries deep in the substance of the lung, *i.e.*, in the smaller bronchi and alveoli which are probably due to the inhalation of poisonous gases which are frequently present whenever there is extensive combustion especially in a closed space. The serious effects produced by these gases are similar to those described in detail later in this chapter under the section devoted to war gases.

The presence of a pulmonary lesion modifies considerably the treatment of thermal burns of the skin. Thus the irritant effect of poisonous gases on the finer bronchi and alveoli may rapidly lead to anoxia, the skin of the patient exhibiting a dusky pallor, which to the uninitiated may suggest surgical shock. While the peripheral circulation is undoubtedly affected, it is important to recognize the pulmonary origin of the manifestations as the primary cause, lest the wrong type of emergency therapy be started. In the first place, morphine must be used with great caution in order to avoid any depressing effect on respiration. Second, plasma transfusions must not be excessive in view of the possible presence or development of pulmonary edema. Third, inhalations of oxygen should be emphasized in the severe cases where respiratory function is seriously impaired. Finally, in the presence of severe edema of the larynx, tracheotomy may be indicated.

Simple Fractures.—Because injuries in military life are usually sustained by flying missiles which penetrate tissues, simple fractures are much less common than compound fractures. Although most of the simple fractures sustained in war time will be similar to those observed in civilian life, a few are peculiar to military casualties; they will be discussed below. The treatment of simple fractures in military casualties differs from similar fractures in civilian life in that there will not be the opportunity to obtain early reduction. Indeed, at the front line stations very little attempt may be made to obtain complete reduction. The primary consideration at this early stage in the treatment of the casualty is immobilization and splinting to enable rapid transportation away from the front lines. In general, skin casts are unsatisfactory for this early treatment; even padded casts should be split to allow for swelling. Although traction is desirable in first aid treatment, one of the serious complications of transportation with traction splints has been the development of pressure sores at the site of application of the hitch which had been applied for traction. Traction on fractures of the upper extremity for immediate fixation and transportation has been abandoned in favor of plaster or simple fixation of the arm to the trunk, because of the complication just mentioned, and because traction on the upper extremity so commonly increases displacement of fragments. Plaster spicas in general are not very satisfactory for transportation. When the injured soldier arrives at a center where controlled anesthesia is possible, efforts then will be made to obtain accurate reduction.

March fracture is located usually in the second or third metatarsal bone of the foot. It is frequently observed in the training period of the recruit and is presumably caused by the continuous trauma of marching or of lifting. However, it has recently been emphasized (Moore and Bracher[19]) that the fracture may be produced by numerous other mechanisms, based on the fact that these bones are somewhat weaker than the others and are subjected to more strain. When it develops following continuous marching, a burning pain which increases in intensity from day to day will be noted in the region of the fracture. Pain is so severe that limping is pronounced, and in fact may result in complete disability. Examination will reveal swelling on the dorsum of the foot in practically all cases, with swelling on the plantar surface in the more severe types. Marked tenderness along the shaft of the metatarsal bone will be elicited, but no crepitus, since the fracture is commonly incomplete, or surrounded with callus by the time the physician sees it. The x-ray will reveal a fracture line, but on certain occasions the line will be so faint as to require two or more views, repeated after an interval of three or four days, for its demonstration. Considerable callus may be observed if the lesion is more than a few days old. At times this callus may be confused with a tumor. Clinically the lesion is also frequently confused with metatarsalgia. The frequent occurrence of March fracture in military personnel makes it mandatory that x-ray films be taken on all occasions when a soldier complains of symptoms such as those described above. Details may be found in an article by Myerding and Pollock [20].

The treatment is simple except that adequate immobilization must be achieved. A plaster cast is usually preferable, thereby obtaining complete immobilization which should be maintained for at least three weeks, with activities limited for an additional two weeks. Very seldom will any attempts at reduction be necessary.

Parachute injuries are fairly common during the early days of training the paratrooper recruit. As training progresses, injury becomes less common. Fortunately, most of the injuries are of the minor type, consisting chiefly of sprains. Most of the fractures are located about the ankle. In a study made by Tobin[21], 50 per cent involved the malleoli. Fractures of the external malleolus are slightly more common than the internal (23 per cent versus 9 per cent). About 12 per cent were fractures of the posterior articular margin or posterior lip of the tibia. Such a fracture is very uncommon in civilian life. Another 4 per cent of his series had a fracture of the posterior lip of the tibia associated with a fracture of one of the malleoli. In about 5 per cent of cases the metatarsals were fractured, and in one per cent the phalanges were the site of fracture. For the most part, the sudden strain thrown upon the foot held in forced plantar flexion is the cause of the fracture. As Tobin remarks, the jumpers often "reach for the ground" and sustain injury largely because oscillation of the parachute causes them to land in an unbalanced position. The majority of these injuries are due to a torsional element in landing, particularly when the weight is not equally distributed to the two lower extremities, rather than due to heavy landing. Jumpers are instructed to land on the balls of the feet equally and to roll forward; these precautions minimize injury.

Treatment consists of reduction of the fragments and immobilization in a plaster cast. Tobin has adopted the principle of utilizing skin plaster with a walking iron incorporated into the cast. Such immobilization will have to be maintained for about four weeks, but jumping should not be resumed for three months. The more severe injuries, particularly those involving the posterior lip and both malleoli, contraindicate continuation in the paratrooper service.

Deck fracture is a classification given primarily to those fractures sustained by naval personnel when explosions (*e.g.,* torpedo) occur below decks. The injuries sustained by explosions forcing the decks upward under the feet will be somewhat similar to injuries sustained in civilian life after a jump from heights, the patient landing on his feet. Thus the classical fracture sustained on board ship as a result of an explosive force underfoot is a bilateral fracture of the os calcis. Fractures of the tibia, femur and compression fractures of the vertebra likewise may occur. In deck fractures it is usually the body of the os calcis which is involved, although occasionally the lower portion with the tendo achilles attached becomes fractured, resulting in a "duck bill" type of fracture. In fractures of the body of the os calcis, there may be a fissure or a crushing of the bone; at times an extreme degree of comminution is present. There will naturally be a derangement of the calcaneo-cuboid-astragalar articulation. The posterior portion of the heel is displaced upward and usually laterally. Moderate shortening of the heel is present, due to forward displacement. Disability is complete, particularly when the fracture is bilateral. The pain is localized in the region of the heel, and examination reveals local swelling with tenderness in this area. Abnormal mobility is frequently demonstrable. Motions of the joint of the ankle produce pain.

Treatment consists of restoration of the position of the bone and the normal tuber angle. To obtain reduction, it will usually be necessary to insert a Steinmann pin through the superior posterior portion of the posterior process of the os calcis. By inserting this pin with the foot in the position of plantar flexion, less tension will be placed upon the skin around the pin. Moulding and manipulation may be necessary to obtain proper position of fragments. The limb is then suspended in some type of traction apparatus (*e.g.,* Böhler frame) with as much as 30 to 40 pounds of traction applied. On certain occasions, particularly in the "duck bill" type of fracture, open reduction with internal fixation may be necessary. Fixation with maintenance of traction should be maintained for 8 to 10 weeks before any weight bearing whatsoever is allowed. After removal of the pin traction, immobilization may be achieved by plaster cast. If the superior articular surfaces are badly injured, poor results may be expected. If the fracture lines extend into the joint surfaces, triple arthrodesis may be advisable.

Compound Fractures.—Among military casualties compound fractures are common, an incidence of about 20 per cent of all wounds being reported from many fronts. The subject is therefore worthy of a great deal of study and thought in order to reduce mortality, avoid disability and shorten convalescence. The mortality rate in World War II has been reduced markedly over that of World War I.

After control of hemorrhage, the first consideration is to determine whether other serious injuries (intracranial, thoracic, etc.) exist. At the same time an estimation of the degree of shock must be made, and shock therapy, including especially blood or plasma transfusions, must be instituted immediately, so that operation can be done at the earliest possible moment. As to operation, the most important decision is whether or not amputation must be performed. In civilian life it is relatively safe to err on the conservative side, since in general, compound fractures are treated early, are associated with a minimum amount of contamination, and do not require further transportation. Such a philosophy is not very safe in military wounds because of the high incidence of serious infections (including gas gangrene) in war wounds when the blood supply is insufficient and devitalization of tissue extensive.

In compound fractures sustained in battle, there are three major indications for amputation:

1. When the popliteal or femoral artery is destroyed.

2. When the lower end of the femur is badly comminuted with destruction of the knee joint.

3. When the muscle and skin of either the anterior or posterior portion of the thigh is destroyed, particularly since the limb will be useless even if it can be saved.

In general more of an attempt is made to save the extremity in the presence of compound fracture of the humerus than in compound fractures of the femur. Wounds of the upper extremity are cleaner, and the collateral blood supply is usually more efficient. Gas gangrene is relatively rare. Shortening of the bone is of relatively minor importance. Moreover, an artificial limb is much less useful from the functional standpoint than prostheses for the lower extremity. All of these factors represent reasons why amputation in the upper extremity is less advisable than in the lower.

Débridement remains the most important procedure in the treatment of compound fractures. No more than a thin edge of skin need be excised, but the excision of necrotic muscle, etc., must be thorough, and all foreign bodies removed. As discussed in the general considerations of compound fractures on page 367, the skin wound must be enlarged adequately and fascia incised to expose all crevices in the depths of the wound, and to relieve subfascial tension by providing drainage. Small detached pieces of bone may be removed, but all fragments which are attached (even though by periosteum only) should be left in place. Bailey[4] very aptly emphasizes the importance of extreme gentleness in the process of débridement, utilizing sharp dissection. Irrigation of the wound should be minimal. Although there is controversy regarding the advisability of local sulfanilamide therapy, the drug is used fairly universally, the powder being sprinkled over the wound after débridement is completed. The wound is left open and packed *lightly* with vaseline gauze. A "booster" dose of tetanus toxoid should be given, along with a heavy dose of anti-gas gangrene antitoxin. If the patient has not been previously immunized against tetanus, the tetanus *antitoxin* should be given.

In compound fractures of the humerus, application of a light cast following débridement is desirable. After the wound is dressed and cotton placed between the arm and chest, the plaster bandage is applied from the shoulder posteriorly under the padded elbow, extending upward along the anterior surface of the arm again to the shoulder. Other turns are made around the arm and chest while the forearm is being held in a cuff and collar sling. This affords a maximum amount of support to the arm with a minimum amount of plaster. While the cast is still wet, it is molded along the margins of the arm and forearm, thereby adding to the 'immobilization.

The Tobruk cast as devised by the British is a splendid method of fixation for transportation of casualties with compound fractures of the femur. After débridement with a dressing in place, skin traction (preferably using one-way elastoplast) is applied to the leg. A plaster cast is then applied around the entire extremity, leaving an opening at the foot for the traction strips. The cast is then split; this procedure may be facilitated by first applying a metal or rubber strip beneath the cast and removing it after the cut has been made. A Thomas or Keller-Blake splint is then applied over the cast, maintaining suspension and traction. This procedure is ideal for transportation.

If the patient is received after infection has already set in, débridement or application of a plaster cast is contraindicated, particularly if the patient is showing evidence of sepsis. Incision to insure adequate drainage is essential, however, as is the lifting out of large foreign bodies. A minimum of manipulation is indicated. Although intensive sulfonamide therapy is important, local chemotherapy is not effective in these cases; the drug, therefore, must be given in other ways.

Amputations.—The principles of amputations vary considerably in military as compared with civilian surgery in that a modified guillotine operation is utilized almost exclusively as the primary procedure in war injuries. After healing has taken place following the guillotine operation, plastic procedures or reamputation may then be indicated. With few exceptions the need for amputations during wartime will be confined to trauma. It should be remembered that its chief purpose at the front is to save life.

To establish definite indications for amputations in military wounds is difficult, because of so many variable factors. However, the indications enumerated under Compound Fractures in this chapter apply well here. In other words, if the major artery is destroyed along with fracture of the bone, if the major mass of muscles on the anterior or posterior surface of the thigh is lost, or if in a compound fracture at the knee the bone comminution is terrific, amputation will be indicated. In addition, it might be stated that if a fracture is not present, severance of the artery alone will usually not be sufficient to demand amputation unless enough soft tissue is destroyed to interfere with the collateral circulation.

Other factors may alter these indications somewhat. For example, if the injured soldier must be evacuated immediately and if transportation involves rough handling in the absence of medical care, the surgeon may decide to amputate an extremity which might have been saved under more ideal conditions. This is explained by the fact that the surgeon is unwilling to risk the possible development of serious infection (perhaps gas gangrene), secondary hemorrhage and shock when medical attention could not be available immediately. Other factors which may lead the surgeon to amputate when the trauma itself is not as severe as described above are the interval since injury and the extent of infection. For example, if 18 hours or more have elapsed since injury, and there is marked swelling and other manifestations of acute infection suggestive of gas gangrene, amputation might be indicated even though the wound is relatively trivial. Under more ideal conditions, of course, gas gangrene itself can now be treated by relatively conservative means, rarely requiring amputation.

As already stated, the guillotine operation is the only type of amputation permissible in war as the primary operation at the front. There is no place for definitive amputations such as the Gritti-Stokes, Callender and Syme's until the wound has healed, and the patient is back at a general hospital or its equivalent. On the other hand, Kirk [22] has very aptly emphasized the fact that the guillotine operation should not be performed literally. In other words, the circular incision of the skin is made, and skin allowed to retract. The fascia is then cut and allowed to retract. Superficial muscles are cut, exposing deeper muscles which are severed still higher. This allows section of the bone at a level much higher than the incision through the skin. However, it should be emphasized that traction on the muscle to expose the bone at a high level must be gentle and limited, lest the periosteum of the bone be torn, and vascular supply throughout the stump be damaged. Such an amputation leaves a concave stump which usually heals satisfactorily requiring a minimum amount of secondary repair.

Sulfanilamide should be placed in amputation wounds and sulfonamide therapy (sulfadiazine or sulfanilamide) by mouth started 8 or 12 hours later and continued until the danger of severe infection is passed. If infection develops, the stump may be irrigated with Dakin's solution or be packed gently with gauze soaked in azochloramid.

As soon as the danger of acute infection has passed, four strips of adhesive are applied on the stump as described on page 235, and traction exerted to prevent further retraction of the skin. The patient can be transported with the skin traction in place by placing the extremity in a Thomas splint. After the wound is healed, reamputation or a plastic operation may be performed, usually in the general hospital away from the front. Detailed consideration of these types of operations will be found in Chapter XI.

Abdominal Injuries.—Only direct injuries of the abdominal wall involving the peritoneal cavity are discussed here. Immersion blast producing abdominal injury is described under a separate heading. Because wounded men suffering from perforative injuries of the abdominal viscera stand transportation so poorly, and because prompt operation is so essential for survival, immediate consideration must be given war wounds of the peritoneal cavity. Numerous surgeons in the armed forces have emphasized the fact that a few beds must be maintained at the front line hospital to furnish 5 to 7 days of postoperative care for intra-abdominal wounds, unless transportation to a stationary hospital can be achieved within a six hour interval and without undue jostling of the patient. Objections that there is not room for this type of postoperative care at the front line hospital are not justified in view of the high mortality rate following transportation immediately after operation. In all abdominal injuries the surgeon must quickly decide whether a perforation is present. This is based on the extent of injury and study of the wounds of entry and exit. He must also determine whether or not the thoracic cavity or other portions of the body have likewise been injured.

The *manifestations* of abdominal wounds which have entered the peritoneal cavity have been discussed in Chapter XXV. However, certain features of war injuries deserve emphasis here, largely because they are dissimilar to the ones encountered in civilian injuries. In the first place, the size of the wound of entry cannot be used in determining the extent of damage within the peritoneal cavity, since long sharp bomb fragments may enter the abdominal wall longitudinally leaving a tiny wound of entrance, but might result in vicious tears after the fragment had rotated 90 degrees. For an hour or two after the wound is inflicted, there may be no muscle spasm and very little tenderness, thereby erroneously giving little evidence that intestine has been injured. After the initial shock associated with infliction of the wound is relieved, muscle spasm, nausea and vomiting become more prominent. Except for the shock produced by the impact of the fragment, manifestations of shock should be considered as an evidence of severe intra-abdominal hemorrhage.

Treatment is surgical and is primarily directed toward (1) the control of hemorrhage, and (2) closure of perforations. Laparotomy is performed if there is *any* likelihood that the peritoneal cavity has been entered (see also page 746). If hemorrhage is severe, it may be impossible to combat shock even with continuous transfusions before the bleeding point has been ligated. Under such circumstances, it becomes necessary to operate as soon as transfusion of plasma or blood is under way. The wound of the abdominal wall should be explored first, and débridement carried out. It is preferable to pack this wound open and make a new incision unless the original wound happened to be inflicted at a location ideal for abdominal exploration. Hemorrhage from lacerations of the liver may be controlled by packs or by sutures. In general the latter method is preferable. With heavy catgut and the proper long, curved needle, most lacerations can be repaired with complete control of hemorrhage. Lacerations of the spleen will usually require splenectomy since the injury is often too extensive and splenic pulp too friable to permit suture. Free blood in the peritoneal cavity must be saved for autotransfusion, and preparations made when hemorrhage is suspected. Basins or bottles containing sodium citrate should be available to salvage blood as soon as the abdomen is opened. Even though a wound of the stomach or the small intestine is present, autotransfusion may be life-saving, particularly if blood or plasma in large quantities is not available immediately. Administration of such contaminated blood after filtering has been used on many occasions, and seldom indeed has it produced deleterious results.

Thorough and systemic exploration of the peritoneal cavity must be made lest intestinal perforations be overlooked. For example, if a wound is found on the anterior surface of the stomach, the surgeon must look thoroughly on the posterior surface to find the wound of exit. However, no time should be wasted looking for small foreign bodies such as bullets. Perforations should be closed by suture without resection, if at all possible. As has been emphasized by Walton [23] and others, it is far safer to close multiple perforations with purse-string sutures than to perform one resection. Perforations of the colon can seldom be closed safely since there is a great tendency for the suture line to break down 4 to 6 days postoperatively. It is advisable, therefore, to exteriorize perforations of the colon if at all possible. Soon after recovery from the operation, the exteriorized colon will usually retract of its own accord; otherwise continuity can be reëstablished after the Mikulicz technic. If the wound occurs in a portion of the colon which cannot be exteriorized, a proximal colostomy must be performed. This principle of doing a colostomy proximal to the repair likewise applies to rectal injuries, which are common in penetrating wounds of the buttocks, a part of the body not infrequently injured by aerial bomb fragments. Even when the wound consists of nothing more than a contusion of the wall of the colon, it may be necessary to perform a proximal colostomy if there is any danger of gangrene and perforation at the injured site. Intestinal contents should be removed by suction, but the abdominal cavity should not be irrigated because this procedure spreads the contaminated material throughout the peritoneal cavity. At the close of the operation 4 to 6 grams of sulfanilamide, sulfathiazole, or sulfadiazine should be placed in the peritoneal cavity and distributed evenly over the contaminated areas.

Postoperative care is, of course, very important in the recovery of these patients; in war injuries of the peritoneal cavity it differs very little from that of civilian injuries as discussed in detail in Chapter XXV. The routine postoperative use of gastric decompression for 2 to 4 days (duration depending upon circumstances) is very important, and has been emphasized in numerous reports from battle fronts. Parenteral nutrition is likewise an essential feature as discussed on page 151. The mortality rate in intra-abdominal wounds still remains high (30 to 35 per cent) although it is markedly improved over that experienced in World War I. The mortality rate will vary directly with the length of time elapsing between infliction of the wound and operation. Indeed, recovery of large perforations can seldom be expected if the time lag is longer than 8 to 10 hours.

Thoracic Injuries.—The seriousness of thoracic wounds inflicted by modern high explosives is exemplified by the observation that 33 per cent of the dead on the battlefield die of thoracic injuries. The mortality at dressing stations and in ambulances has been cited at 20 to 30 per cent [24]. Thoracic injuries are no exception to the general rule discussed previously that the mortality rate of war wounds depends to a large extent upon the speed of evacuation and the manner of transportation. Doubtless lowering of mortality will be achieved by improvements along these lines. However, until transportation can be accelerated greatly, attempts to reduce mortality must be made by appropriate therapy within the combat zone. This means more specialized first aid treatment which implies, of course, that those administering such aid possess accurate physiological knowledge and ability in diagnosis of the systemic and local conditions present in the individual patient. Moreover, it implies that facilities be available for immediate therapy of certain lesions which are peculiar to thoracic wounds.

Inasmuch as many thoracic wounds are associated with severe pneumothorax and hemothorax and therefore an impaired vital capacity, airplane travel is poorly borne by these patients particularly at altitudes of 5000 feet or above. The advantages achieved by speed in transportation may be more than outweighed by the increased anoxia induced, unless adequate apparatus for oxygen inhalation is available.

In the following discussion numerous first aid procedures are mentioned but many of them can scarcely be carried out by non-medical personnel unless they are particularly trained to do so. The *arrest of hemorrhage* from the chest wall by pressure dressings is similar to that exerted in most other wounds except when there is severe bleeding from intercostal or internal mammary arteries. These lesions may require an incision over the bleeding point with the application of pressure or ligature to both ends of the severed vessel. Occasionally aspiration of blood from the thoracic cavity with reinjection of air may be indicated to control hemorrhage from the lung, but in general hemothorax is treated conservatively. In pericardial hemorrhage, however, aspiration of blood as a first aid measure may be life-saving where cardiac tamponade is present. This procedure may relieve the tamponade in a few cases permanently or at least temporarily until the patient can be evacuated to a hospital where operation can be performed.

In thoracic wounds the *position of the patient* may be of great importance. In general the sitting rather than the recumbent posture permits easier breathing in the case of dyspnea. When a massive atelectasis is present, however, it is best to place the patient on the uninjured side in order to help him expectorate the plug in the opposite involved lung. On the other hand, in the case of an intercostal hemorrhage or indeed with any penetrating wound of the chest the patient is placed on the injured side in order to exert pressure and to permit dependent drainage to the outside. Although the usual forms of *dressing* may be used in chest wounds, a circular bandage is extremely important particularly with some compression applied in fractured ribs or other lesions in which breathing is painful, in order to immobilize the chest wall and control pain. In the presence of severe pain it may be also advisable to inject the appropriate intercostal nerves with procaine. In regard to the use of *drugs* morphine is of importance in shock and for the control of pain except that its depressant effect on respiration must be borne in mind. Atropine should be used with caution because it makes bronchial secretions more viscid and hard to cough up. *Oxygen inhalations* are an important measure in the treatment of thoracic injuries particularly when there is respiratory difficulty and cyanosis. Such treatment is often available for use rather close to the combat area. *Transfusions* are used in thoracic injuries for the treatment of surgical shock just as in other conditions. However, the danger of pulmonary edema introduces an element of caution in its use. Indeed, in the presence of an injured lung the too liberal use of any intravenous infusion may precipitate or aggravate pulmonary edema. The situation is thus similar to that mentioned elsewhere in lung injuries due to inhalation of irritant gases. Where hemoconcentration is present plasma is more advisable than whole blood. *Aspiration* of the chest is a first aid procedure which may be very important in the case of *pressure pneumothorax*. This condition, also called "tension" or "valvular" pneumothorax, is more frequent in crushing injuries than in penetrating wounds and produces a high pressure on the injured side because air is forced through a valve-like rupture of the lung whenever the patient coughs or strains. On examination, the mediastinum is displaced toward the normal side as shown by palpation of the trachea in the suprasternal notch and of the apex impulse as well as percussion of cardiac dullness and auscultation of heart sounds. Treatment is urgent and is carried out by introducing a large bore needle in the second anterior interspace one inch from the sternal border; it is left in place only as long as air is escaping. It is then removed and a firm dressing applied. In case of a pneumothorax associated with a *"sucking wound"* closure of the opening is urgent and often life-saving. A tight pack occluding the edges of the wound is preferable to actual suture which is carried out later as definitive therapy. Other emergency procedures which may be important during the first aid period are *mediastinal decompression* in the case of *mediastinal emphysema* in order to relieve the pressure on the large veins created by the air in the mediastinum. This pressure interferes with the return of blood to the heart and may result in circulatory failure and death. The procedure is simple and consists of adequate incision in the suprasternal space. In addition to this decompression of the mediastinum, *tracheotomy* or intubation may be necessary if there is any evidence of laryngeal obstruction.

The definitive treatment of thoracic injuries is described in some detail in Chapter XXX. However, a particularly excellent description of this subject as applied to the war has been prepared and edited by the Subcommittee on Thoracic Surgery of the Committee on Surgery of the Division of Medical Sciences of the National Research Council. This clear, concise and brief monograph is now available and should be read for further information [24].

Craniocerebral War Injuries *.—Head injuries rank highest among causes of death on the battlefield. Of all wounded entering a hospital, perhaps 4 or 5 per cent will have suffered craniocerebral injury and about half of these will require a major surgical procedure. Neurological findings should be recorded at once. In no other way can a progressive lesion caused by hemorrhage be differentiated from a primary destructive one. The administration of morphine or other sedatives, sulfonamides, tetanus toxoid or antitoxin, and so forth, must be noted.

Patients with injury to the skull and brain should have priority for transport to a neurosurgical unit. It has been shown that transportation by air as high as 8,000 feet in altitude does not increase intracranial pressure. For proper surgical management, x-ray facilities and ancillary services are necessary, and until these are available no treatment of the wounds should be attempted. Experience has shown that the management of severe head injury requires specially trained personnel. Under such organization, the percentage of primary wound healing has been greater and the mortality less (even though treatment is delayed up to 72 hours after injury), than if such casualties are treated earlier by less skilled surgeons. Also contrary to earlier teaching, it has been established that patients who are doing well postoperatively may be transported without harm on the second or third day.

Injuries to the Scalp.—Most important is the determination of associated cranial or intracranial damage. Knowing the mode of production of the wound

---

* Submitted by Dr. H. C. Naffziger.

aids the examiner in judging this. Neurological examination and, in doubtful cases, x-ray studies are required. Hemorrhage may be severe and too often, uncontrolled vessels continue to bleed after bandages are applied. Control of bleeding, shaving if possible, use of sulfanilamide in the wound, and the application of a sterile dry dressing are first aid measures. Careful inspection for fracture and for foreign material between the scalp and skull is made. Shaving of the surrounding scalp is followed by preparation of the skin with soap, water, a fat solvent, and skin anti-septic. If anesthetic is needed, 0.5 to 1 per cent procaine hydrochloride with 4 drops of adrenalin to the ounce is injected with a fine needle, vertically to the skin and between it and the skull. The injection is made 3 cm. or more from the edges of the wound. This will raise the scalp in a large welt, lessen bleeding and will anes-thetize in 10 minutes. No intradermal injection is required in the scalp. Shredded and devitalized margins are then trimmed and dirt and foreign material carefully removed. Fine interrupted sutures of silk or cotton in two layers for the galea and the skin control bleeding and secure approximation. The fewest sutures that accom-plish this and secure coaptation should be used. Interrupted figure-of-eight sutures can often be employed to advantage. In relatively old and badly contaminated wounds the use of a rubber drain through a separate stab wound 2 cm. or so from the wound is justified and is essential in patients who are not to be under con-tinuous observation.

Open Wounds with Fracture of the Skull but No Penetration of the Dura.— In addition to the customary management of the scalp wound, fissured fractures with indriven dirt must be guttered. Contaminated periosteum is sparingly trimmed. One especially directed x-ray film made to show the injured area in true profile (with the rays tangential to the skull) will show more exactly the extent of depres-sion. With a burr opening at the margin of a depression, it may occasionally be carefully levered up. The elevated depressed bone, if contamination is not great, is left in place and the scalp closed. In the presence of increasing symptoms, a purple dura under tension, indicating a clot or pulped brain beneath it, may require open-ing. Evacuation of such material by irrigation and suction, and arrest of bleeding with immediate tight closure of the dura are in order. If bone is replaced, which implies a relatively clean field, the scalp is closed without drainage.

Open Wounds with Fracture of the Skull and Penetration of the Dura.—The first aid treatment is the same as that of scalp wounds. Fragments of bone should not be disturbed until definitive care is undertaken. Premature manipulations may release a torn sinus. Shock is unusual except when associated injuries are present. Evidences of intracranial pressure must not be mistaken for shock. Persistence of coma or unconsciousness after injury is a very unfavorable sign, the rate of recovery being directly proportional to the mental clarity of the patient. Comatose patients should be placed on the side or in the Sims position to permit free inspira-tion and to allow drainage from the mouth. Neurological examination and detailed studies of the x-ray films are essential. Complete facilities for treatment and simi-lar preparation of the operative field are required as for all other skull and brain injuries (vide supra). For the anesthetization of restless or irritable patients intravenous sodium pentothal is favored. Induction must be slow, otherwise arti-ficial respiration and oxygen will be needed. The scalp wound, after trimming and then changing to fresh instruments, is made part of a curved flap incision to expose the opening in the bone, or a tripod incision may be required. The opening in the bone is enlarged to expose the dural area of penetration. The craniectomy may be begun from a burr opening nearby. Only exceptionally is the dural opening enlarged. Suction, gentle irrigation and careful removal of all fragments of bone with forceps must be painstaking and these procedures are time-consuming. Vessels are controlled with silver clips and the electro-surgical unit. Metallic foreign bodies, unless readily accessible, are not sought for. They infrequently harbor infection as compared with fragments of bone. In the absence of a mechanical suction apparatus, a catheter and syringe can be used as makeshifts. The dura is left open and the scalp wound is closed. In the presence of serious contamination, a rubber drain through a separate stab wound is used. Closure up to 72 hours is usual. The closure of the scalp is the most difficult portion of the operation, particularly in tangential wounds in which loss of tissue has been considerable. If possible the scalp should be mobilized sufficiently to be closed without tension. Relaxing incisions may be helpful but extensive plastic operations should not be undertaken. Covering the exposed dural defect with vaseline gauze and partial closure of the scalp are preferable. Sulfathiazole applied to an intact cortex produces convulsions.

Sulfadiazine should be administered intravenously to all patients with penetrating head wounds or with involvement of accessory sinuses. Concentration in the cerebrospinal fluid should be brought up to 10 mg. per 100 cc. or more. This usually requires the use of from 4 to 5 grams intravenously twice in 24 hours and should be continued for at least three days. Sodium bicarbonate should be given. For unconscious or dehydrated patients, 6 grams of sulfadiazine may be used in 500 cc. of glucose-saline solution, alternating with salt and sodium citrate solution. Increased cells in the spinal fluid indicate infection such as encephalitis or meningitis; increased protein accompanies abscess. The dosage of sulfadiazine should be increased to 18 grams in 24 hours in cases of meningitis and outspoken infection; obviously, when such large doses of the drug are used, the fluid intake must be adequately maintained. Pain in the kidneys is usually the first sign of renal complications.

Penetrating wounds of the brain involving the accessory sinuses present many special problems. Separation of the intracranial contents from the sinuses by closure of the soft tissues, the use of vaseline gauze, gutta percha or other protective substance should be accomplished and the mucous membrane of the sinus removed. Cerebrospinal rhinorrhea or insufflation of air into the cranial cavity requires early craniotomy and occlusion of the openings in dura and bone by a fascial graft. In such cases chemotherapy is of the greatest value, both prophylactically and in treatment.

Injuries to the Spinal Cord.—In general, injuries to the spinal cord are sustained by one of two methods: (1) fracture dislocation of the vertebra, and (2) direct trauma with a missile. Fracture dislocation of the vertebra is more common in civilian life, and injury by bullets, shrapnel, and fragments of shells are naturally more common in military life. Injuries to the cauda equina, resulting from trauma to the lumbo-sacral spine, are a separate problem and are not covered here.

All members of the medical units, including stretcher bearers, etc., should be well coached in making a sincere effort to identify spinal cord injuries before the wounded soldier is lifted from the ground. The importance of this precaution cannot be overemphasized since injurious handling might result in a complete transverse lesion of a cord in which the initial injury had merely produced a partial lesion. If the patient is conscious and there is the slightest possibility of spinal cord injury, the attendant should try to obtain specific information by two or three questions. Simple questions inquiring into the presence of paralysis, paresthesia, or numbness of the extremities, particularly the lower, require less than a minute and may save the patient from a state of permanent invalidism.

Transportation.—As remarked above, patients with injuries of the spinal cord must be handled and lifted very gently. Preferably it should be done by two or more persons lifting in unison, being careful not to twist the body. Occasionally the wounded soldier can actually be rolled over onto a stretcher with less damage than would be sustained by lifting. Opinions may differ as to the choice of position of the body during transportation, in that some authorities favor transportation in the prone position and others in the supine position. In either case it must be established that the patient's airway is adequate. If he is transported in the supine position and is semicomatose, he must be watched carefully, lest vomiting result in aspiration. Sometimes it is preferable to transport the patient in the same prone position as that in which he was found. In general, however, it will be more comfortable and perhaps more desirable to transport the patient in a supine position. However, if this position is maintained, it is essential that a pad such as a folded towel or blanket be placed under the back at the site of the injury, to prevent severe trauma from motion incident to transportation. The first aid care of the wound, if present, would consist of nothing more than application of a sterile dressing if the patient can be seen by a physician in a relatively short time.

When seen by a physician, as at an advanced dressing station, the skin around the wound may be cleansed with soap and water, foreign bodies removed from the wound, and large blood clots extracted. A large quantity of powdered sulfanilamide, up to 6 or 8 grams, should be placed in the wound, and a sterile dressing applied. Naturally, the patient should be examined for shock and other vital injuries. It may be essential to institute shock therapy, including, particularly, administration of plasma or blood, before transportation for definitive care is carried out. In any event, patients with spinal cord injuries must receive definitive care at the *earliest possible moment*. In other words, like patients with brain, thoracic, and abdominal wounds, they should receive priorities in transportation.

Careful examination must soon be made, determining sensory and motor disturbances as well as changes in the reflexes. Accurate records of these abnormal findings must be kept, so that any changes can be detected. An increase in the amount of positive findings might be indicative of progression of hematoma formation. The x-ray may be very helpful in determining the extent of injury. However, it must be realized that vertebrae may snap back into relatively good position, whereas severe displacement with severe damage of the cord may have momentarily taken place at the time of injury [25].

If a wound is present, débridement should be carried out as with any other wound, and closed if less than 12 hours have elapsed since injury. Nothing can be done about the presence of a severed cord or major nerve trunks. The chief aim is to prevent infection and obtain relief from compression by bone fragments and blood clots. If the patient states that he became paralyzed at the instant the wound was sustained, there is usually little hope that much can be done to prevent a permanent paralysis.

Use of the Queckenstedt test, etc., in determining the need for decompression of the cord are discussed on page 576. As emphasized by Oldberg[42] and others, in the absence of an open wound, immediate operation is performed only for actual mechanical pressure on the cord or cauda equina.

Outside of the care of the wound and the position of the patient, the most important item in the care of the patient is the care of the skin and bladder.

As far as the bladder is concerned, an inlying catheter may as well be instituted immediately, if there has been a marked injury to the cord producing sphincter loss. When the soldier finally reaches more or less permanent hospitalization, such as that afforded by a General Hospital, tidal drainage with a Y tube should be instituted. In some chronic cases, cystotomy may eventually become necessary, if an automatic bladder cannot be developed over a period of months, or if the urethra cannot stand prolonged catheterization.

In caring for the skin, fracture boards should never be used, but as soft a mattress as possible (live rubber sponge is best) should be obtained and placed upon stiff springs. The patient should be kept dry at all times, and the bed linen smooth. Frequent alcohol rubbing, powdering of the skin, and change of position should be insisted upon, especially for the first six weeks.

Injuries to Peripheral Nerves *.—*War injuries* to peripheral nerves include those associated with extensive wounds as well as the usual varieties seen in civil life. Damage to major nerves occurs in some 20 per cent of wounds of the extremity, though not all of these injuries to nerves will require operative repair.

As in civil life, primary suture of the nerve occasionally is feasible after cleanly incised wounds with a minimum of contamination, treated early; but these rarely occur in military service. Dysthesias, severe pain and causalgia in partial lesions of the nerve are common. These, or the presence of a foreign body, sometimes make urgent some sort of operation to free the nerve, remove an irritating agent or block the sympathetic chain. Not infrequently such operative measures are justified before healing of the wound is complete; the approach sometimes can be made through intact skin and a clean field. For the most part, however, immediate repair of war injuries to nerves should not be done.

In lacerated wounds with contamination and a time lag between injury and treatment, associated injuries to tendons and other tissues, and difficulty in judging the amount of resection necessary to assure normal tissues for suture are usual factors. To permit suture of the nerve without tension, extensive incisions and mobilization are the rule but this is not permissible in such contaminated wounds as occur in war. For all of these reasons, as well as because of the time-consuming character of surgery of the nerves, immediate repair is not feasible. If at the time of debridement the severed ends of the nerve can be identified, their approximation

* Submitted by Dr. H. C. Naffziger.

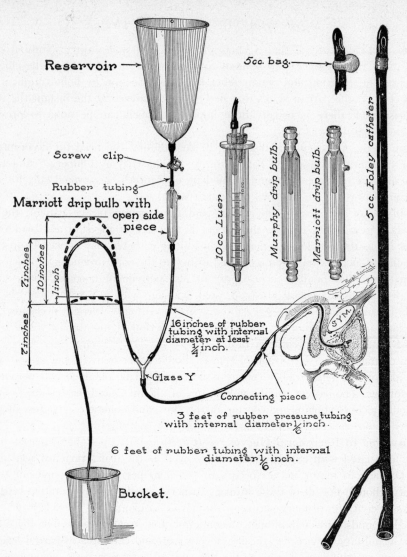

Reservoir →

5cc. bag. →

Screw clip

Rubber tubing

Marriott drip bulb with
open side
piece

10cc. Luer

Murphy drip bulb

Marriott drip bulb

5cc. Foley catheter

2 inches
10 inches
1 inch

2 inches

16 inches of rubber
tubing with internal
diameter at least
¼ inch.

Glass Y

Connecting piece

3 feet of rubber pressure tubing
with internal diameter⅛ inch.

6 feet of rubber tubing with internal
diameter⅙ inch.

Bucket.

SYM.

FIG. 559.—APPARATUS FOR CONTINUOUS TIDAL IRRIGATION (MODIFIED FROM LAWRIE-NATHAN,
1939).

Either a 10-cc. Luer syringe or a Murphy or Marriott drip bulb, as illustrated, may be used to provide a continuous drip. An air vent is essential in this unit. Sixty drops per minute is a suitable rate of flow from the antiseptic solution, as regulated by the screw clip. Since the solution is in contact with the vesical mucosa continuously a mild antiseptic, such as a 1.5 per cent solution of boric acid which is isotonic with the tissues, should be used. The height of the overflow tube above the symphysis pubis is adjusted according to the state of the neurogenic bladder. A height of about 2 inches is recommended for the atonic stage with gradual elevation to 10 inches or more as the hypertonic stage is reached. It is important to exclude all air in assembling the apparatus. This can be accomplished by connecting the rubber tubing to the catheter after the air bubbles have been evacuated from the tubing and while fluid is still running through the system and at the same time escaping from the bladder through the catheter. The reservoir must always contain fluid, and the end of the drainage tube must always be kept above the level of the fluid in the drainage bucket. As the bladder fills, the intravesical pressure rises until it reaches the level of the overflow tube, at which time siphonage takes place and the bladder empties. The cycle then starts again. To maintain proper asepsis the reservoir should be a bottle with a small mouth which can be plugged with sterile gauze. (From *Military Surgical Manual* III, National Research Council, W. B. Saunders Co., Philadelphia.)

with one suture—preferably of wire—and without sacrifice of tissue, is desirable. This suture helps later to identify the injured structure, prevents retraction and displacement of the ends of the nerve, and facilitates eventual resection and suture.

Early secondary suture should be made before irreversible changes have occurred as a result of atrophy and fibrotic changes in muscles and about joints. The time of this repair is governed by the degree of infection, wound healing and associated conditions. Wounds entirely healed may, after two or three weeks, be subjected to hot packs and massage. In the absence of inflammatory reaction, the likelihood of a recrudescence of infection after an open operation is small.

For the later repair of divided nerves, long incisions, wide exposure through muscle planes and isolation of the nerve trunks both proximal and distal to the point of injury are essential before the involved area is isolated. Otherwise valuable branches are often sacrificed and much time is lost in endeavoring to identify the ends of the nerves in scar tissue. In mobilization of the nerve, muscular branches can be dissected and spared and freeing of the nerve must be sufficient to permit adequate resection and suture of the sheath without tension. Complete interruptions of the nerve or complete blockage by scar tissue and neuroma require resection and suture. Partial lesions require experienced judgment for determination of the proper course of procedure. In many cases neurolysis will secure a better result than resection.

Splinting of the extremity to prevent overstretching of muscles is important but, in this connection, splinting does not mean immobilization. Elastic and spring contrivances are preferred and, at least twice daily, the parts should be removed from the splint and the joints be put through their complete range of motion. Splinting which maintains immobility is often more harmful than none. Continued use of the part is often possible if it is protected against injury to anesthetic areas. The value of galvanic stimulation to paralyzed muscles is still in debate. It is not harmful, nor is it important enough to interfere with other activities or occupation.

Injuries of the Intervertebral Disks.—It is becoming evident that injuries of the intervertebral disks are common in military life. For the most part, introduction of mechanized warfare has been responsible for the increase in this type of injury. Personnel in certain of the services are more susceptible than others. It can readily be understood that men in armored cars (particularly "jeeps") or on motorcycles, occupants of tanks, pilots of planes landing on carriers, parachute troops, and members of cavalry units would be most susceptible to injury of a disk, since in all these cases the men are subject to falls or to a sudden impact which throws a strain on the vertebral column. Naturally, effort should be made to minimize the incidence of such injuries by prophylactic measures, which is of course being done by the military authorities.

Falling or jars upon the buttocks with the body in a sitting (slightly flexed) position is a common mechanism producing disk injuries Obviously, any impact putting excessive strain on the spine would likewise tend to produce the injury. Inasmuch as drivers of armored cars or pilots of planes landing on carriers are subjected to such injuries which are obviously frequent and unavoidable, it appears that the use of an especially devised seat might aid in absorbing the impact. It is probably true that occupants of tanks other than the driver have opportunity to protect themselves by standing up, and bracing themselves against supports, so as to absorb part of the shock with their bended knees. As Love [26] has suggested, wearing a snug-fitting canvas corset might protect the spine against flexion injuries by furnishing firm support. Combat troops who are subject to falls (*e.g.,* parachute troops) go through rigid training in learning how to fall or land. Tumblers and football players are taught to minimize injury of all kinds by "rolling" on their bodies rather than absorbing all the impact of the fall on one part of the body.

At the time of injury the patient may feel a sudden snap that results in severe pain in the lumbar region which may or may not radiate down the sciatic nerve immediately after the injury. Ultimately this sciatic pain, frequently with paresthesias, develops. The manifestations of injuries to the intervertebral disks, and the routine therapy are discussed on page 577.

At the present time there is some difference of opinion as to the status of disability in such injuries sustained in military life. Some surgeons are of the opinion that in spite of adequate therapy, including successful operation, the injured soldier should be discharged or assigned to a type of inactive duty. However, most neurosurgeons are of the opinion that following the institution of proper operative therapy, a large portion of these men might be returned to duty. It is obvious that a minimum convalescent period of 8 or 10 weeks will be necessary following operation.

Maxillo-facial Injuries.—Injuries of this type are extremely common because of the frequency of fighting from trenches and "fox holes". Life frequently depends upon proper *first aid treatment* which might be furnished by a fellow soldier. The chief threats to life are suffocation, aspiration of blood, and shock due to hemorrhage. Intelligent first aid care, consisting of immediately turning the injured man on his side or abdomen to prevent aspiration of blood, and assist in maintaining an open pharyngeal airway, is necessary. Obviously, effort should be made to stop the hemorrhage by compression bandages. If there is persistent danger of suffocation by the tongue falling backward against the posterior wall of the pharynx, it may be pulled forward after piercing the tip with a safety pin, suture, or towel clip and anchoring it to some fixed object. Such complicated first aid treatment can probably be rendered only by members of the Medical Corps, who will likewise be more effective in controlling massive hemorrhage. The need for immediate care is made more necessary by the fact that most of these men will be unconscious, at least for a time, although a great many of them may have no significant cerebral damage. During transportation, the wounded man must obviously be kept in a prone or semiprone position to maintain an airway and prevent aspiration of secretions, etc.

Definitive treatment consists of débridement, which, however, need not be extensive. The excision of tissue should be minimal, because the extreme vascularity permits survival of even severely damaged tissue. Large bone splinters which are attached by nothing more than periosteum should be left in place, particularly in the mandible, since defects here would require extensive plastic work later. In a fracture of the mandible, the teeth should be removed on each side adjacent to the fracture line. Wiring of the mandible or fixation of fragments as discussed on page 382 should be performed under local anesthesia, since administration of a general anesthetic (particularly ether) would encourage postoperative vomiting, which might result in immediate suffocation of the patient or aspiration pneumonia because of inability to evacuate the pharynx effectively. Even under local anesthesia, this danger still exists, particularly if the patient has eaten a full meal shortly preceding injury and repair. Likewise, wiring of the upper and lower jaw together is permissible only when good hemostasis has been obtained.

No plastic procedures are attempted during this definitive treatment. The patient is put on sulfonamide therapy (perhaps including local use of the drug), and dressings applied, waiting for the time when sufficient healing has taken place to permit plastic repair, which obviously is done in a general hospital far away from the front line.

CRUSH SYNDROME

Although crushing injuries in significant numbers are seen only during war time, they are much more common in civilian than in military personnel, because such injuries usually occur in those extricated from beneath the debris of bombed buildings. The effect of crushing injury is serious and demands special thought and consideration; the major effect is initial physical shock but there is in addition evidence of a "toxic" factor, *i.e.,* delayed renal damage. Inasmuch as the crush syndrome involves loss of viability of muscle tissue, much of the information concerning this injury can be applied to two other conditions also associated with extensive damage to muscle, *i.e.,* tourniquet shock, which is described later, and extensive muscle damage from bomb fragments.

Pathogenesis.—The mechanism of the initial shock is readily explained by the fall in blood volume from loss of blood and plasma into the injured area. The crushing of the tissue results in obvious damage and anoxia which affects the permeability of the capillaries. After the victim is released from the crush, plasma is lost through the capillary walls, thereby leading to a fall in blood volume which is aggravated by the hemorrhage resulting from laceration of tissues. As would be expected, these shock symptoms develop only after the victim is extricated, since the local plasma loss cannot take place while compression is still exerted and circulation interrupted.

Besides this well known mechanism, the crush syndrome involves another pathological change which is somewhat delayed. This change is due to a serious renal damage which is apt to develop a few days after injury and appears to be the result of toxins arising from the local area. Blalock [27] has demonstrated that the thoracic duct lymph collected after removing animals from a press crushing the lower extremity, was definitely toxic when administered to normal animals. Such animals developed hemoconcentration with casts and blood in the urine; some of them died as the result of injection. Bywaters [28] attributes the renal damage to myohemoglobin liberated from the injured muscle which has a toxic effect on the kidney, perhaps through blockage of the tubules or glomeruli.

Clinical Manifestations.—*Examination* of the victim while still under the debris reveals relatively no symptoms of impending shock; initial pain may even have disappeared. However, within a few hours after release, there is a grave tendency for marked swelling to develop in the crushed extremities. As this swelling appears, manifestations of shock develop which are similar to other types of surgical shock due to loss of plasma or to hemorrhage. A variable amount of ecchymosis develops over the injured area, depending upon the amount of subcutaneous injury. Manifestations of fractures, injury to nerves and other complicating injuries may also be present and search should be made for them. Adequate shock therapy may eliminate all manifestations of shock, but a few days later a still more serious complication, namely renal damage, is apt to develop. Blood, albumin and casts appear in the urine; later, oliguria and finally anuria with resultant uremia develop, commonly terminating in death.

Treatment.—Therapy is directed toward prevention first, of the edema, and second, of the serious renal complications. To combat the rapid development of swelling with consequent loss of circulating plasma Patey and Robertson [29] have recommended compression bandages for the crushed extremities immediately after the victim is extricated. Theoretically the application of cold to the extremity would appear logical, but Duncan and Blalock [27] observed that this therapy in animal experiments was not effective unless it was instituted with onset of the compression. At any rate, it is well known that such extremities should be kept cool and not subjected to the deleterious effects of hot applications. Bywaters [28] has advised administration of large quantities of alkalies (30 to 40 grams of sodium citrate and sodium bicarbonate) by mouth to maintain an alkaline urine, thereby holding the myohemoglobin in solution and preventing its precipitation in the kidney tubules. Atropine or papaverine are indicated to eliminate vaso-constriction; sympathetic block by paravertebral injection of novocaine may be still more effective. If the trauma is severe enough amputation may be imperative.

Crush Syndrome in Other Injuries.—Investigation of the crush syndrome has aroused a good deal of interest in the old "toxic" theory of shock, *i.e.,* the possibility that shock may be due to the presence and perhaps absorption of toxic substances in an injured area. In the case of crush injuries the evidence is clear that such a factor is actually present. Indeed, a similar factor, though developing more rapidly, is probably present in so-called *tourniquet shock,* produced experimentally 25 years ago by Cannon and Bayliss [31] but studied in more detail in recent years [32, 33]. In this condition, which is also seen clinically when a tourniquet is left on too long, there is loss of plasma and blood into the occluded leg when the tourniquet is removed after being in place for several hours. However, the manifestations of shock will persist, though not as severely, if transudation is prevented by compression of the extremity or if the lost plasma is replaced with a transfusion, thus suggesting that a "toxic" factor is superimposed on the loss of plasma. Indeed, in the experiments of Wilson and Roome [32] survival could be achieved by amputation followed by transfusion, but not by either procedure alone. The information obtained in tourniquet shock may be applied to other traumatic conditions in which tissue becomes so damaged that metabolic changes occur presumably due to cellular autolysis. For example, in extensive muscle damage from bomb fragments, large masses of necrotic muscle autolyze and unless promptly removed will result in metabolic changes, leading probably to absorption of the products of its disintegration. Clinical shock developing under such circumstances is well known and often responds but slightly to large plasma transfusions; this last observation adds further evidence to the idea that an additional factor (besides loss of plasma and blood) is present. Another example is the probable existence of manifestations of toxemia in extensive burns. Not often, but occasionally, severely burned patients die in shock, though usually exhibiting so-called "toxic" manfestations as delirium and high fever, even though the hemoconcentration has been controlled with massive plasma transfusions. In burns it is possible for large areas of skin to become necrotic, to disintegrate and produce by autolysis products which, by absorption or otherwise, will be responsible for deleterious effects. Further study is needed, but the observations on the crush syndrome have pointed to the probable existence of a "toxic" factor in shock associated with extensive tissue damage in various injuries entirely apart from the actual loss of blood or plasma into the injured area. Practical inferences from these considerations have been applied to muscle trauma due to bomb fragments by prompt excision of the damaged muscle during débridement; further study is required before therapeutic implications can be drawn in the case of the other conditions mentioned. In regard to tourniquet shock, the lesson is obvious; extremities must not be left with their circulation occluded for more than short periods at a time.

BLAST INJURIES

Blast is a term which is usually applied to the waves produced by a severe explosive force; injuries due to such a force were observed in significant numbers first in World War I in soldiers close to the scene of a bursting bomb. Many died soon afterwards with extensive internal but no external evidence of injury. Other soldiers similarly exposed in which fatalities did not ensue showed mental symptoms which were known by the name of shell shock. However, this term was later applied to a large group of functional neuroses not necessarily connected with exposure to severe blast. During the present conflict there has, of course, been a tremendous increase in the number and size of bombs particularly due to the increased use of aerial combat. Aerial bombs have increased steadily in size, leading to greater and greater detonating effects. In addition to large aerial bombs, depth charges and other explosions at sea have also led to severe and similar forces under water. Injuries resulting from the latter type of blast are usually referred to as immersion or water blast.

Blast will, of course, be indirectly responsible for many common external injuries when the individual is thrown, or objects strike him, producing lacerations, fractures, etc. On the other hand, injuries directly due to the blast wave itself involve in general the three body cavities, but not the extremities, i.e., the head, thorax and abdomen. Blast injuries affecting the head are in reality similar to concussion (see page 563). Indeed, in the early study of the effects of exploding bombs these injuries were referred to as concussion injuries. Although most blast injuries may exhibit evidence of central nervous system involvement, only injuries to the chest and abdomen will be considered in this discussion. Of the two, blast from aerial bombs above ground in general produces lung injuries, whereas immersion blast tends more to produce lesions in the abdominal cavity. In both instances, however, systemic effects, notably severe surgical shock, are frequently present. Much clinical and experimental study has been devoted to this new type of injury and numerous publications on blast have appeared, which should be consulted for further details [4, 5, 34, 35].

Mechanism of Blast.—The physics of the blast wave has been investigated considerably, from which it is evident in general that any body finding itself in the path of such a wave is subject to rapidly changing pressures of which the first is a rapid positive followed by a slower negative phase. Differences in the density of the body tissues and the contents of viscera compared to the surrounding air or water undoubtedly play an important part in the injuries sustained by sudden and violent changes in pressure. The damage inflicted is obviously in direct proportion to the closeness of the body to the center of the explosion. Indeed, only those really close to the detonation are injured inasmuch as the explosive wave is dissipated rapidly. This is particularly true of aerial bombs; depth charges, because of the relatively incompressibility of water, become dissipated much more slowly. On the other hand, the super bombs of one or two tons, often called block busters, undoubtedly create a blast wave which is capable of producing injuries for some distance.

Pathology of Blast.—Multiple and extensive though often minute injury to tissue is the characteristic effect of blast. Undoubtedy nervous tissue and nerve trunks sustain a violent physical blow (concussion) which produces severe but transient functional changes without demonstrable anatomical lesions. However, even in nervous tissue and certainly in the abdomen and lung, tiny hemorrhages have nearly always been found. A sufficiently large number of such minute hemorrhages may account for enough loss of blood to produce shock, although other factors such as actual tissue necrosis may be responsible for later effects (see Crush Syndrome). Hemorrhages, however, may be so large as to produce hematomas. Moreover, in the case of the lung, the hemorrhages plus disruption of alveoli may be sufficiently extensive to interfere with normal pulmonary function. In the abdomen additional injury may be produced entirely apart from hemorrhage; tearing of the omentum, liver or spleen may occur, but of greatest significance is the actual perforation of intestine which undoubtedly is due to a mechanism similar to that illustrated on page 747 (Fig. 451 D).

Lung Injuries Due to Blast.—The symptoms of lung injury from blast consists of respiratory distress which may be severe enough to produce complete cessation of breathing. Cough and hemoptysis may also occur and surgical shock may accompany the dyspnea. Symptoms referable to the central nervous system and abdomen may also be present but are described elsewhere. In examining the injured it should be emphasized that although blast injuries of the lung are not necessarily accompanied by evidence of thoracic trauma, the presence of wounds elsewhere does not mean that lung damage is not present. On many occasions lung injury is not detected, being overshadowed by other and often less serious injuries (see also Lung Injuries in Burns, page 1041). A history of blast plus the presence of blood-stained sputum or hemorrhage in the throat as well as dyspnea should always suggest involvement of the lung. X-ray of the chest if available will be of great diagnostic aid.

Although prevention is obviously of greater importance than treatment, recognition of the injury promptly will enable saving of life. Patients with blast injuries of the lung should be put completely at rest, and inhalations of oxygen of high concentration employed in addition to general measures for surgical shock including judicious use of intravenous blood and plasma; to minimize pulmonary edema fluids are given sparingly.

Immersion Blast.—Momentary neurological symptoms are common, such as paralysis, tingling and anesthesia in the legs. Following this, abdominal pain, nausea and vomiting, diarrhea and distention develop. Passage of blood per rectum or hematemesis, when they occur, are of great diagnostic value. Abdominal injury is much more likely to occur when the victim faces the source of the explosion or is swimming prone; less severe injuries are apt to occur if he finds himself with his back toward it or is floating on his back. Examination reveals evidence of more or less severe intra-abdominal injury including variable tenderness, muscle spasm and distention.

Treatment is to a large extent conservative,—rest in bed and intravenous blood and plasma for shock, nothing by mouth and parenteral nutrition. An indwelling nasal catheter for continuous gastric decompression is of great value. This regime must be carried out until evidence of intra-abdominal injury subsides as shown by local and systemic manifestations. Inasmuch as some of these patients sustain an actual perforation, the question of immediate operation is serious, but difficult to answer dogmatically, and requires all of the judgment of a well qualified abdominal surgeon. It obviously increases the risk of recovery if a needless abdominal operation is carried out in these severely ill patients. On the other hand, if a perforation is present a fatality is almost sure to occur unless the perforation is closed and this can occur with certainty only by operation. X-ray in the upright position will be of value if it shows a pneumoperitoneum. Otherwise, the decision must rest upon a complete evaluation of all the clinical manifestations. In general, if there is any doubt as to whether a perforation exists, it is probably a better policy to operate, particularly if adequate facilities are available for the control of surgical shock, than to take a chance of a general peritonitis. This policy, of course, will necessarily involve operation upon many patients in whom no perforation will be found, but in doing so the likelihood of missing a perforation will be minimized. If operation is performed it is obvious that a thorough exploration will be required in order to find the perforations (see also discussion on Traumatic Peritonitis on page 748 and Abdominal Injuries on page 1047).

WAR GASES

Although war gases have not as yet been used in the present conflict, knowledge regarding them is of great importance when, as and if the enemy decides to employ this particularly treacherous and inhuman method of warfare. To a large extent the use of war gases is based upon the idea of striking fear and terror into opposing troops or civilians, thus lowering morale. This possible effect is, of course, largely lost when complete knowledge is available and adequate equipment and training, particularly with gas masks, have been provided. Such knowledge and preparation is sufficiently adequate, it is hoped, to discourage the enemy from using this method of combat.

There are other reasons, however, why knowledge of war gases is of value to surgeons. Many details which have been worked out can be applied to certain injuries which occur both in war and in civilian life, notably chemical burns and lung injuries due to inhalation of irritant gases resulting from fires, explosions and accidents. Moreover, the inhalation of poisonous gases resulting from incomplete combustion such as carbon monoxide is also important not only in war but in civilian life and will be discussed under the heading of systemic poisons.

The term chemical warfare is preferable to the term gas warfare inasmuch as the agents used include liquids and solids as well as gases. However, the liquid agents prepared in solution as a spray may be dispersed widely in the air. The liquid and solid agents may also be dispersed by shellfire or dropped as bombs from planes. Nevertheless, there are certain general features characteristic of all of them. For example, they are all heavier than air and hence tend to collect in low places close to the ground, a fact which is of obvious importance in protection from exposure against them. Movement of air tends to dissipate the gases rapidly and therefore the agents which are true gases are called *non-persistent*. On the other hand, the solids and liquids which cannot become so dispersed tend to remain for days or weeks and therefore are called *persistent*. In the last war the various chemical agents were disseminated by explosive shells (with various detonating mixtures), or by discharge from cylinders. With the advance in aerial combat newer methods for their dispersion have undoubtedly been developed and may be tried by the enemy.

In presenting the various types of chemical agents in this section, the following classification will be used. In the first group are the persistent agents which produce burns of the skin, often called vesicants, a typical example being mustard gas. In the second group will be the gases which are inhaled and produce evidence of pulmonary damage, a typical example of which is phosgene. In the third group are the harassing agents, a typical example being the lacrimators or tear gases. The fourth group will be the systemic poisonous gases such as carbon monoxide and the fifth group incendiaries. Further details will be found in other publications [36, 37, 41].

The Vesicants or Blister Agents.—These are toxic, dangerous chemicals and may produce a fatal outcome not only because of their local but also because of their systemic effects. These agents include mustard gas, nitrogen mustards, ethyldichlorarsine and lewisite, the last two producing systemic manifestations due to the absorption of arsenic. In reality they are liquids but are usually encountered in the form of vapor. They produce serious lesions upon contact with the skin or mucous membranes either as a liquid or as a spray. Serious burns result after a short latent period. There is no sensation at the time of contact so that little warning is experienced in the case of the mustard group. Ordinary clothing offers no protection to the vapor which clings to and penetrates it. Protection is afforded by specially prepared fabrics. The persistence of these chemicals makes it necessary to eliminate the substance completely lest it spread from individual to individual long after the attack. The process of removing the agent from clothing or other objects is called decontamination and must be elaborately carried out in order to prevent unnecessary spread and involvement of additional personnel.

The lesions in the skin produced by the vesicants vary somewhat, but the destruction of tissue is definite and may be extensive, leading eventually to a second or third degree burn which heals slowly. The effect on the eyes is especially pronounced and the same is true of the mucous membrane of the respiratory tract.

The Lung Irritants.—As used in the last war, these agents were nearly always phosgene, chloropicrin or chlorine. All of them are true gases; low concentration of phosgene has a very faint odor of green corn and therefore may be inhaled without any knowledge thereof and severe systemic manifestations produced insidiously, often leading to the death of the soldier within 16 to 24 hours and without many premonitory signs. These effects are very striking and are due largely to the development of pulmonary edema and a severe degree of anoxemia. The skin of these individuals exhibits a remarkable appearance; they present either a blue cyanotic stage or a gray pallor which may be mistaken for surgical shock. The changes in the lungs have been well studied but no remedy thus far has been found. In treating these patients it is important to remember that no exertion must be expected of them, and they must be placed completely at rest in the horizontal position, and that inhalations of oxygen be started as soon as possible. Spasms of smooth muscle may accompany the edema. Indeed, antispasmodic drugs to control bronchial spasm may prove of some benefit when paroxysms of spasm occur. Morphine must be used with great caution if at all in view of its depressing effect upon respirations. Plasma or other intravenous fluids must always be used with caution in view of the danger of aggravating the pulmonary edema. Indeed, it may be advisable to bleed these patients if there is any evidence of embarrassment to the right heart from pulmonary edema. This picture of anoxemia may be seen in civilian life in patients suffering from cutaneous burns; in such instances it is probable that the inhalation of similar irritant gases may be responsible for similar effects.

In actual warfare the prompt use of gas masks will, of course, prevent the above mentioned effects from pulmonary irritant gases and all army, naval and marine personnel who will likely be exposed to its effects are provided with such equipment and taught the technic of using it promptly.

Harassing Agents.—These chemicals are often called irritant smokes, lacrimators or sternutators, but they all have in common the fact that they are not lethal, their use being only one of harassment or to get opposing troops to don their gas masks which while offering complete protection, does cut down the efficiency of the soldier, interfering with sleep and comfort. All of these chemicals are liquids or solids hence form persistent agents.

The lacrimators are perhaps the most commonly used and are known as tear gases, such as chloracetophenone and brombenzylcyanide. These are used in civilian life in mob control, in warfare in sudden harassing effects. The sternutators include adamsite and diphenylchlorarsine, which are popularly known as sneeze gases, and produce in addition irritation of the eyes, headaches, burning in the throat, tightness of the chest, nausea and vomiting. They have no odor, are very insidious, but the effects are transient. The screening smokes, used in another phase of chemical warfare, are non-toxic, but may produce symptoms when present in heavy concentrations at the immediate site of dispersion. The three agents most commonly used are sulphur trioxide, a zinc mixture, and white phosphorus. White phosphorus is particularly important because it may produce dangerous chemical burns of the skin and lead to absorption of the chemical.

Systemic Poisonous Gases.—These gases are usually formed under conditions of fire or explosion, particularly in closed spaces where there is an insufficient quantity of oxygen, the common examples being carbon monoxide and the nitrous fumes. These gases may be met with under a variety of conditions, both in warfare and in civilian life, and the surgeon must be prepared to recognize them when they occur. The effect of carbon monoxide is largely a physical one in displacing the oxygen-carrying capacity of hemoglobin. It is usually recognizable by the cherry-red color of the mucous membranes. Treatment consists of artificial respiration and use of oxygen inhalations as soon as available. The nitrous fumes have a different effect which is similar in many respects to that of phosgene, symptoms being produced by pulmonary damage and anoxemia. Treatment is the same as for phosgene.

Incendiaries.—Incendiary bombs have been used extensively in the present conflict and have been responsible for many injuries. Incendiary bombs contain either thermite oil or white phosphorus. The injuries in most cases are similar to those produced by fire or molten metal, *i.e.,* they are thermal injuries which are usually treated as already described. White phosphorus is of special interest in that it burns when in the presence of oxygen and therefore its effect will be removed by the use of water or solutions of copper sulphate. However, when bits of white phosphorus become imbedded in the tissues the burn is apt to be deep and complicated by the absorption of phosphorus itself which in a few instances has led to systemic evidence of phosphorus poisoning. Surgical removal is therefore essential.

WAR LESIONS OF THE FEET

Aside from immersion foot, which is a serious lesion, most of the conditions discussed in this section are minor in nature but extremely important in the medical care of large numbers of troops. As would be expected, acute complaints referable to the feet are more common among trainees than in soldiers under battle conditions (exclusive of war wounds themselves). Although most of the acute lesions developing in training camps are not serious, they are nevertheless so common and so disabling (temporarily), that serious attention must be devoted to them.

Immersion Foot.—This condition, which has been described by numerous observers in World War II, is similar to and perhaps identical to the "trench foot" of World War I. The chief manifestation is swelling of the feet which develops several hours or a few days after exposure to wet cold. It is encountered primarily in shipwreck survivors, particularly those who have been forced to sit in a lifeboat for several days with their feet dangling in cold water which has washed aboard from the sea. The condition has been described in detail in the excellent article by Webster, Woolhouse and Johnston [38]; it develops only when the temperature of the water is in the neighborhood of 55 degrees F. or below, although it may occur in less severe forms with exposure to warmer water.

Clinical manifestations develop a day or so after exposure; symptoms consist of pain, numbness and tingling in the feet. Upon examination they are found to be swollen and pallid, with scattered areas of cyanosis. After removal from the cold environment, swelling tends to increase and the pallid color changes to an erythematous color. The feet become unusually warm but do not sweat. The pulse remains palpable except when edema obliterates it. Blisters of variable size containing straw-colored or sanguinous fluid may appear. Local patches of gangrene may develop, but are not extensive and usually require no more than local amputation (*e.g.*, toes). However, if infection develops in the blisters, abrasions, fissures, etc., as it may do, definite threat may be made upon life, and amputation may become necessary. The exudate of fluid (plasma) into the swollen feet may be so extensive as to lead to shock and therefore may actually be a primary cause of death in shipwrecked personnel.

Treatment is simple, but perhaps the most important feature is maintenance of a cool temperature about the feet. They should first be washed gently with soap and water to remove dirt, etc., thereby minimizing the danger of infection. The feet should be kept uncovered and dry. Ice bags placed alongside with a towel intervening will aid in maintaining a low temperature. The maintenance of a low temperature is essential because the increased oxidation created by elevated temperature takes place so rapidly that the metabolic demands in the injured extremities cannot be met. Before the patient is allowed out of bed, he should be given graduated exercises. If pain remains, the peripheral nerves may be crushed, as recommended by White [39]; such a procedure interrupts nerve function but temporarily inasmuch as regeneration will take place in about three months. However, the condition usually clears up within a few weeks, thereby making radical therapy unnecessary. *Prophylactic treatment* is very effective in preventing development of the condition. The most effective method would be for the shipwrecked victim to wear rubber boots which would keep the feet dry and warm. Unfortunately this precautionary measure cannot be made available to all of those likely to be set adrift at sea. In addition to keeping the feet dry, application of grease or heavy oil also aids in preventing the disease by acting as a protective covering. Frequent exercises of the extremity is likewise very helpful as a preventive measure. When victims are rescued, they should not be allowed to walk lest the trauma of weight bearing result in serious damage to the already edematous and damaged tissues of the feet.

A similar disease, consisting of painful swelling of the feet, also occurs in men who are shipwrecked in warm waters. The process does not proceed to such a severe state as in the typical immersion foot syndrome, but may become quite serious when the victim has been shipwrecked for several weeks. After a study of several cases, White [39] concluded that one of the chief causes of the swelling occurring under such circumstances was a vitamin and protein deficiency. It is assumed that the excess heat, continued exercises (created by bailing, rowing, etc.) along with dehydration and starvation, result in a vitamin deficiency and hypoproteinemia within a relatively short time.

Acute Arch Strain.—At least 75 per cent of foot complaints in the army during the training period are probably due to disturbances in function of either the longitudinal or the transverse plantar arch. It should be emphasized that it is by no means necessary for the arch to be flat before serious symptoms are produced. Acute strain of ligaments and muscles supporting the arch may be the chief factors in the production of symptoms; this strain may later result in flat feet. The condition is due to several etiologic factors including the sharp increase in exercises, overweight, trauma, and ill-fitting shoes. In such acute strains there may be moderate swelling of the feet with a burning sensation on the plantar surface. Pain may extend up into the leg. The feet may be cold and pale. There may be tenderness over the central portion of the longitudinal arch or under the first metatarso-phalangeal joint. If the condition is neglected, the peroneal muscles may become spastic, resulting in the so-called spastic flat foot. If the transverse arch is primarily involved, the tenderness may be localized to areas beneath either of the several metatarsal heads. The heads of these bones may likewise be prominent; in chronic cases calluses may develop beneath them.

Treatment for the serious cases consists of bed rest for at least a few days. Hot baths or contrast baths followed by a massage are helpful. If the longitudinal arch is involved, it may be supported by adhesive strips, or a felt pad may be anchored to the medial side of the foot. A Thomas heel, which projects anteriorly on the medial side and is elevated over the lateral side, will be helpful. It is essential that any misfit in the shoes must be corrected. If the transverse arch appears to be primarily involved, application of a metatarsal bar to the sole of the shoe just behind the metatarsal heads, as utilized by Frankel and Funsten [40] and others, will be helpful.

Metatarsalgia.—This condition may be associated with an acute strain of the anterior or transverse arch. It has been designated as metatarsalgia by many orthopedists who claim that the anterior-transverse arch is theoretical and not real, since the heads of all the metatarsals are pressed against the ground by the body weight while walking. Under such circumstances, the symptoms have been explained by some on the basis that the nerves underlying the heads of the metatarsals are compressed. Regardless of the etiologic factor involved, complete rest, application of a metatarsal bar and other methods of treatment advised above will be found helpful.

Bursitis.—Traumatic inflammation of the *retrocalcaneal bursa* lying between the Achilles tendon and the posterior surface of the os calcis may result from undue pressure of shoes and increased exercise. Flexion or extension of the foot becomes very painful. Rest is essential in treatment; release of pressure from the counter of the shoe will also be necessary. A *subcalcaneal bursa* may form on the plantar surface of the heel, particularly if a bony spur is present. Application of a felt pad hollowed in the center will be helpful. However, it may be necessary to remove the spur and the bursa by operation. Bursae may form at various other parts of the foot and present local symptoms, depending upon the severity and site of affection. In general, rest for a few days is essential. Any errors in fitting of the shoe must be corrected. Occasionally, infection will develop in bursae; however, rarely does it progress to the stage where incision is necessary.

Lesions of the Achilles Tendon.—*Traumatic tenosynovitis* of the Achilles tendon is observed occasionally and may be very disabling. Pain, swelling, and even redness develop over the tendon, extending up to the muscular attachment. In addition to bed rest, application of heat, etc., the heel should be elevated to relieve tension on the tendon. *Rupture of the Achilles tendon* may develop in trainees who previously had been leading a sedentary life, and suddenly enter into the strenuous activities of military training. The chief disability is inability to flex the foot. Operative repair should be performed immediately.

Miscellaneous Conditions.—*Epidermophytosis* is extremely common in army camps, and becomes disabling and even dangerous when secondary infection develops. Cleanliness of the feet and well-fitting shoes minimize the incidence of infection. Attempt should be made to eliminate exposure from the floors of shower baths, etc., although this factor in pathogenesis is no doubt exaggerated. The feet should be washed with soap and water daily and dried thoroughly, particularly between the toes. Application of resorcinol lotion (bichloride of mercury 1, resorcinol 30, 50 per cent alcohol Qs. 1000) is quite effective in therapy. Numerous other agents, including Whitfield's ointment, dilute formaldehyde, etc., have been used and may be effective (see also page 490).

Blisters will be encountered frequently in trainees, and result from over-exercise or ill-fitting shoes. The chief danger is that of infection. They should be covered with sterile dressings, and if distended may be opened after application of an antiseptic to the surface. They may be protected by a thin felt pad with a hole cut in the center. *Ingrown toenails* may be the subject of considerable pain and discomfort, and usually produce symptoms because of shoes which are pointed or too narrow. In mild cases, application of cotton under the nail may be sufficient to prevent significant pain. Filing down the center from the tip of the nail to the cuticle will relieve mild cases. The more serious types of ingrown toenails should be treated by resection of the edge of the nail and the matrix. *Corns* are extremely common in trainees, but relatively few will produce significant symptoms. With few exceptions they are the result of ill-fitting shoes. Corns growing between the toes may result from narrow shoes or from exostoses on the plantar surface of one of the metatarsal bones as can be demonstrated by x-ray. Excision of this exostosis may be necessary (see also page 488).

Fitting of Shoes.—Unfortunately, not all feet can be fitted with a universal last. However, a shoe with a broad toe and a straight last with a wide lateral curve for the toes will be most appropriate as a universal type. The sole must be thick enough to prevent "stone bruise", but sufficiently pliable to allow flexion. The shank should be slightly higher on the medial side than on the lateral side. The shoe should be fitted for full weight bearing. There must be at least one-half inch space between the tip of the great toe and the end of the shoe. Before long marches are taken, the shoe must be "broken in". Rubbing the leather with some type of heavy oil will minimize the development of acute traumatic lesions of the foot.

BIBLIOGRAPHY

1. JOLLY, D. W. *Field Surgery in Total War,* Haniesh Hamilton Medical Books, London, 1942.
2. TRUETA, J. *Principles and Practice of War Surgery,* Mosby, St. Louis, 1943.
3. ELOESSER, L.   Treatment of Compound Fractures in War, *J. Am. M. Ass.,* 115:1848, 1940.
4. BAILEY, HAMILTON. *Surgery of Modern Warfare,* The Williams and Wilkins Co., Baltimore, 1942.
5. PUGH, W. S., editor. *War Medicine,* F. Hubner & Co., Inc., N. Y., 1942.
6. GALLAGHER, J. L.   A New Multi Purpose War Dressing, *Military Surgeon,* 92:609, 1943; Definitive Treatment of Severe Wounds, Large Surface to Small Area (in press).
7. ELMAN, R.   Russian War Surgery; Military Medical Reports from Russia, *Surg., Gynec. & Obst.,* 77:93, 1943.
8. KIRK, N. T. *J. Am. M. Ass.,* 115:522, 1943.
9. SMIRNOV, Y. I.   (Quoted by Elman, R.), *Surg., Gynec. & Obst.,* 77:93, 1943.
10. KIRK, MAJ. GEN. N. T. Quoted in *Science News Letter,* page 387, June 19, 1943.
11. PHEMISTER, D. B., and SCHACHTER, R. I.   Neurogenic Shock: Effects of Prolonged Lowering of Blood Pressure by Continuous Stimulation of Carotid Sinus in Dogs, *Ann. Surg.,* 116:610, 1942.
12. STERN, L. S.   Treatment of Shock by Direct Action on Vegetative Nervous Centres, *Brit. Med. J.,* 2:538, 1942.
13. KAYE, GEOFFREY.   Impressions of Anesthesia in a Military Base Hospital, *Anesthesiology,* 3:247, 1942; 3:379, 1942.
14. HALFORD, F. J.   Gas Gangrene and Tetanus, *Hawaii Med. J.,* 1:169, 1942.
15. MITCHELL, G. A. G., and BUTTLE, G. A. H.   Proflavine Powder in Wound Therapy, *Lancet,* 2:416, 1942.
16. CLARK, A. M., COLEBROOK, L., GIBSON, T., THOMSON, M. L., and FOSTER, A.   Penicillin and Propamidine in Burns, Elimination of Haemolytic Streptococci and Staphylococci, *Lancet,* May 15, 1943, page 665.
17. WAKELEY, C. P. B.   The Treatment of War Burns, *War Medicine,* F. Hubner & Co., N. Y., 1942, page 41.
18. AUB, J. C., PITTMAN, H., and BRUES, A. M.   The Pulmonary Complications: A Clinical Description, *Ann. Surg.,* 117:834, 1943.
19. MOORE, P. L., and BRACKER, A. N.   March Fracture: Report of Three Cases, *War Med.,* 1:30, 1941.
20. MYERDING, H. W., and POLLOCK, G. A.   March Fracture, *Surg., Gynec. & Obst.,* 67:234, 1938.
21. TOBIN, CAPT. W. J.   Paratrooper Fracture, *Arch. Surg.,* 46:780, 1943; Parachute Injuries, *Army Med. Bull.,* 66:202, 1943.
22. KIRK, N. T.   Amputations in War, *J. Am. M. Ass.,* 120:13, 1942.
23. WALTON, JAMES.   Abdominal Wounds in War: Treatment of Individual Lesions, *Brit. Med. J.,* 1:61, 1943.
24. *Neurosurgery and Thoracic Surgery,* W. B. Saunders Co., 1943.
25. MUNRO, D.   Thoracic and Lumbosacral Cord Injuries, *J. Am. M. Ass.,* 122:1055, 1943.
26. LOVE, J. G.   Injuries of the Intervertebral Disk in Military Life, *War Med.,* 2:403, 1942.
27. BLALOCK, A.   A Study of Thoracic-Duct Lymph in Experimental Crush Injury and Injury Produced by Gross Trauma, *Bull. Johns Hopkins Hosp.,* 72:54, 1943.
28. BYWATERS, E. G. L.   Crushing Injury, *Brit. Med. J.,* page 643, Nov. 28, 1942.
    BYWATERS, E. G. L., and POPJAK, G.   Experimental Crushing Injury, *Surg., Gynec. & Obst.,* 75:612, 1942.

29. PATEY, D. H., and ROBERTSON, J. D. First Aid Prophylactic Treatment of ·the Compression Syndrome, *Brit. Med. J.,* page 212, Aug. 22, 1942; Compression Treatment of Crush Injuries of Limbs, *Lancet,* 1:780, 1941.

30. DUNCAN, G. W., and BLALOCK, A. The Uniform Production of Experimental Shock by Crush Injury: Possible Relationship to Clinical Crush Syndrome, *Ann. Surg.,* 115:684, 1942; Shock Produced by Crush Injury, *Arch. Surg.,* 45:183, 1942.

31. CANNON, W. B., and BAYLISS, W. M. Quoted in Cannon, W. B., *Traumatic Shock,* D. Appleton and Co., 1923, page 153.

32. WILSON, H., and ROOME, N. W. The Effects of Constriction and Release of an Extremity, *Arch. Surg.,* 32:334, 1936.

33. MYLON, E., WINTERNITZ, M. C., and DE SATO-NOGY, G. J. Studies on Therapy in Traumatic Shock, *Am. J. Physiol.,* 139:313, 1943.

34. FULTON, J. F. Blast and Concussion in the Present War, *War Medicine,* F. Hubner & Co., N. Y., 1942, page 226.

35. Editorials. Further Experimental Studies of Blast Injuries, *J. Am. M. Ass.,* 121:1220, 1943; Abdominal Injury from Blast, *Lancet,* 1:244, 1943.

36. LEAKE, C. D., and MARSH, D. F. Mechanism of Action of Ordinary War Gases, *Science,* 96:194, 1942.

37. *Medical Manual of Chemical Warfare,* Chemical Publishing Co., Brooklyn, 1941.

38. WEBSTER, D. R., WOOLHOUSE, F. M., and JOHNSTON, J. L. Immersion Foot, *J. Bone & Joint Surg.,* 24:785, 1942.

39. WHITE, J. C. Vascular and Neurologic Lesions in Survivors of Shipwreck, *New Eng. J. of Med.,* 228:211, 223, 1943.

40. FRANKEL, C. J., and FUNSTEN, R. V. *Painful Feet in War Medicine,* Philosophical Library, New York, 1942.

41. COLE, W. H., and PUESTOW, C. B. *First Aid, Surgical and Medical,* 2nd edition, 1943, D. Appleton-Century Co., New York.

42. OLDBERG, ERIC. The Neurosurgical Consideration of Fracture of the Spine, *Surg. Cl. N. A.,* 16, 291, 1936; The Reflexes in the Prognosis of Transverse Lesions of the Spinal Cord, *J. Am. M. Ass.,* 110:104, 1938.

INDEX OF AUTHORS

SUBJECT INDEX

(8)